A Comprehensive Textbook of
Community Health Nursing

A Comprehensive Textbook of Community Health Nursing

As per Revised Nursing Syllabus

Second Edition

Bijayalaskhmi Dash
MSc (Community Health Nursing)
Assistant Professor and Principal In-Charge
SCB College of Nursing
Cuttack, Odisha, India

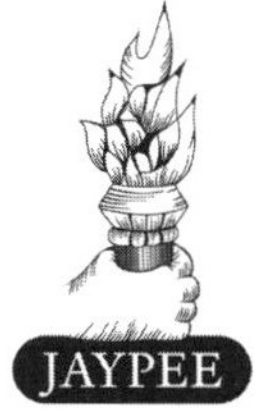

JAYPEE BROTHERS MEDICAL PUBLISHERS
The Health Sciences Publisher
New Delhi | London

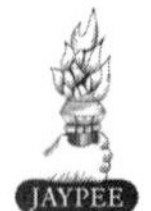
Jaypee Brothers Medical Publishers (P) Ltd.

Headquarters
EMCA House
23/23-B, Ansari Road, Daryaganj
New Delhi 110 002, India
Landline: +91-11-23272143, +91-11-23272703
+91-11-23282021, +91-11-23245672
E-mail: jaypee@jaypeebrothers.com

Corporate Office
Jaypee Brothers Medical Publishers (P) Ltd.
4838/24, Ansari Road, Daryaganj
New Delhi 110 002, India
Phone: +91-11-43574357
Fax: +91-11-43574314
E-mail: jaypee@jaypeebrothers.com

Overseas Office
JP Medical Ltd.
83, Victoria Street, London
SW1H 0HW (UK)
Phone: +44-20 3170 8910
E-mail: info@jpmedpub.com

EU GPSR Authorised Representative
Logos Europe, 9 rue Nicolas Poussin
17000, La Rochelle, France
Phone: +33 (0) 6 67 93 73 78
E-mail: Contact@logoseurope.eu

Website: www.jaypeebrothers.com
Website: www.jaypeedigital.com

Inquiries for bulk sales may be solicited at: jaypee@jaypeebrothers.com

A Comprehensive Textbook of Community Health Nursing

First Edition: 2017

Second Edition: 2023 Reprint : 2024, **2025**

ISBN: 978-93-5696-360-3

Printed at K.K. Printers, Kundli, Haryana-131 028..

Dedicated to

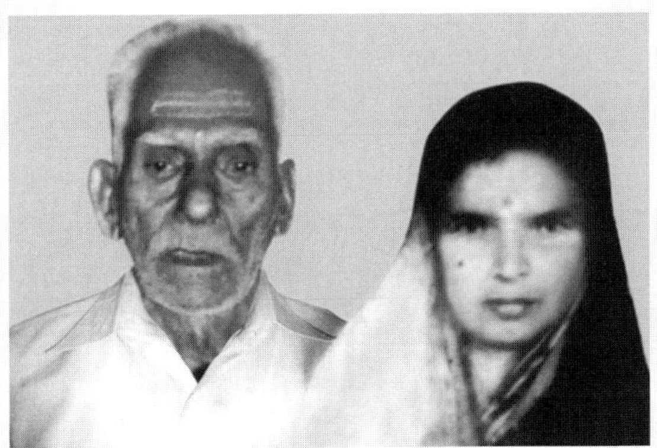

This book is dedicated to my parents Late Rama Chandra Panda and Late Nayana Sundari Panda for their revered memory.

PREFACE TO THE SECOND EDITION

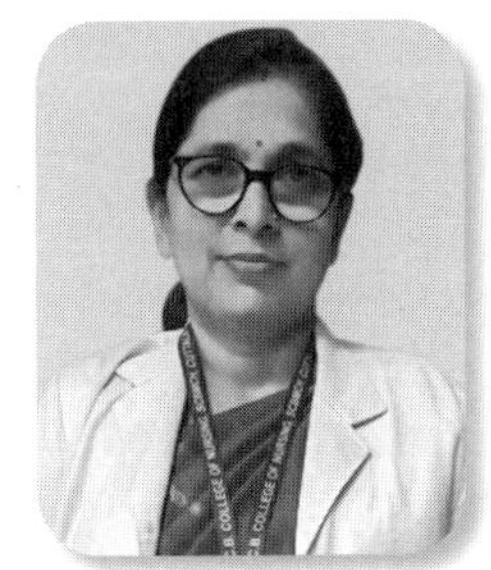

I am delighted to present to you the second edition of *A Comprehensive Textbook of Community Health Nursing*. The overwhelming response and appreciation I received for the first edition have inspired me to develop this book further, incorporating the invaluable suggestions and feedback from our readers and experts. The landscape of healthcare is constantly evolving, with policies, programs, and the delivery of services undergoing continuous changes. Recognizing the need to stay updated, I have extensively revised and updated this textbook to make a valuable, a relevant and indispensable resource for nursing students and professionals.

One of the highlights of second edition is the addition of new chapters that align with the revised BSc and MSc nursing syllabus. I have meticulously curated the content to include all the latest concepts, policies, and programs such as the Sustainable Development Goals (SDGs), Comprehensive Primary Health Care (CPHC), Behavior Change Communication (BCC), Social and Behavior Change Communication (SBCC), and Integrated Management of Neonatal and Childhood Illness (IMNCI). In recognition of the growing significance of disaster management in community health nursing, I have also introduced a new chapter dedicated to this critical area. It is my belief that equipping nurses with the necessary knowledge and skills to effectively respond to emergencies and disasters is essential for the well-being of individuals and communities. This extraordinary textbook comprises nineteen self-sufficient chapters, each addressing a specific area of community health nursing. I have taken great care to comprehensively explain all aspects of this subject, providing readers with a thorough understanding of the principles, practices, and challenges involved.

Furthermore, I understand that community health nursing extends beyond theoretical knowledge. It necessitates a deep understanding of current affairs and emerging trends. Therefore, this edition includes all the latest information desired by the curriculum and our esteemed readers. My goal is to empower students and professionals with the most up-to-date knowledge, enabling them to navigate the complexities of community health nursing in our ever-changing world.

I would like to express my heartfelt gratitude to all the readers and experts who shared their feedback and suggestions, which have greatly contributed to the improvement of this second edition. Your insightful inputs have played a pivotal role in ensuring that this textbook meets the evolving needs and expectations of the nursing community.

In conclusion, I believe that this revised edition of *A Comprehensive Textbook of Community Health Nursing* will serve as an invaluable resource for nursing students, educators, and professionals. My hope is that it will inspire and empower individuals to excel in the field of community health nursing, making a positive and lasting impact on the health and well-being of the communities they serve.

Bijayalaskhmi Dash

PREFACE TO THE FIRST EDITION

It gives me immense pleasure to write the book *A Comprehensive Textbook of Community Health Nursing* and this first edition of the textbook has evolved to reflect the continuous advancements in the field of nursing education, to meet the growing information source required for nursing students. This extraordinary textbook contains all the aspects of community health nursing comprehensively. It covers almost all the chapters as per the latest syllabus of Indian Nursing Council (INC) for BSc, MSc and General Nursing and Midwifery course. This textbook will prove to be an unceasing source of information.

'Gaining knowledge is a never-ending process'. The core subject **community health nursing** in nursing syllabus requires information and knowledge in current affairs. This textbook contains eighteen chapters written in simple language and all the chapters are well-defined with updated knowledge, information and data findings. This book will supply all the updated information like **NITI Aayog**, **new emerging and re-emerging diseases (Ebola virus and Zika virus)**, **new changing policies and National Health Programmes** in details. Separate chapters based on community mental health, international health, occupational health and quality assurance in community health nursing and rehabilitation which are rarely available are emphasized.

I have been encouraged to write this book because of the fact that the students of community health nursing speciality will be highly benefitted by this book. I hope, this book will benefit nursing students. This is my first endeavor of short steps towards contributing my knowledge and experience with the students who are encouraged to move forward. I welcome healthy comments and suggestions from readers which will help me to improve the book.

Bijayalaskhmi Dash

ACKNOWLEDGMENTS

Although, I have invested considerable amount of efforts to make it efficacious and insightful, yet, I would like to acknowledge my indebtedness and render my warmest thanks to people who gave me the necessary support and helped me to make this venture a success.

To begin with, I would like to offer my sincere gratitude for the contributions made by all the editors and readers who applied their expertise and valuable comments guiding me throughout, till the completion of this book.

I would like to express my gratitude to Shri Jitendar P Vij (Group Chairman), Mr Ankit Vij (Managing Director), Mr MS Mani (Group President), Dr Madhu Choudhary (Director–Educational Publishing), Ms Pooja Bhandari [Director–Production (Books and Journals)], Ms Sunita Katla (Executive Assistant to Group Chairman and Publishing Manager), who are the continual source of inspiration throughout this journey.

I would also like to thanks Ms Jitika Royal (Content Strategist) whose constant feedback pushed me to move forward and I am able to complete this second edition within stipulated period of time.

I extend my heartfelt thanks to Ms Samina Khan (Executive Assistant to Director–Educational Publishing) and Mr Sabyasachi Hazra (Associate Director–Publishing and Digital Sales) for helping me through my idea. I also express my gratitude to them, for helping me throughout and encouraging me to complete this book by providing me timely corrections.

I owe my thanks to M/s Jaypee Brothers Medical Publishers(P) Ltd, New Delhi, India, especially Mr Ajay Sharma [DGM–Production (Books and Journals)] Mr Rajesh Sharma (Production Coordinator), Ms Seema Dogra (Cover Visualizer), Mr Akshay Thakur (Typesetter), Ms Geeta Barik (Proofreader), Mr Nitesh Jain (Graphic Designer) and their team members for their brilliant editorial support and guidance.

Last but not the least, I extend my thanks to my husband Mr Pravash Ranjan Dash, my daughter Ms Sayanshree Dash and my son Subhasatya Dash for their support and encouragement.

Finally, I am thankful to all my friends, and my colleagues for their support and encouragement.

CONTENTS

SYLLABUS

BSc NURSING

COMMUNITY HEALTH NURSING-I
Including Environmental Science and Epidemiology

THEORY: 5 Credits (100 hours) include Lab hours also

PRACTICUM: Clinical: 2 Credits (160 hours)

DESCRIPTION: This course is designed to help students develop broad perspectives of health, its determinants, about community health nursing and understanding about the healthcare delivery services, healthcare policies and regulations in India. It helps the students to develop knowledge and understanding of environmental science. It further helps them to apply the principles and concepts of BCC and health education for health promotion and maintenance of health within the community in wellness and illness continuum. It helps students to practice community health nursing for the individuals, family and groups at rural, urban and tribal settings by applying principles of community health nursing and epidemiological approach. It also helps the students to develop knowledge and competencies required to screen, assess, diagnose, manage and refer clients appropriately in various healthcare settings. It prepares the students to provide primary healthcare to clients of all ages in the community, DH, PHC, CHC, SC/HWC and develop beginning skills in participating in all the national health programs.

COMPETENCIES: On completion of the course, the students will be able to:

- Explore the evolution of public health in India and community health nursing.
- Explain the concepts and determinants of health.
- Identify the levels of prevention and health problems of India.
- Develop basic understanding about the healthcare planning and the present healthcare delivery system in India at various levels.
- Locate the significance of primary health care and comprehensive primary health care as part of current healthcare delivery system focus.
- Discuss healthcare policies and regulations in India.
- Demonstrate understanding about an overview of environmental science, environmental health and sanitation.
- Demonstrate skill in nutritional assessment for different age groups in the community and provide appropriate nutritional counselling.
- Provide health education to individuals and families applying the principles and techniques of behavior change appropriate to community settings.
- Describe community health nursing approaches and concepts.
- Describe the role and responsibilities of community health nursing personnel.
- Utilize the knowledge and skills in providing comprehensive primary health care across the life span at various settings.
- Make effective home visits applying principles and methods used for home visiting.
- Use epidemiological approach in community diagnosis.
- Utilize the knowledge of epidemiology, epidemiological approaches in caring for people with communicable and non communicable diseases.
- Investigate an epidemic of communicable diseases.
- Assess, diagnose, manage and refer clients for various communicable and noncommunicable diseases appropriately at the primary health care level.
- Identify and perform the roles and responsibilities of nurses in implementing various national health programs in the community for the prevention, control and management of communicable and noncommunicable diseases particularly in screening, identification, primary management and referral to a health facility/first referral unit (FRU).

COURSE OUTLINE
T – Theory

Unit	Time (Hrs)	Learning outcomes	Content	Teaching/learning activities	Assessment methods
I	4 (T)	Define public health, community health and community health nursing Explain the evolution of public health in India and scope of community health nursing Explain various concepts of health and disease, dimensions and determinants of health Explain the natural history of disease and levels of prevention Discuss the health problems of India	**Concepts of Community Health and Community Health Nursing** • Definition of public health, community health and community health nursing • Public health in India and its evolution and scope of community health nursing • *Review:* Concepts of health and illness/disease: Definition, dimensions and determinants of health and disease • Natural history of disease • Levels of prevention: Primary, Secondary and tertiary prevention – Review • Health problems (profile) of India	• Lecture • Discussion • Explain using chart, graphs • Community needs assessment (Field survey on identification of demographic characteristics, health determinants and resources of a rural and an urban community) • Explain using examples	• Short answer • Essay • Objective type • Survey report

II	8 (T)	Describe health planning and its steps, and various health plans, and committees
		Discuss healthcare delivery system in India at various levels
		Describe SDGs, primary health care and comprehensive primary health care (CPHC)
		Explain healthcare policies and regulations in India
			Health Care Planning and Organization of Health Care at Various Levels
			• Health planning steps
			• Health planning in India: various committees and commissions on health and family welfare and Five Year plans
			• Participation of community and stakeholders in health planning
			• Healthcare delivery system in India: Infrastructure and health sectors, delivery of health services at subcenter (SC), PHC, CHC, district level, state level and national level
			• Sustainable development goals (SDGs), primary health care and comprehensive primary health care (CPHC): elements, principles
			• CPHC through SC/health wellness center (HWC)
			• Role of MLHP/CHP
			• National Health Care Policies and Regulations
			  ▪ National Health Policy (1983, 2002, 2017)
			  ▪ National Health Mission (NHM): National Rural Health Mission (NRHM), National Urban Health Mission (NUHM), NHM
			  ▪ National Health Protection Mission (NHPM)
			  ▪ Ayushman Bharat
			  ▪ Universal Health Coverage
				• Lecture
				• Discussion
				• Field visits to CHC, PHC, SC/Health Wellness Centers (HWC)
				• Directed reading
					• Short answer
					• Essay
					• Evaluation of field visit reports and presentation

III	15 (T)	Identify the role of an individual in the conservation of natural resources Describe ecosystem, its structure, types and functions	**Environmental Science, Environmental Health, and Sanitation** • *Natural resources:* Renewable and non- renewable resources, natural resources and associated problems: Forest resources, water resources, mineral resources, food resources, energy resources and land resources	• Lecture • Discussion • Debates on environmental protection and preservation • Explain using charts, graphs, models, films, slides • Directed reading • Visits to water supply and purification sites	• Short answer • Essay • Field visit reports

Unit	Time (Hrs)	Learning outcomes	Content	Teaching/learning activities	Assessment methods
		Explain the classification, value and threats to biodiversity Enumerate the causes, effects and control measures of environmental pollution Discuss about climate change, global warming, acid rain, and ozone layer depletion Enumerate the role of an individual in creating awareness about the social issues related to environment List the acts related to environmental protection and preservation Describe the concept of environmental health and sanitation Describe water conservation, rain water harvesting and watershed management Explain waste management	• Role of individuals in conservation of natural resources, and equitable use of resources for sustainable lifestyles • *Ecosystem:* Concept, structure and functions of ecosystems, types and characteristics–forest ecosystem, grassland ecosystem, desert ecosystem, aquatic ecosystem, energy flow in ecosystem • *Biodiversity:* Classification, value of biodiversity, threats to biodiversity, conservation of biodiversity • *Environmental pollution:* Introduction, causes, effects and control measures of air pollution, water pollution, soil pollution, marine pollution, noise pollution, thermal pollution, nuclear hazards and their impact on health • *Climate change, global warming:* e.g., heat wave, acid rain, ozone layer depletion, wasteland reclamation and its impact on health • *Social issues and environment:* sustainable development, urban problems related to energy, water and environmental ethics • Acts related to environmental protection and preservation **Environmental Health and Sanitation** • Concept of environmental health and sanitation • Concept of safe water, sources of water, waterborne diseases, water purification processes, household purification of water • Physical and chemical standards of drinking water quality and tests for assessing bacteriological quality of water • Concepts of water conservation: rainwater harvesting and watershed management • Concept of pollution prevention • Air and noise pollution • Role of nurse in prevention of pollution • Solid waste management, human excreta disposal and management and sewage disposal and management • Commonly used insecticides and pesticides	• Observe rainwater harvesting plants • Visit to sewage disposal and treatment sites, and waste disposal sites	
IV	7 (T)	Describe the various nutrition assessment methods at the community level Plan and provide diet plans for all age groups including therapeutic diet	**Nutrition Assessment and Nutrition Education** • *Review of Nutrition* ▪ Concepts, types ▪ Meal planning: aims, steps and diet plan for different age groups ▪ Nutrition assessment of individuals, families and community by using appropriate methods	• Lecture • Discussion • Demonstration • Role play • Market visit • Nutritional assessment for different age groups • Lecture • Discussion	• Performance assessment of nutrition assessment for different age groups

Unit	Time (Hrs)	Learning outcomes	Content	Teaching/learning activities	Assessment methods
		Provide nutrition counseling and education to all age groups and describe the national nutrition programs Identify early the foodborne diseases, and perform initial management and referral appropriately	• Planning suitable diet for individuals and families according to local availability of foods, dietary habits and economic status • General nutritional advice • Nutrition education: purpose, principles and methods and rehabilitation • *Review:* Nutritional deficiency disorders • National nutritional policy and programs in India **Food Borne Diseases and Food Safety Foodborne diseases** • Definition and burden, causes and classification • Signs and symptoms • Transmission of food borne pathogens and toxins • Early identification, initial management and referral **Food poisoning and food intoxication** • Epidemiological features/clinical characteristics, types of food poisoning • Food intoxication—features, preventive and control measures • Public health response to foodborne diseases	• Field visits to milk purification plants, slaughterhouse • Refer Nutrition module-BPCCHN Block 2-unit I and unit 5	• Evaluation on nutritional assessment reports • Short answer • Essay • Field visit reports
V	6 (T)	Describe behavior change communication skills Counsel and provide health education to individuals, families and community for promotion of healthy lifestyle practices using appropriate methods and media	**Communication Management and Health Education** • Behavior change communication skills ▪ Communication ▪ Human behavior ▪ Health belief model: concepts and definition, ways to influence behavior ▪ Steps of behavior change ▪ *Techniques of behavior change:* Guiding principles in planning BCC activity ▪ Steps of BCC ▪ *Social and behavior change communication strategies (SBCC):* Techniques to collect social history from clients ▪ Barriers to effective communication, and methods to overcome them • *Health promotion and health education:* Methods/techniques, and audio-visual aids	• Lecture • Discussion • Role play • Demonstration: BCC skills • Supervised field practice • Refer: BCC/SBCC module (MoHFW and USAID)	• Short answer • Essay • Performance evaluation of health education sessions to individuals and families
VI	7 (T)	Describe community health nursing approaches and concepts Describe and identify the activities of community health nurse to promote and maintain family health through home visits	**Community Health Nursing Approaches, Concepts, Roles and Responsibilities of Community Health Nursing Personnel** • *Approaches:* ▪ Nursing process ▪ Epidemiological approach ▪ Problem-solving approach ▪ Evidence-based approach	• Lecture • Discussion • Demonstration • Role plays • Supervised field practice	• Short answer • Essays • Assessment of supervised field practice

Unit	Time (Hrs)	Learning outcomes	Content	Teaching/learning activities	Assessment methods
			▪ Empowering people to care for themselves • *Review:* Primary health care and Comprehensive Primary Health Care (CPHC) **Home Visits:** • *Concept, principles, process,and techniques:* bag technique • Qualities of community Health Nurse • Roles and responsibilities of community health nursing personnel in family health services • *Review:* Principles and techniques of counseling		
VII	**10 (T)**	Explain the specific activities of community health nurse in assisting individuals and groups to promote and maintain their health Provide primary care at home/health centers (HWC) using standing orders/protocols as per public health standards/ approved by MoHandFW and INC regulation Develop skill in maintenance of records and reports	**Assisting individuals and families to promote and maintain their health** *A. Assessment of individuals and families* (Review from Child health nursing, Medical surgical nursing and OBG Nursing) • Assessment of children, women, adolescents, elderly etc. • Children: Monitoring growth and development, milestones • Anthropometric measurements, BMI • Social development • Temperature and blood pressure monitoring • Menstrual cycle • Breast self-examination (BSE) and testicles self- examination (TSE) • Warning signs of various diseases • Tests: Urine for sugar and albumin, blood sugar, hemoglobin *B. Provision of health services/primary health care:* • Routine check-up, Immunization, counseling, and diagnosis • Management of common diseases at home and health centre level ▪ Care based on standing orders/protocols approved by MoHandFW ▪ Drugs dispensing and injections at health centre *C. Continue medical care and follow up* in community for various diseases/ disabilities *D. Carry out therapeutic procedures* as prescribed/required for client and family *E. Maintenance of health records and reports* • Maintenance of client records • Maintenance of health records at the facility level • Report writing and documentation of activities carried out during home visits, in the clinics/centers and field visits	• Lecture • Discussion • Demonstration • Role plays • Document and maintain • Individual records	• Short answer • Essay • Assessment of clinical performance in the field practice area • Assessment of procedural skills in lab procedures • Evaluation of records and reports

Unit	Time (Hrs)	Learning outcomes	Content	Teaching/learning activities	Assessment methods
		Develop beginning skills in handling social issues affecting the health and development of the family Identify and assist the families to utilize the community resources appropriately	*F. Sensitize and handle social issues affecting health and development of the family* • Women empowerment • Women and child abuse • Abuse of elders • Female feticide • Commercial sex workers • Substance abuse *G. Utilize community resources for client and family* • Trauma services • Old age homes • Orphanages • Homes for physically challenged individuals • Homes for destitute • Palliative care centres • Hospice care centres • Assisted living facility	• Family records • Health center records • Field visits	• Evaluation of field visit reports
VIII	**10 (T)**	Describe the concepts, approaches and methods of epidemiology Investigate an epidemic of communicable disease	**Introduction to Epidemiology–Epidemiological Approaches and Processes** • Epidemiology: Concept and Definition • Distribution and frequency of disease • Aims and uses of epidemiology • Epidemiological models of causation of disease • Concepts of disease transmission • Modes of transmission: Direct, indirect and chain of infection • Time trends or fluctuations in disease occurrence • Epidemiological approaches: Descriptive, analytical and experimental • Principles of control measures/levels of prevention of disease • Investigation of an epidemic of communicable disease • Use of basic epidemiological tools to make community diagnosis for effective planning and intervention	• Lecture • Discussion • Demonstration • Role play • Field visits: communicable disease hospital and entomology office • Investigation of an epidemic of communicable disease	• Short answer • Essay • Report on visit to communicable disease hospital • Report on visit to entomology office • Report and presentation on investigating an epidemic of communicable disease
IX	**15 (T)**	Explain the epidemiology of specific communicable diseases Describe the various methods of prevention, control and management of communicable diseases and the role of nurses in screening, diagnosing, primary management and referral to a health facility	**Communicable Diseases and National Health Programs** *1. Communicable Diseases: Vector borne diseases (Every disease will be dealt under the following headlines)* • Epidemiology of the following vector borne diseases • Prevention and control measures • Screening, and diagnosing the following conditions, primary management, referral and follow up ▪ Malaria ▪ Filaria ▪ Kala-azar ▪ Japanese encephalitis ▪ Dengue ▪ Chickungunya	• Lecture • Discussion • Demonstration • Role play • Suggested field visits • Field practice • Assessment of clients with communicable diseases	• Field visit reports • Assessment of family case study • OSCE assessment • Short answer • Essay

Unit	Time (Hrs)	Learning outcomes	Content	Teaching/learning activities	Assessment methods
		Identify the national health programs relevant to communicable diseases and explain the role of nurses in implementation of these programs	*2. Communicable diseases: Infectious diseases (Every disease will be dealt under the following headlines)* • Epidemiology of the following infectious diseases • Prevention and control measures • Screening, diagnosing the following conditions, primary management, referral and follow up ▪ Leprosy ▪ Tuberculosis ▪ Vaccine preventable diseases – diphtheria, whooping cough, tetanus, poliomyelitis and measles ▪ Enteric fever ▪ Viral hepatitis ▪ HIV/AIDS/RTI infections ▪ HIV/AIDS, and Sexually Transmitted Diseases/ Reproductive tract infections (STIs/RTIs) ▪ Diarrhea ▪ Respiratory tract infections ▪ COVID-19 ▪ Helminthic–soil and food transmitted and parasitic infections – Scabies and pediculosis *3. Communicable diseases: Zoonotic diseases* • Epidemiology of zoonotic diseases • Prevention and control measures • Screening and diagnosing the following conditions, primary management, referral and follow up ▪ Rabies: Identify, suspect, primary management and referral to a health facility • Role of a nurses in control of communicable diseases **National Health Programs** 1. UIP: Universal Immunization Program (Diphtheria, Whooping cough, Tetanus, Poliomyelitis, Measles and Hepatitis B) 2. National Leprosy Eradication Program (NLEP) 3. Revised National Tuberculosis Control Program (RNTCP) 4. Integrated Disease Surveillance Program (IDSP): Enteric fever, Diarrhea, Respiratory infections and scabies 5. National AIDS Control Organization (NACO) 6. National Vector Borne Disease Control Program 7. National Air Quality Monitoring Program 8. Any other newly added program		

Unit	Time (Hrs)	Learning outcomes	Content	Teaching/learning activities	Assessment methods
X	15 (T)	Describe the national health program for the control of non-communicable diseases and the role of nurses in screening, identification, primary management and referral to a health facility	**Noncommunicable Diseases and National Health Program (NCD)** • National response to NCDs (Every disease will be dealt under the following headlines) • Epidemiology of specific diseases • Prevention and control measures • Screening, diagnosing/identification and primary management, referral and follow up care **NCD-1** • Diabetes mellitus • Hypertension • Cardiovascular diseases • Stroke and obesity • **Blindness:** Categories of visual impairment and national program for control of blindness • **Deafness:** National program for prevention and control of deafness • Thyroid diseases • **Injury and accidents:** Risk factors for road traffic injuries and operational guidelines for trauma care facility on highways **NCD-2 Cancers** • Cervical cancer • Breast cancer • Oral cancer • Epidemiology of specific cancers, risk factors/causes, prevention, screening, diagnosis – signs, signs and symptoms, and early management and referral • Palliative care • Role of a nurse in non-communicable disease control program **National Health Programs** • National program for prevention and control of cancer, Diabetes, Cardiovascular Diseases and Stroke (NPCDCS) • National Program for Control of Blindness • National Program for Prevention and Control of Deafness • National Tobacco Control Program • Standard treatment protocols used in National Health Programs	• Lecture • Discussion • Demonstration • Role play • Suggested field visits • Field practice • Assessment of clients with noncommunicable diseases • Participation in national health programs	• Field visit reports • Assessment of family case study • OSCE assessment • Short answer • Essay
XI	3 (T)	Enumerate the school health activities and the role functions of a school health nurse	**School Health Services** • Objectives • Health problems of school children • Components of school health services • Maintenance of school health records • Initiation and planning of school health services • Role of a school health nurse	• Lecture • Discussion • Demonstration • Role play • Suggested field visits • Field practice	• Short answer • Essay • Evaluation of health counseling to school children • Screen, diagnose, manage and refer school children • OSCE assessment

Note: Lab hours less than 1 Credit is not specified separately.

COMMUNITY HEALTH NURSING – II

PLACEMENT: VII SEMESTER

THEORY: 5 Credits (100 hours) – includes lab hours also

PRACTICUM: Clinical: 2 Credit (160 hours)

DESCRIPTION: This course is designed to help students gain broad perspective of specialized roles and responsibilities of community health nurses and to practice in various specialized healthcare settings. It helps students to develop knowledge and competencies required for assessment, diagnosis, treatment, and nursing management of individuals and families within the community in wellness and illness continuum.

COMPETENCIES: On completion of the course, the students will be able to:

- Demonstrate beginning practice competencies/skills relevant to provide comprehensive primary health care/community-based care to clients with common diseases and disorders including emergency and first aid care at home/clinics/centres as per predetermined protocols/drug standing orders approved by MOHandFW
- Provide maternal, newborn and child care, and reproductive health including adolescent care in the urban and rural health care settings.
- Describe the methods of collection and interpretation of demographic data.
- Explain population control and its impact on the society and describe the approaches towards limiting family size.
- Describe occupational health hazards, occupational diseases and the role of nurses in occupational health programs.
- Identify health problems of older adults and provide primary care, counseling and supportive health services.
- Participate in screening for mental health problems in the community and providing appropriate referral services.
- Discuss the methods of data collection for HMIS, analysis and interpretation of data.
- Discuss about effective management of health information in community diagnosis and intervention.
- Describe the management system of delivery of community health services in rural and urban areas.
- Describe the leadership role in guiding, supervising, and monitoring the health services and the personnel at the PHCs, SCs and community level including financial management and maintenance of records and reports.
- Describe the roles and responsibilities of Mid-Level Health Care Providers (MHCPs) in Health Wellness Centers (HWCs)
- Identify the roles and responsibilities of health team members and explain their job description.
- Demonstrate initiative in preparing themselves and the community for disaster preparedness and management.
- Demonstrate skills in proper biomedical waste management as per protocols.
- Explain the roles and functions of various national and international health agencies.

COURSE OUTLINE
T – Theory

Unit	Time (Hrs)	Learning outcomes	Content	Teaching/learning activities	Assessment methods
I	10 (T)	Explain nurses' role in identification, primary management and referral of clients with common disorders/conditions and emergencies including first aid	**Management of Common Conditions and Emergencies Including First Aid** • Standing orders: Definition, uses **Screening, diagnosing/identification, primary care and referral of gastrointestinal system** • Abdominal pain • Nausea and vomiting • Diarrhea • Constipation • Jaundice • GI bleeding • Abdominal distension • Dysphagia and dyspepsia • Aphthous ulcers **Respiratory system** • Acute upper respiratory infections: Rhinitis, sinusitis, pharyngitis, laryngitis, tonsillitis • Acute lower respiratory infections: Bronchitis, pneumonia and bronchial asthma • Hemoptysis, Acute chest pain	• Lecture • Discussion • Demonstration • Role play • Suggested field visits • Field practice • Assessment of clients with common conditions and provide referral	• Short answer • Essay • Field visit reports • OSCE assessment

Unit	Time (Hrs)	Learning outcomes	Content	Teaching/learning activities	Assessment methods
			Heart and blood • Common heart diseases: Heart attack/coronary artery disease, heart failure, arrhythmia • Blood anemia, blood cancers, bleeding disorders **Eye and ENT conditions** • Eye—local infections, redness of eye, conjunctivitis, stye, trachoma and refractive errors • ENT—epistaxis, ASOM, sore throat, deafness **Urinary system** • Urinary tract infections—cystitis, pyelonephritis, prostatitis, UTIs in children **First aid in common emergency conditions–Review** • High fever, low blood sugar, minor injuries, fractures, fainting, bleeding, shock, stroke, bites, burns, choking, seizures, RTAs, poisoning, drowning and foreign bodies		
II	20 (T)	Provide reproductive, maternal, newborn and childcare, including adolescent care in the urban and rural healthcare settings	**Reproductive, maternal, newborn, child and adolescent Health (Review from OBG Nursing and application in community setting)** • Present situation of reproductive, maternal and child health in India **Antenatal care** • Objectives, antenatal visits and examination, nutrition during pregnancy, counseling • Calcium and iron supplementation in pregnancy • Antenatal care at health centre level • Birth preparedness • High-risk approach: Screening/ early identification and primary management of complications—antepartum hemorrhage, pre-eclampsia, eclampsia, anemia, gestational diabetes mellitus, hypothyroidism, syphilis • Referral, follow up and maintenance of records and reports **Intranatal care** • Normal labor–process, onset, stages of labor • Monitoring and active management of different stages of labor • Care of women after labor • Early identification, primary management, referral and follow up–preterm labor, fetal distress, prolonged and obstructed labor, vaginal and perennial tears, ruptured uterus • Care of newborn immediately after birth • Maintenance of records and reports	• Lecture • Discussion • Demonstration • Role play • Suggested field visits and field practice • Assessment of antenatal, postnatal, newborn, infant, preschool child, school child, and adolescent health • Screen, manage and refer adolescents • Counsel adolescents	• Short answer • Essay • OSCE assessment

Unit	Time (Hrs)	Learning outcomes	Content	Teaching/learning activities	Assessment methods

		Promote adolescent health and youth friendly services	• Use of safe childbirth checklist
			• SBA module—review
			• Organization of labor room
			Postpartum care
			• Objectives, postnatal visits, care of mother and baby, breastfeeding, diet during lactation, and health counseling
			• Early identification, primary management, referral and follow up of complications, Danger signs—postpartum hemorrhage, shock, puerperal sepsis, breast conditions, postpartum depression
			• Postpartum visit by healthcare provider
			Newborn and child care
			• Review: Essential newborn care
			• Management of common neonatal problems
			• Management of common child health problems: Pneumonia, diarrhea, sepsis, screening for congenital anomalies and referral
			• Review: IMNCI module
			• Under five clinics
			Adolescent health
			• Common health problems and risk factors in adolescent girls and boys
			• Common gynecological conditions—dysmenorrhea, premenstrual syndrome (PMS), vaginal discharge, mastitis, breast lump, pelvic pain, pelvic organ prolapse
			• Teenage pregnancy, awareness about legal age of marriage, nutritional status of adolescents national menstrual hygiene scheme
			• Youth-friendly services:
			  ▪ SRH service needs
			  ▪ Role and attitude of nurses: Privacy, confidentiality, nonjudgemental attitude, client autonomy, respectful care and communication
			• Counseling for parents and teenagers (BCS–balanced counseling strategy)
			National Programs
			• RMNCH+A approach—aims, health systems strengthening, RMNCH+A strategies, interventions across life stages, program management, monitoring and evaluation systems
			• Universal Immunization Program (UIP) as per Government of India guidelines—Review
			• Rashtriya Bal Swasthya Karyakaram (RSBK)—children
			• Rashtriya Kishor Swasthya Karyakram (RKSK)—adolescents
			Any other new programs		

Unit	Time (Hrs)	Learning outcomes	Content	Teaching/learning activities	Assessment methods
III	4 (T)	Discuss the concepts and scope of demography	**Demography, Surveillance and Interpretation of Data** • *Demography and vital statistics:* Demographic cycle, world population trends, vital statistics • Sex ratio and child sex ratio, trends of sex ratio in India, the causes and social implications • *Sources of vital statistics:* Census, registration of vital events, sample registration system • *Morbidity and mortality indicators:* Definition, calculation and interpretation • Surveillance, Integrated Disease Surveillance Project (IDSP), Organization of IDSP, flow of information and mother and child tracking system (MCTS) in India • Collection, analysis, interpretation, use of data • *Review:* Common sampling techniques—random and nonrandom techniques • Disaggregation of data	• Lecture • Discussion • Demonstration • Role play • Suggested field visits • Field practice	• Short answer • Essay
IV	6 (T)	Discuss population explosion and its impact on social and economic development of India Describe the various methods of population control	**Population and its Control** • Population explosion and its impact on social, economic development of individual, society and country. • *Population control:* Women empowerment; social, economic and educational development • *Limiting family size:* Promotion of small family norm, temporary spacing methods (natural, biological, chemical, mechanical methods etc.), terminal methods (tubectomy, vasectomy) • Emergency contraception • Counseling in reproductive, sexual health including problems of adolescents • Medical termination of pregnancy and MTP Act • National Population Stabilization Fund/JSK (Jansankhya Sthirata Kosh) • Family planning 2020 • National Family Welfare Program • Role of a nurse in Family Welfare Program	• Lecture • Discussion • Demonstration • Role play • Suggested field visits • Field practice	• Short answer • Essay • OSCE assessment • Counseling on family planning
V	5 (T)	Describe occupational health hazards, occupational diseases and the role of nurses in occupational health programs	Occupational Health • Occupational health hazards • Occupational diseases • ESI Act • National/State Occupational Health Programs • Role of a nurse in occupational health services: Screening, diagnosing, management and referral of clients with occupational health problems	• Lecture • Discussion • Demonstration • Role play • Suggested field visits • Field practice	• Essay • Short answer • Clinical performance evaluation

Unit	Time (Hrs)	Learning outcomes	Content	Teaching/learning activities	Assessment methods
VI	6 (T)	Identify health problems of older adults and provide primary care, counseling and supportive health services	**Geriatric Health Care** • Health problems of older adults • Management of common geriatric ailments: counseling, supportive treatment of older adults • Organization of geriatric health services • National Program for Health Care of Elderly (NPHCE) • State level programs/Schemes for older adults • Role of a community health nurse in geriatric health services: Screening, diagnosing, management and referral of older adults with health problems	• Lecture • Discussion • Demonstration	• Visit report on elderly home • Essay • Short answer
VII	6 (T)	Describe screening for mental health problems in the community, take preventive measures and provide appropriate referral services	**Mental Health Disorders** • Screening, management, prevention and referral for mental health disorders • *Review:* ▪ Depression, anxiety, acute psychosis, schizophrenia ▪ Dementia ▪ Suicide ▪ Alcohol and substance abuse ▪ Drug deaddiction program ▪ National Mental Health Program ▪ National Mental Health Policy ▪ National Mental Health Act • Role of a community health nurse in screening, initiation of treatment and follow up of mentally ill clients	• Lecture • Discussion • Demonstration • Role play • Health counseling on promotion of mental health • Suggested field visits • Field practice	• Essay • Short answer • Counseling report
VIII	4 (T)	Discuss about effective management of health information in community diagnosis and intervention	**Health Management Information System (HMIS)** • Introduction to health management system: data elements, recording and reporting formats, data quality issues • *Review:* ▪ Basic Demography and vital statistics ▪ Sources of vital statistics ▪ Common sampling techniques, frequency distribution ▪ Collection, analysis, interpretation of data • Analysis of data for community needs assessment and preparation of health action plan	• Lecture • Discussion • Demonstration • Role play • Suggested field visits • Field practice • Group project on community diagnosis—data management	• Group project report • Essay • Short answer
IX	12 (T)	Describe the system management of delivery of community health services in rural and urban areas	**Management of Delivery of Community Health Services** • Planning, budgeting and material management of CHC, PHC, SC/HWC • Manpower planning as per IPHS standards • **Rural:** Organization, staffing and material management of rural health services provided by Government at village, SC/HWC, PHC, CHC, hospitals – district, state and central • **Urban:** Organization, staffing, and functions of urban health services provided by Government at slums, dispensaries, special clinics, municipal and corporate hospitals	• Lecture • Discussion • Visits to various healthcare delivery systems • Supervised field practice	• Essay • Short answer • Filed visit reports

Unit	Time (Hrs)	Learning outcomes	Content	Teaching/learning activities	Assessment methods
			• Defense services • Institutional services • *Other systems of medicine and health:* Indian system of medicine, AYUSH clinics, Alternative health care system referral systems, Indigenous health services		
X	**15 (T)**	Describe the leadership role in guiding, supervising, and monitoring the health services and the personnel at the PHCs, SCs and community level including financial management Describe the roles and responsibilities of Mid-Level Health Care Providers (MHCPs) in Health Wellness Centers (HWCs)	**Leadership, Supervision and Monitoring** • Understanding work responsibilities/ job description of DPHN, Health Visitor, PHN, MPHW (Female), Multipurpose health Worker (Male), AWWs and ASHA • Roles and responsibilities of Mid-Level Health Care Providers (MLHPs) • Village Health Sanitation and Nutrition Committees (VHSNC): Objectives, composition and roles and responsibilities • Health team management • Review: Leadership and supervision—concepts, principles and methods • Leadership in health: leadership approaches in healthcare setting, taking control of health of community and organizing health camps, village clinics • Training, Supportive supervision and monitoring–concepts, principles and process, e.g., performance of frontline health workers **Financial Management and Accounting and Computing at Health Centers (SC)** • Activities for which funds are received	• Lecture • Discussion • Demonstration • Role play • Suggested field visits • Field practice	• Report on interaction with MPHWs, HVs, ASHA, AWWs • Participation in training programs • Essay • Short answer
			▪ Accounting and bookkeeping requirements– accounting principles and policies, book of accounts to be maintained, basic accounting entries, accounting process, payments and expenditure, fixed asset, SOE reporting format, utilization certificate (UC) reporting ▪ Preparing a budget ▪ Audit **Records and Reports** • *Concepts of records and reports*—importance, legal implications, purposes, use of records, principles of record writing, filing of records • *Types of records*—community related records, registers, guidelines for maintaining • *Report writing*—purposes, documentation of activities, types of reports • *Medical Records Department*—functions, filing and retention of medical records		

Unit	Time (Hrs)	Learning outcomes	Content	Teaching/learning activities	Assessment methods
			• *Electronic Medical Records (EMR)*—capabilities and components of EMR, electronic health record (EHR), levels of automation, attributes, benefits and disadvantages of HER • **Nurses' responsibility in record keeping and reporting**		
XI	**6 (T)**	Demonstrate initiative in preparing themselves and the community for disaster preparedness and management	**Disaster Management** • Disaster types and magnitude • Disaster preparedness • Emergency preparedness • Common problems during disasters and methods to overcome • Basic disaster supplies kit • Disaster response including emergency relief measures and life-saving techniques Use disaster management module	• Lecture • Discussion • Demonstration • Role play • Suggested field visits, and field practice • Mock drills • Refer Disaster module (NDMA) National Disaster/INC – Reaching out in emergencies	
XII	**3 (T)**	Describe the importance of biomedical waste management, its process and management	**Biomedical Waste Management** • Waste collection, segregation, transportation and management in the community • Waste management in health center/ clinics • Biomedical waste management guidelines—2016, 2018 (Review)	• Lecture-cum-discussion • Field visit to waste management site	• Field visit report
XIII	**3 (T)**	Explain the roles and functions of various national and international health agencies	**Health Agencies** • International: WHO, UNFPA, UNDP, World Bank, FAO, UNICEF, European Commission, Red Cross, USAID, UNESCO, ILO, CAR, CIDA, JHPIEGO, any other • National: Indian Red Cross, Indian Council for Child Welfare, Family Planning Association of India, Tuberculosis Association of India, Central Social Welfare Board, All India Women's Conference, Blind Association of India, any other • Voluntary Health Association of India (VHA)	• Lecture • Discussion • Field visits	• Essay • Short answer

MSc NURSING

CLINICAL SPECIALITY- I
COMMUNITY HEALTH NURSING

Placement: 1st Year

Hours of Instructions
Theory: 150 hours
Practical: 650 hours
Total: 800 hours

Course Description

The course is designed to assist students in developing expertise and in- depth understanding in the field of Community Health Nursing. It would help students to appreciate holistic lifestyle of individuals, families and groups and develop skills to function as Community Health Nurse specialist/practitioner. It would further enable student to function as an educator, manager and researcher in the field of community health nursing.

Objectives

At the end of the course, the student will be able to:

- Appreciate the history and development in the field of Community Health and Community Health Nursing.
- Appreciate role of individuals and families in promoting health of the community.
- Perform physical, developmental and nutritional assessment of individuals, families and groups.
- Apply the concepts of promotive, preventive, curative and rehabilitative aspects of health while providing care to the people.
- Apply nursing process approach while providing care to individuals, families, groups and community.
- Integrate the concepts of family-centered nursing approach while providing care to the community.
- Recognize and participate in the management of emergencies, epidemics and disasters.
- Apply recent technologies and care modalities while delivering community health nursing care.
- Appreciate legal and ethical issues pertaining to community health nursing care.
- Conduct community health nursing care projects.
- Participate in planning, implementation and evaluation of various national health and family welfare programs at local, state and the national level.
- Incorporate evidence-based nursing practice and identify the areas of research in the community settings.
- Participate effectively as a member of community health team.
- Coordinate and collaborate with various agencies operating in the community by using intersectoral approach.
- Teach community health nursing to undergraduates, in-service nurses and the community health workers.
- Demonstrate leadership and managerial abilities in community health nursing practice

Course Content

Unit	Hours	Content
I	10	**Introduction** • Historical development of community health and community health nursing—World and India, various health and family welfare committees • Current status, trends and challenges of community health nursing • Health status of the community-community diagnosis • Scope of community health nursing practice • Ethical and legal issues • Sociocultural issues in community health nursing • National policies, plans and programs ▪ National Health Policy ▪ National Population Policy ▪ National Health and Welfare Programmes ▪ National health goals/indicators/Millennium developmental goals (MDG)/strategies ▪ Planning process: Five-year plans ▪ National Rural Health Mission ▪ Panchayat Raj Institutions

Unit	Hours	Content
II	10	**Health** • Concepts, issues • Determinants • Measurements • Alternate systems for health promotion and management of health problems • Health economics • Health technology • Genetics and health • Waste disposal • Ecosystem
III	15	**Population dynamics and control** • Demography • Transition and theories of population • National population policy • National population programs • Population control and related programs • Methods of family limiting and spacing • Research, Census, National Family Health Survey
IV	30	**Community health Nursing** • Philosophy, Aims, Objectives, Concepts, Scope, Principles, Functions • Community health Nursing theories and models • Quality assurance: Community health Nursing standards, competencies, Monitoring community health nursing, nursing audits • Family nursing and family-centered nursing approach • Family health nursing process ▪ Family health assessment ▪ Diagnosis ▪ Planning ▪ Intervention ▪ Evaluation • Nursing care for special groups: Children, adolescents, adults, women, elderly, physically and mentally challenged—urban and rural population at large • Community nutrition • Concept, role and responsibilities of community health nurse practitioners/nurse midwifery practitioners-decision making skills, professionalism, legal issues
V	45	**Maternal and neonatal care** • IMNCI (Integrated Management of Neonatal and Childhood Illnesses) module • Skilled Birth Attendant (SBA) module
VI	15	• Disaster nursing (INC module on reaching out: Nursing care in emergencies)
VII	10	**Information, education and communication** • IEC/BCC: Principles and strategies • Communication skills • Management information and evaluation system: Records and reports • Information technology • Tele-medicine and telenursing • Journalism • Mass media • Folk media
VIII	15	**Healthcare delivery system: Urban, rural, tribal and difficult areas** • Health organization: National, State, District, CHC, PHC, Subcenter, village—functions, staffing, pattern of assistance, layout, drugs, equipments and supplies, roles and responsibilities of DPHNO • Critical review of functioning of various levels, evaluation studies, recommendations and nursing perspectives • Alternative systems of medicine • Training and supervision of health workers

CHAPTER 1

Introduction to Community Health Nursing

INTRODUCTION TO HEALTH

Health is the level of functional or metabolic efficiency of a living organism. In humans it is the general condition of a person's mind and body, usually meaning to be free from illness, injury or pain. Generally we know, health is absence of disease. Individuals describe health in their own way. From the immemorial time man has been interested in trying to control disease. In ancient time health and illness were interpreted in an anthropological perspective. Primitive people also believed that health is a God gift.

Health is a common theme in most culture. In fact all communities have their concept of health apart of their culture. Among definitions still used probably the oldest is that health is absence of disease. The determinants of health are not yet clear. The current meaning or definition of health is elusive and there is no single yardstick for measuring health. In some culture health and harmony are considered equivalent, harmony is being defined as being at peace with the self the community, God and Cosmos. During the past few decades there has been a preawakening that health is a fundamental right and a worldwide social goal which is essential to satisfy the basic human needs to an improved quality of life and that it is to be attained by all people.

So in 1977, 30th World Health Assembly decided that the main social target of government and WHO in the coming decades should be the attainment by all citizens of the world by the year 2000 of a level of health that will permit them to lead a socially and economically productive life called health for all. So, health is an integral part of socioeconomic development by United Nations 1979 and it has also become a major instrument of overall socioeconomic development and the creation of a new social order.

CHANGING CONCEPT OF HEALTH

Health is perceived as different within different communities. An understanding of health which is a basis of all health care is not perceived in same way by all members in a community including various professional groups (e.g., biomedical scientists, social science specialist, health administrator, ecologists, etc.) being giving rise to confusion about the concept of health. In a world of continuous changes new concepts are bound to emerge based on new pattern of thought. Primitive people believed that health is a God gift and it cannot be earned. Health has evolved over the centuries as a concept form an individual concern to world wide social goal and encompass the whole quality of life.

Biomedical Concept

According to the biomedical model, health constitutes the freedom from disease, pain, or defect, thus making the normal human condition 'healthy'. The model's focus on the physical processes, such as the pathology, the biochemistry and the physiology of a disease, does not take into account the role of social factors or individual subjectivity. Traditionally health has been viewed as an absence of diseases and if one is free from diseases that the person was consider as healthy. This biomedical concept is based on the germ theory of disease. According to this theory, the medical profession viewed the human body as a machine. Disease break down the machine and doctor repair it. The criticism that is leveled against biomedical concept is that this concept has minimized the role of environmental, social, psychological and cultural determinant of health. The biomedical model is only for treating diseases but also inadequate to solve some of major health problems of mankind (e.g., malnutrition, accidental, mental illness).

By elaborating the medical technology development in medical and social sciences the conclusion is that biomedical concept of health was inadequate.

Ecological Concept

Inadequacy in biomedical model concept gave rise to other concept. The word ecology derived from Greek word *Oikos*—means house. The ecologist put forward a hypothesis that health is a dynamic equilibrium between man and his environment. The disease is due to maladjustment of human organism to the environment. Ecology is defined as the science of mutual relationship between living organisms and their environment. Dubas defined 'Health implies the relative absence of pain and discomfort and maladaptation and adjustment to the environment to ensure optimal function'. The ecological concept raises two issues. Imperfect man and imperfect environment, history argues and also accept this. The human ecosystem includes—natural environment and manmade environment. The dimensions of environment are, physical, chemical, biological, psychological and also our cultural and its product. Disease is embedded in the ecosystem of man. In a greener pasture, where people inhale fresh air, no black smoke emitted from factory chimneys, the general health condition of local inhabitants is bound to be noteworthy. With global warming, we have experienced erratic rain, drought accompanied by famine. Not only that, with holes in ozone layer, injurious ultraviolet rays are coming into the atmosphere, which may eventually cause skin cancer. These negative aspects arising from ruining the ecosystem by mankind are all will affect to our Health. With good counsel, we can save Mother Earth, by not further damaging the ecosystem, thus not jeopardizing the health of its inhabitants. Health according to ecological concept is visualized as a state of dynamic equilibrium between man and his environment. By instantly altering of ecosystem or environment by such activities: urbanization, industrialization, deforestation, land reclamation, construction of irrigation canals and dams, man has created himself new health problems. Today the greatest threat to human health in India is ever increasing due to unplanned urbanization, growth of slum and deterioration of environment. The changes of ecological cycle of disease has resulted in zoozatic diseases like yellow fever, monkey pox, etc. Ecological factors are the root of the geographic distribution of diseases. Therefore good public health is good ecology.

Psychosocial Concept

Contemporary development in social sciences revealed that health is not only a biomedical phenomenon and ecological phenomenon but one which is influenced by social, psychological, cultural, economic and political factors of the people concerned. These factors must be taken into consideration in defining and measuring health.

Psychosocial well-being is a multidimensional construct consisting of psychological, social, and subjective components which influence the overall functionality of individuals in achieving their true potentials as members of the society. Proper psychological health involves a normal emotional, behavioral, and social maturity to a person. This means such a person is in a healthy state of mental well-being, one that they can use to function normally in society and during everyday events. The psychosocial concept is defined as 'Those factors affecting personal healthcare and community well-being that stream from the psychosocial make up the individuals and it structure avoid and functions within the social group'. The factor includes cultural value, habits, attitudes, religion, lifestyle, health services, customs beliefs, moral education, community life and social and political organization.

In addition to this broad aspect of psychosocial environment, man is constant interaction with the part of social environment as people. He is a member of family, caste, community and nation. Between the individual and other member of group there can be harmony and disharmony. There can be started conflict. The individual behavior can effect on the other members of group. The custom attitude belief tradition all regulates the interaction among group of individual and families. It develops through the process of socialization. Lifestyles are learnt through social interaction with parent, pear group, friends, school and mass media. So, the favorable social environment can improve the health and fulfillment and provide quality of life. Many current health problem especially in the developed countries are due to associated with changes of lifestyle. Coronary heart disease, hypertension, drug addiction, handicapped, emotional symptoms such as feelings of anxiety, depression, anger, frustration, etc., and road accidents are now the principal cause of death in young people, which is related to psychosocial anxiety, frustration, preoccupation which are related to the changes of psychological factors. Social factors include the custom attitude belief tradition all regulate the interaction among group of individual and families. It develops through the process of socialization. Lifestyles are learnt through social interaction with parent, pear group, friends, school and mass media. So, the favorable social environment can improve the health and fulfillment and provide quality of life. Malnutrition, hookworm infestation, diarrhea and cancer can occur due to the influence of social factors.

Holistic Concept

The holistic model is the synthesis of all models or concepts. It recognizes the strength of physical, psychological, social, economic, political and environmental influences of health. Holistic concept of health has been variously defined as a unified multidimensional process involving the well-being of whole person in the contest of his environmental. In ancient time it is stated that health impulse a sound mind in a social body in a sound family in sound environment. The holistic approach implies that all sectors of society have an effect on health in particular. Agriculture, animal husbandry, food industry, education, housing, public work communication and a good social system, all these are emphasis on promotion and protection of health.

By following the holistic concept WHO gave a definition in 1948 'Health is a state of complete physical, mental and social well-being and not merely an absence of disease or infirmity'. Operational definition of Health by WHO—a condition or quality of the human organism expressing the adequate functioning of the organism in given conditions, genetic or environmental dimensions of health and wellness.

DIMENSIONS OF HEALTH

The WHO definition of health has been criticized as being to broad. Some argue that health cannot be defined as a state of all but must be seen as a process of continuous adjustment to the changing demand of living and of the changing meaning, we give to life, it is a dynamic concept. It helps people live well, work well and enjoy themselves so there is some new philosophy of health. In broad sense health can be seen as a condition or quality of the human organism expressing the adequate functioning of the organism in a given condition, genetic or environment. Overall good health and wellness are interdependent on five dimensions, namely physical, intellectual, emotional, social and spiritual.

Physical Dimensions

Physical dimension of health relates to the efficient functioning of the body and its systems, and includes the physical capacity to perform tasks and physical fitness. A person is considered as physically healthy if his/her every system of body functions optimally. He/she is free from any type of physical illness and his/her every tissue and cells functions normal. A healthy body maintained by good nutrition, regular exercise, avoiding harmful habits, making informed decisions about health and seeking medical assistance when necessary. A person who enjoys good physical health is one who:

- Is energetic
- Has good posture
- Weighs normal for age and height
- Has all body organs functioning normally
- Has a clear and clean skin
- Has bright eyes
- Has good textured and shining hair
- Has a clean breath
- Has a good appetite
- Gets sound sleep.

Mental Dimension

A person is mentally healthy if he or she is relaxed and free from any worries. Mental dimensions has two branch, intellectual dimension and emotional dimension.

Intellectual Dimension

Intellectual dimension is a state in which mind is engaged in lively interaction with the world. It involves continued learning, problem solving and creativity. It also involves ability to learn and use information effectively for personal, family, and career development striving for continued growth and learning to deal with new challenges effectively, encompasses cognitive abilities, educational background and past experiences, positive sense of purpose. These influence a client's response to teaching about health and reactions to health care during illness.

Emotional Dimension

Emotional dimension is the ability to understand own feelings, accept own limitations, achieve emotional stability and become comfortable with his/her emotions. It refers to feelings, affect and person's ability to express these, includes belief in one's worth. Long-term stress affects the body systems and anxiety affects health habits; conversely, calm acceptance and relaxation can actually change body responses to illness.

Mental health can be achieved by control on emotions, sensitive to the needs of others, confidence in one's own abilities, freedom from unnecessary tensions, anxieties and worries, accept one's limitations, recognize, accept, and express feelings and ability to manage stress and express emotions appropriately.

Social Dimension

Social dimension concerns the sense of having support available from family and friends; practices, values and beliefs that determine health. The ability to relate well to others, both within and outside the family unit. It encourages contributing to a healthy community by supporting a healthy living environment and initiating better communication with other. It is the ability to interact successfully with people and within the environment of which each person is a part and develop and maintain intimacy with significant others develop respect and tolerance for those with different opinions and beliefs.

Spiritual

Spiritual dimension denotes the sense that life is meaningful and has a purpose; the ethics, values and morals that guide us and give meaning and direction to life. The spiritual dimension is understood to imply a phenomenon that is not material in nature, but belongs to the realm of ideas, beliefs, values and ethics that have arisen in the minds and conscience of human beings, particularly ennobling ideas have given rise to health ideals which have led to a practical strategy for Health for All which aims at attaining a goal that has both a material and nonmaterial component. If the material component of the strategy can be provided to people, the nonmaterial or spiritual one is something that has to arise within people and communities in keeping with their social and cultural patterns. The spiritual dimension plays a great role in motivating people's achievement in all aspects of life.

POSITIVE HEALTH

A positive concept of health refers to the aspect of physical emotional, intellectual and social well-being of a person in terms of being free from any ailments or diseases, it also implies a state of physical, mental and social well-being with the harmonious balance of this state of human individual integrated into his environment. In short, the notion of 'perfect functioning' of the body and mind. A positive healthy individual should be:

Biologically

As a state in which every cell and every organ is functioning at optimum capacity and in perfect harmony with the rest of the body.

Psychologically

As a state in which the individual feels a sense of perfect well-being and of mastery over his environment.

Socially

As a state in which the individual's capacities for participation in the social system are optimal.

Dubos said, 'The concept of perfect positive health cannot become a reality because man will never be so perfectly adapted to his environment that his life will not involve struggles, failures and sufferings. Positive health will therefore always remain a mirage, because everything in our life is subject to change. Health is the ability of an individual or social group to modify himself or itself continually.'

The face of changing condition of life health fluctuates within a range of optimum well-being to various levels of dysfunction, including the state of total dysfunction namely the death. Health of an individual is not static, it is dynamic phenomenon and a process of continuous change. There are degrees or levels of health as there are degrees or severity of illness.

CONCEPT OF WELL-BEING

Individuals functions according to their needs for physical, emotional and social well-being. Well-being is the state of being healthy and happy and living a full life. How individuals might describe their feelings about physical, emotional and social well-being.

Examples

Types of well-being	*Description*
Health	I am usually pretty healthy. I never miss work because of sickness
Energy	I have enough energy to do the things I should do every day
Comfort	I can eat a variety of foods without having stomach problems
Emotional	Everyone says I am a healthy, cheerful person. I am even tempered, but certain things make me a little anxious
Social	Playing on the football team helps me make a lot of friends

Well-being of an individual or group of individuals have objective and subjective components. The objective components relate to such concerns generally known by the term 'Standard of living or level of living'. It referred to as quality of life.

1. **Standard of living:** Refers to usual scale of our expenditure, the goods we consume and the services we enjoy. It includes the level of education, employment status, food, dress, house, amusements and comforts of modern living.

   According to WHO—Income and occupation standards of housing, sanction and nutrition, the level of provision of health, educational, recreational and other services collectively as an index of the standard of living.
2. **Level of living:** It consists of nine components health, food consumption, education, occupation and working condition, housing, social security, clothing, recreation and leisure and human rights. Health is the most important component of the level of living because its impairment always means impairment of the level of livings.
3. **Quality of life:** Quality of life was defined by the condition of the effects of the complete range of factors such as those determining health, happiness (including comfort in the physical environment and a satisfying occupation), education, social and intellectual attainments freedom of action, justice and freedom of expression. The quality of life can be maintained by maintaining harmony to all factors.

The different aspects of quality of life are:

- **Having a purpose in life:** The absence of purpose in life leads to alcoholism, drug, dependence, suicide and depression.
- **Maintaining positive attitudes:** If you keep a journal for one week, of all your attitudes towards life, you will become aware of how much you pollute the environment with your negative attitudes, the positive attitude can be developed by the person's inner motivation. Keep up the journal writing until the positive attitudes are predominant and a part of your thinking process.
- **Using one's abilities fully:** A person may have a lot of hidden qualities which may be ignore to himself/herself. By using one's abilities fully an individual can improve his/her quality of life.
- **Having the will to be whole and healthy:** If you program yourself to be sick, you will be sick constantly telling yourself you are not strong, you catch cold easily, you are allergic to this and that will maintain your body in ill health. Activate your warrior, listen to positive programming and you will reach a high level of wellness.
- **Being adaptable:** If we stay stuck like old cement we will crack and break from the winds of change. It is better to be flexible and adapt to the wind like the reels and the swaying bamboos we need to have lots of give.
- **Cooperating with other people:** This leads to harmony and greater achievement of peace and prosperity.
- **Accepting responsibility for one's thought and action:** It is so easy to blame others, but it is a sign of maturity to see that all your thoughts, feelings, words and actions are under your control. Take self-responsibility and to be a power for good in the world.

Health is a dynamic state that fluctuates a person adapts to changes in the internal and external environments to maintain a state of well-being. Illness is a process in which the functioning of a person is diminished or impaired when compared with the person's previous condition. High level wellness and severe illness are at opposite ends of the continuum. There are a variety of risk factors which are important in identifying level of health. Risk factors include genetic, physiological, environmental, age and lifestyle factors.

CONCEPT OF ILLNESS

Illness is any change, temporary or long lasting in a person's physical and emotional health and social well-being. An illness may be acute, chronic and terminal.

Illness shows positive and negative behavior. It can make persons feel helpless and defenseless. Sick people are unable to do anything for themselves even though they want to during illness. We should respond to patient's need for comfort and safety. A back rub or an extra blanket make patient comfortable, be sure side rails are raised for any patient who is weak or unconscious.

The person who is not healthy has expects and deserves competent care may choose to assume the sick role.

Webster defines disease as a condition in which body health is impaired a departure from a state of health and alternation of the human body interrupting the performance of vital function.

The Oxford English Dictionary defines disease as a condition in which the functions are disrupted or deranged.

From an ecological point of view, disease is defined as maladjustment of the human organism to the environment.

From sociological point of view, disease is considering a social phenomena occurring in all societies and defined and fought in terms of particular cultural forces prevalent in the society.

The simplest definition in disease is opposite to health.

THEORIES AND MODELS OF DISEASE CAUSATION

Epidemiological aspects of diseases: Disease is a dynamic process and it is just the opposite of health. Health denotes perfect harmony and normal functioning of all the body systems, i.e., state of complete well-being. Whereas disease denotes the disharmony and deviations from normal functioning of various body systems, i.e., state of illness. Perfect health and severe disease or wellness and illness are the two end points of health and disease continuum. The disharmony and deviations range from biochemical disturbance to severe disability culminating to death. There are various causative factors which cause the occurrence of a disease. These factors are related to human being and their environment.

The concept of disease causation differed from time to time with the progress of civilization. It changed from supernatural causes during primitive period to multifactorial causes during modern time. It is very important to understand the concept of disease causation and disease progress because it can help in identifying public health measures to prevent and control diseases. The aims of epidemiological studies are to acquire knowledge about the nature of disease/health problems, their etiological factors and then utilize that knowledge in planning community health services to prevent and control diseases/health problems.

Before the discovery of microorganisms (bacteria by Louis Pasteur, 1822–1895), the French scientist in 1860, several theories explaining the causes of diseases were put forward from time to time. The earliest attempt to attribute a cause to illness occurred during the religious era (2000 BC to 600 BC). During this period, disease was thought to be caused by divine power as punishment for sins as bad deeds or considered as fate. This theory is referred as supernatural theory. With the discovery of microorganisms by Louis Pasteur and Roberkoch (1843–1910), the bacteriologic era commenced in the late 1870, which was the turning point in disease causation. The germ theory was put forward by these scientists.

The Germ Theory

The germ theory became popular during the 19th and early part of 20th century. This theory attributes microorganisms as the only cause of diseases. According to this theory, there is one single specific microorganism (causative agent) to every disease. This refers to one relationship between the causative agent and the disease. This is also called as single cause theory **(Fig. 1.1)**.

For example diphtheria due to *Corynebacterium diphtheria*, cholera due to *Vibrio cholerae*, tuberculosis due to tuberculosis bacilli. This theory is limited to infectious disease only. The single cause theory was further supported by the identification of other specific agents as causative agents for certain health problems, i.e., lack of vitamin 'C' was found to cause survey.

Theory of Epidemiological Triad (Fig. 1.2)

The germ theory or single cause theory has many limitations. It was experienced that everyone exposed to disease agent did not contract the disease. For example—tuberculosis, all those who were exposed to the tuberculosis organism did not suffer from tuberculosis. Only those who were under nourished, lived in dark places and who did not have immunity against tuberculosis got the disease. This means it was not only the causative agent that was responsible for causing disease but there were other factors related to man (host) and environment which contributed to the occurrence of a disease **(Fig. 1.2)**.

State of Health Equilibrium (Fig. 1.3)

This model is also called as ecological model. It is evolved through the study of infectious diseases. According to this model there are three elements or major factors which are responsible for a particular disease causation. These are agent, host and environment. The agent is considered to be the primary factor (e.g., amoeba, bacteria, fungi, virus) without which a particular disease cannot occur. The host refers to human beings who come in contact with the agent. The host related factors which play an important role are genetic make up, age, sex, race, immunity, health behavior, etc. The environment includes all that is external to the host and agent but that may influence interaction between them.

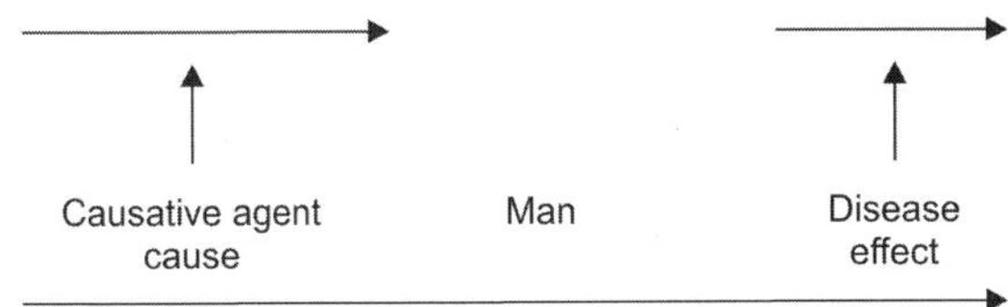

Fig. 1.1: Single cause theory.

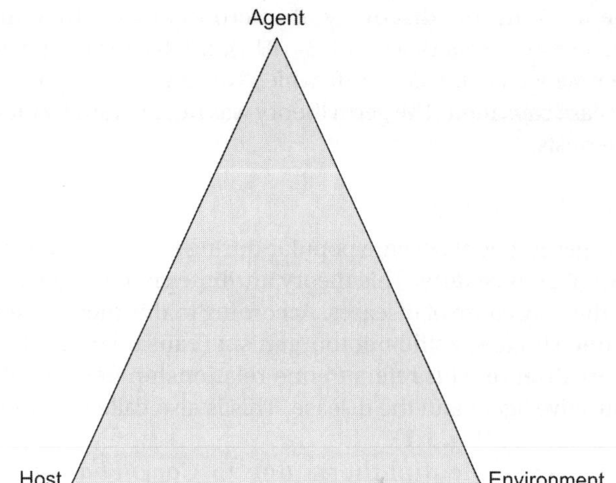

Fig. 1.2: Epidemiological triad.

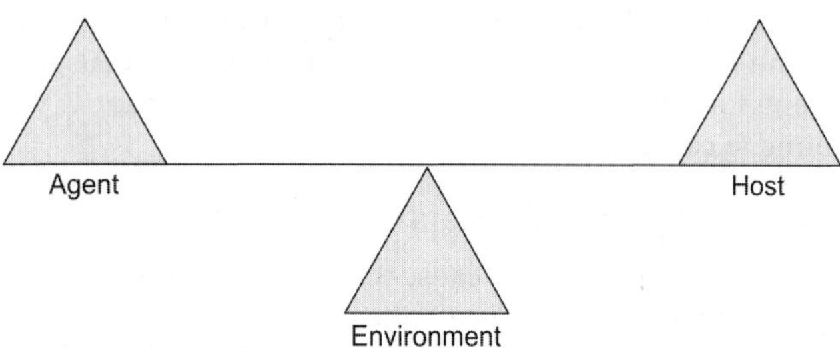

Fig. 1.3: Ecological model of health equilibrium.

As long as they remain in equilibrium or in balance disease will not occur and is referred as state of health equilibrium.

The disease will occur when equilibrium is disturbed due to change or disruption in any of these factors. For example—poor environmental sanitation, open defecation, contamination of water, foods, etc., all these environmental conditions increase the possibility of getting people infected with disease producing organisms.

Other examples of disruption that could increase the possibility of disease occurrence include:

- Conditions in the host such a severe malnutrition, disturbed immune system, poor specific resistance, etc., which increases susceptibility to disease.
- The increased number and mutation of virus which may increase their virulence and ability to infect the human host.

In fact, there has to be optimal interaction of all the three factors to cause a disease in a man. It implies that disease will occur only when the agent is strong and enters the host through the right channel and in sufficient amount, the host is susceptible and when environmental conditions facilitate the interaction of host and agent **(Fig. 1.4)**.

For example, the causation of pulmonary tuberculosis, the live tuberculosis bacilli must enter through respiratory tract and insufficient amount, the host must be susceptible, i.e., has no specific resistance and weak general body resistance and the environment must facilitate interaction of host and organisms, i.e., environment is crowded, dark and dingy.

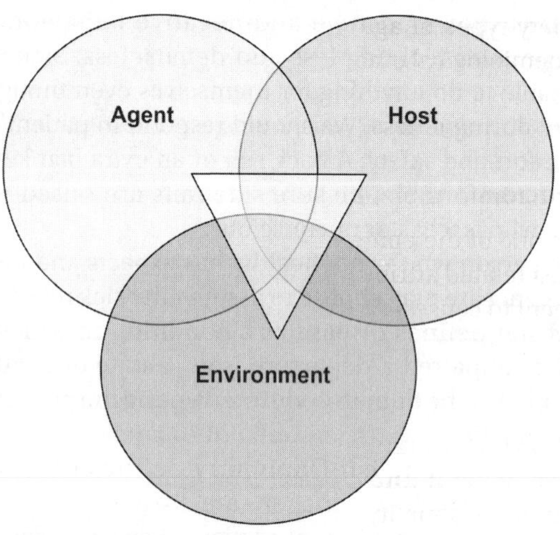

Optimal interaction: Agent, Host, Environment

Fig. 1.4: Epidemiological concept of interaction of host, agent and environment.

Elements of Epidemiological Triad and Related Risk Factors

Agent Factors

A disease agent is the primary link in the development of disease. The disease agent is defined as an element, a substance living or nonliving, or a force tangible or intangible, the presence or absence of which may follow the effective contact with susceptible human host under proper environmental conditions serve as a stimulus to initiate or perpetuate a disease process. The disease agents are usually classified as under:

- **Biological agents:** Biological agents are living agents and include arthropods and helminths, protozoa, fungi, bacteria, rickettsial and viruses.
- **Physical agents:** Physical agents include abnormalities in atmospheric pressures temperature and humidity, unusual intensity of sound, abnormalities of radiation and electricity. These agents are usually associated with certain occupational exposure.
- **Chemical agents:** Chemical agents may include useful substances like iodide and fluoride and harmful substances like noxious gases, volatile drugs and fumes, airborne solid particles. Some chemicals may also be produced in the body as a result of malfunctioning of body systems, for example, urea, bilirubin, ketones, calcium carbonate, uric acid, etc.
- **Mechanical agents:** It include chronic friction and mechanical forces that result in crushing, tearing or penetrating wounds, sprains, dislocation and other accidental injuries and even death.
- **Nutrient agents:** It include fats, carbohydrates, proteins, vitamins, minerals and water. Intake of these elements either in excess or in deficiency results in nutritional disorders, for example, anemia, night blindness, protein energy malnutrition (PEM), goiter. Though there are

variety types of agents responsible for diseases still in epidemiological triad, agent means microbial agent which is responsible for communicable diseases. Epidemiological triad is applicable to communicable diseases.

Host Factors

Host is one of the epidemiological determinants of disease. The host related attributes predispose the interaction of host and agent to cause a disease are:

- Demographic characteristics, i.e., age, sex, race, marital status, etc.
- Biological factors include genetic factors, blood chemistry, blood groups, immune system.
- **Psychosocial and economic characteristics:** These include personality traits, education, occupation, social class and status, mental status, emotional make up health knowledge and attitude, etc.
- **Lifestyle:** These include daily living and cultural practices including customs and traditions, health habits and health seeking behaviors such as physical exercise, nutrition practices, sexual practices, use of alcohol, drugs and smoking, etc.
- **Past history of exposure:** Exposure can range from infectious diseases to smoke in the environment, exposure to various occupational hazards.

Environmental Risk Factors

It is third important epidemiological determinant of disease. The various environmental factors influence the life and development of agents and host and their interaction to cause various diseases. The environment has three component. These are:

1. **Biological environment:** It includes all the living beings like animal kingdom, plants and microorganisms. Among of them some are infectious agents, reservoir of infection, intermediate host and vectors that transmit diseases.
2. **Physical environment:** It includes the nonliving chemical agents and physical factors. These are air, water, soil, environmental sanitation, housing radiation, gravity, atmospheric pressure, noise, electricity, television, radar, etc.
3. **Psychosocial environment:** It include over all socio-economic and political organization that affects health care and its delivery system, health legislation, sociocultural customs, traditions, belief and attitude, lifestyle, family and community life.

Multifactorial Causation

According to this theory, disease is due to multiple factors. As a result of advances in public health chemotherapy and vector control, communicable disease began to decline and replaced by new type of disease called modern disease of civilization, e.g., lung cancer, coronary heart disease, chronic bronchitis, mental illness, etc. These disease could not explained by germ theory and they will neither be prevented by the traditional methods of isolation, immunization or improvement sanitation. The realization began to dawn that the single cause idea was an over simplification and that there are other factors in etiology of disease—social, economic, cultural, genetic and psychological which are equally important for coronary heart disease and cancer due to multiple factors. For example, excess cigarette smoking, obesity, lack of physical exercises all are involved in disease condition. Therefore new model of disease causation have been developed which de-emphasize the concept of disease agent and stress multiplicity of interaction between host and environment. This theory of multifactorial causation was put forth by Pettenkofer of Munich (1819–1901). It is now known that most of these factors are much linked to lifestyle and human behavior that they are considered as 'Risk Factors', in the web causation of disease.

Web of causation (Fig. 1.5): This epidemiological concept of disease etiology is given by Mac Mohan and Pugh. According to this concept, disease (effect) never depends upon single isolated cause. Rather it develops as a result of chains of causation in which each link itself is the result of complex interaction of preceding events. These chains which may be fraction of the whole complex known as web of causation. The web of causation considers all the predisposing factor of any type and their complex inter-relationship with each other. The web of causation does not imply that the disease cannot be controlled unless all multiple factors should changed. It may cause by changes of causation at least a number of them approximately controlled or removed. This model is particularly applicable to chronic diseases where the causative agent is unknown and which are due to interaction of multiple factors, e.g., cardiovascular diseases, cancer.

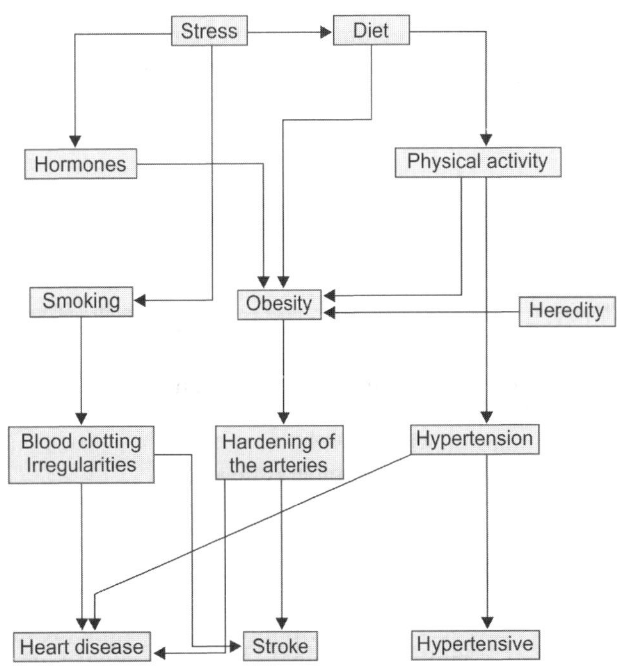

Fig. 1.5: Web of causation of disease.

Dever's Epidemiologic Model

This model is composed of four major categories of factors responsible for diseases such as human biology, lifestyle, environment and healthcare system. This four factors include all factors in its subcategories, for example, human biological factors are all host related factors of epidemiological triad and include genetic inheritance, complex physiologic systems, factors related to maturation and ageing. Similarly lifestyle factors include daily living activities, customs, traditions, health habits and behavior, etc., which influence the quality of life. Environmental factors include physical, biological, psychosocial components of environment. Healthcare system factors include availability, accessibility, adequacy and use of healthcare services at all levels. All these factors influence health status either positively or negatively.

THE HEALTH SICKNESS SPECTRUM

The high level wellness model developed by Halber Dunn in 1997 focuses on maximizing the health potential of an individual, family or community. It requires the individual to maintain a continuum of balance and purposeful direction within the environment.

Halbert Dunn defined high level wellness as an integrated method of functioning which is oriented towards maximizing the potential of which an individual is capable within the environment where he is functioning. Dunn stressed that wellness is an ongoing process directed towards higher potential, not a static goal and that high level wellness is a feeling of being alive to the tips of the fingers with energy to burn tingling with vitality.

The spectrum represented on the left side of the **Figure 1.6** bring the client back from illness or disease to a neutral point. The right side represents the potential for high level health and wellness. The objective of this model is to demonstrate how people can move from the point of illness or neutralize into the realm of high level wellness and to reduce the occurrence or recurrence of illness and disease.

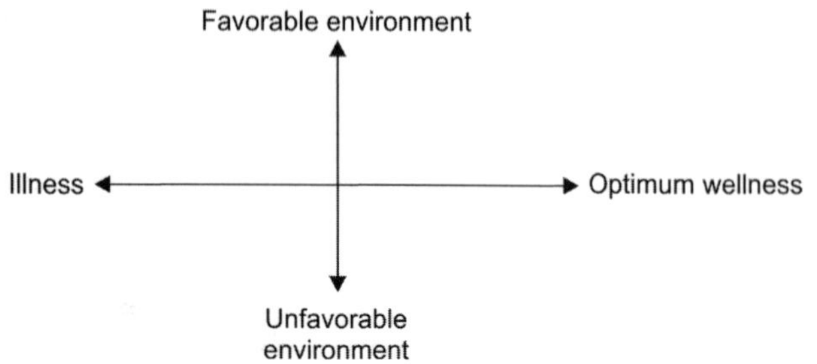

Fig. 1.6: Health illness spectrum.

HEALTH ILLNESS CONTINUUM (FIG. 1.7)

Health always involves a continuum, a range of degrees from optimal health at one end to death or total disability at the other. The health of an individual moves back and forth along this continuum throughout life, according to health illness continuum model-health is a dynamic state that fluctuates as a person adapts to changes in the internal and external environment to maintain a state of total well-being'. Internal environment refers to physiological system, body temperature, blood pressure, humidity, dust, etc.

High level wellness and severe illness at opposite ends of continuum. According to Newman (1990), health on a continuum is the degree of client's wellness that exists at any point in time, ranging from an optimal wellness condition, with available energy at its maximum to death, which represents total energy depletion. A nurse can determine a client level of health at any point on the health illness continuum.

Health and disease lie along a continuum and there is no single cut off point. The lowest point on the health disease spectrum is death and highest point corresponds to the WHO definition of positive health.

Health care directed a helping a client achieve high level wellness emphasizes health promotion and illness prevention rather than treatment. High level wellness is a dynamic process not a passive static state. No one ever reaches the point of perfect health, but there is constant attempt to achieve at optimal level of health a possible. Health is a dynamic process that varies as interaction between the individuals and their environment changes.

NATURAL HISTORY OF DISEASE

The natural history of diseases denotes the evolution of a disease process in an individual, from its early stage to final stage of recovery or death, in the absence of any intervention such as prevention or treatment. The natural history of an infectious disease occurs in two phases:

1. Prepathogenesis phase
2. Pathogenesis phase

Prepathogenesis Phase

This phase refers to the period before the onset of disease. During this phase, interaction is taking place among the three components of epidemiological triad namely agent, host and environment, each representing the angle of a triangle respectively. As long as there equilibrium among these three interacting factors, so long the person will be healthy. Once the equilibrium is disturbed, disease

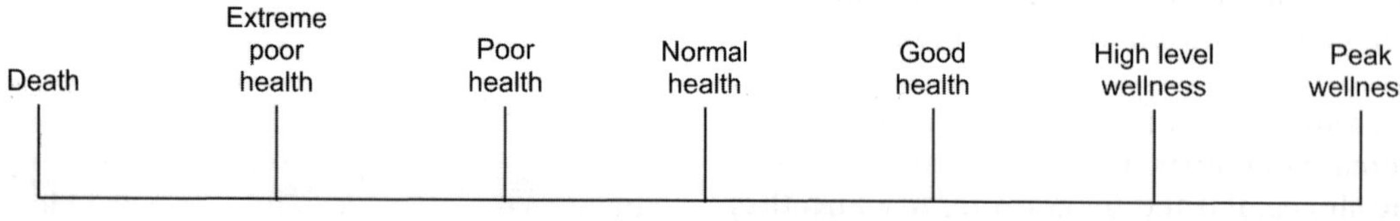

Fig. 1.7: Health illness continuum.

process starts. Here the disease agent has not yet entered man, but the factors which favor its interaction with the human host are already existing in the environment.

Pathogenesis Phase

This phase begins with the entry of the disease 'Agent' in the susceptible human host and multiplies and induces tissue causing physiological changes, the disease progresses through a period of incubation and later through early and late pathogenesis The final outcome of the disease may be recovery, disability or death.

The pathogenesis phase is divided into:

- Stage of subclinical disease
- Stage of clinical disease
- Stage of disability

Stage of Subclinical Disease

Stage of subclinical disease denoted by presymptomatic stage. A period of subclinical or in apparent pathologic changes follows exposure, ending with the onset of symptoms. The characteristic incubation period has a range for every disease. For example, for hepatitis A: 2 to 6 weeks and for HIV/AIDS it become 6 months to 8 years.

Stage of Clinical Disease

This phase starts with onset of sign and symptoms which may be mild to severe or fatal. The onset of symptoms marks the transition from subclinical to clinical disease. The clinical spectrum also depends on infectivity which refers to the proportion of exposed persons who become infected and pathogenicity which refers to the proportion of infected persons who develop clinical disease and virulence which refers to the proportion of persons with clinical disease who become severely ill or die.

Stage of Disability

Some diseases resolve completely but some may leave residual effect of short-term or long-term duration, leaving a person disabled to lesser or greater extent. Here tertiary level of prevention can be applicable.

DISEASE CYCLE

After an infectious agent invades a host (patient), it undergoes a series of phases (stages) that will eventually lead to its multiplication and release from the host.

Stage 1: Incubation Period

This refers to the time elapsed between exposure to a pathogenic organism, and from when symptoms and signs are first apparent. It may be as short as few minutes to as long as many years in various cases. Depending on the disease, the person may or may not be contagious during the incubation period. During clinical latency, an infection is subclinical. With respect to viral infections, in clinical latency the virus is actively replicating. This is in contrast to viral latency, a form of dormancy in which the virus does not replicate.

Stage 2: Prodromal Period

In this phase, the numbers of the infectious agents start increasing and the immune system starts reacting to them. It is characterized by early symptoms that might indicate the start of a disease before specific symptoms occur. Prodromes may be nonspecific symptoms or, in a few instances, may clearly indicate a particular disease. For example, fever, malaise, headache and lack of appetite frequently occur in the prodrome of many infective disorders. It also refers to the initial in vivo round of viral replication. It is the second stage of illness and the period in which signs and symptoms of a disease first appear. Transmission is greatest during this period because of the high communicability of the disease at this stage because the symptoms are not evident.

Stage 3: Fastigium

Fastigium the period when the disease is at its max severity or intensity. In this stage all sign and symptoms are clearly visible. Diagnosis is easiest at or directly after the differential point. In the fastigium period even though the disease is highly communicable, patients do not spread it much. If disease is not controlled in this stage, there is chance of disability or may leads to death.

Defervescence

The period starts when the symptoms of the illness are declining. As patients feel better, they may stop taking their medicine. If the immune system is weakened and cannot fight off the pathogens, a relapse may occur. This is also when transmission of the disease is quite high because the patients may be up and around, despite still being infectious.

Convalescence

Convalescence period is the recovery period. Those affected in infectious disease may still be infectious at this point but are feeling much better. They may be out of danger but act as a source of infection. Changes of lifestyle may be needed. A better lifestyle and complete rest allows our body for complete recovery.

Defection

Is the period during which the pathogen is killed off or brought into remission by the immune system and the human being returns to his normal stage. In some diseases, defection and convalescence may be the same stage.

ICEBERG PHENOMENON OF DISEASE (FIG. 1.8)

According to this concept, the disease in the community is compared to an iceberg. When a piece of ice is allowed to float on water, a small portion is visible and a major portion is submerged in the water. The visible tip of ice is compared to clinical cases, which the physician sees in the community.

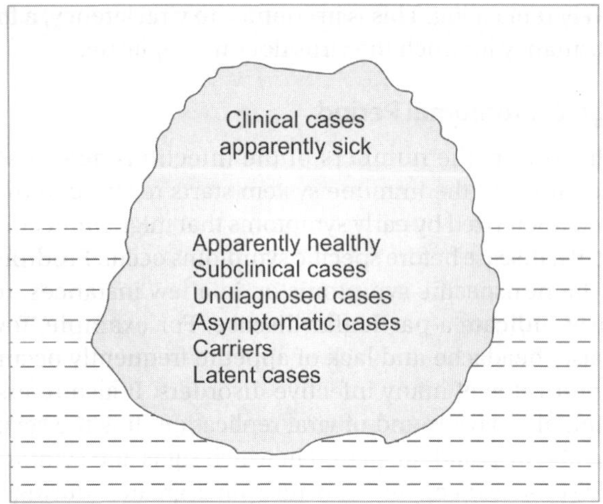

Fig. 1.8: Iceberg phenomenon of disease.

The major submerged portion of ice corresponds to hidden mass of unrecognized diseases such as latent cases, in apparent, carriers, asymptomatic and undiagnosed cases in the community, which are responsible for the constant prevalence of the disease in the community. In some diseases like HTN, diabetes, anemia, malnutrition, mental illness, etc., the unknown morbidity is more than the known morbidity in the community and constitutes an important, undiagnosed reservoirs of disease in the community.

INDICATORS OF HEALTH

Indicator also termed as index or variable is only an indication of a given situation or a reflection of that situation. Health indicator is a variable, susceptible to direct measurement, that reflects the state of health of persons in a community. Health indicator means health measurement. Health cannot be measured in exact measurable forms. Measurement have been framed in terms of illness (or lack of health), consequences or condition of ill-health (morbidity, mortality) and economic, occupation and domestic factors that promote ill health. WHO defines indicators as 'variables which measure change'. Health indicators help to measure the extent to which the objectives and targets of a program are being attained. Health index is a numerical indication of the health of a given population derived from a specified composite formula. **Figure 1.9** shows health belief model.

Characteristics of Health Indicators

1. **Valid:** They should actually measure that they are supposed to measure.
2. **Reliable:** The results should be the same when measured by different people in similar circumstances.
3. **Sensitive:** They should be sensitive to changes in the situation concerned.
4. **Specific:** They should reflect changes only in the situation concerned.
5. **Feasible:** They should have the ability to obtain data when needed.

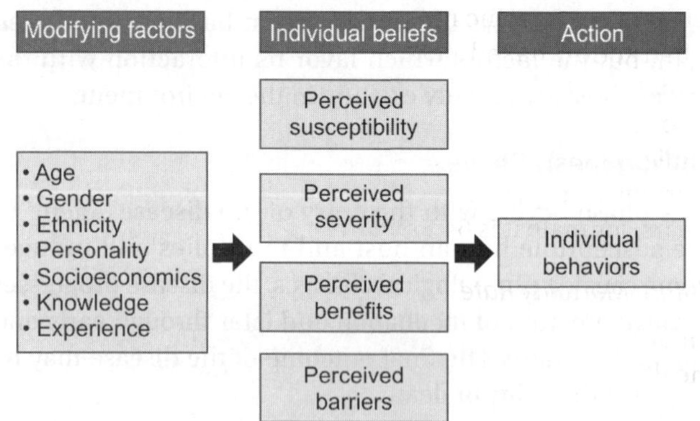

Fig. 1.9: Health belief model.

6. **Relevant:** They should contribute to the understanding of the phenomenon of interest.

Uses of Indicators of Health

- Measurement of the health of the community.
- Description of the health of the community.
- Comparison of the health of different communities.
- Identification of health needs and prioritizing them.
- Communicating critical information about population health.
- Support planning (identify priorities, develop and target resources, identify benchmarks) and track progress toward broad community objectives and allocation of health resources.
- Concurrent evaluation and terminal evaluation of health services.
- Inform policy and policy makers, and can be used to promote accountability among governmental and non-governmental agencies.

Indicators are powerful tools for monitoring and indicators are used to engagement of partners into civic and collaborative action by build awareness of problems and trends, generate interventions.

Types of Health Indicators

Mortality Indicators

Crude Death Rate

Crude death rate (CDR) is considered as a fair indicator for the comparison of the health status of the people. It is defined as the number of deaths per 1,000 population per year in a given community, usually the midyear population. The usefulness is restricted because it is influenced by the age-sex composition of the population, socioeconomic and sociocultural environment of the communities. Current CDR is 7.48 deaths/1,000 population.

$$\frac{\text{Total death of population in a given calendar year}}{\text{Estimated midyear population of the same calendar year}} \times 1{,}000$$

Expectation of Life

Expectation of life is the average number of years that will be lived by those born alive into a population if the current age specific mortality rates persist. It is a statistical abstraction based on existing age-specific death rates which is estimated for both sexes separately. Longer life expectancy is the indicator of good health. It is a good indicator to measure the socioeconomic development. Now current life expectancy at birth for general population is 65.2 years, for male it is 64.3 years, for female it is 66.1 years.

Infant Mortality Rate

Infant mortality rate (IMR) provides a complete picture of the health status of not only infants but also whole population, socioeconomic conditions, availability of health services utilization and effectiveness of health care, particularly perinatal care, etc. The formula for IMR is the ratio of deaths under 1 year of age in a given year to the total number of live births in the same year, usually expressed as a rate per 1,000 live births. The Current IMR - 67/1,000 live birth.

Child Mortality Rate

The child mortality rate (CMR) is the number of deaths at ages 1–4 years in a given year, per 1000 children in that age group at the mid-point of the year which is correlates with inadequate MCH services, malnutrition, low immunization coverage and environmental factors (current rate—18/1000). Other indicators are perinatal mortality rate, neonatal mortality rate, stillbirth rate, etc. are also correlates with inadequate antenatal care and perinatal care.

Maternal Mortality Rate

Ratio of number of deaths arising during pregnancy or puerperal period per 100,000 live births. It is also term as Maternal Mortality, ratio which accounts for the greatest number of deaths among women of reproductive age in developing countries. Current MMR in India is 212/100000 live.

Disease Specific Death Rate

Disease specific death rate is mortality rate which is computed for specific diseases, e.g., TB mortality is 23 per 1,00,000 population per year (*Source:* TB INDIA 2011, RNTCP Annual Report 2011). Proportional mortality rate is the proportion of all deaths attributed to the specific disease, e.g., coronary heart disease causes 25 to 30% of all deaths in developed world.

Morbidity Indicators

Morbidity indicators reveal the burden of ill health in a community, but do not measure the subclinical or inapparent disease states.

Incidence

The number of new events or new cases of a disease in a defined population, within a specified period of time. For example, incidence rate of TB is 168 per 1,00,000 population for the year 2022 in India. From this definition it is clear that incidence rate refers:

- Only to new cases
- During a given period
- In a specified population or population at risk.

Two types of incidence are commonly used: **'incidence proportion'** and **'incidence rate'.**

Incidence proportion, risk or cumulative incidence refers to the number of new cases in your population during a specified time period. It can be calculated using the following equation:

$$\frac{\textit{Number of new cases during a specified time period}}{\textit{Size of population at start of time period}}$$

Incidence rate incorporates time directly into the denominator and can be calculated as follows:

$$\frac{\textit{Number of new cases during a specified time period}}{\textit{Person years at risk during the same time period}}$$

Person years at risk means the total amount of time (in years) that each person of the study population is at risk of the disease during the period of interest.

Prevalence

Prevalence rate is defined as the total number of all individuals who have disease at a particular time divided by population at risk of having disease at this point of time. It reflects the chronicity of the disease, e.g., prevalence of TB (sputum positive in population) is 249 per 1,00,000 population in 2022. It means total number of TB cases present in 2022 during survey. It may include the number of old cases plus new cases minus death and cure cases. It is the cross sectional measurement of any disease or condition.

The Prevalence rate can be calculated by:

$$\frac{\textit{The total number of people suffered sample with characterstics}}{\textit{Total number people studied or total number sample}}$$

The total number of people suffered or the sample having characteristics.

Notification Rates

Notification rate, is calculated from the reporting to public authorities of certain disease, yellow fever, poliomyelitis, cholera, plague. They provide information regarding geographic clustering of infections, quality of reporting system.

Some Other Ways also we can Measure Morbidity Status Like

- Attendance rates at OPDs and at health centers.
- Admission, readmission and discharge rates.
- Duration of stay in hospital—reflects the virulence and resistance developed by the etiological factor.
- Spells of sickness or absence from work or school—
  - Reflects economical loss to the community.
- Hospital data constitute a basic and primary source of information about diseases prevalent in the community.

Disability Rates

Disability rates are of two categories they are event type indicators which is measured by number of days of restricted activity (bed disability days, work-loss days within a specified period) and person type indicators measure by limitation of mobility, e.g., confined to bed, confined to house, special aid in getting around and limitation of activity, e.g., limitation to perform the basic activities of daily living (ADL), e.g., eating, washing, dressing, etc.

Disability rates Sullivan's Index refers to 'expectation of life free of disability.' Sullivan's Index = life expectancy of the country—probable duration of bed disability and inability to perform major activities from. It is considered as one of the most advanced indicators currently available.

Health adjusted life expectancy (HALE) is based on the framework of WHO's ICIDH. It is based on life expectancy at birth but includes an adjustment for time spent in poor health. It is the equivalent number of years in full health that a newborn can expect to live based on current rates of ill-health and mortality.

Disability rates disability adjusted life years (DALYs) is defined as the number of years of healthy life lost due to all causes whether from premature mortality or disability. It is the simplest and the most commonly used measure to find the burden of illness in a defined population and the effectiveness of the interventions. Two things needed to measure DALYs are—life table of that country, to measure the losses from premature deaths—loss of healthy life years resulting from disability; the disability may be permanent (polio) or temporary (TB, leprosy), physical or mental. Disability rates, uses of DALYs to assist in selecting health service priorities to identify the disadvantaged groups targeting health interventions measuring the results of health interventions providing comparable measures for planning and evaluating programmes to compare the health status of different countries. DALY express years of life lost to premature death and years lived with disability for the severity of the disability. One DALY is one lost year of healthy life.

Disability Rates Premature Death

It is defined as one that occurs before the age to which a dying person could have expected to survive if he or she was a member of a standardized mode population with a life expectancy at birth equal to that of world longest surviving population, e.g., Japan.

Quality Adjusted Life Year

Quality adjusted life year (QALY) is the most commonly used to measure the cost effectiveness of health interventions. It estimates the number of years of life added by a successful treatment or adjustment for quality of life.

Nutritional Status Indicators

Nutritional status is a positive health indicator. Newborns are measured for their: (i) birth-weight, (ii) length, (iii) head circumference. They reflect the maternal nutrition status. Anthropometric measurements of preschool children: weight—measures acute malnutrition, height—measures chronic malnutrition, mid-arm circumference—measures chronic malnutrition. Growth monitoring of children is done by measuring weight-for-age, height-for-age, weight-for-height, head and chest circumference and mid-arm circumference. In adults underweight, obesity and anemia are generally considered reliable nutritional indicators.

Healthcare Delivery Indicators

These indicators reflect the equity of distribution of health resources in different parts of the country and of the provision of health care. Doctor-population ratio—1/1700 (sug. norm 1/3500) Nurse-population ratio—0.8/1000 (sug. norm 1/500) Population-bed ratio—8.9/10,000 Population per PHC/subcenter is 20,000—30,000 in Karnataka while in some states, it is more than 50,000. Population per traditional birth attendant—0.47/1000.

Utilization Rates

Utilization rates or actual rates is expressed as the proportion of people in need of a service who actually receive it in a given period, usually a year. It depends on availability and accessibility of health services and the attitude of an individual towards healthcare system. Their direct attention towards discharge of social responsibility of the organization in delivery services, e.g., proportion of infants who are fully immunized—43%, proportion of pregnant women who receive antenatal care (ANC) or have institutional deliveries,%age of population who adopt family planning, bed occupancy ratio, bed-turn over ratio, etc.

Indicators of Social and Mental Health

The indicators of social and mental health include rates of suicide, homicide, other crime, road traffic accident, juvenile delinquency, alcohol and substance abuse, domestic violence, battered-baby syndrome, etc. These indicators provide a guide to social action for improving the health of people. Social and mental health of the children depend on their parents, e.g., substance abuse in orphan children.

Environmental Indicators

The **environmental indicators** reflect the quality of physical and biological environment in which diseases occur and people live. The most important are those measuring the proportion of population having access to safe drinking water and sanitation facilities. These indicators explains the prevalence of communicable diseases in a community. The other indicators are those measuring the pollution of air and water, radiation, noise pollution, exposure to toxic substances in food and water.

Socioeconomic Indicators

Socioeconomic indicators do not directly measure health but are important in interpreting health indicators. These are per capita income, level of unemployment, literacy rate, per capita caloric availability, total fertility rate, family size contraceptive use.

Health Policy Indicators

The single most important indicator of political commitment is allocation of adequate resources. The relevant indicators are proportion of GNP spent on health services, proportion of GNP spent on health-related activities like water supply and sanitation and housing and nutrition proportion of total health resources devoted primary health care.

Indicators of Quality of Life

Physical quality of life index consolidates infant mortality, life expectancy at age of 1 year and literacy. For each component the performance of individual country is placed on a scale of 1 to 100. The composite index is calculated by averaging the three indicators giving equal weight to each of them. The scale is between 0 to 100. The PQLI does not consider the GNP.

It is defined as a composite index combining indicators representing three dimensions—longevity (life expectancy at birth), knowledge (2/3 adult literacy rate and 1/3 mean years of schooling), income (real GDP per capita in purchasing power parity in US dollars).

Other Indicators Series

Social indicators as defined by the UN Statistical Office has been divided into 12 categories: (1) population, (2)family formation, (3) families and households, (4) learning and educational services, (5) earning activities, (6) distribution of income, consumption and accumulation, (7) social security and welfare services, (8) health services and nutrition, (9) housing and its environment, public order and safety, (10) time use, (11) leisure and culture, (12) social stratification and mobility. Basic needs indicators are used by ILO and include calorie consumption, access to water, life expectancy, deaths due to disease, illiteracy, doctors and nurses per population, rooms per person, GNP per capita.

Other indicators series health for all indicators for monitoring the progress towards the goal of health for all (HFA) by 2000, the WHO has listed the following four categories of indicators. Health policy indicators political commitment to HFA resource allocation degree of equity of distribution of health services community involvement organizational framework and managerial process.

It also include 40 social and indicators related to health rate of population growth GNP or GDP income distribution, work conditions, adult literacy rate, housing food availability, indicators for the provision of health care, availability, accessibility, utilization, quality of care.

DETERMINANTS OF HEALTH

See **Figure 1.10**.

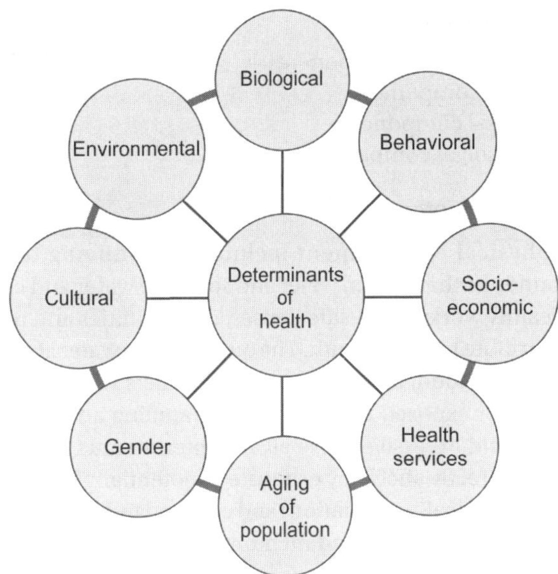

Fig. 1.10: Determinants of health.

Biological Determinants

It is also known as human biology. It encompasses those aspects of health (both mental and physical) which are determined by the organic structure and physiological functioning of the human body. The genetic makeup of the individual determines the likelihood of inherited disorders and the predisposition to later acquired diseases. The transmission of genetic characters from parents to offspring is dependent upon the segregation and recombination of genes, chromosomal anomalies, errors of metabolism, and mental retardation are the examples of genetic disorders. The individual's constitution is also a determinant of susceptibility to risk factors arising from certain lifestyles and environments. Changes in the human body due to maturation and aging are also important factors that can interact with the other three Health Field elements in determining the individual´s state of health. The human biology elements has many facets, only a few of which are adequately understood. The medical and allied sciences have made great progress in understanding the complex process of the human body and mind, but much remains to be elucidated.

Environmental Determinants

Environmental factor is classified into two types: (1) Internal environment and (2) external environment.

Internal environment (cells, tissues, organs): The environment inside an organism is called internal environment in animal Internal Environment In order for cells of the body to function optimally, the physical factors and the chemical factors within the internal environment must be maintained at a relatively constant level. Example: Temperature for human, the internal environment need to be maintain around 37°C. At this temperature, the enzymes give the optimal enzyme activity. If the temperature too high, enzymes denatured—so lose ability to function. If the temperature too low, enzymes become inactive. The harmonious functioning should be maintained.

External Environment

It has mainly three components:
1. Physical component
2. Biological component
3. Psychosocial component.

Physical Environment

The physical environment include all nonliving things surrounds us that are air, water and soil. Safe water and clean air, healthy workplaces, safe houses, communities and roads all contribute to good health. The quality of air, water and soil, the safety of food, drugs, and other products which human consume or exposed to, the physical handling and disposal of waste and excessive noise all are determinants to health. They are directly affects by exposure to potentially hazardous agents (chemicals or radiation) and etc., and indirectly affects by global warming, redundant hunt of animals, etc.

Biological Environment

Biological environment include all animals, plants including microorganism, so many animals can directly create zoonotic disease and, spread different vector borne diseases also. Some of the disease can spread by eating the meat and drinking the milk of infected animals. Similarly different plants can spread different diseases. Microorganism are the agents and that are directly responsible for diseases.

Psychosocial Environment

The social environment also act as determinants of health. In a community social environment include custom, culture and tradition of society, social organization and stress. The WHO's world health report 2002 identified five important risk factors for noncommunicable disease in the top ten leading risks to health. These are raised blood pressure, raised cholesterol, tobacco use, alcohol consumption, and overweight. Other factors associated with higher risk of NCDs include a person's economic and social conditions, also known as the advance life, the social gradient, social determinants and due to imbalance social environment. It also include labor market, unemployment, non-employment, job insecurity, psychosocial environment at work, transportation, social support and social cohesion, poverty, social exclusion, and minorities, social patterning of individual health behaviors, the social determination of ethnic/racial inequalities in health, the social determinants of health in older age, neighborhoods, housing, sexual behavior, and sexual health social vulnerability and inequality.

Behavioral and Sociocultural

Behavioral and sociocultural lifestyle (the way people live) culture, behavior, personal habits, parents, peer groups, friends, siblings, schools, mass media greater support from families, friends and communities are linked to better health. Culture—customs and traditions, and the beliefs of the family and community all affect health. Adequate nutrition, enough sleep, sufficient physical activity are consider as healthy lifestyles, lack of sanitation, poor nutrition, poor personal hygeine elementary human habits, harmful customs and cultural patterns are harmful lifestyles. Some of the disease are linked with lifestyles are coronary heart diseases, obesity lung cancer, drug addiction.

Socioeconomic Conditions

Poor socioeconomic conditions leads to inadequate education or illiteracy poor nutrition. Illiteracy also leads to poor health. Employment, housing, Political system, higher income and social status are linked to better health. The greater the gap between the richest and poorest people leads to the greater differences in health.

Health Services

Though Government of India made differ health schemes, still health services are not accessible to all population and also not acceptable due to lack of motivation. Immunization of children still also incomplete in urban slums, some rural area and also tribal area. Doctor population and nurse population ratio is inadequate to provide health services properly. Provision of safe drinking water for all and proper care of pregnant and children till now in half way.

Aging of the Population

Aging of the population by 2020—1 Billion are aged > 60, 2/3 are living in developing countries. The reasons for increase in the size of elderly people are decrease of mortality from infection and chronic disease during this century and improvement in sanitation, housing, nutrition and medical innovations, including vaccination and the discovery of antibiotics which prevent disease and increases longevity of life. Aging process leads to a number of changes in human being. It acts as a determinants of health as it acts on the health of individual.

Gender

Men and women suffer from different types of diseases at different ages. Women are more vulnerable than men and more prone to different diseases like malnutrition and anemia, etc. Some of the aspects we should more careful for women like reproductive health, violence, nutrition and occupational health but women health is especially neglected in developing country like India. Women's health is closely related to the economic and political position of women in society, the division between productive and reproductive labor, and cultural values in relation to motherhood, sexuality and decent.

HEALTH ECONOMICS

Health economics has developed into discipline itself due to size and differential characteristic of health sector in economy. Health economics is a branch of economics concerned with issues related to scarcity in the allocation of health and health care. In developing countries like India where less than two%age of GDP is invested for delivering healthcare services, health economics is very much essential. The main focus of health economics is to provide the maximum benefits for the money invested in health care. Benefits refers to the reduction in the disease burden of community and improvement in people's health and welfare. Health economics is the application of the principle and tools of economics to health services. The goods and services with which health economics is concerned include medical, surgical, cold chain equipment, drugs, vaccines, diagnostic and therapeutic services, environmental sanitation, family planning, school health and reproductive and child health.

Definitions: Health economics is the study of distribution of health care. It is a branch of economics concerned with issue related to efficiency, effectiveness, value and behavior in the production and consumption of health and health care.

Concepts in Health Economics

Resources: Resources are the inputs, factors of production, i.e., land, labor, capital. It covers all the inputs used to produce goods and services, have health stock in order to improve the health status of individuals in terms of healthy days or quality of life.

Scarce resources: Resources are considered scarce when society demands more resources and good services than are available.

Scarcity: It has two sides, the infinite nature of human wants and the finite or limited nature of resources available to produce goods and services as depicted by:

Scarcity = **Infinite wants vs. Limited resources available to produce services**

Opportunity: It means the value of forgone benefit which could be obtained from a resource in its next-best alternative use.

Need for Health Economics

There is a need to study health economics due to increasing demand and rising cost of health care services. The reason are:

- Medical advances, such as organ transplants and gene therapy, have provided new treatments and therefore greater hopes and new needs arise among public.
- Due to increase in life expectancy, more resources are required for medical treatment and continuing care for the elderly.
- Changes in the family structure and norms, i.e., more likely the elderly may not be cared for by their families.
- Higher expectation among general people about their levels of the health and demanding more and better health care.
- Public awareness about their rights for their health and its facilities.
- Advance in health research and concern for cost effectiveness programs in the health market.

Hence the health economics need to understand the relationship between resources used and health outcomes achieved by alternative options and compare them in order to balance between demand and cost of health services.

Importance of Health Economics

- To formulate heath services policy, might be in the form of demand studies, or by trying to discover what policy makers preferences are.
- To established the true cost of delivering health care or to estimate all real costs like the use of patients' time, loss of output elsewhere in the system, etc.
- To evaluate the relative costs and benefits of particular policy options.
- To estimate the effects of certain economic variables like user charges, time and distance costs of accessibility, etc., on the utilization of health services.
- To evaluate planning and budgeting systems and make possible changes therein in healthcare delivery system.

Major Tasks of Economics in Health Care

- **Descriptive quantification:** It refers to the identification, definition, and measurement of phenomena. It also concerned with determining the nature of the phenomena as well as obtaining estimates of their magnitude.
- **Explanatory or predictive:** It means identifying impact of change. It involves explaining and predicting certain phenomena, conducting an analysis in a cause effect format and performed with the aid of models that classify various causal factors in a systematic framework.
- **Evaluative:** This means relative preference over situations. It involves judging or ranking alternative phenomena according to some standard. An acceptable standard must be obtained. Based on the standard, alternative ways of using scarce resources are then ranked. In choosing the standard, one major criterion is acceptability.

Features of Health Economics

- Health and medical care is considered as economics goods
- Health is a private or public good
- Measurement of health is also considered in economics
- Stock of health
- Investment aspects of health
- Loss due to ill health
- Planning of health and medical care
- Choice of technology in healthcare system
- Provision of equity in health outcomes and health care
- Resource costs of different diseases, effects of health and medical care provision.

Areas of Health Economics

- Economic aspects of relationship between health status and productivity
- Financial aspects of healthcare services

- Economic decision making in health and medical care institutions
- Planning of health development and such other related aspects.

Factors Influencing Health Economics

Extensive Government Intervention

Generally the government intervention are the regulatory actions taken by a government in order to affect or interfere with decisions made by individuals, groups or organizations regarding social and economic matters. Extensive government intervention like changing health policies frequently can affect the health economics.

Intractable Uncertainty in Several Dimensions

Intractable means not easily controlled or managed and uncertainty is the situation which involves imperfect and/ or unknown information. So intractable uncertainty is some predicted unknown situation which is difficult to manage. For example lack of IPR skill among health personnel can reduce the output which cannot predicted before.

Information Asymmetric

Asymmetric information is a situation in which one party in a transaction has more or superior information compared to another. This often happens in transactions where the seller knows more than the buyer, although the reverse can happen as well. Potentially, this could be a harmful situation because one party can take advantage of the other party's lack of knowledge. Sometime market failure may results.

Barriers to Entry

Barriers to entry are the existence of high start-up costs or other obstacles that prevent new competitors from easily entering an industry or area of business. Because barriers to entry protect incumbent firms and restrict competition in a market, they can contribute to distortionary prices and are therefore are most important when discussing antitrust policy.

Externalities and the Presence of a Third Party Agent

An externalities is a consequence of an economic activity experienced by unrelated third parties; it can be either positive or negative. Pollution emitted by a factory that spoils the surrounding environment and affects the health of nearby residents is an example of a negative externalities. The effect of a well-educated labor force on the productivity of a company is an example of a positive externalities.

The presence of third party agent may also influence the business without direct involvement in costs for example: in health care, the third party agent is the physician, who makes purchasing decisions (lab test, treatment prescription, etc.) while being insulated from the price of the product or services.

GENETICS AND HEALTH

Although there are many possible causes of human disease, family history is often one of the strongest risk factors for common disease complexes such as cancer, cardiovascular disease (CVD), diabetes, autoimmune disorders, and psychiatric illnesses. A person inherits a complete set of genes from each parent, as well as a vast array of cultural and socioeconomic experiences from his/her family. Family history is thought to be a good predictor of an individual's disease risk because family members most closely represent the unique genomic and environmental interactions that an individual experiences. Inherited genetic variation within families clearly contributes both directly and indirectly to the pathogenesis of disease. A community health nurse must have to know the genetic factors affecting health condition and eugenics.

EUGENICS

The word eugenics was coined by Francis Galton in 1883. This word has been derived from two Greek word; *Eu*-good or well and genes means born. It is considered as the study of improving the genetic qualities.

Definition

- Eugenic is mainly concerned with the decrease of hereditary diseases and improvement of the overall health status of the people or community. Eugenics results in reducing genetic morbidity.
- Eugenics is the science which deals with all influences that improve inborn qualities of a race also with that develop them to utmost advantage. **—F. Gaton, 1940**
- Eugenics is the way by which a healthy society, community can be created. Nurse can reduce the human suffering through education among the community.

Goals

To improve the genetic composition of population.

Aim

- To save the resources
- To create healthy community
- To have intelligent people or to have the community to free from mentally retarded people.
- To decrease the human suffering
- To reduce economic burden on nation due to disease.

How Eugenic Measures Reducing Health Problem

Eugenics is helpful in reducing morbidity due to hereditary diseases among the community by:

- **Positive eugenics:** Positive eugenics encourages reproduction among genetically advantages population. Various ways of positive eugenics are *in vitro* fertilization, cloning. Positive eugenics is difficult to achieve due to complexity of the trait, multifactorial causes and unawareness regarding which gene to be transmitted or which not to be transmitted.

- **Negative eugenics:** It is mainly concerned with decreasing or lowering the fertility among genetic disadvantages. The various ways of negative eugenics are abortion, sterilization, adoption of family planning methods. It is considered as immoral because it:
  - Enforces sterilization among genetically defective
  - Allows to kill institutionalized population.

The various ways to achieve healthy community by eugenics are:

- **Euthenics:** Euthenics is manipulating the environment in order to improve the genotype. As environmental factors are involved such as smoking, diet, obesity, lack of exercise in reducing diseases such as cancer, hypertension, DM which can cause abnormalities in genetic constitution. So it is required to provide stable environment to achieve normal genetic constitution. Community health nurses can take appropriate steps to provide safe environment to people to achieve euthenics. As man is adopting the environment it leads to increased chances of having healthy population.
- **Genetic counseling:** It includes screening of the cases and informing them the risk of having the affected children. It helps to provide information by nurses regarding the cost of correction of diseases, prognosis and burden of care on the family members will help them to take decision and prevention of further occurrences of genetic diseases.
- **Marriage restriction:** Genetically disadvantaged people is considered one of the way to achieve genetic endowment among population. Marriages if restricted among the people who can produce affected children will help in achieving the genetic health among the populations.

  In following cases marriages need to be restricted:
  - Marriages among the individuals suffering congenital abnormalities, mental retardation, gout, thalassemia, sickle cell anemia may increase the risk of the defective children.
  - Consanguineous marriages can cause increased risk in the off-spring of the recessive trait, even premature deaths due to consanguineous marriages are also noted.
  - Late marriage increases the risk of genetic disease such as Down syndrome.

  As a community health nurse it is necessary to understand the prevailing marriage system in the community.
- **Birth control:** The aim of birth control measures as eugenics is to reduce the frequency of hereditary disease and disabilities in the community to the low level due to adoption of birth control measures. So as no child born with defective genotype.
  - Community health nurse teaches the community for adoption of birth control measures (temporary/permanent) to limit size of family.
- **Early diagnosis and treatment:** Some of the genetic diseases which has diagnosed earlier can be corrected such as congenital hip dysplasia.
  - Early diagnosis can be made by identifying the carriers of genetic disorders by investigations, such as serum creatinine kinase level to identify the carriers of muscular dystrophy.
  - It assists the community health nurse for teaching the appropriate measures for correction of some of hereditary diseases among community.
- **Segregation of mentally ill from normal:** There is need to segregate mentally ill from normal so as to prevent birth of mentally ill child in community. For example, a mentally ill person who is living in community gets married to either a mentally ill or a normal genetically healthy person. In such case the offspring will have abnormal genes and if this continued it will lead to more of hereditary diseases in the community.

Methods of Application of Eugenics

- **At government level:** Government should make policies and legislation to achieve healthy community.
- **At population level:** Eugenics should be promoted among general population through education using democratic approach.
- **At individual level:** Eugenics should be practiced by individual on the basis of decision so as to reduce economic burden of disease in the family.

Role of Community Health Nurse

- Nurse's knowledge on genetic diseases will be helpful in identification of hereditary diseases, need of care to be provided to family and to provide support to the persons affected by or at risk of genetic diseases.
- She provides education to people about risk factors for hereditary diseases such as DM, HTN which occur due to multifactorial reason. She should provide information about diseases which occur due to chromosomal abnormalities.
- She must identify the hereditary diseases among the population, refer and motivate them to seek medical treatment.
- She informs the community about risk and benefits associated with genetic testing.
- She analyzes the data and develops plan to address the genetic concerns.
- Plan to manage the hereditary diseases, to control and reduce the chances of genetic diseases and will prevent further occurrence of abnormality in family.
- She teaches the people about eugenics methods such as birth control, genetic counseling, etc.
- She identifies the carriers and diseased person in the community and refers them.

LEVEL OF PREVENTION

Prevention is always better than cure. As per the natural history of disease, epidemiology has derived four levels of prevention.

Primordial Prevention

Primordial prevention is defined as prevention of risk factors themselves, beginning with change in social and environmental conditions in which these factors are observed to develop, and continuing for high risk children, adolescents and young adults. It is a relatively new concept, is receiving special attention in the prevention of chronic diseases. Many adult health problems like obesity, hypertension have their origins in the childhood, because this is the time when lifestyles are formed (e.g., smoking, eating patterns, physical exercise). In primordial prevention efforts are directed towards discouraging children towards adopting harmful lifestyles. Primordial prevention is achieved in part through health promotion, which includes health education programs in general, marriage counseling, sex education, and provision of adequate housing. It is important to change the milieu that promotes major risk factor development. Primordial prevention calls for changing the socioeconomic status of society. A better socioeconomic status correlates inversely with lifestyle factors like smoking, abnormal food patterns and exercise.

Primary Prevention

Primary prevention is true prevention—it precedes disease or dysfunction and its applied to clients considered to be physically and emotionally healthy. It includes all health promotion efforts as well as wellness activities that focus on maintaining and improving the general health of individuals, families and communities. Health promotion includes: health education programs, immunization, physical and nutritional fitness activities. Primary prevention means measures designed to promote positive general health—development of good health habits and hygiene—proper nutrition—proper attitude towards sickness—proper and prompt utilization of available health and medical facilities. Primary prevention also includes specific protection which means the use of measures adopted against specific disease agents like protection of the individual by increasing resistance of the individual through specific immunization, the establishment of barriers against agents in the environment, i.e., control of means of spread of vector such as control, sanitation of food, milk, water, and air, proper sewage disposal, proper disposal and or disinfection of soiled articles or clothing, eradication of animal reservoir, handwashing technique, etc.

Secondary Prevention

Secondary prevention includes early diagnosis and prompt treatment. Regular health checkup of community, check up of children, pregnant mothers and elder people. Health checkup of high risk groups like smokers, obese, alcoholic, sedentary worker and factory workers. Examples of secondary prevention include public education to promote breast self-examination, use of home kits for detection of occult blood in the stool specimens, screening programs for hypertension, diabetes, uterine cancer (Pap smear), breast cancer, glaucoma and sexually transmitted diseases. Focuses on individuals who are experiencing health problems or illness and who are risk for developing complications or worsening condition. Activities are directed at diagnosis and prompt intervention thereby reducing the severity and enabling the client to return to a normal level of health as early as possible. Includes screening techniques and treating early stages of disease to limit disability.

Tertiary Prevention

Tertiary prevention means disability limitation and rehabilitation. Tertiary prevention begins early in the period of recovery from illness. It consists of such activities as consistent and appropriate administration of medications to optimize therapeutic effects moving and positioning the patient to prevent complications of immobility and active and passive exercises to prevent disability, minimizing residual disability and helping the client learn to live productively with limitations through proper exercise, physiotherapy and occupation therapy and corrective, plastic surgery can improve mobility, which is otherwise known as rehabilitation. Rehabilitation may be physical mental and occupational which make the individual productive. Occupational therapy depending on the nature and extend of disability can provided. By rehabilitation clients achieve as high a level of functioning as possible, despite the limitations caused by illness or impairment. It involves preventing further disability or reduced functioning.

HEALTH PROMOTION

It is the science aiming at reaching optimal (perfect) health. All activities aiming at increasing well-being, prevention of disease and health hazards, or control of disease are included under health promotion. Health promotion is to add "life into the years" and not just add years onto life'. Health promotion is an important component of nursing practice. It is a way of thinking that revolves around a philosophy of wholeness, wellness and well-being. Health promotion enables people to increase control over their own health. In public health it covers a wide range of social and environmental interventions that are designed to benefit and protect individual people's health and quality of life by addressing and preventing the root causes of ill health, not just focusing on treatment and cure. Health promotion programs aim to engage and empower individuals and communities to choose healthy behaviors, and make changes that reduce the risk of developing chronic diseases and other morbidities.

Definition

Health promotion as a "behavior motivated by the desire to increase wellbeing and actualize human health potential".

—Pender, Murdaugh and Parsons, 2006

Health promotion is a process of enabling people to increase control over the determinants of health and their by improve their health.

Health promotion may be defined as any combination of educational and social efforts designed to help people take greater control of and improve their health.

'Enables people to increase control over their own health. It covers a wide range of social and environmental interventions that are designed to benefit and protect individual people's health and quality of life by addressing and preventing the root causes of ill health, not just focusing on treatment and cure'.

—According to World Health Organization

Key Elements of Health Promotion

There are three key elements of health promotion:

Good Governance for Health

The policy makers across all government departments should make health a central line of government policy for health promotion. This means the government policies should be formulated in giving importance on healthy practices and other health related activities. Health implications into all the decisions they take, and prioritize policies that prevent people from becoming ill and protect them from injuries.

These policies must be supported by regulations that match private sector incentives with public health goals. For example, by aligning tax policies on unhealthy or harmful products such as alcohol, tobacco, and food products which are high in salt, sugars and fat with measures to boost trade in other areas. And through legislation that supports healthy urbanization by creating walkable cities, reducing air and water pollution, enforcing the wearing of seat belts and helmets.

Health Literacy

People need to acquire the knowledge, skills and information to make healthy choices, for example about the food they eat and healthcare services that they need. They need to have opportunities to make those choices. And they need to be assured of an environment in which people can demand further policy actions to further improve their health.

Healthy Communities

Cities have a key role to play in promoting good health. Strong leadership and commitment at the municipal level is essential to healthy urban planning and to build up preventive measures in communities and primary health care facilities. From healthy cities evolve healthy countries and, ultimately, a healthier world.

Programs or Health Promotion

Health promotion and disease prevention programs often address social determinants of health, which influence modifiable risk behaviors. Social determinants of health are the economic, social, cultural, and political conditions, in which people are born, grow, and live that affect health status. Modifiable risk behaviors include, for example, tobacco use, poor eating habits, and lack of physical activity, which contribute to the development of chronic disease. The programs include:

- Information dissemination.
- Health risk appraisal and wellness assessment.
- Lifestyle and behavioral change.
- Environmental control programs.
- Health education programs
- Immunization, physical and nutritional fitness activities

Nurses Role in Health Promotion

- Model healthy lifestyle behaviors and attitudes.
- Facilitate client involvement in the assessment, implementation and evaluation of health goal.
- Teach client healthcare strategies to enhance fitness improve nutrition, manage stress and enhance relationships.
- Assist individuals, families and communities to increase their levels of health.
- Educate client to be effective healthcare consumers.
- Assist clients, families, and communities to develop and choose health promoting options.
- Guide clients development in effective problem solving and decision making
- Reinforce client's personal and family health promoting behaviors.
- Advocate in the community for changes that promote a healthy environment.

Health Promotion Aspect for Infants

- Infant parent attachment/bonding
- Breastfeeding
- Proper complementary feeding
- Hygiene
- Sleep patterns
- Playful activity to stimulate development
- Immunization
- Safety promotion and injury control

Health Promotion Aspects of Children

- Nutrition
- Immunization
- Dental checkup
- Rest and exercise
- Diet
- Safety promotion and injury control

Health Maintenance

- Health maintenance refers to activities that preserve an individual's present state of health and that prevent disease or injury occurrence.
- Examples of these activities include screening or surveillance, providing immunizations to prevent illnesses, and health education. The various aspects of maintaining good health are:
    - Proper nutrition required to maintain energy balance and other body requirements.
    - Exercise needed for physical and mental fitness.

- Taking adequate rest and sleep to maintain mental balance and calm.
- Take care of skin and personal; hygiene, other things include better housing, clean environment and sanitation.
- Yoga helps to overcome stress, tones up the body, calms down the mind and also help to relieve many chronic ailments.
- Relaxation and entertainment through music, games, dancing, reading, etc., are vital for physical and mental health.
- Avoidance of addictions and over indulgence to anything.

Screening

Definition

It is active detection of disease in apparently asymptomatic individuals by application of tests, examinations or other procedures which can be applied rapidly.

Screening is aiming for early detection of the disease that can be better controlled if detected early in apparently healthy individuals.

Types of Screening

- **Mass screening:** Means screening of the whole population.
- **Multiple or multiphasic screening:** The use of variety of screening tests on the same occasion.
- **Prescriptive screening:** For early detection of disease in apparently healthy individuals which can be better controlled if it is detected early.

Criteria of Screening Program

A. Criteria of the disease:

1. Should be important one.
2. Should be common enough to warrant a search for its risk factors and latent stages.
3. The morbidity and mortality of the untreated conditions must be substantial.
4. An effective treatment must exist and should be more beneficial when applied to the presymptomatic stage.
5. The natural history of the disease should be understood.

B. Criteria of the test:

1. Should be accepted by the population and suitable for application.
2. Should be easy, inexpensive, quickly done and free from hazards.
3. Sufficiently sensitive to detect disease during the asymptomatic stage.
4. Sufficiently specific to minimize the false positive test results.

C. Criteria of the screened populations:

1. Agreement should be obtained from people who will be screened.
2. Patients will benefit from further investigations and treatment.
3. High prevalence of the disease to justify screening.

INTRODUCTION TO COMMUNITY HEALTH NURSING

Community means a group of people living in a certain locality such as a village, who have common interests. They meet and react with one another. A community consists of people living together in some form of social organization and cohesion. Its members in varying degrees share political, economical, social and cultural characteristics as well as interests and aspirations including health.

In biological terms, a community is a group of interacting organisms sharing a populated environment. With regard to humans, a 'community' is understood as a group of interacting people, possibly living in close proximity, and often refers to a group that shares some common values, and is attributed with social cohesion within a shared geographical location, generally in social units larger than a household. The word can also refer to the national community or international community.

Concept of Community

The word "community" is derived from the Latin word communitas (meaning the same), which is in turn derived from communis, which means "common, public, shared by all or many". A community is a small or large social unit (a group of living beings) who have something in common, such as norms, religion, values, or identity. Communities often share a sense of place that is situated in a given geographical area (e.g., a country, village, town, or neighborhood). It is a social group sharing an environment, normally with shared interests. In human communities, intent, belief, resources, preferences, needs, risks and a number of other conditions may be present and common, affecting the identity of the participants and their degree of cohesiveness. Human beings, like many other species, are essentially social beings, and naturally form communities which often develop into more structured societies.

Communities are the building blocks that allow us to make sense of the world in which we live, participate and share experiences. They provide a sense of identity and purpose, a sense of being a part of and belonging.

Definitions

The WHO expert committee on CHN in their report agreed in following definition 'A community is a social group determined by geographical boundaries and or common values and interest'. Its member know and interact with each other. Its function within a particular structure and exhibits and create certain norms, values and social institutions. Many authors have tried to analyze various definitions to identify common aspects and those common factors are highlighted. Those are:

Community as Collection of People

Community is collection of people who are social interact with each other within same type of organized structure for mutual benefit. It is collection of people where the people identify themselves as a separate group and the people included both healthy and sick. The people may be from a small hamlet to a large metropolitan city implying the variability size of community.

Community as Place

Community as a place refers to specific location, geographical area and boundaries within which group of people with common culture, beliefs values, and customs, etc., are live together, the geographical area comprise the physical and biological; environment, housing and transportation, etc.

Community as a Social System

Community as a social system organize itself to meet the needs of its members by the joint efforts of the members of specific community. It is the combination of all social units and systems which have been developed to carry out its major functions by interaction. A number of ways to categorize types of community have been proposed; one such breakdown is:

Geographic Communities

Range from the local neighborhood, suburb, village, town or city, region, nation or even the planet as a whole. These refer to communities of location.

Rural Community

Rural community is a simple community of primary relation with low population based on primarily on agriculture life. The village socially did not spring all of a sudden, so they developed slowly and adjustment with society. Property is likely to be thought as a family possession. The second control in the rural community is exercised with minimum of formally and maximum command. The groups are more reflecting a commonly share of values, they effective themselves with social pressure by the support of specialized agencies.

Urban Community

It is different from village rural community. The social control system is urban or cities life the social behavior complex are informal. The relation are contractual. The mechanism of social control are largely legal and exercised by state and secondary institution.

Communities of Culture

Communities of culture range from the local clique, subculture, ethnic group, religious, multicultural or pluralistic civilization, or the global community cultures of today. They may be included as communities of need or identity, such as disabled persons, or frail aged people.

According to the bonding relation with the community people the community is classified as:

- **Gemeinschaft:** Characterized by implicit bonds that relate all community members to each others.
- **Gesellschaft:** Characterized by bonds that are both formal and specific.

Nowaday's different communities are formed to fulfill different needs of the peoples:

- The spiritual community
- The family community
- The living community
- The recreational community
- The learning community
- The employment community
- The health community
- The internet community.

Characteristics of a Community

Roles/Goals of Communities

Each community has a particular role that fulfills a particular need.

The role of the community provides the members with a sense of belonging and purpose. Community roles can be active in providing a service, supportive, where the members support the activities of another community, or a mixture where the members share experiences, resources, skills and knowledge with each other. Communities can be recreational, and provide a social role in enabling its members to participate in various activities, or provide an educational role in providing its members with knowledge, skills and resources, or fulfill any other role that is valued in society as well as other communities that it is a part of.

Valued community roles provide a common cause or focus for the community. The members develop a sense of pride and purpose in being a part of the community that bond and strengthen the community. The role is valued in a sense that it brings something to the wider community that it is a part of, as well as the members of the community. Valued roles are also about community leadership that is in touch with the community and can create a feeling of importance within the members.

Community is an Institution

Community is compared with an institution as it is having all characteristics of an institution. Institution define the way we interact with each other within the community. They are determined by the formal and informal cultures and values of the society in which the community participates, and provide order and stability within the community. Social role valorization provides valued roles for ALL members of the community. In doing this, a positive environment is created where all members have valued roles in supporting each other as a group. The characteristics of an institution are culture, values, hierarchy, roles, expectations and behaviors.

Culture

'The set of shared attitudes, values, goals, and practices that characterizes an institution, organization or group' is termed as culture.

The culture of the institution is the way the institution is organized. This is generally determined by its role in society.

For example, while the institutions of a hospital, nursing home or prison are similar, the culture of each is quite different.

Values

Institutional values (or social values) are different to our personal values in that they allow the members to function within the institution.

Hierarchy

Institutions are all about a means of coordination and cooperation. The hierarchy defines the agenda and purpose, and the way things get done.

Roles

Leadership is probably the most important role, and provides the identity and purpose within the institution. Other roles are determined by the hierarchy and the members in fulfilling the agenda and purpose of the institution.

Expectations

The members are expected to fulfill their assigned role within the institution.

Behaviors

The way the members treat each other or interact with each other is determined by the culture, values, hierarchy, roles and expectations of the members within the institution.

Community have Geographical Boundaries

All communities need a way to determine what the community does and how it does. Boundaries can be physical, virtual or psychological. They define the identity of the community. Without boundaries, the roles of the community become meaningless. Does a sporting community focus on transportation or scientific research? While transportation or scientific research may be a part of the community, they are not a part of the role of the community in society.

Without boundaries the community may:
- Become unfocused
- Become too diversified and uncoordinated
- Not adequately provide for its own needs, or the needs of its members
- Create tensions within communities that it is a part of, or a part of it
- Create layers of bureaucracy that become communities in their own right.

Boundaries are often defined by the:
- The institutions of the community
- The members of the community
- The settings (physical, virtual or psychological)
- Government (local state and federal) policy and practice
- Other communities that it is a part of, or are a part of it.

Members

Communities are about caring and sharing. All members share a common cause and have a sense of identity. A sense of belonging is created where the members are connected to, and interact with each other.

Just as the members of the community have ownership of their lives and property, the community has ownership of its members and property through the various mechanisms put in place by the community.

The community has ownership of its members through:
- May involve some formal/informal induction or rite of passage.
- **Commitment:** Members have a sense of obligation towards the community.
- **Loyalty:** Members give up a certain amount personal autonomy for the greater good.
- **Respect:** Members have respect for each other.
- **Responsibility:** Members take on responsibilities (and feel responsible for others) within the community.
- **Safety and security:** Members feel that they can call on other members in times of need or when threatened.
- **Resources:** Community resources are owned by the community on behalf of its members. Personal resources are sometimes shared between the members.

All members have the opportunity to participate in the activities of the community.

Social Role Valorization Provides Valued Roles for All Members of the Community

Communication

The community needs to be able to communicate with its members in order to achieve its goals.

The members communicate with each other to share thoughts, feelings, experiences, skills and knowledge. Clear thinking and expression of thoughts are essential to effective communication.

The community also needs to communicate with others outside the community. To function effectively as a community, the community needs to be able to respond to events that are outside the community and have an impact on the community.

'Communication is the process of exchanging information, beliefs and feelings among people; it may be oral, written, or nonverbal. Information may travel up, down, or horizontally.'

The Skills and Resources of the Community Provide for the Needs of its Members

A community needs a set of skills and resources in order to achieve its goals. They provide an available source of wealth that can be drawn upon when needed. If the community does not have the skills and resources to look after the needs of its members, those skills and resources need to come from somewhere else.

NEEDS OF COMMUNITY

Balance the needs of the community with the needs of its members.

Community Leadership

- Understanding the changing internal and external environments and how they relate to the community
- Involving all members
- Effective communication between all members
- Understanding what members need
- Aware of relevant research and the evidence base for practice
- Data gathering, analysis and reporting mechanisms
- Informed decision making processes
- Coordinating internal and external services.

Teams and Groups

Teams and groups are an important part of any community in providing for the needs of its members.

Communities have rights and responsibilities:

- The right to its own identity
- The right to set its own agenda, constitution and institutions
- The right to participate within the wider community
- The right to access skills and resources within the wider community
- The right to support its members within the wider community
- The right to protect its members from influences that disadvantage its members
- The right to refuse entry to members that do not fit into the community
- The right to evict members that do not accept the agenda, constitution and institutions of the community
- The right to refuse skills and resources to the wider community, where its members are disadvantaged
- The right to determine its own destiny.

Responsibilities

- Ensure the agenda, constitution and institutions of the community, protect and support its members, as well as other communities and their members. Provide a safe, secure environment for its members, as well as other communities and their members.
- Facilitate the development of valued roles and relationships for the community, its members, as well as other communities and their members.
- Ensure that the community communicates with its members as well as other communities and their member.
- Ensure the community does not disadvantage other communities or their members.
- Responsibility use, and share, skills and resources to the advantage of its members, as well as other communities and their members.
- Respect, protect and promote the rights, cultures and institutions of other communities and their members.
- Engage with other communities in an interdependent relationship.

COMMUNITY HEALTH

The concept of community is defined as 'a group of people who share some important feature of their lives and use some common agencies and institutions.' The concept of health is defined as 'a balanced state of well-being resulting from harmonious interactions of body, mind, and spirit.' The term community health is defined by meeting the needs of a community by identifying problems and managing interactions within the community.

The healthy community is one that makes wide use of its resources and is prepared to meet threats and dangers. In assessing the health of any community, it is necessary to collect information not only about variables specific to location but also about relationships between the community and its location. Do groups cooperate to identify threats? Does the community make certain that its members are given available information about resources and dangers? The location perspective of the community profile inventory, including the six location variables: community boundaries, location of health services, geographic features, climate, flora and fauna, and the human-made environment.

Location

Every physical community carries out its daily existence in a specific geographic location. The health of a community is affected by location, because placement of health services, geographic features, climate, plants, animals and the human-made environment are intrinsic to geographic location. The location of a community places it in an environment that offers resources and also poses threats (Skelly, et al., 2002; Neuman and Fawcett, 2001).

Community health is a field of public health, is a discipline which concerns itself with the study and improvement of the health characteristics of biological communities. While the term community can be broadly defined, community health tends to focus on geographical areas rather than people with shared characteristics. The term 'community health' refers to the health status of a defined group of people, or community, and the actions and conditions that protect and improve the health of the community. Those individuals who make up a community live in a somewhat localized area under the same general regulations, norms, values, and organizations. For example, the health status of the people living in a particular town, and the actions taken to protect and improve the health of these residents, would constitute community health. In the past, most individuals could be identified with a community in either a geographical or an organizational sense. Today, however, with expanding global economies, rapid transportation, and instant communication, communities alone no longer have the resources to control or look after all the needs of their residents or constituents.

The actions and conditions that protect and improve community or population health can be organized into three areas.

1. Health promotion
2. Health protection
3. Health services.

This breakdown emphasizes the collaborative efforts of various public and private sectors in relation to community health. Health promotion may be defined as any combination of educational and social efforts designed to help people take greater control of and improve their health. Health protection and health services differ from health promotion in the nature or timing of the actions taken. Health protection and services include the implementing of laws, rules, or policies approved in a community as a result of health promotion or legislation. An example of health protection would be a law to restrict the sale of hand guns, while an example of health services would be a policy offering free flu shots for the elderly by a local health department. Both of these actions could be the result of health promotion efforts such as a letter writing campaign or members of a community lobbying their board of health.

Concept of Community Health Nursing

Definition of community health nursing (CHN) must be based on an understanding and appreciation of the whole spectrum of nursing and its contribution to the individual sickness and health, to his family and to his community with this change of thought, the role of community health nurse has became complex and dynamic. Every nurse should be a community health nurse in practice.

Meaning

Community health nursing is concern with the people who are sick as well the healthy, young and old, male and female. At the same time from the above points it is clear that community health nurse is responsible for family centered care rather than an individual oriented one. Community health and CHN draw knowledge and practices from other disciplines such as medicine, surgery, pediatrics, obstetrics, dentistry, health education and vital statistics.

Definitions

- Community health nursing has been defined by the Division of CHN Practice of ANA as a field of nursing practice for which there exists a body of knowledge and related skills which is applied in meeting the health needs of communities, families and individuals in their normal environment such as at home, at school and at place of work.
- As defined by Ruth Freeman, service rendered by a professional nurse with the communities, groups, families, individuals at home, in health centers, in clinics, in schools, in places of work for the promotion of health, prevention of illness, care of the sick at home and rehabilitation.
- 1982, APHA (American Public Health Association) defines public health nursing as follows: Public health nursing synthesizes the body of knowledge from the public health sciences and professional nursing theories for the purpose of improving the health of the entire community. This goal lies at the heart of primary prevention and health promotion and is the foundation for public health nursing practice. To accomplish this goal, public health nurses work with groups, families, and individuals as well as in multidisciplinary teams and programs. Identifying subgroups within the population which are at the high risk of illness, disability or premature death, and directing resources towards these groups, is the most effective approach for accomplishing the goal of public health nursing.
- As explained by ANA (American Nurses Association) 1980, The CHN is defined as a synthesis of nursing and public health practice applied to promoting and preserving the health of people. The practice is general and comprehensive. It is not limited to a particular age group or diagnoses and is continuing, not episodic.

Goals of Community Health Nursing

- To increase the capability of families, groups and communities to cope with health and illness problems.
- To support and supplement the efforts of other professional restoration and preservation of health.
- To control or counteract as much as possible physical and social environmental conditions that threaten health or decrease the enjoyment of life.
- To contribute to the refinement and improvement of nursing practice and of public health practice and service.

Scope of Community Health Nursing

Scope means the extent and the areas the CHN can spread. They can work in variety settings like home, industry, health clinics, community health centers, school, rehabilitation centers, geriatric homes, hospice centers. They are providing a lots of services mainly preventive and primary curative services by dealing with all types of clients. They work with individuals and families in a setting that interacts with various healthcare providers, community organizations and county departments. Their duties involve the full scope of CHN activists. Community health nurses work as a part of the community that conducts home visits as well as special clinic like MCh clinic, immunization, mental health clinics, counseling centers and health education activities. The scope of CHN is vast. It is not limited to certain workspaces and responsibilities. Community health nurses work in many different locations with many different populations. Some of the examples are described below.

1. **Community health centers:** This is a setting where the community health nurses work with the members of the community to discuss their medical needs. They also run campaigns and develop resources around important topics like family planning, sexual health and other

preventative care. They are in contact with the member of the community only. Community health nurses may also work outside the community health center to have contact with a wider cross-section of the community.

2. **Correctional facilities:** This is a setup where many people are held in close proximity. Community health nurses work to limit the spread of various communicable diseases. They also run programs for the staff and inmates and implement various disease control protocols. They work very closely with the state and local health departments.
3. **Schools:** The scope of CHN expands at school level as it can help children lead healthier lives and manage their problems better. Community health nurses provide education on good health and illness prevention to students in schools. They also help students overcome any health issues the students might be facing. In case any student is experiencing abuse or neglect, these nurses help them address such issues as well.
4. **Aid organizations:** Organizations such as the Red Cross and Doctors without borders have many community health nurses working for them. These nurses work with disaster relief, access to clean drinking water, and how to counter contagious disease along with other needs similar to the work at any community health center.
5. **Government agencies:** Community health nurses working in a government agency setup have minimal direct contact with the members of the community. They work on the development of policies and their implementation. They aim at creating a change on a large scale for different groups.

COMMUNITY HEALTH NURSING APPROACHES

To accomplish community health goals and its aim the following aims are to be utilized by community health professionals, i.e.

Persuasive approach: The persuasive approach implies convincing people through dialogue and educate them to change or modify their health behavior. Community health nurse make use of this approach in all types of nursing interventions related to health promotion and specific protection, early recognition, diagnosis and treatment and disability limitation and rehabilitation. It is through education that self-care competencies of individual, family and community can be developed which is essential to achieve the goal of health for all.

Enforcement: The enforcement implies the use of more coercive measures such as use of legislation, e.g., prohibition of drug abuse, child abuse, immunization as a condition to school admission, etc., and the use of authority, e.g., giving strict instructions or orders to do certain things especially when it is a question of life and death during emergency situations such as child labor, acute bronchopneumonia, etc. Community health nurses make use of such measures in life-threatening emergency situations.

Team approach: Community health is a problem solving process and a team approach is very necessary to deal with varied and complex health needs and problems at large. It is just not possible for any one profession or discipline to provide such care. CHN is one of the professions and community health nurses along with auxiliary nurses and female health supervisors help to meet nursing needs of the community as a whole. Other members of the team who are usually there include physicians, clinical specialists, public health engineers, health statistians, epidemiologists, health educationalists, counselors, social workers, clinical psychologists, pharmacologists, lab technicians, village health workers. Community health nurses working in the community health settings needs to identify the health teams and their roles, functions and team dynamics so as to participate effectively in providing compressive healthcare services to people in the community and accomplish community health goals and aims.

Community involvement: Health of individual living in a defined community is not only their 'right' but also their 'responsibility' to take of their own health and also of community at large. Without people's help, participation or cooperation, it is neither possible to make healthcare services accessible and acceptable to them nor it is feasible to achieve community health goals and aims. Community involvement and participation is recognized as one of the crucial supportive approach for successful implementation of community healthcare services. But it is all the more important for the primary healthcare component which is given greatest emphasis at the grass root level. The extent of community involvement may vary from one community to another. It may depend upon their socioeconomic and cultural aspects, health attitude, health knowledge, etc. It ranges from true or active participation, i.e., people are knowledgeable and have a positive attitude and get involved in planning and implementing their health care to passive recipient of care provided, i.e., the major responsibility of community involvement lies with health personnel who directly deal with people at the community level. They need to encourage and promote them for their participation. Community health nurse working with individuals, families, groups within the community as a whole for CHN services need to mobilize, encourage, organize and prepare them to take greater interest and responsibilities, develop self-reliance for their own health matters.

Intersectoral approach: Health of people at large cannot be attained by health sector alone because there are many factors which affect people's health but they are not under the purview of the health sector, e.g., food production and distribution, water, sanitation, housing, environmental protection and education, etc., each one is dealt by separate sector and socioeconomic development and health. It is felt necessary to have proper coordination between the health and all other sectors concerned at all levels. Health workers including community health nurses working at the grass root level for primary health care need to identify these sectors and coordinate with them to provide desired services which serve as entry points for the development and implementation for primary care services. Community health nurses can also educate on nutritional status of the family, food storage through programs in the agriculture and health economics, proper use and maintenance of houses and the areas surrounding them through respective programs, etc. Health workers including community health nurse who can also involve personnel from these sectors at community level to promote health activities, e.g., agricultural workers can promote production of appropriate food stuff and their consumption by families; teachers in schools can promote good sanitation, encourage healthful behavior in students, conduct courses on nutrition and first aid; mass media personnel can popularize various primary healthcare services by disseminating authentic in different communities, etc. Evidence-based practice (EBP) entails making decisions about how to promote health or provide care by integrating the best available evidence with practitioner expertise and other resources, and with the characteristics, state, needs, values and preferences of those who will be affected. This is done in a manner that is compatible with the environmental and organizational context. Evidence is comprised of research findings derived from the systematic collection of data through observation and experiment and the formulation of questions and testing of hypotheses.

Epidemiological approach: Epidemiological analysis and measurement allow researchers to measure health status and measurement of disease occurrences in a population. Surveillance of disease yields epidemiological intelligence data by providing systematic count of disease frequency. These data can be in turn used to estimate the magnitude of health problems in the community, detect epidemics and understand natural history of a disease or detect potential emerging infectious disease threats. Another use of this approach is case finding to identify health status of people who are at risk.

Nursing Process Approach

The nursing process is a modified scientific method. Nursing practice was first described as a four stage nursing process by Ida Jean Orlando in 1958. The nursing process uses clinical judgement to strike a balance of epistemology between personal interpretation and research evidence in which critical thinking may play a part to categorize the clients issue and course of action. Nursing offers diverse patterns of knowing. The nursing process is goal-oriented method of caring that provides a framework to nursing care. It involves five major steps: (1) A: Assess (what data is collected?) (2) D: Diagnose (what is the patient's problem) (3) P: Plan (how to manage the problem) (4) I: Implement (putting plan into action) (5) E: Evaluate (did the plan work?). Assessing phase: The nurse completes an holistic nursing assessment of the needs of the individual/family/community, regardless of the reason for the encounter. The nurse collects subjective data and objective data using a nursing framework, such as Marjory Gordon's functional health patterns. Nursing assessments provide the starting point for determining nursing diagnoses. It is vital that a recognized nursing assessment framework is used in practice to identify the patient's problems, risks and outcomes for enhancing health. The use of an evidence-based nursing framework such as Gordon's Functional Health Pattern. Diagnosing phase: Nursing diagnoses represent the nurse's clinical judgment about actual or potential health problems/life process occurring with the individual, family, group or community. The accuracy of the nursing diagnosis is validated when a nurse is able to clearly identify and link to the defining characteristics, related factors and/or risk factors found within the patient's assessment. Multiple nursing diagnoses may be made for one client.

Nursing Theories Approaches

A nursing theory is a conceptualization of some aspects of nursing communicated for the purpose of describing, explaining, predicting, and or prescribing nursing care. There are lot of theories identified by different theorist which can be applied in community field during providing care, developing IPR and giving health education. Health belief model can be applied to change behavior during community education program to motivating the people.

HOME VISIT

The home visit is a family-nurse contact which allows the health worker to assess the home and family situations in order to provide the necessary nursing care and health related activities. In performing this activity, it is essential to prepare a plan of visit to meet the needs of the client and achieve the best results of desired outcomes. It is a purposeful interaction in a home (or residence) directed at promoting and maintaining the health of individuals and the family (or significant others). A major distinction of a home visit is that the health professional goes to the client rather than the client coming to the health professional. Home visiting involves a process of initiating relationships with family members, negotiating and implementing a family-focused plan of care, and evaluating health outcomes and family satisfaction.

Definition

The home visit is a family-nurse contact which allows the health worker to assess the home and family situations in order to provide the necessary nursing care and health-related activities.

A home visit is a purposeful interaction in a home directed at promoting and maintaining the health of individuals and the family. Home visit is the process of providing nursing care to the client's own setting. The setting may be in a single or multiple unit structure and may be located in a rural or urban setting.

A comprehensive range of community nursing services is provided by community health. The main focus of this service is to enable people to be cared for in their own homes rather than as patients in hospitals.

Aims of Home Visit

- To assess the family
- To provide nursing care
- To treat according to the need
- To rendered health education
- To provide referral services (if care fails).

Objectives

- Promoting support systems that are adequate and effective and encouraging use of health-related resources.
- Promoting adequate, effective care of a family member who has a specific problem related to illness or disability.
- Encouraging normal growth and development of family members and the family and educating the family about health promotion and illness prevention.
- Strengthens family functioning and relatedness.
- Promoting a healthful environment.

Principles

- A home visit must have a purpose or objective.
- Planning for a home visit should make use of all available information about the patient and his family through family records.
- In planning for a home visit, we should consider and give priority to the essential needs if the individual and his family.
- Planning and delivery of care should involve the individual and family.
- The plan should be flexible.

Guidelines

- The physical needs, psychological needs, and educational needs of the individual and family.
- The acceptance of the family for the services to be rendered, their interest and the willingness to cooperate.
- Take into account other health agencies and the number of health personnel already involved in the care of a specific family.
  - Careful evaluation of past services given to the family and how the family avails of the nursing services.
  - The ability of the patient and his family to recognize their own needs, their knowledge of available resources and their ability to make use of their resources for their benefits.

Procedure of Home Visit

Greet the patient and introduce yourself.
- State the purpose of the visit.
- Observe the patient and determine the health needs.
- Put the bag in a convenient place.
- Perform the nursing care needed and give health teachings.
- Record all important date, observation and care rendered.
- There is no easy access to emergency equipment or consultation with.

Advantages

- These visits cost less than hospital care, with better outcomes, especially when chronic health issues are involved.
- Clients have greater control over their health and lives.
- The community health nurse gains access to families to provide health education and other prevention strategies. Individuals and family members may be more receptive to learning because they are less anxious in their own environment and because the immediacy of needing to know a particular fact or skill becomes more apparent.
- Home visits allow for primary intervention, to prevent disease or injury from occurring.
- Home setting provides more opportunities for comprehensive care.
- Most people prefer to be cared for at home for getting better psychological support.
- Environmental factors impinging on health, such as housing condition and finances, may be observed and considered more readily.
- Information collection and understanding lifestyle values are easier in families' own environment.
- Participation of family members is facilitated.
- Care to ill members in the home can reduce overall costs by preventing hospitalizations and shortening the length of time spent in hospitals or other institutions.
- A family focus is facilitated.

Disadvantages

- The nurses skills, personality, or physical ability may not be compatible with providing home visit.
- Home visits are time consuming; travel time is required to get to the persons needing care.
- There is no easy access to emergency equipment or consultation with other health professionals if needed.
- Home visits may present issues regarding the nurse personal safety in some community or family settings.
- The nurse has less control over the care setting (for example, cleanliness, noise, privacy, or distractions).

BAG TECHNIQUE

Home visiting is very essential and back bone of public health nursing because majority of client are found in the home. While home visit community health nurse should carry community health bag. The community health bag is designed to carry equipments and material needed during a visit to the home, school or factory. Equipment and materials are needed to make test, demonstrate patient care and perform dressing, etc.

The bag should be made up of canvas, leather or light metal. This is stitched in such a way that it can be carried either by hand or over shoulder.

Ideally the CHN bag should have four pockets, 2 outer pocket and 2 inner pocket.

1st outer pocket: 1st outer pocket contained hand washing articles (soap, soap dish, towel, nailbrush), note book, pen, plastic sheet and news paper, etc.

2nd outer pocket: 2nd outer pocket is used to keep used articles.

N.B: Ideally it should be opposite to first outer pocket.

1st Inner Pocket

1st inner pocket contain:
- **The articles for physical assessment** such as torch, spring balance, weighing cloth, BP instrument, stethoscope, fetoscope, tape measure, thermometer.
- **Articles for urine testing** such as test tube, test tube holder, match box, litmus paper, dropper, filter paper, Benedict's solution, spirit lamp.
- **Articles for dressing** such as Betadine solution, adhesive tape, gloves, spirit.
- **Articles for injection** like syringe and needle cotton swab, gauze piece, etc.
- **Other** articles like slides, lancet, drugs, ORS, contraceptives.

2nd Inner Pocket

2nd inner pocket contains all sterile materials (dressing instruments, sterile instrument and swab stick for culture, sterile artery forcep.

Principles of Bag Technique

1. **Cleanliness:** The bag and its contents are all designed for efficiency and cleanliness. The content and bag also must kept clean and ready to use for all time.
2. The hand should be washed every time before touching the bag.
3. For doing any dressing the surgical aseptic technique should follow.
4. During giving care or doing any procedure the name most avoid to touch the bag.
5. Contaminated article should be separately properly.
6. Sterilized articles aseptic principle should be maintained.
7. Maintain bag technique properly.
8. Bowl contaminated instrument and equipment before returning them to the bag. The article should be autoclaved.
9. Protect and take care of the bag.

Preprocedural Responsibility

- Check the bag before leaving for home visit.
- Bag should be kept at proper place, out of reach of children.
- Personal equipment should not be kept inside the bag.

After Procedure

- Wash hand with soap under tap water
- Return articles to the bag. Use a cotton must and swab with spirit wipe outside used bottles
- Washable articles should be properly washed

Table 1.1: Steps of procedure of bag technique.

Sl. No.	*Steps*	*Rationale*
1.	Select a work area where the bag may be setup without danger of being contaminated by children or domestic animal	Children and domestic animal can contaminate the bag
2.	Spread a plastic sheet or new paper on surface to place the bag	For creating clean surface area
3.	Remove hand washing material and wash hand under tap water with bacteria static soap if available	Running water help to remove dirty easily and antiseptic soap reduce the bacterial growth
4.	Remove apron from the bag put it on grasp the apron at the neck line and shake out	For less contamination
5.	Setup paper bags	For collecting dry wastes
6.	Remove basin, scale, thermometer, dressing cotton swabs, urine and kit dressing sets as per needed and place on clean area	Removing all needed articles at a time to save time
7.	Wash hands again if you are going to do any surgical procedure	For creating or maintaining surgical asepsis
8.	Close the bag securely	Some time small children can take article and handle it
9.	Give nursing service as indicated	To fulfill our purpose
10.	When the procedure in over wash the hands over soap under top or poured water	For keeping own free from danger

- Fold used proper with used side inside and ask the family members for next visit
- Close the bag
- Write the report of what are observed and what are done, etc.

Steps of procedure of bag techniques is discussed in **Table 1.1.**

CURRENT STATUS OF COMMUNITY HEALTH NURSING

Community health nursing has evolved into a focus on care of individuals, families and communities. The focus and orientation are different to other nurses in their work areas.

Community health nursing is a specific and specialized orientation to the care that embodies principle of public health as guiding concepts.

Primary health care is one aspect of CHN. CHN focuses on the physical, biological, social, psychological and environmental health of a population group. While primary care is a 'coordinate system of personal health care, emphasizing first contact care and continuously.'

—Ruth, 1978

Primary care emphasizes ambulatory care that addresses total client needs both for curative and preventive services. CHN is population based.

School nurses have played a significant part in school health programs. They need to be flexible, creative, and involved in revising their role to fit with new directions, otherwise, the role of the school nurse may be jeopardized. Economic justification for services is necessary and therefore, the value of the school nurse must be ascertained.

National health objectives for the year 2000 seek to increase school based education to prevent human immunodeficiency virus infection, alcohol and other drug use, tobacco use, injury and sexually transmitted diseases.

Health education has proven to be effective at reducing risk behaviors associated with the leading causes of death that is heart diseases, cancer stroke, COPD, unintentional injuries, AIDS, etc., responsibility needs to be a fundamental components of health care reform.

Trends Influencing CHN

Community health nursing practice today has been affected by several newer developments in the field of medicine, nursing and other scientific disciplines. Several trends currently influencing community health and nursing. They are:

- **Demographic trends:** Increase population, greater%age of elderly people, suburbanization of society, etc.
- **Technological trends:** Knowledge explosion, environmental pollution, use of nuclear energy, etc.
- **Sociocultural trends:** Woman liberalization, health insurance, mass communication techniques.
- **Economic trends:** Rising cost of health care, independent nurse practitioner, self-care by individuals.
- **Political trends:** Research in CHN field, more specialization in community health.

ISSUES AND CHALLENGES OF COMMUNITY HEALTH NURSE

India is the second most populous country in the world. The death rate has declined but birth rates continue to be high in most of the states. Healthcare structure in the country is over-burdened by increasing population. This country has highly affected by the pandemics like COVID-19 and other types of emerging and re-emerging diseases. India also faces the epidemic of continuing/emerging infectious diseases as well as chronic degenerative diseases. These all required proper implementation of public health programmes with mass awareness in community which is a major challenge for community health nurse to keep her community healthy.

Community nursing is the coming together of primary health care and nursing profession with public health nursing. A community nurse not restricted to providing care to particular group or age but is encouraged to participate in all aspects of social life activities for the promotion of health and education. Community nursing as we know has come a long way in the last ten years with the change in the demography and diversity, technical advancement, educated consumers, use of alternative therapies and palliative care. Nurses are a major player towards building a healthier community, so they have to make their presence felt in each and every way possible for a healthier and disease free society. People involved in nursing profession have also been affected by the rise of electronic media and social networks like Facebook (Meta) and Twitter which now has a become a major factor in how a community nurse operates for the healthier society.

The common issues and challenges in CHN are discussed below.

Advance Technology in Medical Education

Advances in healthcare bring significant social and economic benefit, increased life expectancy and improved quality of life. Medical explorations in the last century has led to people live longer with high expectations. So community nurses are required to be ready to meet the expectation of community people. A community nurse must encourage and promote healthier living, build an cooperating environment and respond as required, give information and support they need for change.

Sociodemographic Context: Demographics Diversity

People live longer due to improvement in health knowledge, and consequent improvements in diagnostic techniques and treatments. The average life expectancy in developed countries has now reached 80 years and continues to lengthen. It has also been observed that, aging population will be increased to 25% of whole populations by 2030. Nowaday people don't have time to take care of parents there is altered in family support for older. So community health nurse must be concern towards taking extra care for geriatric people by regular health check-up, health education and counseling.

Service is in Demand

There is increasing demand on the healthcare delivery organizations. Community people become more concern regarding their own health. There is increasing expectation for quality, efficient and effective healthcare service of every people which is also a challenge for community health nurse to meet this.

Epidemiological Context

India is the second most populous country in the world. The death rate has declined but birth rates continue to be high in most of the states. Healthcare structure in the country is over-burdened by increasing population. With a view of epidemiological context it has been observed that increasing prevalence of chronic conditions requiring long-term care. India also faces the twin epidemic of continuing/emerging infectious diseases as well as chronic degenerative diseases. Due to change in lifestyle and other factors there is multiple chronic diseases and comorbidities are prevalent among peoples and also psychosocial problems become emerging problems in every part of community. Increase prevalence of noncommunicable diseases and psychosocial illness require continuous health education and counseling in community. This country has highly affected by the pandemics like COVID-19 and other types of emerging and re-emerging diseases. These all required proper implementation of public health programmes with mass awareness in community which is a major challenge for community health nurse to keep her community healthy.

Peoples are Stakeholders in their own Healthcare

As a society, we are changing rapidly, and this is apparent in the relationship between care providers and the citizen. Patients are increasingly becoming stakeholders in their own care journeys; they demand transparency in access and information about their care and importantly, about the quality of service provided. Citizens are now demanding access on their terms. In community we are encouraging people participation during any programme planning and implementation by which the community people becoming more demanding in nature which is a challenge for community health nurse.

Healthcare Context

Patients discharge from hospitals quicker and sicker and they are no longer interested to stay in hospital, requiring considerable interventions in the community. Nowadays health services become health oriented not disease oriented and more focus is given in preventive aspect rather than curative aspects. So it is a major task and challenge of community health nurse how to promote and maintain health status of community people.

Economic Development, Education and Health

Though there is economic development still a large segment of population suffered due to economic deprivation which results in poor access to health care. Poor educational status leads to non-utilization of scanty health services which increase the avoidable risk factors, decrease life expectancy and increase morbidity and mortality rate. Though advances in medicine are responsible for improvement in health indices but it is not sufficient. Here door to door community services can only help in improvement of health indices which can be possible by a community health nurse.

Inequity in Health Care

Almost everywhere, the poor suffer poor health and the very poor suffer appallingly. In addition, the gap in health between rich and poor remains very wide. Addressing this problem, both between countries and within countries, constitutes one of the greatest challenges of the new century. Failure to do so properly will have dire consequences for the global economy, for social order and justice, and for the civilization as a whole. The important principle in primary healthcare is equity in health care services which can be provided by a community health nurse.

High Burden of Disease

India faces high burden of disease because of lack of environmental sanitation and safe drinking water, under-nutrition, poor living conditions, and limited access to preventive and curative health services. Lack of education, gender inequality and explosive growth of population contribute to increasing burden of disease. Full impact of the HIV epidemic and tobacco-related diseases is yet to be felt. Despite incredible improvements in health since 1950, there are still a number of challenges, which have to be solved. Here health education and behavior change communication can play a major activity and community health nurse can act as a change agent. This is a great challenge for community health nurse.

Other Challenges

- Inadequate and unsupportive working condition and environment
- Financial and supplies are limited in delivering CHN services
- Community health nursing workforce is inadequate in delivering essential CHN services
- Accommodation and transportation facilities are insufficient
- Absence of educational standard at entry to public health setting
- Training exposure to international or regional updates in CHN services are limited
- Lack of consensus on the scope of practice for CHNs
- Complete autonomy in performing CHN activities is not permitted.
- Role conflict exists
- Service recognition from community residents is unavailable
- Lack of research for developing evidence-based practice in CHN
- Community health nursings should involve in members of policy makers and health leaders
- Lack of empowerment

PRINCIPLES OF COMMUNITY HEALTH NURSING

- Community health nursing is an established activity based on recognized needs and functioning within the total health programmes.
- The CHN agency has clearly defined objectives and purposes for its services.
- An active organized citizens group, representative of the community is an integral part of the community health programme, e.g., mandals, school teachers act as the community representative to share in the health programs. Their knowledge and experience shared with professional workers.
- Community health nursing services are available to the entire community regardless of origin, culture or social and economic resources and also it should be available to

people irrespective of age, sex, creed, nationality, political affiliation.
- Community health nursing recognized the family and community as units of service.
- Health education and counseling for individual, family and community are the integral part of CHN.
- Recipients of health care should participate in planning relating to goals for the attainment of health.
- The community health nurse is a qualified as a full-fledged nurse.
- The CHN service should be based on the needs of the patient and there will be proper continuity of services to patients. Periodic and continuing appraisal and evaluation of the health situation of the patients are basic to the CHN.
- The community health nurse should function or serve as an important member of the health team.
- The community health nurse does not provide material relief to patients, but directs the patient to appropriate community resources for necessary financial and social assistance.
- The community health nurse should not accept gifts or bribes from the patients.
- The community health nurse should not belong to any one section or any political group.
- The nurses assume responsibilities of their own continuing professional development through acquiring higher and higher education and forming and strengthening the professional associations.
- The CHN services must develop proper guidelines in maintaining records and reports which are very essential for community health.
- There must be proper facilities and job conditions.
- The community health nurses will maintain professional relationship with all the leaders in the community and maintain ethics at all times.
- Community health nursing is based on recognized needs of communities, families, groups and individuals.
- The community health nurse must fully understand the objectives and policies of the agency she represents.
- Community health nursing must be available to all regardless of race, creed and socioeconomic status.
- Health teaching is a primary responsibility of community health nurse.
- Community health nurse works as a member of the health team.
- There must be provision for periodic evaluation of CHN services.
- Opportunities for continuing staff education programs for nurses must be provided by the CHN agency. She has a responsibility for his/her own professional growth.
- The community health nurse makes use of available community health resources.
- Community health nurse utilizes the already existing active organized groups in the community.
- There must be provision for educative supervision in CHN
- Clients of the community health nurse are Individual, family and community.

ETHICS INVOLVED IN COMMUNITY HEALTH NURSING

Every profession makes provision to raise its status and to safeguard its own interest and that of its clients there is no legal binding for the acceptance of a particular ethic. It is a self-imposed discipline. There are some moral rules and principles adopt in nursing profession after conducting many conferences and meetings from time to time professional ethics governing CHN practices are essentially the same as applied to nursing in other fields.

In 1973 The International Council of Nurses Code of Ethics had resulted in clear and broader standards which can be applied in any culture and anywhere in the world. Some of the standards given in the code for nurses are also stated in the Nightingale Pledge which is universally known and used in the nursing profession.

- The fundamental responsibility of the nurse is fourfold: to promote health, to prevent illness, to restore health and to alleviate suffering.
- Inherent in nursing is respect for life, dignity and rights of man.
- It is unrestricted by considerations of nationality, race, creed, color, age, sex, politics or social status.
- Nurses render health services to the individual, the family and the community and coordinate their services with those of related groups. These are discussed in the following order:
    - *Nurses and people:* The earlier term patient has been replaced by client. The code directs the nurse to respect a person's values, customs and religious beliefs. Each country and different areas within a country has certain values and customs. The nurse is expected to learn the accepted patterns of behavior of the community and not insult the people knowingly or unknowingly by behavior that is not acceptable to them. Any personal information must be held in confidential or shared only with careful judgement. Careless talk about a person is always unethical conduct. The religious beliefs must be respected and spiritual advisers should be provided.
    - *Nurses and practice:*
        - The nurses must maintain at all times the highest standards of nursing care and professional conduct.
        - She should maintain at all times the highest standards of nursing care and of professional conduct.
        - She should maintain up to date scientific knowledge and skills and have the right attitude in using this knowledge.
        - She must give medical treatment without medical orders only in emergency and reports such action to the physician at earliest possible movement.
        - She must carry out the physicians orders intelligently and loyally and to refuse to participate in unethical procedures.
        - A nurse is entitled to just remuneration and accepts only such compensation as the contract, actual or implied, provides.

- She should not permit her name to be used in connection with the advertisement of products or with any form of self-advertisements.
- *Nurses and society:*
  - Nurse should participate and share responsibility with other citizens and other health professions in promoting efforts to meet the health needs of the public, local, state, national and international.
  - The code states the responsibility of the nurse for positive promotion of health for the community by birth initiating and supporting action to meet the health and social needs. Social needs are closely link with the health needs. Poor housing, sanitation, nutrition, unemployment and illiteracy affect the health of the people.
  - The nurse has an important role to play in education and referral work.
- *Nurse and coworkers:*
  - The nurse should cooperate with and maintain harmonious relationship with members of other professions and his nursing colleagues.
  - The nurse is one member of the health team who can serve and meet the health needs of the people.
  - She should understand her own responsibilities on the health team with others.
- *Nurses and profession:*
  - The code points out the role of a nurse as a leader and active participant.
  - The nurse should take the leadership role in setting up desirable standards of nursing education and practice.
  - She should enlarge the care of professional knowledge and take interest in research.
  - She should setting up and maintaining fair social and economic working conditions in nursing. This should be done in the right way by peaceful negotiations and not by means of strike which is very unethical. Action should be initiated through professional organizations.

Application of Ethics to Community Health Nursing Practice

The priority of ethical principles in CHN, ethical principles direct and guide nursing actions with individuals and aggregate groups. The professional ethic, in general, places a greater emphasis on the observance of the principles of autonomy and beneficence than the principles of justice in most nursing actions but in community action is directed towards group, that is why autonomy of individual has less importance. The ethical principle of beneficence is given slightly less emphasis in the code for nurses but it is given more importance in CHN. The principle of justice is also not strongly emphasized in the professional code of ethics but justice can strongly emphasized in CHN it is noted in passing that nursing practice is not influenced by age, sex, race, color, personality or other personal attributes or individual differences in customs, beliefs, or attributes. The code estates that nursing care is delivered without disease detection and prevention and in health maintenance. Accountability: In CHN Moral accountability in nursing practice means that nurses are answerable for how they promote, protect, and meet the health needs of clients while respecting individual rights to self-determination in health care. She should accountable for client and employing agency. In CHN, where the greater emphasis is on aggregates rather than individual clients, moral accountability means being answerable for how the health of aggregate groups justice are still important in CHN. Yet they are less important than the principle of beneficence in CHN the emphasis of the professional ethic is slanted toward benefit to aggregates, which implies following a rule of utility in planning, implementing, and evaluating of CHN services.

SOCIOCULTURAL ISSUES IN COMMUNITY HEALTH NURSING

The definition of sociocultural is something that involves the social and cultural aspects. Social problems are the general factors that affect and damage society. A social problem is normally a term used to describe problems with a particular area or group of people in the world. Social problems often involve problems that affect real life even though world advances a lot, people in the community still have lot of social issues.

Major Social Issues

- Child abuse
- Elderly abuse
- Female feticide
- Prostitution
- Food adulteration
- Substance abuse
- Women abuse
- Women empowerment.

Child Abuse

There is clear evidence that child abuse is a global problem. It occurs in a variety of forms and is deeply rooted in cultural, economic and social practices. It has observed that two out of every three children were physically abused. Out of 69% children physically abused, 54.68% were boys and among them physically abuse in family situations, 88.6% were physically abused by parents. Before defining 'child abuse' it's crucial to get informed about 'children's rights' in the first place because so many children prohibited to enjoy their rights.

Rights of Children

Right to Education

- Access to quality, free, compulsory primary education.
- Non-discrimination in access to education (gender gap).
- Right to leisure, recreation and cultural activities.

Right to Health

- Access to quality health services
- Rights of children with disabilities
- Adolescents and reproductive health knowledge
- Right to benefit from social security
- Right to an adequate standard of living.

Right to Special Protection

- Protection from all forms of exploitation (economic, sexual).
- Violence against children (physical, psychological and sexual).
- Female genital mutilation and early marriage.
- Torture and deprivation of liberty for juvenile in conflict with the law
- Hazardous occupations.
- Smoking, substance abuse, and trafficking.
- Protection of street children.

Definition of Child Abuse

Child abuse can be defined as a variety of abnormal behaviors directed against children which can take many forms.

Types of Child Abuse

Physical Abuse

Physical abuse is any nonaccidental injury to a child under the age of 18 by a parent or caretaker. These injuries may include beatings, shaking, burns, human bites, strangulation, or immersion in scalding water or others, with resulting bruises and welts, fractures, scars, burns, internal injuries or any other injuries. The term 'battered child syndrome' was coined to characterize the clinical manifestations of serious physical abuse in young children. This term is generally applied to children showing repeated and devastating injury to the skin, skeletal system or nervous system. It includes children with multiple fractures of different ages, head trauma and severe visceral trauma, with evidence of repeated infliction.

Another form is the 'The shaken infant'. Shaking is a prevalent form of abuse seen in very young children (less than 1 year). Most perpetrators of such abuse are males. Intracranial hemorrhages, retinal hemorrhages and chip fractures of the child's extremities can result from very rapid shaking of an infant.

Corporal Punishment

In the form of hitting, punching, kicking or beating is socially and legally accepted in most countries. In many, it is a significant phenomenon in schools and other institutions and in penal systems for young offenders.

Emotional Abuse

It includes the failure of a caregiver to provide an appropriate and supportive environment, and includes acts that have an adverse effect on the emotional health and development of a child. Such acts include restricting a child's movements, denigration, ridicule, threats and intimidation, discrimination, rejection and other nonphysical forms of hostile treatment. The consistent failure of a parent or caretaker to provide a child with appropriate support, attention, and affection also act as emotional abuse. It also include a chronic pattern of behaviors such as belittling, humiliating, and ridiculing a child.

Neglect

It refers to the failure of a parent to provide for the development of the child where the parent is in a position to do so in one or more of the following areas: health, education, emotional development, nutrition, shelter and safe living conditions. Neglect is thus distinguished from circumstances of poverty in that neglect can occur only in cases where reasonable resources are available to the family or caregiver.

Child Sexual Abuse

Child sexual abuse is the exploitation of a child or adolescent for the sexual gratification of another person, e.g., child prostitution, pornography, intercourse.

Risk Factors for Child Abuse

Individual Risk Factors

- Parents' lack of understanding of children's needs, child development and parenting skills
- Parents' history of child maltreatment in family of origin
- Substance abuse and/or mental health issues including depression in the family
- Parental characteristics such as young age, low education, single parenthood, large number of dependent children, and low income
- Nonbiological, transient caregivers in the home (e.g., mother's male partner)
- Parental thoughts and emotions that tend to support or justify maltreatment behaviors.

Family Risk Factors

- Social isolation
- Family disorganization, dissolution, and violence, including intimate partner violence
- Parenting stress, poor parent-child relationships, and negative interactions.

Community Risk Factors

- Community violence
- Concentrated neighborhood disadvantage (e.g., high poverty and residential instability, high unemployment rates, and high density of alcohol outlets), and poor social connections.

Indicators of Child Abuse

Type of abuse	Physical indicators	Behavioral indicators
Physical	Unexplained bruises, welts, burns, fractures, or bald patches on scalp	Wary of adult contact, frightened of parents or afraid to go home, withdrawn or aggressive, moves uncomfortably, wears inappropriate clothing for weather
Sexual	Difficulty walking or sitting; torn or stained/ blood underclothes; pain, itching, bruises, swelling in genital area; frequent urinary or yeast infections	Advanced sexual knowledge, promiscuity, sudden school difficulties, self-imposed social isolation, avoidance of physical contact or closeness, depression
Emotional	Speech or communicative disorder, delayed physical development, exacerbation of existing conditions, substance abuse	Habit disorders, antisocial or destructive behaviors, neurotic traits, behavior extremes, developmental delays
Neglect	Consistent hunger, poor hygiene, inappropriate dress, unattended medical problems, underweight, failure to thrive	Self-destructive behaviors, begging or stealing food, constant fatigue, assuming adult responsibilities or concerns, frequently absent or tardy, states no caretaker in home

Role of a Community Health Nurse in Prevention and Management of Child Abuse

Identification of child abuse: The community health nurse can identify by observing the child in day to day life their normal childhood development, conditions that may be confused with abuse, unintentional vs intentional injury, human bite marks, hair loss, falls, head, facial, oral injuries, shaken baby syndrome, abusive burn patterns, scald, flexion burns, contact burns or pseudoabusive' burns, etc. When observing injury she should check the color of the injury. Or any other indicators of psychological or sexual abuse. The community health nurse can report to child abuse help line.

Educating the family: She can educate the family regarding:
- Nurturing parenting skills
- Stable family relationships
- Household rules and child monitoring
- Parental employment
- Adequate housing
- Access to health care and social services.

Her supportive role is also:
- Strengthen family and community connections and support.
- Treat parents as vital contributors to their children's growth and development.
- Create opportunities for parents to feel empowered to act on their own behalf.
- Respect the integrity of the family.
- Enhance parents' capability to foster the optimal development of their children and themselves.
- Establish links with community support systems.
- Provide settings where parents and children can gather, interact, support and learn from each other.
- Enhance coordination and integration of services needed by families.
- Enhance community awareness of the importance of healthy parenting practices.

Female Feticide

Female feticide is the abortion of a female fetus outside of legal channels. It occurs in India for assumed cultural reasons that span centuries. Ultrasonography and fetoscopy helps determine abnormalities in the fetus. But it is misused to find out sex of the fetus and abortion is done if it is a girl. The child sex ratio is calculated as number of girls per 1000 boys in the 0–6 years age group. According to 2011 census the girls sex ratio is 940/1000 boys. Though the condition is improving still it needs special attention to stop female feticide.

Causes of Female Feticides

- Strong male child preference
- Gender inequity
- Easy availability of sex determination test, abortion services
- Child marriage
- Economic dependence
- A low status of the women in the family
- Dowry system
- Cultural preference (one male child must)
- Illiteracy.

Preventive Measures

Legal Initiatives

The Prenatal Diagnostic Test Act (PNDT Act): The Prenatal Diagnostic Techniques (Regulation and Prevention of Misuse) Act, 1994, was enacted and brought into operation from 1st January, 1996, in order to check female feticide. Rules have also been framed under the Act. The Act prohibits determination and disclosure of the sex of fetus. It also prohibits any advertisements relating to prenatal determination of sex and prescribes punishment for its contravention. The person who contravenes the provisions of this Act is punishable with imprisonment and fine.

The Medical Termination of Pregnancy (MTP) Act: This Act was enacted by the Indian Parliament in the year 1971 and came into force in 1972. As per India's abortion laws only qualified doc stipulated conditions, can perform abortion on a woman in an approved clinic or hospital. The Medical Termination of Pregnancy (MTP) Act of India clearly states the conditions under which a pregnancy can be ended or aborted.

The Dowry Prohibition Act, 1961: As dowry is considered to be an important cause of female feticide, the Dowry

Prohibition Act should be made more stringent by proper amendments and should be implemented strictly. According to this act, if any person, after the commencement of this Act, gives or takes or abets the giving or taking of dowry, he shall be punishable with imprisonment for a term which shall not be less than five years, and with fine which shall not be less than fifteen thousand rupees or the amount of the value of such dowry, whichever is more.

Other Measures

- The related social malaises such as dowry, poverty, women's unemployment and exploitation, lack of proper education to girl child and their dropouts, early marriage, etc., are to be dealt with sternly by enacting proper laws and implementing them in true spirit.
- Affirmative action on part of the government and the corporate sector by providing security for parents and granting financial aid to the girl child can help in changing the mindset of the society of treating the girl as a burden.
- Corporate initiatives, such as 'Beti Ek Anmol Ratan' scheme in which the donations are invested in mutual funds, Kisan Vikas Patras and National Savings Certificates in the name of newborn girls and on maturity (age of 21 years) to be utilized for higher education or marriage; has found favor with the parents and the scheme is yielding positive results.
- Government schemes like 'LADLI' have created gender revolution in national capital, and impacted sex ratio in favor of the girl child. Banks need to be encouraged to give loans for female child's higher education at lower rates of interest.
- Awareness programs should be launched to make the woman aware about their rights and about the ill effects of abortions. Women should know their rights regarding adoption, maintenance, marriage, property, employment, education, etc.
- In order to make the females independent, women should be imparted skill and training through various vocational programs. Free and compulsory education should be provided to female children so that they can support themselves during exigency. Also it would remove the attitude that investing in girls is unnecessary.
- Medical termination of pregnancy should only be permitted after approval of PNDT authority/committee/ gazetted female officer/Mahila Panchayat members/ NGOs on proof of the existence of medical condition necessitating such termination.
- A social audit of all documents received from sonography clinics and making the data regarding sale of ultrasound machines, which are used for illegal sex determination tests, should be made available online. Information received will help governmental and non-governmental organization in estimating the targets for proper implementation of the Acts and for suggesting remedial measures to combat the problem. By involving all the stakeholders, a comprehensive social audit can be conducted to launch a crusade against female feticide.

Prostitution

Prostitution is the sale of sexual services, such as oral sex or sexual intercourse for money. Prostitution the word itself speaks about the plight of a women. It is not a problem which exists in India but exists throughout the world. Prostitution was a part of daily life in ancient Greece. In the more important cities, and particularly the many ports, it employed a significant proportion of the population and represented one of the top levels of economic activity. In the ancient city of Heliopolis in Syria, there was a law that stated that every maiden should prostitute herself to strangers at the temple of Astarte.

Definition

A prostitute may be defined as an individual (male or female) who for some kind of reward (monetary or otherwise) or for some other form of personnel satisfaction and as a part of full time profession engage in normal or abnormal sexual intercourse with various persons who may be of the same sex or opposite sex to the prostitute.

Causes of Prostitution

- Poverty
- Broken homes
- Mental illness
- Uneducated women
- Widows and divorces
- Easy way to income money
- Over sexual desires
- Indebtedness
- False hope of marriage
- Influence of peer group.

Types of Prostitution

Street Prostitution

Street prostitution who typically find their customers, or are found by their customers, somewhere on a street. They then have a quick act of sex in the customer's car, in an alleyway or other secluded spot, or in a cheap hotel.

Escort or Out Call Prostitution

Call girls work as independent operators in their homes or fairly fancy hotels and charge a lot of money for their services, which include sex but also talking and dining. Their clients are typically businessmen or other wealthy individuals. Many call girls earn between $200 and $500 per hour, and some earn between $1,000 and $6,000 per hour or per session. Call girls and escorts rank at the top of the prostitution hierarchy.

Brothel Workers

As the name implies, are prostitutes who work in brothels. The only legal brothels in the United States today are found in several rural counties in Nevada, which legalized prostitution in these counties in 1971. Workers in these brothels pay income tax. Because their employers require regular health exams and condom use, the risk of sexually transmitted disease in Nevada's brothels is low.

Massage Parlor Workers

Massage parlor workers, as their name also implies, work in massage parlors. Many massage parlors, of course, involve no prostitution at all, and are entirely legal. However, some massage parlors are in fact fronts for prostitution, where the prostitute masturbates a man and brings him to what is often termed a 'happy ending.'

Bar or Casino Workers

A final category of prostitution involves prostitutes who work in bars, casinos, or similar establishments (bar or casino workers). They make contact with a customer in these settings and then have sex with them elsewhere.

Theoretical Perspective

Functionalism

Prostitution is functional for several parties in society. It provides prostitutes a source of income, and it provides a sexual alternative for men who lack a sexual partner or are dissatisfied with their current sexual partner. According to Kingsley Davis, prostitution also helps keep the divorce rate lower than it would be if prostitution did not exist.

Conflict theory prostitution arises from women's poverty in a patriarchal society. It also reflects the continuing cultural treatment of women as sex objects who exist for men's pleasure.

Symbolic Interactionism

Prostitutes and their customers have various understandings of their behavior that help them justify why they engage in this behavior. Many prostitutes believe they are performing an important service for their customers, and this belief is perhaps more common among indoor prostitutes than among street prostitutes.

Impact of Prostitution

Personal Disorganization

Prostitutes are almost social outcast. Though men use them in order to satisfy their lust they are otherwise looked down upon and condemned. The prostitute losses all their self-respect and acts merely as a machine. They lack normal emotions and moral value.

Family Disorganization

The person habitually visit to a prostitute loses interest in his own family. Harmonious relationship with his family affected. Husband wife relationship scattered. If the father behavior is known to the children he loses esteem in their eyes too. Similarly the family life of the women also affected. If a married women entered also to prostitution by the permission of her husband then also tensions and conflicts can be unavoidable.

Economic Problem

The man who goes to a prostitute regularly loses a lot of money in this manner.

Health Hazards

Both the prostitution and customer are at a risk of Sexually transmitted diseases including HIV AIDS.

Moral Degradation

Prostitution defines their results in moral degradation of the entire society.

Degradation of Women

With increasing trend of prostitution women are losing respect in the society. Women are more and more looked upon as sex symbols. The unhealthy environment in which the prostitute are living are demoralizing.

Community Disorganization

The prostitute community will may have different types of STI or STDs which is created in sanitary condition in the community. The general people will hate that community and may be isolate that.

Children Born to Prostitute

The children born to prostitute are called offspring of unwanted mother. Generally they are not accepted in society. Such type of children in later life turn to antisocial works.

Prevention and Control of Prostitution

The measures against this can be grouped under four heading:

1. Preventive
2. Prohibitory
3. Prophylaxis
4. Legislation

Preventive

- Facilitate vocational or moral training to lower socioeconomic groups
- More job facility and vocational training
- Rescue home, shelter home or other facility should be provided to the poor and destitute women
- Male should be taught to respect women folk not explore them sexually
- Unhealthy social custom 'devdasi' should abolish completely
- Social education propaganda are important measure
- Pornographic literature or obscene film should be completely banned.

Prohibitory

- Medical examination of all prostitute.
- Segregate the infected person.

- Medical personnel dealing with them should be especially trained sympathetic, efficient and free care should be provided.
- Many brothels are situated near the market place or industrial area. In such cases no prostitute should allowed in or near the residence of men or educational institutions.
- The term brothel should be adequately defined in order to facilitate the enforcement of law.

Prophylaxis

The prophylactic measure include prevention of communicable diseases and improvement of hygienic condition. It can be possible by using condom, isolation of infected person and sex education in the brothel.

Legislation

According to law, prostitution is legal where both parties to the acts are adult and no fraud or force has been used, but a number of related activities, including soliciting in a public place, kerb crawling, owning or managing a brothel, prostitution in a hotel, pimping and pandering, are crimes. Prostitution is legal only if carried out in the private residence of a prostitute or others. The Immoral Trafficking Prevention Act, 1956 can help in preventing prostitution.

The Immoral Trafficking Prevention Act, 1956 ('ITPA')

The main statute dealing with sex work in India, does not criminalize prostitution or prostitutes per se, but mostly punishes acts by third parties facilitating prostitution like brothel keeping, living off earnings and procuring, even where sex work is not coerced.

Section 3: Punishment for Keeping a Brothel or Allowing Premises to be Used as a Brothel

Any person who keeps or manages, or acts or assists in the keeping or management of a brothel, shall be punishable on first conviction with rigorous imprisonment for a term of not less than one year and not more than three years and also with fine which may extend to two thousand rupees and in the event of a second or subsequent to conviction with rigorous imprisonment for a term of not less than two years and not more than five years and also with fine which may extend to two thousand rupees.

- **Any person who:**
  - Being the tenant, lessee, occupier or person in charge of any premises, uses, or knowingly allows any other person to use, such premises or any part thereof as a brothel, or
  - Being the owner, lessor or landlord of any premises or the agent of such owner, lessor or landlord, lets the same or any part thereof with the knowledge that the same or any part thereof is intended to be used as a brothel, or is willfully a party to the use of such premises or any part thereof as a brothel, shall be punishable on first conviction with imprisonment for a term which may extend to two years and with fine which may extend to two thousand rupees and in the event of a second or subsequent conviction, with rigorous imprisonment for a term which may extend to five years and also with fine.

Section 5: Procuring, Inducing or Taking Person for the Sake of Prostitution

- **Any person who:**
  - Procures or attempts to procure a person whether with or without his/her consent, for the purpose of prostitution; or
  - Induces a person to go from any place, with the intent that he/she may for the purpose of prostitution become the inmate of, or frequent, a brothel; or
  - Takes or attempts to take a person or causes a person to be taken, from one place to another with a view to his/her carrying on, or being brought up to carry on prostitution; or
  - Causes or induces a person to carry on prostitution; shall be punishable on conviction with rigorous imprisonment for a term of not less than three years and not more than seven years and also with fine which may extend to two thousand rupees, and if any offence under this subsection is committed against the will of any person, the punishment of imprisonment for a term of seven years shall extend to imprisonment for a term of fourteen years:

Provided that if the person in respect of whom an offence committed under this subsection:

- Is a child, the punishment provided under this subsection shall extend to rigorous imprisonment for a term of not less than seven years but may extend to life; and
- Is a minor; the punishment provided under this subsection shall extend to rigorous imprisonment for a term of not less than seven years and not more than fourteen years.

So it can be seen that both the sections namely section 3 and section 5 punishes only the acts of the 3rd party and same does the other sections in the Act and so new legislation shall be passed as to punish the client who are visiting the prostitutes.

Substance Abuse

Substance abuse refers to the harmful or hazardous use of psychoactive substances, including alcohol and illicit drugs. Psychoactive substance use can lead to dependence syndrome—a cluster of behavioral, cognitive, and physiological phenomena that develop after repeated substance use and that typically include a strong desire to take the drug, difficulties in controlling its use, persisting in its use despite harmful consequences, a higher priority given to drug use than to other activities and obligations, increased tolerance, and sometimes a physical withdrawal state. Drug abuse is also inextricably linked with adverse effects such as infectious diseases, crime, accidents, and teenage pregnancies. Approximately half of those suffering from a chronic alcohol or drug disorder also suffer from a chronic psychiatric disorder.

Definition

Substance abuse can be defined as using a drug in a way that it is inconsistent with medical or social norms and despite negative consequences.

Using of substances for pleasure is increasing day by day in the modern society, as a mark of fashion.

The chronic usage of addictive substances creates chronic physical and psychological problems among individuals and also has an impact on society.

Causes of Substance Abuse

- Biological causes
- Psychological causes
- Social causes

Biological Causes

- Family history of substance abuse
- Personality disorders
- Comorbid medical disorders
- Re-enforcing effects of drugs
- Withdrawal effects and craving
- Biochemical factors.

Psychological Causes

- Curiosity
- Poor impulse control
- Low self-esteem
- Poor stress management skills
- Childhood trauma
- Psychological distress
- Reaction to neglect

Social Causes

- Peer group pressure
- Modeling
- Easy availability of alcohol and drugs
- Familial conflicts
- Religious reasons
- Unemployment
- Poor social support

Consequences of substance abuse: Substance abuse leads to disturb marriage/relationships, home/family life, poor performances in education and also leads to confusion, mental tension, shoplifting, violence, stealing and trafficking, etc. The health effects of substances abuse are unsafe sex, sex in exchange of substances, unwanted pregnancy, depression and other psychiatric diseases, comorbid illnesses, self-injurious behavior and suicidal ideation and suicide.

Commonly used Substances

- Alcohol
- Opioids
- Cannabinoids
- Cocaine
- Amphetamine
- Hallucinogens
- Barbiturates
- Inhalants
- Nicotine
- Other stimulants.

Control of Substance Abuse

Primary Prevention

- Provision of happy and healthy family life
- Establishment of healthy parent-child relationship
- Provision of love and care to the children
- Show interest towards the child's activities
- Offer counseling to the teenagers
- Reduce the availability of drugs
- Legislation.

Secondary Prevention

- Closely monitor the changes in the behavior of an individual.
- Early detection and treatment of addicts.
- Establishment of de-addiction centers, after care centers and day care centers.
- Proper treatment and specific therapies should be given to prevent complication of disease.

Tertiary Prevention

- Provision of treatment in the state of severe dependence.
- Provision of rehabilitation measures for the drug addicts.
- Involvement of family in the restorative and rehabilitative activities.
- Involvement of social agencies for the rehabilitation.

Women Abuse

Definition

Women abuse is define as any act of gender based violence that result in, as is likely to result in physical, sexual as psychological harm, as suffering to a women, whether occurrence in public or private life. **—Gomez, 1996**

Forms of Women Abuse

Physical Abuse

Physical abuse is the intentional infliction of pain or injury by:

- Slapping, shoving, punching, strangling, kicking, burning, stabbing and/or shooting
- 'Caring' in an abusive way including giving too much medication, keeping confined, neglecting or withholding care
- Using a weapon or other objects to threaten, hurt or kill
- Sleep deprivation—waking a woman with relentless verbal abuse
- Poisoning.

Sexual Abuse

Sexual abuse is any form of forced sexual activity, including unwanted sexual touching, sexual relations without voluntary consent and the forcing or coercing of degrading, humiliating or painful sexual acts, including:

- Rape
- Forcing a woman to watch or take part in pornography
- Forcing a woman to watch partner engage in sexual acts with others
- Being compared to other lovers
- Ridiculing sexual performance or sexual organs
- Using weapons or other objects to penetrate
- Touching or acting in any way that a woman does not want
- Forcing or pressuring a woman into sexual acts
- Forcing a woman into prostitution
- Preventing a woman from receiving information or education about sexuality
- Forcing a woman to become pregnant, have an abortion or have an operation to prevent pregnancy
- Infecting a woman with HIV or other sexually transmitted diseases (STDs).

Psychological/Emotional Abuse

Psychological or emotional abuse is the use of systematic tactics and behavior intended to control, humiliate, intimidate, instill fear, or diminish a person's sense of self-worth, including:

- Verbal aggression
- Forcing a woman to do degrading things (e.g., eating cigarette butts or licking the floor)
- Forcibly confining a woman against her will
- Stalking or harassing
- Threatening to harm or kill children, other family members, pets or prized possessions
- Threatening to remove, hide or prevent access to children
- Threatening to commit suicide
- Controlling a woman's time, actions, dress, hairstyle, etc.
- Preventing a woman from seeing a dentist or doctor
- Not respecting a woman's privacy
- Denying affection or personal care
- Belittling a woman through name-calling or descriptions such as 'stupid,' 'crazy' or 'irrational'
- Accusing a woman of cheating or being promiscuous
- Leaving a woman without transportation or any means of communication, especially in isolated or rural communities
- Attacking a woman's self-esteem in other ways.

Social Abuse

- Putting her down or ignoring her in public
- Not letting the woman see her friends or family, making a scene, being charming with others and aggressive with her
- Embarrassing the woman in front of her children, using children as a weapon, not taking responsibility for children
- Placing limits on a woman about the people with whom she can talk on the phone or visit
- Cutting a woman off from friends and family
- Forcing a woman to be part of illegal/criminal acts (e.g., welfare fraud, drug operations, etc.)

Stalking/Harassment

Stalking includes repetitive harassing or threatening behavior done in a way that creates physical or emotional fear or apprehension in the person being stalked. A stalker may be trying to get his partner back or may wish to harm her as punishment for her departure. Regardless of the form, the victim fears for her safety or even her life.

Stalking includes:

- Harassing her at work
- Repeated phone calls, sometimes with hang-ups
- Following, tracking (possibly even with a global positioning device)
- Finding her through public records, online searching, or paid investigators
- Watching with hidden cameras
- Suddenly showing up where she is, at home, school, work, in the grocery store, at a movie, or in a restaurant
- Sending emails, communicating in chat rooms, or with instant messaging
- Sending unwanted packages, flowers, cards, gifts, or letters
- Monitoring her phone calls or computer use
- Contacting her friends, family, coworkers, or neighbors to find out about her
- Going through her garbage
- Threatening to hurt her or her family, friends or pets
- Damaging her home, car or property
- Using the children as an excuse to repeatedly contact the woman or to show up where she and the children are (at the children's school or day care, at their extracurricular activities)
- Engaging in legal bullying during family court proceedings.

Legal Bullying

Legal bullying is a very common kind of separation violence since this is one of the few remaining ways he can attempt to control and harass her. Legal bullying includes dragging out support and custody proceedings, refusing to pay support or alimony, withholding assets, and fighting for custody solely to maintain control over the woman. The abuser may:

Economic Abuse

Economic abuse includes any act or behavior that maintains control of financial resources or maintains a woman's financial dependence. It can include the following:

- Withholding money for basic necessities (e.g., food, clothing, diapers, medication, transportation, etc.) or for emergencies
- Forcing her to pay a disproportionate share of household expenses
- Preventing a woman from getting to work, controlling where she works, not allowing a woman to work, forcing her to work
- Spending or mismanaging family income, including a woman's earned income and/or savings, and leaving her and the children with little or no money

- Controlling a woman's spending, including where purchases are made, what is purchased, etc., and forcing her to account for and justify all spending
- Using credit cards without her permission and destroying her credit rating
- Obtaining credit or incurring bills in her name without her knowledge or consent
- Forcing her to turn over benefit payments or entitlements
- Denying access to education/training opportunities (e.g., upgrading, ESL) that may lead to increased earnings or employment
- Threatening to make false allegations about fraud to Ontario Works.

Spiritual Abuse

The use of a belief system to control, degrade or punish a woman. Spiritual abuse may include:

- Using religion to control a woman's behavior
- Punishing or ridiculing a woman for her religious beliefs
- Preventing a woman from practicing her religious beliefs
- Forcing a woman to practice certain beliefs and engage in rituals
- Putting down or attacking her spiritual beliefs
- Preventing a woman from going to church, synagogue, temple or other religious institution of her choice
- Forcing a woman to join and/or stay in a cult.

Prevention of Women Abuse

Violence against women and girls is rooted in gender-based discrimination and social norms and gender stereotypes that perpetuate such violence. Given the devastating effect violence has on women, efforts have mainly focused on responses and services for survivors. However, the best way to end violence against women and girls is to prevent it from happening in the first place by addressing its root and structural causes. Prevention should start early in life, by educating and working with young boys and girls promoting respectful relationships and gender equality. Giving importance on woman empowerment can helps in prevention and control of women abuse.

Domestic Violence Act

The Protection of Women from Domestic Violence Act 2005 is an Act of the Parliament of India enacted to protect women from domestic violence. It was brought into force by the Indian government from 26 October 2006. The Act provides for the first time in Indian law a definition of 'domestic violence', with this definition being broad and including not only physical violence, but also other forms of violence such as emotional/verbal, sexual, and economic abuse. It is a civil law meant primarily for protection orders and not meant to penalize criminally. The act does not extend to Jammu and Kashmir, which has its own laws, and which enacted in 2010 the Jammu and Kashmir.

Women Empowerment

Over the past decade, gender equality and women's empowerment have been explicitly recognized as key, not only to health of Nations, but also to social and economic development. India's National Population Policy 2000 has 'empowering women for health and nutrition' as one of its crosscutting strategic themes. Additionally, the promotion of gender equality and empowering of women is one of the Millennium Development Goal (MDG) to which India is a signatory. MDG recognizes that gender equality and women empowerment are two sides of the same coin.

Definition

Empowerment: Development must be by people, not only for them. People must participate fully in the decisions and processes that shape their lives. Investing in women's capabilities and empowering them to exercise their choices is not only valuable in itself but is also the surest way to contribute to economic growth and overall development.

Women empowerment means strengthening the capacity of women in order to identify, understand and control their lives. Women due to lack of control have little to say in decisions, so they need to be empowered to achieve control and to participate in decision making related to their health matters.

According to Arrow (1995) women empowerment is the process by which women strengthens their capacity individually and collectively to identify, understand and overcome gender discrimination, thus taking control of their lives.

Women empowerment can be achieved by changing policy and programs of actions and directing these policies and programs that will improve women's access to secure livelihood and economic resources, alleviating their extreme responsibility with regard to house work, remove legal impediments to their participation in public life and raising social awareness through effective programs of education and mass communication. Even improving the status of women also enhances the decision making capacity at all levels in all spheres of life.

The women need to be developed socially, educationally and economically in order to achieve empowerment among them.

Social Development

Social of women development of women means raising the status of women in society. Women in male dominating society, i.e., patriarchal form of society do not get the same status as men especially in decision making. As a result, they are facing threats to their lives, health and well-being.

Social legislation has brought a change by developing the women socially. Nowadays, if women compared with the women of earlier ages, they are having more privileges. This is due to certain social legislations.

- In 1950, New constitutions of India accorded equal rights to women. All women now enjoy political equal rights with men. They have the right to vote and have right to hold public offices.
- In 1955, Hindu marriage Act and Divorce Act have removed several disabilities. No Hindu can marry second time unless wife or husband is dead or divorced.

- In 1976, the equal remuneration Act, 1976 provide for equal payment of remuneration to men and women workers.
- In 1978, the child marriage restraint amendment Act, has raised the marriage of girls from 15 to 18 years of for boys 18 to 21 years.

All the legislative measures help in bringing awareness among women and removing social prejudices and inequalities; thereby bringing social development.

Educational Development

Women need to be educationally developed. It has been seen that women receive less formal education than men and at the same time, women's knowledge, abilities and coping mechanisms often go unrecognized. Education will help them in creating awareness regarding demerits and merits of large and small family size as well as other aspects of health. If she is educated, then she can educate the whole family and can care the family adopting appropriate measures.

Lack of education has been an obstacle in the development of women. So there is need to take all special efforts to raise the literacy rate among women and girl's education. Government is making the efforts to raise the educational level of women. The Central Government is providing financial assistance under the plan schemes to establish schools and colleges exclusively for girls in backward states. Special programs have been started for improving girl's education level. Other incentives are also provided such as clothing, free tuition.

Eliminating gender differences in access to education and educational attainment are key elements on the path to attaining gender equality and reducing the disempowerment of women.

The grants are provided by central social welfare board to voluntary organization to conduct courses of two or three years duration for having education. In order to achieve increased literacy rate, there is need to bring changes in policies and programs.

Economic Development

Educational development and social development will bring a change in economic condition of the women. Women can be empowered economically by:

Implementing Income Generating Schemes

By these schemes rural and poor women come together and develop an understanding of their problems and fulfill their need. Under these schemes:

- Technical information is imparted and strategies to plan action towards development and against injustice.
  - Vocational courses for women
  - Opening of women polytechnics
  - Rehabilitation of women by providing vocational training cum employment and residential care to old widows, deserted women.
- To raise the economic level of women, women's development corporation are playing an important role in providing employment opportunities to women so it is essential for the sustainable development of community that the women should be empowered and developed socially, educationally, politically and economically. Experience shows that population and development programs are effective if overall development occurs in women.
- In 2000, the Government of India adopted a national policy for the empowerment of women. This was to bring about gender justice. National Health Policy was under consideration in 2005 for implementation and it to be reviewed twice a year. The aims of the policy are:
  - Women equality in power sharing and active participation in decision making.
  - Comprehensive economic and social empowerment of women.
  - The advancement, development and empowerment of women in all spheres of life.
  - Strengthening and formation of relevant institutional mechanisms.
  - Partnership with community based programs.
  - Implementation of international obligations and co-operation at international, regional and subregional levels.
  - More responsive judicial legal systems that are sensitive to woman's need.
- To review laws and legislation related to women, a task force for women headed by deputy chairperson of planning commission has been constituted. The laws related to divorce, marriage and succession were amended to empower the women. National Commission on women has formulated a code of conduct for preventing sexual harassment at place of work. Tenth five year plan (2002–2007) is concerned towards promotion of gender equality and empowering women which include three strategies of empowering women. These are social empowerment, economic empowerment and gender injustice.

Programs and Schemes for Women Empowerment

The ministry of women and child development launched different schemes for over all empowerment of girls and women. They are listed as follows:

- Beti Bachao Beti Padhao Scheme
- One Stop Center Scheme
- Women Helpline Scheme
- UJJAWALA which is a comprehensive scheme for prevention of trafficking and rescue, rehabilitation and reintegration of victims of trafficking and commercial sexual exploitation
- Working Women Hostel
- Rajiv Gandhi National Creche Scheme for the children of working mothers
- SWADHAR Greh (A scheme for women in difficult circumstances)

- Revision under IGMSY in accordance with national Food Security Act, 2013 in12th Plan
- Support to Training and Employment Programme for Women (STEP)
- Nari Shakti Puraskar
- Rajya Mahila Samman and Zila Mahila Samman awards
- Indira Gandhi Matritva Sahyog Yojana (IGMSY)—A conditional maternity benefit scheme
- Release of 2nd installment of grant for 2015—2016 for all the States under IGMSY.

CONCEPT OF PUBLIC HEALTH

The CDC Foundation defines public health as "the science of protecting and improving the health of people and their communities." Public health professionals work to prevent the spread of illness in a particular population, which can be as small as a single neighborhood or as large as an entire country. Their work is largely preventive, as they take steps to ensure that a population has clean food and water, and design informational campaigns to teach the public about health and wellness.

However, preventive action is not all that public health professionals do. They also work to understand the spread of disease in certain populations, particularly after a health-related outbreak. By studying the patterns of various diseases and how they can affect a population, public health professionals provide vital information to key decision-makers, both in the healthcare sphere and in government. In this way, public health plays a vital role in making sure that a population is as healthy as possible.

The public health nurse's scope of practice includes policy reform, system-level changes, and health promotion. This nursing practice includes advocacy, policy development, and planning. Dr Gayol adds, "It is the balance where health professionals work toward health promotion and illness prevention with a focus on identifying the origins of disease then determining how policy, education, and health systems can work together toward improved health outcomes."

For example, if an illness outbreak such as measles, tuberculosis, or hepatitis B occurs, the public health nurse will evaluate the need and develop a program for an immunization clinic.

Public health nurses often work for the government—usually county though can be state or federal. They work in health departments, correctional facilities, worksites, and other locations where population-specific nursing care is in need. For example, they monitor for trends in disease outbreak and prevention, run flu clinics, and work to reduce illnesses like heart disease by providing education to their town.

Community Health Nurse

Community health nurses maximize the health status of individuals, families, groups, and the community through direct approach with them. A community health nurse combines facets of direct care and public health practice to a target population of patients who may not have access to—or be able to afford—health services. The community health nurse's scope of practice includes educating and developing intervention plans for individuals, families, or groups about illness and disease prevention, safe health practices, nutrition, and wellness, among other topics. For example, a community health nurse might meet with young mothers to provide valuable immunization information or teach a new diabetic how to give insulin injections by practicing with an orange.

Community health nurses work within the community. This can be for a public entity such as a school district or community clinic. The types of communities these nurses serve will vary; economic situation, school, and culture all play a part in dictating community needs. "What may be a health issue in downtown Atlanta, GA may not be a health issue in rural Tennessee—therefore community health is specific to a location, as well," says Dr Gayol.

Difference between Public Health and Community Health (Table 1.2)

Public health is "the science and art of preventing disease, prolonging life and promoting health through the organized efforts and informed choices of society, organizations, public and private, communities and individuals". It is concerned with threats to health based on population health analysis. Public health incorporates the interdisciplinary approaches of epidemiology, biostatistics and health services, environmental health, community health, behavioral health, health economics, public policy, insurance medicine and occupational health (respectively occupational medicine) are other important subfields. Community health is a discipline concerned with the study and improvement of the health characteristics of different communities. Community health tends to focus on geographical areas, and includes primary, secondary and tertiary healthcare. Because public health and community health share the same ultimate goal, some of their efforts are similar. For example, professionals in both fields may be involved in developing health education programs or health plans.

Historical Development of Public Health in India

Ancient India (3000 BC): Ancient India was among the pioneer countries where knowledge of public health existed. As early as 3000 BC Indus Valley Civilization showed practice of public health. The relics excavated at the site of two cities Mohenjodaro and Harappa showed water supply, public baths and drainage system. It was also found that these cities were built with adequate planning.

Vedic period (1400 BC–600 BC): People during Vedic period were conscious of health and hygiene. The book Manu Samhita written during this period. This book prescribed rules for personal hygiene, diet and rituals to be followed during birth and death. Susruta, who is considered as the father of surgery in India lived during this period.

Table 1.2: Difference between public health and community health.

Aspects	*Public health*	*Community health*
Focuses	Public health focuses on the scientific process of preventing infectious diseases	Community health focuses more on the overall contributors to a population's physical and mental health
Tend to work	In the United States, most public health initiatives fall under the jurisdiction of federal departments of public health, such as the CDC or the Food and Drug Administration. Many public health professionals work in offices and laboratories with local or state health departments, hospitals, and colleges and universities	The community health professionals often work on a more localized scale, from state and county jobs to local hospitals (though some community health professionals also work at the CDC)
Careers	Those interested in public health's scientific aspects can pursue jobs such as: • Epidemiologist • Public health engineer • Biostatistician Those more interested in policy development and legislation can pursue careers such as: • Medical writer • Health promotion program coordinator • Hospital administrator	Students interested in community health also have numerous options and can work for various health-related organizations following graduation. • Health coach (a mentor who helps promote wellness and healthy living, either as a private business or through a healthcare facility) • Community health worker (a professional who works to improve population health—particularly those who've been historically underrepresented—through outreach, education and community advocacy) • Healthcare analyst (a professional who evaluates medical data to better understand and improve local hospitals and other healthcare centers)
Scope of practice	Policy reform, system-level changes, and health promotion. This nursing practice includes advocacy, policy development, and planning	The community health nurse's scope of practice includes educating and developing intervention plans for individuals, families, or groups about illness and disease prevention, safe health practices, nutrition, and wellness, provide preventive care, immunizations, treat urgent illnesses, education, and medication refills
Work area	They work in health departments, correctional facilities, worksites, and other locations where population-specific nursing care is in need	Community health nurses work within the community. This can be for a public entity such as a school district or community clinic, community health centers. The types of communities these nurses serve will vary; economic situation, school, and culture all play a part in dictating community needs

600 BC–600 AD: During this period there were two famous universities namely Nalanda and Taxila, which started systematic medical education. Buddhism became popular during this period and these universities came out of Buddhist religious movement.

Ayurvedic system of medicine which originated in India, was widely accepted during this period. Charak, who has been considered as the father of Indian medicine, also practiced during this period.

268 BCE–232 BCE: King Ashok ruled, during which period, prevention of disease was given importance and hygienic practices were adopted. Cleanliness of body considered as a religious duty. Doctors and midwives were to be trustworthy and skillful. Lying in room for delivery was kept clean and it was well ventilated.

Mughal period (1650–1857 AD): The Mughal emphasis on physical fitness and encouragement of out-of-door mainly games for maintaining their general standard of health. Though the medical services were inadequate for the people, still the local physicians were able to deal with normal problems. Public hospitals had been provided in Muslim India, at least since the days of Firuz Tughluq (1351–1388). As early as 1616 they knew the important characteristics of the bubonic plague and suggested suitable preventive measures. A crude form of vaccination against smallpox seems to have been employed by Eastern doctors, for it was vaguely realized that the introduction of a mild form of cowpox prevented the virulent form of smallpox. In this period the use of medicines had been well developed among the Hindus, but dissection was considered to be irreligious. The Muslims, who did not have this restriction, performed a number of operations. With the invasion of Mughals, Unani system of medicine, which originated in Arab countries, also came to India.

During British Rule (1757–1947): Concern for public health was established in India with commencement of British rule. British soldiers stationed in India, died in large numbers due to unhygienic conditions and contagious diseases prevailing at that time. So the British Government felt concerned about the poor condition of public health in the country.

1825 – Quarantine Act was promulgated.

1839 – A Royal Commission was appointed to investigate the causes of death of British Soldiers in India. Florence Nightingale who had experience in Military Barracks of Scutari and recommended corrective measures for improvement of sanitary conditions in India. The Royal Commission recommended supply of safe drinking water, construction of proper drainage system and prevention of epidemics among the civil population where British soldiers are stationed.

1864 - Sanitary Commissioners were appointed in Mumbai, Madras, and Bengal. At the same time many actions were initiated and public health acts were passed to improve the existing condition of health in India. Some of these are:

1869 - Public Health Commissioner and a Statistical Officer were appointed with the Government of India.

1873 - Birth and Registration Act. The different phases of public health

1880 - 1920 Disease Control Phase

1880 - Vaccination Act was passed.

1881 - First Indian factories act was passed and first All India Census was taken.

1885 - Local self government act was passed.

1886 - The idea of training females for maternity care came. Missionaries felt the need of training the Dais who assisted in the delivery of mothers at home.

1888 - Government of India directed that local bodies should be responsible to look after the sanitation but no local public health staff was appointed to carry out that task.

1891 - First All India Census

1896 - Government of India awoke to improve the public health of India, subsequent to an outbreak of plague. The Plague Commission was appointed.

1897 - The Epidemic Disease Act was promulgated.

1904 - Plague Commission recommended in its report that:
- Public Health Departments should be reorganized and expanded
- There should be laboratory facilities established for purposes of research and production of Sera and Vaccine.

1907 - Central Malaria Bureau at Kasavli was established.

1911 - Indian Research Fund Association was established for the purpose of research.

1917 - Government of India sanctioned the appointment of Deputy Sanitary Commissioners and Health Officers. Also grants were sanctioned to local bodies.

1918 - Lady Reading Health School in Delhi was established. The Nutrition Research Laboratory at Coonoor was established.

1919 - The Public Health sanitation and vital statistics responsibilities were transferred to provinces under the control of an elected minister. This is the first step taken in decentralizing the health administration of India.

Health Promotional Phase (1920–1960)

1920 - In several provinces, Municipality and Local Boards Act were passed.

1921 - The act providing legislation for the advancement of public health was passed. First confined their efforts to control of small pox, cholera and plague. Priority was given to small pox vaccination.

1924 - A subsidized rural practitioner scheme was introduced.

1926 - Madras Nursing Council was the first one to pass the act to train nurses in midwifery to replace the dais in 1926 - Missionaries established the Lady Reading Health School for training the health visitors to carry out public health nursing along with midwifery care. Then few other states also established schools for health visitors.

1930 - At Kolkata, an All India Institute of Hygiene and Public Health was established with aid from the Rockefeller Foundation.

1931 - A Maternal and Child Welfare Bureau was established by Indian Red Cross Society.

1935 - The health activities in the country were grouped as under the control of Central or Central-cum-provincial or Provincial government.

1937 - A Central Advisory Board of Health was setup. The public health commissioner was the secretary and states were members to coordinate the public health activities in the country.

1939 - Madras Public Health Act was passed. Indian Tuberculosis Association was established.

1940 - The Drug Act was passed and for the first time were brought under control.

1943 - In October 1943, Bhore Committee was appointed by the Government of India to make survey of the existing health conditions and to formulate a comprehensive plan for administration.

1946 - Bhore Committees' report was submitted and recommended the establishment of health centers for providing integrated curative and preventive services. Recommended the posts of PHN in PHC. So two colleges of Nursing at Vellore and New Delhi were established to train graduate nurses undergoing an integrated course of theory and practice of public health nursing along with GNM.

One of the main objectives of preparing BSc Nurses was to prepare PHN to function with a high level of efficiency in the community health setup. But due to shortage of teachers in newly opened schools of nursing, most of the BSc Nurses were absorbed as teachers.

Post Independence Era

1947 - India established the concept of Welfare State at the time of independence. The National Government took up the responsibility of improving the health of people by covering all aspect of community, i.e., administration, training, expansion of health services, research.

1948 - India joined as a member state of World Health Organization. Employees State Insurance Act was passed. Report of environment hygiene committee was published.

1950 - The Constitution of India came into force in 1950. The Planning Commission was setup by the Government of India, which immediately drafted the first five year plan.

1951 - Beginning of First Five Year Plan. BCG vaccination programme was launched. Central Drug Research Institute launched at Pune.

1952 - Constitution of Central Council Health. Primary Health Centers setup. To train the GNM Nurses as Public Health Nurse, however, a diploma course of one academic year was introduced and started at College of Nursing, New Delhi. The training was transferred to All India Institute of Hygiene and Public Health, Kolkata, Lady Reading Health School in Delhi, LHV training was also started. GNM Nurses were given theory and practical training in public health to become PHN.

1953 - National Malaria Control Programme was initiated. Nationwide family planning research and programme committee was setup.

1954 - Contributed health services scheme was initiated in Delhi. Central social welfare board was setup.
- National water supply and sanitation scheme was inaugurated
- National Leprosy Control programme was started
- VDRL antigen production was setup in Kolkata
- Food Adulteration Act was passed by Parliament.

1955 - National Filaria Control Programme was started. Central Leprosy Training and Research Center was established at Chengalpattu in Tamil Nadu. National Tuberculosis survey commenced.

1956 - Second Five Year Plan begun. Central Health Education bureau was established. Director for family planning was appointed at the Union Ministry of Health. Chemotherapy center at Madras was started.

1958 - National Malaria Control Programme was changed to National Malaria Eradication Programme. National Tuberculosis survey was completed.

1959 - Mudaliar Committee was appointed to review the progress made in health since the Bhore Committee recommendation. The National Tuberculosis Institute at Bengaluru was established. The Nutrition Research Laboratories at Coonoor was shifted to Hyderabad.

Social Engineering Phase (1960–1980)

1960 - Mudaliar Committee report was published and recommended. Training of auxiliary nurse midwives should be continued and extended to have a second line of trained personnel to meet the needs of the country and one auxiliary nurse will be for 500 population by the end of 15 years. There should be a public health nurse with a basic nursing qualification and one year training in domiciliary care and other public health aspects of community work.
Male nurses should be trained only for certain types of work, i.e., mental hospital, army hospital, etc.

1962 - The central family planning institute was established. National Smallpox Eradication Programme, National Goiter Control Programme, National School Health Programme and District Tuberculosis Programme Were Established.

1963 - Applied Nutrition Programme started by Government of India and WHO. National Institute for Communicable Disease was established in Delhi. The Chadha committee was established a norm of one Basic Health Worker for every ten thousand people. A drinking water board was setup.

1964 - National Institute for Health Administration and Education was established in Delhi.

1965 - IUCD was introduced. Direct BCG vaccination programme without tuberculin test was introduced.

1966 - Minister for Family Planning was appointed under Ministry of Health. A separate department of Family Planning was constituted to coordinate family planning programme at central and state.

1968 - Medical Education Committee was appointed by Government of India.

1970 - All India Hospital Family Planning Programme was started. Birth and death registration act came into force.

1971 - Medical Termination of Pregnancy bill was passed by Parliament.

1972 - Medical Termination of Pregnancy bill was came into force. National Institute of Nutrition was setup at Hyderabad.

1973 - Government plans to setup 30 bedded rural hospital one for every four primary health centers.
A new cader of health workers called multipurpose health workers was formed on the basis of the recommendation of Kartar Singh Committee report who will eventually replace auxiliary nurse midwives, family planning workers and basic health workers.

1974 - The fifth five year plan came into operation. It was the year of world population by the United Nations. The term community health is replaced in place of public health.

1975 - India was declared as smallpox free in July. Integrated Child Development Scheme was launched in India. National Children's Welfare Board was setup.

1976 - A three tier plan of healthcare delivery system to rural areas was proposed by Central Council of Health. National Programme for Prevention of Blindness was formulated. The Prevention of Food Adulteration Act of 1975 was amended and passed.

1977 - International Commission declared that India has eradicated smallpox. National Institute of Health and Family Planning was formed. Community Health Workers Scheme was begun by the Union Ministry of Health.

1978 - The slogan Health for All by 2000 AD came into light by the International Conference on Primary Health Care in Alma-Ata Declaration in USSR.

1979 - The year, was observed a The Year of Child all over the world.

1980 - Small pox was officially declared eradicated worldwide by WHO.

Health for All Phase (1981–2000 AD)

1981 - The 1981 census was taken up. India is committed to the goal of providing safe drinking water and adequate sanitation for all by the year 1990. Emergence of AIDS as a life-threatening infection. First recognized in United States of America. AIDS had already appeared in several areas of the world by late seventies posing a serious international health problem of extraordinary urgency.

1982 - The new 20-point programme was announced. The Government of India announced its National Health Policy. WHO experts committee meeting organized in Geneva on the training of nurse teachers and managers with special regard to primary health care.

1983 - Common Wealth Nurses Federation South Asian Seminar on the Role of Nurse in the Delivery of Primary Health Care Programme was conducted in the college of Nursing, Madras, Tamil Nadu from 5th to 7th December. This was organized by Trained Nurses Association of India (TNAI) and Tamil Nadu State branch was the hot. Nurses from India and other countries participated. This was the first of its kind in India. The TNAI was initiated various programmes for primary health care at National, Regional level.

1984 - Bhopal Gas Tragedy was occurred on the night of December. The ESI Amendment Bill, 1984 was passed by Parliament.

1985 - Seventh Five Year Plan was launched and universal immunization programme was launched. A separate department of women and child development was setup under Ministry of Human Resource Development. INC prescribed a Diploma in Nursing Education and Administration Course for General Nursing and Midwifery nurses with 2 years experience. This courses along with teachers training and administration course curriculum also includes training in public health to make them suitable to act as public health nurse as well as PH instructors in schools of nursing. The introduction of MPHW scheme.

1986 - The Environment Protection Act, 1986 promulgated.

1987 - The Government of India appointed a High Power Committee on Nurses and Nursing Profession to go into the working conditions of nurses, nursing education and other related matters.

1988 - New 20-Point Programme was launched. India Standards Institution was renamed as Bureau of Indian Standards. Safe motherhood programme was launched. National Diabetes Control Programme and National AIDS Control Programme was initiated.

1989 - Blood Safety Programme was launched.

1990 - Control of Acute Respiratory Infections Programme was initiated.

1992 - Eighth Five Year Plan was launched. Child Survival and Safe Motherhood Programme was launched.

1993 - Revised National TB Programme with DOTS was introduced.

1995 - ICDS was renamed as Integrated Mother and Child Development Services.

1996 - Pulse Polio Immunization was initiated.

1997 - Reproductive and child health programme was launched. Ninth five year plan was launched.

1998-99 - National Family Health survey was undertaken. National Malaria Eradication Programme was renamed as National Antimalaria Programme.

2000 - Government of India announced National Population Policy.

2002 - National Health Policy (2002) was announced. Government announced National AIDS Prevention and Control Policy.

In September 2000, Representatives from 189 countries met at the Millennium summit in New York to adopt the United Nations Millennium Declaration. The leaders made specific commitments in seven areas: peace, security, disarmament, development and poverty eradication, protecting our common environment, human rights, democracy and good governance, protecting the vulnerable, meeting the special needs of Africa and strengthening the United Nations. The Road Map established goals and targets to be reached by year 2015 in each of seven areas. The goals in the area of development and poverty eradication are known as Millennium Development Goals.

COMMUNITY DIAGNOSIS

Concept

When a person in a community is sick or ill, the people are able to find the illness and take steps to help his get well.

Similarly, can we tell when, a community is ill, the question that naturally arises whether a community can get ill. What do you mean by the health of a town or a community? In a community at any point in the same persons are ill and others are well. If many persons are ill, we say that the health of the community is poor. If many persons are well, we say that the health community is good. On the other hand in a 'healthy' community there will be ill and in 'sick' community there will be some persons who are healthy. Can anyone find out the total numbers of ill persons in a community? How does one identify any measure of health diseases? It also involves the social, economical, political living conditions and the attitude and beliefs of people on their health status. A person will be found ill when he is diagnosed by the doctor. In the same way community diagnosis will help in identifying the health status of a community.

Definition

Community diagnosis is a comprehensive assessment of the state as an entire community in relation to its social, political, economic, physical and biological environment, A process by which the nurse collects data about the community in order to identify factors which may influence the deaths and illnesses of the population, to formulate a CHN diagnosis and develop and implement CHN interventions and strategies.

The purpose of this diagnosis is to determine problems and to set priorities for planning and developing programmes of care for the community.

Purpose of Community Diagnosis

- It helps to identify community needs and problems.
- It is a prerequisite for planning, implementing and evaluation of successful community-based health and development programmes.
- It helps to decide strategies for community involvement.
- It helps to match project organizations and services with community needs.
- It can be used to help the community become conscious of its existing problems and finding solutions.

Assessing the Health Status of the Community

The process of community diagnosis is critical for the following reasons:

- It is an opportunity for the community to learn about itself.
- It is an opportunity for outsiders, such as health workers and personnel from other sectors, to learn about the community.
- It will generate information to be used for planning.

Ideally, the process of community assessment should aim to find out all information relevant to the health and all information relevant to health and well-being of entire community nor the health workers may have sufficient time available to devote to data collection. Another important reason is that the community may not at first see the need for detailed collections of information. They may feel, with justification that they know all by virtue of their day-to-day experiences. For this reason it may be a better approach to begin by asking the community, through its leaders, to describe its present circumstances in the following terms:

All of this information can usually be obtained at least roughly through conversation. It should be recorded systematically, in writing, in terms that the people can understand and constantly refer to. Any gaps should be noted for future information gathering. This initial conversation is also good means of assessing the knowledge of the leaders concerning their community, which in turn is a useful indication of their or concern with community as a whole.

Objectives of Community Diagnosis

- To find about all information relevant to the health and well-being of the community
- To identify and quantity of the health problems in a community in a term of mortality morbidity
- To evaluate health services
- The qualification of health problems can be a source of new knowledge about disease distribution, causation and prevention
- To understand about the social, cultural and environmental characteristics of the community.

Content of Community Diagnosis

A programme coordinator should know the following facts about the community:

Hard Measurable Facts

- Age
- Sex distribution
- Literacy status
- Prevalence of disease
- Land holdings
- Sanitary conditions
- Irrigation facilities
- Others

Overall organization pattern of the community within which there are several suborganizations, e.g., castes with their own values and pattern of conduct. Each suborganization is intricately interrelated to the other and to the overall community, thereby affecting its entire behavior.

The process of community diagnosis is a continuous learning experience both for the programmer and community, when considered in all its aspects community. Diagnosis a simple process that develops gradually and only requires keen perceptiveness, observations and study of the facts obtained.

Steps in Community Diagnosis

- **Defining area–who and what:** This is an area of intensive study from which it is gathered the data for community diagnosis and in which health action is most easily evaluated. The data should be gathered and health action evaluates unless it is limited and defined in this way.

- **Identifying the needs from the community perspective:** The identification of needs as perceived by the community is a useful means of assessing the priorities and values of the people. It is quite possible that directly health related needs may not feature high on a list of overall community needs in order to obtain such information, it is important that the outsiders enquires about needs do not pressurize the community, to include health needs they do not consider important.

  Numbers of approach are needed to elicit reliable data. In other cases an additional enquiry will be usually required, either as apart of a community survey on all respect of the community or as a separate enquiry.
- **Specifying priority health needs of the community:** Specifying priority health needs is a delicate process requiring a lot sensitivity on the part of the health worker who may be receipted to regard this as his particular field of expertise with the consequence danger of dictating to the people what their problems are. This must be registered at all costs and genuine community involvement is to succeed.
- **Identifying community resources for facilitating health problems:** Resources available for health care, particularly in developing countries, are limited. It follows that countries must strive to identify and then to mobilize all potential resources and ensure that they are used as effectively as possible. Community involvement in PHC makes possible the mobilization of plenty of resources, which might otherwise remain unutilized.

  The individual and collective actions of the people constitute one of the most important types of community resources for achieving better health. The people should be motivated to provide facilities such as drugs, building, equipment, money, or contributions in terms of money and materials.
- **Setting priorities for action:** The priorities may vary greatly, reflecting local judgement as far as possible. However, it must be recognized that certain national health priorities already, have been established, for example with respect to immunization and control of malaria, TB and AIDS/STD. The health consequences for the country as a whole may be such that these cannot be postponed until all communities have explicitly endorsed the national programmes. Thus, communities are likely to be faced with a number of health's initiators which are already being implemented their approval being sought. It will be important for the local health workers, to explain the existence and relevance of such initiatives, so that communities can incorporate them into their agreed priorities for action.
- **Community needs in proportion to national capacity:** Closely associated with the setting of priorities at community level is the capacity of the country as a whole to support this implementation. One striking example is the construction of a clinic or health center rather common community felt need. In almost all countries, there are insufficient resources. To finance such projects every community taking into account not only the costs of constructions but of training staff, paying their salaries and keeping them supplied with medicines and equipment. In such circumstances, where community felt needs cannot be met, it is as possible to prevent to be building up and enable them to adjust their expectations to realistic levels.
- **Mechanisms for intersectional cooperation in planning:** No sector involved in community development can work effectively in isolation. Interdependence in such those activities in one sector have an impact on the goals of another. For maximum benefit it is essential that all sectors fully appreciate their roles in overall community development and their relationships with one another. Thus, there is an essential need for effective coordination at all levels between health and all other sectors.'

  At local level the mechanism established for adequate in providing for intersectional cooperation, for example, the CD committees just like the local health worker, the school teacher, the agricultural worker, and the social worker will act as a technical adviser to the community as well as provider of logistical support where appropriate.

HEALTH FOR ALL

Definition

Health for all (HFA) has been defined as attainment or a level of health that will enable every individual to lead a socially and economically productive life. Health for all means simply the realization of WHO's objective of attainment by all people the highest possible level of health. HFA means that health is brought within reach of everyone in a given country. It enables a person to lead a socially and economically productive life. The stress is on the provision of the treatment, promotion and prevention to the people representing a shift from medical care to health care and from urban population to rural population.

HFA is thus a holistic concept calling for efforts in agriculture, industry, education, housing and communications, medicine and public health. The basis for HFA strategy is primary health care (Halfdan Mahler, 1981).

History and Evolution of HFA

In 1977, the World Health Assembly decided that the major social goal of governments and WHO should be the attainment by all people of the world by the year 2000 of a level of health that would permit them to lead a socially and economically productive life.

In 1981, the Assembly unanimously adopted the global strategy for health for all by the year 2000. This was the birth of the 'Health for All' movement.

'Health for All' does not mean an end to disease and disability, or that doctors and nurses will care for everyone. It means that resources for health are evenly distributed and that essential healthcare is accessible to everyone.

It also means that health begins at home, in schools, as well as the workplace, and that people use better approaches for preventing means that people recognize that ill health is not inevitable and that they can shape their own lives and those of their families from the avoidable burden of disease.

In 1994, WHO's member states acknowledged that significant global changes had occurred since that time, and called for a strategy renewal to meet challenges, expand opportunities, and overcome obstacles at the dawn of the 21st century.

The concept of HFA conceived and practiced in India during Vedic civilization in the cherished value of health is enshrined in an ancient Sanskrit verse **'SARVE SANTU NIRAMAYAH'** which means 'let all be free from disease.' Let all be healthy used to express good wishes. Factors led to the evolution of goal for HFA - 2000:

- Inaccessibility of and nonequitability of essential health care of life saving measures to majority of people in developing countries.
- Gross inequalities in healthcare system and distribution of health facilities.
- Failure of existing healthcare system to cope with primary healthcare problems.
- Unresolved emerging healthcare problems in developed countries.

The term primary health care was first used to mean the care given to the patient by health worker who saw him first. It was also called FIRST CONTACT CARE.

Central Theme for HFA

- Universal coverage with primary health care that is relevant effective, acceptable and affordable in terms of the need, culture interest and resources of each community.
- Community participation in the planning, provision and evaluation of health services.
- Integration between health and other health related sectors.

Global Targets for HFA

- All people in every country will have at least a ready access to essential health care and to first level of referral facility.
- All people will be actively involve in care for themselves and their families as far as come in first level of care and in community action for health.
- Countries throughout the world will share with government responsibility for health care of the members.
- All government will have assumed overall responsibility for the health of their people.
- Availability of safe drinking water and basic sanitation for all.
- Adequate nourishment for all people.
- Full coverage of children for vaccine prevented diseases.
- Communicable disease in the developing countries will be of no greater significance in the year 2000 than they are in developed countries in the year 1980.
- All possible ways will be applied to prevent and control on communicable diseases and promote mental health through influencing lifestyle and control of physical; and psychological environment.
- Provide essential drugs for all.

MILLENNIUM DEVELOPMENT GOALS

In September 2000, representatives from 189 countries met at the Millennium summit in New York to adopt the United Nations Millennium declaration. The leaders made specific commitments in seven areas; peace security and disarmament, development and poverty eradication; protecting our common environment, human rights, democracy and good governance, protecting the vulnerable; meeting the special needs of Africa and strengthening the United Nations.

Government set a date of 2015 by which they would meet the Millennium development goals. The Millennium Development Goals place health at the heart of development and represent commitments by government throughout the world to do more to reduce poverty and hunger, and to tackle ill-health, gender inequity, lack of education, access to clean water and environmental degradation.

Millennium development goals have been set by the United Nations and health has been identified as a significant area of concern. MDGs are as follows:

- **Goal 1: Eradicate Poverty and Hunger**
  - *Target-1:* Halve hunger between 1990 and 2015 the proportion of people whose income is less than one dollar a day.
  - *Target-2:* Achieve full and productive employment and decent work for all, including women and young people.
  - *Target-3:* Halve between 1990 and 2015 the proportion of people who suffer from hunger.
- **Goal-2: Universal Primary Education**
  - *Target-1:* Ensure that, by 2015 every children where boys and girls a like, will be able to complete a full course of primary schooling.
- **Goal-3: Promote Gender Equity and Empower Women**
  - *Target-1:*Eliminate gender disparity in primary and secondary education, preferably by 2005 and to all levels of education no later than 2015.
- **Goal-4: Reduction of Child Mortality**
  - *Target-1:* Reduce under five mortality by two third.
- **Goal-5: Improve Maternal Health**
  - *Target-1:* Reduce maternal mortality by three quarters.
- **Goal-6: Combat HIV/AIDS, Malaria and Other Diseases**
  - *Target-1:* Have halted by 2015 and began to reverse the spread of HIV/AIDS.
  - *Target-2:* Have halted by 2015 and begun to reverse the incidence of Malaria and other major diseases.
- **Goal-7: Ensure Environmental Sustainability**
  - *Target-1:* Integrate the principles of sustainable development into country policies and programs and reverse the loss of environmental resources.
  - *Target-2:* Reduce biodiversity loss, achieving by 2010 a significant reduction in the rate of loss.

- *Target-3:* Halve by 2015, the proportion of people without sustainable access to safe drinking water and basic sanitation.
- *Target-4:* By 2020, to have achieved a significant improvement in the lives of a least 100 million slum dwellers.

- **Goal-8: Development of a Global Partnership for Development**
  - *Target-1:* Develop further an open, rule based, predictable, nondiscriminatory trading and financial system.
  - *Target-2:* Address the special needs of the least developed countries.
  - *Target-3:* Address the special needs of the land locked countries and small island developing states.
  - *Target-4:* Deal comprehensively with the debt problems of developing countries through national and international measures in order to make debt sustainable in the long-term.
  - *Target-5:* In cooperation with the developing countries, develop and implement strategies for decent and productive work for youth.
  - *Target-6:* In cooperation with pharmaceutical companies provide access to affordable, essential drug in developing countries.
  - *Target-7:* In cooperation with the private sector make available the benefits of new technologies especially information and communication.

Societal Influences

Many factors influenced the growth of CHN. These are:

- Advanced technology shaping the practice of health care, nutrition, lifestyle transportation, job mobility, free products, equipment, computer technology and treatment for other technology.
- Progress in causal thinking. In the health science, particularly in epidemiology significantly affected the nature of CHN.
- Changes in education
- Changing role of women has profoundly affected CHN—nurse still struggle for equality.
- Consumer movement—demanding their rights in many areas.
- Economic forces.

CHN has evolved into a focus on care of individuals families and communities. The focus and orientation are different to other nurses in their work areas. CHN is a specific and specialized orientation to the care that embodies participles of public health as guiding concepts.

Primary health care is one aspect of CHN. CHN focuses on the physical, biological, social, psychological and environmental health of a population group. While primary care is a coordinated system of personal health care, emphasizing first contact care and continuously. Primary care emphasizes ambulatory care that addresses total client needs both for curative an preventive services. CHN is population based.

At the beginning of the new millennium, in 2000, world leaders gathered at the UN to shape a broad vision to fight poverty in its many dimensions, that vision was translated into 8 Millennium Development Goals (MDGs). The MDG framework has guided development work across the world for the year 2000–2015. In millennium development goals significant achievements have been made, but many people are being left behind. The gaps are gender inequality persists, big gaps exist between poorest and richest households, rural and urban areas. Climate change and environmental degradation undermine any progress achieved and poor people suffer the most. It was observed that millions of people still live in poverty and hunger, without access to basic services. The successes of the MDG agenda prove that global action can work. It is argues that global action is the only path to ensure that the new development agenda leaves no-one behind. However the new agenda should be "truly universal and transformative" as the human race, we seek a sustainable future.

The United Nations Conference on Sustainable Development - or Rio +20—took place in Rio de Janeiro, Brazil on 20–22 June 2012. It resulted in a focused political outcome document which contains clear and practical measures for implementing sustainable development. In Rio, Member States decided to launch a process to develop a set of Sustainable Development Goals (SDGs), which will build upon the Millennium Development Goals and converge with the post 2015 development agenda.

For scoping the goals all the member states of the UN were involved and the cooperation with major NGOs and civil society agencies are obtained, open forums and regional consultations around the world obtained, 4.5 million people were surveyed about the most important goals and how they might be achieved. Collaborative wish for the world to create a better and more equal place to live in and around 5 million people involved in the process.

On September 25, 2015, 193 Heads of State at the United Nations General Assembly on it's 17th anniversary setup a collection of 17 goals which are known as the Sustainable Development Goals (SDGs) or otherwise called as Global Goals. These **goals** are a collection of 17 interlinked goals designed to be a "blueprint to achieve a better and more sustainable future for all". The SDGs and their 169 targets form the core of Resolution 70/1 of the United Nations, which is a breakthrough agreement called AGENDA 2030. The SDGs are intended to be achieved by all member states by the year 2030. Though the goals are broad and interdependent, after two years on 6th July 2017 the SDGs were made more "actionable" by a United Nation Resolution adopted by the General Assembly. The resolution identifies specific targets for each goal, along with indicators that are being used to measure progress toward each target. The year by which the target is meant to be achieved is usually between 2020 and 2030. For some of the targets, no end date is given. To facilitate monitoring, a variety of tools exist to track and visualize progress towards the goals. All intend to make data more available and more easily understood. For example, the online publication SDG-Tracker, launched in June 2018, presents available data across all indicators. The goals are a universal call to action to end poverty, protect the planet and ensure all people enjoy peace and prosperity. The goals are broad, interdependent and cover social, economic and social issues and making them work is everyone's responsibility.

The 2030 Sustainable Development Goals focus on the 5 Ps

1. **People:** The wellbeing of all people
2. **Planet:** Protection of the earth's ecosystems
3. **Prosperity:** Continued economic and technological growth
4. **Peace:** Securing peace
5. **Partnership:** Improving international cooperation

These five aspects are interdependent. Therefore, the SDGs demand integrated thinking as well as integrated approaches to achieving the goals.

1. **The focus on People:**
   - End poverty in all its forms everywhere
   - End hunger, achieve food security and improved nutrition and promote sustainable agriculture
   - Ensure healthy lives and promote well-being for all at all ages
   - Ensure inclusive and equitable quality education and promote lifelong learning opportunities for all
   - Achieve gender equality and empower all women and girls
2. **The focus on the Planet and on Prosperity:**
   - Ensure availability and sustainable management of water and sanitation for all
   - Ensure access to affordable, reliable, sustainable and modern energy for all
   - Promote sustained, inclusive and sustainable economic growth, full and productive employment and decent work for all
   - Build resilient infrastructure, promote inclusive and sustainable industrialization and foster innovation
   - Reduce inequality within and among countries
   - Make cities and human settlements inclusive, safe, resilient and sustainable
   - Ensure sustainable consumption and production patterns
   - Take urgent action to combat climate change and its impacts
   - Conserve and sustainably use the oceans, seas and marine resources for sustainable development
   - Protect, restore and promote sustainable use of terrestrial ecosystems, sustainably manage forests, comat desertification, and halt and reverse land degradation and halt biodiversity loss
3. **The focus on Peace:**
   - Promote peaceful and inclusive societies for sustainable development
   - Provide access to justice for all and build effective, accountable and inclusive institutions at all levels
4. **The focus on Partnerships:** Strengthen the means of implementation and revitalize the global partnership for sustainable development

Sustainable Development Goals Targets and Indicators (Table 1.3)

Each goal typically has 8–12 targets, and each target has between 1 and 4 indicators used to measure progress toward reaching the targets. The targets are either "outcome" targets (circumstances to be attained) or "means of implementation" targets. The latter targets were introduced late in the process of negotiating the SDGs to address the concern of some Member States about how the SDGs were to be achieved. Goal 17 is wholly about how the SDGs will be achieved.

The numbering system of targets is as follows: "Outcome targets" use numbers, whereas "means of implementation targets" use lower case letters. For example, SDG 6 has a

Table 1.3: Sustainable development goals targets and indicators.

Goal 1: End poverty in all its forms everywhere	The five outcome-related targets by the year 2030 are: 1.1 : The eradication of extreme poverty where the people living on less than $1.25 a day 1.2 : Reduction of all poverty by half 1.3 : Implementation of social protection systems 1.4 : Ensuring equal rights to ownership, basic services, technology, and economic resources 1.5 : The building of resilience to environmental, economic and social disasters The two targets related to means of achieving SDG 1 1. Call for mobilization of resources to end poverty 2. The establishment of poverty eradication policy frameworks at all levels
Goal 2: End hunger, achieve food security and improved nutrition, and promote sustainable agriculture	The five "outcome targets" are: 2.1 : Ending hunger and improving access to food 2.2 : Ending all forms of malnutrition 2.3 : Agricultural productivity 2.4 : Sustainable food production systems and resilient agricultural practices 2.5 : Genetic diversity of seeds, cultivated plants and farmed and domesticated animals investments, research and technology The three means for achieving SDG 2 include: a. Invest in rural infrastructure, agricultural research, technology and gene banks b. Addressing trade restrictions and distortions in world c. Agricultural markets and food commodity markets and their derivatives.

Contd...

Contd...

Goal 3: Good health and well-being	Out of total 13 targets, the first nine targets are "outcome targets". By 2030 these are: 3.1 : Reduce the global maternal mortality ratio to less than 70 per 100,000 live births 3.2 : End preventable deaths of newborns and children under 5 years of age, with all countries aiming to reduce neonatal mortality to at least as low as 12 per 1,000 live births and underfive mortality to at least as low as 25 per 1,000 live births 3.3 : End the epidemics of AIDS, tuberculosis, malaria and neglected tropical diseases and combat hepatitis, water-borne diseases and other communicable diseases 3.4 : Reduce by one third premature mortality from noncommunicable diseases through prevention and treatment and promote mental health and well-being 3.5 : Strengthen the prevention and treatment of substance abuse, including narcotic drug abuse and harmful use of alcohol 3.6 : Ensure universal access to sexual and reproductive healthcare services, including for family planning, information and education, and the integration of reproductive health into national strategies and programs 3.7 : Achieve universal health coverage, including financial risk protection, access to quality essential healthcare services and safe, effective, quality and affordable essential medicines and vaccines for all 3.8 : Reduce the number of deaths and illnesses from hazardous chemicals and air, water and soil pollution and contamination 3.9 : By 2020, halve the number of global deaths and injuries from road traffic accidents The four "means to achieving" SDG 3 targets are: a. Implement the who framework convention on tobacco control b. Support research, development and universal access to affordable vaccines and medicines c. Increase health financing and support health workforce in developing countries d. Improve early warning systems for global health risks
Goal 4: Ensure inclusive and equitable quality education and promote lifelong learning opportunities for all	The UN has defined 10 targets and 11 indicators for SDG 4. The seven "outcome-oriented targets" by the year 2030 are: 4.1 : Ensure that all girls and boys complete free, equitable and quality primary and secondary education leading to relevant and effective learning outcomes 4.2 : Ensure that all girls and boys have access to quality early childhood development, care and preprimary education so that they are ready for primary education 4.3 : Ensure equal access for all women and men to affordable and quality technical, vocational and tertiary education, including university 4.4 : Substantially increase the number of youth and adults who have relevant skills, including technical and vocational skills, for employment, decent jobs and entrepreneurship 4.5 : Eliminate gender disparities in education and ensure equal access to all levels of education and vocational training for the vulnerable, including persons with disabilities, indigenous peoples and children in vulnerable situations 4.6 : Ensure that all youth and a substantial proportion of adults, both men and women, achieve literacy and numeracy 4.7 : Ensure that all learners acquire the knowledge and skills needed to promote sustainable development The three "means of achieving targets" are: a. Build and upgrade inclusive education facilities and safe schools b. Expand higher education scholarships for developing countries c. Increase the supply of qualified teachers in developing countries
Goal 5: Achieve gender equality and empower all women and girls	Out of the nine targets, six are "outcome-oriented" 5.1 : Ending all forms of discrimination against all women and girls everywhere 5.2 : Ending violence and exploitation of women and girls 5.3 : Eliminating harmful practices such as child, early and forced marriage and female genital mutilation 5.4 : Increasing value of unpaid care and promoting shared domestic responsibilities 5.5 : Ensuring full participation of women in leadership and decision-making
	5.6 : Ensuring access to universal reproductive rights and health. The three "means of achieving" targets are: a. Fostering equal rights to economic resources, property ownership and financial services for women b. Promoting empowerment of women through technology c. Adopting, strengthening policies and enforcing legislation for gender equality
Goal 6: Clean water and sanitation	The six "outcome-oriented targets" include by the year 2030 are: 6.1 : Achieve universal and equitable access to safe and affordable drinking water for all 6.2 : Achieve access to adequate and equitable sanitation and hygiene for all and end open defecation. 6.3 : Improve water quality by reducing pollution, eliminating dumping and minimizing release of hazardous chemicals and materials. 6.4 : Increase water use efficiency across all sectors and ensure sustainable withdrawals and supply of freshwater to address water scarcity. 6.5 : Implement integrated water resources management at all levels, including through transboundary cooperation as appropriate 6.6 : By 2020, protect and restore water related ecosystems, including mountains, forests, wetlands, rivers, aquifers and lakes The two "means of achieving" targets are: a. Expand international cooperation and capacity building and sanitation support to developing countries b. Support and strengthen the participation of local communities in improving water and sanitation management

Contd...

Contd...

Goal 7: Affordable and clean energy	SDG 7 has five "outcome targets" by 2030 are: 7.1 : Ensure universal access to affordable, reliable and modern energy services 7.2 : Increase substantially the share of renewable energy in the global energy mix 7.3 : Double the global rate of improvement in energy efficiency: a. Enhance international cooperation to facilitate access to clean energy research and technology, including renewable energy, energy efficiency and advanced and cleaner fossil fuel technology. b. Expand infrastructure and upgrade technology for supplying modern and sustainable energy services for all in developing countries, least developed countries, small island developing. States and landlocked developing countries, in accordance with their respective programmes of support
Goal 8: Decent work and economic growth	SDG 8 is to "Promote sustained, inclusive and sustainable economic growth, full and productive employment and decent work for all". 8.1 : Sustain per capita economic growth in accordance with national circumstances 8.2 : Achieve higher levels of economic productivity through diversification, technological upgrading and innovation, including through a focus on high value added and labor intensive sectors 8.3 : Promote development oriented policies that support productive activities, decent job creation, entrepreneurship, creativity and innovation, and encourage the formalization and growth of enterprises, including through access to financial services 8.4 : Improve progressively, through 2030, global resource efficiency in consumption and production and endeavor to decouple economic growth from environmental degradation, in accordance with the 10 Year Framework of Programmes 8.5 : By 2030, achieve full and productive employment and decent work for all and equal pay for work of equal value 8.6 : By 2020, substantially reduce the proportion of youth not in employment, education or training 8.7 : Take immediate and effective measures to eradicate forced labor, end modern slavery and human trafficking and by 2025 end child labor in all its forms 8.8 : Protect labor rights and promote safe and secure working environments for all workers. 8.9 : By 2030, devise and implement policies to promote sustainable tourism that creates jobs and promotes local culture and products 8.10: Strengthen the capacity of domestic financial institutions to encourage and expand access to banking, insurance and financial services for all: a. Increase aid for trade support for developing countries b. By 2020, develop and operationalize a global strategy for youth employment and implement the Global Jobs Pact of the International Labour Organization
Goal 9: Industry, Innovation, and Infrastructure	SDG 9 is to: "Build resilient infrastructure, promote inclusive and sustainable industrialization, and foster innovation 9.1 : Develop quality, reliable, sustainable and resilient infrastructure, to support economic development and human wellbeing, and equitable access for all 9.2 : Promote inclusive and sustainable industrialization and, by 2030 9.3 : Increase the access of small scale industrial and other enterprises, in particular in developing countries, to financial services, including affordable credit, and their integration into value chains and markets 9.4 : By 2030, upgrade infrastructure and retrofit industries to make them sustainable, with increased resource 9.5 : Enhance scientific research, upgrade the technological capabilities of industrial sectors in all countries, in particular developing countries, including, by 2030: a. Facilitate sustainable and resilient infrastructure development in developing countries through enhanced financial, technological and technical support to least developed countries. b. Support domestic technology development, research and innovation in developing countries. c. Significantly increase access to information and communications technology in least developed countries by 2020
Goal 10: Reducing inequalities	SDG 10 is to: "Reduce income inequality within and among countries". Progress toward SDG 10 targets: 10.1 : By 2030, progressively achieve and sustain income growth of the bottom 40% of the population at a rate higher than the national average 10.2 : By 2030, empower and promote the social, economic and political inclusion of all, irrespective of age, sex, disability, race, ethnicity, origin, religion or economic or other status 10.3 : Ensure equal opportunity and reduce inequalities of outcome, including by eliminating discriminatory laws, policies and practices and promoting appropriate legislation, policies and action in this regard 10.4 : Adopt policies, especially fiscal, wage and social protection policies, and progressively achieve greater equality 10.5 : Improve the regulation and monitoring of global financial markets and institutions and strengthen the implementation of such regulations 10.6 : Ensure enhanced representation and voice for developing countries in decision making in global international economic and financial institutions in order to deliver more effective, credible, accountable and legitimate institutions 10.7 : Facilitate orderly, safe, regular and responsible migration and mobility of people, including through the implementation of planned and well managed migration policies: a. Implement the principle of special and differential treatment for developing countries, in particular least developed countries, in accordance with World Trade Organization agreements b. Encourage official development assistance and financial flows, including foreign direct investment, to States where the need is greatest, in particular least developed countries, African countries, small island developing States and landlocked developing countries, in accordance with their national plans and programmes c. By 2030, reduce to less than 3% the transaction costs of migrant remittances and eliminate remittance corridors with costs higher than 5%

Contd...

Contd...

Goal 11: Sustainable cities and communities	SDG 11 is to: "Make cities and human settlements inclusive, safe, resilient, and sustainable" 11.1: By 2030, ensure access for all to adequate, safe and affordable housing and basic services and upgrade slums 11.2: By 2030, provide access to safe, affordable, accessible and sustainable transport systems for all, improving road safety, notably by expanding public transport, with special attention to the needs of those in vulnerable situations, women, children, persons with disabilities and older persons 11.3: By 2030, enhance inclusive and sustainable urbanization and capacity for participatory, integrated and sustainable human settlement planning and management in all countries 11.4: Strengthen efforts to protect and safeguard the world's cultural and natural heritage 11.5: By 2030, significantly reduce the number of deaths and the number of people affected and substantially decrease the direct economic losses relative to global gross domestic product caused by disasters, including water-related disasters, with a focus on protecting the poor and people in vulnerable situations 11.6: By 2030, reduce the adverse per capita environmental impact of cities, including by paying special attention to air quality and municipal and other waste management 11.7: By 2030, provide universal access to safe, inclusive and accessible, green and public spaces, in particular for women and children, older persons and persons with disabilities a. Support positive economic, social and environmental links between urban, periurban and rural areas by strengthening national and regional development planning b. By 2020, substantially increase the number of cities and human settlements adopting and implementing integrated policies and plans towards inclusion, resource efficiency, mitigation and adaptation to climate change, resilience to disasters, and develop and implement, in line with the Sendai Framework for Disaster Risk Reduction 2015 to 2030, holistic disaster risk management at all levels c. Support least developed countries, including through financial and technical assistance, in building sustainable and resilient buildings utilizing local materials
Goal 12: Responsible consumption and production	12.1: Implement the 10' Year Framework of Programmes on Sustainable Consumption and Production Patterns, all countries taking action, with developed countries taking the lead, taking into account the development and capabilities of developing countries 12.2: By 2030, achieve the sustainable management and efficient use of natural resources 12.3: By 2030, halve per capita global food waste at the retail and consumer levels and reduce food losses along production and supply chains, including post-harvest losses 12.4: By 2020, achieve the environmentally sound management of chemicals and all wastes throughout their life cycle, and significantly reduce their release to air, water and soil in order to minimize their adverse impacts on human health and the environment 12.5: By 2030, substantially reduce waste generation through prevention, reduction, recycling and reuse 12.6: Encourage companies, especially large and transnational companies, to adopt sustainable practices and to integrate sustainability information into their reporting cycle 12.7: Promote public procurement practices that are sustainable, in accordance with national policies and priorities 12.8: By 2030, ensure that people everywhere have the relevant information and awareness for sustainable development and lifestyles in harmony with nature: a. Support developing countries to strengthen their scientific and technological capacity to move towards more sustainable patterns of consumption and production b. Develop and implement tools to monitor sustainable development impacts for sustainable tourism that creates jobs and promotes local culture and products c. Rationalize inefficient fossil fuel subsidies that encourage wasteful consumption by removing market distortions, in accordance with national circumstances, including by restructuring taxation and phasing out those harmful subsidies, minimizing the possible adverse impacts on their development in a manner that protects the poor and the affected communities
Goal 13: Take urgent action to combat climate change and its impacts	13.1: Strengthen resilience and adaptive capacity to climate-related hazards and natural disasters in all countries 13.2: Integrate climate change measures into national policies, strategies and planning 13.3: Improve education, awareness-raising and human and institutional capacity on climate change mitigation, adaptation, impact reduction and early warning a. Implement the commitment undertaken by developed country parties to the United Nations Framework Convention on Climate Change to a goal of mobilizing jointly $100 billion annually by 2020 from all sources to address the needs of developing countries in the context of meaningful mitigation actions and transparency on implementation. b. Promote mechanisms for raising capacity for effective climate change related planning and management in least developed countries and small island developing States, including focusing on women, youth and local and marginalized communities
Goal 14: Conserve and sustainably use the oceans, seas and marine resources for sustainable development	14.1: By 2025, prevent and significantly reduce marine pollution of all kinds, in particular from land-based activities, including marine debris and nutrient pollution 14.2: By 2020, sustainably manage and protect marine and coastal ecosystems to avoid significant adverse impacts, including by strengthening their resilience, and take action for their restoration in order to achieve healthy and productive oceans 14.3: Minimize and address the impacts of ocean acidification, including through enhanced scientific cooperation at all levels 14.4: By 2020, effectively regulate harvesting and end overfishing, illegal, unreported and unregulated fishing and destructive fishing practices and implement science-based management plans, in order to restore fish stocks in the shortest time feasible, at least to levels that can produce maximum sustainable yield as determined by their biological characteristics

Contd...

Contd...

	14.5: By 2020, conserve at least 10% of coastal and marine areas, consistent with national and international law and based on the best available scientific information 14.6: By 2020, prohibit certain forms of fisheries like overfishing, illegal, unreported and unregulated fishing and refrain from introducing new such subsidies, recognizing that appropriate and effective special and differential treatment for developing and least developed countries should be an integral part of the World Trade Organization fisheries subsidies negotiation. 14.7: By 2030, increase the economic benefits to small island developing States and least developed countries from the sustainable use of marine resources, including through sustainable management of fisheries, aquaculture and tourism. a. Increase scientific knowledge, develop research capacity and transfer marine technology, taking into account the Intergovernmental Oceanographic Commission Criteria and Guidelines on the Transfer of Marine Technology, in order to improve ocean health. b. Provide access for small scale artisanal fishers to marine resources and markets c. Enhance the conservation and sustainable use of oceans and their resources by implementing international law as reflected in the sea, it is also called Law of The Sea Treaty.
Goal 15: Protect, restore and promote sustainable use of terrestrial ecosystems, sustainably manage forests, combat desertification, and halt and reverse land degradation and halt biodiversity loss	15.1: By 2020, ensure the conservation, restoration and sustainable use of terrestrial and inland freshwater ecosystems and their services, in particular forests, wetlands, mountains and drylands, in line with obligations under international agreements 15.2: By 2020, promote the implementation of sustainable management of all types of forests, halt deforestation, restore degraded forests and substantially increase afforestation and reforestation globally 15.3: By 2030, combat desertification, restore degraded land and soil, including land affected by desertification, drought and floods, and strive to achieve a land degradationneutral world 15.4: By 2030, ensure the conservation of mountain ecosystems, including their biodiversity, in order to enhance their capacity to provide benefits that are essential for sustainable development 15.5: Take urgent and significant action to reduce the degradation of natural habitats, halt the loss of biodiversity and, by 2020, protect and prevent the extinction of threatened species 15.6: Promote fair and equitable sharing of the benefits arising from the utilization of genetic resources and promote appropriate access to such resources, as internationally agreed 15.7: Take urgent action to end poaching and trafficking of protected species of flora and fauna and address both demand and supply of illegal wildlife products 15.8: By 2020, introduce measures to prevent the introduction and significantly reduce the impact of invasive alien species on land and water ecosystems and control or eradicate the priority species 15.9: By 2020, integrate ecosystem and biodiversity values into national and local planning, development processes, poverty reduction strategies and accounts: a. Mobilize and significantly increase financial resources from all sources to conserve and sustainably use biodiversity and ecosystems b. Mobilize significant resources from all sources and at all levels to finance sustainable forest management and provide adequate incentives to developing countries to advance such management, including for conservation and reforestation c. Enhance global support for efforts to combat poaching and trafficking of protected species, including by increasing the capacity of local communities to pursue sustainable livelihood opportunities
Goal 16: Promote peaceful and inclusive societies for sustainable development, provide access to justice for all and build effective, accountable and inclusive institutions at all levels	16.1 : Significantly reduce all forms of violence and related death rates everywhere 16.2 : End abuse, exploitation, trafficking and all forms of violence against and torture of children 16.3 : Promote the rule of law at the national and international levels and ensure equal access to justice for all 16.4 : By 2030, significantly reduce illicit financial and arms flows, strengthen the recovery and return of stolen assets and combat all forms of organized crime 16.5 : Substantially reduce corruption and bribery in all their forms 16.6 : Develop effective, accountable and transparent institutions at all levels 16.7 : Ensure responsive, inclusive, participatory and representative decision-making at all levels 16.8 : Broaden and strengthen the participation of developing countries in the institutions of global governance 16.9 : By 2030, provide legal identity for all, including birth registration 16.10 : Ensure public access to information and protect fundamental freedoms, in accordance with national legislation and international agreements: a. Strengthen relevant national institutions, including through international cooperation, for building capacity at all levels, in particular in developing countries, to prevent violence and combat terrorism and crime b. Promote and enforce nondiscriminatory laws and policies for sustainable development
Goal 17: Strengthen the means of implementation and revitalize the global partnership for sustainable development	The targets are classified on finance, technology, capacity building, trade and other systemic issues. *Finance* 17.1 : Strengthen domestic resource mobilization, including through international support to developing countries. 17.2 : Developed countries to implement fully their official development assistance commitments. 17.3 : Mobilize additional financial resources for developing countries from multiple sources 17.4 : Assist developing countries in attaining long-term debt sustainability through coordinated policies aimed at fostering debt financing, debt relief and debt restructuring, as appropriate, and address the external debt of highly indebted poor countries to reduce debt distress 17.5 : Adopt and implement investment promotion regimes for least developed countries

Contd...

Contd...

	Technology 17.6 : Enhance triangular regional and international cooperation on and access to science, technology and innovation and enhance knowledge sharing on mutually agreed terms, including through improved coordination among existing mechanisms. 17.7 : Promote the development, transfer, dissemination and diffusion of environmentally sound technologies to developing countries on favorable terms, including on concessional and preferential terms, as mutually agreed 17.8 : Fully operationalize the technology bank and science, technology and innovation capacity building mechanism for least developed countries by 2017. *Capacity building* 17.9 : Enhance international support for implementing effective and targeted capacity building in developing countries to implement all the Sustainable Development Goals. *Trade* 17.10 : Promote a universal, rules based, open, non discriminatory and equitable multilateral trading system under the World Trade Organization. 17.11 : Significantly increase the exports of developing countries, in particular with a view to doubling the least developed countries' share of global exports by 2020. 17.12 : Realize timely implementation of duty free and quota free market access on a lasting basis for all least developed countries, consistent with World Trade Organization decisions. *Systemic issues* 17.13 : Enhance global macroeconomic stability, including through policy coordination and policy coherence 17.14 : Enhance policy coherence for sustainable development 17.15 : Respect each country's policy space and leadership to establish and implement policies for poverty eradication and sustainable development 17.16 : Enhance the global partnership for sustainable development, complemented by multistakeholder partnerships that mobilize and share knowledge, expertise, technology and financial resources. 17.17 : Encourage and promote effective public, public private and civil society partnerships, building on the experience and resourcing strategies of partnerships 17.18 : By 2020, enhance capacity building support to developing countries, including for least developed countries and small island developing States, to increase significantly the availability of high quality, timely and reliable data to all. 17.19 : By 2030, build on existing initiatives to develop measurements of progress on sustainable development that complement gross domestic product, and support statistical capacity building in developing countries

total of 8 targets. The first six are outcome targets should be reached by 2030 and are labeled Targets 6.1 to 6.6. The final two targets are "means of implementation targets" that have no specified date and are labeled as Targets 6.a and 6.b and two that have no specified date.

PRIMARY HEALTH CARE

Primary health care is the first level of contact between the individual and the health system where 'essential' health care (primary health care) is provided. A majority of health complaints and problems can be satisfactorily managed. This level of care is closest to the people. This care is provided by the primary health centers and their subcenters, within community participation.

Primary health care is a practical and key approach to making essential healthcare accessible to all in the universe and helping them to attain acceptable of health. It is equally valid for all the countries from most developed to the least developed countries.

Primary health care addresses the main health problems in the community, providing promotive, preventive, curative and rehabilitative services accordingly within the economic conditions.

Concept of Primary Health Care (Fig. 1.11)

After three decades of trial and error and dissatisfaction in meeting peoples' basic health needs, the World Health Assembly, in May 1977, the Government of India launched a Rural Health Scheme, based on the principle of 'placing people's health in people's hands. It is a three tire system of healthcare delivery in rural areas based on the recommendation of the Shrivastav committee in 1975. Close on the heels of these recommendations, an international conference at Alma-Ata in 1978; jointly WHO and UNICEF introduce primary healthcare approach to achieve the goal of an acceptable level of Health for All the people of the world by the year 2000 AD.

The conference declared (PHC) as the key approach to achieve the 'HFA' goal. It also stated that PHC shall be the part of overall development of the nation and should be the spirit of social justice.

Definition

The Alama Ata Conference defined Primary Health Care as:

'Primary health care is essential health care made universally accessible to individual and acceptable to them, through their full participation and a cost the community and country can afford.'

History of Primary Health Care

The concept of primary health care was born in India during postindependent era. In 1947 the Bhore committee recommended for the integration of preventive health services along with the curative services in offering health

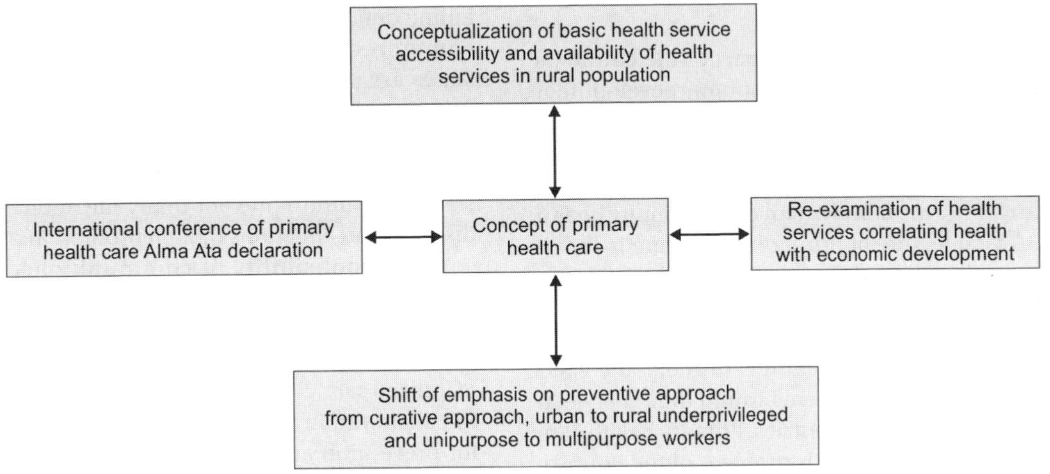

Fig. 1.11: Concept of primary health care.

care to the people in rural and remote area through the organization of health center. The Bhore committee recommendation highlighted on:

- To provide comprehensive and preventive, curative and promotive health services to the people in the rural areas through the network of PHC and the health care to be accessible to all.
- Another short-term plan was proposed to establish a PHC for a population of forty thousand and a secondary unit to supervise thirty PHC with 650 bedded hospital. A distinct hospital which will serves as a referral center with specialties. These recommendations were not satisfactorily implemented because: (1) distance from PHC to district hospital became greater from 8 to 160 km which become impossible for the people to get immediate medical help. Now there are nearly 5,886 PHC operating in India.
- The health needs of the people in India are varied. The population is increasing at the rate of 18 million annually. MMR (3–4) and IMR (120) are very high. Nutritional status and hygienic conditions are very poor and all these may vary from urban to rural areas state to state, religion to religion and region to region, etc. life expectancy was low. Literacy rate was only 30%. The PHC was not covered with doctor with all regions. The health services is mostly urban oriented only curable in nature since 1952. The emphasis was on preventive concept which integrated in GNM curriculum to prepare nurses for health orientation in meeting the need of the people. But in many states the thought are not implemented and lost gradually.

Now the concept of primary health care has become a global level with Alma-Ata declaration at the USSR to the grassroots level with increasing recognition of failure of existing health services to provide health care. Alternative ideas and methods have been tried.

In 1947 the World Health Assembly gave the call for HFA by 2000 AD. Health for all basically meant that individual should attained a level of health which will enable them to earn their livelihood and lead a socially congenial life. So, at the joint venture of WHO and the UNICEF executive in the national conference at Alma-Ata USSR, the capital of Kazakhstan from 6 to 12 September, 1978 with the Governments of 134 countries and many volunteer agencies called for a revolutionary approach to healthcare and the topic was the existing gross inequality is the health status of the people particularly between developed and developing countries as well as within countries politically, socially and economically unacceptable. The conference emphasizes that the key to attain the HFA by 2000 AD was through implementation of primary health care and this is put forcefully in the declaration of Alma-Ata to which all the participating countries were signatory and India was one of these countries.

The 30th health assembly decided in 1977 May that the main social target of government and WHO should be the attainment of HFA by 2000 AD, i.e., the attainment by all the people of the world of the level of health that will permit them to lead socially and economically productive life.

In 1978, an international conference on PHC held at Alma-Ata USSR issued a declaration which stated that PHC is key to attaining the HFA by 2000 AD.

In May 1979, the World Health Assembly endorsed declaration of Alma-Ata on primary health care and invited member states to proceed immediately to formulate their own national policy strategy and plan to attain the target the HFA by 2000 AD.

The global strategy of WHO for the goal of health for all was endorsed by the WHO in 1981. There is now a growing national and international movement to attain HFA.

Planner in every countries have develop their own strategy for achieving the goal. Milestones set by the WHO for achieving the goal for HFA are:

- Right kind of food for all by 1985
- Provide essential drugs for all by 1986
- Providing an adequate supply of safe drinking water and basic sanitation by 1990
- Immunizing children against six killer diseases by 1990
- Other cardinal features of movements are to ensure.

Concept of Primary Health Care

Primary health care form an integral part of the country's health system and overall social and economic development of the community. It is the first level of contact of individual, family, and community with the national health system bringing health care as close as possible where people live and work. It constitute the first element of a continuity health care process. A vital feature of primary health care is that it is based upon participation of the people themselves. Many health programs have failed because they were perceived by the people not as their own program but rather as government program, primary health care is equally valid for all countries though the problems would differ between the developing and developed countries. Primary health care is concerned with the main health problem of the country providing promotive, preventive, curative and rehabilitative services as required.

Characteristics of Primary Health Care

- It is the essential health care based on practically sound and socially acceptable technology.
- It should be rendered universally.
- Acceptable by individual and form in the community by their full participation.
- Its availability to a cost which the community and country can afford to maintain in a spirit of self reliance and self develop.
- It requires joint efforts of health sector and other health related sectors like education, food, agriculture, social welfare, animal husbandry and housing, etc.

Elements of Primary Health Care

- **Education regarding existing health problems and methods of preventing and controlling them:** Health education is an integral part of all health services and all health personnel, including nurses and nurses are responsible for educating people as to how they can improve their own health. Public education is the first, and one of the most essential, component of primary health care. By educating the public on the prevention and control of health problems, and encouraging participation, WHO works to keep disease from spreading on a personal level. The community health nurse has to play an important role in organizing appropriate health educational programs according to the needs of the community, collaborating and coordinating with intra-disciplinary and inter disciplinary teams. The promotion, maintenance and restoration of health requires that patient understand healthcare requirements.
- **Promotion of food supply and proper nutrition:** Nutrition is another essential component of health care. In India, available statistics indicate that 65% of our children are malnourished about 1 lakh die due to it every year, dominating among under fives. Vitamin A deficiency increases vulnerability to respiratory infections, gastrointestinal infections and xerophthalmia, iodine deficiency resulting in hypothyroidism is another common deficiency disease. Nutritional deficiency states are particularly noticeable among pregnant and lactating mothers and in infants and children. This may be due to sociocultural/economic factors prevailing in the community. WHO works to prevent malnutrition and starvation and to prevent many nutritional deficiencies diseases and afflictions though promotion of food supply.

  The responsibility of community health nurse in this regard is to provide essential health services. This include surveillance and case finding through use of growth charts in children, making provisions for supply of iodized salt. Vitamin A supplements, food supplements in collaboration with other members of the health team for prevention and treatment of malnutrition. She takes suitable measures for prevention and treatment of diarrheal diseases, intestinal parasites and other diseases affecting ability to utilize food.
- **An adequate supply of safe water and basic sanitation:** In India, safe and potable water is not available to a major section of the population. Many water-borne diseases prevalent in the country are preventable, but the importance of the use of pure and safe water as well as the personal hygiene do not properly appreciated. The environmental sanitation also is very poor due to so many reasons, particularly in rural areas and in urban slums. There are no proper arrangements for disposal of human excreta and animal wastes, sewage, garbage and sullage, etc. A supply of clean, safe drinking water, and basic sanitation measures regarding trash, sewage and water cleanliness can significantly improve the health of a population, reducing and even eliminating many preventable diseases.
- **Maternal and child health care, including family planning:** In India maternal mortality rate is quite high as compared to other countries. The main causes for increased MMR are sepsis, hemorrhage, toxemia, illegal abortions and malnutrition. Maternal morbidity is also increasing for malnutrition, anemia, infections, malaria, hepatitis, urinary tract infections, tuberculosis, etc., during the child-bearing year. Ensuring comprehensive and adequate health care to children and to mothers, both expecting and otherwise, is another essential element of primary health care. By caring for those who are at the greatest risk of health problems, WHO helps future generations have a chance to thrive and contribute to globally. Sometimes, care for these individuals involves adequate counseling on family planning and safe sex. CHN are assigned to carry out maternal and child health care, which includes antenatal, prenatal perinatal and postnatal care.
- **Immunization against major infectious diseases:** Immunization is to prevent endemic and epidemic diseases. India has a long history of vaccination programmes. In the sixties, this vaccination against smallpox and tuberculosis was started. Now universal immunization programme is in operation in India. Nurses

and nursing team plan immunization programmes for adults and children, particularly infants and pregnant women. Encouragement and persuasion are strategies in monitoring and scheduling immunization. By administering global immunizations, WHO works to wipe out major infectious diseases, greatly improving overall health globally.

- **Prevention and control of locally endemic diseases:** In India, the government has launched various national programmes for the control or eradication of these endemic diseases like leprosy eradication programme, tuberculosis control programme for controlling TB, malaria, eradication programme and others prevention and control of local diseases is critical to promoting primary health care in a population. Many diseases vary based on location. Taking these diseases into account and initiating measures to prevent them are key factors in efforts to reduce infection rate. Nurses and nursing team collect data care of the ill, offer health education, visit and follow up cases, and provide surveillance over the target population to ensure that communicable diseases are eradicated or controlled.
- **Appropriate treatment of common diseases and injuries:** Another important component of primary health care is access to appropriate medical care for the treatment of diseases and injuries. By treating disease and injury right away, caregivers can help avoid complications and the expense of later, more extensive, medical treatment. First aid measures may be taken at village level. Treatment of common diseases and injuries are to be provided at the subcenter, and primary health center and appropriate referral services are to be organized. Nurses have been trained to treat patient under a doctor's standing order. The emergency treatment and primary care provided by nurses help to reduce morbidity and mortality rates.
- **Provision of essential drugs:** By providing essential drugs to those who need them, such as antibiotics to those with infections, caregivers can help prevent disease from escalating. This makes the community safer, as there is less chance for diseases to be passed along. The community health nurse has to procure, keep and also utilize whenever necessary essential drugs to treat minor ailments, etc. Also she should be aware of the resources and facilities for getting essential drugs to inform the client within a short distance.

Principles of Primary Health Care

Equitable Distribution

Equitable distribution means health services must be shared equally by all people irrespective of their ability to pay (rich or poor, urban or rural must have access to health services).

Previously health services mainly concentrated major towns and cities resulting in a inequality of care to the people in rural areas. The worst hit are the needy and vulnerable groups of the population in rural areas and urban slums. This is termed social injustice. Primary health care aims to redress this imbalance by shifting the center of gravity of the health care system from cities (where three quarters of the health budget was spent) to the rural areas (where three quarters of the people lived) and bring these services to the door step level.

Community Participation

The involvement of individuals, family and communities in promotion of their own health and welfare is an essential ingredient of primary health care. Countries are now conscious of the fact that universal coverage by primary health care cannot be achieved without involvement of the local community. There should be continuing effort to involve the community in the planning implementation and maintenance of health services, maximum reliance on local resources such as manpower, money and materials. Primary health care must be built on the principle of community participation.

One approach that has been tried successfully in India is by health guides and trained dais, being selected and trained by local community in delivery of primary health care free of charge. By overcoming cultural and communication barrier they provide primary health care in community acceptable way.

Focus on Prevention

Vigorous action to be taken to ensure availability of adequate number of appropriate self-health personnel required to devise and implement plan of action, preventive measures such as safe water, sanitation, immunization was emphasized. The focus is on disease prevention.

Intersectoral Coordination

The declaration of Alma-Ata states that primary health care involves in addition to health sector, all related sectors and aspects of national and community development, such as agriculture, animal husbandry, food, industry, education, housing, public works, communication and other sectors.

Agriculture

Agricultural policies can help improve nutritional status of vulnerable sections. Appropriate agricultural technology can lighten the work load and increase work productivity. The person from agriculture, irrigation and engineering can help farmers grow more food (cereals, pulses, oil seeds, vegetables, fruits, etc.) locally, can provide seeds for kitchen garden and community garden, can educate people for composting, can also motivate people in family welfare activities, etc.

Animal Husbandry

The personnel from animal husbandry can help people to develop farms for poultry, fisheries, fruits, vegetables, etc., can help in immunization of domestic animals, and can also help in prevention of zoonotic diseases, etc.

Housing

Housing structure need to be built up considering the climatic and environmental conditions; the basic facilities, etc., so as to have wholesome effect on health; and be easy to clean and maintain. Education is very important to ensure healthful living in the house. Housing department can play an important role in this to promote healthy house/building structure, etc.

Water Supply

Adequate safe drinking water supply need to be there both in urban and rural areas within easy reach of people to reduce morbidity, mortality due to water-borne diseases.

Sanitation

Sanitary facilities are equally important to control such problems. It is also necessary to educate people regarding the proper use and maintenance of water and sanitary facilities.

Public Works

For public workers, it is very important to have good roads connecting villages with each other and the town and cities to have easier reach to villages, market places, health agencies, etc. It requires coordination with departments which deals with these services.

Communication (Education and Mass Media)

Mass media, two way radio communications can help in disseminating valid primary health care information to people living in remotest areas. It can also help in establishing contacts between isolated areas and centrally located administrative levels.

Education sector can play a very important role in developing instructional material on primary health care aspects to educate people at large in the communities. Primary health care activities can be planned and organized by the teachers and parents—Teachers Association in the school for school children and also in the community for different groups.

Social and Women's Welfare

The personnel from social and women's welfare can help in: mobilizing women, mahila mandals, etc., for propagation of various aspects of healthy living in the community, education of mothers regarding maternal and child care, prevention and control of locally endemic diseases, etc.

Panchayats

Panchayats can play very important role in providing funds and administrative support for infrastructure, various health programs, health education, propagating messages, mobilizing transport, etc.

Cooperatives and Banks

Cooperatives and banks can provide funds for community garden, community composting, soak pit etc., making farms for poultry, fisheries, vegetables, fruits, milk, etc., health insurance.

Appropriate Technology

Appropriate technology has been defined as technology that is scientifically sound, adaptable to local needs, and acceptable to those who apply it and those for whom it is used, and can be maintained by the people themselves, in keeping with the principle of self-reliance with resources the community can afford is emphasized. The term appropriate because in some countries, large luxurious hospitals that are totally inappropriate to the local needs, are built, which absorb a major part of the national health budget, effectively blocking any improvement in general health services.

This also applies to using costly equipment, procedures and techniques when cheaper, scientifically valid and acceptable ones are available, viz. oral rehydration fluid, stand pipes which are socially acceptable, and financially more feasible than house to house connections, etc.

Primary health care is qualitatively a different approach to deal with the health problems of community. Unlike the previous approaches, e.g., basic health services, integrated health care, vertical health services to the doors of the people, primary health care approach starts with the people themselves. This approach signifies a new dynamism in health care and has been described as health by the people, placing peoples health in people hands.

The ends of the primary health care approach are the same of those of earlier approaches (i.e., attainment of an acceptable level of health by every individual) but the means adopted are different that is more equitable distribution and nationwide coverage, more intersectoral coordination and more community involvement in health-related matters. Primary health care forms part of the larger concept of human resources and development.

WHO strategies of primary health care:

- **Reducing excess mortality of poor marginalized populations:** Primary Health Care must ensure access to health services for the most disadvantaged populations, and focus on interventions which will directly impact on the major causes of mortality, morbidity and disability for those populations.
- **Reducing the leading risk factors to human health:** Primary health care, through its preventative and health promotion roles, must address those known risk factors, which are the major determinants of health outcomes for local populations.
- **Developing sustainable health systems:** Primary health care as a component of health systems must develop in ways, which are financially sustainable, supported by political leaders, and supported by the populations served.

Primary Health Care Approach

In 1978 WHO at a meeting at Alma-Ata, Russia declared the new concept of primary health care. India being a member country of WHO was committed to implement the new method of approach. The approach came into existence in 1978. Primary health care delivery first proposed by Bhore Committee in 1946 and before Alma-Ata Primary Health Care was regarded as synonymous with **Basic Health Care Services, First Contact Care, Health Accessible Care, Services provided by Generalists**, etc.

Although specific services provided will vary in different countries and communities, the Alma-Ata Declaration has eight essential components for patient care.

Roles of Nurse in Primary Health Care

In 1981, International meeting was convened by WHO to consider the role of nursing in contributing to the achievement of the goal of HFA-2000 through primary health care. The development in each country of a corps of nurses that is well-informed about health care and ready to bring necessary changes in the nursing system. The inclusion of nursing personnels at all levels of policy making and administration so that the profession can contribute to determine the action plan. The involvement of nurse and use of their skills in initiating an extending primary health care. Fundamental changes at all levels of nursing education, basic, post-basic and continuing to ensure that priority needs of population are functionally integrated into the education and in the nursing practice. Research into nursing administrations, practice and education that will demonstrate nurses contribution to primary health care. The focus and core of all registered nursing practice is to provide care to patients/clients. Using the nursing process of assessment, diagnosis, planning, implementation and evaluation registered nurses are skilled and competent professionals who provide holistic nursing care to individuals, families, communities or populations. The registered nurse's practice is guided by essential interventions that are considered fundamental to primary health care and can occur in any practice setting from acute care to community care to continuing care. WHO study group 1985 identified four main self-explanatory role of nurse including the eight essential elements.

1. Nurse as a direct care provider
2. Nurse as a teacher and educator
3. Nurse as a supervisor and manager
4. Nurse as a researcher and evaluator health promotion

Nurse as a Direct Care Provider

Nurse as a direct care provider provide curative service at clinic camp in the home also provide emergency service first aid during disaster. The care should be client as the center of care using community involvement approaches. As a direct care provider, she can provide maternal and child healthcare, i.e., antenatal care delivery care, postnatal care, managing complication during pregnancy, delivery or postnatal period. In home or clinic she is providing direct care to the people who are sick or ill. She will assist in the arranging of, and participate in specialty clinics with physician specialists or other health care provider whenever needed and maintain client and administrative records following professional and legal guidelines in a confidential, concise and accurate manner. Assist patients to achieve their optimum level of health in situation of normal health, illness, injury, or through the process of dying. Assess the patient for physical and psychological needs, knowledge of their health, disease process and learning needs during giving care. Apply and promote principles of equity and fairness to assist patients in receiving unbiased treatment and a share of health services and resources proportionate to their needs.

Nurse as a Teacher and Educator

Nurse as a teacher and educator should not miss any opportunity to provide health education. As primary health care main focusing preventive approach rather than curative approach the nurse can use health education as a weapon to achieve her goals. Provide counseling during any personal or family problems, teaching patient and family, providing guidance for restoration and maintenance of their health. She can educate the people regarding a safe and healthy environment in homes, schools and throughout the community. Not only this in every home visit she can educate the pupil regarding existing health problems and methods of preventing and controlling them MCH and family planning hygiene, proper nutrition safe water and basic sanitation prevention of common communicable diseases.

Nurse as a Supervisor and Manager

Supervision is a process by which the supervisor is in constant daily touch with the operation, teach and motivate the subordinates to achieve the objectives hold the key to effective direction of human beings. Through the influence of the supervisor on work environment and their adoption of wholesome attitudes, can tremendously contribute towards enlisting the full support and collaboration of employees. In providing primary health care the community health nurse can supervise ASHA or AWW or other co-worker to achieve the goal of MDG like reduction IMR, MMR, and TFR (total fertility rate), etc.

Nurse as a Researcher and Evaluator Health Promotion

The nurse can act as a researcher by identifying unsolvable problems of the people and try to solve them through scientific research process. The researcher's role is an integral part of the CHN practice. The nurse in providing primary health care can act as a researcher to determine needs, evaluate effectiveness of care and develop theoretical basis for CHN. As a evaluator she evaluates the effectiveness of care provided to individuals, families and groups. She also evaluates the effectiveness of the services in the health programs in special settings.

Community health nursing has evolved into a focus on care of individuals families and communities. The focus and orientation are different to other nurses in their work areas. CHN is a specific and specialized orientation to the care that embodies principles of public health as guiding concepts. Primary health care is one aspect of CHN. CHN focuses on the physical, biological, social, psychological and environmental health of a population group while primary care is a coordinated system of personal health care, emphasizing first contact care and continuously. Primary care emphasizes ambulatory care that addresses total client needs both for curative an preventive services but is population based.

COMPREHENSIVE PRIMARY HEALTH CARE

In 1978, at an international conference convened by the World Health Organization (WHO) and UNICEF (United Nations Children's Fund) in Kazakhstan, the 134 members of the World Health Assembly of World Health Organization ratified the Declaration of Alma-Ata (World Health Organization, 1978). The declaration committed member states to supporting Primary Health Care (PHC) as a policy to achieve the WHO definition of health as a "state of complete physical, mental and social well-being and not merely the absence of disease or infirmity" (WHO, 2006A).

The declaration's lack of concrete guidelines resulted in an attempt by the recognized authorities in the health field to give some shape and form to the concept of Primary Health Care to lead to a definition for global health policy. The Alma-Ata declaration defined eight elements of PHC (World Health Organization), however, no guidance on how to pursue these elements was provided. In an article in the prestigious New England Journal of Medicine, Julia Walsh and Kenneth Warren, who was then the director of health sciences at the Rockefeller Foundation, stated that though the vision and values of PHC were unquestionable, translating policy into practice needed refining. They put forward the concept of "selective primary health care" (SPHC) focusing on implementing policy for the diseases that had the highest prevalence and morbidity, highest risk of mortality, and greatest possibility of control in terms of the cost and effectiveness of the intervention. The advantages of selective PHC include: a rational, cost-effective way to prioritize disease problems; narrow scope, making it affordable for developing countries; and readily detectable results in the short-term. Rejecting an interpretation of health as holistic and reflective of social justice and social determinants, SPHC put forward a view of health as dependent on vertical delivery of health services. It challenged the alternative "comprehensive Primary Health Care" (CPHC) approaches to health improvements, which included community participation, intersectoral collaboration, and appropriate technology. While WHO struggled with how to pursue a holistic approach to health, the cosponsor of the Alma-Ata conference, UNICEF, chose to focus on specific interventions, referenced by the acronym GOBI-FFF (Growth Monitoring, Oral Rehydration, Breast Feeding, Immunizations, Family Planning, Female Literacy, and Food Technology; United Nations Children's Fund, 2016). The Child Survival Revolution, the umbrella for GOBI, was considered a Selective Primary Health Care (SPHC) approach. It focused on maternal and child health and ignored the health of the wider population, including males and seniors. The debate over SPHC versus CPHC became a consistent theme in translating PHC into practice.

The National Health Policy, 2017 recommended strengthening the delivery of Primary Health Care, through establishment of "Health and Wellness Centers" in place of subcenters and PHCs as the platform to deliver comprehensive primary health care (CPHC) and policies called for a commitment of two thirds of the health budget to primary health care. Keeping view on this in February 2018, the Government of India declared that 1,50,000 Health and Wellness Centers (HWCs) would be created by transforming existing subhealth centers and primary health centers to deliver CPHC and declared this as one of the components (between two) of Ayushman Bharat. This was the first step in the conversion of policy articulations to a budgetary commitment. Based on the Report of the Primary Health Care Task Force, Ministry of Health and Family Welfare, Government of India, while reiterating that as primary health care is the only affordable and effective path for India to universal health coverage, it is also required to provide valuable insights to structure and processes required health systems which will enable to provide Comprehensive Primary Health Care (CPHC). It was also decided to construct health wellness center for delivering CPHC. The delivery of CPHC through HWCs rests substantially on the institutional mechanisms, governance structures, and systems created under the National Health Mission (NHM). NHM, as part of health system reform in the country, in its nearly 12 years of implementation, has supported states to create several platforms for delivery of community-based health systems, expanding human resources for health and infrastructure towards strengthening primary and secondary care. Though largely limited to a few conditions, NHM created mechanisms for expanded coverage and reach, and developed systems for improved delivery of medicines, diagnostics and improved reporting. About five years ago, these components were also introduced in urban areas. Thus, although the delivery of universal CPHC, through HWCs builds on existing systems, it will need change management and systems design at various levels, to realize its full potential. The other component of Ayushman Bharat, namely the Pradhan Mantri Jan Arogya Yojana (PMJAY) aims to provide financial protection for secondary and tertiary care to about 40% of India's households. Its success and affordability rests substantially on the effectiveness of provision of CPHC through HWCs. Together, the two components of Ayushman Bharat will enable the realization of the aspiration for universal health coverage.

Primary Health Care to Comprehensive Primary Health Care

- Currently the primary health Care is selective: Limited to RCH and communicable diseases—addresses about 20% of healthcare needs.

- Low utilization of public health facilities—NSSO data (71st round): 28% in rural areas and 21% in urban areas sought care in the public sector; of which only 11% and 3% respectively sought any form of care at a level below the CHC (other than child birth related services).
- Health care is fragmented—disrupts continuity of care and impacts on clinical outcomes and leads to high out-of-pocket (OOP).
- High costs are incurred because of lack of gate keeping function—raises the load on secondary and tertiary facilities and compromises quality.
- Epidemiologic transition: Death from the four major NCDs—cancer, CVD, diabetes, and respiratory diseases accounts for nearly 62% of all mortality among men and 52% among women—of which 56% is premature.
- Unfinished agenda of RCH and communicable diseases:
  - Persistent challenge—high levels of maternal and child mortality with inter and intrastate variations
  - High TFR: States of Bihar, Uttar Pradesh, Rajasthan, Madhya Pradesh, Jharkhand and Chhattisgarh (56% of India's population increase)
  - High proportion of underweight children—38% children under five are stunted and 36% continue to have low weight for age.
  - Challenge of communicable diseases: Tuberculosis including multidrug-resistant TB (MDR TB), hepatitis and rising burden of dengue, chikungunya

Challenges to CPHC and Design Principles

• Selective primary health care: limited to RCH/few infectious diseases; not in consonance with changes in demography and disease burden • Growing burden of NCDs—62% of mortality due to NCDs; 55% is premature, requires prevention, early detection, and long- term follow up	• Provision of 12 essential PHC packages • Prioritize universal screening and management of common noncommunicable diseases: Leverage NPCDCS • Transform subcenters/PHC to Health and Wellness centers by increasing human and financial resources to increase footfalls—close to community
• Low use of primary health care facilities: 11% of people in rural areas and 3% in urban areas, reported seeking care below CHC • Only 8% of outpatient care is provided by primary care facilities in public sector • Fragmented care: Increases burden on secondary and tertiary facilities: compromises quality • Exclusion and marginalization	• Increase in service package, backed by availability of drugs for chronic diseases and point of care diagnostics will enable increased use of ambulatory care • Develop referral protocols, and IT solutions to strengthen continuum of care • Population enumeration and registration: learning from MCTS

Development of Guidelines

Guidelines have been developed after consultation with policy makers and practitioners at national and state level and with technical experts. It also draws on implementation experiences of government, NGO and private sector in the delivery of primary health care. These guidelines are developed to serve as a framework for operationalizing the multiple components required for the delivery of CPHC services through the Health and Wellness Centers. These guidelines are anticipated to support programme managers at state and district levels in rolling out CPHC. This guideline provide an overview of the systems requirements and strategies for change management to deliver CPHC. The use of these guidelines would enable the states to put in place the necessary design elements and subsystems required for Health and Wellness Centers to be created and deliver the health services expected of them. However, states have the flexibility to make necessary modifications based on their specific needs and capacities. The implementation of CPHC would require substantial change management in processes for planning, service delivery, monitoring and financing and will require the active participation of several stakeholders including civil society, NGOs, academic and research agencies development partners, the private sector and the community. Operationalizing HWCs will be incremental in nature with contextual variations in models and processes evolving in different states. These guidelines highlight areas in which transformation and change management is needed, besides clarifying key concepts related to CPHC and Health and Wellness Centers. These guidelines are envisaged to be reviewed periodically and revised based on implementation lessons from the field so that they continue to provide meaningful and updated guidance to programme implementers and inform policy adaptation and modification.

Development of Health-wellness Center

In order to ensure delivery of CPHC services, existing subhealth centers which is only manned by one HWM and one HWF covering a population of 3,000–5,000 would be converted to Health and Wellness Centers (HWC), with the principle being "time to care" to be no more than 30 minutes. Primary health centers in rural and urban areas would also be converted to HWCs. Similarly, in the urban context, the Urban Primary Health Centers would be strengthened as HWCs to deliver CPHC. The norm of One MPW-(F) per 10,000 population supported by four to five ASHAs, will enable outreach services, preventive and promotive care and home and community-based services. Therefore, in the urban context, the team of MPWs (F) and ASHAs would be considered equivalent to a front-line provider team with the first point of referral being the UPHC catering to about at 50,000 population.

Key Principles of Health and Wellness Centers for Provision of Comprehensive Primary Health Care

1. Transform existing subhealth centers and primary health centers to HWCs to ensure universal access to an expanded range of CPHC services.
2. Ensure a people centered, holistic, equity sensitive response to people's health needs through a process of

population empanelment, regular home and community interactions and people's participation.

3. Enable delivery of high quality care that spans health risks and disease conditions through a commensurate expansion in availability of medicines and diagnostics, use of standard treatment and referral protocols and advanced technologies including IT systems.
4. Instill the culture of a team-based approach to delivery of quality health care encompassing: preventive, promotive, curative, rehabilitative and palliative care.
5. Ensure continuity of care with a two way referral system and follow up support.
6. Emphasize health promotion (including through school education and individual centric awareness) and promote public health action through active engagement and capacity building of community platforms and individual volunteers.
7. Implement appropriate mechanisms for flexible financing, including performance-based incentives and responsive resource allocations.
8. Enable the integration of Yoga and AYUSH as appropriate to people's needs.
9. Facilitate the use of appropriate technology for improving access to healthcare advice and treatment initiation, enable reporting and recording, eventually progressing to electronic records for individuals and families.
10. Institutionalize participation of civil society for social accountability.
11. Partner with not for profit agencies and private sector for gap filling in a range of primary health care functions.
12. Facilitate systematic learning and sharing to enable feedback, and improvements and identify innovations for scale up.
13. Develop strong measurement systems to build accountability for improved performance on measures that matter to people.

All the key principles of HWCs indicated above will be applicable to PHCs in urban areas. Initial action for upgrading UPHCs to HWCs would require capacity building of staff and field functionaries in the expanded range of services. Population enumeration, empanelment, disease screening would also be required. In many cities, where specialists' consultation is currently being made available through evening OPDs on prefixed days, these could be leveraged as a strategy for ensuring continuity of care. However, states are free to undertake modifications that best fit their contexts.

Key Elements of Comprehensive Primary Health Care through Health and Wellness Centers (Fig. 1.12)

The H and WC would provide preventive, promotive, rehabilitative and curative care for RMNCH+A, communicable diseases, noncommunicable diseases, ophthalmology, ENT, dental, mental, geriatric care, palliative care, treatment for acute simple medical conditions and emergency and trauma services. Of these services, several are already being provided through the NHM.

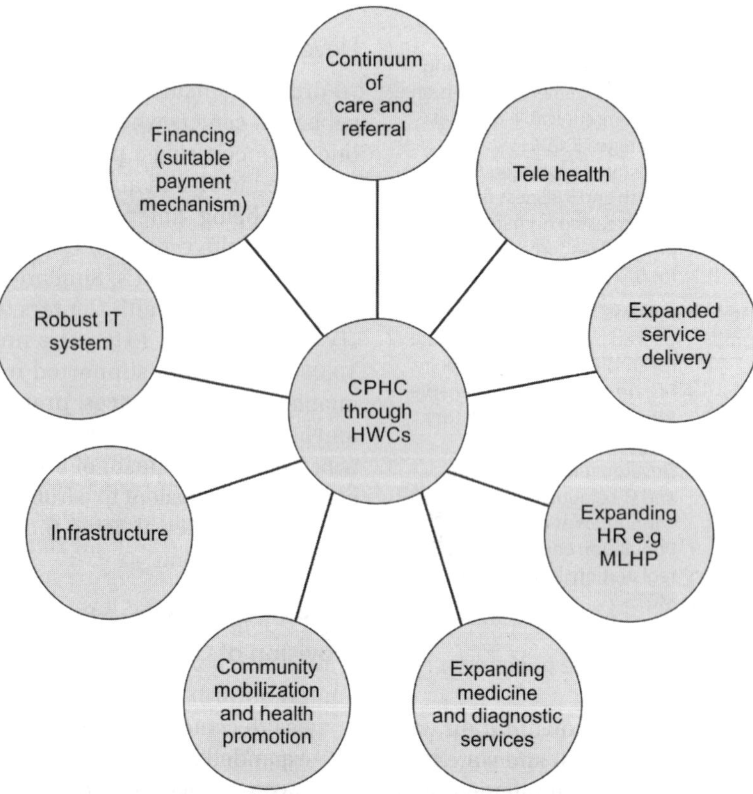

Fig. 1.12: Key elements of CPHC through HWCs.

- **Expanded service delivery:** HWCs enable the expansion of the package of services that go beyond maternal and child health to include care for non-communicable diseases, palliative and rehabilitative care, oral, eye and ENT care, mental health and first level care for emergencies and trauma. The services envisaged at the HWC level will include early identification, basic management, counseling, ensuring treatment adherence, follow up care, ensuing continuity of care by appropriate referrals, optimal home and community follow up, and health promotion and prevention for the expanded range of services. The primary health care team led by the mid level health provider would be trained to provide first level of management and triage, i.e., refer the patient to the appropriate health facility for treatment and follow up. Care provision at every level would be provided as per clinical pathways and standard treatment guidelines. Delivery of an expanded range of services, closer to the community at HWCs would require reorganization of the existing workflow processes. The delivery of services would be at three levels, i.e., (i) family/household and community levels, (ii) HWCs and (iii) and referral facilities/sites. Delivery of services closer to the community and close monitoring would enable increased coverage and help in addressing issues of marginalization and exclusion of specific population groups.
- **Continuum of Care-Tele-health and referral:** The delivery of comprehensive primary health care through HWCs envisages a gatekeeping function, and a two-way referral system—that links to secondary and tertiary care and also follow up care. At all levels, teleconsultation are being done to improve referral advice, seek clarifications, and undertake virtual training including case management support by specialists. Continuum of care spans for the individuals from the same facility to her/his home and community, and across levels of care—primary, secondary and tertiary. Care must be ensured from the level of the family through the facility level.
- **Community/household:** The ASHA would undertake home visits to ensure that the patient is taking actions for risk factor modification, provides counseling and support, including reminders for follow up appointments at HWC and collection of medicines.
- **Health and Wellness Centers (HWC):** Dispensation of medicines, repeat diagnostics as required, identification of complications and facilitating referrals at a higher-level facility/teleconsultation with a specialist as required are undertaken at the HWC, including maintenance of records. The last activity would enable HWC team to identify stable patients, and to organize community level supportive activities to improve adherence to care protocols and reduction of exposure to risk factors. The referring HWC uses a clear referral format to provide information on reason for referral and care already being provided and other details as necessary (especially on insurance coverage). The referring HWC also ensures that the appropriate specialists are available in that facility and to the extent possible, facilitate the referral appointment.
- **Higher-level facility:** The referred medical officer or specialists would examine the patient and develop/modify the treatment plan, including instructions for the patient as well as a note to the HWC provider, indicating the need for change. Systems need to be in place so that a medicine prescribed by a specialist is made available to the patient at the HWC where she/he is empaneled. Periodic meetings (whether in person or through virtual platforms) between HWC team and the specialists/medical officers referred to, are also essential to ensure that they all function as one team and ensure care continuum.
- **Developing referral linkages:** In effect, every existing HWC providing the expanded range of services, would manage the largest proportion of disease conditions and organize referral for consultation and follow up with an MBBS doctor at the linked Primary Health Center-HWC, (one per 30,000 population/20000 in hilly areas) that would also provide a similar set of services as the subcenter HWC, but of a higher order of complexity. The Block PHCs and CHCs would now need to provide referral services beyond emergency obstetric care, to include general medical and specialist consultation. Strengthening of health facilities as FRUs and first level of hospitalization would need to be done in a phased manner based on the availability of infrastructure, equipment and Human Resources for Health at the identified health facilities. For example, cases of acute simple illness need not be referred to DH/FRU but can be handled at PHC itself. On the other hand, high-risk pregnancy, sick newborn, care for serious mental health ailments may be referred directly to a District Hospital.
- **Expanding HR–CHO and multiskilling:** A new cadre of worker Community Health Officer, trained in competencies of public health and primary health care has been posted at SHC-HWC. The Community Health Officer is expected to improve clinical management, continuum of care, dispensation of drugs and close follow up for those with chronic illness/patients discharged from health facilities. CHO leads the team of multipurpose workers, and ASHAs. All the service providers at HWCs are being trained appropriately to deliver the expanded package of services to the community. Frontline workers, and service providers posted at all levels would also be multiskilled to address the mismatch in the services to be provided and present levels of training of primary care team members. The key principle is that as many skills as possible and appropriate at that level should be available within the team at the HWC, so that the services are assured to the population and the team is able to resolve more at their level including through telehealth with fewer referrals.
- **Medicines and expanding diagnostics:** Adequate availability of essential medicines and diagnostics enable medicine dispensation and necessary tests close to community. A total of 105 free and essential medicines

at HWC-SHC and 172 medicines at HWC-PHC; and 14 diagnostic tests at HWC-SHC and 63 at HWC-PHCs are available for the community. Diagnostic services as per the Guidelines for National Free Diagnostic Initiative need to be available at HWC (SHC-7 and PHC-19 investigations). In addition, a peak flow meter and Snellen's and near vision chart are recommended for inclusion at SHC-HWCs
- **Community mobilization and health promotion:** Health promotion and information provision at the community level is an integral part of the expanded range of services under CPHC. Health is affected by various social and environmental determinants and actions to address these issues often do not fall in the purview of health systems alone and therefore requires intersectoral convergence and people's participation. Health promotion at HWCs is facilitated through engagement of community level collectives such as: VHSNCs, MAS and SHGs. Community mobilization, for action on social and environmental determinants, build on the accountability initiatives under NHM ensure that there is no denial of health care and universality and equity are respected. For action on social and environmental determinants, would require intersectoral convergence and build on the accountability initiatives under NHM so that there is no denial of health care and universality and equity are respected. As envisioned in the policy, States should plan for a coordinated action on seven priority areas for improving the environment for health as part of CPHC:
  - The Swachh Bharat Abhiyan.
  - Balanced, healthy diets and regular exercises.
  - Addressing tobacco, alcohol and substance abuse.
  - Yatri Suraksha—preventing deaths due to rail and road traffic accidents.
  - Nirbhaya Nari—action against gender violence.
  - Reduced stress and improved safety in the work place.
  - Reducing indoor and outdoor air pollution

Infrastructure for Health and Wellness Centers

Ensuring adequate infrastructure for the delivery of CPHC and HWCs would need to cater to a population size as per IPHS norms for subhealth centers—one per 5,000 population in all areas and one per 3,000 in tribal, hilly and desert areas. Where currently subcenters are catering to much larger population, their numbers need to be increased. Essential requirements for strengthening a SHC to serve as a HWCs are:
- A well-ventilated clinic room with examination space and office space for Midlevel Health Provider/Community Health Officer.
- Storage space for storing medicines, equipment, documents, health cards and registers.
- Designated space for laboratory/diagnostic.
- Separate male and female toilets.
- Deep burial pit for biomedical waste management.
- Proper system for drainage.
- Assured water supply that can be drawn and stored locally.
- Electricity supply linked to main lines or adequate solar source, inverter or back-up generator as appropriate.
- Patient waiting area covered to accommodate at least 20–25 chairs.
- Repairs of roofs and walls, plastering, painting and tiling of floors to be undertaken as per requirement.
- Space/room for Yoga if adequate space for expansion is available.
- Adequate residential facilities for the service providers.
- Rain water harvesting facilities may be planned if required.
- Once the numbers of SHC to be upgraded as HWCs are final the identified blocks will need to systematically map SHCs: with and without buildings.
- For a PHC-HWC, infrastructure would be as per current Indian Public Health Standards.

Robust IT system: HWC team are equipped with IT equipment—Tablets at SCs and Laptop/Desktop at PHC level to create electronic health record of the population covered by HWCs. Developing a robust IT system will support HWC team to track patients for treatment adherence and follow up. The key functions of the IT system are:
- Registration individuals and families
- Record all services that are delivered at the HWC under different programs.
- Enable follow up of services that individual patients are receiving by recording relevant parameters, diagnostic results, medication given, etc.
- Facilitate clinical decision making for the service providers (based on standard treatment protocols).
- Track and support upward and downward referrals to support continuity of care.
- Ability to print key summary and prescription based on individual's requirement.
- Ability to provide standardized prescription, discharge summary and/or referral note which can be scanned/photographed or printed and uploaded as per requirement.
- Capture, store and transmit images to support teleconsultation, referral and follow up.
- Support inventory management and regular supply of medicines, vaccines and consumables by linking with Drug Vaccine Distribution and Management System (DVDMS).
- Used for reporting and monitoring and teleconsultation

Service Packages

- Care in pregnancy and child birth.
- Neonatal and infant health care services
- Childhood and adolescent healthcare services
- Family planning, contraceptive services and other reproductive healthcare services
- Management of communicable diseases: National health programs
- General out-patient care for acute simple illnesses and minor ailments
- Screening, prevention, control and management of noncommunicable diseases

- Care for common ophthalmic and ENT problems
- Basic oral health care
- Elderly and palliative healthcare services
- Emergency medical services including burns and trauma
- Screening and basic management of mental health ailment

Organization of Comprehensive Primary Health Care

The service delivery including preventive, promotive, curative, rehabilitative health care has been organized at three levels, i.e., family/household and community levels through outreach OPDs, Health Mela, Village Panchayat, Village and Home Visits, School and Anganwadi visits, at HWCs by midlevel healthcare providers and MPWs and at first Referral Facilities sites like general medical consultation at PHC/UPHC, specialist consultation and first level of hospitalization at CHC/SDH/DH. Each service package is delivered at different levels in different ways for ex. At community level pregnancy can be diagnosed by ASHA or AWW which will be registered in HWC. Similarly follow up to ensure compliance with IFA in normal and anemic cases will be managed at village level but screening, referral and follow up care in cases of gestational diabetes and syphilis during pregnancy will be done at SHCs level and surgical interventions like cesarean section will be managed at FRU level. In prevention, screening and management of noncommunicable diseases service. Health promotion activities like to promote healthy lifestyle and address risk factors will be educated and guided by village level workers like ASHAs and AWWs and diagnosis and management of occupational diseases such as silicosis, fluorosis and respiratory disorders will be taken care at the referral site.

COMMUNITY HEALTH NURSING PROCESS

The nursing process is the framework for providing professional, quality nursing care. It directs nursing activities for health promotion, health protection, and disease prevention and is used by nurses in every practice setting and specialty. 'The nursing process provides the basis for critical thinking in nursing'. The nursing process is dynamic and requires creativity for its application. The steps remain the same, but the application and results will be different in each client situation. It can be applied to individual family and community. Based on its application in hospital and community it is classified as Individualized nursing process, family health nursing process and CHN process. Though the same steps of nursing process (assessment, nursing diagnosis, planning, implementation and evaluation) can be followed at each level (individual, family and community) but there is a vast difference between the institutional level and community level of nursing process. The steps of family health nursing process and CHN process are same but the main variation is in nursing diagnosis.

Community is the client or target of service in CHN practice. The focus is on the health of community at larger rather than an individual or family health. The community directly influences the health of individuals, families, groups, subpopulations, and populations who are a part of it. The individual's families are the units of services. The services are rendered not only to any specific individual families but to the whole community. For example, for eradication of malaria we are changing the whole environment of the community, provision of most health services occurs at the community level. Community agencies help develop specific health programs and disseminate health information to many types of groups and populations. In community the community health nurse gives care to the whole community not particular individual or group. The services pertaining to primary, secondary and tertiary level of prevention are rendered to entire community and not to any selected individuals/families or groups in the community.

Definitions

- **Nursing process:** Nursing process generally defined as a designated series of actions intended to fulfill the purposes of nursing to maintain the patient's wellness and, if this state changes, to provide the amount and quality of nursing care the situation demands to direct the patient back to wellness, and if wellness cannot be achieved, then contribute to the patient's quality of life, maximizing his resources as long as the life is a reality.'
- **Community health nursing process:** It is a problem-solving process that addresses community health problems at every aggregate level with the goals of preventing illness and promoting public health.

It is a management process that requires situational analysis, decision-making, planning, organization, direction and control of services, and outcome evaluation.

It is a process for implementing changes that improve the function of various health-related systems and the ways that people behave within those systems.

Community health nurse, must consider community as the client. Understanding of the community is a prerequisite for providing effective services to the community as the client. Community identification is the first phases of community assessment. Through community identification the community health nurse can assess the size of the population, density of the population, composition of the population, rate of growth or decline, cultural characteristics, social class and educational level mobility pattern of the population.

Community identification is the beginning of community health and nursing care process. It refers to 1st level 'Assessment Phase'. This phase is fundamental to 'Planning of Community Health Actions' which is followed by 'Implementation of Plan' and 'Evaluation of Actions and Outcomes'. Altogether there are four phases of the CHN practice process which have been discussed.

Steps of CHN Process

The nursing process is a series of steps or acts that lead to accomplishment of some goal or purpose. The purpose of the nursing process is to provide care for clients that is individualized, holistic, effective, and efficient but in CHN process the whole community is an individual. The steps of the nursing process are same like general nursing process which build upon each other, but they are not linear. There is overlap of each step with the previous and subsequent steps.

Assessment phase	Community identification	Date review and update
1st level	• Planning of data collection; categories of information • Method and techniques • Data collection • Data analysis • Community profile and diagnosis	
Planning phase	**Community health planning**	**Review/ revise**
2nd level assessment	• Analyzing health problems • Establishing priorities • Setting goals and objectives • Formulating community health actions	Goals and objectives and actions
Action phase	**Implement actions plan**	
	• Considering nursing interventions • Review and revise if needed • Mobilization of resources—health facilitating working environment • Implementing and documentation	
Evaluation phase	**Evaluation**	
	• Concurrent quantitative • Terminal qualitative	

Community Identification (Assessment Phase)

Definition

A community assessment is basically a description of a community and its people. The purpose is to identify the needs of a community in order to provide services appropriate to those needs. Community identification refers to 'systematic process of knowing and exploring the defined community for assessing its health status and determining the possible factors affecting the health of people in the community.'

It helps to know all the three dimensions of community, i.e., geographical area, the people and the social system and also helps to identify determinants of community health (biological characteristics of people, their lifestyle, the environment in which they live and the resources available to them) which affect their health. Community identification is the first step of CHN practice process and it is also otherwise termed as the first level of assessment or initial assessment.

Benefits of Community Identification

- **Provides comprehensive knowledge about the profile of the community:** Community identification provides information about health status of community, its health problems and the factors that interfere to their health. These information form the baseline date for planning community health services and determining their effectiveness.
- **Helps to develop good working relationship with the community:** Community identification provides opportunity for establishing working relationship and gaining acceptance of the community. The community health nurse is a part of healthcare system. Some of the people may not accept this system or some of its health services. So the community health nurse should work in coordination with various formal and informal leader in the community for implementation of healthcare activities. She talks to them about her functions and explains to them about her willingness to help in meeting their health needs/health problems as perceived by them. Hence she gain entry in the community and be accepted by the leaders and people.
- **Make community diagnosis:** This is a statement that defines the health strength, health problems or health risks of the community. The community health nurse arrange and analyze the collected data and make community diagnosis and organize community development programs. The problems could be with reference to people, their environment, lifestyle and resources. For example, inadequate ANC r/t inadequate health information or service accessibility as evidenced by 70% of female delivering at hospital with no antenatal care.
- **Designing community health actions plan:** Community identification act as an instrument for community health planning. Community identification forms community diagnosis which forms the basis for designing community health actions plan according to priorities and goals and objectives and available resources/health services.
- **Promotes community participation:** Community identification improves community participation. It gives an opportunity to mix with people and the leaders informally and meet them formally. As we mix and meet with the people and leaders, we come to know each other, get informed about each other's intentions and expectations, strengths and weaknesses, etc. This will help not only in developing confidence, trust and faith in each other's abilities but also help in communicating people's contributions in dealing with their health needs/health problems individually and unitedly.

The other benefits are:

- There is increased understanding within the community about its needs, why they exist, and why it is important for the needs to be addressed.
- Community members have the opportunity to share how the needs impact the quality of life for the larger community.
- Community engagement is increased because members from different parts of the community are included in discussions about needs, assets, and the community's response.
- The community's strengths and weaknesses are identified.

- There is an inventory of the resources currently available within the community that can be leveraged to improve the quality of life for community members.
- Communities identify the asset gaps that exist in their communities.
- Community members have an increased awareness of how they can contribute to their community's assets.
- Community organizations can use the information about community needs to assess their service delivery priorities.
- There is data for making decisions about the actions that can be taken to address community needs and how to use the available assets.
- Data can be used to inform strategic planning, priority setting, program outcomes, and program improvements.

Planning of Data Collection

Before data collection understanding the community is very important in CHN process. Understanding the community means what a community is, and the specific nature of the communities we work in. Anything we do in a community requires us to be familiar with its people, its issues, and its history. Carrying out an intervention or building a coalition is far more likely to be successful if they are informed by the culture of the community and an understanding of the relationships among individuals and groups within. Understanding the community entails understanding it in a number of ways. Whether or not the community is defined geographically, it still has a geographic context, a setting that it exists in. Getting a clear sense of this setting may be key to a full understanding of it. At the same time, it's important as a community health nurse to understand the specific community she is concerned with.

After understanding the community, the community health nurse will plan to collect the data by deciding what type of data will be collect, where to collect data, what are the major source of information. It is impossible for a community health nurse to get all the information from a single source or one method. Therefore different methods will be used to collect data from different source. For collecting data establishing working relationship is very essential.

Establishing Working Relationship

Building and sustaining relationships are at the heart of organizing community development program. The strength of community lies in the strength of the connections that we have with each other. With strong connections, people have the power to make real change. Building these connections takes time. But it is worth it.

A working relationship makes the client and nurse to know each other and work together, by this the problems can be easily identified and solved. Community involvement is the main aspect of community care for that a good trusting working relationship is essential. It promote the acceptance and interest by the client to accept things and also asking questions. Some tips to develop good interpersonal relationship are as follows:

- **Be friendly and tactful:** A community health nurse should be friendly with the community people for developing working relationship. She should have a smiling face and tactfully she should try to develop good IPR.
- **Ask people to questions:** People love to talk about them and about what they think. If a community health nurse ask people about themselves and then take time to listen attentively, they can become her fast friend.
- **Tell people about yourself:** People will not trust you unless you are willing to trust them. Tell them what you genuinely care about and what you think. Explain the benefits of your care.
- **Accept people the way they are:** Before going to modify their behavior we should be accept them the way they are. If they are doing wrong also first we should be non-judgmental.
- **Overcome your fear of rejection:** Before development of trust among community people the chance of rejection is more. A CHN should be mentally prepared for that and plan how to overcome it and develop trust among community people.
- **Be persistent:** People are often shy and suspicious. It takes a while to win trust. A health worker can almost always form a relationship if he/she stick with it.
- **Invite people to involved:** During organizing any community development program more participation from the people should be initiated. The CHN should encourage more involvement of the people by which the program will be fruitful.
- **Learn about the person's culture:** Learning about the person's culture is very much essential because for providing comprehensive care not only learning about the person's culture is sufficient. The CHN should put herself at the center of another person's culture for developing a strong IPR.
- **Hang in there even if you feel rejected:** It means sometimes people do not accept us and trust us. In that case we should not lose our hope and we will stick with them to make them understanding even if we feels rejected also.

The community assessment is required at all levels of its geographical organization and setup, because assessment and planning of health services are necessary at each level. According to the definition of community, a community can be very small as like small helmet or as large as the state, country, etc. Republic of India has a federal structure consisting of 30 states and 7 union territories. Each state and union territory has a number of districts. Each district is organized into a number of blocks depending upon the population and the area coverage. Altogether there are 466 districts and 6000 blocks. Each block has 80–100 villages and a population of 80,000–1,00,000 or even more in some places.

Categories of Informations Required

For community identification a variety of information required like geographical characteristics, population composition, environmental and social factors. Community organization, communication pattern, etc. The information needs to be collected for community assessment are described below. A community health nurse should have detail idea about her community.

Geographical Characteristics

Every physical community carries out its existence in a specific geographic location. The health of a community is affected by this location including the placement of health services, the geographic features, plants, animals and animals and the human made environment.

- **Geographical area:** Every community has a defined geographical area in which people live and carry out their existence. It is very important for the community health nurse to study and familiar with the topography of any community which includes the study of its location and geographical boundaries; physical setup, natural resources such as land area, forest and jungles, minerals, water; important landmarks, important institutions, etc. The geographical area only does not reflects, geographical location and geographical boundaries physical setup, etc., but also it depicts the followings:
  - Levels of population density in different parts of a city
  - Where different ethnic or racial groups are concentrated
  - Income levels in different areas
  - Increases in housing starts for various areas
  - Current ranges of endangered species
  - The frequency of particular diseases or conditions in various regions, towns, neighborhoods, or even city blocks
  - The proportion of children under 18 in different school districts.
- **Geographical location/boundary of a community:** Geographical location of a community determines its climate, resources, health threats and dangers, e.g., communities in the mountain areas in the Northern India will be entirely different from communities in Southern India. The most obvious type of geographical boundary is a physical boundary which is a naturally occurring barrier between two areas. Rivers, mountain ranges, oceans, and deserts can all serve as physical boundaries.

  The incidence and prevalence of various diseases, mortality and morbidity of a community is measured and compared with other community locally, nationally or internationally and sometimes with whole world, which determines health action to be taken for the community.
- **Physical setup:** Each community has its own physical setup which includes pattern of settlement, arrangements of dwellings and other buildings, streets, connecting roads, important landmarks and institutions, etc. It is important to know the community's size, its topography (the lay of the land– the hills, valleys, rivers, roads, and other features you would find on a map), and each of its neighborhoods. Also you would important are how various areas of the community differ from one another, and the CHN should assess whether the community is one of clean, well-maintained houses and streets, or one of shabbiness, dirt, and neglect.

  The physical setup of a town is differ from the physical setup of a village. If it is a city or a town, the community health nurse have to see whether the facilities of the town are sufficient to meet their need, town is properly planned, housing structure, overcrowding, drainage facility, water supply and presence of industries, etc. If it is a village, the CHN should have to find out the arrangement of houses, the type of houses, facilities available, whether the village is self-sufficient in fulfilling the basic needs of the people or not.

  The pattern of settlement and arrangement of dwellings and the basic amenities available will influence the environment and the lifestyle of the people which will have an impact on the health status of the community. The people of urban community are exposed to stress, overcrowding, pollution, development of slum beggary, poverty, crime, prostitution, delinquency, alcoholism, air and water-borne diseases, etc., in the other hand in rural community they are exposed to agricultural environment, lack of electricity and potable water facility. So the community health nurse must study the physical setup, boundaries, draw a map of a community and identify factors that influences their health status influences on the health status of the people.
- **The natural resources:** Natural resources are also very important to the economy of a community. A natural resource is anything that people can use which comes from nature. People do not make natural resources, but gather them from the earth. They are useful raw materials that we get from the Earth. We use and modify natural resources in ways that are beneficial to us. Different communities around the world use the natural resources around them to make their lives better. Natural resources are trees, minerals, water, and animals. Without them, we would have no food, clothing, or shelter.

  Land area (cultivable and noncultivable) determines the bulk of crops and types of crops as a source for self-consumption and for generating income which is sufficient or not.

  Water is the most important natural resource and is vital for life. The CHN has to see that the water should be safe and potable because there are so many water-borne diseases are there.

  Flora and fauna: Poisonous plants and disease carrying animals can affect community health.

  Forests, jungles and animals: Plays very important role in maintenance of ecosystem.

  Minerals are good source of income for the community. So, the community health nurse also have to identify the availability of natural resource in that area which can helps to make solution of so many problems. Natural resources are the foundation from which rural poor people can overcome poverty.
- **Important landmarks and institutions:** It is very important to know the important landmarks and

institutions such as community center, panchayat ghar, school, post office, anganwadi, religious centers, village pond, bank, health center, etc. These places will be helpful in searching and locating the houses, etc.

- **Environmental sanitation:** Environmental sanitation is defined by WHO refers to 'control of all those factors in man's physical environment which exercise or may exercise a deleterious effect on his physical development, health and survival'. It includes control of housing, food, water, refuse and excreta, waste water, air, soil, vectors, insects and rodents, etc. Environmental sanitation is one of the essential measures of healthcare service to promote the health of the people. It is essential for community health nurse to identify factor that alter environmental sanitation which will help her to implement health community health actions.
- **Climate:** Climate has a direct effect on health of a community, e.g., extreme heat and cold.

Population Characteristics

The total number of inhabitants living in a particular geographical area called as population. Population is another very important component of the community which influence there health. Health in the group depends upon the dynamic relationship between the member of people, the space they occupy and the skill that they have acquired in meeting their need. The scientific study of human population is termed as demography. It focuses attention on population size, composition and distribution of population in space. These demographic characteristics of people helps to identify their health problems and needs and helps health planner for selection of health services.

Size

The size of the community refers to the total number of people staying in that community. The size of a population influences the number and size of healthcare institutions and bulk of health services need to be rendered. The smaller the size, the easier it will be to identify cases, trace the source of infection and causes of infection and plan and provide the services and the same will be difficult if the size of the community will be large. Knowing community size provides important information for planning.

Thus it is very important to study the size of the population and its impact on the health of the community.

Density

It refers to number of persons living per square kilometer of area. It is the ratio between total population and surface area. The more the people, the more dense it becomes. For the year 2014 the density of population per square kilometer in India was 394. It is very high especially in towns and cities. The increased population density may increase stress and so many health problems like development of slum, insanity, water and air borne diseases. Similarly when people are spread out healthcare provision may become difficult. The rural areas are much less dense than urban areas which affect allocation of health resources in these areas.

Composition

It refers to distribution of population by age, sex, education and occupation, etc. Understanding of population's composition is very important because it helps in assessing health problems and health needs by different age groups, sex, occupation and education. There may be some common health problems for all the people by virtue of common environmental factors, resources and lifestyle. But, there are specific health problems and health needs of each age group by virtue of their growth and development and physiological status. Health needs and health problems also vary in males and females, more so during various stages of child bearing period in women. A healthy community is one that takes full account of and provides for differences in age, sex, educational level, and occupation of its members, all of which may affect health concerns. Determining a community composition is an important early step in determining its level of health.

Occupation is another variable which influences the health status of people depending upon its nature and risk involved, e.g., industrial occupations, agriculture, managerial occupations, health and science related occupations etc. Education and literacy level is still another variable of population composition which would determine health related attitude, behavior and competency and in turn affect the health status of people.

Vital Events

Some of the vital events which determine community health status are live birth, death, fetal death, marriage, divorce, adoption, legal separation, etc. These are like vital signs of human being as it serves as a reliable source of community health information. Death rates and morbidity rate are the most easily available and accessible indicators which can be used to determine health status of community and plan for services. Morbidity refers to the state of being diseased or unhealthy within a population, In addition to mortality and morbidity statistics, it is important to study the growth in population. Community population changes over time. It changes in size and composition. Some communities grow rapidly and place great demands on the provision of health services whereas some others may grow very slowly or some may even decline because of socioeconomic developments and changes. Any significant change in population can affect the health of community.

Vulnerable/High-risk Groups

Vulnerable population includes the economically disadvantaged, racial and ethnic minorities, children, elderly, homeless person with HIV, those with other chronic conditions like mental illness, one living in abusive family, the homeless, immigrants and refugees. So, it is important to identify high-risk groups in the community as they form the target group for providing health service.

Social Structure

The notion of social structure as relationship between different entities or groups or as enduring and relatively stable pattern of relationship. According to social science, social structure is the patterned social arrangements in society that are both emergent from and determinant of the actions of the individuals. On the macro scale, social structure is the system of socioeconomic stratification (class structure), social institution or other patterned relations between large social group. On the macro scale, it is the structure of social network ties between individuals or organizations. On the micro scale, it can be the way norms shape the behaviors of individuals within the social system. So it include social stratification, social control system, community organization and group dynamics, leadership pattern, sociocultural practices (lifestyle) and communication system. The community health nurses need to study these elements of social structure of the community as it will help to understand attitude, health behavior and health competencies and abilities to deal with health situations. These structural elements are social stratification, social control system, community organization and group dynamics, leadership pattern, lifestyle and communication system which are briefly discussed here.

Social Stratification

Social stratification is a division of society into permanent or temporary groups or categories. The group are interlinked with each other by the relationship of superiority and subordination. Social class is determined on the basis of certain acquired characteristics, e.g., economic condition, individual attainment, wealth and social status, or derived power. Traditionally stratification is done on the basis of caste system. There are four such classes: Brahmins, Kshatriyas, Vaishyas and Shudras. Each caste is governed by certain rules and regulations relating to cultural practices. The caste system is on the basis of occupation and each caste group is supposed to provide specific services to the community.

People also have been grouped into three classes on the basis of income they have. These are upper income, middle income and lower income groups. This can determine standard of life.

It is important for the community health nurse to know the social stratification of community because each social group will have some different health problems, resources to cope with health problems and ways of using health services. In general, people in lower classes have poor health and multihealth problems because of lack of education, poverty and ignorance. Health services are mostly needed by this strata of population but, services should be available to all social groups.

Social Control System

Social control is a concept that refers to the ways in which people's thought, feelings, appearance and behavior are regulated in social systems. It mainly consists of formal and informal rules and regulations. Informal means of control is internalization of norms and values by a process known as socialization, i.e., the process by which an individual born with behavioral potentialities and formal means of social control is by external sanctions which is enforced by government to prevent the establishment of chaos or anomie in society. The social control system may vary from one community to another community and from one social strata to another in the same community. Community health nurse must try to know the social control system as it may be helpful in carrying community health programs.

Community Organization and Group Dynamics

Community organization covers a series of activities at the community level aimed at bringing about desired improvement in the social well-being of individuals, groups and neighborhoods. It is being often used synonymous to community work, community development and community mobilization. Every community has social groups based on a variety of common factors such as culture, beliefs, mores and codes, religion, caste, occupation, political beliefs, functions, common ailments, etc. Each group has a leader members work together under the leadership. Each group has definite goals and objectives and program activities which are taken care of by members working together in the group.

Community health nurse needs to identify such groups in the community, their integrating and disintegrating factors.

Leadership Pattern

For organizing a community health program the community health nurse should organize formal meetings with the leader because by this it will become for a CHN to enter the community easily. So it is very important for a CHN to know the leadership pattern of the allotted community. Leader means not only formal leader like Sarapancha or ward members but also informal member like priest, school teacher, lawyers, doctors or the people who will be accepted and obeyed in the community. They may help in approaching the community, developing and maintaining working relationship with the people, organizing them into working groups, seeking their help and cooperation in dealing with their health needs and health problems and mobilizing community resources, etc.

Lifestyle

Lifestyle is a way of living of individual, families and societies which they manifest in coping with their physical, psychological, social and economic environment on a day to day basis. Lifestyle is expressed in both work and leisure behavior pattern and attitude, opinion, values, beliefs and attitude; religion, education, political and administrative system, socioeconomic status, caste, interest and allocation of income. Lifestyle varies from community to community and sometime from one social strata to another strata in a same community.

Lifestyle has a strong association with health status of people. Healthy lifestyle promotes optimum health. Unhealthy lifestyle and behaviors like smoking, excessive alcohol consumption, misuse of elicit drugs, excess consumption of sugary foods, rituals and taboos during illness, pregnancy, natal and postnatal period alters health. Other factors like social norms, price and legality promotes good lifestyle. Community health nurses need to study the lifestyle of community and identify health practices, unhealthy practices that affect their health.

Communication System

Communication is the process by which ideas, facts, impression, feelings, informations and knowledge facilitate through the process of social interaction. It helps the individual to understand various forms of social relationships and to make necessary adjustments. It moulds personality of individual, fulfills need, exchange information through the process of social interaction and the person develops bondage and leads effective social life. The ultimate aim of communication is to socialize its members, make them knowledgeable, inculcate positive attitude in them and develop behavior which is useful and acceptable by the society.

As a community health nurse, it is very essential to identify their channel of communication (formal and nonformal), common meeting places for the people in the community; informal communicators like barbers, numberdar, etc.; mechanism of communication of cultural heritage, e.g., fairs and festivals, political and religious gatherings, etc. and modern media of communication. The community health nurse can use these communication channels for dissemination of health information and motivation of people for acceptance of healthy behavior.

Sources of Information

These are various sources for attaining information relevant to three dimensions of community.

1. **The sources of information regarding geographical aspects** of the community are maps; local administrative bodies like municipalities, panchayati raj organizations; development department, like block development office, area development committees, school, temple, flora and fauna, minerals, etc.
2. **The source of information relevant to population aspects:** Census, registration of vital events, notifications of diseases, health survey, records of hospitals and health centers, sample registration system (SRS), record linkage, epidemiological surveillance, other health service records, environmental health data, health manpower statistics. The department of health intelligence and annual reports; the epidemiological surveillance and notification records and reports at the local health departments; health service records and reports maintained at the center and other allied agencies if any in the community.
3. **Sources of information about social system are:** Local, political and administrative bodies; local development departments; local directory and organization literature if available; key informants from various systems.

   In addition to these specific sources for each category of information there are common sources for all these categories of information. These include community environment; community people in general and formal and informal leaders in particular; village level workers like birth attendants, village health guides, anganwadi workers; health officials and officials from other organizations, health records and reports.
4. **Community people:** Community people are also a major source of information in all aspect. The can provide information about their lifestyle, customs, culture, environmental data, etc. The data can be collected from them is mainly survey method.

Approach and Methods for Data Collection

Community identification is done by descriptive survey approach. This approach provides broad range of data about all the dimensions of community, community health problems and the associated factors. But it is neither feasible nor advisable to gather all possible data because it is laborious, time-consuming, expensive and is not required. It needs to be planned carefully. There are various methods to get informations about the community. These are as under:

Listening Sessions and Community Forum

Listening sessions are forums used to learn about the community's perspectives on local issues and options. They are generally fairly small, with specific questions asked of participants. The CHN can get a sense of what community members know and feel about the issues, as well as resources, barriers, and possible solutions. Public forums tend to be both larger in number of participants and broader in scope than listening sessions. They are gatherings where citizens discuss important issues at a well-publicized location and time. They give people of diverse backgrounds a chance to express their views, and are also a first step toward understanding the community's needs and resources. A good public forum informs the group of where the community is and where the members would like to go. By this method a CHN can arrange formal and informal meeting with community people, leaders and organized groups which may include panchayat members, school teachers, mahila mandals, youth club/groups, young innovators, traditional leaders, professionals, etc.

The initial meetings need to be organized properly. One needs to spell out the purpose and specific objectives indicating the informations to be sought or issues to be discussed. Invitation should be given ahead of the time in person. Date, time and venue should be fixed which is convenient to all. All the principles of conducting group meetings should be considered. Keep in mind the agency's policies, goals and objectives.

Community forum approach is useful and relatively less expensive method of gathering data.

Observation Method

Observation offers a distinct way of collecting data. It does not rely on what people say they do, or what they say they think. It is more direct than that. Instead, it draws on the direct evidence of the eye to witness events first hand. It is a more natural way of gathering data. Whenever direct observation is possible it is the preferable method to use. Here the CHN gathering data by watching the physical characteristics of community in their natural setting. More over observation is a method of data collection that can be used together either information or characteristics and conditions of individual. This method depends upon nonverbal communication. Observation visits to community can help gain a lot of information about geographical area of the community, environmental sanitation, socioeconomic conditions, population density, population stratification and their interaction, social mobility, etc. These observatory visits can be informal and formal.

Informal visits are done to get familiar with the area, to know its general pattern of setup whereas the formal observation visits are done with specific objectives to attain specific data, e.g., mapping of the area, observation of land area, the natural resources, pattern of settlement, environmental sanitation, health problems, contributing factor and uses of health services, etc. These visits need to be planned, specific objectives need to be outlined and an observation checklist required to be prepared to collect and record information.

Interview

Interviews are an attractive proposition for collection of data. Interviews are something more than conversation. They involve a set of assumptions and understandings about the situation which are not normally associated with a casual conversion. Interviews are also referred as an oral questionnaire by some people. Interview data is collected directly from others in face to face contact. It is a method to elicit needed information by asking relevant questions. In community interviews can be in the form of informal conversation with people; face to face interview of key informants, the entire population, sample population Informal conversation with people can provide many information which can be validated through other methods. A carefully planned conversation can be very useful.

The face to face interview of key informants can provide valuable information about social structure, lifestyle, health problems, health services and allied services. The key informants can be formal and informal leaders and the representatives from social system's organizations and institutions in the community. The interviews can be formal and informal. These interviews need to be planned properly like community forum meetings. Generally the interview method may be structured or unstructured. Structured interview involves fight control over the format of questions and answers. It is like a questionnaire which is administered face to face with a respondent. The researcher has a predetermined list of questions. Each respondent is faced with identical questions. The choice of alternative answers is restricted to a predetermined list. This type of interview is rigidly standardized and formal.

The unstructured interviews are sometimes referred to as 'discovery interviews' and are more like a 'guided conservation' than a strict structured interview. They are sometimes called informal interviews. An interview schedule might not be used, and even if one is used, they will contain open-ended questions that can be asked in any order. The questions can be changed to meet the respondent's intelligence, understandings and beliefs. Hence, the interviewer encourages the respondents to talk freely about given topic with minimum prompting. In this, no preplanned schedule is used. These interviews are also known as non-standardized interview generally this method is used in community setting.

Self-answering questioning is useful for collecting data from a large sample but it is feasible for literate population only. Moreover, the return rate is very less. Hence, it has its limited use in the community health settings.

Physical Examination

Just as physical examination is important to individual patients, so is examination of the community physical environment. Five senses are used in physical assessment: inspection, auscultation, vital signs, system review, and laboratory studies. Inspection uses all sense organs and is done by walking survey in the community, or microassessment of housing, open spaces, boundaries, transportation service centers, markets places, meeting street people, signs of decay, ethnicity, religion, health and morbidity, political media. Auscultation is listening to the community residents about the physical environment. Vital signs can be observed the climate, terrain, natural boundaries such as rivers and hills. Community resources can assessed by looking the signs of life such as notices, posters, new housing and buildings. System review can done on housing age, architecture, building materials used, signs of disrepair, running water, plumbing, sanitation, windows (glasses), etc. Also business facilities and churches. Laboratory studies depicts the census data or planning studies for community mapping.

Record Review Method

It is one of the important means to gather data in short period of time. Data can be gathered from secondary sources like records, documents, and other previously collected information from schools, departments of health at the city and state levels, county data, private foundations, and state universities. Secondary data provides the statistics that are the vital signs of the community. Much of community identification informations such as housing conditions, vital events, morbidity, health services, etc., are available in the records maintained in health agencies. These informations can be collected by record review through the use of record review checklist. Record review checklist needs to be developed based on the informations to be obtained from records.

Conversation/Discussion Method

Conversation/discussion with health personnel can generate information on community health problems in the past and present, services rendered, difficulties encountered, etc. Similarly discussion with representatives from other organizations can help to attain information about functioning of their organizations and about establishing working relationships etc. Like community forum method, these meetings need to be planned and informed and guidelines are to be prepared to conduct discussion session.

Questioning

It is done by asking formal questions. It may be informal conversation or face to face interview. Question method requires the well planned interview schedule and questionnaire to obtain proper information.

Case Study

The case study is a way of organizing social data for the purpose of viewing social reality. It is an in depth study of social unit. It examines a social unit as a whole. The unit may be a person, a family, a social institution or a community. It analyzes limited number of events or conditions and their interrelations. Main advantages of this method is; it enables to understand the total behavior pattern of the concerned unit, it helps to obtain real record of personal experience and great number of interesting insight can be developed. But it has also some drawback like; it is expensive, time consuming, generalization and comparison may not be possible and subjective bias may be there.

Other Methods

Other methods which can be used for data collection clinical examination, investigation, etc. These methods involve the use of standard screening instrument like sphygmomanometer, audiometer, weighing scale, Snellel's chart, thermometer, laboratory test protocol, etc.

Listening is yet another very good method of data collection in community health. Attentive listening can help to gather many information which otherwise might not have been possible. It gives many verbal and nonverbal clues.

No single method can be used for gather information rather a combination of techniques required to be used to get complete data. The instruments which need to be developed and procured are: community forum guidelines, observation checklist, interview schedule, questionnaire, opinionnaire, record review checklist, discussion guidelines, health record form, screening instruments and laboratory test protocol.

Data Collection

Data collection is a systematic approach to gather information from a variety of sources to get a complete and accurate picture of an area of interest. The community health nurse must possess strong cognitive, interpersonal, and technical skills to gather appropriate information and make relevant observations during the data collection process. This process often begins prior to initial contact, i.e., plan for data collection, development of tool/checklist etc. The community identification survey needs to be planned carefully to ensure systematic and appropriate collection of valid information.

The following steps need to be considered.

- **Define the community to be studied:** Mention the name of community, address, level of community, i.e., whether it is a village, villages under subcenter or primary health center or community health center, whole area or part of the area covered by maternal and child health and family welfare center, etc.
- **Set tentative community goal:** This is where the community planning process begins to bring a real road map for the future. Determine the general goals first before getting bogged down in wordsmithing.
- **Determine specific information:** Determine specific information/data to be collected and identify the sources from where these information can be obtained. Specify the measurement of data.
- **Identify the population and sampling unit under study:** It will depend upon the sources of information. These can be: people in the community, key informants, health and allied officials, records, etc., or all of these. Identify the sampling unit, e.g., when study-population is 'people' in the community, the sampling unit could be an individual, family or a house hold. Select the respondent when family and household is the sampling unit.
- **Decide on the sample size and sampling method:** As we know the size of the community may vary from a small hamlet to a big metropolitian city. During data collection sometimes the CHN has to select sample to collect the data. In this stage the CHN will decide what type of sampling technique will be followed to collect the data.
- **Decide on the methods and instruments of data collection:** This will depend upon nature and sources of information and population under study, etc. It is advisable to work out the blue print based on these steps which can serve as guidelines for collection of desired data.
- **Develop the instruments decided:** These may include interview schedule, observation checklist, community forum guidelines, etc.
- **Organize and conduct survey:** Organize and conduct survey by collecting data using various methods as decided and planned. In order to gain acceptance, cooperation and confidence of people it is important to

follow the principles of community approach and data collection.

Some of the tips which are important from practical point of view are listed here:

- Before visiting a community find out any kind of customs which are expected from a visitor. Develop working relation sheep with them
- Identify leaders, develop a good relationship make them understood the purpose of your visit.
- Dress up appropriately in a manner acceptable by the local people.
- Do not act as a stranger or a superior. Empathize with them. Appreciate what they are and their cultural practices and customs.
- Mix up with the people, accept their hospitality. Participate in their cultural events. Play and joke with them as and when necessary.
- Watch and listen to them attentively, answer their queries and consider their point of view.
- Make only those commitments which can be fulfilled.
- Avoid unnecessary arguments, criticism and comments.
- Be neutral in any kind of dispute in the family or in the village.
- Maintain confidentiality.

It is very important to hold initial informal and formal meetings with community people and their representatives. These meetings help in gaining entry in the community, earning their trust, confidence and cooperation. The people get involved and informed about what is happening or going to happen, etc.

It is not difficult to arrange such meetings. Thematic film is a film on relevant subject (10–15 min.) can precede the meeting to draw and sensitize the people. The meeting should not be too long and be arranged at a time and place convenient to them. Agenda must be drawn. Guidelines must be prepared to steer the discussion towards the purposes, i.e., community identification, its purposes, strategy their help and cooperation, etc.

Community identification requires collection of large and variety of data from various sources using variety of methods and instruments. It will be difficult for any one health worker to carry on such huge task.

It requires the efforts of health team to share the task. The team members need to be trained in data collection and recording information. Confidentiality of the date collected from individual/family needs to be maintained. Schedule for data collection needs to be worked out and implemented as feasible.

Data Analysis

Data analysis is a process of extracting, compiling and modeling raw data for purposes of obtaining constructive information that can be applied to formulating conclusion, predicting outcome or supporting decision. It provides a way of drawing inductive inferences from data and distinguishing the signal (the phenomena of interest) from noise (statistical fluctuation) present in the data. Analysis of data consists of putting all the factual information collected into an order, compile and summarize according to variables studied. It reveals relationship, trends. This step is very important and essential to make the collected data meaningful, understandable and be able to describe the community profile, identify health problems and their possible associated factors. The phases of analysis include:

- Data categorization (demographic, geographic, socioeconomic, health resource and services...etc.) then organizing by Coding, key punching then arranging of data for tallying.
- Data summarization (rates, charts graphs...etc.)
- Comparing data (compared with similar data, identification of data gaps, incongruence...etc.)
- Draw inferences (draw logical conclusions from the evidence) that lead to community diagnosis.
- Reporting of the findings: It includes describing the community profile, making community profile, making community diagnosis, i.e., stating health problems and their associated/underlying possible causes, implications and recommendations.

Community Profile and Diagnosis

Community identification process helps to determine community profile and helps in drawing conclusions or make diagnosis of its health needs and health problems from interpretation of data collected. The health problems during community assessment can be identified from their lifestyles (e.g., poor dietary habits, sedentary lifestyle, substance abuse), environmental condition, (e.g., unsafe drinking water, substandard housing conditions), inadequate healthcare system (e.g., insufficient primary care providers, lack of prenatal care services, etc. The community health nurse can identified possible risk factors as high infant mortality rate, lack of prenatal care and delivery services, available care not affordable/accessible, available care not culturally sensitive, lack of transportation to health care, high percentage of teenage mothers, low education levels of mothers (high school drop outs), poor maternal nutrition, maternal smoking during pregnancy, family and neighborhood stress, multiple pregnancies (twins, triplets, etc.), high unemployment incomplete immunization, early marriage high fertility and growth, malnutrition, unsafe water supply, improper collection and disposal of garbage, field defection, prevalence of communicable diseases, nutrition deficiency diseases, poor personal practices, traditional cultural practices regarding antenatal, postnatal and child rearing practices, etc. A nursing diagnosis has three parts:

1. Description of the problem (specific target or groups)
2. Identification of factors/etiology related to (r/t) the problem
3. The sign and symptoms (the manifestations) that characteristics of the problem.

Example: Poor nutritional status of under five children in the community r/t knowledge deficit regarding weaning diet as evidenced by growth monitoring chart.

Community Health Planning (Planning Phase)

In general planning is the third step of the nursing process and includes the formulation of guidelines that establish the proposed course of nursing action in the resolution of nursing diagnoses and the development of the client's plan of care. Once the nursing diagnoses have been developed and client strengths have been identified, planning can begin. The planning phase involves several tasks. Here the plan will be developed for a community or country Community health planning is very important to determine the course of action to be implemented to meet community health needs and resolve community health problems. It is based on community diagnosis. Community health planning is a systematic process and involves logical decision making at each step of its process. The process includes four steps.

1. Analyzing health needs/health problems.
2. Establishing priorities.
3. Setting goals and objectives.
4. Formulating community health action plan to achieve the objectives.

Community health planning process requires collaborate functioning of the team including community people so that they get interested, informed, involved and feel responsible.

Analysis of Health Problems

A problem is the difference between what and what should be. The cause of community problem may be inside or outside the community. The identified problems of community required to be analyzed further to clarify the nature and extent of problems, the factors associated with problems and its consequences. It may required further collection of some specific information regarding identified problems (if already collected data does not provide such information), e.g., health and illness status, etc. This is known as problem-oriented assessment and it is *second level of assessment*. After further assessment it is required to find out the community's comprehension of problems, perception and evaluation of the problems in terms of seriousness and urgency of attention needed and resources available to resolves the problems.

Why to analyze a problem:

- To know facts about a disease
- Helps in making specific diagnosis which becomes the basis for setting goals and objectives
- To formulating community health action plan
- To credible communicate this information to other
- To raise community awareness of the importance and seriousness of this health issues.
- To able to compare the data with local, state, national and with the world.

Establishing Priorities

Establishing priorities refers to ranking of health problems identified by determining their relative importance on the basis of predetermined criteria.

Prioritization is necessary because of limited resources available and many problems to deal with which is not feasible. Priorities require consideration of nature of problems, their impact and consequences, community's readiness to resolve the problems and the resources available to deal with the problems. The criteria must be decided by the team. The following criteria have been suggested by many Public Health Nursing experts and may be used to rank the problems:

Type of Health Problems

According to Ruth Freeman, there are three types of health problems which can be grouped as:

- **Health deficits:** It is the gap between actual and achievable health status. For example, illness state, failure to thrive, disability, amputation.
- **Health threats:** Conditions that are conducive to disease, accident or failure to realize one's potential. For example, family history of hereditary disease, faulty eating habits, unhealthy lifestyle, threat of cross infection, etc.
- **Foreseeable crises or stress points**, i.e., anticipated periods of unusual demands on the individual or family in terms of adjustment/family resources. For example, marriage, pregnancy, parenthood, divorce, loss of job, death, etc.

Extent of Problems (Who all in the Community are Affected?)

This refers to the extent of prevalence of the problems. This may range from high prevalence to low prevalence depending upon the number of people affected, timing of prevalence and seriousness of the problem.

Severity of the Consequences of the Problems (How Serious or Significant are the Consequences/ Outcome of this Problem in this Community?)

This refers to the nature and magnitude of the resultant problems, i.e., the impact of the problems, if problems concerned are not resolved on time. It is the mortality, morbidity, disability from the disease, injury, accidents, violence and crime associated with the problem.

Salience (How does the Community Perceives this Problem?)

It refers to the community's perception and evaluation of the problems in terms of seriousness and urgency of attention needed.

Modifiability of the Problems (Whether the Problem can be Resolved?)

It refers to the possibility of resolving problems. It will depend upon the availability of resources relevant to resolve the problems.

Three points rating scale may be prepared to evaluate each problem against these criteria and give a score accordingly.

Setting Goals and Objectives

Goal is an aim, intent, or end. Goals are broad statements that describe the intended or desired change in the client's behavior. Goal statements refer to the diagnostic label (or problem statement) of the nursing diagnosis. Once the priorities are established, relevant goals and objectives are setup.

It is very important to setup goals and objectives because goals and objectives not only give directions and determine relevant actions but also help in sustaining and evaluating the actions planned and implemented. They also help community understand about what is happening and what is expected of them. The goals and objectives must be acceptable to the community, i.e., the client.

Characteristics of good objectives: The good objectives always follow SMART.

- **Specific:** Target specific population
- **Measurable:** When the results are stated
- **Achievable:** Within the capacity of the available resources
- **Relevant:** Fits with the general police
- **Time bound:** That is achieved within specified time frame.

Formulating Community Health Action Plans

An important step of CHN process is to develop effective community health strategies. A community action plan is a road map for implementing community change by identifying and specifying what will be done, who will do it, and how it will be done. In other words the community action plan describes what the community wants to accomplish, what activities are required during a specifies timeline and what resources (money, people, materials) are needed to be successful. It is critical that the activities selected seem feasible to implement. The point is not to become overwhelmed with the process, but rather to clearly define the health priorities, actions, and expected results. The key to developing successful plans is to begin with health priorities identified by the community, develop measurable objectives to address these priorities, use evidence-based interventions, and plan realistic evaluation methods. Formulation of community health action plans refers to identification of appropriate community health and nursing intervention and preparing an operational plan to be implemented to achieve the established goals and objectives. The interventions are identified on the basis of objectives. For any objective to be achieved there will be more than one possible course of action that appear suitable to the problem under consideration. All the possible alternative interventions must be listed and evaluated to select the most suitable one.

The criteria for formulating community action plan:

- Agency policy.
- The resources available.
- The nature of problem.
- The community's interest and feasibility.
- Competencies of health personnel.
- Practicability and efficiency, etc.

Principles

- It is a process for action not a blue print for future development.
- The solution of problem comes from the community itself.
- Avoid activities like lecturing or teaching to people, concentrate more on workshops as a form of discussion with the community.
- Avoid too many picture and text.
- Use simple language and avoid difficult term.

Steps for developing community action plan:

1. **Opening (Introduction and socialization):** It provides a common understanding of the importance of having a good action plan.
2. **Social environmental mapping and financing:** Collect latest information on community life (social, economic, environmental condition). By developing a map the community will be able to get a better picture of problem and priorities.
3. **Identifying the problems, needs and resource potentials:** This stage defines the problem that are actually faced by the community, financial resources available to accomplish the needs.
4. **Determining priority in the need:** In this stage problem and needs are ranked by the community member according to their level of urgency, their importance for development of community life.
5. **Formulating the choice of strategy:** The strategy is developed and the approach chosen that is the most feasible to be used in overcoming the problems and fulfilling the needs on the priority list.
6. **Formulating the implementation plan:** This stage is used to formulate a schedule and the division of tasks in carrying out the action chosen.
7. **Formulating the monitoring and evaluation plan:** Formulate a plan and system of monitoring and evaluating the execution of activities.
8. **Implementing, monitoring and evaluation:** The final stage consists of carrying out the action and at the same time monitoring and evaluating.

Alternative Interventions

An intervention is a process or action intended to address an existing or potential problem. The alternative activities need to be listed for all objectives and enlisting those which are appropriate considering the criteria mentioned. This way it can help clubbing the common activities and strategies and can help in formulating a plan for a particular health problem/health situation, say, e.g., in this case tackling of malnutrition problem. Likewise it can be done for other problems and together it can help formulating a comprehensive plan. Explain how the intervention addresses health disparities, individual, policy, or environmental change. The interventions can be classified as dependent, independent and collaborative interventions. Independent interventions are actions that the nurse is able to initiate independently. Dependent interventions will require an order from another healthcare provider such as a physician or any higher person. Collaborative interventions means the intervention is done by the effort of whole team which is specially applied to the CHN process.

The elements of comprehensive plan thus include general goals, specific objectives, planned actions, general strategy and schedule including when, where, how, by whom and in how much durations, etc.

Criteria for judging best strategy/solution to a problem:

- Costs involved
- Time required
- People required
- Driving forces and obstacles for taking action
- Possible impact of taking/not taking action
- Community preference of problem as priority
- The likelihood of successful solution.

Planning with the Community

It is very important that what is being planned for the community is planned with them. This will not only add to their self-esteem but also create interest in them, develop sense of responsibility and autonomy. It is therefore useful to meet community after identification of community profile and community health problems/health needs.

If feasible, meet the whole community and share the findings and the ideas and then or else meet the village leaders/village health committee/planning groups to discuss and draw up some general plan. All the health workers involved in community identification and diagnosis need to participate and make joint presentation and lead the discussions.

The community would be interested to know the findings of the questions they were asked during the survey. But keep these information simple. Explain to them the main problems found in a manner which is understandable to them. The purpose is not only to give the information but also to sensitize and motivate the people so that they understand and feel the seriousness of their problems and realize the importance of finding solutions to the problems. Tell them the number of people having a particular problem and the consequences of the problem, e.g., children suffering from malnutrition and their chances for contracting other illnesses like diarrhea, measles, pneumonia and resulting mortality. Help people to understand the preventive nature of the problem, e.g., malnutrition can be prevented and controlled by proper and nutritious feeding.

Present the problems in order of priority as worked out but at the same time be flexible to change the priority as felt by the people or there may be some other problem expressed by them. After presenting the problems, discuss the actions that can be planned. If feasible in the same meeting or have a separate meeting after working out some plan that can be presented, discussed and finalized. All this will depend on their level of comprehension and readiness for such kind of approach.

Implementation of Community Health (Action Phase)

Implementation refers to putting the plan into action to achieve the set goals and objectives of community health. In this phase, carrying out the activities delineated in the plan, either by nurse or other professionals. It is the action phase of the nursing process which refers to the translation of the planning into practice according to principles of nursing. Community interventions are the therapeutic actions designed to promote and protect the community, health, treat and remediate community health problems and support the community as it changes over time. The implementation is feasible through the collaborative efforts of the entire health team.

The general purpose/goal of community health action plan is to help people learn to help themselves in solving their health problems, in meeting their own health needs, using their resources so as to attain and maintain optimum level of health. This implies constant involvement of community people, families and groups to develop a sense of responsibility and autonomy. It also lays emphasis on educating people for whatever is done for them. The community health nurse along with her other nursing personnel is in a better position to achieve this general goal.

According to Ruth-Freeman there are three types of nursing interventions which a nurse can make use of while implementing community health actions which she as a nurse is supposed to do. These are:

- **Supplemental**, i.e., doing things for the families, groups and community at large which they are not able to do, e.g., nursing care of the sick at home or in the center or in any other setting. Also, preparing them to do so in her absence by training and supervision and guidance. The direct nursing care can be given by the PHN herself or by ANM under her supervision and guidance.
- **Facilitative**, i.e., removing barriers, obstacles, etc. She helps them to mobilize and develop their resources. The nurse needs to know community resources-health and health allied, know their functions and establish functional relationship.
- **Developmental**, i.e., helping families, groups and people at large to develop and improve their capacities. She educates members to recognize their health problems, health needs, find solutions, mobilize and develop their resources and abilities to implement actions, etc.

Most of the times all the three types of nursing interventions are implemented because one without the other is unable to bring desired outcomes. But, any one of these may predominate depending upon the situations and health problems/health needs.

The process of implementation requires review of the overall plan, understanding of the strategy and the schedule, i.e., What ?, When?, How? and Who ? Clarify any doubt for smooth implementation.

It also requires mobilization of resources and establishing working relationship with the community and their active participation. Regular and periodical contacts and meetings should be arranged for the same. The plan is implemented as it is or modified and implemented depending upon the resources available, community's readiness to participate, the environmental conditions, urgency of the existing conditions and conditions which may emerge, etc.

Above all, it is very essential to do the recording of all the interventions implemented and progress made, difficulties and constraints encountered. It is both descriptive and analytical. This alone can help in evaluation which is the next step.

Evaluation of Community Health Actions and Feedback (Evaluation Phase)

Evaluation, the final step of the nursing process which involves determining whether the client goals have been met, have been partially met, or have not been met. Even though it is the final phase of the nursing process, evaluation is an ongoing part of daily nursing activities that determines the effectiveness of those activities in helping clients achieve expected outcomes. It begins with assessment phase when decisions are made while preparing community identification guidelines for collection of data. Evaluation is then done in the planning phase when problems are analyzed, priorities are established, goals and specific objectives are set and alternative actions are planned to achieve the goals and objectives. Evaluation is finally done when actions are implemented and results are observed and recorded.

Evaluation Process

Structure (Include the physical settings, instrumentalities and conditions through which nursing care is given)	**Process** (Includes all the steps of nursing process)	**Outcome** (changes in clients health status that results from nursing intervention)
• Philosophy • Objective • Building • Organizational structure • Financial resources (Budget, equipment and staff)	• Taking the family health data base • Performing physical examination • Making a nursing diagnosis • Determining nursing goal • Writing nursing care plan • Performing nursing intervention • Coordination of services • Measuring of success of nursing action	• Modification of sign and symptom • Knowledge • Attitude • Satisfaction • Skill level of client • Compliance with treatment regimen

The evaluation is a two part process: The first part of the evaluation is the determination of what is of value or in simple terms the identification of the objective or goals towards which nursing process is aimed. The second part of evaluation is the judgement of whether these goals are being achieved or the event to which they are being achieved. So evaluation is a systematic process of determining the extent to which objectives are achieved.

Evaluation is an ongoing decision making process: Evaluation is done at each step of the process to get feedback so as to make accurate decisions as far as possible. Observations are also done of the difficulties encountered, time spent and actions which were not feasible and intended results not achieved. So far, it is concurrent or formative evaluation which is the evaluation of resources (structure evaluation) and the process (process evaluation). It helps in taking remedial measures and appropriate decisions throughout the community health process as far as possible.

Terminal evaluation is done at the end of determined period with set goals (standards) and objectives (criteria). Evidence of effectiveness are: reduction in morbidity rates, decrease in birth rates, increase in population coverage for various services, clinic attendance, change in knowledge, attitude and health practices and degree of self-dependence etc. This is the outcome of evaluation. It shows evaluation is both quantitative and qualitative. Outcomes will depend upon goals and objectives setup, base line information available, maintenance of accurate and complete record of services rendered, compiling and computing of results, observation of changes in health knowledge, health behavior, health practices and competencies etc. This also refers to terminal evaluation.

The terminal evaluation helps in determining the achievements and intended outcomes, difficulties and constraints encountered and help identify associated problems and new emergent problems, etc. It promotes rethinking, data review and its update, review and revisions of goals and objectives, reformulation of action plan and activating of the plan considering various requirements, etc. This evaluation is also known as summative evaluation.

Evaluation in CHN process is a long-term process. In achievement of the some of the targets it may be take one year two year or more. As per the time determined during goal setting the achievements will be evaluated how much the goal is achieved. The community health nurse will do the evaluation of her contributions and responsibility throughout the CHN process. She will also participate as one of the members of team to evaluate the whole community health action plans. During terminal evaluation she will also follow some specific steps as:

- Determine what is to be evaluated
- Establishment of standards and criteria
- Planning the methodology
- Gathering information
- Analysis of results.

Evaluation is both individual member activity and team activity. It is done by individual team member of his/her share of contribution and responsibility, e.g., community health nurse will do the evaluation of her contribution and responsibility, e.g., community health action outcomes

Table 1.4: Differences between community health nursing process, family health nursing process, and nursing process at hospital for individual patient.

Criteria	*Nursing process for individual patient*	*Family health nursing process*	*Community health nursing process*
Meaning	Nursing process which is applied for individual patient	Nursing process which is applied for family	Nursing process which is applied for whole community
Categories of informations required	Patient personal history, medical and surgical history, patient' present condition, investigation about diseases, etc.	Family characteristics, family history of diseases, family environment, family risk and threats and family abilities to solve the family health problems	Geographical area, geographical location/boundary of a community, physical setup, environmental sanitation, population characteristics, social system, communication pattern
Data collection methods	Individual interview, physical examination, lab investigation and other biophysiological measurements	Interview, observation, review of family health records, physical examination of family members	Interview, observation, record review method, community forum method, conversation/discussion method
Nursing diagnosis priority	Based on the seriousness of individual problems	Depends upon five different factors of family, type of health problems, extent of problems, modifiability of the problems, consequences of problems, preventive potential, salience	Depends upon five different factors of the community, type of health problems, extent of problems, modifiability of the problems consequence and available resource
Nursing diagnosis format	Diagnosis consists existing individual problem related factors, and signs and symptoms	Diagnosis consists any risk threat or foreseeable crises situation of the family, during development of family profile	Total mortality and morbidity conditions of the community, development of community profile
Client	Individual	Family	Community
Characteristic of care plan	Based on only the individual patient problems	Based on over all family health problems	Based on whole community health problems
Implementation	By following individual care plan	By following family healthcare plan	By following community healthcare action plan
People involvement	People will be informed and permission will be taken	More involvement of family members because the care is given in their own house	The community people will be only organizing community development program
Evaluation	Evaluation can be done then and there to assess the outcome of nursing procedure. It is a short-term process	Evaluation may be a long-term process sometimes. Some of the goals can be achieved in short period of time	Evaluation is generally a long-term process

are due to the contributions of entire health team and it is difficult and may not be feasible to determine outcomes due to nursing intervention alone.

Table 1.4 shows differences between community health nursing process, family health nursing process, and nursing process at hospital for individual patient.

CHAPTER 2

Family Health Nursing

INTRODUCTION

The family is the most important primary group in society. It is a group of biologically-related individuals living together and eating from a common kitchen. It is the first and the most immediate social environment to which the child is exposed the most basic of all social groupings. Family is the most pervasive and universal social institution. It plays a vital role in the socialization of individuals and is regarded as the first society of human-being. It is also known as the first school of citizenship. Family is the backbone of social structure which occupies a nuclear position in society. As the family is the basic significant unit of society, the changes in social behavior can affect the family's development in relation to structure, functions and interactions both within the family and within the community. Family is the most stable, enduring and universal cultural form.

The importance of family and family considerations become important for a nurse while practicing in community health setting because family is the unit of Community Health Nursing service. Family usually involves a residence in which family members, friends, relatives interact with each other.

The family health work is the basis upon which all factors rest. The family is the unit of service in all generalized community health nursing programme. The health of one member affects the welfare of every other member in the family. Though every family is some how different in structure still the culture of a particular community makes the uniqueness in that community. So the community health nurse must know the family ways, traditions and customs of people. The families are attended by every aspect of community life.

Concept of Family

Family refers to the group comprising parents and children, it may also refer in some cases, to a group of relatives and their dependents forming one household. All these refer to the compositional aspect of this institution. Another aspect is that of residence of its members. They usually share common residence, at least for some part of their lives. There is rational aspect of the family. Family members have reciprocal rights and duties towards each other. Finally, the family is also an agent of socialization. All these aspects make this institution different from all other units of social structure.

Definition

Family is a group of persons whose relations to one another are based upon consanguinity and who are therefore, kin to another. **—Kingsley Davis**

Family is a group defined by a sex relationship sufficiently precise and enduring to provide for the procreation and upbringing of children.

Family is a socially recognized unit of people related to each other by kinship, marital and legal ties.

MF Nimkoff says that family is a more or less durable association of husband and wife with or without children, or of a man or woman alone, with children.

According to Burgess and Locke, family is a group of persons united by ties of marriage, blood or adoption constituting a single household interaction and inter-communicating with each other in their respective social roles of husband and wife, father and mother, son and daughter, brother and sister creating a common culture.

Eliot and Merrill, defines the family is the biological social unit composed of husband, wife and children.

MacIver addressed family as a group defined by sex relationship sufficiently precise and enduring to provide for the procreation and upbringing of children. National Center for Health Statistics, 1990 has defined the family as a group of two or more persons related by birth, marriage, or adoption and residing together in a household.

According to Stanhope, Lancaster, 1992, family is represented by two or more individuals belonging to the same or different kinship groups, who are involved in a continuous living arrangement, usually residing in the same household experiencing common, emotional bonds and sharing certain obligations towards each other and towards others.

Characteristics of Family

A Mating Relationship

A family comes into existence when a man and woman establish mating relation between them.

A Form of Marriage

Mating relationship is established through the institution of marriage. The society regulates sexual behavior between opposite sexes through the institution of marriage. Through the institution of marriage, mating relationship is established. Without marriage family is not possible. Hence, family is a form of marriage.

A Common Habitation

A family requires a home or household for its living. Without a dwelling place the task of child-bearing and child-rearing cannot be adequately performed. The members of a family have a common habitation or household.

A System of Nomenclature

Every family is known by a particular name. It has own system of reckoning descent. Descent may be recognized through male line or through mother's line. In patrilineal families descent is recognized through male line. Similarly in matrilineal families descent is recognized through mother's line.

An Economic Provision

Every family needs an economic provision to satisfy the economic needs. The head of the family carries on certain profession and earns to maintain the family.

System of Interaction and Communication

The family is composed of person who interact and communicate with each other in their social roles such as husband and wife, mother and father, son and daughters, etc. It is important to mention that the family is composed of persons united by ties of marriage, blood or adoption, the family maintains a common but a distinctive culture.

Other than this every family has some characteristics, these are:
- Family is a small social system.
- Family has its own cultures, value and rules.
- Family has its own structure.
- Family performs extreme basic function.
- Family moves through stages of the life cycle.
- Family has a sense of togetherness that promotes capacity to change.
- Family has a balance between mutual and independent action in the part of family members.
- Family nurturance and provide resources for growth.
- Stability and integrity of structure.
- Mastery of developmental tasks and ability to meet demand for survival and development.

Nature of Family

Besides the characters mention above a family as possessed of several distinctive features. It influences the entire life of people in memorious ways. It differs from other group in the following respects.

Universality

There is no human society in which some form of the family does not appear. Malinowski writes the typical family a group consisting of mother, father and their progeny is found in all communities, savage, barbarians and civilized. The irresistible sex need, the urge for reproduction and the common economic needs have contributed to this universality.

Emotional Basis

Family is a fundamental unit of human society. The family is grounded in emotions and sentiments which is based on our impulses of mating, procreation, maternal devotion, fraternal love and parental care. It is built upon sentiments of love, affection, sympathy, cooperation and friendship.

Limited Size

The size of a family is of necessity limited for it is defined by biological condition which it cannot transect. Other groups may be smaller than a family but they are not so because of biological conditions.

Formative Influence

The family exercise the most profound influence over the member. It mold the character of individuals and influence in infancy determines the personality structure of the individual. Parents are better at teaching the social niceties of more formal settings—how to act in public, how not to embarrass oneself at the dinner table, for etc.

Nuclear Position

The family is the nucleus of all other social groups. The distinctive characteristic of marriage is parental obligation and sibling. Family is the primary institution call of a society. The whole social structure is built of family unit.

Responsibility of Member

In the family the child learns the meaning of social responsibility and the necessary for cooperation. As MacIver aptly describe, the child develops his basic attitudes and ideals. It is a great agency of the socialization of the child.

Social Regulation

The family is peculiarly guarded by social customs and legal regulations. It is not easy to violet them. The children after birth, from their families only learning what are the rules and regulations of society and how to abide them.

Permanent and Temporary

Family is an institution is permanent and universal while as an association. It is temporary and transitional. When the son marries he goes out of the family and start another family which again may give rise to more families.

TYPES OF FAMILY

Though family is an universal institution, its structure or form vary from one society to another. Sociologists and anthropologists have mentioned about different types of families found in different cultures. Classification of families is generally done on the basis of organization—Nuclear and Joint and three generation family. Forms of marriage—monogamous or polygamous. Authority—matriarchal or patriarchal and residence, etc.

On the Basis of Organization or Family Structure

On the basis of organization or family structure classification of families is generally done as Nuclear and Joint and three generation family.

Nuclear Family

The nuclear family is a unit composed of husband, wife and their unmarried children. This is the predominant form of modern industrial societies. This type of family is based on companionship between parent and children. The husband and wife relationship is likely to become intimate in the nuclear family than in the joint family. The size of the nuclear family is very small. It is free from control of elder. In this family the children gets maximum care, love and affection from the parents. The nuclear family is independent and economically self-sufficient. The members of nuclear family also enjoy more freedom than the members of joint family.

Extended/Joint Family

The joint families is a kind of family grouping which is common in India, Africa and the Middle East. The orthodox kind of family in India is a joint family. Due to raise of education, urbanization and industrialization, we were losing the joint family system. The main characteristic of this family are—it consists of a number of married couples and their children who live together in the same household. All the authority is vested in a senior male member of the family. He is the most dominant member and controls the internal and external affairs of the family. The senior female members by virtue of her being the wife of the male head shares his power so far as the women of the family are concerned. The familiar relations enjoy privacy over marital. Union is strength relation, early and arranged marriage is advocated toward off any threat from marital relationship. The merits of the joint family system is that it is based on the motto. There is a sharing of responsibilities practically in all matters which give the family a greater economic and social security. It provides economic and social security to the old, the helpless and the unemployed.

Three Generation Family

The three generation family confused with the joint family. It is fairly common in the West. This tends to be a household where there are representatives of three generations. It occurs usually when young couples are unable to find separate housing accommodation and continue to live with their parents and have their own children. Thus, relatives of three generation related to each other by direct descent live together.

On the Basis of Authority

Patriarchal Family

It is a type of family in which all authority belongs to the paternal side. In this family the eldest male or the father is the head of the family. He exercises his authority over the members of the family. He presides over the religious rights of the household. He is the guardian of the family goods. In the developed patriarchal system of the past, the patriarch had unlimited and undisrupted authority over his wives, son and daughters.

Matriarchal Family

It is a form of family in which authority is centered in the wife or mother. The matriarchal family system implies rule of the family by the mother, not by father. In this type of family women are entitled to perform religious rites and husband lives in the house of wife. Matriarchal family is also called mother right family or maternal family under which the status, name and sometimes inheritance is transmitted through the female line. This type of family is now found among the Khasi and Garo tribes of Assam and Meghalaya, among Nayars of Malbar in Kerala.

On the Basis of Residence

In terms of residence, there are also different types of families described below:

Patrilocal Family

When the wife goes to live with the husband's family, it is called the patriarchal family.

Matrilocal Family

When the couple after marriage moves to live with the wife's family, such residence is called matriarchal, the husband has a secondary position in the wife's family where his children live.

Neolocal Residence

When the couple after marriage which is neither attached to the bride's family of origin nor bride groom's family of origin is called neolocal residence and staying separately.

Avunculocal Family

In this type of family the married couple moves to the house of the maternal uncle and live with his son after marriage.

Matri-patrilocal Family

In matri-patrilocal family, immediately after marriage the bridegroom moves to the house of bride and temporarily settles there till the birth of the first child and then move with the child for permanent settlement.

On the Basis of Descent

On the basis of descent, families may be divided into two type such as patrilineal and matrilineal.

Patrilineal Family

When descent is traced through the father it is called patrilineal family. In this type of family inheritance of property takes place along the male line of descent. The ancestry of such family is determined on the basis of male line or the father. A patrilineal family is also patriarchal and patrilocal. This is the common type of family prevalent today.

Matrilineal Family

In this type of family descent is traced along the female line and inheritance of property also takes place along the female line of descent.

On the Basis of Marriage

On the basis of marriage, family has been classified into two types such as monogamous and polygamous.

Monogamous Family

A monogamous family is one which is consisted of one husband and one wife. In this type of family one man has one wife or one woman has one husband at a given time. Hence a husband and a wife living together, constitute a monogamous family. It is an ideal form of family prevalent widely.

Polygamous Family

When one man marries several women or one woman marries several men and constitute the family, it is polygamous family.

On the Basis of Blood Relationship

Consanguine Family

A consanguineal family consists of a husband and wife, their children, and other members of either the husband's and/or wife's family. This kind of family is common in cultures where property is inherited. In patriarchal societies where important property is owned by men, the consanguine family otherwise termed as extended families commonly consist of a husband and wife, their children, the husband's parents, and other members of the husband's family. In societies where fathers are absent and mothers do not have the resources to rear their children on their own, the consanguineal family may consist of a mother and her children, and members of the mother's family.

Conjugal Family

The conjugal family is a nucleus of the husband, the wife and their off spring, who are surrounded by a fringe of relatives only incidental to the functioning of the family as an unit.

FAMILY CYCLE

The institution of the family is so permanent and universe and is an association which is the most temporary and the most transitional of all important organizations within society. The family is an ever-changing association. A family as an association has a life of its own and family sociology adopts the life cycle perspective to through to old age. The life cycle perspective seeks to explore the passage of an individual through the successive stages of life, from birth to death through childhood, adolescence, adult life and old age. Likewise each family passes through various phases, formation, growth, maturation and dissolution. To quote MacIver and Page again, each individual family is, in part, the story of the life together of the original partners, a story that ends with their life.

A key concept of research studies in the life cycle of families is family time which addresses the timing and sequence of transitions such as marriage and parenthood and how such timings are precipitated by individual family members and by society at large. The timings of earlier events (such as age of first marriage) are shown to have a great impact on later outcomes (such as birth of first child or loss of spouse or divorce). Research concerned with the life cycle of families have also analyzed the sudden shifts in economic status, migration, uprooting, disasters, physical change or incapacity of a family member and impact of crisis at various stages of family life.

Stages of Family Life Cycle

A typical nuclear family which constitutes the core of traditional extended or joint families is generally conceived as having four phases.

First Phase

The first phase begins with the marriage, i.e., living together of a male and female, creating the environment of the home. This is a highly valued stage living together, as husband and wife does not concern mere satisfaction of the sexual needs. As parents they share a home, with its combination satisfaction. The sharing of home evokes new experiences, develops new attitudes of the partners towards each other and towards society and of society towards the partnership. It is a partnership in which as Wordsworth put it, we live by admiration, hope and love. This stage ends with coming of the first child.

Second Phase

The second phase begins with the birth of the first child, except one child family. It is regarded as the next important phase of the family life cycle, with the birth of the child the fruit of the sexual union brings above a transformation of man, woman relationship. The child acts as a child-rearing evokes new interests and attitudes and sentiments among the parents.

Third Phase

This is the stage of maturation when the biological functions of the parents have been fulfilled and when the children become less and less dependent upon parental care liberated from the responsibility of child rearing. New interest, new activities replace the old ones, parent child relationships undergo changes as grown up children begin independent life of their own.

Fourth or Final Phase

The family life cycle ends with the dissolution of the family. This phase begins with the death of the first spouse and end with the death of the survivor.

All families may not pass through all these phases. There are a number of variations and exceptions to the typical life cycle such as the early death of children or one spouse, death or separation or divorce before the final stage is reached. The length of each stages also varies as social conditions and culture vary.

FUNCTIONS OF THE FAMILY

All families have certain functions that are performed to maintain the integrity of the family unit needs, the individual family members needs and society's expectations. Duvall and Miller identified seven family functions that are generally applicable to all types of family structures:

1. **Generating affection:** Affection is generated between spouses, between parents and children and among members of the generations.
2. **Providing personal security and acceptance:** The family provides a home base with a stability that allows the family members to develop naturally in their own way and their own pace.
3. **Giving satisfaction and sense of purpose:** In the family setting the family members enjoy life with each other through satisfying activity.
4. **Ensuring continuity of companionship:** In most cases family associations that provides sympathetic companionship and encouragement can be expected to endure.
5. **Providing social placement and socialization:** The family serves as the transmitter of culture from one generation to the next and prepare family members for their place in the social hierarchy.
6. **Imposing control and sense of what is right:** Within the family, members first learn the rules, rights, obligations and responsibilities characteristics of human society.
7. **Protect the health of the family members:** A basic family function is to protect the health of the family members and to provide supportive nurturing care during illness. The individual family members and to provide supportive nurturing care during period of illness. The family contributes to the health of the individual family members by supporting the biophysical and psychosocial developments of the members.

It is within the family unit that member of the family develop their concept of health and establish their health habits. The family as a social unit develops a system of values, beliefs and attitudes about health and illness behavior of the family members. The family also functions as the primary intermediary for transmitting health-related cultural traits to the next generation. It is through family that practices of the larger society concerning health and illness. The way in which the family carries out healthcare responsibilities and the ability of the family to do so, will be influenced by factors such as the family structure, division of labor, socioeconomic status and ethnicity.

Besides these the corelated social functions are:

- Regulation of sexual behavior and reproduction
- Care and training of children
- Cooperation and division of labor
- Primary group satisfaction. Develop personality of individual.

According to WHO, family functions categorize under six major headings, these are:

Biological

Family provide a field for fulfillment of all biological activities like reproduction and childbearing, rearing of children, nutrition of family members, protection of health at all ages by preventing developmental crises, recreation for its members, etc. Sexual activities are approved by social manner in family. The child enjoy a lot of recreational activities within its family.

Psychological

Man is a social animal. Safety and security is a basic need of individual. Mental health is as essential dimension of health. All psychological needs of an individual is fulfilled by its family members. Family provides emotional security and a sense of identity for the family members. It helps maturation of personality and develop ability to make relationship outside the family.

Sociocultural

Family impart the knowledge of social customs, culture, values. It exercises social control over its members, which helps in the maintenance of a well-organized society. Family is an important agency of social control. It is also custodian of culture. Family maintain discipline and decorum in the society. Individual with society learns various skills and develops appropriate value system in which he lives. Family is the first social agency to operate any individual and it act as a major role in transfer of values relating to behavior, tradition, language, socialization of children and formulation of norms of behavior at all stages in development. The process of socialization begins within the family. The influence of the family upon the child is older and childhood playmate then he find out the schoolmates. Family as primary group, the members are bonded with feeling which is helpful in transmitting the attitude and sentiment.

Economic

Family members are taking responsibility of distribution of resources, expenditure, the member of modern family do not work together. They are engaged in different outside activities. Family member helps economic adjustment in the family. Economic protected and maintenance by the family savings.

Educational

Family is an important educational agency. A child learn all developmental and social activities like talking, behaving, communicating, identifying and fulfilling his needs, etc., from his family. Family is the vocational education center, because the children from early childhood were associated with the family. Educational function include inculcation of skills, attitude and knowledge relating to other functions, preparation for other life situation, modification of behavior and fulfillment of adult role.

Health-related Functions

A family was fulfilling all health-related functions of a family like provision of adequate food shelter and clothing, maintenance of health supporting physical psychosocial environment, provision of resources for maintenance of personal hygiene, provision for meeting spiritual needs, health education, health illness, decision-making, recognition of health disruption, seeking illness care, and health care and providing first aid, etc.

FAMILY AS A UNIT OF COMMUNITY HEALTH NURSING

Family as a Unit of Service

The family performs various health-related functions like prevention of diseases, promotion restoration of health and by which it act as a agency for providing of health services. Family as a unit of service by rediscovery of the human social and cultural aspects of health and disease and recognition of family is a focal part of health care and formulating the right place for integrating preventive, promotive and curative and rehabilitative services. Ruth Freedman said, the family system is a basic unit within which health behavior like health values, health habits and health risk perceptions are developed, organized and performed. It was also observed that the interrelationship between health, health behavior and the family is a highly dynamic one on which each may have a dramatic effect on the others.

Family is a Natural and Fundamental Unit of Society

Family is a natural and fundamental unit of society because every individual of the community belongs to the family and society has responsibilities of taking care of all its members in various aspects. Family is a primary social institution based on enduring relationship defined by marriage, birth or adaptation, etc. Health is one of the important aspects of every individual. Therefore, it is one of the responsibilities of nurse to provide health services to the family.

Family as a Group

Family generates, prevents, tolerates and corrects all the problems including health problems. Health problem may be caused by family behaviors and their style of living, lack of knowledge and emotional imbalance, which can be corrected and prevented by them.

Health Problems of Family are Interlocking

The health of any family member may affect health of others. For example, if anybody becomes sick it disturbs to whole function of family. Some infectious disease spread to other members of family. An interaction of family members reinforces the members to maintain conducive environment to maintain good health. The family provides crucial environmental force, each member of the family constantly interacts with other members of the family and environment. The individual responds in his own way and affects family environment by his own presence.

Family Acts as a Central Point of Decision-making

In all aspects of family affairs including taking care of health of its members and provides family nursing care to the individual members who required. Hence, the ability of family to provide nursing care for its member is an important factor in health care.

The family is an effective and available channel for most of the community health nursing services. So the community health nurse may consider family as a unit of service just as a clinical nurse in the hospital setting may consider an individual patient as a unit of service.

Family is an Effective and Available Channel for Community Health Nursing Service

The health data of individual is generally available from families. In family setup a community health nurse will get the individual client including different risk groups to provide care. It is the unit for whom a community health nurse will provide all types of comprehensive care. In family a community health nurse can provide all type of health services like preventive, promotive, curative and rehabilitative service to a group of people.

Characteristics of a Family as a Unit

Family is a Product of Time and Place

Family is a universal phenomenon. Family type, size, organization structure value and behavioral pattern will vary with the time and place. In modern time, increasing technology and urbanization will encourage both parents as wage earners. Economic functions may be subordinated based its social functions. Family size and style also affected by social condition. It increases in good time such as rise in economic level, and falls in poor times such as war or death of wage earner. The families of developed area is different from the families of developing areas in type, size, organization structure and value also.

The Family Develops its Own Lifestyle

Each family develops its own values, its own pattern of behavior and its own style of life. Families have full rights to develop their own power system in decision-making, etc.,. which may be balanced. Sometimes the family can influenced from society in decision-making. Some of the families have balanced power system. In balanced power system the father, mother and children have their own areas of decision and control. Some of the families do not have balanced power system. In that type of families one of the member gain dominance over the others. Some of the families are male dominated whereas some others are female dominated. These may reflect their role in family.

The Family Operates as a Group

The family members are depends upon each other. Generally the family develops its own ways of operation and dealing with common problems. During any problematic crises situation, the family members are taking decision. Some family may give up when trouble strike and wait helplessly for something to happen or someone to care and help them.

Family Accommodates to the Needs of the Individual

Each individual is a unique human being. Sometimes individual needs, group needs and family needs find a natural balance. In some families, members accommodate each other's needs. From childhood the individual depends on other family members to fulfill their needs. In some families, the family members do not easily accommodate with their needs and conflict results.

The Family Relates to the Community

Family is a unit of community. The family utilizes community resources and contribute whatever it can do for Community's betterment. The development of community helps in developing the lifestyle of family members and vice versa. The families with their joint efforts can develop a healthy community and a healthy environment. The community can take care of families of that community and families have rights and duties for the community to the community.

Family has its Growth Cycle

Families have their own growth cycle. Each family follows a particular path of growth for increasing or decreasing the size of the family:

- When a couple gets married, generally children are born and new parental task arise.
- They provide guidance and enable their children to live independently.
- After children have grown and moved away and create their own families.
- The parents readjusts to difficult period.
- They face retirement and try to cope with special problems of ageing.
- Some parents may or may not stay with their children.

The family is the unit to which community health nursing is most often addressed. Family is the group in which action of any family member may set off a whole series of reactions within a group. These reactions may be a supportive factor towards members who are sick or in need of health care.

THE DETERMINANTS OF FAMILY HEALTH

Family health is determined by the interaction of so many factors.

Environmental Factors

Physical Environment

Safe water and clean air, healthy workplaces, safe houses, communities and roads, all contribute to good health. Man made physical environment, i.e., building, space, noise, sewage, disposal, etc., are the factors affecting family health.

The Biological Environment

The biological environment includes all animals, plants, insects and all living beings including microorganism. Animals can directly create zoonotic disease and spread, different vector borne diseases also. The disease can spread by eating the meat and drinking the milk of infected animals, and by animal biting. Similarly different diseases can spread through different plants. All of us know, microorganisms are directly responsible for diseases.

The Social Environment

The Social Environment also act as determinants of health. In a community, social environment include custom, culture and tradition of society, beliefs of the family, social organization and stress can directly affect the lifestyle of family members and affect the health of family. Greater support from families, friends and communities is linked to better health.

Family Factors

Family structure and type, number, age, relationship, family type which influence family health included in family factors. Health problems of the family are interlocking, a healthy mother can give birth a healthy child. Biological characteristics of family members, cultural patterns, family dynamics and roles, coping and behavior patterns, social class or status, value systems, religious beliefs, occupation of wage earners, skills, education, social habits and economic status of the family also influencing on family health.

Ethnic and Geographic Factors, Migration, Racial Minorities

The Ethnic and geographic factors, migration and racial minorities, this total environmental system forms the framework of families needs. Knowledge of these factors can help the nurse to identify the health illness factors that affect family health. These factors can affect the health of the family members directly.

The factor influencing family health may be external or internal.

External environment: Includes physical environment like climate, water supply, air, and manmade physical environment, i.e., location and construction of house space, surroundings, etc., and biological environment that include insects, rodents and others which surrounding human being.

Internal environment: Includes family size, structure, type, members relationship, biological characteristics and each member's cultural patterns, values, etc. Information regarding these factors can help nurse to plan family care in better way.

FAMILY DEVELOPMENT AND ITS TASKS

Family development refers to the process of progressive structural differentiation and transformation over time. A family developmental task is defined as a 'growth responsibility that arises at a certain stage in the life of a family, the successful achievement of which leads to present satisfaction, approval and success with later tasks'. Failure in completing the tasks can lead to family unhappiness, societal disapproval and difficulty with later developmental tasks.

The healthy family performs all roles appropriately according to family members, ages, competencies and needs during the family life cycles. Family life cycle dimensions provide the basis for the study of families over time, emphasises family members and families developmental tasks at every stage of development, identifies family, stresses on critical developmental periods and recognizes the need for services and programs for families throughout the life cycles. Duvall and Miller categorized the family life cycles into eight stages. He developed a theory which is known as Duvall developmental theory. He explains eight stage of life with specific functions in each stage.

In brief the family is expected to perform certain tasks during illness of its members which continue to be met in various ways described below:

- Provide for physical safety, daily routines, and economic needs of its members and obtain enough resources to survive.
- Create a sense of family loyalty and security and a mentally healthy environment for the family's well-being.
- Reproduce and socialize the children teaching values, and appropriate behavior.
- Teach members to effectively communicate their needs, ideas, feelings, and respect for each other.
- Provide social togetherness simultaneously with the division of labor, patterning of sexual roles, and performance of family roles with flexibility and cooperation.
- Help members to develop physically, emotionally, intellectually and spiritually and to develop a personal and family identity while adjusting to the demands of family life.
- Release family members into the larger society—school, church, temples, organizations, employment and eventually another family unit.

Health Tasks of the Family

The health tasks of the family are the primary concern for the nurse. These are:

- **Recognizing interruptions of health development:** The family monitors illness and this recognition will facilitate healthful development.
- **Making decisions for seeking health care:** Family members must take decision about utilizing health are system when there is deviation of health of any member.
- **Dealing with health crisis:** Crisis are inevitable in any family like:
  - Severe illness
  - Death
  - Childbearing
  - Hospitalization situations affect the health of the family.
- Providing nursing care to sick or dependant members of the family.
- Maintaining healthy home environment:
  - Home should be clean.
  - Safe from hazards like fire, falls.
  - Place for play and recreational activities.

The family health tasks are of great importance for CHN as she is deeply concerned with increasing the capability of each family to be responsible for their own health. This is called safe care approach.

NURSING CARE FOR SPECIAL GROUPS

PHYSICALLY HANDICAPPED

The term impairment, disability and handicap are closely related. The sequence of events leading to disability and handicap have been stated as follows:

Disease → impairment → disability → handicap.

Impairment

'Any loss or abnormality psychological, physiological, or anatomical structure or functions', e.g., missing limb, paralysis after polio, mental retardation, etc.

Impairment may cause functional limitations which may be partial or total, visible or invisible, temporary or permanent.

Disability

'Any restriction or lack (resulting from an impairment) of ability to perform an activity in a manner within the range considered normal for a human being'.

Disability is the inability to carry out certain activities due to impairment.

Handicap

'A disadvantage for a given individual resulting from an impairment or a disability, that limits or prevents the fulfillment of a role that is normal (depending on age, sex, social and cultural factors) for that individual'.

Types of Disability

Disabilities are broadly divided into following 4 groups:

Locomotor Disability

It occurs when movements in our body are affected due to disease, injury, any absence or deformities in the joints, bones and muscles, or an injury of the nerves, spinal cord or brain.

Locomotor impairment can lead to paralysis (paraplegia, monoplegia, and hemiplegia), weakness, spasticity, sensory loss, pressure ulcer, incontinence, urinary retention, deformities and contractures, hearing or speech impairment, visual loss, mental retardation, limitations in the Activities of Daily Living (ADL), etc.

Hearing and Speech Disability

Hearing Disability

Hearing impairment or disability indicates deafness. Deafness is a condition in which the child/adult suffers from hearing difficulties. The extent of deafness depends upon the (i) type, and (ii) degree of hearing impairment.

Definition of Hearing Impairment

According to the Persons with Disabilities (equal opportunities, protection of rights and full participation) Act-1995, hearing impairment means 'loss of 60 decibels or more in the better ear in the conversational range of frequencies'.

Speech and Language Disability

The ability to speak well is an asset. If one's speech is defective, it may become very difficult to manage many situations in life. There are large number of persons/children suffering from speech and language disorders.

Visual Disability (Visual Impairment and Blindness)

Visual impairment affects all aspects of life, and blindness is counted as a disgrace of the God.

Definition of Blindness

- According to Persons with Disability Act-1995 Blindness refers to a condition where a person suffers from any of the following conditions:
  - Total absence of sight
  - Visual acuity not exceeding 6/60 or 20/200 (Snellen) in the better eye with correcting lenses
  - Limitation of the field of vision subtending an angle of 20 degree or worse.

Role of Community Health Nurse in Care of Handicaps

- Prevention from disability at all levels of care.
- Early identification of risk factors and impairment/disability.
- Assessment of extent of handicap.
- Referral to specialists of concerning discipline, seeking advice.
- Coordination between the efforts and team members, NGOs, agencies, etc.
- IEC activities for handicaps.
- Arrangement for helping devices/aids for handicaps, minor repairs.
- Check on further complications/deterioration.
- Rehabilitation: Medical and physical, social, psychological and vocational.
- Nursing research for the care of handicapped.

Coping with Disability/Handicaps

The nurse will educate the community people how to cope with the disability.

Personal Priorities/Objectives

- Maintain priorities in order, eliminate non-essential activities.
- Plan your activities:
  - Keep work in front of yourself.
  - Plan each day.
  - Distribute heavy work load throughout week.
  - Organize work routine.
- Rest before undertaking difficult job/task and stop the activity before fatigue sets in.
- Follow daily exercise program.

Environmental Adjustments

- Try to be well organized.
- Place articles/possessions in same place, to save time and energy.
- Place equipment in box/basket, essential for personal care, use self-help aids/equipment as and when needed.
- Use work simplification and energy conservation techniques.
- Take safely precautions.

Life Philosophy

- Face the reality of your disability/handicaps.
- Remain outward and positive looking/approach.
- Seek innovative ways to tackle problems.
- Maintain and improve general health/strength.
- Plan for recreation/humor.

CARE OF MENTALLY CHALLENGED

Challenged condition makes the normal function of individual very difficult and leads to dependency. These conditions are increasing day by day due to changing lifestyle and complicated environment. Challenged children is one who deviated from normal health status either physically, mentally or socially and requires special care, treatment and education. According to WHO the sequence of events leading to disability and handicapped OR challenged conditions are as follows like:

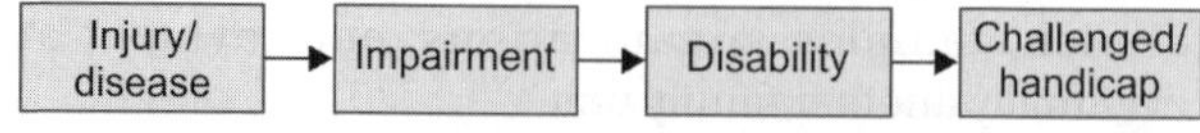

Physically challenged Grouped according to affected part of the body, e.g., orthopedically handicapped, sensory handicapped, neurologically handicapped and handicapped due to systemic diseases. Socially challenged Social disturbances are found in the form of broken family, loss of parents, poverty, lack of educational opportunities, environmental deprivation and emotional disturbances as lack of tender loving care. Socially challenged Social disturbances are found in the form of broken family, loss of parents, poverty, lack of educational opportunities, environmental deprivation and emotional disturbances as lack of tender loving care. Mentally challenged is now used for the condition mental retardation.

Intellectual disability (ID)/intellectual development disorder (IDD)/mental retardation (MR).

Intellectual disability (ID), also called intellectual development disorder (IDD) and formerly known as mental retardation (MR). Mental retardation (MR) is a developmental disability that first appears in children under the age of 18. It is characterized as a level of intellectual functioning (as measured by standard intelligence tests) that is well below average and results in significant limitations in the person's daily living skills (adaptive functioning). It is a generalized disorder, characterized by significantly impaired cognitive functioning and deficits in adaptive behaviors with onset before the age of 18. IQ Score under 70. The term MR as offensive and the term intellectual disability or intellectually challenged is now preferred by most advocates in most English speaking countries.

Definition of mental retardation (MR):

- Mental retardation refers to significantly sub-average general intellectual functioning (BELOW 70) resulting in or associated with concurrent impairments in adaptive behavior and manifested during the developmental period.
- American Association on Mental Deficiency,1983, retardation means a condition of arrested or incomplete development of mind of a person which is specially characterized by subnormal intelligence'.

In other words, we can say that mental retardation or mental handicap is a state of sub-average intellectual function combined with deficits in adaptive behavior. (The term idiot, moron, imbecile are now not used).

Etiology

- **Genetic factor:** Chromosomal abnormalities, cranial malformation, gross disease of brain
- **Prenatal factor:** Infections, endocrine disorders, physical damage and disorders, intoxication, placental dysfunction
- **Perinatal factors:** Birth asphyxia, prolonged or difficult birth, prematurity, kernicterus, instrumental delivery
- **Postnatal factors:** Encephalitis, measles, meningitis, septicemia, accidents, lead poisoning
- **Environmental and sociocultural factors:**
  - Cultural deprivation
  - Low socioeconomic status
  - Inadequate caretakers
  - Child abuse.

Predisposing Factors

- Low socioeconomic strata or poverty.
- Low birth weight of children.
- Advanced maternal age.
- Consanguinity.
- Extreme malnutrition.
- Lack of stimulating environment and poor sensory experience.
- Defective low standard education due to defective scholastic environment.
- Parental deprivation, prolonged isolation of caretakers during developmental period.
- Sensory deprivation and social deprivation.

Types of mental retardation: Types of IQ range in mental retardation:

1. Mild (Educable) 50–70
2. Moderate (Trainable) 35–50
3. Severe (Dependent retarded) 20–35
4. Profound (Life support) <20

Mild retardation (IQ 50–70) (Educable): 85–95% of total mental retardation cases belong to mild mental retardation. They have deficient in intellectual skills, studies up to 6–8th standard, problem in reading and writing, difficult in academic school work, normative living skills, walking, talking, toilet training, language abilities, and development of domestic skill, behavior, social and emotional adjustment like a normal person. They can fully adjust educable, finds difficulty in complex ideas, drawing generalization, can learn motor skills better than verbal skill and writing, emotionally they are stable, overactive, temper tantrum is common, can understand simple terms, they can be trained in special school. In adult life most of them lead independent life in normal surroundings.

Moderate retardation (Trainable) (IQ 35–50): 10% of mental retardation cases belong to moderate mental retardation. Children can be trainable, aimed at self-help skills, they can speak and support themselves, able to perform semi-skilled or unskilled work under supervision can learn few basic skills. Communication skills develop much slowly, limited progress in scholastic work, studies up to 2nd grade, unaware of needs, have less neuropathological complications, partially depends on others for their care.

Severe retardation (Dependent) (IQ 20–35): 7% of total mental retardation cases, belong to severe MR. Slow motor development in preschool years, trainable for normal living activities, allow them to do daily living activities under supervision, contributes partially to self-maintenance, some children may learn social behavior, able to communicate in simple way, engaged in limited activities, delayed speech and communication skills.

Profound retardation (Life support) (IQ <20): 1–2% of mental retardation cases are profound type. Considerable organic pathology, nervous system is noticed, associated conditions are—blindness, deafness, seizures are common, delayed milestones, motor impairment, totally dependent, cannot do anything on their own. Death may occur due to variety of problems or complications.

Prevention of Mental Retardation

Primary Prevention

Preconception

- Genetic counseling
- Immunization for maternal rubella.
- Blood tests for marriage licenses can identify the presence of venereal disease.
- Adequate maternal nutrition can lay a sound metabolic foundation for later childbearing.
- Family planning in terms of size, appropriate spacing and age of parents can also affect a variety of specific causal agents.

During Gestation

Prenatal care:

- Adequate nutrition, fetal monitoring and protection from diseases.
- Avoidance of teratogenic substances like exposure to radiation and consumption of alcohol and drugs.
- Analysis of fetus for possible genetic disorder by amniocentesis, fetoscopy, fetal biopsy and ultrasound.

At Delivery

- Delivery conducted by expert doctors and staff, especially in cases of high-risk pregnancy.
- Apgar scoring done at 1 to 5 minutes after the birth of the child.

During Childhood

- Proper nutrition throughout the developmental period and particularly during the first 6 months after birth.
- Dietary restriction for specific metabolic disorders until no longer needed.
- Avoidance of hazards in the child's environment to avoid brain injury from causes such as lead poisoning, ingestion of chemicals, or accidents.

Secondary Prevention

- Early detection and treatment of preventable disorders. For example phenylketonuria, hypothyroidism can be effectively treated at an early stage by dietary control or hormone replacement therapy
- A delay in diagnosis may cause unfortunate delay in rehabilitation.
- Psychiatric treatment for emotional and behavioral difficulties.

Tertiary Prevention

- This includes rehabilitation in vocational, physical and social areas according to the level of challenged.
- Rehabilitation is aimed at reducing disability and providing optimal functioning in a child with mental retardation.

Care and Rehabilitation of Mental Retardation

- The prevention and early detection of mentally handicaps.
- Regular assessment of the mentally retarded persons attainments and disabilities.
- Advice, support, and practical measures for families.
- Provision for education, training, occupation, or work appropriate for each handicapped person.
- Housing and social support to enable self-care.
- Medical, nursing, psychiatric and psychological services those who require them as outpatients, day patients or inpatients.

Role of a Community Health Nurse in Prevention of Mental Retardation

Tasks of the community nurse are:

- Coordination of services for the mentally retarded
- Education of public and professionals
- Assessment and planning
- Counseling and support
- Training and rehabilitation of the mentally retarded for community living
- Placement in the community and supervision.

In order to facilitate the aforementioned optimum care the nurse should function as a member of a multidisciplinary team, which includes a psychologist, psychiatrist, social worker, occupational therapist, physiotherapist and teacher.

The nurse must educate and guide the community regarding prevention of mental retardation.

Alcoholism in the mother and malnutrition of the infant are two high-risk medical conditions. Social stress, e.g., poor housing, insufficient income, may cause emotional problems in the family resulting in rejection, emotional deprivation and mental and physical abuse, any of which may contribute to mental retardation.

So the nurse must aware the community in this regards.

Acceptance by the Community: Acceptance of the mentally retarded child by the community is very essential by which they may live within their potential, enjoy the rights accorded to others. The first and most important group is the parents of the newly born retarded child. The immediate effects of this trauma are feelings of shock, disbelief and grief. The nurse must be aware of this and give immediate support. The support is firstly to disclose the problem to, ideally, both parents simultaneously and as soon after birth as possible. Once the parents feel that they are not alone in the world to carry this heavy burden and that people with knowledge, empathy and willingness to help are at hand, they can begin to accept this child and the all-important bonding with the mother is assured. Acceptance by the general public is essential for facilitating normalisation. The public can also be motivated to provide funds for special facilities such as schools, recreation clubs, playgrounds, etc.

Mobilization of the Community: The nurse must familiarize herself with the community and make herself known to them. She must work with the community, not for them, or they for her. A pleasant personality and appearance go a long way to "sell" mental retardation to the public. The needs of the mentally retarded and their families must be assessed. The type of assistance given will depend on what these individuals find the most acceptable and feasible. Priority needs must be established, and short, medium and long-term goals planned. Resources in the community need to be identified. These might be existing service clubs and organizations, student groups, parents of retardates etc. There might be existing facilities in the community which can be used for the mentally retarded or where the mentally retarded can participate in the activities of normal people, e.g., coffee mornings for the aged, horse riding schools, public swimming pools, seaside camps. The support of community leaders, e.g., city councillors, school principals, clergymen, etc., can stimulate projects aimed at normalisation for the mentally retarded.

CARE OF CHILDREN

Child health refers to a state of complete physical, mental and social well-being and not merely the absence of disease or infirmity in matters relating to growth and development of fetus during antenatal period and from birth of the baby till five years of age. It implies health care of the fetus during antenatal period, which refers to antenatal pediatrics, health care of neonates from birth to 28 days, care of infants up to one year, care of toddler from one year up to two years, care of preschool child from two years to five years of age. The health of the children is also very important not only because they are the asset and future of their families and the nation but also because health status, health behavior and lifestyle thus form during childhood determine the quality of life during the following years of life.

Different Aspects of Child Health

Breastfeeding

Breast milk contains all types of nutrients which are essential for normal growth and development of child up to six months of age and should continue up to at least 2 years of age. It also provides high immunity power which can protect the child from many diseases. So, it is important for the mother to give breastfeeding to the baby soon after the child's birth and continue it exclusively for six months, which will prevent malnutrition and other diseases in the later life. Although exclusive breastfeeding prevents malnutrition on a large scale, many mothers are not practicing exclusive breastfeeding and colostrum feeding till now. The community Health Nurse should educate all the mothers regarding breastfeeding, its importance, good attachment and positioning, etc.

Weaning

For the first 6 months, the breast milk is sufficient for the baby's normal growth and development, but after 6 months, the baby requires additional food to meet the body's requirements as the breast milk alone cannot meet the requirements of the child. Therefore, supplementary feeding is essential along with breastfeeding.

Principles of introducing supplementary feeding to the child should be explained by the community health nurse.

Immunization

Immunization is a process of protecting an individual from a disease through introduction of live or killed and attenuated organisms in the individual. Immunization against vaccine—preventable diseases is essential to reduce the child mortality, morbidity and handicapped condition. It is the means of protecting the largest number of people from various diseases. It gives resistance to an infectious disease by producing or augmenting the immunity. The main role of a CHN is to observe that all the children should complete every immunization by following the National Immunization Schedule.

Growth Monitoring

The growth sprout is the highest during the first five years of life. Weight and height increase with age. In a normal child, the birth weight can double by the age of 5 to 6 months and triple by the age of 1 year. During the second year of life, the weight gain is about 2 to 2.5 kg from the period of infancy. During 3 to 5 years of age, the weight gain for the baby is 1.5 kg to 2 kg. Similarly, the length of the newborn is approximately 50 cm (20") at birth, which increases to 75 cm (29") at the age of one year. During the second year of life, the increase in height is about 10 cm (4–5") and the height increases to 6–7 cm (3") during 3–5 years. Regular weight-checking and comparison to the normal standard help to identify the degree of malnutrition and its related factors. The weight-checking can be done in the nearer hospitals, PHCs, subcenters or Anganwadis. Normally, every month, the weight of the child should be checked during the first year, and later, weight can be recorded at 3 months interval. The doctor should be consulted when the child's weight is reducing without any reason, weight is static for continuously 3 months or if there is any continuous illness.

GERIATRIC CARE

Healthy aging depends on genetic, environmental and behavioral factors as well as broader environmental and socioeconomic determinants. Some of these factors are within the control of the individual, usually referred to as lifestyle factors and others are outside the individual control. Social determinants of health, such as income and education, influences the choices that individual can make and create life circumstances which limit opportunities for healthy lifestyle and create health inequalities.

At all the stages of life course the adoption of healthy lifestyles and actively participating in one's own care are of great importance. The WHO active aging states that engaging in appropriate physical activity, healthy eating, not smoking and drinking alcohol, medication wisely in old age can prevent disease and functional decline, extend longevity and enhance one's quality of life.

The individual grows old and older; various changes take place in the body with time under the influence of biological factors within the individual, the external factors in the environment and kind of his/her lifestyle. But many of the changes can be prevented and/or delayed by modifying various influencing factors such as diet, exercise, lifestyle, etc., leading to healthy aging.

Different Aspects of Geriatric Care

Nutrition

As old age, physical changes impact nutrient needs and can result in deficiencies, nutritional care is an important aspects of geriatric care. The daily energy requirements for old ages are 1,600–2,200 calories. Geriatric people are more susceptible to medical problems, such as disability and disease, which can impact appetite, the ability to plan and prepare food, chewing and swallowing, self-feeding, and general nutrient intake. During selecting cooking and serving, the caretaker should keep in mind all things.

A nutrient-dense, plant-based diet can help prevent or support the healing of a number of disorders that impact the elderly, including macular degeneration and arthritis. A low-fat, high-fiber diet is not appropriate for all elderly people, especially those with repeated infections, generally poor health or a poor appetite. It is important that older people choose a nutrient rich diet, high in foods providing protein, vitamins and minerals such as milk and dairy products, meat, eggs, fish, bread, cereals, and fruit and vegetables. A varied diet will also help to ensure adequate nutritional intake. Soft healthy diet in small amount should be provided.

Recreation

There are many fun activities elderly people can take part in to keep their minds sharp, bodies strong and spirits high. Whether it's spending time outdoors, playing games with friends, or spending time working on a favorite hobby, doing things they love can benefit the overall well-being of all seniors. Some other outdoor activities are picnic, fishing, gardening, listening music, singing song, reading and listening mythology book, watching TV, etc.

Spirituality

The spirituality of aging varies among individuals, but some generalizations include a need to review life events, face the certainty of death and process the emotional aspects of multiple chronic diseases and losses, mental peace. We gain spirituality from pray to god, yoga, exercise, etc.

Yoga practice benefits people of all ages, younger or older. Yoga is beneficial for older people, unfit people and unhealthy people too. Yoga helps all. Yoga aids and assists in healthy retirement. Yoga is not only for the young, fit and healthy.

Exercise

Exercise is very essential for the normal growth and development of the body and perfect maintenance of health. It is also required to excite the demand for oxygen required for utilization of food and to promote the repair of worn out tissues.

Exercise should be done in early hours of the morning or in the evening. It should not be taken within two hours of every meal. One should not eat too soon either before or after exercise. Games should be encouraged since they combine recreation with exercise. Morning walk with proper yoga and pranayam is the best exercise for elderly people. The benefit of morning walk is reduced weight, blood pressure, cardiovascular risk and increased blood circulation in the body.

Sleeping

Sleep disturbances are very common in older people. Changes in sleep pattern may be a normal part of aging, but many other factors common in this age group contributes to sleep problem. These include physical illness or symptoms, medication, side effects, changes in activity or social life and death of a spouse or loved one. Sleep disorders decrease quality of life in older people by causing daytime sleepiness, tiredness and lack of energy. Poor quality sleep can also lead to confusion, difficulty concentrating and poor performance on tasks. 6 to 7 hours of sleep required in night during this age. Daytime sleeping is another cause of night time wakefulness. Older people are more likely to be sleepy during the day but too much sleepiness during the day is not a part of normal aging.

FAMILY HEALTH NURSING

Definition of Family Health

Family health can be defined as possessing the abilities and resources to accomplish family developmental tasks.

In other words family health can be defined as the continuing ability to met defined functions in interaction with other social, political, economic and health systems.

Definition of Family Health Care

Family health care is for providing comprehensive care to family. It is the functions of a community health nurse to provide healthcare services to families and their members.

Objectives of Family Health Care

For providing nursing care to family, the main objectives which are kept in mind:

- To identify and appraise health problems of the family.
- To ensure family's understanding and acceptance of the problems. The family should recognize and accept the health problems.
- To provide nursing services according to the health needs of the family, which cannot provide by themself.

- To develop the competence of each individual member of the family to think through and cope with his or her own problems.
- To contribute to personal and social development of the family members.
- To promote full and intelligent use of available facilities and services for medical care, health promotion, illness, prevention and for related social and educational facilities.
- To provide health education and necessary information to use resources wisely and fully.

Principles of Family Health Care

Community health nurse should keep the following principles in mind when planning and implementing family health care:

- Establishing good professional relationship with family and members, in which the role of nurse and each family members in health development should be clear, unambiguous and accepted by everyone.
- Proper health education and guidance should be provided to family to take care of themselves according to their needs, intelligently.
- Collect information about the size, occupation, education, religion, custom and tradition of the family.
- Identify the health problems of the family and set priorities.
- Provide need-based support to the family to improve their health status instead of routine services.
- Health care services should be provided to the family irrespective of sex, age, income, religion, etc.
- Duplication of health services should be avoided and there is need to coordinate services with other disciplines providing health service, to save time, energy, manpower and financial resources.
- Provide service, which are preventive in nature so, that the family members are maintaining good health and this would help to minimize the need for curative services.
- Proper health messages to be communicated to family in every contact.
- Knowledge of basic facts, e.g., size, occupation, customs, rituals, and education standard is required by the Nurse during providing care.
- Problem identification and priority: Need-based support and services to family can be provided.
- Problem discussion with family and possible solution to drawn out.
- Encourage family to be self-sufficient to fulfill their needs.
- Encourage the participation of family members during providing any care.

Advantages of Family-based Health Care

- The family-based health care provide a lot of advantage. Through Family-based Health Care the Community Health Nurse can provide preventive, promotive and curative services to a number of people.
- By gaining knowledge of family background, it become easy to assess and understand the health care needs of each member.
- The community (family health nurse) get cooperation easily from family member for planning, implementing and evaluating health care in their home .
- Family-based health care provides opportunity to give health care to an individual as per predetermined schedule.
- It is economical as it saves time, man, money, material and resources of health services.
- Family-based health care helps family in self reliant of meeting health needs, improving health, welfare, and nutrition of the family.
- The individual feels more secure and comfortable in home with their family members rather than hospital during treatment.
- Overlapping of services and deficient services can be avoided.
- Through family health care the CHN can easily address the barriers for assessing health services and provide necessary guidance.
- Family is the best field for health education.

Aims of Family Health Service

Four main aims are:

1. Reduction of maternal, infant and childhood mortality and morbidity rate.
2. Family planning to space out children and ensure planned parenthood.
3. Improve nutritional status of all family members.
4. Health education of family in all preventive, promotive, curative and rehabilitative aspects of health care.

Scope of Family Health Service

Maternal Child Health Services

Maternal health is the health of women during pregnancy, childbirth, and the postpartum period. It encompasses the health care dimensions of preconception, prenatal, and postnatal care in order to reduce maternal morbidity and mortality. Preconception care can include counseling on health promotion, screening and other interventions among women of reproductive age to reduce risk factors that might affect future pregnancies. Similarly prenatal care is the care provided from conception to delivery of baby which is an important aspect for a healthy mother and baby and care during labor is consider as natal care. Postnatal care issues include recovery from childbirth, concerns about newborn care, nutrition and breastfeeding. Family is a vast field to provide all types of maternal and child health care.

Family Planning Services

Family planning services are defined as 'educational, comprehensive medical or social activities which enable individuals, including minors, to determine freely the number and spacing of their children and to select the means by which this may be achieved. The goal of family planning services can be achieved through family approach.

Nutrition

The nutritional status of the individual can be improved through family health care. A community health nurse can directly assess the nutritional status of family members through direct and indirect method and can provide health education regarding selection, purchase and consumption of foods. She can also educate the mothers regarding food hygiene, preservation of nutrients and can demonstrate the different methods of cooking.

Health Education

Health education is a process of providing information and advice related to healthy lifestyle and encouraging the development of knowledge, attitudes and skills aimed at behavior change of individuals or communities. It is a process which affects changes in the health practices of people and in the knowledge and attitude related to such changes. Family health nursing primarily depends upon Health Education because it emphasize preventive approach rather than curative approach.

Geriatric Care

Geriatric nursing is the nursing care and the services provided to older adults. The aim of geriatric nursing is to safeguard and increase health to the extent possible and to provide comfort and care to the extent necessary. For a healthy aging family-centered approach is very much essential. Family provide a perfect field to provide geriatric care.

Care of Adolescence

Adolescence is a time of moving from immaturity childhood to maturity adulthood by unfolding a set of transitions that touch upon many aspects of the individual's behavior, development, and relationships. These transitions are biological, cognitive, social, and emotional which also affect the health condition of adolescents if they are not coping properly. With that there are a variety of health problems of adolescents can be solved by family-centered approach.

FAMILY HEALTH NURSING PROCESS

It refers to a series of planned step and interventions directed at meeting the health needs and solving the problems of family. The component of nursing process are same but focus become family rather than individual.

- It requires long-term, continuous care to solve the problem.
- The process provides systematic need-based comprehensive care to the entire family within the given resources.
- It helps to achieve the desired goal, i.e., health promotion, prevention and control of health problems.

Purpose of Family Health Nursing Process

Main: To provide a systematic methodology for nursing practice in family.

Others

- It Unifies, standardizes and directs Nursing Practice in community.
- Nursing roles and functions in family are defined.
- Communication, Collaboration and Synchronization of health team members in community are enhanced.
- Health promotion, maintenance and restoration of family health or a peaceful death depending on the client's situation can be achieved.
- Facilitate documentation of data, diagnoses, plans, client responses and evaluation.
- Evaluate the efficiency and effectiveness of family health care.
- Give direction, guidance of nursing care in families.
- Provide continuity of family health care and to reduce omissions.
- Enhance client and family members involvements in health care.
- Promote creativity and flexibility in community health nursing practice.
- Accountability and responsibility to clients and nursing professions care be demonstrated.
- Enhance professional growth and competence.
- Increases job satisfaction of nursing personnel.
- Fulfill professional and legal responsibilities.

Characteristics of Family Health Nursing Process

- Goal-directed toward family-centered health care.
- Systematic and provides an organized approach to family health care.
- Dynamic by focusing on the changing responses of the family members during the ongoing process.
- Applicable to families and community groups at any level of health.
- Interpersonal and based on the nurse-client and family members relationship.
- Useful for family diagnosis and community diagnosis.

Phases of Family Health Nursing Process

There are five distinct phases of family health nursing process (**Fig. 2.1**):

1. Assessment phase
2. Family health diagnosis
3. Planning phase
4. Implementation phase
5. Evaluation phase.

Assessment Phase

It is continuous, systematic, critical, orderly and precise method of collecting, validating, analyzing and interpreting information about physical, psychological and social needs

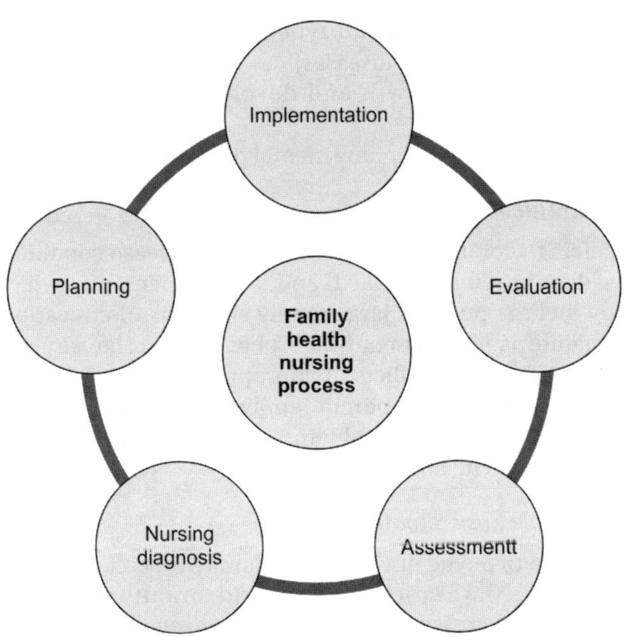

Fig. 2.1: Phases of family health nursing process.

of an individual family and community. It is the first major phase of family health nursing process which helps to explore the family as a client, its health needs/problems. It also finds the possible underlying factors that affect their health. It also helps to explore families ability to maintain wellness, prevent, control and resolve problem. Data about present condition of family are compared against standard, norms of personal, social and environmental health. These standards are derived from values, beliefs, principles, etc.

Types of Assessment

a. **First Level Assessment:** It is a process whereby existing and potential health problems of the families are determined. It establishes productive working relationship with each other and promotes participation of family member in taking care of their own health. It also provides opportunities to know each other, work together, develop faith and confidence.
b. **Second Level Assessment:** It defines the nature and type of nursing problem that family encounters in performing health task with respect to given health condition or problem and etiology or barriers to the family assumption.

Planning for Data Collection

It depends upon purpose and scope of family health care, i.e., the purpose is to find the health deficit, then data to be collected regarding acute/chronic illness, poor growth and development, etc. During data collection the nurse should observe the normal/optimum health of individual members, family lifestyle conducive to family's health. Family environment conducive to family's health family structure characteristic and functioning conductive to family health and development. During data collection, there is a wide range and variety of data which can be collected for doing health assessment, these are: Family structure and characteristics—family size/type, composition, genogram, family's development, family's power system, family's interactions, Family's lifestyle and culture—dietary practices, sleep, rest and exercise practices, leisure time activities, cultural practices, etc., Socioeconomic factors—religion, social class, income, monthly expenditure, family's perception about their income, socioeconomic status, family's relationship with other, family's participation in community activities. Health and medical history, present health and illness status, history of past significant illness and accident, immunization status of each member, family's attitude towards health personnel and agencies, family's expectation from CHN, fertility behavior and vital health events. During data collection environmental status of the family should be assessed which include housing condition, ventilation, lighting kitchen condition and maintenance of food hygiene, source and preservation of water supply, disposal of excreta, disposal of solid and liquid waste, presence of any domestic animal and maintenance of hygiene, etc. Data regarding transportation and communication is also important.

Data Collection Method and Techniques

Data collection requires certain skills like judgement, effective communication and investigation/measurements.

Observation

Observation is a technique for collecting all the data or acquiring information through occurrences that can be observed through senses with or without mechanical devices. The nurse gathers information about the family's state of being and behavioral responses. Observation of home environment, interaction, communication among family member gives information about family characteristics, dynamics, socioeconomics, ability to cope, etc. Observation are mainly two types: Formal observation and informal observation when the purpose, of observation visit is informed to family members it is called Formal observation

One can also participate in some of the family activities/ cultural events and observe the cultural pattern is an example of informal observation.

Interview

An interview is a conversation between two or more people (interviewer and interviewee) where questions are asked by interviewer to obtain information from the interviewee. It is done by asking formal questions. It may be informal conversation or face to face interview. This method requires the well planned interview schedule and questionnaire to obtain proper information. In collecting data from a community, generally we are following non structure interview schedule.

Listening

This is very useful method during informal conversation, when more chance is given to the client to talk express views and feelings. During listening the nurse can show her response by nodding her head or saying yes, etc.

Review of Family Record

Gather information through reviewing existing records and reports pertinent to the client. Individual's clinical records, laboratory and diagnostic reports, immunization record, report about home and environmental conditions.

Physical Examination

Significant data about the health status of individual members can be obtained through direct examination, measurement of specific body parts, etc. Through physical examination directly health condition can assessed. Different methods of physical examinations are inspection, palpation, percussion, auscultation and manipulation, etc.

Guideline for Data Collection

During data collection, in order to gain acceptance, co-operation and confidence of family, the Community Health Nurse has to follow some of the relevant principles of data collection:

- Inform the family members before head the date of data collection by which they can easily spare time for you
- Develop trust with family members
- Developing good interpersonal relationship
- Explain reason for home visiting
- Do not give wrong information to the family members
- Make sure the tools being used for measurements are calibrated and in good condition
- Be systematic
- Do not pressurize the family members to get information
- Ensure confidentiality
- Do not let the family feel small or embarrassed
- Make them comfortable
- Listen attentively
- Record data as planned on the interview schedule/ observation check list.

Analysis of Data

Steps of data analysis includes:

- Sorting of data
- Clustering of related cues
- Distinguishing relevant from irrelevant cues
- Identifying patterns
- Comparing patterns
- Interpreting inferences and drawing conclusions.

By analysis and interpretation, the family health problems are driven out. Family health problems are different than individual problems. According to ruth freeman the family health problems is explained as:

Health Deficit

Health deficit generally occurs due to failure of health maintenance and development or otherwise it is called as disease condition which includes:

- Disease condition (all types of communicable and noncommunicable diseases)
- Deviation in growth and development (nutritional deficiencies)
- Personality disorder (any mental problems).

Health Threats

It refers to conditions that predispose to disease condition, accident or retarded growth and development, etc., which may include poverty, large family size, lack of education, immature pattern, poor nutrition, poor quality of life, strained family relations, conflicts in appropriate role distribution. Broken family, single parent family, and family history of congenital hereditary problems, etc., the problems which may affect the health condition.

Foreseeable Crisis Situation

There are two type of crises from family we can observed, these are: Maturational Crisis and situational crises. Maturational crisis also called as the expected crisis, which should be addressed. The expected are these periods that occurs with some degree of predictability as the result of matuaration, e.g., stage of growth and development of an individual. It occurs during transition from phase of life to the next such as from childhood to adolescence and from adolescence to adulthood. For example, adolescent issues such as dating, sexual activity, carrier choice, etc. The situational crisis though it is unexpected or an accidental occurrence called situational crisis. Still it should be addressed. These crisis follow an anticipated sudden events over when no control can be exerted, e.g., diverse, death, etc.

Family Profile and Diagnosis

It is the 2nd step of nursing process. It is a clinical judgment about individual, family or community response to actual or potential health problem. It provides the bases for selection of nursing intervention.

Activities of Nursing Diagnosis

a. Interpret and analyze patient data
b. Identify patient strength and health problem
c. Formulate and validate nursing diagnosis
d. Develop a prioritized list of nursing diagnosis
e. Detect and refer signs and symptoms that may indicate a problem beyond the nurses experience.

Once the data are analyzed, it is necessary to describe the family profile and make diagnosis to communicate these findings to family and concerned health personnel. After identifying the problems it is the role of a community health nurse to assess the patient strength and weakness to solve the problem which is known as second level assessment. Formulation of family profile includes family structure, environmental factor, lifestyle and culture, socioeconomic condition, health and medical history. Family health diagnosis is the written statement of family health problem/ health needs which are assessed from analysis of data collected.

Planning Phase

In this phase family health nursing care plan is formulated to meet family health need and resolve the problem. It involves some steps like:

- Analysis of diagnosed health problems
- Establishing priorities
- Setting goal and objectives
- Formulating family health and nursing care plan.

Analysis of Diagnosed Health Problems

Analysis of health problem and assessment of families ability. The diagnosed problem should be further reassessed to understand nature of their problem and the ability of family members to solve the problem, such as Recognition of own health problem, Ability to take decision and appropriate health action, Ability to provide desired care to sick/dependent member of the family and Ability to maintain conducive living environment, etc. The nursing care plan will be prepared, based the ability of the family to solve their own health problem. Second level assessment helps to develop proper **(Table 2.1)**.

Table 2.1: Comparison between first and second level assessment.

First level assessment	*Second level assessment*
Large family size (health threat) (husband, wife, four children and mother)	Inability to: • Recognize presence of large and associated health problem • Make decision about suitable action Due to: • Ignorance of its impact • Their belief that children are God gift and asset to the family • Misconception about family planning
Two children: Aged 5 and 3 years having malnutrition: health deficit (under weight, look paled, lethargic and weak)	Inability to: • Recognize presence of malnutrition • Make decision about the care of children • Gives desired care to children Due to: • Lack of comprehension of nature and extent of malnutrition • Ignorance of dietary requirement of children • Ignorance of care needed for malnourished children
Mother suspected of having PTB: Health deficit • Chronic cough with expectoration more than 2 month • Evening rise of temperature • Night sweating • Taking treatment from quack	Inability to: • Recognize the presence of pulmonary tuberculosis • Decide for suitable medical assistance • Provide desired and proper care Due to: • Lack of knowledge about PTB • Ignorance about care needed • Lack of competency • Fatalistic attitude
Insanitary home environment: Health threat • Unsafe water supply • Improper collection and removal of refuse • Poor drainage system and collection of waste water • Inadequate space and poor ventilation	Inability to: • Make decision about handling these problems • Maintain home environment conducive to health promotion and maintenance Due to: • Inadequate knowledge regarding sanitary environment • Inadequate resources • Fatalistic attitude

Priorities of Problem

Prioritize establishment: According to relative importance of health problem, rank order of health problem to be done. For priority setting, following steps are used: Types of health problem, i.e., health deficit, health threat, foreseeable crisis, severity of the consequence of problem. Modifiability of the problem: Possibility of resolving the problem through nursing intervention within the available resources of both family and nurse. Salience: Seriousness and urgency of attention needed and preventive method.

- Study medical and nursing records including care plan, family folder antenatal and postnatal card.
- Briefly enlist the total condition: Health deficit, health threat and foreseeable crises situation.
- Determine any problems that need to be resolve immediately and take appropriate actions.
- List the problems including nursing association and problems and ask oneself questions like what problems must be resolved today, what happens if I wait later? Which problem can I realistically work on today, etc.
- Determine the interventions that must be done to prevent, resolve, or control the problems listed. List these interventions along with routine tasks of bath, meal.
- Determine the thing that the patient and his significant others can do on their own and those that require your assistance include the patient in making these decisions.
- Make a detailed personal work sheet for getting things done for the day and refer to it frequently. Be sure to consider the daily routine of the unit.

In community setting prioritization among nursing process is depends upon not only the severity of the problems but also the five characters are taken into consideration, these are as such, Type of problem, Severity, Modifiability, Salience and Preventive potential.

Through the scoring process the rank can be determine which is described below. The rank one problem will get first priority followed by other ranks **(Table 2.2)**.

Setting of Goal

Goals are general statement of the desired outcomes and directions to resolve identified problems.

Objectives

It is the specific statements determining actions and/or desired targets.

NB: Objectives are stepping stones to achieve goal.

- Goal/Objectives should be measurable, time bound and clearly stated.

Table 2.2: Comparison between first and second level assessment.

Problem situation	Type of problem (3–2-1)	Severity (3–2-1)	Modifiability (3–2-1)	Salience (3–2-1)	Preventive potential (3–2-1)	Total score	Rank
Large family size	2	3	3	1	3	12	3
Suspected PTB and spread of infection to other	3	3	3	2	3	14	1
Malnutrition	3	3	3	1	3	13	2
Insanitary home environment	2	3	2	2	3	12	3
Postnatal mother	1	3	3	1	3	11	4
Newborn baby	1	3	3	1	3	11	4

Types

Goal has two types: 1. Client focussed
2. Nurse focussed

- Immediate
- Intermediate
- Long-term.

Goal and objectives should be acceptable to the family and therefore should be set up with the family.

Factors Influencing Formulation of the Goal

- Interpersonal relationship
- Family's perception of its health problem and its seriousness
- Family's felt need
- Family's ability to face the reality.

Implementation Phase

- While making decision about intervention, it is important for nurses to recognize that the family has the right to make its own health decision.
- While selecting alternative nursing intervention for dealing with health problem/needs, it is very important to consider available resources, i.e., family resources, community resources and nursing resources.
- The nurse may assist the family by:
  - *Supplemental:* Direct care by CHN
  - *Developmental:* To prepare family member for giving care
  - *Facilitative:* Improve physical facilities by modifying old facilities and adopting new one.

Approaches in Family Health Nursing Interventions

- Compensating approach
- Teaching approach
- Supporting and counseling approaches
- Preparing for report and getting report
- Setting daily priorities
- Assessing and reassessing
- Performing interventions and making necessary changes
- Giving report.

The role of nurse is:

- To offer guidance to the family
- To provide information
- To assist the planning process
- Implementation of care and documentation.

Barriers that may Interfere with Accomplishing Family Client Outcomes

- Family apathy
- Family indecision about the outcome or actions
- Nurse imposed ideas
- Negative labeling
- Overlooking family strengths
- Neglecting cultural or gender implications
- Family perception of hopelessness
- Fear of failure
- Limited access to resources and support
- Limited finances
- Fear and distrust on health care system.

Evaluation Phase

Evaluation means measures the degree to which the objectives and the targets are fulfilled and the quality of the results obtained. It measures the productivity of available resources in achieving clearly defined objectives. It measures how much output or cost effectiveness achieved. It makes possible the reallocation of priorities and of resources on the basis of health needs.

There are different types of classification for evaluation like Structure evaluation, process and outcome evaluation, Summative and formative evaluation, etc.

Structure evaluation: In nursing process Structure evaluation tends to evaluation of total care plan which include assessment, care plan and adequate resources to meet the plan.

Process evaluation: Process evaluation relate to evaluation of implementation whether it is carried out properly whether any intervention left.

Outcome evaluation: Outcome evaluation is the actual evaluation. It is the evaluation of result whether goals are met properly.

Formative evaluation: It evaluates family health and nursing care plan as it is planned and implemented to determine its strength and weaknesses at each stage and its progress towards meeting the objectives.

Summative evaluation: It concludes progress or lacks of progress towards the goal after several objectives-based action are implemented. The reasons are identified and modified and further action suggested.

It is the last steps of nursing process. The family nursing care plan will be incomplete if it is not judged or appraised to ascertain their achievement. Here the CHN should compare actual outcomes with the intended goals and objectives. Care should be evaluated against some standard and criteria. The crucial step of evaluation and its accompanying reassessment and revision processes.

Nurse will observed weather the degree to which objectives and targets are fulfilled and quality of the result obtained, the productivity of available resources in achieving clearly defined objectives and how much output or cost effectiveness is achieved in evaluation the Nurse will assess whether the goal is fully met or partially met or sometimes not met at all. In that cases once again she will assess and change her planning and makes possible for the reallocation of priorities and of resources on the basis of changing health needs. During any evaluation, there are some fix standards and criteria which should be met. Standard means expected level of performance and criteria means indicator of expected level of performances which helps to facilitate additional decision-making, conclude what had been done, what could not have been done to reach to goal, identify the alterations that are needed in the plan of care to make effectively reach the desired outcomes and to know the cost effectiveness in terms of money, time and other resources. During evaluation community health nurse will plan for next visits, making referral to the needed cases and making provision for resources.

Tools for Evaluation

- Direct observation
- Questioning
- Record review.

FAMILY NURSING THEORY

It is derived from three traditions, family social science, family therapy and nursing. The family social science theories is best developed and informative with respect to how families function, the environment family interchange, interaction within the family, how the family changes over time, and the family's reaction to health and illness.

Structure Function Theory

It defines family as social system which is open to outside that influence it.

Assumptions are:

- Family is social system with functional requirement
- A family is a small group that has basic features common to all subgroups
- Individual act within a set of internal norms and values that are learned primarily in the family socializing process.

System Theory

The system approach to understanding families was influenced by theories derived from biology and physics. A system is composed of a set of interacting elements: each system can be identified and is different from the environment in which it exists.

Assumptions are:

- Family system is greater than and different from the sum of their parts.
- There are many hierarchies within a family and logical relationship between subsystem.
- Boundaries in the family system can be open, closed or random.
- Family system changed constantly in response to stress and strains from within and outside environments.
- Change in one part of family system affects the total system.

Interactionist Theory

It views family as unit of interacting personalities and examines symbolic communications by which family member relates to one another. Within the family, each member occupies positions to which a number of roles are assigned. Members decides their role expectations in each situation through their perceptions of the role demands. This theory emphasizes that interaction between and among family members and family communication patterns about health and illness behaviors appropriate for different roles.

FAMILY SOCIAL SCIENCE THEORIES

- Duvall's family developmental theory.
- von Bertalanffy's systems theory.
- Friedman's structural-functional theory.
- Aguilera and Messick's crisis intervention theory.

DUVALL'S FAMILY DEVELOPMENTAL THEORY (MAJOR CONCEPTS)

Evelyn Duvall's (1977) family developmental framework provides guide to examine and analyze the basic changes and developmental tasks common to most families during their life cycle. Although each family has unique characteristics, normative patterns of sequential development are common to all families. These stages and developmental tasks illustrate common family behaviors that may be expected at specific times in the family life cycle. The stages are marked by the age of the oldest child however some overlapping occurs in families with several children.

According to Duvall's family developmental theory there are eight stages of family life cycle which started from beginning families (married couple without children) to aging families (retirement to death of both spouses) having different developmental task at each stages. Duvall's Developmental Theory addresses family change over time in life cycle based on predictable changes in structure, function and roles of the family. Age of the older child is the marker for stage transition, arrival of first child marks the transition from Stage I to Stage II. As the first child grows and develops, the family enters subsequent stages. At every stage family is at a developmental task. At the same time, each member of the family must achieve individual developmental task.

Stage I

Beginning families (married couple without children) involves merging of values brought into the relationship from the families includes adjustments to each other's routines (sleeping, eating, chores, etc.), sexual and economic aspects. Members work to achieve and separate identifiable tasks:

- Establish a mutually satisfying relationship
- Learn to relate well to their families of orientation
- If applicable, engage in reproductive life planning.

Stage II: Early Childbearing

This stage starts with birth or adoption of a first child which is 30 months of age. Which requires economic and social role changes the family. Families with infants, Integrate infants into family unit, Accommodate to new parenting and grand parenting roles, Maintain marital bond. The task in this stage are:

- Stabilizing the family unit.
- Reconciling family members conflicting developmental tasks.
- Facilitating developmental needs of mother, father and infant.

Stage III: Families with Preschoolers

In stage III the family members having at least one preschool child who is between 3 to 5 years of age. In this stage the children mingles with others like playmates, school teachers, socialize children, parents and children adjust to separation are happening in this. The basic task in this stage includes division of labor, income, managing household tasks, maintaining home, care for young and care for old, nurturing and socializing children and maintaining a stable marriage.

Stage IV: Families with School Children (Oldest of 6–13 Years of Age)

Children develop peer relations, parents adjust to their children's peer and school influence. The major task in this stage includes Socialization of family members. The family assumes responsibility for guiding development of nature and acceptable patterns of socially acceptable behavior in eating, elimination, sleeping, sexuality, aggression and intervention with others. Promoting school, environment is also very important for proper development of child.

Stage V: Families with Teenagers (Oldest 13–20 Years)

Adolescence is the transitional period from childhood immaturity to maturity and this is the most important period in human life. Adolescents develop increasing autonomy. Parental role focus on midlife marital and career issues. Parents begin shift toward concern for older generation. The developmental task in this stage include:

- Balance teenage freedom and responsibility.
- Maintaining open parent child communication.
- Maintaining a stable marital relationship.
- Building a foundation for future family stages.

Stage VI: Launching Center Families (Young Adult–Time)

Families as launching centers, parents and young adults establish independent identities, renegotiate marital relationship. It is the time when the young adult leaving home. The major tasks in this stage are:

- Releasing children as young adults.
- Readjusting with situation.

Stage VII: Middle-aged Families

Reinvest in couple identity with concurrent development of independent interests. The task in this stage are Placement of members in the larger society. Family members establish roots in society through relationships in church, school, political and other organization which will protect the family members from undesirable outside influences and it may prohibit membership in objectionable groups.

- Strengthening the marital relationship.
- Sustaining relationship with parents and children.
- Providing a healthy environment.
- Cultivating leisure time activities.

Stage VIII: Aging Families

Aging families shift from work role to leisure and semi-retirement or full retirement. Maintain couple and individual functioning while adapting to the aging process. Prepare for own death and dealing with the loss of spouse and/or siblings and other peers include in-laws and grand children. Deal with disabilities and death of older generation. The task is maintenance of motivation and morale. Family members reward each other for their achievements and provide for an individual's needs of acceptance, encouragements and affection. The family develops a philosophy of life and sense of family unity and loyalty, thereby enabling members to adopt to both personal and family crises.

Uses of Duvall's Family Developmental Theory

- It can be used an excellent guide for assessing, analyzing and planning around basic family tasks at a specific developmental stage.
- Applicable for nuclear families with growing children and families who are experiencing health-related problems.
- The nurse must first determine the family's stage of development then examine the tasks that are appropriate for respective stage.

STEVENSON'S FAMILY DEVELOPMENTAL MODEL

She views family tasks as maintaining a common household rearing children and finding satisfying work and leisure. It also includes sustaining appropriate health patterns and providing mutual support and acculturation of family members **(Table 2.3)**.

This model is useful for nuclear families because it examines psychosocial patterns to specific stage of development, however, it also does not include family structure, nor it addresses health promotion and health-related concerns that the family may face.

FRIEDMAN'S STRUCTURAL-FUNCTIONAL THEORY

Friedman's Structural-Functional Family Model was developed from sociological frameworks and systems theory by Marilyn Friedman (1986). The family is the focus of this model as it interacts with suprasystems in the community and with individual family members in the subsystem. This model provides a broad framework for examining the interactions among family and within the community. This incorporates physical, psychosocial and cultural aspects of the family along with interacting relationships. According to him the families had some structural and functional components.

Structural Components

It examines the family composition, how it is organized and how members relate to one another in terms of their values, communication, network, role system and power. Structural component examines the family unit, while functional components refers to the interaction outcomes resulting from family organizational structure. The structural-functional components and parts all intimately related. The structural components consist of role structure, power structure, value system and communication pattern.

Role Structure

Family composed of different family members adopting varying roles that may change over time. Role can be formal (or) informal and adopted or assigned. There are conflicts between role expectations of others and roles adopted by members. Sometimes there is flexibility of family members in changing roles as needed according to situations.

Table 2.3: Joanne Stevenson (1977) describes the basic tasks and responsibilities of families in four stages.

Stages	*Health tasks*
Emerging family (from marriage for 7 to 10 years)	Couple strives for independence from their parents and to develop a sense of responsibility for family life
Crystallizing family (with teenage children)	To assume responsibility for growth and development of individual members and outside organizations
Interacting family (children grown and small grandchildren)	Assumption of responsibility for 'continued survival and enhancement of the nation.'
Actualizing family (aging couple alone again)	Assume the responsibility for sharing the wisdom of age, reviewing life and putting affairs in order

Power Structure

Power structure in the family is determined by various influencing factors—social, ethic class, family, communication pattern, interpersonal and financial resources, family coalitions, and implementation to decision. To identify the family power structure the Community Health Nurse should find out who is really incharge of the family and why, who makes the major decision and rules? Who is consulted about family plans/ changes. Based on the family power structure the family may be classify as authoritarian or democratic and paternalistic or maternalistic families.

Value Systems

Value systems developed by exposure to and experience with influential groups and individuals such as parents, culture, religion and ethnic groups. Values leads to chosen behaviors, which are reinforced by others and expressed by family members behaviors, how they allocate resources and where time and energy are invested. These values are related to health care, education, independence, productivity and cleanliness.

Communication Patterns

Communication patterns in the family means the way of interaction with each other. As family evolve they develop communication patterns which is ways of relating to each other. It may be functional or dysfunctional. It involves verbal and nonverbal behaviors including tone, intent and message. How they are interacting with each other and also interacting with community.

Functional Components

Affective

The affective function is one of the most vital functions for the formation and continuation of the family unit. This function refers to the family meeting the needs for love and belonging of each member. The family is a home base where the individuals can express their true feelings and thoughts without fear of rejection.

Physical Needs

In a family the adult family members responsible for fullfilling the physical needs of family members by providing, food, clothing, shelter, health care and also responsible for protect from danger.

Socialization and Social Placement

Socialization and social placement function refers to teaching children how to function and assume adult social roles. This function involves the acquisition of internal controls needed for self-discipline and values such as what is right and wrong according to society. Socialization is a process of learning the rules and expected behaviors of a society. One goal of parenting is to socialize children, which includes teaching which behaviors are expected and appropriate, and fostering the development of self-control. This is also the goal of discipline. The social and emotional development needs of family members must be recognized and met by family members. The emotional needs are reduce tension, maintaining morale, conveying esteem and love for family members.

The Health Care Function

The health care function includes provision of physical necessities to keep the family healthy, such as food, clothing, and shelter as well as health care (Friedman, 1998). The family keeps its members well by passing on attitudes, values, and behaviors that promote health and by caring for them in times of illness.

Economic

Economic function mainly deals with financial allocation for different purpose to complete the household task. It also include allocating other resources like material goods to family members. In some families the head of the family member is responsible, for this task. Where as in some other families it is based on the joint decision of family.

Reproduction

Reproduction function depends upon the eligible couple whether they use contraception or not. Sometime it depends upon the decision of whole adult family members in the family. They assume responsibility for conception and contraception.

Family Coping

For family stability and growth, the members need adaptive patterns and problem-solving abilities to respond to demands and expectations outside the family that create changes within the family. The structural functional components and parts all intimately interrelate and interact each component and part is affected by the others.

Uses

This theory is used to assess for modification of structure or function of the family. It is used to assess the normal and health problems of family member. For example, Head of the family met an accident, Family with handicapped children, Head of the family suffering with paralysis.

AGUILERA AND MESSICK'S CRISIS INTERVENTION THEORY

Major Concepts

Aguilera and Messick consider a stressful event or change in the individual's life involving loss or threat of loss, which disturbs the individual's equilibrium. Crises are categorized as maturational or situational.

Maturational Crises

It is also called as the expected crisis. The expected are these periods that occurs with some degree of predictability as the result of matuaration, e.g., stage of growth and development of an individual. It occurs during transition from phase of life to the next such as from childhood to adolescence and from adolescence to adulthood. For example, Adolescent issues such as dating, sexual activity, carrier choice, etc.

Situational Crises

The unexpected is one accidental occurrence called situationl crisis. These crisis follow anticipated sudden events over when no control can be exerted. For example, diverse, death, failing an examination, losing a job, receiving a promotion and sustaining an injury.

In Crisis Intervention Model, Aguilera and Messick identified three balancing factors and these factors reduce the risk of crises and help the individual to maintain equilibrium. The factors are as follows:

Realistic Perception of the Event

The realistic perception of the event means actual understanding of the events. Sometimes past experiences, evoke feelings unrelated to the event, when an individual attaches to an event, that influences the perception. These feelings may distort the individuals perception and magnify the consequences of the event. When an individual attaches great significance to an event, a distorted perception is likely to occur. The individual's feelings and emotions may create an unrealistic picture of the present and future, which hinders effective decision-making and may lead to crisis. With a realistic perceptions of the event are able to view the situation in perspective, which reduces the chance that their emotions will be decision-making. A realistic perception of the event may avert a crisis. The individual's feelings and emotions may create unrealistic picture of the present and future, which hinders effective decision-making and may lead to crisis. Those with a realistic perception of the event are able to view the situation in perspective, which reduces the chance that their emotions will be decision-making. A realistic perception of the event may avert a crisis.

Adequate Situational Supports

After providing the realistic perception of the event, the nurse focuses on who will be available to support the client. Questions such as the following can help identify the client's support systems: 'Whom do you trust ?' 'Who is your best friend ?' 'Is there a member of your family with whom you are particularly close?' The nurse also should inquire to the client's religious beliefs. For many families, God is a source of comfort and strength. It is best to have several supportive people involved with the client.

Because a crisis period lasts for a brief time and the nurse will be involved only temporarily, the client needs others on whom to rely for continued support. When the individual faced with a loss or threat of loss, individuals share the meaning of the event with significant others. Individuals rely an others to assist them in times of need. This sharing helps the individuals place the event in perspective. Situational supports are considered adequate when individuals feel they can share the concern with and receive support from significant others. Sometimes an individual cannot share the concern with others for fear of losing respect or esteem. When individuals lack others with whom to share the events or concerns, their situational supports are inadequate. This may cause disequilibrium and lead to crisis.

Adequate Coping Mechanisms

The nurse must encourage the client to describe coping methods as specifically as possible. Then the nurse should determines whether the client's coping mechanisms are adaptive or maladaptive. From life experiences, individuals learn a repertoire of coping responses or pattern. These patterns assist individuals in reduce tension, adapting to daily stressful events and maintaining equilibrium. Occasionally a stressful event occurs that overwhelms the individual. There may be a unfamiliar situation. When usual coping responses are ineffective, disequilibrium and crisis may occur. Aguilera and Messick's crisis intervention model describer, three balancing factors. Each factor must be adequately present to maintain equilibrium and avoid crisis.

Uses of Aguilera and Messick's crisis intervention model:

- This model is used for individuals or families experiencing situational or maturational crises
  - Pregnancy and childbearing strains
  - Illness and Family 'Care' strains
- Marital strains
- Family legal violations
- Intrafamily strains
- Work family transitions and strains
- Transitions 'in' and 'out'
- Losses.

FAMILY HEALTH RECORDS

Definition of Record

Records are written documents/information kept in notebook or folder, register, file or card, etc. In other words records are the administrator memory and also essential for administrative matters.

In every institution some kinds of record are maintained. In health care set up records contain not only the information regarding health but also the general information of individual and family. It include the information about socioeconomic, physiologic and environmental factor, heredity, and geographic factor. So it is the aid to doctor, nurses and paramedical personnel in giving the best possible services to individual, family and to the community.

Purposes of Records

- **Communication:** The record is a means by which health care team members communicate with each other and with the client regarding needs and problems of the client, treatment progress, therapies changes, client education and discharge planning, etc.
- **Legal documentation:** Accurate documentation is one of the best defenses for legal claims associated with nursing care. Nursing documentation must be written clearly and comprehensively which indicate that individualized, goal directed nursing care was provided to client based on the nursing assessment.
- **Financial billing:** Diagnosis related groups have become the basis for establishing reimbursement for client care, e.g., the nurse's contribution to documentation can help clarify the type of treatment a client receives and help support the reimbursement to the health care agency. Medical records are also audited to review financial charges used in client care, client behaviors. The nature of illness and the client response is to read from the client care record.
- **Research:** A nurse may use clients records during a clinical research study to investigate a new nursing intervention.
- **Auditing monitoring:** Nurses monitor or review records throughout the year to determine the degree to which quality improvement standards are met. Deficiencies identified during monitoring and corrections in place can be made.
- **Education:** A client's record contains a variety of information including diagnosis, signs and symptoms of disease, therapies, findings and client behviors. The nature of illness and the client response is to read from record.

Principles of Writing Health Records

Community health nurse must clarify her own thinking about the uses to which the record is put to. She also needs to develop her own expression. The health record should be:

- Focus on the needs and problems of the individuals family and community.
- Present the problem in, explicit and dynamic terms.
- Written clearly, appropriately and legibly.
- Contain health-related facts based on observation, conversation and action.
- It should be brief and accurate, neat, complete and uniform, based on the relevant facts.
- Records are valuable legal documents and so it should be handled carefully, and accounted for.
- Record systems are essential for efficiency and uniformity of services.
- The wording should be easily understand and using of common abbreviation can only acceptable.

- Record should provide for periodic summary to determine progress and to make future plans.
- Records should be written immediately after data collection.
- Records are confidential documents.
- Record should be written concise and neatly.

Legal Guidelines for Recording

- Do not erase, apply correction fluid, or scratch out errors made while recording. Draw single line through error, write word error above it and sign your name or initials. Then record note correctly.
- Record all facts. Record must be accurate and reliable.
- Do not leave blank space in nurse's note. Another person can add incorrect information in space.
- Record all entries legibly and in black ink. Never erase entries or use correction fluid, and never use pencil.
- Begin each entry with time, and end with your signature and title.

Criteria for Recording in Family Health Records

The criteria should reflect both the purpose and process of community health nursing practice.

- Record should concentrate on the family and community as focus of care. It should reflect not only the health of the members of the family but also the ways in which the functioning of the family a unit has an impact on the health of the family as a whole. It should also specify the ways in which family functions within its physical and social environment.
- Family health records should serve as guides for comprehensive care. These should include health threats and health behaviors that have significance for family health.
- An apparently healthy family may have poor nutritional habits and poor housekeeping practice inviting accidents. It is important that records show the potential problems which can be developed in future.
- The record should indicate the expected outcomes and also the degree to which outcomes are achieved. This means that the goals of care to a family are also defined in the records.
- The family health record should have specific actions planned for the family actions actually taken and distribution of responsibility to family and other community resources so that necessary activities are carried out. Action taken should be recorded in such a way that it can be easily located and future planning can be done.
- The family record should indicate family response to nursing action.
- Since initial planning and implementation can redefine a problem the record must show revision in the status of the problem so that further planning can be done accordingly.
- Record system should posses sufficient uniformity to make recording, tabulation and collection easy and to permit in her unit in service comparisons and easy reference.
- Maintenance of records should require minimal amount of time. Unimportant and irrelevant data reading may also require more time and lengthy records may result in errors.
- Family records should be quickly available to the user. Accessibility is not always easy to achieve. Compiled individual and family records can be made available at a central location for easy reference, only for professional use.
- Family records require reasonable storage space. A number of individuals are added the records also increase and require more storage space and facilities.
- Depending upon the number of years records should be retained, according to agency, policies and storage space will be required.
- Family record system should provide confidentiality of record content. For example, sometimes a mother in the family may not like information about family planning methods she has adopted to be shared with other members of the family or her neighborhood women. There should be provision for such confidential information and sometimes official records in the agency do not have provisions for such recording. The community health nurse must find her own ways to incorporate such summarization into her recording so that priority needs can be attend to first.

Types of Records

Based on some characteristics the records are classified.

According to 'Periodical'

- Permanent records (cumulative)
- Temporary records (casual/daily records).

According to 'Unit Based Records'

- Individual (individual health cards)
- Related to family (family folders)
- Related to community (community folders)
- National (national health programmes records).

According to 'Subject Based'

- Economical (financial structure of family, village)
- Social (records of social structure)
- Political
- Medical and nursing (treatment and medicine records).

According to 'Collection Place Based'

Collected at institutions:

- Records of hospitals/health centers
- Records to be kept with the individual (immunization cards, disease cards)
- Records to be kept with the patient
- Records related to community.

Records related to community are:

- Cumulative or continuing records
- Family Records

- Anecdotal records
- Individual health records
- Village records.
- Charts, maps, graphs.

Cumulative or Continuing Individual Records

Cumulative health record is a continuing record which contain all the health-related facts of an individual from childhood to life long. It is found to be time saving, economical and also it is helpful to review the total history of an individual and evaluate the progress of a long period. It also provide the past medical and surgical history for a person when the individual suffers from any new diseases.

Family Records

The basic unit of service is the family. All records, which relate to members of family, should be placed in a single-family folder. This gives to the picture of the total services and helps to give effective, economic service to the family as a whole.

Separate record forms may be needed for different types of service such as tuberculosis maternity, etc. All such individual records which relate to members of one family should be placed in a single family folder.

The family folder consists of different family health records which are commonly used are grouped in different ways. These may be grouped according to age of family member for whom records are used such as:

- Newborn care
- Road to health card
- Toddler card
- Adult card
- Old age or elderly card
- Mother child link card.

Health care requirement cards as per health conditions and morbidity status.

- Pregnant woman or antenatal card
- Intranatal care card or labor record
- Person with illness for example:
  - Tuberculosis record
  - Diabetic record
  - Hypertension care card
  - Malaria record.
- Drug addicts or alcoholic record
- Any chronic care record
- Immunization record.

Usually for family health services a family folder including different card is maintained. This includes sociodemographic information, children health status (including height, weight, immunization and feeding habits) maternal records, morbidity records and observations of general health status of family and the environment of the family.

These records have individual formats and styles of recording which is prescribed for each agency. The method of recording is usually a standard one and general instructions are provided. Examples of records for infant, toddler, antenatal women, immunization and family planning are shown in end of the topic.

Functions

Records have different functions in different persons and place also.

Record for Nurses are:

- Record provides basic facts for service.
- Record shows the patients and families.
- It provides analyzing needs.
- It provides basis for short and long-term planning.
- It prevent duplicity and helps follow-up service effectively.
- It helps to evaluate teaching.
- It helps to organize the work in an orderly ways and make effective ways of time.
- It guides to professional growth.
- It judges the quality and quantity of work done.

Record for Family and Individuals are:

- Helps them to become aware and to recognize their health needs.

For doctors:

- Records are guidelines for diagnosis treatment and evaluation of services.
- Indicates progress.
- Used in research purpose.

For paramedicals:

- It helps to identify families needs.

For organization and community:

- Records help the authority to evaluate the services given teaching done, actions and reactions of other staff members for giving reward and punishments.
- It helps in the guidance of staff and students as an evaluate tool.
- It helps to administrator accessing the health needs of the community.
- It helps in making studies and research.
- Useful for legislative purpose.
- For planning budget.
- It is legal evidence of the services rendered by each worker.
- It provides justification for expenditure of funds.

Records use in family planning:

- Family records—within it:
  - Number of lining children male/female
  - Age of the last child
  - Couple eligible for family planning
  - Use of a family planning method.
- **Individual health cards:** Services delivered to individuals who became family planning acceptors are recorded as follows:
  - Family planning method
  - Regularity of use
  - Side effect or complications
  - Treatment for problems
  - Prenatal records
  - Infertility.

- **Eligible couple register:** This has been following particulars:
  - Serial number
  - House number
  - Names of husband and wife, and address
  - Age of husband and wife
  - Number of living children, male and female
  - Age of the youngest child with sex
  - Is the woman pregnant now
  - Use of family planning method.
- **Village record:** This is a list of the different family planning methods. You should fill in the number of couples at present practicing each method, with number of living children.
  Depot holders are also listed with name, sex, address, occupation and designation of each.
- **Monthly report:** This includes:
  - Total number of eligible couples
  - Number of vasectomy was performed
  - Number of tubectomy done
  - Number of IUD inserted cases
  - Number of nirodh distributed
  - Number of diaphragms fitted
  - Number of packets of oral contraceptives distributed
  - Total number of depot holders.

Anecdotal Records

It means short narrative facts or records. Narrative documentation is the traditional method for recording nursing care. It is simply the use of a story like format to document information specific to client conditions and nursing care. Narrative charting, however has many disadvantages.

Disadvantages

- Time consuming
- Chance of repetitions
- Difficult to locate desired data.

Guide to Secure Information

Recording requires all of the basic skills of nursing itself, such as communication, listening, observation and analysis. The nurse's task here is to elicit and evaluate information not simply to receive and record it. The community health nurse and family should sit together and:

- Explore the problems, assuring privacy while securing information.
- Not to force information.
- Ask questions in a friendly, definite and direct manner, e.g., about diet, vaccination.
- After every visit, make relevant notes of visit such as purpose, what was done, attitude of family, plan for next visit and any referrals. Community health nurse should discipline herself in her record writing.

The nurse needs to have pleasant expression while securing information. If she appears to be very serious and authoritative in questioning, she may not get accurate information from the family. At one visit all the required information cannot be obtained and so the community health nurse needs to pay frequent visits to obtain the necessary data from the family.

Characteristics of Record and Reports

It have five important characteristics those are factual, accurate, complete, current and organized.

1. **Factual:** A record must contain descriptive, objective information about a nurse sees, hears, feels and smells. An objective description is the result of direct observation and measurement, e.g., objective signs of anxiety may include increased pulse rate, increased respiration and increased restlessness. When recording subjective data, document the client's exact words within quotation marks, e.g., a client exhibits anxiety the nurse may record, client states, 'I feel very nervous'.
2. **Accurate:** The use of exact measurement establishes accuracy, e.g., in take 350 mL is more accurate than client drank an adequate amount of fluid.
3. **Complete:** Record should be complete containing appropriate and essential information.
4. **Current:** Timely entries are essential in the client's ongoing care. Many health care agencies use records kept near the client's bedside to increase accuracy and decrease unnecessary duplication, e.g., vital signs of administration of medication, surgery, diagnostic test, etc.
5. **Organized:** The nurse communicates information in a logical order. For example, an organized note describes the client's pain, nurse's assessment and interventions.

Filing of Records

The records could be arranged:

- **Alphabetically:** Record should be filing according to alphabets, e.g., family folder according to name of the head.
- **Numerically:** When numerical filing is used 3" × 5" card, alphabetical file is needed.
- **Geographically:** Family folder is filed as per geographical location or as per house no. or village record.
- **Index cards:** Each file have index card, e.g., just like library books.
- **Chronologically:** Records should be arranged according to number, e.g., 1, 2, 3, 4... etc.

Method of Recording

Narrative documentation: It is the traditional method for recording nursing care. It is simple use of a story like format to document information specific to client conditions and nursing care. It is time consuming.

POMR (Problem Oriented Medical Record): It gives emphasis on client's problems. Data are organized by problem or diagnosis. The POMR has the following major sections—Data Base, Problem List, Care plan and Progress notes.

- **Data base:** History and physical examination. Laboratory report, radiological test.

- **Problem list:** After data are analyzed, problems are identified and a single list is made. The problem list includes physiological, psychological, social, cultural, spiritual, developmental and environmental needs.
- **Nursing care plan:** A care plan is developed for each problem by the nurse.
- **Progress notes:** Health care team members monitor and record the progress of a client's problems. One method is the soap charting.

SOAP are:

S: Subjective data—verbalizations of the client.
O: Objective data (which is measured and observed).
A: Assessment—diagnosis based on the data.
P: Plan (caregiver's plan to do).
An I and E sometimes added.

SOAPIE—I stands for Intervention and E stands for Evaluation. It is similar as nursing process.

Storage of Records

If a record is preserved for a long period of time and needs frequent handling.

- They should be kept in the proper filing space or in a shelf with labels so it can be easily traced.
- When cards are maintained as per age groups or type of morbidity conditions, these may be filed under these headings.
- Record are storage according to agency's policy, often the period of retention is as low as five years.

How to Maintain Records

- Record must be kept carefully and in clean conditions, safe form rats and insects.
- Records are not last or invalid. They are confidential and should be shown only to authorized persons.
- Have a good system of filing.
- Records must be readily available and kept up-to-date.

How to Write Records

- Write promptly, and keep them up-to-date.
- Write legibly, to be understood by others.
- Keep sentences short and clear.
- Be accurate and complete in details.
- Replace records in their proper place.
- Consult your supervisor in case of difficulty.

HEALTH ASSESSMENT OF INDIVIDUAL AND FAMILIES

Introduction

A health assessment is a plan of care that identifies the specific needs of a person and how those needs will be addressed by the healthcare system or skilled nursing facility. Health assessment is the evaluation of the health status by performing a physical exam after taking a health history. It is done to detect diseases early in people that may look and feel well. It is the evaluation of the health status of an individual along the health continuum. Health assessment helps to find out if anybody have any particular disease or condition even if he/she feel perfectly well, without any symptoms and/or signs of disease. Early detection, followed by treatment and good control of the condition can result by proper health assessment, and it lowers the risk of serious complications are the first step of nursing process which involves critical thinking skills and data collection. Assessment involves the systematic and continuous collection of data; sorting, analyzing, and organizing that data; and the documentation and communication of the data collected. It generally include history-taking and physical examination though the component of history-taking and physical examination is differ according to age, disease condition, sex, etc., but the overall steps are nearly same. A short, rapidly obtained history of the events of the immediate past may suffice temporarily, but as soon as the crisis is controlled, a more complete history is necessary.

Definition

Assessment refers to the collection and interpretation of clinical information. Its focuses on gathering the data about a client's state of wellness, functional ability, physical status, strengths and responses to actual and potential health problems. **—Gordon, 1987; 1994**

Health assessment is a systematic, deliberative and interactive process by which nurses use critical thinking to collect, validate, analyze and synthesize the collected information in order to make judgment about the health status and life processes of individuals, families and communities.

It is systematic and continuous collection, validation and communication of client data as compared to what is the standard/norm. It includes the client's perceived needs, health problems, related experiences, health practices, values and lifestyles.

Purpose

- Health assessments provide benefits for all those who are interested in understanding their own health and health risks.
- Establish data base for members of family and communities to assist in order to make nursing judgment
- Obtain data that will help the nurse in nursing diagnosis for individual families and communities.
- To evaluate appropriate nursing intervention
- To determine client's normal function and to know any deviation from normal and discover problems and factors that affect the health of individual.
- Holistic data collection can be possible
- Assess how health status affect family, daily activity and community
- To identify client's strength and weakness to solve their problems.
- To identify need for health teaching.

Types of Health Assessment

In general, there are four fundamental types of assessments that nurses perform.

1. **A comprehensive or complete health assessment:** Comprehensive or complete health assessment usually begins with obtaining a thorough health history and physical exam. This type of assessment is usually performed in acute care settings upon admission, once your patient is stable, or when a new patient presents to an outpatient clinic.
2. **An interval or abbreviated assessment:** Nurses perform an interval or abbreviated assessment at this time. This type of assessment is not as detailed as the complete assessment that occurs at admission. The advantage of an abbreviated assessment is that it allows you to thoroughly assess your patient in a shorter period of time.
3. **A problem-focused assessment:** The problem-focused assessment is usually indicated after a comprehensive assessment has identified a potential health problem. The problem-focused assessment is also indicated when an interval or abbreviated assessment shows a change in status from the most current previous assessment or report you received, when a new symptom emerges, or the patient develops any distress. An advantage of the focused assessment is that it directs you to ask about symptoms and move quickly to conducting a focused physical exam.
4. An assessment for special populations, e.g., the special population means the population in special age group like under five children, infants, school going children, elderly assessment.

History-taking

History-taking is an important aspect in assessing the health status of individual, family and community. The history collection include personal history, family history, past medical or surgical history, present chief complains, past obstructive history if the individual is an antenatal or postnatal mother, etc.

- **Personal history:** Personal history include the personal habits affecting health condition like smoking, tobacco chewing or any birth injury etc.
- **Family history:** Record the chief complaint as a brief statement of whatever is troubling the patient and the duration of time the problem has existed. The chief complaint is the signs and symptoms causing the patient to seek medical attention. Record his reason for the visit and the date of his last contact with a medical treatment facility.
- **Past medical history:** This provides background for understanding the patient as a whole and his present illness. It includes childhood illnesses, immunizations, allergies, hospitalizations and serious illnesses, accidents and injuries, medications, and habits.
- **Family health history:** This enhances your understanding of the environment in which the patient lives. Obtaining this information identifies genetic problems, communicable diseases, environmental problems, and interpersonal relationships. Specific inquiry should be made regarding the general state of health of parents, grandparents, siblings, spouse, and children. Record if the patient is adopted and has no access to his biological family's history.

Method of Examination

Inspection: Visual examination of the body is called inspection. It is the observation with the naked eyes to determine the structure and function of the body. Inspection is seeking physical signs by observing the patient. Of the several methods of examination inspection is the least mechanical the hardest to learn, but it yields most physical signs. More diagnoses are probably made by inspection than by all other methods combined. The method is the most difficult to learn because no systematic approach can encompass the variety of signs. More than any other method, inspection depends entirely upon the knowledge of the observer. Practice is required to learn inspection. The inspection may be general or local.

- **General inspection:** The initial act of physical examination is the inspection of the body as a whole. In looking at the patient as a whole, many facts can be noted. General inspection include motor activity, body builds, outstanding anatomic malformation, behavior, speech, nutrition, and appearance of illness.
- **Local inspection:** Focusing observation on a single anatomic region. When there is any surgical wound or any other local wound, local infection, the condition of the wound or infection can be assessed in detail by local inspection.

For inspection different audiovisual aids can be used like ophthalmoscope, slit lamp, gonioscope, otoscope nasoscope, laryngoscope, bronchoscope, gastroscope, thoracoscope, peritoneoscope, cystoscope, anoscope, and sigmoidoscope. The pathologist uses the microscope; the radiologist inspects the fluoroscopic screen and photographic films.

Palpation: It is the felling of the body or a part with the hands to note the size and positions of the organs. In palpation the finger pads and note the finger tips are used. Palpation is widely used in the physical examination especially in the abdomen examination. The tips of the fingers are the most sensitive for fine tactile discrimination, and temperature sense. The dorsa of the hands or fingers can be used as the skin is much thinner than elsewhere on the hand for vibratory sense. Palpation is employed on every part of the body accessible to the examining fingers and pam.

Percussion: It is the examination by tapping with the fingers on the body to determine the condition of the internal organs by the sounds that are produced. It is done by placing a finger of the left hand firmly against a part to be examined and tapping with the fingers tips of the right hand. In physical diagnosis, percussion is the method of examination in which the surface of the body is struck to emit sounds that vary in quality according to the underlying tissues.

Auscultation: It is the listening to sounds within the body with the aid of a stethoscope, fetoscope and directly with the ear place on the body. Although auscultation might literally imply the act of hearing to obtain physical signs, usage restricts it almost solely to hearing through the stethoscope, i.e., rales and friction rubs. Crepitus can be heard in joints tendon sheaths, muscles, fractured bones, and in subcutaneous emphysema. The heart makes its various valve sounds with their splitting, murmurs, rhythm disturbances, pericardial rubs and knocks. Auscultation of the abdomen reveals bowel sounds, murmurs from aneurysms and stenotic arteries, especially the renal. The stethoscope is applied to the scrotum to detect bowel sounds in a scrotal hernia.

Manipulation: It is moving of a part of the body to note it flexibility, limitation of movements is observed by this method. This is mainly performed in orthopedic cases.

Testing of reflexes: The response of the tissues to external stimuli is tested by; means of percussion hammer, safety pin, wisp of cotton hot and cold water etc.

Conduction of Physical Examination

Preparation of the Environment

Maintenance of Privacy

- A separate examination room is needed.
- Keep the doors closed.
- The relative are not allowed.
- Drape the patient according to the parts that are exposed.

Lighting

As per as possible allowed natural light for examination, for better assessment.

Comfortable Bed for Examination

The patient should be placed in a comfortable position throughout examination.

For examination of genitalia its need special examination table.

Preparation of equipment: The equipment needed as per the purpose of examination or the condition of patient. All instruments are not essential for every cases. The equipment are sphygmomanometer, stethoscope, fetoscope, TPR tray, tongue depressor, pharyngeal retractor, laryngoscope, tape measure, flash light, weighing machine, ophthalmoscope, otoscope, nasal speculum, percussion hammer, vaginal speculum, protoscope and so on.

Preparation of the patient:

- Keep the patient in a comfortable position which is convenient for examinationt
- Empty the bladder and bowel prior to the examination if needed.
- Loosen the garments and drape the patient with extra sheets and expose only the need area to avoid necessary exposure
- Explain the sequence of the procedure to the patient to gain his confidence and cooperation.

Carry out of physical examination and identification of abnormality: In physical examination the person should be assessed from head to toe with measurement of anthropometry and vital signs and any deviation which can be noted. During measuring of anthropometry and vitals there is a normal range. Above or below that range is considered as abnormal. The following parameters will be assessed during physical examination.

Anthropometry

- Height
- Weight
- BMI

Vital Signs

- Temperature
- Pulse rate
- Respiration rate
- Blood pressure

General Appearance

- Nourishment—well-nourished or under-nourished
- Body build—thin or obese
- Health—healthy or unhealthy
- Activity—active or dull

Mental Status

- Consciousness—conscious, unconscious, delirious, taking incoherently.
- Look—anxious or worried depressed, etc.

Posture

- Body curves—lordosis hypnosis,scoliosis.
- Movement—any limp.

Skin Conditions

- Color—pallor, jaundice, cyanosis, flushing, etc.
- Texture—dryness, flaking wrinkling or excessive moisture.
- Temperature—warm, cold and clammy
- Lesions—macules, papules, vesicles, wounds, etc.

Head and Face

- Shape of the skull and fontanel.
- Skull circumference.
- Scalp—cleanliness, condition of the hair, dandruff, pediculi, infections like, ringworm.
- Face—pale flushed, puffiness, fatigue, pain, fear, anxiety, enlagement of parotid glands etc.

Eye

- Eyebrows—normal or absent
- Eyelashes—infection, sty
- Eyelids—edema, lesion

- Eyeballs—sunken or protruded
- Conjunctiva—pale, red, purulent
- Sclera—jaundice
- Cornea and iris—irregularities and abrasions
- Pupils—dilated, constricted, reaction to light
- Lens—opaque or transparent
- Fund us—congestion, hemorrhagic spots.
- Eye muscles—strabismus (squint)
- Vision—normal, myopia, hypermetropia.

Ears

- External ear discharge, cerumen obstructing the ear passage
- Tympanic membrane—perforations, lesions, bulging
- Hearing—acuity.

Nose

- External nares—crusts or discharge
- Nostrils—inflammation of the mucus membrane, septal deviations.

Mouth and Pharynx

- Lips—redness, swelling, crusts, cyanosis, angular stomatitis
- Odor of the mouth—foul smelling
- Teeth—discoloration and dental carries
- Mucus membrane and gums—ulceration and bleeding, swelling, pus formation.
- Tongue—pale, dry, lesions, furrows, tongue, tie, etc.
- Throat and pharynx—enlarged tonsils, redness and pus.

Neck

- Lymph nodes—enlarged, palpate
- Thyroid gland—enlarged
- Range of motion—flexion, extension and rotation
- Chest—thorax-shape, symmetry of expansion.
- Breaths sounds—sigh, swish, rusted, wheezing/posture, rales, crepitations, pleural rub, etc.
- Breaths—enlarged lymph nodes.

Abdomen

- Observation—skin rashes, scars, hernia, ascites, distention, pregnancy, etc.
- Auscultation—bowel sounds, fetal heart sounds.
- Palpation—liver margin, palpable spleen, tenderness at the area of appendix, inguinal hernias.
- Percussion—presence of gas, fluid or masses.
- Back—spina bifida curves.

Genitalia and Rectum

- Inguinal lymph glands—enlarged, palpable
- Patency of urinary meatus and rectum (in infants)
- Descent of the testes
- Vaginal discharge
- Presence of sexually transmitted diseases.
- Hemorrhoids enlargement of the prostate gland
- Pelvic masses.

Neurologic Tests

- Coordination tests reflexes
- Equilibrium tests
- Tests for sensations.

Aftercare of the Article

- Wash hand
- Replace the articles after cleaning
- Record the procedure in the nurse's record sheet.

Characteristics Healthy Individual

WHO given the definition of health as "Health is a state of complete physical, mental and social well-being and not merely the absence of disease or infirmity." From the definition it is clear that overall the health has major two aspects Physical and Mental. Though social aspect of health is included in definition but it has very less effect and it is associated with psychological aspect.

- Clear skin
- Steady heartbeat that is neither too fast nor too slow
- Blood pressure in range
- Symmetrical features
- Clear eyes with even pupils that track together
- Appropriate flexibility in the joints
- Expected reflex responses
- Weight in the expected ranges, neither too high nor too low
- A reasonable amount of endurance and strength.

The important components to evaluating physical fitness are cardiovascular capability, muscle strength and endurance, joint flexibility, and body composition, according to Functional Fitness Facts. A physically fit individual, regardless of weight, has a strong heart, vascular system and lungs

The healthy individual has a strong sense of self, the capacity for successful interpersonal functioning and the ability to function well occupationally. Such an individual possesses an awareness of having a unique identity, grounded in personal history, with well-delineated interpersonal boundaries leading to a firm sense of self. The ability to experience, think about, and make sense of internal sensory, affective, and cognitive experience is present. The individual's identity remains intact, interactive and spontaneous in the context of relationships. This identity, however, is not static but open to growth and change. The self-concept is associated with a relatively consistent and self-regulated level of positive self-esteem and self-respect. One's self-appraisal is accurate and based in reality, neither grandiose nor deprecating. The person has the ability to identify, set and attain satisfying and rewarding personal goals. The healthy individual can analyze what a situation requires, selects an appropriate goal, decides how best to implement that goal and proceeds to carry out the plan and achieve the goal. The person has a sense of direction, meaning, and purpose resulting in a sense of fulfillment in life. Essential to being a healthy individual is the capacity for effective interpersonal functioning. The healthy individual possesses the essential social skills to recognize, interpret, and respond constructively to emotions in oneself and others. This is reflected in the ability to understand and appreciate the mental state of others and to comprehend and appreciate the effect of one's personal actions on others.

ASSESSMENT OF CHILDREN

Pediatric History

Complete history of the child is necessary which leads to the correct diagnosis usually is obtained from the parent, the older child, or the caretaker of a sick child. During the interview, it is important to convey to the parent interest in the child as well as the illness. Allow the parent/caretaker to talk freely at first and to express concerns in his or her own words. The nurse when collecting history should look directly either at the parent or the child intermittently and not only at the writing instruments as they will feel the concern of the nurse. The nurse should always be a sympathetic listener who addresses the parent and child by name frequently obtains more accurate information than does a harried, distracted interviewer. Careful observation during the interview frequently uncovers stresses and concerns that otherwise are not apparent.

As many components in pediatric history and the history of an adult are same, some of the differences are prenatal and birth history, developmental history, history of immunization must be collected from children which are not necessary in case of adults. Here we can collect the history from parents or caretakers who are attending the patient. If the child is 4 years or more may be able to provide some of their own history which can be confirm from their parents.

Outline of the Pediatric History

General Information

General Information needed for the client include, name, age, date of birth, sex, referral source if pertinent—relationship of the child and informant contacts—address, and telephone numbers of the informants.

Chief Complaint

- Chief complaint are the overall major problems explained by the parents or patient. These are the brief statement of primary problem (including duration) that caused family to seek medical attention.
- The information given by informant's or patient's own words, the chief complaint is a brief statement of the reason why the patient was brought to be seen. It is not unusual that the stated complaint is not the true reason the child was brought for attention.
- During data collection, Expanding the question of "Why did you bring him?" to "What concerns you?" allows the informant to focus on the complaint more accurately.

History of Present Illness

- Details of the present illness are recorded in chronologic order. Initial statement identifying the historian, that person's relationship to patient and their reliability.
- During history-taking it is helpful to begin that, the child was apparently well until "X" number of days before this visit and this is followed by a daily documentation of events leading up to the present time, including signs, symptoms, and treatment.
- Statements should be recorded about the chronological account of the illness, including any previous treatment with full description of symptoms in number of days before the visit.

Past Medical History

Past medical history includes:

- Major medical illnesses
- Major surgical illnesses—list operations and dates
- Trauma—fractures, lacerations
- Previous hospital admissions with dates and diagnoses
- Current medications
- Known allergies (not just drugs)
- Immunization status—be specific, not just up to date.

Pregnancy and Birth History

For a child it is important to take the history of pregnancy and birth which might be included:

- Maternal health during pregnancy: Bleeding, trauma, hypertension, fevers, infectious illnesses, medications, drugs, alcohol, smoking, rupture of membranes
- Gestational age at delivery
- Labor and delivery—length of labor, fetal distress, type of delivery (vaginal, cesarean section), use of forceps, anesthesia, breech delivery
- Neonatal period—Apgar scores, breathing problems, use of oxygen, need for intensive care, hyperbilirubinemia, birth injuries, feeding problems, length of stay, birth weight.

Developmental History

- Ages at which milestones were achieved and current developmental abilities—smiling, rolling, sitting alone, crawling, walking, running, 1st word, toilet training, riding tricycle, etc. (see developmental charts)
- School—present grade, specific problems, interaction with peers
- Behavior—enuresis, temper tantrums, thumb sucking, pica, nightmares, etc.

Feeding History

- Breast or bottle fed, types of formula, frequency and amount, reasons for any changes in formula
- Solids—when introduced, problems created by specific types
- Fluoride use.

Review of Systems

Usually very abbreviated for infants and younger children

- Weight—recent changes, weight at birth
- Skin and Lymph—rashes, adenopathy, lumps, bruising and bleeding, pigmentation changes
- HEENT (Head, Eyes, Ears, Nose, and Throat)—Headaches, concussions, unusual head shape, strabismus, conjunctivitis, visual problems, hearing, ear infections, draining ears, cold and sore throats, tonsillitis, mouth breathing, snoring, apnea, oral thrush, epistaxis, caries
- Cardiac—cyanosis and dyspnea, heart murmurs, exercise tolerance, squatting, chest pain, palpitations
- Respiratory—pneumonia, bronchiolitis, wheezing, chronic cough, sputum, hemoptysis, TB
- GI—stool color and character, diarrhea, constipation, vomiting, hematemesis, jaundice, abdominal pain, colic, appetite
- GU—frequency, dysuria, hematuria, discharge, abdominal pains, quality of urinary stream, polyuria, previous infections, facial edema
- Musculoskeletal—joint pains or swelling, fevers, scoliosis, myalgia or weakness, injuries, gait changes
- Pubertal—secondary sexual characteristics, menses and menstrual problems, pregnancies, sexual activity
- Allergy—urticaria, hay fever, allergic rhinitis, asthma, eczema, drug reactions.

Family History

- Illnesses—cardiac disease, hypertension, stroke, diabetes, cancer, abnormal bleeding, allergy and asthma, epilepsy
- Mental retardation, congenital anomalies, chromosomal problems, growth problems, consanguinity, ethnic background.

Social

- Living situation and conditions—daycare, safety issues
- Composition of family
- Occupation of parents.

Physical Examination

Examination of the infant and young child begins with observing him or her and establishing rapport. The order of the examination should fit the child and the circumstances. It is wise to make no sudden movements and to complete first those parts of the examination that require the child's cooperation and painful or disagreeable procedures should be deferred to the end of the examination which should be explained to the child before proceeding. For the older child and adolescent, examination can begin with the head and conclude with the extremities. This procedure should start with gentle approach by following tender loving care.

General Approach to be Followed

- Gather as much data as possible by observation first
- Position of child: Parent's lap vs. exam table
- Stay at the child's level as much as possible. Do not tower!!
- Order of exam: Least distressing to most distressing
- Rapport with child
  - Include child—explain to the child's level
  - Distraction is a valuable tool
- Examine painful area last-get general impression of overall attitude
- Be honest. If something is going to hurt, tell them that in a calm fashion. Do not lie or you lose credibility!
- Understand developmental stages' impact on child's response. For example, stranger anxiety is a normal stage of development, which tends to make examining a previously cooperative child more difficult.

Vital Signs

Normal vital signs differ from adults, and vary according to age. The nurse has to see the "code card" for charts of age-adjusted normals

- **Temperature:** Tympanic vs. oral vs. axillary vs. rectal
- **Heart rate:**
  - Auscultate or palpate apical pulse or palpate femoral pulse in infant
  - Palpate antecubital or radial pulse in older child
  - The normal rate varies from 70 to 170 beats per minute at birth to 120 to 140 shortly after birth, and ranges from 80 to 140 at 1 to 2 years, from 80 to 120 at 3 years, and from 70 to 115 after 3 years
- **Respiratory rate:** Infants normally have periodic breathing so that observing for only 15 seconds will result in a skewed number but respiratory rate should be determined by counting while observing the movement of the chest for complete one minute
  - Blood pressure: Should be measured with a cuff, with the bladder completely encircling the extremity and the width covering one half to two thirds of the length of the upper arm or upper leg.
- Growth parameters—must plot on appropriate growth curve
  - Weight
  - Height/length
  - Occipital frontal circumference (OFC): Across frontal-occipital prominence so greatest diameter.

Emergency Signs

Triage of patients involves looking for signs of serious illness or injury. These emergency signs are connected to the Airway-Breathing-Circulation/Consciousness and Dehydration which are easily remembered as "ABCD". Each letter refers to an emergency signs which, when positive, should alert you to a patient who is seriously ill and needs immediate assessment and treatment.

Outline of a Pediatric Physical Examination

- **Vitals:** Already explained in above points.
- **General status:**
  - Statement about striking and/or important features. Nutritional status, level of consciousness, toxic or

distressed, cyanosis, cooperation, hydration, dysmorphology, mental state
    - Anthropometric measurements: These include Length/Height, Weight, Head circumference (OFC) and MUAC which already measured.
- **Skin and lymphatics:**
    - Birthmarks—nevi, hemangiomas, Mongolian spots, etc.
    - Rashes, petechiae, desquamation, pigmentation, jaundice, texture, turgor
    - Lymph node enlargement, location, mobility, consistency
    - Scars or injuries, especially in patterns suggestive of abuse
- **Head:**
    - Size and shape
    - Fontanelle(s)
        - Size
        - Tension—calm and in the sitting up position
    - Sutures—overriding
    - Scalp and hair
- **Eyes:**
    - General
        - Strabismus
        - Slant of palpebral fissures
        - Hypertelorism or telecanthus
    - EOM
    - Pupils
    - Conjunctiva, sclera, cornea
    - Plugging of nasolacrimal ducts
    - Red reflex
    - Visual fields—gross exam
- **Ears:**
    - Position of ears
        - Observe from front and draw line from inner canthi to occiput
    - Tympanic membranes
    - Hearing—Gross assessment only usually
- **Nose:**
    - Nasal septum
    - Mucosa (color, polyps)
    - Sinus tenderness
    - Discharge
- **Mouth and throat:**
    - Lips (colors, fissures)
    - Buccal mucosa (color, vesicles, moist or dry)
    - Tongue (color, papillae, position, tremors)
    - Teeth and gums (number, condition)
    - Palate (intact, arch)
    - Tonsils (size, color, exudates)
    - Posterior pharyngeal wall (color, lymph hyperplasia, bulging)
    - Gag reflex
- **Neck:**
    - Thyroid
    - Trachea position
    - Masses (cysts, nodes)
    - Presence or absence of nuchal rigidity
- **Lungs/thorax:**
    - Inspection
        - Pattern of breathing
            - Abdominal breathing is normal in infants
            - Period breathing is normal in infants (pause <15 seconds)
        - Respiratory rate
        - Use of accessory muscles: Retraction location, degree/flaring
        - Chest wall configuration
    - Auscultation
        - Equality of breath sounds
        - Rales, wheezes, rhonchi
        - Upper airway noise
    - Percussion and palpation often not possible and rarely helpful
- **Cardiovascular:**
    - Auscultation
        - Rhythm
        - Murmurs
        - Quality of heart sounds
    - Pulses
        - Quality in upper and lower extremities
- **Abdomen:**
    - Inspection
        - Shape
            - Infants usually have protuberant abdomens
            - Becomes more scaphoid as child matures
        - Umbilicus (infection, hernias)
        - Muscular integrity (diasthasis recti)
    - Auscultation
    - Palpation
        - Tenderness—avoid tender area until end of exam
        - Liver, spleen, kidneys
            - May be palpable in normal newborn
        - Rebound, guarding
            - Have child blow up belly to touch your hand
- **Musculoskeletal:**
    - Back
        - Sacral dimple
        - Kyphosis, lordosis or scoliosis
    - Joints (motion, stability, swelling, tenderness)
    - Muscles
    - Extremities
        - Deformity
        - Symmetry
        - Edema
        - Clubbing
    - Gait
        - In-toeing, out-toeing
        - Bow legs, knock knee
            - "Physiologic" bowing is frequently seen under 2 years of age and will spontaneously resolve
        - Limp
    - Hips
        - Ortolani's and Barlow's signs

- **Neurologic**—most accomplished through observation alone
  - Cranial nerves
  - Sensation
  - Cerebellum
  - Muscle tone and strength
  - Reflexes
    - DTR
    - Superficial (abdominal and cremasteric)
    - Neonatal primitive
- **Genitourinary system:**
  - External genitalia
  - Hernias and Hydrocoeles
    - Almost all hernias are indirect
    - Can gently palpate; do not poke finger into the inguinal canal
  - Cryptorchidism
    - Distinguish from hyper-retractile testis
    - Most will spontaneously descend by several months of life
  - Tanner staging in adolescents—see Tanner Staging handouts
  - Rectal and pelvic exam not done routinely—special indications may exist.

ASSESSMENT OF ADOLESCENTS

Growth and development occur in an individual as she or he transitions from childhood to adulthood. Adolescence is generally understood as the period of transition from childhood to adulthood. It is distinguished by significant physical changes culminating in sexual maturity. It begins in the second decade of human life and is accompanied by marked biophysical changes towards sexual maturity and attainment of psychological independence. Adolescence is marked by rapid physical, psychological and social maturation, a need to extend relationships beyond the immediate family, a sense of idealism, curiosity and adventure and willingness to take greater risks and experiment. Assessment of adolescents include history-taking and physical examination.

Points to remember during assessment of adolescents:
- Do not treat adolescents like children
- Be honest and show respect
- Display genuine interest and concern
- Avoid criticism and judgment
- Be casual and give friendly responses
- Ensure privacy and confidentiality
- Interview should be held in a quiet and comfortable environment
- Initiate with small talk relevant to the interviewee's interests, e.g., asking about his/her academic progress, home life, relationships and favourite pastimes
- Explain every step and give the rationale
- Use open-ended questions
- Encourage the adolescent to talk freely in order to gather more information.
- Questions should be asked one by one and the counsellor should refrain from pushing the client too hard.

History-taking: A comprehensive health history is a precursor before performing any health assessment. Health history includes subjective and objective data. Subjective data are the information exposed by the adolescent; objective data are the information from the physical examination and laboratory studies. A combination of both types of data provides health workers with a clear picture of the health status of an adolescent.

Health history from parents
- General data
- Name:
- Age:
- Sex:
- Religion:
- Education
- Occupation if any:
- Marital Status
- Relationship with siblings and Parent.

Personal History

- Staying with—parents/alone/friends
- Is she feeling neglected...yes/no
- Sharing of emotions and feelings with whom
- Faith on divine.... yes/no
- Any addiction: Yes/No
  - If yes, type
  - Age of initiation of addiction:
  - Reason for initiation of addiction:
  - Knowledge of parents regarding addiction of daughter.

Immunization history: Include all the immunizations starting from 0 to 18 years of age.

Past medical history: Parents are usually most familiar with the adolescent's perinatal period, early developmental milestones, serious or chronic illnesses, hospitalizations, accidents and immunizations.

Family history: This provides a genetic and familial medical history, and may also give a clue as to the residential "health environment" of the adolescent.

Psychosocial history: Parents can provide information on the adolescent's personality, strengths, weaknesses and school life.

Chief complaint: Chief complaint are the major cause for which the adolescent have brought. During assessment a nurse should first focus on chief complain.

Psychological History

- Assessing the adolescent's establishment of independence, sexual development and future role in society
- Health habits and health risks: Activities, feelings or experiences that involve health risks
- Family functioning
- Social and school situation: Socioeconomic, cultural and spiritual factors.

In Case of Girl (Menstrual History)

- Regularity: Regular/Irregular
- Maintenance of hygiene:
  - Regular bath during menstruation: Yes/No
  - Use of diaper - type - Sanity napkin/old clothes/washed and reused/not reused
- Any social restriction during menstruation (if yes mention)
- Knowledge about contraception: Yes/No
- If yes, mention the name
- Source of information about contraceptive
- Knowledge of contraceptive which will also protect from RTI, STD, HIV—Yes/No:
- If yes mention the name
- Knowledge about RTI/STD: Yes/No.

"HEADSS" (Cohen, 1991) is a valuable screening framework for exploring psychosocial functioning with adolescents. Health care professionals use HEADSS (Cohen, 1991) to screen for the potential psychosocial problems of adolescents before they mature into serious disorders. HEADSS allows us to organise and remember the important elements of adolescents' psychosocial history; it also provides a natural pattern of progression in history-taking.

Example of HEADSS (Cohen, 1991) Psychosocial Screening Questions

H–Home

- Where do you live and who lives with you?
- How do you get along with each member of your household?
- Who could you go to if you needed help with a problem?

E–Education/employment

- What do you like about school (or work)?
- What are you good and not good at?
- How do you get along with your teachers and other students (or work colleagues)?

A–Activities

- What sort of things do you do in your spare time out of school?
- Do you belong to any clubs, groups, etc.?
- What sort of things do you like to do with friends?

D–Drugs

- Many young people at your age are starting to experiment with cigarettes or alcohol. Have you tried these or other drugs like opiates, ecstasy, and injecting drugs?
- How much are you taking and how often?

S–Sexuality

Some young people are getting involved in sexual relationships. Have you had a sexual experience with a guy or girl or both?

S–Suicide/depression Screen

- What sort of things do you do if you are feeling sad/angry/hurt?
- Some people who feel really down often feel like hurting or even killing themselves. Have you ever felt this way?
- Have you ever tried to hurt yourself?

Preparation for Physical Examination

- The examination can be conducted in a room with adjustable lighting
- All procedures should be explained clearly
- A well-lit room is needed for the visual acuity test
- A darkened room is better for pupillary reflexes assessment and ophthalmoscopic examination.

Allow to undress in private:
- Give gown
- Expose only area to be examined
- Respect need for privacy
- Explain findings during examination.

Physical Examination

The physical examination for an adolescent follows a head-to-toe direction to provide a general guideline for assessing each body area in order not to omit segments of the examination. The examination of adolescents uses developmental and chronological age as the main criteria for assessing each body system, which accomplishes several goals. Before head to toe examination vitals like temperature, pulse, respiration, blood pressure must be assessed.

General condition	• Height weight Affect/behavior/anxiety • Level of hygiene • Body position
Skin, hair, and nails	• Inspect for lesions, bruising, and rashes. • Palpate skin for temperature, moisture, and texture. Condition of nails
Head and neck	• Inspect eyes for drainage • Nose for DNS
Chest and breast	• Expansion/retraction of chest wall/work of breathing • Breast palpation
Abdomen	Abdomen for distension, asymmetry or any other abnormality
Extremities	Arms and legs for pain, deformity, edema,
Genital organ	To assess growth maturity or any symptom of STI
Back area	• Inspect back and spine. • Inspect coccyx/buttock for any types of abnormalities

The following findings can be assessed:
- **Nutrition and eating disorders**
  - Anorexia nervosa
  - Bulimia nervosa
  - Obesity
- **Skin problems in adolescence**
  - Acne vulgaris
  - Seborrhoeic dermatitis
- **Psychosomatic disorders and somatic complaints**
  - Headache
  - Back pain
  - Abdominal pain.

Assessment of geriatrics and woman has given in different chapters.

ASSESSMENT OF VITALS

Blood Pressure Assessment

Blood Pressure is defined as the lateral force exerted by blood on the arterial walls, blood pressure depends on the force of ventricular contractions, arterial wall elasticity, peripheral vascular resistance, and blood volume and viscosity. Systolic, or maximum, pressure occurs during left ventricular contraction and reflects the integrity of the heart, arteries, and arterioles. Diastolic, or minimum, pressure occurs during left ventricular relaxation and directly indicates blood vessel resistance.

Pulse pressure, the difference between systolic and diastolic pressures, varies inversely with arterial elasticity. Rigid vessels, incapable of distention and recoil, produce high systolic pressure and low diastolic pressure. Normally, systolic pressure exceeds diastolic pressure by about 40 mm Hg.

Frequent blood pressure measurement is critical after serious injury, surgery, or anesthesia and during any illness or condition that threatens cardiovascular stability. (Frequent measurement may be performed with an automated vital signs monitor.) Regular measurement is indicated for patients with a history of hypertension or hypotension, and annual screening is recommended for all adults.

Equipment

Aneroid sphygmomanometer, stethoscope and alcohol pad.

The sphygmomanometer consists of an inflatable compression cuff linked to a manual air pump and an aneroid gauge. A recently calibrated aneroid gauge should be used. To obtain an accurate reading, rest the gauge in any position but view it directly from the front. Cuffs come in sizes ranging from newborn to extra-large adult.

Preparation of Equipment

Carefully choose a cuff of appropriate size for the patient; the bladder should encircle at least 80% of the upper arm. An excessively narrow cuff may cause a falsely high pressure reading; an excessively wide one, a falsely low reading. If you are not using your own stethoscope, disinfect the earpieces with an alcohol pad before placing them in your ears to avoid cross-contamination.

Procedure

- Perform hand hygiene and put on gloves if appropriate or indicated.
- Close curtains around bed and close door to room if possible.
- Select the appropriate arm for application of cuff.
- Have the patient assume a comfortable lying or sitting position with the forearm supported at the level of the heart and the palm of the hand upward.
- Expose the brachial artery by removing garments, or move a sleeve, if it is not too tight, above the area where the cuff will be placed.
- Palpate the location of the brachial artery. Center the bladder of the cuff over the brachial artery, about midway on the arm, so that the lower edge of the cuff is about 2.5 to 5 cm (1″ to 2″) above the inner aspect of the elbow. Line up the artery marking on the cuff with the patient's brachial artery. The tubing should extend from the edge of the cuff nearer the patient's elbow.
- Wrap the cuff around the arm smoothly and snugly, and fasten it. Do not allow any clothing to interfere with the proper placement of the cuff.
- Check that the needle on the aneroid gauge is within the zero mark. If using a mercury manometer, check to see that the manometer is in the vertical position and that the mercury is within the zero level with the gauge at eye level.
- Estimating systolic pressure
- Palpate the pulse at the brachial or radial artery by pressing gently with the fingertips.
- Tighten the screw valve on the air pump.
- Inflate the cuff while continuing to palpate the artery. Note the point on the gauge where the pulse disappears.
- Deflate the cuff and wait 15 seconds.
- Obtaining blood pressure measurement.

Assessment of Temperature

Body temperature represents the balance between heat produced by metabolism, muscular activity, and other factors and heat lost through the skin, lungs, and body wastes. A stable temperature pattern promotes proper function of cells, tissues, and organs; a change in this pattern usually signals the onset of illness. Temperature can be measured with an electronic digital, chemical-dot, or tympanic thermometer. Oral temperature in adults normally ranges from 97°F to 99.5°F (36.1° to 37.5°C); rectal temperature, the most accurate reading, is usually 1°F (0.6°C) higher; axillary temperature, the least accurate, reads 1° to 2°F (0.6° to 1.1°C) lower; and tympanic temperature reads 0.5° to 1° (0.3° to 0.6°) higher.

Temperature normally fluctuates with rest and activity. Lowest readings typically occur between 4 and 5 AM; the highest readings occur between 4 and 8 PM. Other factors also influence temperature, including gender, age, emotional conditions, and environment. Keep the following principles in mind: Women normally have higher temperatures than men, especially during ovulation. Normal temperature is highest in neonates and lowest in the elderly. Heightened emotions raise temperature; depressed emotions lower it. A hot external environment can raise temperature; a cold environment lowers it.

Articles Required

- A clinical glass thermometer
- Disinfectant or an alcohol wipe
- A watch or clock
- Tissue or dry swab
- Record chart/patient's notes
- Pen.

Preparation

- Wash and dry your hands—this will help to prevent cross-infection.
- Explain to the patient what you are going to do. This will help the patient to understand and will make it easier for them to cooperate.
- Disinfect the thermometer by wiping with an alcohol wipe, or use a swab moistened with the disinfectant. Dry with a tissue or swab.

Procedure

- Ask the patient to open the mouth and place the thermometer under the tongue, ask the patient to hold the thermometer in place by closing the lips and not biting on thermometer
- Read the level of mercury in good light. To read the level of mercury in thermometer, hold thermometer with fingers of right hand, very slowly rotating back and forth until the silver mercury measurement to the nearest line
- Shakes the thermometer if mercury level is above 35°C or 95°F. Shake it with quick movement of wrist. To shake thermometer, hold it firmly by its stem and move away from the wall, furniture and equipment.

In Axillary Method

- Ask the patient to loosen any tight clothing or remove long-sleeved garments so it is possible to access the axilla. Before placing the thermometer, dry the axilla
- Place the bulb of thermometer in the axilla so that the bulb is in touch with two skin folds of axilla
- Keep thermometer in position by placing the arm over chest
- Do not allow clothing to come in contact with bulb of thermometer
  - Have thermometer in place for 2 minutes, in axillary method leave thermometer in position for 5 minutes
  - Remove the thermometer after two minutes (after 5 minutes in case of axillary method). Wipe the thermometer from stem to bulb with a clean cotton swab, using a rotating movement. Discard the swab
  - Read level of mercury
  - Return thermometer to bottle, shaking it down again
  - Wash hands.

If you are checking pulse and respiration along with temperature then

- Count the pulse and respirations while thermometer is in place
- Place patient's hand over his chest with wrist extended and the palm downwards. Place the finger tips over pulse point
- Holding watch in left hand, start to count the pulse rate with zero then 1, 2, etc.
- If pulse is regular, count the number of pulsations for half minute and multiply it by two. If pulse is not regular, count for one full minute
- Continue palpation of pulse to assess rhythm, volume, tension, and irregularity
- With the right hand still on the pulse count respiration by watching the rise and fall of chest, without knowledge of patient
- If the respirations are normal, count the number of respirations in the 30 second and multiply by two. If respiration is abnormal, count the rate for one full minute and note pattern of breathing
- Record the temperature, pulse and respiration.

GROWTH AND DEVELOPMENT

Growth

Growth is the process of physical maturation resulting an increase in size of the body and various organs. It occurs by multiplication of cells and an increase in intracellular substance. It is quantitative changes of the body.

Development

- It is the process of functional and physiological maturation of the individual. It is progressive increase in skill and capacity to function.
- It is related to maturation and myelination of the nervous system.
- It includes psychological, emotional and social changes.
- It is qualitative aspects.

Many people use the terms 'growth' and 'development' interchangeably. In reality they are inseparable and neither takes place alone.

Growth	*Development*
Growth refers to increase in physical aspects of change or increase in structure and size	Development refers to overall changes in the whole of the organism
Growth is quantitative	Development is qualitative
Growth is structural	Development is functional
Growth stops when the organisation reaches the stage of maturity	Development involves changes from origin to maturity
Growth involves body changes	Development may or may not involve bodily change. It can occur without growth

Principle of Growth and Development

- **Cephalocaudal direction:** Growth directs the development from the head downward. The head region starts growth at first, following by which other organs starts developing. The child gains control of the head first, then the arms and then the legs. Infants develop control of the head and face movements at first two months. In next few months they are able to lift themselves up by using their arms. Next gain control over leg and able to crawl, stand, walk, run, jump, climb, day by day.
- **Proximodistal direction:** The directional sequence of development during both prenatal and postnatal stages may either be (i) from head to foot, or (ii) from the central axis to the extremities of the body. The spinal cord develops before outer parts of the body. The child's arms

develops before the hands, the hands and feet develops before the fingers and toes. Fingers and toe muscles are the last to develop in physical development.

General to Specific

- **Orderly or sequential process:** Every species, whether animal or human, follows a pattern of development peculiar to it. This pattern in general is the same for all individuals. All children follow a development pattern with one stage leading to the next. For example, Infants stand before they walk, draw circles before they make squares.
- **Development is a continuous process:** Growth and Development is a continuous process from conception to death. In the early years of life, development consists of changes that lead the child to maturity not only of body size and functioning, but also of behavior. Even after maturity has been attained, development does not end. Changes continue which lead to the period of life known as senescence or old age. These changes continue until death ends the life cycle.
- **Development proceeds at different rate:** Development proceeds from simple to complex. Children use their cognitive and language skills to reason and solve problems. Children at first are able hold the big things by using both arms, in the next part able to hold things in a single hand, then only able to pick small objects like peas, cereals etc. Children when able to hold pencil, first starts draw circles then squares then only letters after that the words.
- **There are individual differences:** The speed of development is not even. Individuals differ in the rate of growth and development. Boys and girls have different development rates. Each part of the body has its own particular rate of growth. Development does not occur at an even pace. There are periods of great intensity and equilibrium and there are periods of imbalance. Development achieves a plateau and this may occur at any level or between levels.
- **Development comes from maturation and learning:** Human development, the process of growth and change that takes place between birth and maturity. The changes in behavior that can occur by maturation process and by learning. Both are equally important. While learning comes from experiences and practice, maturity comes from individual growth without any external stimuli. In fact, we can say that maturation is essential for learning skills.
- **Early development is significant than the latter:** Early child development sets the foundation for lifelong learning, behavior, and health. The experiences children have in early childhood shape the brain and the child's capacity to learn, to get along with others, and to respond to daily stresses and challenges. This is a crucial time in a child's development because this period lays the foundations for the child's learning and well-being throughout their life. It is therefore considered early development is more significant than the latter.

Factor Influencing Growth and Development

Genetic Factors

- Genetic predisposition
- Sex, race

Prenatal Factors

- Maternal malnutrition
- Maternal infection
- Substance abuse

Postnatal Factors

- Nutrition
- Childhood illness
- Physical environment

Developmental Age Periods

Infancy:

- Neonate: Birth to 1 month
- Infant: 1 month to 1 year

Early childhood:

- Toddler: 1–3 years
- Preschool: 3–6 years

Middle childhood

- School age: 6–12 years

Late childhood

- Adolescent: 13–18 years

Aspects of Growth

- Biologic
- Sensory
- Motor

Biologic Growth

Changes of body due to growth of different parts of the body.

Weight

- Normal wt at birth: 2.5–3.5 kg
- 10% wt. loss in 1st week which is regained by 10th day.
- Weight gain @25–30 g/day for 1st 3 month and 40 gm/month till one year of age.
- Birth weight doubles by 5 month of age.
- Trebled by one year.
- Fourth time by two years, five times by three year, six times by five year, 7 times by 7 year and 10 times by 10 year.

Length

- Increase in height indicates skeletal growth.
- At birth average length is 50 cm.
- It increases to 60 cm at 3 months

- 70 cm of 9 month
- 75 cm at one year of age.
- 85 cm at 2 year
- 95 cm at 3 year
- 100 cm at 4 year
- Thereafter 5 cm each year till puberty.

N.B: Height doubles at 4 year and triples at 13 year of age.

Head Circumference

- It represents the growth of brain.
- ½ inch/month in first 6 month then ¼ inch/month in next 6 month.
- It is 30 cm at birth, 40 cm at 3 month, 43 cm at 6 month, 45 cm at 1 year, 48 cm at 2 year, 50 cm at 7 year.
- Method: Place the tape over the occiput at the back and just above the supraorbital ridge.

Chest Circumference

- At birth it is barrel-shaped, gradually it increases transversely.
- At birth it is 31 cm
- By 6 month to 1 year it becomes equal with HC.
- Method: Placing the tape measure around the chest at the level of the nipple, in between inspiration and expiration.

Body Mass Index

It is an important criteria which helps to assess the normal growth or its deviation, i.e., malnutrition or obesity. BMI remains constant up to the age of 5 years. If the BMI is more than 30 kg/m^2, it indicates obesity and it is less than 15 kg/m^2, it indicates malnutrition.

$$\text{BMI} = \text{Weight in kg}/\text{Height in m}^2$$

BMI Categories

- Underweight = <18.5
- Normal weight = 18.5–24.9
- Overweight = 25–29.9
- Obesity = 30 or greater.

Fontanelle Closure

- At birth, anterior and posterior fontanelle are usually present.
- Posterior fontanelle closes early (6–8 week) of age.
- The anterior fontanelle normally closes by 12–18 months of age.
- Early closure of fontanelle indicates craniostenosis due to premature closure of skull sutures.

Mid Upper Arm Circumference (MUAC)

- The average MUAC **at birth is 11 to 12 cm**
- At one year of age it is 12–16 cm
- 1 to 5 years = 16–17 cm
- 12 years = 17–18 cm
- 15 years = 20–21 cm

Eruption of Teeth

- First teeth erupt is **lower central incisior** in 6 to 7 months of age.
- It can be delayed even up to 15 months.

Motor Growth

It depends on maturation of muscular, skeletal and nervous system. It follows proximodistal and cephalon-caudal pattern.

- **Gross motor:** It is the acquisition of mobility and independent movement, e.g., sitting, turning.
- **Fine motor:** This growth leads to acquisition of motor dexterity, Finger/pincer/palmer grasp.

Sensory Growth

- At birth only taste and smell
- Gradually learn perception of stimulation.
- As per myelination of nervous system baby perceive to different stimulus.
- Visual system mature at last.

GROWTH MONITORING

- Growth monitoring is a screening tool to diagnose nutritional, chronic, systemic and endocrine disease at an early stage.
- **Growth Chart:** The growth of the child is monitored by recording the weight of the child periodically and plotting against the age, in a specially designed chart called Growth Chart.
- It was 1st designed by David Morley.
- The chart is a visible display of a graph, showing horizontal X-axis and longitudinal Y-axis.

Importance of Growth Monitoring

Growth monitoring helps detect three main problems:

- Feeding difficulties, particularly in the younger child
- Chronic ill health from whatever cause, including respiratory infection, malaria, tuberculosis, and growth hormone deficiency.
- Social deprivation, where poverty and home circumstances are such that one outcome is poor nutrition as depicted in **Figure 2.2**.

Growth Chart

Many biophysiologic and psychosocial problems can adversely affect growth, and aberrant growth may be the first sign of an underlying problem. The most powerful tool in growth assessment is the **growth charts**.

In 2006 the WHO released growth charts based on the Multicenter Growth Reference Study. Six study sites representing 5 continents were included: USA, Brazil, Norway, Ghana, Oman, and India **(Fig. 2.3)**.

How to Maintain this Chart

- All the points on the growth chart should be marked only as dots and not circles around the dot.

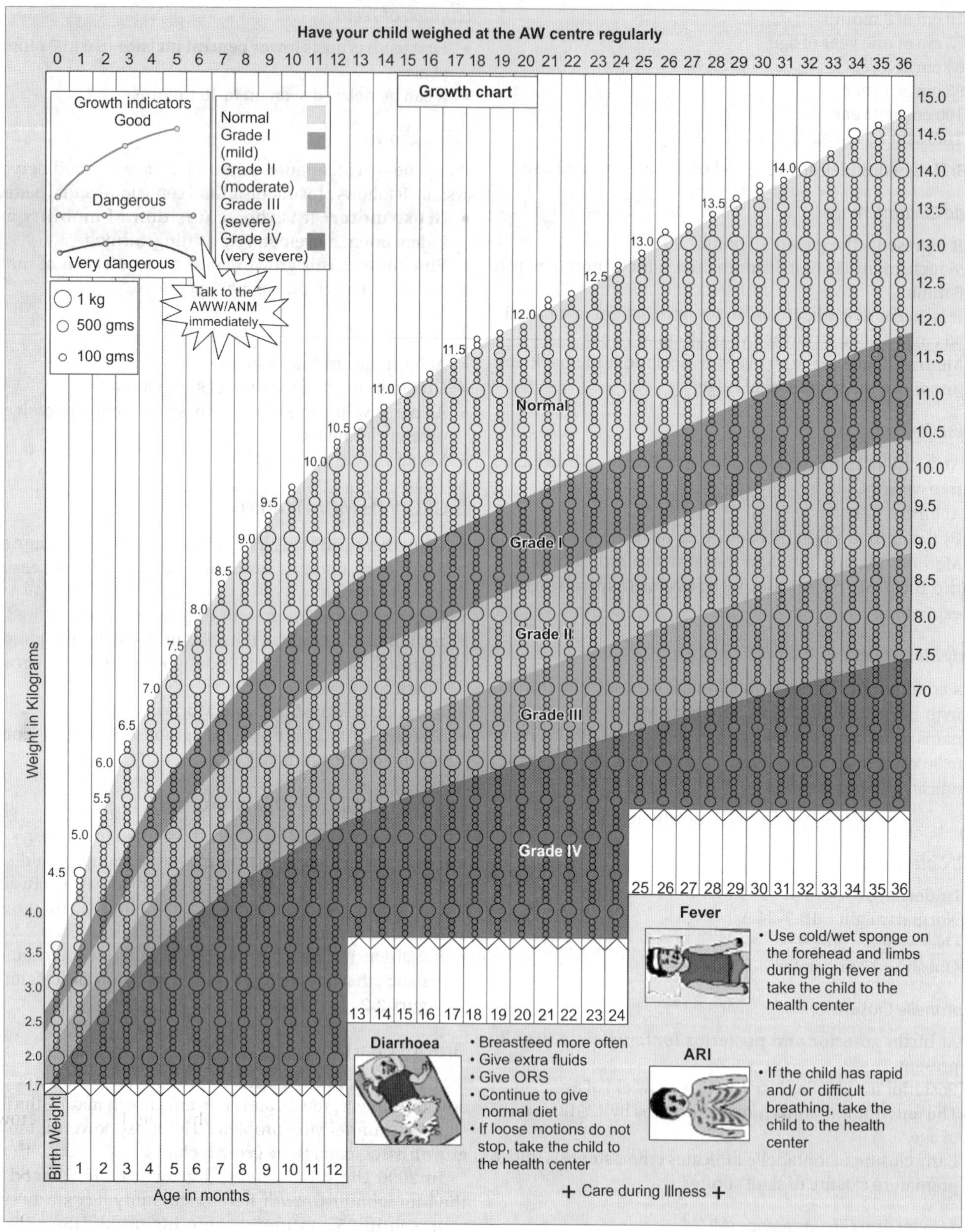

Fig. 2.2: Schedule of growth monitoring as per National Institute of Public Cooperation and Child Development.

- The height and weight should be recorded (and head circumference till 3 years) and plotted on the chart.
- At all subsequent visits join the dot up to the previous dot.
- Remind parents of the time for the next measurement.
- The growth should be monitored:
    - From birth—1 month weekly

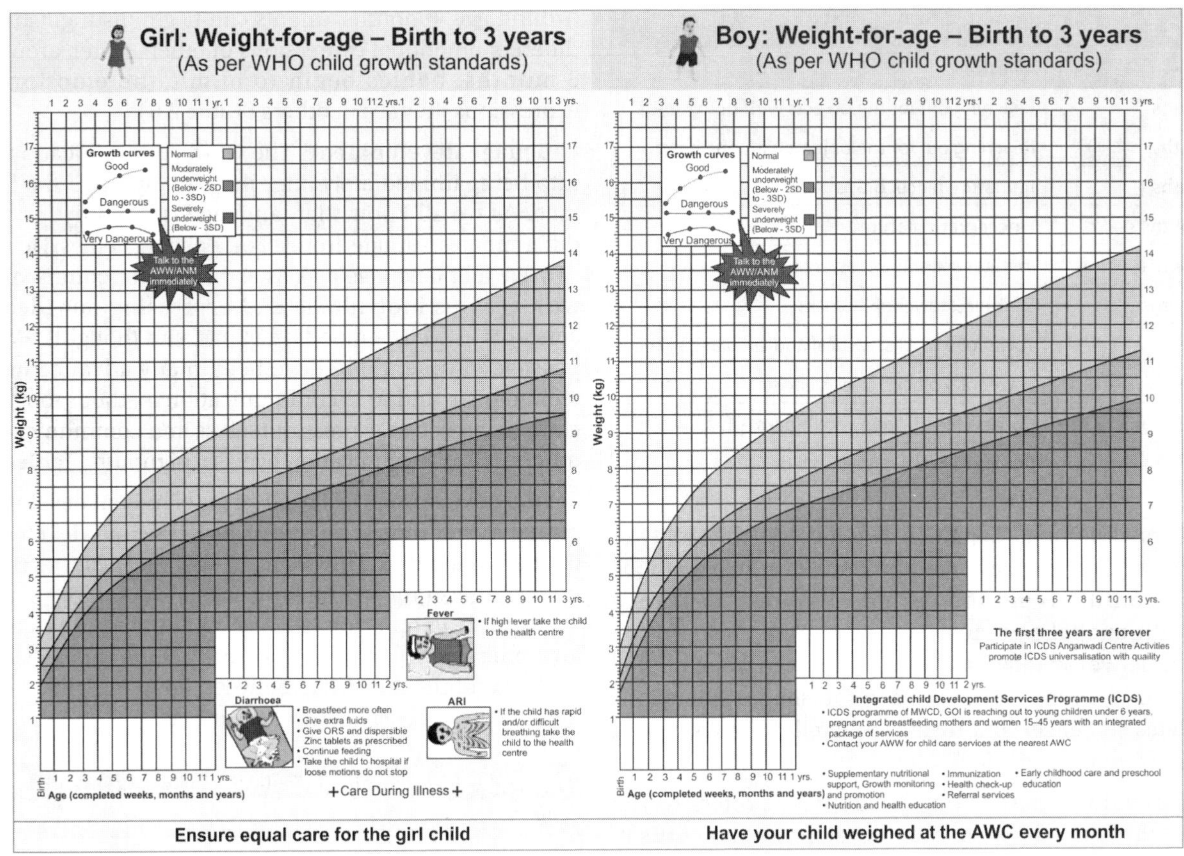

Fig. 2.3: WHO growth chart.

- One month—3 years every month and
- 3–5 years at every three months.

NB: However, children who are severely underweight, or who have not gained weight for 2 months, or who are "at risk" of under nutrition, should be weighed frequently preferably every month.

Limitations

- It does not reflect current feeding practices
- The rapid gain demonstrated in breastfed infants first six months may not be appropriate for all breastfed babies.
- Slower than the expected growth rates may be interpreted as neglect especially in aboriginal communities.

DEVELOPMENT

Aspects of Development

- Physical
- Intellectual
- Moral
- Emotional
- Social
- Sexual

Physical aspect: Physical development is also known as physical growth and it refer to physiological and psychomotor changes of an individual. It is basically related to the growth of a child's height, weight, and physique. The rate of growth is different in every individual depending upon his/her age group. Children belonging to the elementary group (6–9 years) tend to grow at a slow pace. It also relate the physiological changes that begins with puberty as depicted in **Tables 2.4 and 2.5**.

Table 2.4: Key gross motor development.

Age	*Milestone*
3 months	Neck holding
5 months	Rolls over
6 months	Sits with own support
8 months	Sitting without support
9 months	Standing, holding on (with support)
12 months	Creep well, stand without support
15 months	Walks alone, creeps upstairs
18 months	Runs
2 years	Walks up and down stairs
3 years	Rides tricycle
4 years	Hops on one foot, alternate feet going downstairs

Intellectual or cognitive development: The meaning of cognition is to know, perceive or comprehend. Hence, it would mean the development of the capability of knowing and understanding things over time, again in interaction

Table 2.5: Key fine motor development.

Age	Milestone
4 months	Reaching out for the objects with both hands
6 months	Reaching out for the objects with one hand
9 months	Immature pincer graps
12 months	Pincer graps mature
15 months	Imitates scribbling, tower of 2 blocks
18 months	Scribbles, tower of 3 blocks
2 years	Tower of 6 blocks, vertical and circular stroke
3 years	Tower of 9 blocks, copies circle
4 years	Copies cross, bridge with blocks
5 years	Copies triangle, gate with blocks

with an environment. Cognition also involves the ability to construct mental images based on one's own imaginations and reasoning. From the period of infancy cognitive development takes place. The examples of cognitive development of an infant are finds things even when hidden under two or three covers, begins to sort shapes and colors, completes sentences and rhymes in familiar books, builds towers of four or more blocks, etc.

Moral development: Moral development refers to the process through which children develop the standards of right and wrong within their society, based on social and cultural norms, and laws. Lawrence Kohlberg describes moral development as a process of discovering universal moral principles, and is based on a child's intellectual development. By the end of the first year, most babies are beginning to learn about right and wrong, and are learning to imitate and communicate feelings and preferences.

Emotional: All emotions play an important role in making adjustments in an individual's life. One of them is the emotional aspect. The ability to respond emotionally is present even in a newborn infant. There are different types of emotions that are demonstrated by an individual at different stages of his life. Joy, anger, fear, anxiety, jealousy, happiness, envy, and curiosity are some of them.

Social: Babies can feel interest, distress, disgust, and happiness from birth, and can communicate these through facial expressions and body posture. Infants begin showing a spontaneous "social smile" around age 2 to 3 months, and begin to laugh spontaneously around age 4 months. In addition, between ages 2 and 6 months, infants express other feelings such as anger, sadness, surprise, and fear. Between ages 5 and 6 months, babies begin to exhibit stranger anxiety. They do not like it when other people hold or play with them, and they will show this discomfort visibly. These are the social development. Previously, they would smile at anyone and allow them to hold them but after that they will show their willingness to their close one to hold them. However, during this time babies are learning not only how to show their own feelings, but also how to notice others' feelings. Around age 4 months, infants can begin distinguishing the different emotional expressions of others. Later, around age 6 months, babies begin to mimic the emotions and expressions they see in others **(Table 2.6)**.

Language development: The word communication came into being immediately after the coming up of the human race. As we all know that language is the only mode that differentiates humans from all other living beings. Hence, we can say that language acts as a channel for communicating with various individuals and expressing our ideas and concepts as well as moods, feelings, and thoughts. With the passage of time, there have been many advancements in technologies and so in communication methods too. It is the code we all use to express ourselves and communicate with others. It is communication by word of mouth **(Table 2.7)**.

Sexual development: Like all forms of human development, sexual development begins at birth. Sexual development includes not only the physical changes that occur as children grow, but also the sexual knowledge. By age 2 or 3, a child starts to develop a sense of being a male or female. This awareness is called gender identity. Kids this age start to understand the difference between boys and girls, and can identify themselves as one or the other.

Table 2.6: Social and adaptive development.

Age	Milestone
2 months	Social smile
3 months	Recognizes mother
6 months	Recognizes strangers, stranger anxiety
9 months	Waves "bye bye"
12 months	Comes when called, plays single ball game
15 months	Jargon
18 months	Copies parents in tasks
2 years	Asks for food, drink, toilet
3 years	Shares toys, knows full name and gender
4 years	Plays cooperatively in a group, goes to toilet alone
5 years	Helps in household tasks, dressing and undressing

Table 2.7: Language.

Age	Milestone
1 month	Alerts to sound
3 months	Coos (musical vowel sounds)
4 months	Laugh loud
6 months	Monosyllables (ba, da, pa) sound
9 months	Bisyllables (mama, baba, dada) sound
12 months	1–2 words with meaning
18 months	8–10 words vocabulary
2 years	2–3 word sentences, uses pronouns "I", "Me", "you"
3 years	Ask question
4 years	Says songs or poem, tell stories
5 years	Asks meaning of words

There are different theories of development given by different scientist.

- Intellectual development theory: Jean Piaget
- Moral development theory: Jean Piaget and Kohlberg
- Psychological development theory: Eric H Erikson
- Spiritual development theory: James W Fowler
- Sexual development theory: Sigmund Freud
- Emotional development theory: Eric H Erikson

THE MENSTRUAL CYCLE

A menstrual cycle (also termed a female reproductive cycle) can be defined as periodic uterine bleeding in response to cyclic hormonal changes or a series of changes that occur on the ovary, uterus, and cervix in response to hormonal change. The average age at which menarche (the first menstrual period) occurs at the average age of 12.8 years. This may occur as early as age 9 or as late as age 17 years. The purpose of a menstrual cycle is to bring an ovum to maturity and renew a uterine tissue bed that will be responsive to its growth should it be fertilized. The average age of onset of menstrual cycles is 21 to 35 days. The accepted average length is 28 days. The length of the average menstrual flow is 1–9 days and the average length is 5 days. Amount of flow is from spotting to 80 mL on average. Four body structures that are involved in the normal physiology of the menstrual cycle are:

- The hypothalamus
- The pituitary gland
- The ovaries and
- The uterus.
- Cervix.

For a menstrual cycle to be complete, all four structures must contribute their part, in activity from any part will result in an incomplete or ineffective cycle. Some women have symptoms of anxiety, fatigue, abdominal bloating, headache, appetite disturbance, irritability and depression in pre-menstrual period. Some women may experience abdominal pain during ovulation and the release of accompanying prostaglandins. Some even notice irritation when a drop or two of follicular fluid or blood spills in to the abdominal cavity of the uterus begins to degenerate (at approximately day 24 or day 25 of the cycle). The capillaries rupture, with minute hemorrhage, the endometrium sloughs off, and menstruation starts.

BREAST SELF-EXAMINATION

Breast self-examination (BSE) is a life-saving habit and screening tool for cancer. In this procedure, women undergo a systematic review of their breasts to look for lumps. BSE can be a valuable tool in diagnosing breast cancer at an early stage. Everyone's breasts are different and that changes can be related to aging, menstrual cycle, pregnancy, menopause or hormone use. Normal breast tissue feels lumpy and uneven. It is normal for a woman's breast tissue to become swollen and tender right before or during her menstrual period.

BSE is one of the easiest detection methods and it is the physical examination of own breast tissue. It is a simple, zero expensive and more effective step for prevention of breast cancer. In this procedure, women undergo a systematic review of their breasts to look for lumps. BSE can be a valuable tool in diagnosing breast cancer at an early stage. Regular BSE will help to identify changes that require further evaluation and possible treatment. Breast self-exams to aid in the detection of breast cancer and its helps to familiar with the normal consistency of breasts and underlying tissue so aware of any abnormal lumps or other changes. The best time to do a breast self-exam is on a monthly basis and usually about three to five days after the end of menstruation, at that time breasts are less tender or swollen. Try to remember to do the exam on the same day every month. More early diagnosis, more advanced treatments, can result in full active life to an woman **(Fig. 2.4)**.

BSE is a check-up a woman does at home to look for changes or problems in the breast tissue. It is a simple, painless procedure that helped to create awareness about female heath. It is preventive health care practice to helped many women diagnose and treat various conditions at an early stage.

BSE should be started at 20 years of age. A breast self-exam involves both looking and feeling. It can be performed while looking in a mirror and when in the shower or lying down. It takes time only 10–15 minute in the detection of breast cancer and it helps to familiar with the normal consistency of breasts and underlying tissue so aware of any abnormal lumps or other changes.

The best time to do a breast self-exam is on a monthly basis and usually about three to five days after the end of menstruation, at that time breasts are less tender or swollen and should be on the same day of every month.

Benefits of BSE

- It is an important step for early detection of breast cancer.
- It is a simple, zero expensive and more effectiveness steps for prevention of breast cancer.
- By early diagnosis prompt and appropriate treatment can be initiated.
- It reduces the chances of complication of breast disorder.
- Early diagnosis, early treatment saves life.
- Much better chance of cure.

The Five Steps of Breast Self-exam

Step 1

- Begin by looking at breasts in front of the mirror with shoulders straight and arms on hips.
- Check both breasts for anything unusual like size, shape, and color.
- Discharge from the nipple, Dimpling or scaling of the skin, puckering or bulging of the skin.
- A nipple that has changed position or an inverted nipple (pushed inward instead of sticking out)
- Redness, soreness, rash, or swelling.

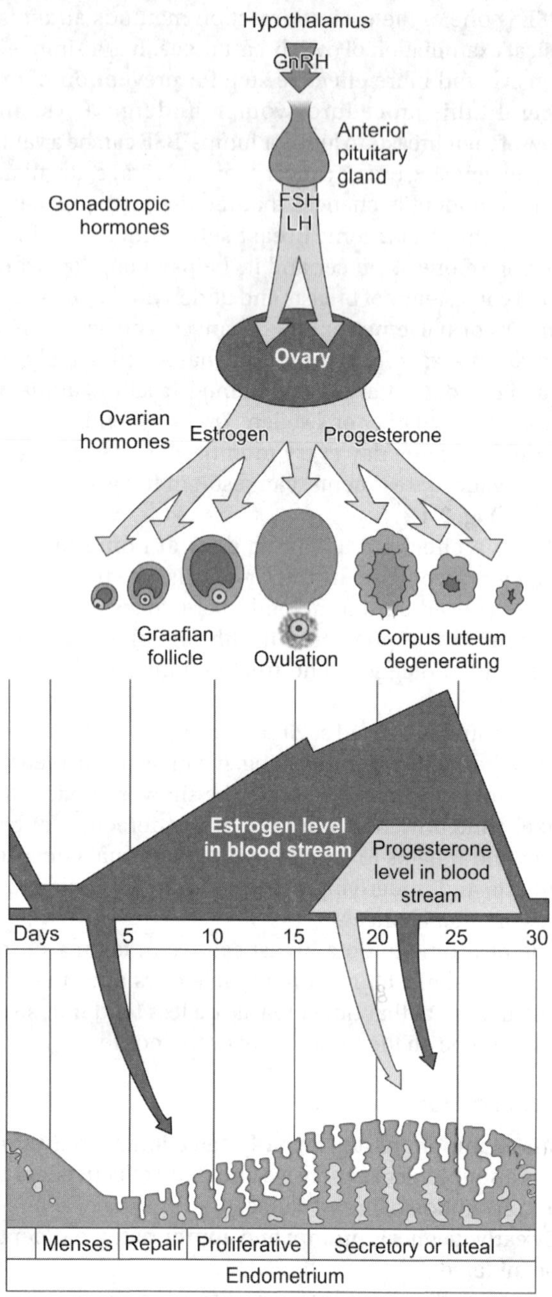

Fig. 2.4: Menstrual cycle.

Step 2

- Now, watch closely in the mirror as you clasp your hands above your head and press your hand forward.
- Note any change in the contour of your breast.

Step 3

Now, press your hands firmly on your hips and bow slightly toward the mirror as you pull your shoulders and elbows forward and note any change in the counter of your breasts. Some women do the next part of the examination in the shower. Your finger will glide easily over soapy skin, so you can concentrate on feeling for changes inside the breast.

Step 4

In this step palpation of breast to find out any abnormalities. It can be done by circular, line wedge method.

- Raise your left arm
- Use three or four fingers of right hand to feel left breast firmly, carefully and thoroughly
- Beginning at the outer edge, press the flat part of fingers in small circles, moving the circle slowly around the breast.
- Gradually move toward the nipple.
- Be sure to cover the whole breast.
- Pay special attention to the area between the breast and the underarm, including the underarm itself.
- Feel for any unusual lumps or masses under the skin.
- If any spontaneous discharge during the month—whether or not it is during BSE-see doctor.
- Repeat the examination on right breast.

Step 5

- In this step breast is palpated as in step-4 but in lying down position.
- So, lie flat on your back with left arm overhead and a pillow or folded towel under left shoulder.
- Use the same circular motion described as above
- Repeat on right breast.

What are the finding we will get like after breast self-exam?

- A lump in the breast or armpit. These can range from marble-sized to tennis ball-sized.
- Increase in the size of one breast.
- Swelling in glands of armpit.
- Enlargement of one arm.
- Dimpling or puckering of the skin.
- Dimpling of or changes to the nipple.
- Discharge from the nipple (Other than breast milk).
- Nipple inversion
- 'Orange peel' appearance to the skin of the breast and/ or nipple.
- Retraction of one or both nipples.
- Dry skin (eczema) of the nipple.
- Irregular thickening of breast tissue
- Swelling
- Redness or scariness of the nipple or breast.

TESTICULAR SELF-EXAMINATION

Testicular self-examination (TSE) is a procedure where a man examines his own testicles and scrotum for possible lumps or swelling. It is usually undertaken at home while standing in front of a mirror and after having a warm bath or shower. Monthly self-examination of the testicles starting at puberty may be an effective way of detecting testicular cancer at an early, potentially treatable stage, which can lead to a 5-year survival rate of 98%. In men aged 15 to 40, testicular cancer is the most common cancer, and the annual rate of increase over the last 10 years in cases of testicular cancer has been shown to be approximately 1% each year. Testicular cancer typically presents with a painless testicular swelling or lump or any change in shape or texture of the testicles.

Indication of TSE

- Family history of testicular cancer
- Men who had undescended testicles at birth, or who are infertile
- Testicular self-exams help an individual to learn how own testicles normally look and feel and identify any changes or symptoms of cancer.

The characteristics of healthy testicles include:
- Each testicle feels like a smooth, firm egg.
- Adult testicles range in size from about 15 mL (similar to a bird egg) to 35 mL (similar to a small chicken egg).
- One testicle may be slightly larger than the other.
- Commonly, one testicle hangs lower than the other.
- There should be no pain or discomfort when the testicles and scrotum are handled gently.

How to perform testicular self-examination?
Generally, the TSE procedure includes:
- Make sure your scrotum is warm and relaxed. You may like to perform TSE after showering or bathing.
- It may help to do TSE in front of the mirror, so you can see as well as feel what you are doing.
- Check one testicle first, then the other.
- Gently roll one testicle using the fingers and thumbs of both hands.
- Feel along the underside of the scrotum to find the epididymis that sits at the back of the testicle. It should feel like a little bunch of tightly curled tubes.
- Perform TSE on the other testicle.

TSE should not be painful or uncomfortable. If one or both testes have become tender or painful, see your doctor.

Symptoms of Testicular Cancer and Testicular Self-examination

Symptoms of testicular cancer include a testicular lump that is usually painless (about one in 10 are painful), a sensation of heaviness in the scrotum, and a persistent ache in the affected testicle.

Take notice of anything unusual, such as:
- A lump or swelling in or on the testicle itself
- Change in testicular size
- Change in testicular shape
- Change in the consistency or feel of the testicle.

Testicular Conditions Other than Cancer

It is important to remember that testicular cancer is relatively uncommon, so do not panic if you find a lump or anything else that seems unusual. See your doctor for a prompt diagnosis.

Some non-cancerous conditions that may affect the testicles include:
- Cyst—an abnormal but harmless collection of fluid
- Varicocele—varicose veins. About 10 to 15 per cent of men have varicose veins of the scrotum
- Hematocele—a blood clot caused by trauma or injury to the testicles or scrotum
- Epididymo-orchitis—infection of the epididymis, testicle or both that causes inflammation and pain. Treatment is usually antibiotics
- Testicular torsion—the cord that attaches the testicle to the body twists and cuts off the blood supply. This extremely painful condition needs urgent medical attention
- Undescended testicles—either one or both testicles are missing from the scrotum and are lodged instead inside the lower abdomen. Premature and low-weight newborn boys are most prone to undescended testicles. This condition is known to increase the chance of testicular cancer later in life and is also linked to infertility.

WARNING SIGNS OF VARIOUS DISEASE

Today the number of persons with heart disease, cancer, and stroke are increasing. These diseases are responsible for majority of deaths. Unhealthy lifestyle is a major contributor for these life-taking diseases. According to Stanford University of School of Medicine in California, "Not only do persons with better health habit survive longer, but in such persons, disability is postponed and compressed into fewer years at the end of life." Warning sign means a sign giving warning of a hazard or risk. By knowing the warning signs any health personnel can identify and make diagnosis of the health problems early and provide early treatment decreases morbidity, mortality.

Warming Signs of Various Diseases in General

- *Unexplained weight loss,* which may signal such things as chronic infection, depression or in serious cases, cancer.
- *Unexplained changes in bowel habits* may be due to inflammatory bowel disease, ulcers, cancers or infections.
- *Chest pain with a pain in the jaw or arm* can be a sign of heart disease.
- *Shortness of breath, breathing trouble* may indicate lung or heart disease.
- *Sudden unexplained headaches,* especially in people over 50. It may be nothing or it may something serious in the brain like an infection or a tumor.
- *Sudden weakness or numbness of the face, arm or leg on one side of the body.*
- Loss of speech or trouble talking or understanding speech or blurring or loss of vision. This may indicate a stroke or a transient ischemic attack.
- *Confusion, changes in behavior or thinking, disorientation, hallucinations* are the warning signs of possible low blood sugar, possible head injury, side effects of drugs.
- *Flashing lights* in someone who has otherwise normal vision may be the beginning of retinal detachment.
- *Hot, red or swollen joints* indicate arthritis or joint infection.
- *Fever (over 37.5°C)* persisting over a week may mean a chronic underlying infection, cancer or some other illness.

Warning Signs of Brain Tumor

Tumors may originate in the brain (the primary brain tumor) or it starts elsewhere in the body such as a lung or breast cancer and spreads to the brain (the metastatic tumors). This depends on whether the tumor is a primary brain tumor, meaning it originates in the brain, or elsewhere. The metastatic tumors are malignant. The causes of primary brain tumors are unknown. Warning signs for brain tumor are:

- Intermittent headaches that come and go, worse in the morning and when exercising or changing position.
- Problems with memory, speech and concentration.
- Deterioration in behavior, temperament and intellectual ability.
- Nausea, drowsiness and vision problems.

Warning Signs of Cancer

In simple terms, cancer is an abnormal growth of body cells. Each one of us is born with a potential for cancer. One cannot "Catch" it as one would an infection or a cold. When the programming of a cell or a group of cells is affected, growth may become uncontrolled. Some of the factors that can alter the code are chronic irritation, tobacco, smoke and dust, radioactive substances, age, sex, race and heredity. Early identification can helps to control the disease at early stage. The seven warning signs of cancer are CAUTION by its acronym.

C: Change in bowel or bladder habits: Everyone has regular pattern of bowel habits. If this changes suddenly, that is, if people have diarrhoea or of they are constipated for days together and if that does not clear it in a day or two, it is better to consult a doctor. This could be a sign of cancer in the abdomen, or colorectal cancer. As for bladder habits, sometimes the urine might be discolored, deep yellow, or have blood in it. These might signify cancer in the kidney or bladder, though extremely rare. Deep yellow urine might indicate jaundice, and jaundice could be an indicator of cancer in the liver or pancreas. In men, difficulty in passing urine, or frequently feeling the urge to urinate could be a sign of an enlarged prostate, a marker of prostate cancer.

A: A sore that does not heal: If there is a wound that does not heal, and continues to pester, it might indicate cancer. In India, where sari wearing is common, there is a unique type which doctors identify as 'sari cancer'. It is a rare type of skin cancer caused by constant irritation and pigmentation that occurs along the waistline of women who drape saris regularly. Repeated trauma can worsen these wounds. If such a sore is present in the mouth, it could indicate oral cancer.

U: Unusual bleeding or discharge: If there is bloody discharge from the nipples, it could be a sign of breast cancer. In women who have already attained menopause, sudden bleeding could be a sign of uterine cancer. Even if she has undergone hysterectomy (surgical removal of uterus), such bleeding could indicate a cancer in the vagina. Colorectal bleeding may be a sign of colon cancer. Any unusual bleeding or discharge may be a sign of cancer.

T: Thickening or lump in the breast or elsewhere: Most common is lump in the breasts. Painful lumps are usually non-cancerous but if it is a painless lump, people tend to ignore and take it lightly, however, what's ironic is that as a thumb rule, most cancers have pain as the very last symptom. A painless lump in the breast is more dangerous than a painful one. The same applies to men, too. One per cent of all breast cancers are in men but due to ignorance and stigma attached, breast cancer in men gets diagnosed late.

I: Indigestion or difficulty in swallowing: This could be passed off as a throat infection or something similar. However, if it is not cured in spite of medications, seek help. It could be a sign of oesophageal or stomach cancer.

O: Obvious changes in warts or moles: If we observe moles or warts growing, or bleeding, it could be an indication of melanoma.

N: Nagging cough or hoarseness: This should raise an alarm especially in smokers. Persistent cough could indicate lung cancer or throat cancer.

All these symptoms need not necessarily signify cancer, but one should watch out for bodily changes and seek medical help at the earliest.

Endocrine System: Diabetes Warning Signs

Early Warning Signs of Diabetes

Both types of diabetes have some of the same tell-tale warning signs.

- **Hunger and fatigue:** When body converts the food into glucose that the cells use for energy. But cells need insulin to take in glucose. If body does not make enough or any insulin, or if cells resist the insulin your body makes, the glucose cannot get into them and patient feels hungrier and more tired than usual.
- **Peeing more often and being thirstier:** The average person usually has to pee between four and seven times in 24 hours, but people with diabetes may go a lot more. Why? Normally, your body reabsorbs glucose as it passes through your kidneys. But when diabetes pushes your blood sugar up, your kidneys may not be able to bring it all back in. This causes the body to make more urine, and that takes fluids. The result: You will have to go more often. You might pee out more, too. Because you are peeing so much, you can get very thirsty. When you drink more, you will also pee more.
- **Dry mouth and itchy skin:** Because your body is using fluids to make pee, there is less moisture for other things. You could get dehydrated, and your mouth may feel dry. Dry skin can make you itchy.
- **Blurred vision:** Changing fluid levels in your body could make the lenses in your eyes swell up. They change shape and cannot focus.
- **Overweight/unexplained weight loss:** Obesity, is a risk for six times more likely to develop Type 2 diabetes. In people with diabetes, insufficient insulin prevents the body from getting glucose from the blood into the body's

cells to use as energy. When this occurs, the body starts burning fat and muscle for energy, causing a reduction in overall body weight.
- **Slow healing wounds:** Over time, high blood sugar can affect blood flow and cause nerve damage that makes it hard for patient's body to heal wounds.
- **Persistent numbness in hands or feet:** This is another result of nerve damage.
- **Yeast infections:** Both men and women with diabetes can get these. Yeast feeds on glucose, so having plenty around makes it thrive. Infections can grow in any warm, moist fold of skin, including:
  - Between fingers and toes
  - Under breasts
  - In or around sex organs.

Warning Signs of Lung Disease

- **Chronic cough:** A cough that you have had for eight weeks or longer is considered chronic. This is an important early symptom that tells you something is wrong with your respiratory system.
- **Shortness of breath:** It is not normal to experience shortness of breath that does not go away after exercising, or that you have after little or no exertion. Labored or difficult breathing—the feeling that it is hard to breathe in out—is also a warning sign.
- **Chronic mucus production:** Mucus, also called sputum or phlegm, is produced by the airways as a defense against infections or irritants. If your mucus production has lasted a month or longer, this could indicate lung disease.
- **Wheezing:** Noisy breathing or wheezing is a sign that something unusual is blocking your lungs' airways or making them too narrow.
- **Coughing up blood:** If you are coughing up blood, it may be coming from your lungs or upper respiratory tract. Wherever it is coming from, it signals a health problem.
- **Chronic chest pain:** Unexplained chest pain that lasts for a month or more—especially if it gets worse when you breathe in or cough—also is a warning sign.

Warning Signs of Cardiovascular System

Warning Signs of Hypertension

- Sweating
- Headache
- Dizziness
- Quick exhaustion
- Rapid pulse or palpitation
- Vision disorder.

Warning Signs of Heart Disease

- Chest pain, chest tightness, chest pressure and chest discomfort (angina)
- Shortness of breath
- Pain, numbness, weakness or coldness in your legs or arms if the blood vessels in those parts of your body are narrowed
- Pain in the neck, jaw, throat, upper abdomen or back.

The signs of heart attack.
- Sweating
- Shortness of breath
- Nausea or vomiting
- Dizziness
- Crushing or squeezing chest pain radiating to the arm, neck or jaw
- Irregular and/or rapid pulse
- Intense pain in the jaw line.

Warning Signs Stroke

Use the FAST test to check for the most common symptoms of a stroke
- **Face:** Smile and see if one side of the face droops.
- **Arms:** Raise both arms. Does one arm drop down?
- **Speech:** Say a short phrase and check for slurred or strange speech.
- **Time:** If the answer to any of these is yes, call ambulance right away and write down the time when symptoms started.

The most warning signs of stroke are:
- Numbness or weakness in your face, arm, or leg, especially on one side
- Confusion or trouble understanding other people
- Difficulty speaking
- Trouble seeing with one or both eyes
- Problems walking or staying balanced or coordinated
- Dizziness
- Severe headache that comes on for no reason.

Warning Signs of Kidney Disease

The most warning signs of kidney diseases are nausea or vomiting, Weakness or fatigue, loss of appetite, trouble sleeping difficulties in concentrating and poor school performance, weight gain, swollen feet and ankles puffiness around eyes and high blood pressure, etc.

URINE TEST FOR GLUCOSE

A urine glucose test is a quick and simple way to check for abnormally high levels of glucose in urine. Glucose is a type of sugar that the body requires and uses for energy.

Preparation of Articles

The articles required to test the urine for sugar by using Benedict solution are as follows:
- Test tube in a test tube rack
- Test tube holder
- Spirit lamp
- Match box
- Kidney tray
- Duster or rag pieces to wipe test tube before heating
- Benedict's solution
- Pipette/filler
- Syringe
- Small bottle brush

Articles required for urine testing by using dipstick:

- Clean container for routine test/sterile container for culture
- Disposable gloves
- Antiseptic solution
- Cotton balls

Preparation of Patient

- Explain the procedure to the patient, the purpose of the test, what specimen to collect, when to collect, how to collect and the amount to be collected.
- Provide appropriate container and demonstrate how to use it
- Instruct patient not to contaminate the outside of the bottle
- Ask patient to wash external genitalia with soap and water before collecting the urine specimen.

Step of Procedure

- Wash hands
- Take 5 mL of Benedict's solution in test tube
- Light the lamp
- Heat Benedict's solution by holding it over spirit lamp
- Bring it to a boil by holding it away from the face
- Let it cool down
- Observe the color and interpret the results.

Procedure using Dipstick

- Remove one strip from the bottle of dipsticks and replace the cap.
- Completely immerse the regent area of the strip in urine and remove immediately to avoid dissolving the reagent.
- When removing the strip from the urine, run the edge against the rim of the urine container to remove excess urine.
- Hold the strip horizontally.
- Compare the color of the reagent area to the color chart on the label of the bottle, after the time specified (usually 60 seconds)
- Document the results in the MCP card and the case sheet
- Provide result specific dietary advice and referral.

Read the result as follows:

- Blue liquid with no deposits—absence of sugar
- Green liquid with no deposit—1%
- Green with yellow, no deposit—2%
- Orange, no deposit—3%
- Brick red—5% or above.

After Care

- Discard the urine and clean the test tube using brush, replace
- Inform patient about result
- Record findings.

URINE TEST FOR ALBUMIN

Articles Required

Prepare the necessary equipment. A tray containing:

- Test tube
- Test tube holder
- Spirit lamp
- Match box
- Kidney tray
- Duster or rag piece
- Acetic acid
- Red and blue litmus paper
- A small bottle brush
- Container for collecting urine.

Articles required for urine testing by using dipstick

- Clean container for routine test/sterile container for culture
- Disposable gloves
- Antiseptic solution
- Cotton balls

Explain to the woman how to collect a clean-catch specimen of urine (Fig. 2.5):

Give her a labeled container and instruct her to clean her vulva with water then:

- Use the fingers of one hand to spread the labia;
- Urinate in a free stream;
- Use the other hand to hold the container to catch the urine in mid-stream; and
- Remove the container before stream of urine stops.

Dipstick Procedure

- Remove one strip from the bottle of dipsticks and replace cap.

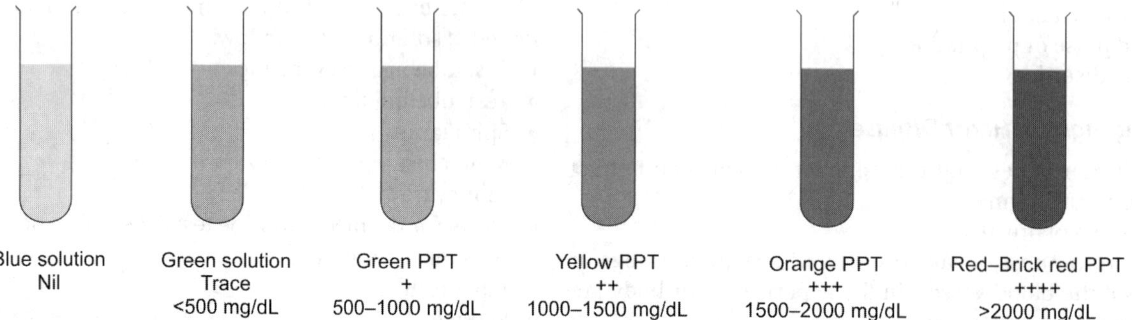

Fig. 2.5: Urine albumin test.

- Completely immerse reagent areas of strip in urine and remove immediately to avoid dissolving reagents:
  - When removing the strip from urine, run the edge against the rim of urine container to remove excess urine.
  - Hold the strip horizontally to prevent possible mixing of chemicals from adjacent reagent areas and/or contaminating the hands with urine.
- Compare reagent areas to corresponding color chart on bottle label, at the time specified (usually 60 seconds):
  - Hold strip close to color blocks and match carefully
  - Avoid placing strip directly on color chart
  - Development of any greenish color is due to presence of protein in urine (color ranges from yellow for negative reactions through to yellow-green and green to green-blue for positive reactions).
  - Place strip in plastic bag or leakproof covered container.

Hot test for detecting protein in urine:

- Place urine in a clean, dry test tube and heat to boiling.
- Allow test tube to stand; a thick precipitate at the bottom of the test tube indicates protein in the urine.
- If acetic acid is available:
  - Add 2–3 drops of 2–3% acetic acid after boiling urine;
  - If urine becomes cloudy, protein is present; and
  - If the urine remains clear, protein is not present.

After Care

- Dispose of urine in toilet or latrine.
- Decontaminate urine container and test tube in 0.5% chlorine solution
- Wash hands thoroughly with soap and water and dry with a clean, dry cloth or allow to air dry.

BLOOD TEST FOR HEMOGLOBIN

Preparation of Articles

- A pair of gloves
- Spirit swabs
- Lancet
- N/10 HCL
- Distilled water
- Dropper
- Hemoglobinometer with a comparator on both sides
- Pippette and stirrer
- **Hemoglobin tube (Sahli-Adams Tube):** It is graduated on one side in g% from 2 to 24 g% and on the other side in percentage from 20% to 40%.

Preparation of Patient and Environment

- Explain the purpose of the hemoglobin test to the woman and encourage her to ask questions.
- Tell the woman how the test will be done.
- Wash hands thoroughly with soap and water and dry with clean dry cloth or allow to air dry.
- Put new examination or high-level disinfected gloves on both hands.
- Fill the Hb tube with N/10 HCl up to 20% or 2 g% with the dropper.

Procedure

- Clean the tip of the woman's index finger with an alcohol swab.
- Prick finger using lancet and discard first drop of blood.
- Allow a large drop of blood to form on the fingertip. Dip the tip of the Hb pipette into the blood drop and suck blood up to the 20 cmm mark on the pipette. Do not squeeze finger tip to collect blood. While sucking the blood, care should be taken to prevent entry of air.
- Wipe the tip of the pipette with cotton. Immediately transfer the 20 cmm (0.02 mL) of blood from the pipette into the Hb tube containing N/10 HCL
- Rinse the pipette two to three times by drawing up and blowing out the acid solution
- Leave the solution in the tube for about 10 minutes (for conversion of Hb into hematin)
- After 10 minutes, dilute the acid by adding distilled water drop by drop. Mix it with stirrer.
- Note down the reading (lower meniscus) when the color of the solution exactly matches that of the comparator on both sides of the hemoglobinometer. This expresses the Hb content as g%.

Hemoglobin Test by using WHO Hemoglobin Color Scale

- Clean the tip of the woman's index finger with an alcohol swab.
- Prick finger using lancet.
- Squeeze blood into capillary tube or collect in pipette
- Place one drop of blood at one end of test paper to form stain of 8–9 mm in diameter:
- Wait 30 seconds
- Compare stain with color scale in good light with open color scale booklet in left hand, avoiding shadow and direct sunlight.
- Slide bloodstain up and down behind color-scale apparatus.
- If bloodstain closely matches one of the shades on the scale, record its hemoglobin value
- If color of stain lies between two of the shades, record the lower value.

After Care

- Dispose of pipette or capillary tube and lancet in puncture proof container
- Immerse both gloved hands in 0.5% chlorine solution:
- Remove gloves by turning them inside out
- If disposing of gloves, place in leak proof container or plastic bag
- If reusing surgical gloves, submerge in 0.5% chlorine solution for 10 minutes to decontaminate
- Discuss the results of the test with the woman.
- If hemoglobin is less than 7 g/dL, refer the woman for treatment. If hemoglobin is 7–11 g/dL prescribe iron/folate one tablet daily and provide nutrition counseling
- Record test results on the woman's record.

CHAPTER 3

Epidemiology

CONCEPT OF EPIDEMIOLOGY

Epidemiology is the basic science of preventive and social medicine. The science of epidemiology deals with the study of health-related states and events occurring in a population. Epidemiology helps in understanding the health concepts, natural history of disease and disease causation. It also helps in planning, implementing and evaluating effective and efficient healthcare services. Epidemiology is a quantitative basic science built on a working knowledge of probability, statistics, and sound research methods, a method of causal reasoning based on developing and testing hypotheses pertaining to occurrence and prevention of morbidity and mortality; and a tool for public health action to promote and protect the public's health based on science, causal reasoning, and a dose of practical common sense.

The term epidemiology is derived from the term epidemic. The literal meaning of the term is study among people Epi = among, demos = people, logus = study.

Definitions

- According to Parkin, 1873 the epidemiology is that branch of medical science which deals with epidemics
- According to Frost, 1927 Epidemiology is the science of mass phenomena of infectious diseases
- Greenwood, 1934 stated that Epidemiology is the study of disease, any disease, as a mass phenomenon
- Epidemiology is the study of distribution and determinants of disease frequency in man. **—MacMohan, 1960**
- Clark, 1965 described the Epidemiology as the study of various factors and conditions that determine the occurrence and distribution of health disease defect, disability and death among groups or individuals
- Epidemiology is concerned with the study of processes which determine or influence the physical, mental and social health of people. **—Cassel, 1965**
- Epidemiology is the study of the distribution of a disease or a physiological condition in human populations and of factors that influence this distribution. **—Lelien Field**

The most acceptable definition of Epidemiology is 'Epidemiology is the study of the distribution and determinants of health-related states or events in specified populations, and the application of this study to the control of health problems.' **—M last,1988**

This definition of epidemiology includes several terms which reflect some of the important principles of the discipline. The description of these terms are given below.

Study

Epidemiology is a scientific discipline, sometimes called 'the basic science of public health.' It has, at its foundation, sound methods of scientific inquiry. It is a highly quantitative discipline based on principles of statistics and research methodologies.

Distribution

Epidemiologists study the distribution of frequencies and patterns of health events within groups in a population. Frequency includes not only the number of such events in a population, but also the rate or risk of disease in the population. The rate (number of events divided by size of the population) is critical to epidemiologists because it allows valid comparisons across different populations. Pattern refers to the occurrence of health-related events by time, place, and personal characteristics.

- Time characteristics include annual occurrence, seasonal occurrence, and daily or even hourly occurrence during an epidemic
- Place characteristics include geographic variation, urban-rural differences, and location of work sites or schools
- Personal characteristics include demographic factors such as age, race, sex, marital status, and socioeconomic status, as well as behaviors and environmental exposures.

Determinants

Epidemiology is also used to search for causes and other factors that influence the occurrence of health-related events. Epidemiology will search for the factors which are responsible for disease may agent, host and environmental factors. Analytic epidemiology attempts to provide the Why and How of such events by comparing groups with different rates of disease occurrence and with differences in demographic characteristics, genetic or immunologic make-up, behaviors, environmental exposures, and other so-called potential risk factors. Under ideal circumstances, epidemiologic findings provide sufficient evidence to direct swift and effective public health control and prevention measures.

Health-related States or Events

Originally, epidemiology was concerned with epidemics of communicable diseases. Then epidemiology was extended to endemic communicable diseases and non-communicable infectious diseases. Now epidemiology deals with any health-related states or events which include any type of accidents, chronic diseases, injuries, birth defects, maternal-child health, occupational health, and environmental health. Now, even behaviors related to health and well-being (amount of exercise, seat-belt use, etc.) are recognized as valid subjects for applying epidemiologic methods. Here, we use the term 'disease' to refer to the range of health-related states or events.

Specified Populations

Specified populations include population in a specific community. Although epidemiologists and physicians in clinical practice are both concerned with disease and the control of disease, they differ greatly in how they view 'the patient.' Clinicians are concerned with the health of an individual; epidemiologists are concerned with the collective health of the people in a community or other area. When faced with a patient with diarrheal disease, for example, the clinician and the epidemiologist have different responsibilities. Although both are interested in establishing the correct diagnosis, the clinician usually focuses on treating and caring for the individual. The epidemiologist focuses on the exposure the number of other persons who may have been similarly exposed, the potential for further spread in the community, and interventions to prevent additional cases or recurrences.

Application

The different health program for control of communicable and noncommunicable diseases are initiated on applying the result of epidemiological investigation. Epidemiology provides data for directing public health action. Using epidemiologic data is an art as well as a science. To treat patient, a clinician must call upon experience and creativity as well as scientific knowledge. Similarly, an epidemiologist uses the scientific methods of descriptive and analytic epidemiology in 'diagnosing' the health of a community, but also must call upon experience and creativity when planning how to control and prevent disease in the community.

Epidemiologic Process

Epidemiological process tells the answer of five questions thats are who was affected? Where were they affected? When were they affected? How they affected and why they affected? Who refers to personal characteristics, i.e., age, sex, race/ethnicity, socioeconomic status and behaviors where refers to place, geographic distribution clustering, uniform, scattered home, work, school and hospital when refers to time, i.e., onset of symptoms, incubation period, infectious period, seasonality, epidemic, interval and long-term trends.

According to different epidemiologist, epidemiology is:
- An inductive method applied to a large group
- A research method of public health
- The science of public health
- The study of statistics of disease in population
- The quantitative science. The measured quantities and descriptive terms used to describe groups
- The measurement of risk of diseases in community
- The study of epidemics of hard to large group
- A method of diagnosing the conditions of the people
- The study of health of population in relation to their environment and ways of living.

Modern Epidemiology Deals with

- Measurement of occurrence of health-related states and events, i.e., health needs, health demands, impact of health services and measurement of frequency of disease, disability or death. The measurement are done in the form of rates, ratios and proportion, i.e., incidence rate, prevalence rate, male-female ratio percentage of children with malnutrition.
- Distribution of disease pattern in a community by time, place and person
- Testing of etiological hypothesis derived from descriptive study of diseases and health-related events
- Planning of healthcare services based on the studies, implementation and evaluation of healthcare services.

Aims of Epidemiology

The basic purposes of epidemiology are:
- To prevent control and eradicate health-related problems
- To minimize the impact of these problems
- To promote health and quality of life of people at large.

Objectives of Epidemiology

1. To describe the distribution and magnitude of health and disease problems in the population
2. To identify the etiological factors—risk factors in the population
3. To provide the data essential to planning, implementation and evaluation of services for prevention, control and treatment of disease and to setting up of priorities for these services.

Scope of Epidemiology

The scope of epidemiology is ever increasing. It is destined grow to further to meet new emerging challenges to health and survival of man on this planet. Now it stresses the concept of excessive prevalence of disease as its basic implication. Epidemiologists are now concerned not only

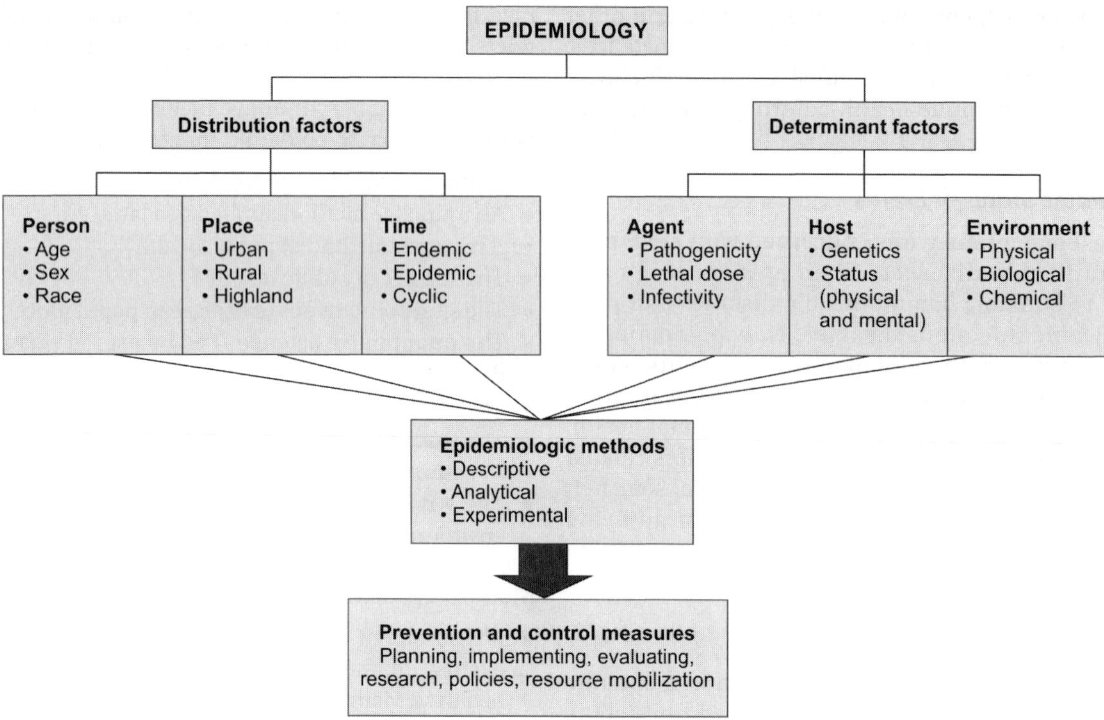

Fig. 3.1: Models of epidemiology.

with infectious diseases but also with noninfectious diseases, i.e., coronary heart disease, diabetes, accidents, injuries, cancer, and mental illness.

Thus, modern epidemiology has taken within its scope all diseases whether acute or chronic, physical or mental, communicable or noncommunicable and health-related states and events occurring in human population.

We have also seen that epidemiology is the study of disease/conditions distribution and determinants. As a science, it utilises rational study methods in identifying the distribution patterns and determinants of diseases. From the studies, recommendations are generated on how to:

- Plan for disease prevention and control
- Predict the disease patterns for effective prevention and control
- Mobilize resources for effective prevention and control
- Evaluate programs for disease prevention and control
- Develop evidence based and practical policies for effective disease prevention and control
- Develop a data base for further studies in epidemiology of diseases and conditions **(Fig. 3.1)**. Epidemiological models of causation of disease is already described in Chapter 1.

HISTORICAL BACKGROUND AND TRENDS OF EPIDEMIOLOGY

Although epidemiologic thinking has been traced from Hippocrates (Circa 400 BC) through Graunt (1662), Farr, Snow (both mid-1800's), and others, the discipline did not blossom until the end of the Second World War. Hippocrates (Circa 400 BC) attempted to explain disease occurrence from a rational instead of a supernatural viewpoint. In his essay entitled 'On Airs, Waters, and Places,' Hippocrates suggested that environmental and host factors such as behaviors might influence the development of disease. Another early contributor to epidemiology was John Graunt, a London haberdasher who published his landmark analysis of mortality data in 1662. He was the first to quantify patterns of birth, death, and disease occurrence, noting male-female disparities, high infant mortality, urban rural differences, and seasonal variations. No one built upon Grant's work until the mid-1800's.

When William Farr began to systematically collect and analyze Britain's mortality statistics, Farr considered the father of modern vital statistics and surveillance, developed many of the basic practices used today in vital statistics and disease classification. He extended the epidemiologic analysis of morbidity and mortality data, looking at the effects of marital status, occupation, and altitude. He also developed many epidemiologic concepts and techniques still in use today. Epidemiology is derived from the word epidemic. (epi - among, demos - people, logos - study). The foundation of morden epidemiology was laid in a 19th century when a few classic studies made a major contribution to the saving of life. In 1850, under the presidency of Earl of Shaft Esbury, an epidemiological society was made. In early 1920 Winslow and Sedgwick both lectured on epidemiology in United States. Although the subject was not given departmental status in 1927. WH Frost become the first professor of epidemiology in US. Later Major Greenwood become first professor of epidemiology and medical studies in the University of London. Epidemiology has grown rapidly during the first three decades. It has now become firmly established in medical education.

On analysis disease condition, there had been considerable reduction in the morbidity and mortality from these diseases, as a result of epidemiological studies and improved methods of diagnosis prevention and control. But still due to poor socioeconomic conditions, ignorance poor health practices and inadequate resources the epidemic is continued. While many communicable diseases continue to be a serious problems of community health, many new problems have emerged in the 20th century. These problems include cardiovascular diseases, mental health problems, cancer, accidents, immunodeficiency diseases and many other problems related to lifestyle, environment, advance technology and stress. These noncommunicable diseases are due to changing environment or ecosystem. Currently the focus of epidemiologists are not only limited to the infectious diseases but also on these new emergent problems. It is expected to have many more new problems and hazards related to computer technology, electric appliances, space travel and increased leisure time and sedentary life, etc. The review of historical traced back to Hippocrates (460-547 BC) who tried to explain the association of lifestyle and environmental factors with the occurrence of diseases. However, the foundation of modern epidemiology was laid down on late 20th century when infectious and communicable diseases like cholera, typhoid, plague, etc., were most prevalent in the world in the form of epidemic and pandemics. Other communicable diseases which were the major concerns of epidemiologists and public health personnel include small pox, TB poliomyelitis, measles, STDs. Epidemiology became a distinct branch of medical science and it flourished as a result of study and control of these communicable infectious diseases. Thus during late 19th century and early 20th century, the primary focus of epidemiologists was to study the prevalence, prevention and control of various infectious and communicable diseases.

Significant Mile Stones in the History of Epidemiology

- **1662 (John Graun):** Used bills of mortality to study patterns of death in various populations in England. Published early form of life table analysis
- **1747 (James Lind):** Study of scurvy using observation and comparison of response to various dietary treatments. Early precursor of clinical trial
- **1760 (Daniel Bernoulli):** Used life table technique to demonstrate that small pox inoculation conferred life long immunity
- **1775 (Percival Pott):** First cancer epidemiologist noted high proportion of patients presenting with cancer of scrotum were chimney sweep
- **1798 (Edward Jenner):** Demonstrated effectiveness of small pox vaccination
- **1798 (Marrie Hospital service):** Fore runner of US Public health services (1912)
- **1836 (Pierre Charles—Alexander Louis):** Comparative observational studies to demonstrate ineffectiveness of bloodletting emphasized the importance of statistical method
- **1840 (William Farr):** Developed for runner of middle vital records system in regular general's office
- **1850 (Lemuel Shattuck):** Report on sanitation and public health in Massachusetts
- **1850 (John Snow):** Epidemiologic research on transmission of cholera
- **1870–1880:** Discovery of casual agents for anthrax, TB and cholera
- **1887 (Joseph Kinyion):** Founded laboratory of hygiene, fore runner of the national institute of health
- **1921 (Wade Hampton Frost):** Founded first US academic program in epidemiology at Johns Hipkins

In fact epidemiology includes the study of all those conditions which affect the health of the people.

METHODS OF EPIDEMIOLOGICAL INVESTIGATION

The epidemiologist and community health workers are interested in the study of health status of the population by which they identifies morbidity and mortality patterns, determines the factors affecting health and disease and utilizes this information in planning to provide need-based health care. The epidemiological investigation requires:

- Systematic collection of data
- Analysis of data
- Description of health needs and problems
- Identification of factors associated with problems and stating the hypothesis which are further explored and tested.

The epidemiologist try to relate the cases to define population and search for the causes of disease and mode of transmission affects the prevention and control and eradication. The methods of epidemiological investigations are:

- Observational method
- Experimental method

The observational method is classified as:

- Descriptive methods
- Analytical methods

Analytical method again classified as:

a. Ecological or correlational study
b. Case-control study
c. Cohort study

Observational Method

In observational studies, the researcher observes and systematically collects information, but does not try to change the people (or animals, or reagents) being observed. In an experiment, by contrast, the researcher intervenes to change something (e.g., gives some patients a drug) and then observes what happens. In an observational study there is no intervention. Here researchers observe the effect of a risk factor, diagnostic test or treatment without trying to influence what happens. Such studies are usually 'retrospective'—the data are based on events that have already happened. Most workplace health research falls into this category.

Examples of Observational Studies

- A survey of drinking habits among students;
- A researcher who joins a biker gang to study their lifestyle (note, as long as the researcher does not try to change their behavior, it is an observational study); taking blood samples to measure blood alcohol levels during to take the blood, but you are not trying to change the blood alcohol level: it is just a measurement (In all epidemiological studies, the disease should be investigated and defined properly. It is very difficult to experience in interpreting the data without clear experience of disease and exposure).

Descriptive Methods

It is the first phase of epidemiological investigation. Descriptive epidemiology deals with the distribution of health-related states and events by time, place and person. The data is collected about the personal characteristics such as age, sex, marital status, occupation, education, income, dietary pattern, etc. Descriptive epidemiology provides a way of organizing and analyzing the data in order to understand variations in disease frequency geographically and over time, and how disease (or health) varies among people based on a host of personal characteristics (person, place, and time). This makes it possible to identify trends in health and disease and also provides a means of planning resources for populations.

It is the study of magnitude and distribution of disease or health status within a population by person, place and time.

- **Time distribution:** When is the disease occurring?
- **Place distribution:** Where is it occurring?
- **Person distribution:** Who is getting disease?

Purpose

- To provide a statistical overview of community health problems and gives clues about the etiological factors
- To provide information about diseases, i.e., incidence, prevalence and mortality rate, etc. by age, sex, occupation, social class
- For planning, organizing and implementation of health care services to deal with these problems.

Steps of Descriptive Epidemiology

- Defining the population to be studied
- Defining the disease under study
- Describing the disease by:
  - Time
  - Place
  - Person
- Measurement of disease
- Comparing with known indices
- Formulation of an etiological hypothesis.

- **Defining the population:** Descriptive studies are investigations of populations. It is based on population. The total number of population, age, sex, occupation, cultural characters and similar information needed for the study. The population needs to be large and stable.
- **Defining the disease under study:** The disease or condition being investigated must be defined. This is to obtain an accurate estimate of disease in a population. The disease will be defined operationally and it will different from their actual definition. For example, Defining TB means the patient should have sputum positive.
- **Describing the disease:** The primary objective of descriptive epidemiology deals with the distribution of health-related states and events by time, place and person.

Distribution by Time

The disease pattern may be described by the time of its occurrence, i.e., by week, month, year, the day of the week, hour of onset, etc. It raised questions whether the disease is seasonal in occurrence, whether it shows periodic increase or decrease, whether it follows a consistent time trend. Disease rates change over time. Some of these changes occur regularly and can be predicted. For example, the seasonal increase of influenza cases with the onset of cold weather is a pattern that is familiar to everyone. By knowing when flu outbreaks will occur, health departments can time their flu shot campaigns effectively. Other disease rates make unpredictable changes. By examining events that precede a disease rate increase or decrease, we may identify causes and appropriate actions to control or prevent further occurrence of the disease.

- Short-term fluctuations or epidemic trends
- Periodic fluctuations or seasonal trends
- Long-term fluctuation or secular trends.

Short-term Fluctuation or Epidemic Trends

The epidemic is defined as 'the occurrence of disease in a community or any region of community. The cases or an illness or other health-related events clearly in excess than the normal expectancy'. The occurrence of disease can last for a short period of time. It can classified as:

I. **Common source epidemics:** When a common source is responsible for spreading any diseases rapidly we can consider as Common source epidemics. The disease can occurred by single source through single exposure or repeated exposure.
   a. *Single exposure or point source epidemics:* The exposure to the disease agent is brief and essentially simultaneous. All develop within one incubation period of disease, for example an epidemic of food poisoning. The epidemic tends to be explosive within a narrow interval of time. All the cases develop within one incubation period of disease. They can result from contamination of the environment (air, water, food, soil) by industrial chemicals or pollutants, for example, Bhopal Gas Tragedy in India.
   b. *Continuous or repeated exposure:* Sometimes the exposure form the same source may be prolonged. The people repeatedly exposing to same source repeatedly,

a prostitute may be a common source in gonorrhea outbreak or the people who are using the same water from pond repeatedly suffered from water-borne diseases.

II. **Propagated epidemics:** A propagated epidemic is of infectious origin and results from person to person transmission of an infectious agent, i.e., epidemics of hepatitis A and polio. Propagated epidemics are more likely to occur where large numbers of susceptible are aggregated.
   a. Person to person
   b. Arthropod vector
   c. Animal reservoir

Periodic Fluctuations or Seasonal Trends

The occurrence of disease for a particular period of time.

Seasonal Trend

Seasonal variation is a well known characteristic of many communicable diseases like measles, varicella, and malaria, etc. Measles is usually at its height in early spring, gastrointestinal infections are prominent in summer month. By graphing the occurrence of a disease by week or month over the course of a year or more, we can show its seasonal pattern, if any. Some diseases are known to have characteristic seasonal distributions; for example, as mentioned earlier, the number of reported cases of influenza typically increases in winter. Seasonal patterns may suggest hypotheses about how the infection is transmitted, what behavioral factors increase risk, and other possible contributors to the disease or condition.

Long-term Fluctuation (Secular Trends)

Secular trends are continuous long-term changes in the frequency of diseases occurring over many years or decades. The secular trend describes the occurrence of disease over a prolonged period, usually years; it is influenced by the degree of immunity in the population and possibly nonspecific measures such as improved socioeconomic and nutritional levels among the population. For example, the secular trend of tetanus in the United States since 1920 shows a gradual and steady decline. The trends may be upward or downward, apparent or real. An apparent upward trend may be due to increased disease awareness improved diagnostic and treatment facilities, and improved recording and reporting of cases. A real downward secular trend may be caused by a favorable change in the epidemiological behavior of a disease. Among noncommunicable diseases, diabetes and heart diseases are upward secular trend. By graphing the occurrence of a disease by week or month over the course of a year or more, we can show its pattern, if any.

Distribution by Place

Studies of the geography of disease is one of the important dimensions of descriptive epidemiology factors that govern the distribution of diseases on this planet are extremely varied such as longitude, temperature, humidity, rainfall, soil, water, air, lifestyle, occupation, urbanization. Depending on their individual requirements, diseases show considerable variability in their geographic distribution. Distribution of diseases may be described as global, regional, national or local. It may examine mortality and morbidity in relation to socioeconomic factors, dietary differences and the differences in culture and behavior.

Global Distribution

Descriptive studies by place have shown that the pattern of disease is not the same everywhere. Global distribution of diseases reflects interesting pattern of endemicity. Malaria and leprosy which are tropical diseases requiring hot and humid climate, are prevalent in South East Asia, Africa and South and Central America. Filarial and hookworm diseases show specific distribution patterns.

National Distribution

National distribution relates to distribution within countries or national boundaries. In a vast country like India, a study of distribution of diseases is not without epidemiological curiosity. Inhabited by a huge population compressing of a variety of religious, cultural, linguistic and ethnic groups. India is an ethnic home to a host of tropical, subtropical and cosmopolitan diseases. For example, the distribution of endemic goiter, leprosy, malaria, nutritional deficiency diseases have all shown variations in their distribution in India. Some parts of country are more affected and some are less affected. The descriptive epidemiology provide data regarding the type of disease problems and their incidence, prevalence and mortality rates. These informations are needed to demarcate the affected areas and for providing appropriate health care service.

Regional Distribution

It is a comparative study of distribution of diseases within climatically homogenous regions of the world. It provides important clues of epidemiological interest. The data base of the six regional organizations of WHO facilitates such comparisons. The most leading types are oropharyngeal cancer in India, cervical cancer in Sri Lanka, breast cancer in Indonesia, and stomach cancer in Mongolia. Rural or urban variations in disease distribution are well known. Chronic bronchitis, accidents, lung cancer, cardiovascular disease, mental illness and drug dependence are usually more frequent in urban than rural areas. Skin and soil transmitted helminths may be more frequent in rural areas. The epidemiologist provides guidelines for disease prevention and control.

Local Distribution

Inner and outer city variations in disease frequency are well known. These are best studied with the aid of spot maps or shaded maps. These maps show at a glance areas of high or low frequency the boundaries and patterns of disease distribution. If there is clustering of cases in an area, it is an indication for further epidemiological enquiry.

Distribution by Person

Diseases are not spread uniformly in human populations. The nature and frequency of diseases is also influenced by host characteristics such as age, sex, occupation, marriage, residence, sociocultural and socioeconomic background, stress migration.

Age

Age is strongly related to disease than any other single host factor. Certain diseases are more frequent in certain age groups like measles in childhood, cancer in middle age and atherosclerosis in old age. Age is associated with maturity of organ systems, efficiency of defense mechanisms and the state of health. Age also influences the attitude of individuals towards personal and community health.

Sex

Sex is a biological reality. It is an important personal attribute, responsible for dissimilar anatomical, physiological and psychological profiles of two gender groups. Disease like thyrotoxicosis, cholecysititis, diabetes, obesity, arthritis, psychoneuroses are more frequent in women while diseases like peptic ulcer, cancer lung, coronary heart disease and various kinds of accident more common in men. Female group shares a greater burden of morbidity associated with pregnancy and childbirth during the reproductive age period.

Occupation

Occupation may alter the habit pattern of employees, i.e., sleep, alcohol, smoking, drug addiction, etc. Distribution of diseases is also influenced by the principal occupation of people. While agriculture is main occupation the diseases like allergic reaction, worm infestation, are more frequent. In industrial towns, cities people suffer from diseases due to hazards of physical and chemical exposures, e.g., coal mines, silicosis sedentary occupation, heart diseases.

Marriage

Marriage is known to promote health and security of individuals. It influences their health habits and lifestyle. Disruption of marriage due to death, separation or divorce has adverse effect on health of spouses. The married people have lowest mortality, the widowed, separated and divorced have the highest mortality rates. Cancer cervix may be associated with multiple sexual contact.

Residence

Residence determines the nature of environment. The infection, infestations, deficiency and zoonotic diseases are common among rural folk, chronic bronchitis, cancer lung, coronary heart disease more frequent among city dwellers.

Sociocultural Milieu

Sociocultural milieu of individual determines their habits, customs, practices, beliefs which influence their health.

Economic Background

Poor class suffers from diseases of poverty associated with hostile environment, inadequate nutrition substandard housing, the rich class suffers from diseases of affluence associated with over nutrition, sedentary occupation and stressful environment.

Measurement of Disease

The disease can be measured by the tools of epidemiology, i.e., Rate ratio and proportions. Rate may be expressed in terms of mortality, morbidity, disability and so on. Descriptive epidemiology may use a cross sectional or longitudinal design to obtain estimates of magnitude of health and disease. Problems in human population. Morbidity has two aspects, i.e., incidence and prevalence. Incidence can be obtained from longitudinal studies and prevalence from cross sectional studies. Cross sectional studies based on a single examination of a cross section of population at one point in time. The results of the study are applied on the whole population. The cross section of the population is sampled carefully, so that it is representative of the whole population. It is also called as prevalence study. Cross sectional studies are useful for detailed community assessment, study of morbidity and underlying factors especially chronic diseases, for example study of diabetes or hypertension by personal characteristics and lifestyle. These studies are economical and comparatively quick to perform.

Comparing with Known Indices

Asking questions and making comparison are the two approaches of epidemiology. We can compare the epidemiological data with the data obtained other known indices like the global data, national data, etc. By making comparisons between different populations, it is possible to find out the disease etiology. By this we can define groups who are at risk.

Formulation of Hypothesis

As per the distribution of disease, utilizing the techniques of descriptive epidemiology, it is possible to formulate hypothesis relating to disease etiology. For example the smoking of 30–40 cigarettes per day causes lung cancer in 10% of smokers after 20 years of exposure.

Analytical Studies

In this second type of observational study, analysis is made to study the relationship between disease or other condition with different variables. There are various subtypes of analytical study.

Ecological or Correlational Study

Groups of population of different countries or geographical areas with different characteristics and values of variables are compared with reference to the frequency of occurrence of a disease associated with differing values of a variable may point towards association and possible cause and effect relationship.

Advantages

- Data collected for some other purpose is readily available for use

- Can carried out without much cost or effort of data collection provide some indication
- It helps in initiation of depth studies
- It may be used to find out marked differences in frequencies of different disease.

Disadvantages

- Interpretation of results difficult as the data on other possible factors influencing occurrence may not be available
- Remain unsettled and the inference inconclusive
- Cause and effect relationship may be suspected but not proved
- Associations of levels of population may not be valid at individual levels.

Case-control Study

A case-control study is a type of study design used widely, originally developed in epidemiology. Although its use has also been advocated for the social sciences. It is a type of observational study in which two existing groups differing in outcome are identified and compared on the basis of some supposed causal attribute. Case-control studies are often used to identify factors that may contribute to a medical condition by comparing subjects who have that condition/disease (the 'cases') with patients who do not have the condition/disease but are otherwise similar the 'controls'. The case-control is a type of epidemiological observational study. An observational study is a study in which subjects are not randomized to the exposed or unexposed groups, rather the subjects are observed in order to determine both their exposure and their outcome status and the exposure status is thus not determined by the researcher.

This type of study known a case reference or retrospective study. It is often used to investigate cause of a disease, if the disease occurs rather infrequently. It starts with cases, i.e., persons who are not suffering from the disease, but would have been included in the study, if they were suffering, are investigated. In case-control study:

- The frequency of occurrence of the possible cause is compared in two groups of persons
- Differences in these two groups suggest association and causation
- These are longitudinal as compared to cross sectional.
- Called retrospective because the investigation goes back into the past of those persons who have developed the disease and compares with the past of the control
- Can be organized in a short time are economical and give results quickly
- They are inexpensive because the starting point is persons who have developed the disease
- Only a small number of person are required.

The case-control approach has emerged as a permanent method of epidemiological investigation case-control method has three distinct features.

1. Both exposure and outcome (disease) have occurred before the start of the study
2. The study proceeds backwards from effect to cause
3. It uses a control or comparison group to support of refute an inference.

Case-control study involves two populations' cases and control. The unit is the individual rather than the group, which focus on a disease or some other health problem that has already developed. Cases and controls must be comparable with respect to known 'confounding factors' such as age, sex, occupation, social status. For example, one can use as 'cases' the immunized children and look for factors of interest in their past histories. Case-control studies have been used for studies of many concerns and other serious conditions such cirrhosis of the liver, lupus erythematosis and congestive cardiac failure.

Steps of Case-control Study

There are four basic steps in conducting a case-control study which are as follows:

1. Selection of cases and controls
2. Matching
3. Measurement of exposure
4. Analysis and interpretation.

Selection of Cases and Controls

Identification of cases is easy, selection of suitable controls may present difficulties.

Selection of cases: A 'case' is crucial to the case-control study. It involves two specification such as (1) Diagnostic criteria and (2) Eligibility criteria.

Diagnostic criteria: The diagnostic criteria of the disease is based on the stage of disease or some characteristics or sign and symptoms of the disease. The criteria to be included in the study must be specified before the study is undertaken. Once the diagnostic criteria are established, they should not be altered or changed till the study is over.

Eligibility criteria: This is second criterion of eligibility. A criterion customarily employed is the requirement that only newly diagnosed cases within a specified period of time are eligible than old cases or cases in advanced stages of the disease.

Sources of cases: May drawn from hospitals or general population.

Hospitals: To select cases from hospitals, cases may be drawn from a single hospital or a network of hospitals admitted during a specified period of time.

General population: In a population based case-control study disease occurring within a defined geographic area during a specified period of time. The entire case series or a random sample of it is selected for study.

Control Group Selection

The controls must be free from the disease under study. They must be similar to the cases as possible, except for the absence of the disease under study. But need not be in good health; inclusion of sick people is sometimes appropriate, as the control group should represent those at risk of becoming a case. Controls should come from the same population as the cases, and their selection should be independent of the exposures of interest.

Controls can carry the same disease as the experimental group, but of another grade/severity, therefore being different from the outcome of interest. However, because the difference between the cases and the controls will be smaller, this results in a lower power to detect an exposure effect.

As with any epidemiological study, greater numbers in the study will increase the power of the study. Numbers of cases and controls do not have to be equal. In many situations, it is much easier to recruit controls than to find cases. Increasing the number of controls above the number of cases, up to a ratio of about 4 to 1, may be a cost-effective way to improve the study.

Difficulties may arise in the selection of controls if the disease under investigation occurs in sub-clinical forms, whose diagnosis is difficult. Selection of an appropriate control group is therefore an important prerequisite, we make comparisons draw inferences and make judgments.

Sources of controls includes:

- **Hospital controls:** The controls may be selected from the same hospital but with different illnesses other than the study disease. For example, if we are going to study cancer cervix patients, the control group may comprise patients with cancer breast, cancer of the digestive tract or patient with non-cancerous lesion and other patients. Many hospital patients may have diseases which are also influenced by the factor under study. For example, if one was studying the relationship of smoking and myocardial infarction and chooses bladder cancer cases as controls, the relationship between smoking and myocardial infarction may not have been demonstrated.
- **Relatives:** Controls may taken up from relatives. Siblings controls are unsuitable where genetic conditions are under study
- **Neighborhood controls:** The controls may be drawn from persons living in the same locality as cases, persons working in the same factory or children attending the same school
- **General population:** Population controls can be obtained from defined geographic areas by taking random sample of individuals free of the study disease.

Matching

Controls may differ from the cases in a number of factors such as age, sex, occupation, social status. Matching defined as the process by which we select controls in such a way that they are similar to cases with regard to certain pertinent selected variables which are known to influence the outcome of the disease. A confounding factor defined as one which is associated both with exposure and disease and is distributed unequally in study and control groups. A confounding factor is one that although associated with exposure under investigation, independently of any such association, a risk factor for the disease.

The study of the role of alcohol in the etiology of esophageal cancer, smoking is a confounding factor because:

- It is associated with the consumption of alcohol.
- It is an independent risk factor for esophageal cancer.

The effects of alcohol consumption can be determined only if the influence of smoking is neutralized by matching.

Age could be a confounding variable. We are investigating the relationship between steroid contraceptive and breast cancer.

If the women taking these contraceptives were younger than those in the comparison group, they would necessarily be at lower risk of breast cancer since this disease becomes increasingly common with increasing age. Matching protects against on unexpected strong association between the matching factor the disease is breast cancer.

Measurement of Exposure

Are important as those used to define cases and controls? Information about exposure should be obtained in the same manner both for cases and controls. This may be obtained by interviews, by questionnaires or by studying past records of cases such as hospital records, employment records.

Analysis

The final step is analysis to find out:

- Exposure rates among cases and controls to suspected factor.
- Estimation of disease risk associated with exposure.

Exposure rates: The exposure rates can be calculated among cases and controls. Example can be taken in a case study to identify the factors associated with tuberculosis.

Exposure	*Cases (with TB)*	*Control (without TB)*
Living in slum dwelling (overcrowded area)	30 (a)	70 (b)
Not overcrowded rural area	5 (c)	95 (d)
Total	(a + c)	(b + d)

$$\text{Exposure rate among cases} = \frac{a}{(a+c)} \times 100 = \frac{30}{35} \times 100 = 86\%$$

$$\text{Exposure rate among control} = \frac{b}{(b+d)} \times 100 = \frac{70}{165} \times 100 = 42\%$$

From the above analysis, it has been observed that the frequency of TB is higher among slum dweller.

Relative risk:

$$\text{Incidences among exposed} = \frac{a}{a+b}$$

$$\text{Incidences among nonexposed} = \frac{c}{c+d}$$

A typical case-control study does not provide a direct estimation of the incidence rate because there is no appropriate denominator or population at risk.

Odd ratio: From a case-control study odd ratio can be derived which is the measure of the strength of the association between risk factors and outcome.

Formula for odd ratio is:

$$\frac{ad}{bc} = \frac{2850}{350} = 8.14$$

In the above example the slum dwellers are 8.1 risk of TB then normal rural population.

Estimation of risk: Estimation of disease risk associated with exposure is obtained by an index known as relative risk or risk ratio which is defined as the ratio between the incidence of disease among exposed persons and incidence among nonexposed.

Advantages of Case-control Study

- Relatively easy to carry out
- Rapid and inexpensive
- Require comparatively few subjects
- Particularly suitable to investigate rare diseases or diseases about which little is known. A disease which is rare in the general population such as leukemia in adolescents may not be rare in the general population.
- No risk to subjects
- Allow the study of several different etiological factor such as smoking, physical activity and personality characteristics in myocardial infarction
- Risk factors can be identified. Rational prevention and control programs can be established
- No attrition problems because case-control studies do not require follow up of individuals into the future
- Ethical problems minimal.

Disadvantages

- Problems of bias e.g., relies on memory or past records, the accuracy of which may be uncertain, validation of information obtained is difficult or sometimes impossible
- Selection of an appropriate control group may be difficult
- We cannot measure incidence and can only estimate the relative risk
- Do not distinguish between causes and associated factors
- Not suited to the evaluation of therapy or prophylaxis of disease
- Another major concern is the representatives of cases and controls, e.g., oral contraceptives and thromboembolic disease who had been admitted to hospitals with venous thrombosis or pulmonary embolism without medical cause and compared the history with that obtained from other women who had been admitted to the same hospital with other diseases who were matched for age, marital status and parity.

Cohort Study

A cohort is a group of people who share a common characteristic or experience within a defined period (e.g., A group of individuals are born, are exposed to a drug or vaccine or pollutant, or undergo a certain medical procedure or a group of people who were born on a day or in a particular period, say 1948, form a birth cohort. Hence, it is clear that the group of individuals sharing some common characteristic is kept under observation prospectively is called cohort study. The cohort must consist of individuals who are not affected by the disease or condition under study. Some of the individuals will have the characteristics which is suspected to be associated with that disease or condition while some individuals will be free of that conditions. Cohort of the individual is then observed and followed up to detect the occurrence of the disease under study. The size depend upon the frequency with which the disease occur. If the disease occur in frequent, a very large sized cohort will have to be kept under observation. For research purposes, a cohort is any group of people who are linked in some way and followed over time. Researchers observe what happens to one group that has been exposed to a particular variable—for example, the effect of company downsizing on the health of office workers. This group is then compared to a similar group that has not been exposed to the variable.

The difference in the incidence rates of the specific disease among those who have or do not have a particular characteristic provides evidence of association. Cohort study is known by a variety of names such as:

- Prospective study
- Longitudinal study
- Incidence study
- Forward looking study

Features of Cohort Studies

- Cohorts are identified prior to the appearance of the disease under investigation
- The study groups so defined are observed over a period of time to determine the frequency of disease among them
- The study proceeds forward from cause to effect.

Types of Cohort Studies

Three types of cohort studies have been observed on the basis of the time of occurrence of disease.

1. Prospective cohort studies
2. Retrospective cohort studies
3. A combination of retrospective and prospective cohort studies.

Prospective Cohort Studies

A prospective cohort study is one in which the outcome has not yet occurred at the time of investigation, e.g., long-term effects of exposure to uranium was evaluated by identifying a group of uranium miner and a comparison group of individuals not exposed to uranium mining and by assessing subsequent deviation of lung cancer in both the groups. The advantage of prospective cohort study data is that it can help determine risk factors for contracting a new disease because it is a longitudinal observation of the individual through time, and the collection of data at regular intervals, so recall error is reduced. However, cohort studies are expensive to conduct, are sensitive to attrition and take a long follow-up time to generate useful data. Nevertheless, the results that are obtained from long-term cohort studies are of substantially superior quality to those obtained from retrospective/cross-sectional studies. Prospective cohort studies are considered to yield the most reliable results in observational epidemiology. They enable a wide range of exposure-disease associations to be studied.

Retrospective Cohort Studies

A retrospective cohort study, also called a historic cohort study, generally means to take a look back at events that already have taken place. For example, the term is used in medicine, describing a look back at a patient's medical history or lifestyle. This type of study is known by a variety of names. Retrospective cohort study, historical cohort study, prospective study in retrospect and nonconcurrent prospective study. Retrospective cohort studies are generally more economical and produce results more quickly than prospective cohort study. In a historical cohort study the data concerning exposure and occurrence of a disease, births, a political attitude or any other categorical variable are collected after the events have taken place, and the subjects (those exposed and unexposed to the agent under study) are assembled from existing records or health care registers. A 'prospective cohort' defines the groups before the study is done, while historical studies, which are sometimes referred to as 'retrospective cohort', defines the grouping after the data is collected. It is a medical research study in which the medical records of groups of individuals who are alike in many ways but differ by a certain characteristic (for example, female nurses who smoke and those who do not smoke) are compared for a particular outcome (such as lung cancer). In retrospective cohort studies, a risk ratio or odds ratio gives an assessment of relative risk.

In the case of a retrospective cohort study, the investigator collects data from past records and does not follow patients up as is the case with a prospective study. However, the starting point of this study is the same as for all cohort studies. The first objective is still to establish two groups—exposed versus non-exposed; and these groups are followed up in the ensuing time period.

In a nutshell, in Retrospective Cohort Study, all the events—exposure, latent period, and subsequent outcome (e.g., development of disease) have already occurred in the past. We merely collect the data now, and establish the risk of developing a disease if exposed to a particular risk factor. On the other hand, Prospective Cohort Study is conducted by starting with two groups at the current point, and following up in future for occurrence of disease, if any.

Combination of Retrospective and Prospective Cohort Studies

Cohort is identified from past records and is assessed of date for the outcome. The somewhat is followed up prospectively into future for further assessment of outcome. The investigator collects data from past records and follow patients up as is the case with a prospective study. The starting point of this study is the same as for all cohort studies. The first objective is still to establish two groups—exposed versus nonexposed; and the back history of the two groups elements of prospective and retrospective cohort are combined.

- The Cohort is identified from past records and assesses of date for the outcome. The same cohort is the followed up prospectively into future for the further assessment of outcome example of Ambidirectional cohort study
- Curt-Brown and Dolls study on effects of radiation began in 1955 with 13,352 patients who received large dose of radiation therapy for ankylosing spondylitis between 1934 to 1954
- Outcome evaluated was death from Leukemia or aplastic anemia between 1934 to 1954
- A prospective component was added up in 1955 and surviving subjects were followed up to identify deaths in subsequent years.

Elements of a Cohort Study

- Selection of study subjects
- Obtaining data on exposure
- Selection of comparison groups
- Follow-up
- Analysis

Selection of Study Subjects

Study subjects are usually assembled in one of two ways:

1. General population
2. Select groups of the population. **For example,** persons with different degrees of exposure to the suspected casual factor.

General Population

When the exposure or cause of death is fairly frequent in population, cohorts may be assembled from the general population residing in well defined geographical, political and administrative areas. The exposed and unexposed segments of the population to be studied should be representative of the corresponding segments of the general population.

Select Groups

These may be special groups or exposure groups:

- **Special groups:** These may be professional groups, e.g., doctors, nurses, lawyers, teachers, civil servants, insured persons, obstetric population, college alumni, government employees, volunteers, etc.
- **Exposure groups:** If the exposure is rare, a more economical procedure is to select a cohort of persons known to have experienced the exposure. Cohorts may be selected because of special exposure to physical, chemical and other disease agents.

Obtaining Data on Exposure

Cohort members through personal interviews, e.g., collect smoking histories, reviewing past records certain kinds of information, e.g., dose of radiation, kinds of surgery or details of medical treatment can be obtained only from medical records, medical examination or special tests like blood pressure, serum cholesterol, ECG and by environmental surveys which is the best source for obtaining information on exposure levels of the suspected factor in the environment where the cohort lived or worked.

Selection of Comparison Groups

- **Internal comparisons:** Internal comparisons means the selection of comparison can be obtained from the same exposure group but the level exposure will be vary. In a single cohort study, the selection of its members may on the basis of information obtained according to the degrees or levels of exposure to risk before the development of the disease in question.
- **External comparisons:** When information on degree of exposure is not available it is necessary to put up an external control, to evaluate the experience of the exposed group with nonexposed group, e.g., smokers and nonsmokers. A cohort of radiologists compared with a cohort of ophthalmologists. The study and control cohorts should be similar in demographic data **(Table 3.1)**.

Comparison with General Population

If none is available, the mortality experience + of the exposed group is compared with the mortality experience of the general population in the same geographical area as the exposed people. For example, comparison of frequency of lung cancer among uranium mine workers with lung cancer in the general population where the miners resided or the comparison of frequency of cancer among asbestos workers with the rate in general population in the same geographic area.

Follow-up

At the start of the study, methods should be devised depending upon the outcome to be determined to obtain data for assessing the outcome. The procedures required:

- Periodic medical examination of each member of the cohort
- Reviewing physician and hospital records
- Routine surveillance of death records
- Mailed questionnaires, telephone calls, periodic home visits.

Analysis

Data are analyzed in terms of:

- Incidence rates of outcome among exposed and nonexposed
- Estimation of risk.

Table 3.1: Association of smoking with lung cancer.

Smoking	*Lung cancer*		*Total*
	Yes	No	
Yes	70	6930	7000
No	3	2997	3000
	73	9927	10000

Incidence Rates of Outcome

Incidence among exposed = a/a + b

Incidence among nonexposed = c/c + d

Relative Risk

$$RR = \frac{\text{Incidence of disease among exposed}}{\text{Incidence of disease among nonexposed}} = \frac{a/a+b}{c/c+d}$$

Attributable Risk

Attributable risk (AR) is the risk difference between exposed and unexposed groups. From above analysis it is clear that attribute risk is the [Risk (exposed) – Risk (unexposed)] = [A/(A+B)] – [C/(C+D)]. It is the quantity of disease that one could hope to avoid by removal of the risk factor in question. Thus, attributable risk is sometimes called the Risk Difference, or Excess Risk. The excess risk is "attributed" to the exposure. Attributable risk (AR) is often described as percentage

$$AR = \frac{\text{Incidence of disease among exposed} - \text{Incidence of disease among nonexposed} \times 100}{\text{Incidence of disease among exposed}}$$

$$AR = \frac{\frac{a}{a+b} - \frac{c}{c+d}}{\frac{a}{a+b}} \times 100$$

Find out RR and AR for above data

- Incidence of lung cancer among smokers
  70/7000 = 10 per 1000
- Incidence of lung cancer among nonsmokers
  3/3000 = 1 per thousand
  RR = 10/1 = 10
  (Lung cancer is 10 times more common among smokers than nonsmokers)

AR = 10 – 1/10 × 100 = 90%

(90% of the cases of lung cancer among smokers are attributed to their habit of smoking).

Among smokers – 70/7000 = 10/100

Among nonsmokers – 3/3000 = 1/1000

Advantages

- Incidence can be calculated
- Several possible outcomes related to exposure can be studied simultaneously, e.g., cohort studies designed to study the association between smoking and lung cancer showed association of smoking with coronary heart disease, peptic ulcer
- Cohort studies provide a direct estimate of relative risk
- Dose response ratios can also be calculated
- Comparison groups are formed before disease develops certain forms of bias can be minimized like misclassification of individuals into exposed and unexposed groups.

Disadvantages

- It involves a large number of people. They are unsuitable for investigating uncommon diseases or diseases with low incidence in the population

Table 3.2: Difference between case-control and cohort study.

Case-control study	*Cohort study*
Proceeds from effect to cause	Proceeds from cause to effect
Starts with the disease	Starts with people exposed to risk factor or suspected cause
Tests whether the suspected cause occurs more frequently in those with the disease than among those without the disease	Tests whether disease occurs more frequently in those exposed than in those not similarly exposed
The first approach to the testing of a hypothesis	Reserved for testing of precisely formulated hypothesis
Involves fewer number of subjects	Involves larger number of subjects
Yields relatively quick results	Long follow up period often needed involving delayed results
Suitable for the study of rare disease	Inappropriate when the disease or exposure under investigation is rare
Cannot yield information about diseases other than that selected for study	Can yield information about more than one disease outcome
Relatively inexpensive	Expensive

- It takes a long time to complete the study and obtain results or more in cancer by which time the investigators may have died or the participants may have changed their classification
- It is difficult to keep a large number of individuals under medical surveillance indefinitely
- Lack of experienced staff, loss of funding and extensive recordkeeping are inevitable
- It is not unusual to lose a substantial proportion of the original abort they may migrate, lose interest in the study or simply refuse to provide any required information
- Selection of comparison groups is difficult which are exposed and unexposed segments of the population
- Changes in the standard methods or diagnostic criteria of the disease
- Cohort studies are expensive.
- The study itself may alter people's behavior
- With any cohort study we are faced with ethical problems of varying importance. **Table 3.2** depicts the difference between case-control and cohort study.
- In a cohort study practical considerations dictate that we must concentrate on a limited number of factors possible related to disease outcome.

Experimental Epidemiology

A study in which a population is selected for a planned trial of a regimen, whose effects are measured by comparing the outcome of the regimen in the experimental group versus the outcome of another regimen in the control group. Such designs are differentiated from observational designs by the fact that there is manipulation of the study factor (exposure), and randomization (random allocation) of subjects to treatment (exposure) groups. Here researchers observe the effect of a risk factor, diagnostic test or treatment without trying to influence what happens. Experimental studies is same as Cohort Studies but it is under the direct control of the investigator. It involves some action or interventions. Investigator intentionally alters one or more factors under controlled conditions to study the effects of doing so. The usual formal epidemiological experiment is the randomized control trial, which is done to test a preventive or therapeutic regimen or diagnostic procedure (clinical trials).

Aims of Experimental Epidemiology

- To provide scientific proof of etiological factor which may permit modification or control of those diseases
- To provide a method of measuring the effectiveness and efficiency of services for the prevention, control and treatment of disease and improve the health of the community.

Advantages

- Provide stronger evidence of the effect (outcome) compared to observational designs, with maximum confidence and assurance
- Yield more valid results, as variation is minimized and bias controlled
- Determine whether experimental treatments are safe and effective under 'controlled environments' (as opposed to 'natural settings' in observational designs), especially when the margin of expected benefit is doubtful/narrow (10–30%)
- Only possible design for some research question (new drug)
- Can sometimes be faster and cheaper.

Disadvantages

- Costly in time and money
- Many research questions are not suitable: ethical barriers or outcome too rare
- Reduced generalizability (standardized interventions may be different than common practice)
- Tend to restrict the scope and narrow the study question.

Types of Experimental Studies

According to the selection of population the Experimental Studies can be classified as animal studies and human studies

Animal Studies

Animal Studies is an emerging field that builds on scholarship in the humanities, social sciences, and sciences to investigate past and present relations between human and nonhuman animals, the representation of those relations, their ethical implications and their social, political, and ecological effects in and on the world. It is a field of critical importance today as the complex 'Animal Studies', or 'Anthrozoology'. Contributions to this field draw upon a wide range of disciplinary formations: sociology, philosophy and history;

studies of literature, the visual arts, cinema and popular culture; bio-behavioral biology like anatomy, physiology, pathology, microbiology, genetic, etc., and other science, technology, and medicine studies.

The important application of animal studies are:

- Experimental reproduction of human disease to confirm etiological hypothesis and to study pathogenic phenomena or mechanisms
- Testing the efficacy of preventive and therapeutic measures such as vaccines, drugs and completing the natural history of disease. Example: Leprosy in armadillos.

Advantages

Despite claims by animal rights activists, it is undeniable that animal-based research has contributed to significant improvement in the length and quality of our lives. By this a lots of life shaving drugs can be prepared to treat the fatal disease. Animal study conducting process is also easy. Generally animals can be bred in lab and can be manipulated easily by the investigator. For experiments in genetics they can multiply rapidly.

Limitations

Not all human diseases can be reproduced in animals. Conclusions derived may not be applicable to humans always.

Human Experiments

Human subject research is a systematic investigation that can be either research or clinically oriented and involves the use of human subjects in any capacity. Systematic investigation incorporates both the collection and analysis of data in order to answer a specific question. Examples of clinically oriented investigation include analysis of biological, specimens, epidemiological and behavioral studies and medical chart review studies. Examples of research oriented investigation include surveys, questionnaires, interviews, and focus groups. In 18th–19th century human subject research experiments were recorded during vaccination trials in the 18th century as doctors struggled to find a preventive of smallpox.

In 20th century Walter Reed experimented on humans (including himself) to develop an inoculation for yellow fever; his work resulted in major advances in medicine. Similarly during World War II several nations conducted experiments on human subjects before and during the war, justifying it on grounds of war exigency.

Human beings have been participating in studies of malaria, syphilis, hepatitis, measles, polio and others but it should be on controlled observation. Thalidomide disaster highlights the unfortunate consequence of therapy on the basis of uncontrolled observations.

According to the types of study design the Experimental Studies are two types—randomized controlled trails, nonrandomized trials. Randomized controlled trails is a type of experimental design where the people being studied are randomly allocated. Randomized controlled trails can be classified as concurrent parallel study designs and crossover type of study designs. A cluster randomized controlled trial is a different type of randomized controlled trial in which groups of subjects (as opposed to individual subjects) are randomized. Cluster randomized controlled trials are also known as cluster randomized trials, group-randomized trials, and place-randomized trials similarly. Nonrandomized control studies can be classified as Uncontrolled Trials and Natural Experiments.

Randomized Controlled Trails

Random allocation means allocating them by chance (e.g., the toss of a coin). As long as you have relatively large groups (50 or more people in each), this means that the two study groups will end up equivalent (comparable) in terms of factors such as age, sex, and even other things that you do not even know about (such as their reaction to the medication).

Randomized controlled trial is a type of scientific (often medical) experiment, where the people being studied are randomly allocated one or other of the different treatments under study. The RCT is the gold standard for a clinical trial. RCTs are often used to test the efficacy or effectiveness of various types of medical intervention and may provide information about adverse effects, such as drug reactions. Random assignment of intervention is done after subjects have been assessed for eligibility and recruited, but before the intervention to be studied begins. To study the effects of a particular intervention, subjects in the study population are randomly allocated to intervention and control groups, and the results are assessed by comparing outcomes.

Study Designs

Concurrent Parallel

In concurrent parallel study designs comparison made two randomly assigned group one is exposed and other is not exposed. A parallel study is a type of clinical study where two groups of treatments, A and B, are given so that one group receives only A while another group receives only B. Other names for this type of study include 'between patient' and 'non-crossover'. The two treatment groups in a parallel study can either consist of two completely separate treatments (i.e., different drugs), or simply different doses of a common drug. One major aspect of a parallel study is randomization–this ensures that the results are accurate and have a lower risk of being biased. Control groups utilizing a placebo, or active control, are often used in this type of study. A parallel study would be more appropriate if any concerns about carryover effects were present. This type of study might also be more beneficial if the disease or disorder being studied has a likely chance of progression during the time in which the study takes place. One significant issue with parallel studies, though, is the concept of intrasubject variability, which is defined as variability in response occurring within the same patient.

Crossover Type of Study Designs

In Crossover type of study designs, study group received consider treatment and other is some alternative treatment. It is also referred to as a crossover study or crossover trial, is a longitudinal study in which subjects receive a sequence of different treatments (or exposures). While crossover studies can be observational studies, many important crossover studies are controlled experiments, which are discussed in this article. Crossover designs are common for experiments in many scientific disciplines, for example, psychology, education pharmaceutical science, and medicine.

Randomized, controlled crossover experiments are especially important in health care. In a randomized clinical trial, the subjects are randomly assigned to different arms of the study which receive different treatments. When the randomized clinical trial is a repeated measures design, the same measures are collected multiple times for each subject. A crossover clinical trial is a repeated measures design in which each patient is randomly assigned to a sequence of treatments, including at least two treatments (of which one 'treatment' may be a standard treatment or a placebo).

A cluster randomized controlled trial is a type of randomized controlled trial in which groups of subjects (as opposed to individual subjects) are randomized. Cluster randomized controlled trials are also known as cluster randomized trials, group-randomized trials, and place-randomized trials.

In statistics, a full factorial experiment is an experiment whose design consists of two or more factors, each with discrete possible values or 'levels', and whose experimental units take on all possible combinations of these levels across all such factors. A full factorial design may also be called a fully crossed design. Such an experiment allows the investigator to study the effect of each factor on the response variable, as well as the effects of interactions between factors on the response variable. For the vast majority of factorial experiments, each factor has only two levels. For example, with two factors each taking two levels, a factorial experiment would have four treatment combinations in total, and is usually called a 2 × 2 factorial design.

Randomized Control Studies

- **Uncontrolled Trials:** Trials without control groups
- **Natural Experiments:** Observation among smokers and nonsmokers for disease in them, e.g., lung cancer, Atomic bombing in Japan
- Before and after comparison study.

Steps of Randomized Control Studies

- Drawing up a strict protocol
- Selecting reference and experimental populations
- Randomization
- Manipulation or intervention
- Follow-up and assessment of outcome.

Drawing a Protocol

The term 'protocol' is defined as a complete written description of, and scientific rationale for, a research activity involving human subjects. In the context 'protocol' means both the written description of the research activity and the activity itself. It should specifies aims and objectives of the study, questions to be answered, criteria for the selection of cases and controls, treatments to be applied.

Selecting a Reference and Experimental Populations

- **Reference or target population:** Population to which findings of trial if found successful are expected to be applicable. The reference population may be as broad as mankind or geographically limited or limited to a specific age group, sex occupational group. Thus the reference population may be comprise of the population of a city or any specific group like mine workers depending on the nature of the study.
- **Experimental or study population:** The **experimental or study population is** randomly chosen from reference population so that both groups have same characteristics. The experimental population should be a stable population by which losses to follow-up can be avoided. The participant must be fulfil three criteria.

1. Informed consent must be obtained.
2. Study population must be the representative to reference population.
3. Should be eligible for the trial which means they must have the diagnostic criteria of diseases.

Randomization

Random allocation means allocating them by chance (e.g., the toss of a coin). As long as you have relatively large groups (50 or more people in each), this means that the two study groups will end up equivalent (comparable) in terms of factors such as age, sex, and even other things that you do not even know about (such as their reaction to the medication). Randomization is the heart of a control trial. Randomization increases the likelihood that unmeasured variables are equally distributed between the two arms. Randomization in assigning the intervention promotes avoidance of bias. Randomization is best done by using a table of random numbers. The entire study population can be stratified into subgroups according to the variable and individuals within each subgroup can then be randomly allocated into study and control groups.

Manipulation or Intervention

The independent variable, also known as the manipulated variable (drug, vaccine a new procedure) and dependent variable (incidence of disease, survival time, recovery time). The independent variable is the factor manipulated by the researcher, and it produces one or more results, known as dependent variables. There are often not more than one or two independent variables tested in an experiment, otherwise it is difficult to determine the influence of each upon the final results.

Follow-up

Loss to follow-up – Attrition Assessment, Positive results. Negative results.

Single blind trial: Participant not aware

- **Double blind trial:** Neither doctor nor participant is aware
- **Triple blind trial:** Doctor, participant and the person analyzing the data are not aware.

The mainstay of experimental medical studies, normally used in testing new drugs and treatments.

- A sample of patients with the condition, and who meet other selection criteria, are randomly allocated to receive either the experimental treatment, or the control treatment (commonly the standard treatment for the condition).
- Occasionally, a placebo or sham treatment will be used in the control group, but where there is already an accepted treatment, it is unlikely to be ethical to use a placebo.
- The experimental and control groups are then followed for a set time, and relevant measurements are taken to indicate the results (or outcomes) in each group.

Steps in an Epidemiologic Investigation

Epidemiologic investigations are usually conducted in outbreak situations. The primary reasons for conducting an epidemiologic investigation are to determine the cause of an outbreak and to implement control measures to prevent additional illness. Though there are different techniques/ methods for epidemiological investigations there are certain steps which will be followed during epidemiological investigation.

A questionnaire is often solicited to assist the investigator in developing better hypotheses about the etiologic agent's identity, source and transmission. The investigators interview ill and well persons, and calculate and compare rates of illness in both groups. They make time, place and person associations and calculate the probability of the risk factors. The investigator incorporates results from epidemiological associations and the environmental and laboratory investigations, and uses these data in forming and testing hypotheses. The steps are as follows:

1. Confirm the Existence of an Epidemic or an Outbreak

An outbreak is essentially the same thing as an epidemic, i.e., an increased frequency of a disease above the usual rate (endemic rate) in a given population or geographic area. To determine if there is an outbreak, one can compare the current number of cases (incidence) with past levels of the same disease over a similar time period. If the number is unusually large or unexpected for the given place and time, you may have an outbreak. For example, in August of 2014, the infection control department of a community hospital noticed an increase in the number of stool specimens which tested positive for *Salmonella* sp. So the first steps in an epidemiologic investigation confirm the existence of an epidemic means there is abnormally increase of any diseases.

2. Confirm the Diagnosis

Confirming the diagnosis is usually done by obtaining appropriate specimens for laboratory study and obtaining clinical histories. In some cases, it is best to actually look at the laboratory report. It is important to establish that the outbreak is real by examining how the cases were diagnosed and by determining what the baseline rate of disease was previously. For reportable diseases, baseline rates of disease can be determined from surveillance data, and can be compared rates during the previous month or weeks with the current rates of disease. For nonreportable diseases or conditions you may be able to find baseline data from state or national vital statistics, from disease registries, or from hospital discharge records.

3. Determine the Number of Cases

The creation of a case definition helps determine the magnitude of the problem and the actual case numbers. A case definition is a set of criteria for deciding whether an individual should be classified as a case or not. The case definition places boundaries on who is considered a case, so the investigation does not include those with illnesses unrelated to the outbreak. The common elements of a case definition include information on symptoms, laboratory results, time, place and person.

4. Orient the Data in Terms of Time, Person and Place

The purpose of data orientation or epidemiological characterizations is to arrange all incoming data so it means something. The investigator is searching for common associations based on time, place and person to strengthen or amend current hypotheses. This step is clearly described in descriptive epidemiology. A common method of data orientation is plotting, on a graph, the cases by time of symptom onset to get an epidemic curve. An epidemic curve is a graph that depicts the association of the time of illness onset of all cases that are associated with the outbreak. It helps to determine whether the outbreak originated from a common source or person to person. Time is plotted on the horizontal axis and the number of cases plotted on the vertical axis.

5. Develop a Hypothesis

One of the most important steps in generating hypotheses when investigating an outbreak is to consider what is known about the biology of the disease, including it's possible modes of transmission, whether there are animal reservoirs of disease, and the length of its incubation and infectious periods. This can be done by using the information gathered from the previous steps, consider the possible source(s) from which the disease may have been contacted.

6. Evaluate and Refine Hypotheses

The next step is to evaluate the hypotheses. In some outbreaks the descriptive epidemiology rapidly points convincingly to a particular source, and further analysis is unnecessary. For example, in 1991 Massachusetts had an outbreak of vitamin D intoxication in which all of the affected cases reported drinking milk delivered to their homes by a local dairy. Inspection of the dairy revealed that excessive quantities of vitamin D were being added the milk. However, in other situations the source is unclear, and analytic epidemiology must be utilized to more formally test the hypotheses. There are two general study designs that can be used in analytical epidemiology: a cohort study or a case control study. Both of these evaluate specific hypotheses by comparing groups of people. If analytical studies do not confirm any of the hypotheses generated by descriptive epidemiology, then you need to go back to the descriptive epidemiology and consider other sources and routes of transmission.

7. Implement Control and Prevention Measures

Before initiating any control measures, one should think about the effectiveness, timeliness, costs, available resources, personnel requirements and possible ramifications of proposed actions. Are the recommendations realistic for the establishment involved? This step is listed toward the end, but, you obviously want to initiate prevention measures as soon as possible if you have identified the source, even if you haven't worked out all of the details.

8. Prepare a Written Report

After analysis of epidemiologic and environmental data, conclusions should be summarized in a report. This is one of the most important steps in the outbreak investigation. Report should identifies a potential source(s) of the outbreak and suggests control measures to prevent future illness. The written report should follow standard scientific guidelines, and it should include an introduction, background, methods, results, discussion, and recommendations. It should be communicated to the local health authorities and to those responsible for implementing control and prevention measures.

USES OF EPIDEMIOLOGY

To Study Historically the Rise and Fall of Disease in the Population

This is the first use of the epidemiology. If we will look back we can plan for the future. By studying the effects of disease state in a population over a long time we can predict future health needs. It is well known that the health and illness pattern in a community is never constant. There are fluctuation over both short and long period of time. But by studying the time trend the epidemiologist can make the useful projections into the future and identify the correlations among different emerging reemerging health problems. By studying historically the rise and fall of diseases an epidemiologist can study the changing behavior of diseases, make future predictions and give early warnings or feedback

Diagnose the Health of the Community

Community diagnosis is generally refers to identification and quantification of health problems in a community in terms of mortality and morbidity and rates and ratios. Community diagnosis otherwise termed as nature and distribution of health and disease among the population and the dimensions of these are incidence, prevalence, and mortality. Taking into account that society is changing and health problems are changing community diagnosis must be dynamic. In a world of change, epidemiologist have a special duty to observe the impact 'upon the people' and the way we live to diagnose where well-being is increasing and where losing out, to probe for unintended consequences, to identify trends and to think ahead. By quantification health problems, we lay down the priorities in disease control and prevention and it can act as a benchmark for evaluation of health services. The data act as a source of new knowledge about disease distribution causation and prevention.

Planning and Evaluation of Health Services

Epidemiological information about distribution of health problems over time and place provides the fundamental basis for planning and developing the needed health services and for assessing the impact on people's health problems. One of the major objective of epidemiology is provide the data essential to planning, implementation and evaluation of services for prevention, control and treatment of disease and to setting up of priorities for these services. The existing health services can be evaluated for appropriate, cost effective, community need based, judicial mix of preventive, promotive, curative, rehabilitative and public health services by using epidemiology. Before, during and after implementing any health programme for prevention and control of health problems must be assessed.

Estimate the Individual Risk from Group

The investigator can estimate, from the common experience, the individual's chances and risks of disease. This can be estimated by identify the individuals for exposure, studying the epidemiological pattern of diseases and identifying the agent host and environmental interaction his/her own risk. The risk of bearing a Mongol child and some of its hereditary disorders are the examples of estimating the individual risk from group.

Syndrome Identification

In identifying syndromes from the distribution of clinical phenomena among sections of the population, it include grouping and dividing the symptom complexes and naming them as syndromes is the starting point for the study of natural history of any disease. Epidemiological investigation can be used to define refine syndrome.

Clinical Picture of Chronic Diseases and their Natural History

Epidemiology can help in completing the clinical picture by including all types of cases in proportion, by relating clinical disease to the subclinical, and observing secular changes in the character of disease, and its picture in other countries.

When studying a disease outbreak, epidemiologists depend on clinical physicians and laboratory scientists for the proper diagnosis of individual patients. But epidemiologists also contribute to physicians' understanding of the clinical picture and natural history of disease. Epidemiology is the study of populations and all cases that can be defined in them. These cases will often include, and in their due proportion, cases differing in type from those presenting to particular clinical attention (early disease, minor, the symptomless cases, and the somehow peculiar). The epidemiological method can also be used to identify subclinical manifestations and again in proper proportion to the clinical. Epidemiology thus helps to complete the clinical picture and natural history of disease.

Search for Causes of Health and Disease

In the search for causes of health and disease, starting with the discovery of groups with high and low rates, studying these differences in relation to differences in ways of living; and, where possible, testing these notions in the actual practice among populations. Most of the times, we may find difficulty in knowing the cause of illness inspite of having lot of known and observed facts. The secret may lie somewhere in the nature (environment). Tact and skill are required to think philosophically to detect this secret. Epidemiologists identifying the cause of the diseases by relating the diseases to inter population difference and other attributes of the population. In this way epidemiology is used to identify the cause or risk factors.

DISEASE TRANSMISSION

Every disease agent follows a series or chain of infectious process to infect others and all disease agents does not follows same mode of transmission. The infectious agents through a receptive portal of entry can infected a normal human being or animal.

Diseases are transmitted from the source of infection to susceptible host. The medical model of infectious disease transmission consists of three interlinked chains. They are:

1. Sources of reservoir
2. Modes of transmission
3. Susceptible host.

Sources or Reservoir

A source of infection is defined as the person, animal, objects or substance from which an infectious agent passes or is disseminated to the host. Reservoirs are sites in which viable infectious agents remain alive and from which infection of individuals may occur. Reservoirs may be either animate or inanimate. They are the natural habitat in which the microorganisms metabolizes and replicates. For example, in typhoid fever the reservoir of infection is human but the source of infection may be feces or urine of patients or contaminated food or water. In hookworm infection, the reservoir is a man, but the source of infection is the soil contaminated with infective larvae. In tetanus, the reservoir and source are the same, which is the soil. There are three types of reservoir:

1. Human reservoir
2. Animal reservoir
3. Reservoir in non-living things.

Human Reservoir

Human himself is the important source or reservoir of infections. Human maybe a case or a carrier.

Cases

- A case is defined as 'a person in the population or study group detected as having the particular disease, health disorder or condition under investigation.'
- The cases are identified by clinical, biochemical and laboratory tests and maybe clinical, sub-clinical or latent.
- The clinical case may be mild or moderate, typical or atypical, severe or fatal.
- The mild cases are more important source of infection as compared to severe cases.
- The subclinical cases are also called inapparent cases. They are important source of infection because they do not show any signs and symptoms of disease and shed infectious agent continuously.
- Subclinical infection can be detected by lab test, isolation of micro-organisms, antibody assay, biochemical and skin sensitivity tests. The host does not shed the infectious agent in latent infection.

Carrier

A carrier is defined as 'an infected person or animal that harbors a specific infectious agent in the absence of the clinical disease and serve as a potential source of infection for others.' Epidemiologically, carriers are more infectious because they are not recognized and live as normal in community. In carriers there must be the presence of disease agent in the body and absence of noticeable signs and symptoms of disease. They are shedding the disease agents in their excretions.

Classification of Carriers: Basis of Classification

On the Basis of Type

- **Incubatory carrier:** Incubatory carrier shed the infectious agents during the incubation period of disease. They are capable of infecting others before the onset of disease. Examples: measles, polio, influenza, hepatitis B, etc.
- **Convalescent carrier:** These carriers continue to shed the infectious agents during recovery. Convalescent carriers pose threat to the unprotected household member, for example Typhoid fever in which patients may excrete the bacilli for 6–8 weeks.
- **Healthy carrier:** These are subclinical cases which have developed carrier state without suffering from disease and shed the disease agent. For example, poliomyelitis, salmonellosis and diphtheria.

On the basis of Duration of Infection

- **Temporary carrier:** Temporary carriers are those who shed the infectious agents for short period of time. Incubatory and convalescent carriers are temporary carriers.
- **Chronic carrier:** Chronic carriers excrete the infectious agents for indefinite period of time, i.e., more than 6 months. The longer the carrier state, the greater is the risk to the community. Some chronic carriers excrete the infectious agents intermittently and some continuously.

On the Basis of Portal of Exit

Carriers are also classified according to the portal of exit to the infectious agents. Therefore, there are urinary carrier, intestinal carriers, nasal carrier etc. In typhoid fever, urinary carrier is more dangerous than an intestinal carrier.

Animal Reservoir

The animal reservoir may also be case or carrier. The disease which are transmitted from animal to man are called zoonotic diseases, e.g., Rabies, Yellow fever, influenza. There are more than 100 zoonotic diseases. Pigs and ducks serve as reservoir for the transmission of influenza virus and pigeons can transmit Chlamydia. The vectors like mosquitos are responsible for transmitting malaria, filaria, etc. The reservoir of plague is usually the rodent population. Similarly rabies is carried by many domestic and wild mammals.

Environment Reservoir (Reservoir in Non-living Things)

- Soil and inanimate matter can also act as reservoirs on infection.
- Soil also serves as a permanent habitat for a few virulent human pathogens.
- These dangerous microbes include *Clostridium tetani*, Clostridium botulinum, and fungi responsible for opportunistic pathogen.
- Water is an important reservoir of human disease when it is contaminated by raw sewage.
- Feces from infected persons are the most common source of water contamination.

Modes of Transmission

Different pathogens have different modes of transmission, which are usually related to the habitats of the organisms in the body. For instance, respiratory pathogens are generally airborne, whereas intestinal pathogens are spread by food or water.

Transmission involves three stages:

1. Escape from the host
2. Travel
3. Entry into a new host

The mode of transmission of infectious disease is classified as direct transmission and indirect transmission:

- Vehicle-borne
- Vector-borne
- Mechanical
- Biological
- Fomite-borne
- Unclean hands and fingers.

Types of Transmission

Direct Transmission

During direct transmission microbes are directly transferred from an infected person to another person. This may be by direct contact as by touching, biting, kissing or sexual intercourse, or by direct droplet spray onto the mucous or conjunctiva membranes of the eye, nose, or mouth during sneezing, coughing, spitting, singing, or talking.

Types of direct contact include:

1. **Person-to-person contact:** Infectious diseases are commonly transmitted through direct person-to-person contact. Transmission occurs when an infected person touches or exchanges body fluids with someone else. This can happen before an infected person is aware of the illness. Sexually transmitted diseases (STDs) can be transmitted in this way.
2. **Droplet spread:** The spray of droplets during coughing and sneezing can spread an infectious disease. Since droplets fall to the ground within a few feet, this type of transmission requires close proximity. Droplet nuclei are usually the small residues that result from evaporation of fluid from droplets emitted by an infected host. During droplet transmission, respiratory droplets carrying infectious pathogens can lead to disease transmission during coughing, sneezing, talking, and even certain medical procedures such as suctioning. Droplets are generally defined as being greater than 5 micrometers and the area of defined risk has been a distance within 3 feet around the infected patient. However, the maximum distance for droplet transmission is currently unresolved and a distance of 3 feet around the patient is best viewed as an *example* of what is meant by "a short distance from a patient" and should not be used as the sole *criterion* for deciding when a mask should be donned to protect from droplet exposure. Examples of diseases that are transmitted through droplet transmission include influenza and pertussis.
3. **Contact with soil:** The disease agent is acquired by direct touch with soil. In addition to tetanus, anthrax, and botulism, soil bacteria may cause gastrointestinal, wound, skin, and respiratory tract diseases.
4. **Inoculation into skin or mucosa:** The disease agent is inoculated directly into the skin, e.g., Rabies by dog bites, Hepatitis B through contaminated needle and syringe, etc. The pathogen enters the body through skin or mucous membranes such as the eyes also. These infections are associated with poor personal hygiene.

Transplacental

Pregnant women can also transmit infectious diseases to their unborn children via the placenta. Some STDs, including gonorrhea, can be passed from mother to baby during childbirth. Vertical transmission is the spread of disease from parents to offspring by an infected sperm or egg, by passage of pathogens across the placenta during fetal development, or during the birth process. These are known as transplacental transmission.

Indirect Transmission

Infectious diseases can also be spread indirectly through the air and other mechanisms. Contaminated inanimate materials or objects (fomites) such as toys, handkerchiefs, soiled clothes, bedding, cooking or eating utensils, surgical instruments or dressings; water, food, milk, biological products including blood, serum, plasma, tissues or organs; or any substance serving as an intermediate means by which an infectious agent is transported and introduced into a susceptible host through a suitable portal of entry. The different mode of indirect contact can be classified as follows.

Vehicle-borne

- Vehicles are non-living materials are capable of transmitting infectious agent.
- If the vehicle is a contaminated inanimate object, it is called a fomite.
- Some organisms can live on objects for a short time. If you touch an object, such as a doorknob, soon after an infected person, you might be exposed to infection. Transmission occurs when you touch your mouth, nose, or eyes before thoroughly washing your hands
- Bedding, clothing, cooking, and eating utensils, surgical instruments are common fomites.
- Vehicles usually become contaminated by contact with either the reservoir or with respiratory droplets, pus, urine, or feces shed from infected person.
- Infectious diseases can be transmitted via contaminated food and water. *E. coli* is often transmitted through improperly handled produce or undercooked meat. Improperly canned foods can create an environment ripe for *Clostridium botulinum*, which can lead to botulism.
- Acute diarrheas, typhoid fever, cholera, polio, hepatitis A are water-borne diseases.
- Those transmitted by blood include Hepatitis B, malaria, syphilis, trypanosomes etc.

Vector-borne

Vector is defined as "an insect or any living carrier that transports an infectious agent from an infected individual or its wastes to a susceptible individual or its food or immediate surroundings." Example: Various species of rodents (rats and mice) and arthropods (mosquitoes, ticks, sand flies, biting midges). They can spread diseases by their biting and also mechanical ways.

- **Mechanical:** It includes simple mechanical carriage by a crawling or flying insect through soiling of its feet or proboscis, or by passage of organisms through its gastrointestinal tract. This does not require multiplication or development of the organism.
- **Biological:** Propagation (multiplication), cyclic development, or a combination of this (cyclopropagative) is required before the arthropod can transmit the infective form of the agent to humans.

Air-borne Transmission

Some infectious agents can travel long distances and remain suspended in the air for an extended period of time. You can catch a disease like measles by entering a room after someone with measles has departed. The small particles of widely varying size that may arise from soil (as, for example, fungus spores separated from dry soil by wind or mechanical agitation), clothes, bedding or contaminated floors.

EPIDEMIOLOGY OF EMERGING AND RE-EMERGING DISEASES

There has been a remarkable progress in the prevention, control and even eradication of infectious diseases with improved hygiene and development of antimicrobials and vaccines. However, infectious diseases still remain a leading cause of global disease burden with high morbidity and mortality especially in the developing world. Furthermore, there have been threats of new diseases during the past three decades due to the evolution and adaptation of microbes and the reemergence of old diseases due to the development of antimicrobial resistance and the capacity to spread to new geographic areas. The impact of the emerging and reemerging diseases in India has been tremendous at socioeconomic and public health levels. Their control requires continuing surveillance, research and training, better diagnostic facilities and improved public health system. Emerging and reemerging zoonotic diseases, food borne and waterborne diseases and diseases caused by multiresistant organisms constitute the major threats in India. This review of bacterial emerging and reemerging diseases should be of critical importance to microbiologists, clinicians, public health personnel and policy makers in India. Though today the world stands on the threshold of a new era in which hundreds of millions of people will be safe from some of the most terrible diseases. Soon poliomyelitis, neonatal tetanus, leprosy, guinea worm disease, river blindness, chagas disease will join small pox as disease of the past but on the other hand, the world also stands on the brink of a global crisis in infectious diseases. No country is safe from them and no country can afford to ignore their threat any longer. Some infectious diseases once through to be all but conquered, have return with a vengeance. Other has developed stubborn resistance to antibiotic drugs. New and previously unknown diseases continue to emerge. Together these trends amount to a crisis for today and the challenge for the future.

Factors Contributing to Emerging and Re-emerging Diseases

Agent

Evolution of pathogenic infectious agents: Increasing virulence of microbes like Influenza A virus, which exhibits frequent changes in its antigenic structure giving rise to new strains with endemic and pandemic propensities. It is due to microbial adaptation and change.

Use of anti-infective drugs in animals and plants: Use of anti-infective drugs in animals and plants may develop drug resistance in them, when the human being act as a primary consumer and consume that food the resistance bacteria may pass to the human being and develop drug resistance.

Development of resistance to drugs: Due to wrong prescribing practice, non-adherence by patients and counterfeit drugs, the Antimicrobial Drug Resistance develops which cause emerging of new pathogenic infectious agents by which there is prolonged hospital admissions, higher death rates from infections.

Resistance of vectors to pesticides: Resistance of vectors to pesticides can creates difficulties in controlling the vectors which result increasing vectors and vector borne diseases. For example mosquitoes now develop resistance to DDT spraying, which is a major step adopted by WHO to eradicate malaria. Similarly ticks, fleas lice and sand flies also develops resistance to their pesticides.

Host

Host factors contributing to emergence are:

- Mass migration of people provoked by natural and manmade disaster with concomitant rehabilitation of displaced people in temporary human settlements under unhygienic conditions.
- Uninhibited and reckless industrialization leading to migration of labor population from rural to urban areas in unhygienic squatter settlements.
- International travel as a result of trade and tourism contributing to global dispersion of disease agents, disease reservoirs and vectors.
- Changes in lifestyle that promote unhealthy and risk prone behavior patterns affecting food habits and sexual practices.
- Declining immunity of as a result of HIV infection, which make him vulnerable to a host of infections.

Environment

Environmental sanitation characterized by unsafe water supply, improper disposal of solid and liquid waste, poor hygienic practices and congested living conditions all contribute to emergence of infection.

Climatic changes resulting from global warming inducing increased surface water evaporation, greater rainfall changes in the direction of bird migration and changes in the habitat of disease vectors are also contributory factors. Breakdown of public health measure (war, unrest, overcrowding), Deterioration in surveillance systems (lack of political will), Poverty, Neglect and Weakening of Health Infrastructure are also the factors increasing the chance.

Emerging Diseases

During the past 30 years, new disease have emerged to threatened the health of hundreds of millions of people. From many of those diseases there is no treatment, cure or vaccine and the possibilities of preventing and controlling them are limited.

Emerging infectious disease are those whose incidence in human has increase during the last two decades or which threaten to increase in near future. The term also refers to new appearing infectious disease, or disease that is spreading new geographical area such as Cholera in South America and yellow fever in Kenya.

The disease in question involve all the major model of transmission—they are spread either from person to person transmission, by insects or animal, or through contaminated food or water. The most dramatic example of new disease is AIDS, caused by HIV virus. The existence of viruses is unknown till 1983. Presently estimated 2.3 cases occur every year worldwide.

The new breed of deadly hemorrhagic fever of which Ebola virus disease known as Ebola hemorrhagic fever is the most notorious. Has struck in Africa. Ebola appear first time in Zaire and Sudan in 1976. Since then it has been appeared periodically. Ebola virus is a member of *Filoviridae* and comprises 5 distinct species: Zaire Ebola virus, Reston Ebola virus, Sudan Ebola virus, Tai Ebola virus, and Bundibugyo Ebola virus. The recent epidemics started in December 2013, Guinea and spread to South Africa by 18 September 2014, a total of 7,192 cases detected with 3,286 death. Case fatality rate may be high 70%. Ebola has incubation period 2–21 days, and is not infect during the period. Transmitted through direct contact with the blood, organ, body secretion or other body fluid of infected animals like chimpanzees, gorillas, monkeys, fruit bats, etc. Human to human transmission through body fluid or blood of an infected symptomatic person or through exposure to objects (needle) that have been contaminated with infected secretion.

It is not transmitted through air, water, food. The ill characterized by sudden unset of fever, intense weakness, muscle pain, headache, sore throat, vomiting, diarrhea, rash, impaired kidney and liver function and both cases internal and external bleeding. Currently there is no specific treatment for this disease. There is no vaccine against Ebola.

The US has been emergence of Hanta virus pulmonary syndrome, characterized by respiratory failure and case fatality rate over 50%. Since it was first recognized in 1993, this Hanta virus infection has been detected in more than 20 states in that country, and has also surfaced in Argentina and Brazil. This Hanta virus is carried by rodent, particularly deer mice. Other Hanta virus is recognized for many years in Asia, where they cause hemorrhagic fever with renal involvement in humans.

Epidemic of food-borne and water-borne disease due to new organism such as cryptosporidium or new strain of bacteria such as *E. coli* have hit industrialized and developing countries alike. The strain of E. Coli was first reported in 1982 and has since then been implicated in many serious outbreaks of diarrheal illness, sometimes leading to kidney failure. The strain has been linked to undercooked hamburger beef and unpasteurized milk. A completely new strain of cholera appeared in South Eastern India in 1992 and has since spread North and West to other areas of India into Western China, Thailand and other part of South East Asia.

The threat of new global influenza pandemic also is increasing. Occur every 20 years or so, triggering large epidemics in many parts of the world, and causing many thousands of deaths. The next such shift is expected to take place very soon. Epidemic strains of influenza virus are carried by ducks, chickens, pigs raised in close proximity to one another on farms. The exchanges of genetic material between these viruses produces new strains, leading to epidemics of human influenza, each epidemic being due to a different strain. Since it might adopt into a strain that is contagious among humans. Since 1997, 478 cases with 286 deaths have been reported to WHO. The first case was from Hong Kong. Other countries involved are Cambodia, Indonesia, Thailand and Vietnam. In late 2002 a new disease called SARS was reported from China with rapid spread to Hong Kong Singapore, Vietnam, Taiwan and Toronto. During 2003, 8,422 SARS cases were reported from 30 countries with 916 fatalities. More recently, pandemic due to influenza A (H1N1) 2009 strain in continuing worldwide involving 214 countries already taking 18,156 lives. New strains such as those of cholera and influenza do not follow the usual pattern of being more common in younger people. They affect all age groups, since older people have not acquired immunity to them from previous infection.

On 10 December 2015, A panel of scientists and public health experts convened by WHO met in Geneva to prioritize the top five to ten emerging pathogens likely to cause severe outbreaks in the near future, and for which few or no medical countermeasures exist. These diseases will provide the basis for work on the WHO Blueprint for Research and development preparedness to help control potential future outbreaks. The initial list of disease priorities needing urgent Research and development attention comprises: Crimean Congo hemorrhagic fever, Ebola virus disease and Marburg, Lassa fever, MERS and SARS coronavirus diseases, Nipah and Rift Valley fever. The list will be reviewed annually or when new diseases emerge.

Re-emerging Diseases

The term re-emerging diseases refers to the diseases which were previously easily controlled by chemotherapy and antibiotics, but now they have developed antimicrobial resistance and are often appearing in epidemic form.

The emergence of drugs-resistant strains of micro-organisms or parasites is promoted by treatments that do not result in cure. The increasing use of antimicrobials worldwide, often in subtherapeutic doses and sometime counterfeit form, indicates that this problem will increase in the foreseeable future. Changes in lifestyle, behavior (including the injecting and non-injecting drug use) and cultural or social values are behind the emergence of some infectious diseases such as syphilis, increases in the number of sexual partners have been the main factor in the spread of HIV infection and other sexually transmitted diseases. Travel including tourism, also plays a role. The spread of syphilis in the 18th and 19th centuries was related to the movement of armies. Today the introduction of HIV in parts of the world is due to greatly increased human mobility. Studies show that whereas only a few generations ago most people in their lifetime travelled no further than 40 kilometers from their birthplace, many today go up to 1,000 times further, traveling the whole world.

The practices of modern medicine also contribute. The spread of viral hepatitis is related in part to techniques such as kidney dialysis and multiple blood transfusions as well as to other form of transmission. Relaxation in immunization practices can quickly result in the resurgence of diseases, as for example, the recent spread of diphtheria in the Russian Federation and other former republics of the USSR.

New animal diseases pose potential food borne risks to human health that are sometimes difficult to evaluate or predict. An example that has caused much public concern in Europe is bovine spongiform encephalopathy ('mad cow disease'). Fears have grown that the infectious agent responsible may be passed through the food chain to cause a variant of the incurable Creutzfeldt-Jakob disease in humans, in which the brain is attacked. The British beef market has been seriously affected and stringent public health safeguards have been introduced.

The reasons for outbreaks of new diseases, or sharp increases in those one believed to be under control, are complex and still not fully understood. The fact is however that the national health has become an international challenge. An outbreak anywhere must now be seen as a threat to virtually all countries, especially those that serve as major hubs of international travel. Despite the emergence of new diseases in the last 30 years, there is still a lack of national and international political will and resources to develop and support the systems that are necessary to detect them and stop their spread. Without doubt diseases as yet unknown, but with the potential to be the AIDS of tomorrow, lurk in the shadows.

EPIDEMIOLOGICAL INVESTIGATION

Epidemiologic investigations are usually conducted in outbreak situations. The primary reasons for conducting an epidemiologic investigation are to determine the cause of an outbreak and to implement control measures to prevent additional illness. The purpose of the epidemiologic investigation is to identify a problem, collect data, formulate and test hypotheses. It involves the collection and analysis of more facts or data to determine the cause of illness and to implement control measures to prevent additional illness. There are certain phases of epidemiological investigation which are described below:

- **Diagnostic phase:** Diagnostic phase, in which the presence of the disease is confirmed. Diagnosis must be confirmed by reviewing the clinical information available. This includes lab results if available. Realize that not every case has to have lab confirmation to be considered part of the outbreak, but some of the initial cases should have lab confirmation. Set of standard criteria for deciding whether an individual should be classified as a case. Create a workable case definition, simple and objective criteria, ideally. The case definition will include most of the actual cases, very few or none of what are called 'false-positive' cases (persons who actually do not have the disease in question but nonetheless meet the case definition).
- **Descriptive phase:** A descriptive phase, which describes the populations at risk and the distribution of the disease, both in time and space, within these populations. This may then allow a series of hypotheses to be formed about the likely determinants of the disease and the effects of these on the frequency with which the disease occurs in the populations at risk.
- **Investigative phase:** Investigative phase, which normally involves the implementation of a series of field studies designed to test these hypotheses. All reasonable hypothesis need to be considered and weighted by comparing the attack rates in various groups for those exposed and those not exposed to each suspected factor.
- An experimental phase, in which experiments are performed under controlled conditions to test these hypotheses in more detail. When divergent theories are presented, it is not easy to distinguish immediately between those which are sound or which are plausible.
- **Analytical phase:** Analytical phase, in which the results produced by the above investigations are analyzed. This is often combined with attempts to model the epidemiology of the disease using the information generated. Such a process often enables the epidemiologist to determine whether any vital bits of information about the disease process are missing.
- **Intervention phase:** Intervention phase, in which appropriate methods for the control of the disease are examined either under experimental conditions or in the field. Interventions in the disease process are effected by manipulating existing determinants or introducing new ones.
- **Decision-making phase:** In decision-making phase, the knowledge of the epidemiology of the disease is used to explore the various options available for its control. This often involves the modelling of the effects that these different options are likely to have on the incidence of the disease. These models can be combined with other models that examine the costs of the various control measures and compare them with the benefits, in terms of increased productivity, that these measures are likely to produce. The optimum control strategy can then be selected as a result of the expected decrease in disease incidence in the populations of livestock at risk.
- **Monitoring phase:** Monitoring phase, which takes place during the implementation of the control measures to ensure that these measures are being properly applied, are having the desired effect on reducing disease incidence, and that developments are likely to jeopardize the success of the control program are quickly detected.

PRESENTATION OF EPIDEMIOLOGICAL DATA

Data analysis is an important component of epidemiologic practice. To analyze data effectively, an epidemiologist must first become familiar with the data before applying analytic techniques. The epidemiologist may begin by examining individual records such as those contained in a line listing, but will quickly progress to summarizing the data with tables.

Sometimes, the resulting tables are the only analysis that is needed, particularly when the amount of data is small and relationships are straightforward. When the data are more complex, graphs and charts can help the epidemiologist visualize broader patterns and trends and identify variations from those trends. Variations may represent important new findings or only errors in typing or coding which need to be corrected. Thus, tables, graphs, and charts are essential to the verification and analysis of the data.

Once an analysis is complete, tables, graphs, and charts further serve as useful visual aids for describing the data to others. In preparing tables, graphs, and charts for others, it must be keep in mind that their primary purpose is to communicate information about the data.

Tables

A table is a set of data arranged in rows and columns. Almost any quantitative information can be organized into a table. Tables are useful for demonstrating patterns, exceptions, differences, and other relationships. In addition, tables usually serve as the basis for preparing more visual displays of data, such as graphs and charts, where some of the detail may be lost. Tables designed to present data to others should be as simple as possible. Two or three small tables, each focusing on a different aspect of the data, are easier to understand than a single large table that contains many details or variables.

A table should be self-explanatory. If a table is taken out of its original context, it should still convey all the information necessary for the reader to understand the data. To create a table that is self-explanatory, follow the guidelines below:

- Use a clear and concise title that describes the what, where, and when of the data in the table
- Precede the title with a table number
- Label each row and each column clearly and concisely and include the units of measurement for the data
- Show totals for rows and columns. If you show percents (%), also give their total (always 100)

- Explain any codes, abbreviations, or symbols in a footnote
- Note any exclusions in a footnote (1 case and 2 controls with unknown family history were excluded from this analysis)
- Note the source of the data in a footnote if the data are not original.

One-variable Table

In descriptive epidemiology, the most basic table is a simple frequency distribution with only one variable. In such a frequency distribution table, the first column shows the values or categories of the variable represented by the data, such as age or sex. The second column shows the number of persons or events that fall into each category, often, a third column lists the percentage of person. The example of one-variable table is given in **Table 3.3**.

Two- and Three-variable Tables

Data can also be cross-tabulated to show counts by a second variable shows the number of cases by both age and sex of the patient. A two-variable table with cross-tabulated data is also known as a contingency table. In example of a common type of contingency table, which is called a two-by-two table because each of the two variables has two categories. Epidemiologists frequently use contingency tables to display the data used in calculating measures of association and tests of statistical significance.

Tables of Other Statistical Measures

Although all the examples used so far show counts (frequency) of the variables, tables can also be used to show other statistical measures. The cells can contain rates, means, relative risks or other measures. Just be sure the titles and row/column headings clearly identify what data is being presented.

Creating Class Intervals

Some variables such have a limited number of possible values, example-sex. Others have a broader range of possible responses, and categories or 'class intervals' are needed to group them. The following rules are important when creating class intervals:

- Class intervals should be mutually exclusive and exhaustive which means include all of the data and ranges should not overlap. For example, if the first category is 0–5, the next one must start with 6, not 5.
- A relatively large number of narrow categories can be used for the initial analysis, which can always combine in later.

Table 3.3: Age-wise distribution of females in reproductive age group present in RTI clinic N = 250.

Age in years	*Number*	*Percentage*
15–25	113	45.2
25–35	75	30
35–45	62	24.8

- Use of standard groupings will be advisable if they are available - for example, age categories used by CDC for a particular disease and for unknowns, a category can created since there will usually be missing information for some of the cases.

Charts

In general charts are a method of organizing and illustrating data using only one coordinate and are best used for comparing data with discrete categories. Several types of charts may be produced using common spreadsheet software such as Excel.

Types of Charts

Bar Charts

Bar charts are used to create a visual display of the data from a table. The bars may be either horizontal or vertical. Bar charts are one of the easiest, graphically attractive and hence most commonly used methods of presenting all types of data. They are especially useful for representing various data series. The data series comprises the continuous variables while the values of the specific instances at which the value of the data series is measured, represents the values of the discrete variables.

Presentation of data as bar charts makes the comparative study of the data very easy. A bar chart consists of a group of bars which are equidistant from each other. The values on the bar charts are read by the measurement of the length or the height of the bars. The width of the bars is largely inessential and is used only for the clarity of the presentation.

Simple Bar Diagram (Fig. 3.2)

The simple bar chart is the 'simplest' bar chart which has one continuous variable charted along with one discrete variables used to display the data from a frequency distribution (one-variable table). Each bar represents one value of the variable. **Figure 3.2** is an example of simple bar diagram. It can be used to compare the relative magnitude of the different values but one of the primary limitations of the simple bar chart is that it can only be used to display a single continuous variable.

Composite Bar Chart (Fig. 3.3)

If two or more sets of continuous variables are to be shown on the same bar chart, we use what is called a composite

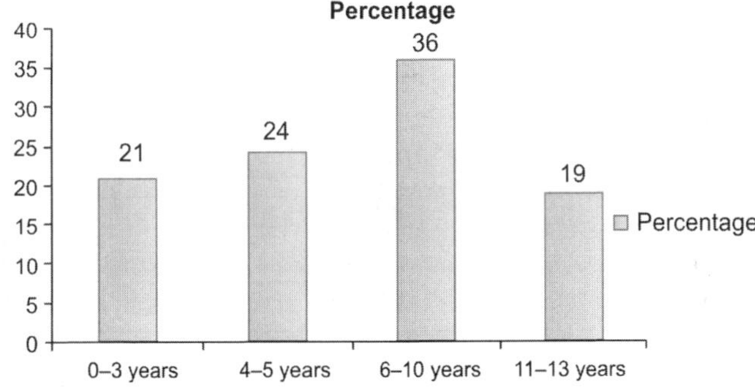

Fig. 3.2: Simple bar chart with a single continuous variable.

bar chart. **Figure 3.3** shows an example of the composite bar chart. This bar diagram depicts the age-wise and sex-wise distribution of children. This composite bar charts is quite convenient for comparing two or more sets of data. This is otherwise known as group bar diagram. A grouped bar chart is particularly useful when you want to compare the subgroups within a group. Bars within a group are adjoining. The bars should be illustrated distinctively and described in a legend.

Stacked Bar Charts (Fig. 3.4)

A stacked bar chart is used to show the same data as a grouped bar chart but divides the subgroups of the second variable into a single bar of the first variable. It deviates from the grouped bar chart in that the different groups are differentiated not with separate bars, but with different segments within a single bar for each category. A stacked bar chart is more effective than a grouped bar chart at displaying the overall pattern of the first variable but less effective at displaying the relative size of each subgroup. The example of a stacked bar diagram is given in **Figure 3.4**, which shows death of people due to different causes in different year.

Percentage Bar Diagram (Fig. 3.5)

Percentage bar diagram is a variant of a stacked bar diagram, in which all of the bars are pulled to the same height (100%) and show the components as percentages of the total rather than as actual values. This type of chart is useful for comparing the contribution of different subgroups within the categories of the main variable.

Pie Charts (Fig. 3.6)

A pie chart is simple and easily understood. Very useful for showing the component parts of a single group or variable. The size of the pie 'slices' shows the percentage for each component part of the whole. Pie diagrams are diagrammatically represented in circles with at angle 360 degree. The segments

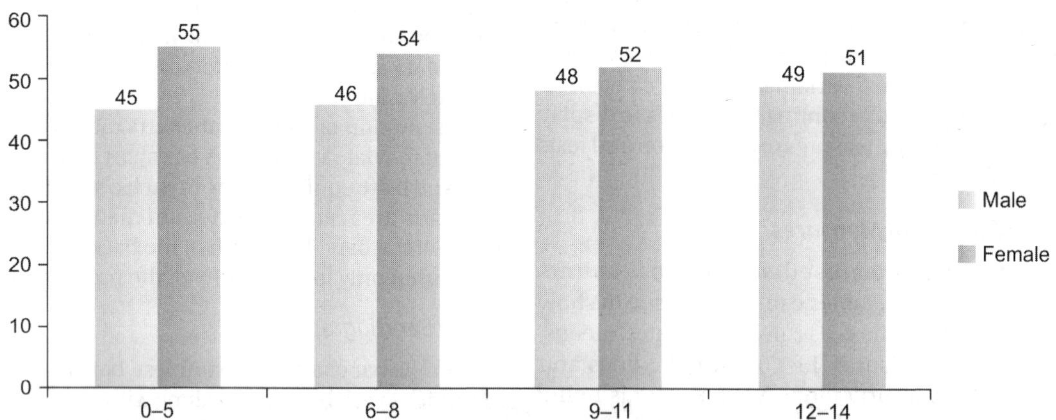

Fig. 3.3: Percentage of children according to their age and sex in a composite bar chart.

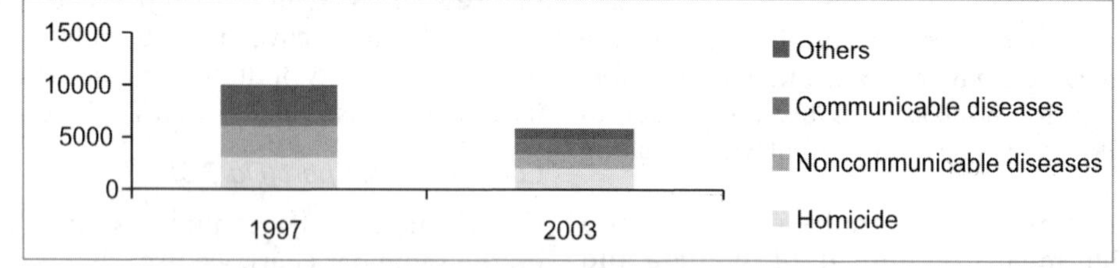

Fig. 3.4: Death of people due to different causes in different years presented in a stacked bar chart.

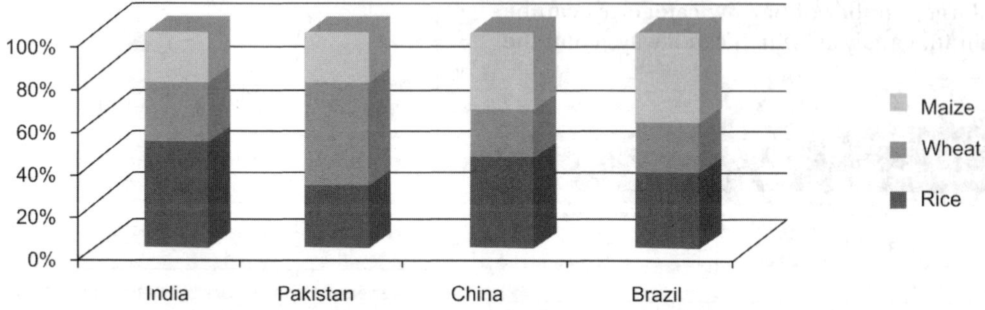

Fig. 3.5: Percentage bar diagram on production of crops in different countries.

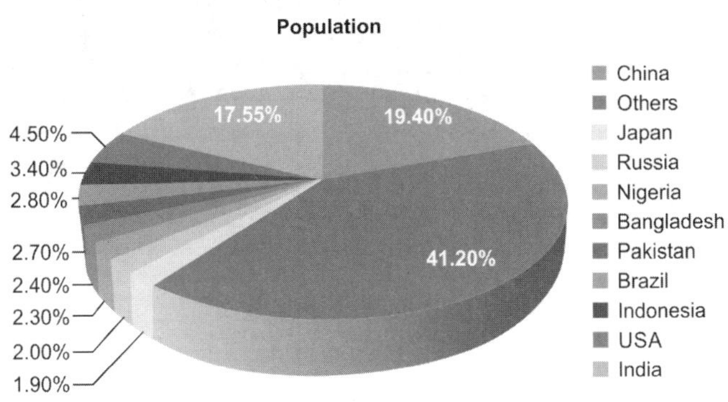

Fig. 3.6: Pie diagram showing population of different countries.

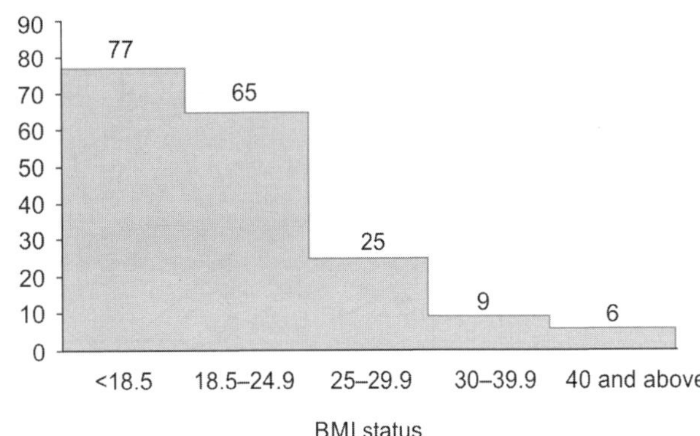

Fig. 3.7: Histograms showing BMI status of under-five children.

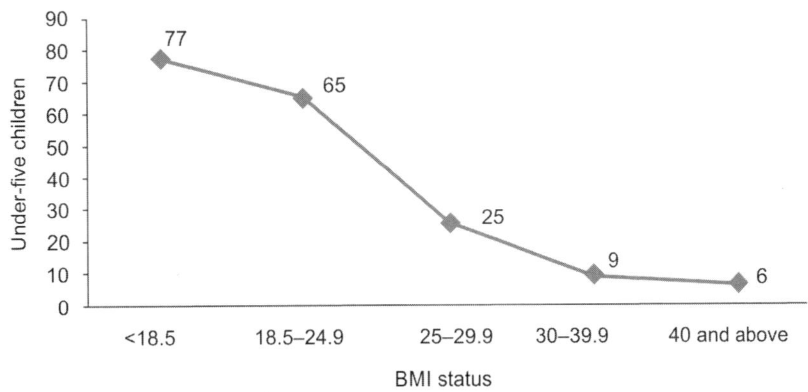

Fig. 3.8: BMI status of under-five children depicted by frequency polygon.

of the circle are comparable, which are indicated in percentage. The angle can be calculated by:

$$\text{Degree to be presented} = \frac{\text{Given \%}}{100} \times 360$$

Histograms (Fig. 3.7)

A histogram is a graph of the frequency distribution of a continuous variable, based on class intervals. It uses adjoining columns to represent the number of observations for each class interval in the distribution. The area of each column is proportional to the number of observations in that interval. Underlying figure shows the BMI of under-five children in a selected community through histograms.

Frequency Polygons (Fig. 3.8)

A frequency polygon, like a histogram, is the graph of a frequency distribution. In a frequency polygon, the number of observations within an interval is marked with a single point placed at the midpoint of the interval. Each point is then connected to the next with a straight line. The above histogram is changed to frequency polygons.

Population Pyramid (Fig. 3.9)

A population pyramid displays the count or percentage of a population by age and sex. It does so by using two histograms—most often one for females and one for males, each by age group—turned sideways so the bars are horizontal, and placed base to base.

Maps

Maps are a very widely used type of chart. They are also called geographic coordinate charts.

Maps are used to show the geographic location of events or attributes. Two types of maps commonly used in field epidemiology are spot maps and area maps. Spot maps use dots or other symbols to show where each case-patient lived or was exposed.

Spot maps use dots or other symbols to show where an event took place, or where a disease condition exists. Spot maps are good for detecting clusters of disease cases. A spot map is useful for showing the geographic distribution of cases, but because it does not take the size of the population at risk into account a spot map does not show risk of disease. Even when a spot map shows a large number of dots in the same area, the risk of acquiring disease may not be particularly high if that area is densely populated.

Area map: An area map, also called a choropleth map, can be used to show rates of disease or other health conditions in different areas by using different shades or colors. When choosing shades or colors for each category, ensure that the intensity of shade or color reflects increasing disease burden areas. Mapping technology has grown very sophisticated in recent years. The widespread availability and use of Global Positioning Systems (GPS) devices and Geographic Information Systems (GIS) software has made it easier to produce accurate, up-to-date maps to aid in epidemiologic investigations.

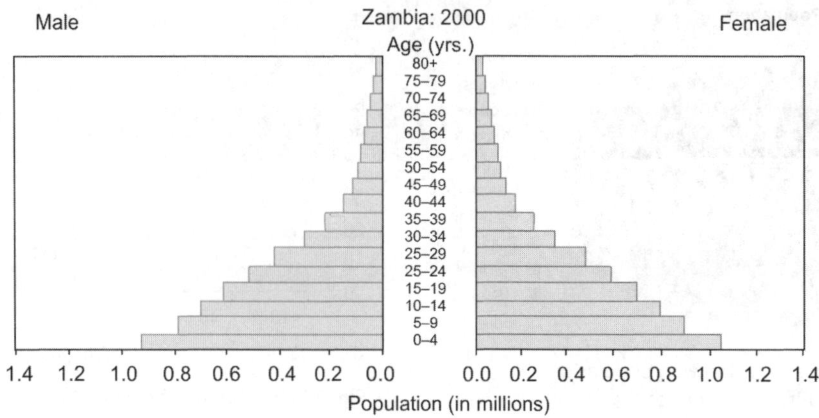

Fig. 3.9: Population pyramid.

APPLICATION OF EPIDEMIOLOGY IN HEALTHCARE DELIVERY

Healthcare Delivery

The ultimate goal of healthcare services are to promote and protect health, to alleviate and minimize sufferings, and disabilities and to regain health so as to lead socially useful and economically productive life. Preventive approach is the best approach to achieve these goals because preventive measures can be implemented with the joint efforts of health personnel and the people at larger at the family and the community level which is satisfied by epidemiology. Epidemiology is the study of distribution and determinants of health-related states or events in a specified community and always stress on preventive approaches.

- In healthcare delivery system, epidemiology helps in prevention of diseases, promotion of health, diagnosing disease and Taking rehabilitative measures in at the rehabilitative state of diseases.
- Emphasizing a population perspective, epidemiology offers a set of tools and principles for the healthcare manager to monitor health states and to evaluate the impact of programs and, hence it forms the scientific basis for policy formulation.
- The use of epidemiologic and other data, e.g., aging of the population can help in the planning of health services is at different level. Similarly, the evaluation of various services can be done by the use of epidemiology study design.
- Epidemiologic indicators can be used to estimate needs and perceived health states and to identify the relation between need and demand. An analogy is drawn between 'classic' or 'etiologic'.
- The quality of health care depends heavily on epidemiology because epidemiology helps in improving the health status of the population at large. The receipt of healthcare procedures and their associations with outcome measures depends upon their study variables such as age, sex, ethnicity, and race, etc., which are also studied in epidemiology. In other hand for the control of communicable diseases which is other area of the management of healthcare quality; epidemiology provides a comprehensive understanding on the magnitude, causes, and consequences.
- Modern epidemiological methods such as 'clinical decision trees' are being increasingly used in clinical practice for taking decision regarding optimum clinical management of individual patients.
- A working knowledge of essential principles of epidemiology, research methodology, and biostatistics is useful for research activities of medical persons who are interested in research.
- The diagnosis of a particular new rare disease can be done by retrospective approach of disease through case control study, e.g., Swine flu, Ebola disease.
- Through epidemiological methods, that we are able to put the pieces of information together and identify 'syndromes' and these etiological factors. For instance, till 1920s, peptic ulcer was thought to be a single entity. Based on collection of large scale epidemiological data (From death certificates and surgical records) and its analysis according to sex, social class, anatomical site and time-related trends, the two entities, viz. duodenal and peptic ulcer were clearly distinguished.
- The above facets, according to which we consider any disease, put together, are nothing but what we call 'Epidemiology'. It is that branch of medicine that answers the issues related to all human health problems and diseases, their magnitude, their distribution according to persons, place and time, the various factors that determine the causation, risk, prognosis, management, and prevention of the diseases.
- Epidemiology provides both the body of knowledge—information on the distribution and determinants of health conditions—and methods for investigating health problems and evaluating services.
- One of the important applications in epidemiology is to provide methodologies used to describe the overall health of a particular community. The resulting description may then provide a key to the types of problems that require attention and also accentuate the need for specific health services. A complete epidemiologic description

would include indices of health as well as indicators of the psychosocial milieu of the community.

- Provides the data on demographic and social variable like (age, sex, distribution, socioeconomic status, racial, ethnic, and religious composition) variables related to community infrastructure or geographical areas, boundaries which can help in organizing community development programs.
- Epidemiology can help in measuring of health outcomes like mortality rates (infant mortality rate, maternal mortality, child mortality rate) morbidity rate specially about chronic and infectious diseases. Teenage pregnancy rates/sexually transmitted diseases which helps in changing health policies formulation of health programs etc.
- Provide data on environmental variables like Numerous adverse environmental factors are implicated in the health of the people like air pollution, water pollution, soil pollution and their implication on health status.
- Epidemiology helps in describing the health of the total community and eliminate health disparities among segments of the population, including differences that occur by gender, race or ethnicity, education or income can be possible.
- Regarding the health of the community, epidemiology is not only a descriptive tool but also plays a role in policy evaluation. The findings of epidemiologic research helps in developing policies to safeguard the public's health. Epidemiologic evidence receives consideration at the national and even global levels, while also directly and indirectly influencing individual decisions concerning lifestyle, work, and family.

Operations Research and Program Evaluation

The term operations research (operational research) is defined as the systematic study, by observations and experiment, of the working of a system (e.g., health services), with a view to improvement.' Epidemiology applied to operations research refers to the study of the placement of health services in a community and the optimum utilization of such services. 'The usual epidemiologic approaches (descriptive, analytic, and experimental) are all used in health services research and, in addition, methods of evaluation have been expanded through their application to problems in health services. A major contribution of epidemiology to operations research is the development of research designs, analytic techniques, and selection of the sample and conducting.

Study of Risks to Individuals

In many instances, epidemiologic research on disease etiology involves collection of data on a number of individual members of different study groups or study populations. Epidemiologists use two main types of observational studies for research on disease etiology: case-control and cohort studies. A case-control design compares a group of individuals who have a disease of interest (the cases) with a group who does not have the disease (the controls). The two groups are compared with respect to a variety of hypothesized exposures (e.g., diet, exercise habits, or use of sunscreens). Differences in exposure that are observed between the two groups may suggest why one group has the disease and the other does not. Another research method is the cohort study. In this approach, a study group free from disease is assembled and measured with respect to a variety of exposures that are hypothesized to increase (or decrease) the chance of getting the disease. Here also the researcher can identify the chances of health problems by exposing a group of particular population to a situation or conditions.

Enlargement of the Clinical Picture of Disease

When a new disease first gains the attention of health authorities, usually the most dramatic cases are the ones observed initially. One may conclude incorrectly that the new disease is an extremely acute or fatal condition; later epidemiologic studies may reveal that the most common form of the new disease is a mild, subclinical illness that occurs widely in the population. To develop a full clinical picture of the disease, thorough studies are necessary to find out about the subacute cases; an adequate study may require a survey of a complete population.

Prevention of Disease

One of the potential applications of research on disease etiology is to identify where, in the disease's natural history, effective intervention might be implemented. The natural history of disease refers to the course of disease from its beginning to its final clinical end points.

ROLE OF A NURSE IN EPIDEMIOLOGY

Epidemiology encompasses the identification of infectious disease, the vectors of transmission, the sources of contamination, the patient population exposed or involved, containment practices, and preventive measures to stop further transmission of the disease. Community health nurse deals with the people in various settings where she can aware about identification of infectious disease, it's management and prevention. The nurses should have epidemiological knowledge to make her practice fruitful. She is the person to interact directly with the individual patient and family. She plays an important role in epidemiological studies. She can interpret the study findings to families, schools, industries and others. In actual practice community health nurse is considered as the "foot soldier" in the army of epidemiology. The epidemiologist is dependent on the local community health nurses for follow up various conditions. Epidemiology is really a community health, problem-solving process, which is similar to other processes used in healthcare. A community health nurse can act as an epidemiologist or help the epidemiologist in any epidemiological investigations and planning, programming for the same.

On dealing with various communicable and non-communicable disease the role of a nurse in epidemiology can be explained in 4 aspects. These are:

1. Preventive role
2. Promotive role
3. Curative role
4. Rehabilitative role

Role in Prevention

Epidemiology is one of the basic sciences which is included in nursing. The community health nurse during working in a community deal with people in various settings and help them solve their health problems. They make the nursing process. They identify and investigate the problem, formulate and test the hypothesis regarding the causal factors, formulate alternative interventions and implement to prevent and control the problem and evaluate effectiveness of intervention.

They have an active role in the prevention and control of communicable diseases which include:

- Identify sources of infection and mode of transmission of infection.
- Health education or creating awareness to people in general.
- Having an important role in the prevention and control of chronic and non-infectious diseases, such as cardiovascular conditions, accident, cancer, etc.
- Notification of certain diseases like measles, diphtheria, tetanus, etc., to health authority.

They can also teach and supervise other workers in surveillance activities.

Role in Promotion of Health

Using knowledge of epidemiology, the community health nurses can set priorities among the health problems and plan for health programs according to the immediate health problems.

Using knowledge of epidemiology, they establish the health resources more effectively, by giving more emphasis to urgent health problems needing attention.

Plan the strategies to meet the new health needs. Nurses in the community as a member to health team participate in surveillance at all levels, which will depend on the existing situation, their preparation, and the level at which they work.

Curative Role

Community health nurse may deal with the problem independently, especially when these are the nursing problems, minor ailments or simply health conditions and they are only the health workers in a healthcare setting. They may participate as them members of team, especially when it is large scale investigation, e.g., occurrence of any epidemic. A community health nurse may participate in data collection, data analysis, planning, implementation and evaluation when an epidemiological investigation is going on or when there is a programme planning and evaluation. They may did early diagnosis and provide treatment before sending them to the hospitals. During epidemic outbreak they traces the contacts and keep them under surveillance. They also identify sources of infection and methods of spread of infection.

Role in Rehabilitation

In a community a CHN can evaluate the effectiveness of measures used to control specific disease or disorder after implementing programme. They may help people in the restoration of family and social life. They can also play a role in psychological rehabilitation by helping in restoring personal dignity and confidence of a person after any epidemiological outbreak. Community health nurse can also teach and supervise other workers in surveillance activities.

CHAPTER 4

Communication and Health Education

INTRODUCTION

Nowadays and importance is being given in preventive aspect of health service than curative aspects. Important aspects of public health service is providing counseling for areas of family planning services, preventing sexually transmitted diseases (STDs), creating awareness of the linkages between resource use and population dynamics, social marketing of contraceptives, addressing adolescent reproductive health and using entertainment to foster awareness. It is very important for a public health nurse to maintain the health status of her community by motivating them to adopt healthy behavior. This could be possible by creating awareness among people not only by using proper IEC material but also through proper behavior change communication. The awareness programme can be successful if health educator have proper communication skills.

CONCEPT OF COMMUNICATION

The word 'communication' is derived from Latin word 'communicare' which means to participate, to inform or impart. Communication can be regarded as a two-way process of exchanging or sharing ideas, feelings and information. That means to the countless ways that human have of keeping in touch with one another.

The communication is a process of sharing and exchange of information ideas/views among people. Without communication an individual could never become a human-being, without mass communication, he could never become a part of modern society.

Communication is part of our normal relationship with other people. Our ability to influence others depends on our communication skill, i.e., speaking, writing, listing, reading and reasoning.

According to John M Brion defines communication is simple and comprehensive way of transmission and receiving of information, feelings and attitudes Communication is a two way process and it is a continuous process involving interaction between two or more people. It takes place between human-beings, because man is a social animal and the only creature who can speak language is used for communication.

PURPOSES/IMPORTANCE OF COMMUNICATION

- Exchanging information regarding health
- Encouraging cooperation, coordination, good-personal relations and motivation among health workers
- Ensuring public participation in health program
- Publicity health policies, action and activities and to remove rumors
- Maintaining continues public contact
- Maintenance of health records and to receive correct reports
- Obtaining feedback from community or health workers
- Making health education effective.

PROCESS OF COMMUNICATION

The main components of communication are message, communicator, audience and the channels of communication.

Communication process passes through the following seven stages:

1. **Source sender:** Individual or article which delivers information to others.
2. **Ideas:** This is the content (message—subject matter) of communication.
3. **Encoding:** To convert content into codes (words, actions, pictures, etc.) is known as encoding.
4. **Channel:** Radio, telephone, speech, television, written message, gesture, etc. can be the channels of communication.
5. **Receiver:** It is the person for whom the message is sent.
6. **Decoding:** The opening of codes is called as decoding. It provides meaning to the received content.
7. **Feedback:** This is an answer from the receiver.

Feedback is necessary to ensure whether the message has reached in the desired form.

Communication process can also be taught through another model, that is S-M-C-R in which

S - Source M - Message C - Channel R - Receiver.

TYPES OF COMMUNICATION (FIG. 4.1)

- **On the basis of relationship:**
  - *Formal:* This is a communication given under the organizational structure

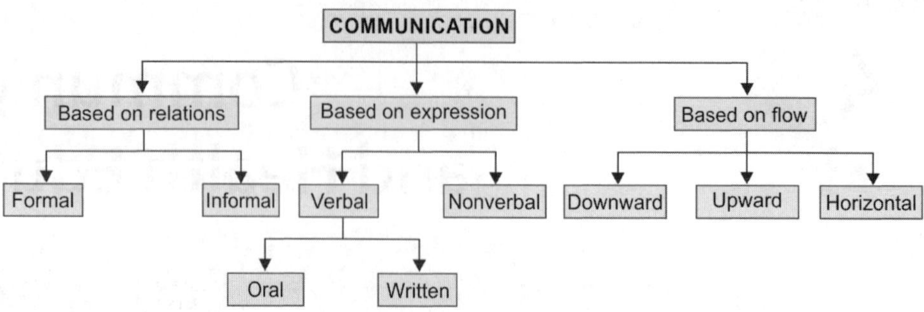

Fig. 4.1: Types of communication.

- *Informal:* This is the process in which individuals carry out social but unscheduled activities within the limits of an organization.
- **On the basis of direction or flow:**
  - *Downward communication:* This communication flows from top to bottom and the main objective is to convey orders, directives, instructions, etc.
  - *Upward communication:* This communication is from the subordinate staff to the superior, which flows in the form of reports, complaints and suggestions message runs from lower level to higher level.
- **On the basis of expression:**
  - *Nonverbal communication:* In this type of communication facial expressions, expression through eyes, touch and bodily gestures, etc., are included. Words are not used in this type of communication.
  - *Verbal communication:* In this type of written or spoken words are used for communication. Verbal communication is of two types:
    - Oral communication: This is done through conversation, telephone, interview, lecture, conference and other means but under words and absence of permanent record can dead to misunderstanding and damage.
    - Written communication: For health education, written communication is done by posters, handbook, booklets, newspaper, magicians, bulletins and notice board, etc. but the readers or viewers should be able to understand the language for effective communication.

PRINCIPLES AND BARRIERS OF COMMUNICATION

Principles of Communication

The principles of communication which should be considered by community health nurses and other health professionals in health education are as under:

- The communicator must perceive their clients health problems from their points of view before planning of health teaching
- Systematic analysis of the message, i.e., the idea, the thought to be communicated, so that one is clear about it
- Clarity of thought with simple and understandable language
- Use of two way communication
- Proper use of audio-visual aids, gestures, words and pictures
- Credibility and genuineness of communication
- Topic for health education according to requirement, feelings, beliefs and experiences of people
- Latest and reliable information
- Correct medium or method for communication
- Appropriate attention to verbal as well as nonverbal messages
- Increase communication skill, for this following steps may be fruitful:
  - Be confident in your ability to relate to people
  - Be honest with your feelings
  - Be sensitive to the needs of others
  - Be consistent and know yourself
  - Recognize symptoms of anxiety
  - Be careful in your nonverbal communication. In this position gestures, touch, physical appearance, facial expression, vocal cues, distance, etc. are included.

Barriers of Communication

Effective communication is necessary for the achievement of objectives of health education. So, many times, obstructed or faulty communication can lead to undesired results. Hence, it is necessary to know the barriers of communication. These can be as follows:

- **Linguistic barriers:** These include incorrect message, faulty translation, use of technical language, etc.
- **Psychological barriers:** These include perceptions, values and emotions, immaturity, haste, carelessness, prejudices, jealousy, lack of interest, failure of communication, poor retention power, fear, phobia, superstition, opposite thinking, etc.
- **Organizational barriers:** These include lack of organizational structure, incorrect policies, and lack of means of communication.
- **Personal barriers:** Lack of interest in communication, false promises, lack of knowledge, confidence and time, fear of criticism, hearing impairment and sensory disorder are included in this.
- **Sociocultural background:** Culture is the sum total of the learned ways of doing, feeling, and thinking. It is a form of conditioning that shows itself through behavior. Language, gestures, values, attitudes reflect cultural origin.

The influence of culture sets limits for the way people act and communicate.

HEALTH EDUCATION

Education is an important instrument of personality building, progress and awareness. Education is a process, the chief goal of which is to bring about change in human behavior. Similarly health education is the pillar of community health. Health education is related to health which provides knowledge about health to individuals and motivate them towards forming healthy habits. Health education is the process of providing information, motivation and help to maintain and adopt healthy habits and lifestyles. Health education is directly related to health behavior. So health education is defined as a part of health care that is concerned with promoting healthy behavior. It is a systematic social educational activity which has plan, organization, and evaluation. Health education spreads the knowledge related to health care to people. It assists people to understand themselves health status, recognize the factors harming health. It makes people change their ill life habits and behaviors, and adopt the behaviors and lifestyles conducive to health actively, and reduce and eliminate the health risk factors in order to prevent illness, promote health and increase the quality of life.

Definitions

Health education is a process of providing information and advice related to healthy lifestyle and encouraging the development of knowledge, attitudes and skills aimed at behavior change of individuals or communities. **—WHO**

It is a process which affects changes in the health practices of people and in the knowledge and attitude related to such changes.

It is the teaching process providing basic knowledge and practice of health, so as to be interpreted into proper health behavior.

Health education enables and influences control over own's health leading to optimalization of attitudes and habits related to lifestyle and increasing quality of life.

According to The National Conference on Preventive Medicine (USA) Health education is a process which informs, motivates and helps people to adopt and maintain healthy practices and lifestyles; advocates environmental changes as needed to facilitate this goal and conducts professional training and research to the same end.

Aims of Health Education

- Health promotion and disease prevention.
- Early diagnosis and management.
- Utilization of available health services.
  - Specific objectives of health education
- To make health an asset valued by the community.
- To increase knowledge of the factors that affect health.
- To encourage behavior which promotes and maintains health.
- To enlist support for public health measures, and when necessary, to press for appropriate governmental action.
- To encourage appropriate use of health services especially preventive services.
- To inform the public about medical advances, their uses and their limitations and adoption of new ideas or practice.

Steps of Health Education

- **Awareness:** Awareness means to know about health-related facts. It is the first step of health education process. In this stage when the health educator will provide health education the client will listen first and then he or she will be well motivated and show the interest to listen more.
- **Interests:** It is the second step of health education process. In this stage when the clients will be well motivated then only they will show the interest to know in details of health-related behavior.
- **Evaluation:** In this stage the client will analyze the advantages and disadvantages of the health education provided. They also analyze the barriers for practicing the health behavior.
- **Trial:** After analyzing the advantages and disadvantages of the health education provided when they feels health behavior has more advantageous, then they will well motivated and try to make it practices.
- **Adoption:** After practicing of health-related behavior the healthy habit will formed.

Stages for Health Education

- **Stage of sensitization:** People are sensitized of an emerging problem, like, 'AIDS causes death.' It is easy to sensitize literate population, rather than illiterate one. If people are sensitized then they become more receptive to health education messages and try to seek more information regarding the health problem.
- **Stage of publicity:** After sensitizing the media and all possible means of advertising are used to provide information to the public. The people who are receptive will absorb and understand the implications of the disease. The idea here is that people discuss among themselves and become more knowledgeable.
- **Stage of education:** This is the stage of real education for the disinterested and illiterate population. Leaders of the local community like religious leaders and teachers should be approached first then after they are convinced the communities can be educated. During this stage, simultaneous messages on TV and the media should be continued.
- **Stage of attitude change:** It is the stage when reformation of attitude takes place. People will motivated to leave their traditional unhealthy practice. This is very important stage because without change attitude the behavior change never takes place.
- **Stage of motivation and action:** In this stage real motivation will takes place.

- **Stage of community transformation:** In this stage really social changes takes places.

Contents of Health Education

- **Personal hygiene:** Personal hygiene involves those practices performed by an individual to care for one's bodily health and well-being, through cleanliness. Motivations for personal hygiene practice include reduction of personal illness, healing from personal illness, optimal health and sense of well-being, social acceptance and prevention of spread of illness to others. What is considered proper personal hygiene can be cultural-specific and may change over time. The practices that are generally considered proper hygiene include bathing regularly, washing hands regularly and especially before handling food, washing scalp hair, keeping hair short or removing hair, wearing clean clothing, brushing one's teeth, cutting finger nails, besides other practices. Some practices are gender-specific, such as by a woman during her menstrual cycle. People tend to develop a routine for attending to their personal hygiene needs. Other personal hygienic practices would include covering one's mouth when coughing, disposal of soiled tissues appropriately, making sure toilets are clean, and making sure food handling areas are clean, besides other practices. Maintenance of proper personal hygiene can help the individual to make them healthy.
- **Proper health habits:** A **habit** is a routine of behavior that is repeated regularly and tends to occur unconsciously. In the American Journal of Psychology (1903) it is defined in this way: 'A habit, from the standpoint of psychology, is a more or less fixed way of thinking, willing, or feeling acquired through previous repetition of a mental experience. Formation of healthy habits is very important in prevention of disease and promotion of health. Healthy habits include eat healthy foods, maintenance of proper hygiene, proper sleeping pattern, regular exercises and avoid stress and strain, etc.
- **Nutrition education:** Nutrition education is any combination of educational strategies, accompanied by environmental supports, designed to facilitate voluntary adoption of food choices and other food- and nutrition-related behaviors conducive to health and well-being. Nutrition education is delivered through multiple venues and involves activities at the individual, community, and policy levels. It Helps people to choose balanced diet—method of preparation, storage, taught nutrient value of food stuffs for prevention of malnutrition.
- **Personal preventive measures:** Personal preventive measures are primary prevention measures are those measures taken by individuals to protect themselves from getting a disease specially when any person suffering from any diseases. The measures includes hand washing, handling of waste and excreta, cough hygiene, etc. This is also an important area of health education.
  - Safety rules
  - Proper use of health services
  - Mental health
  - Sex education
  - Special education (occupation, mothers ...., etc.).

Principles of Health Education

Interest

It is a psychological principle that pupils do not listen to those things which are not to their interest. That is why health teaching should relate to the interests of the pupils. The pupils are not interested in health slogans such as 'take care of your health' or 'be healthy'. Health educators must find out the real health needs of the pupils.

Psychologists call them 'felt needs', i.e., 'needs', the pupils feels about themselves. If a health program will be based on 'felt needs' pupils will gladly participate in the program and only then it will be a pupils' program. The health educator will have to bring about recognition of the needs before he proceeds to tackle them.

Participation

Participation is based on the psychological principle of active learning and group discussion, panel discussion, workshop—all provide opportunities for active learning. Health education must include not only the personal element but also social. However the personal and community health are closely interlinked and interdependent. 'To live must and to live best' may be a very desirable motto for health education.

Comprehension

In health education one must know the level of understanding for which the teaching is directed. One barrier to communication is the use of words which cannot be understood. Especially in the lower grades children do not understand the meaning of health. They are not interested in it as adults.

Therefore, they should be led to practice certain health habits through concrete goals than to be imparted certain abstract rules of health which are difficult to comprehend. In community there are different levels of understanding people. So the health education should be based on their individual difference.

Reinforcement

Reinforcement is an important principle of health education repetition at intervals is extremely useful. It assists comprehension and understanding of individuals. Health education program needs reinforcement for better understanding of clients. Reinforcement not only means repetition. It may be in the form of encourage, appraise or praise for giving answer well.

Motivation

In every person there is a fundamental desire to learn. Awakening of this desire is called motivation. There are two types of motives—primary and secondary. Primary motives are sex, hunger, survival which initiate people into action. These motives are inborn desires! But secondary motives are based on desires created by the outside forces or incentive.

Some of the secondary motives are praise, love, rivalry, rewards, punishment and recognition. In health education motivation is an important factor. The incentives may be positive or negative, but the positive must be emphasized as against the negative. The people are motivated to learn by awakening them about the importance of healthy behavior you taught. Once they recognize the importance they will not only remember it but also follow it in their day to day life.

The important thing is 'what to do' and not 'what not to do' for imparting health education fear as a motive should not be used invariably. Because conduct controlled by fear is the conduct of a slave Fear of disease cannot be a goal, but to live most effectively and to serve society in the best possible way should be set up as an ideal.

Learning by Doing

Learning is an action process; not a 'memorizing' one in the narrow sense. The Chinese proverb 'If I hear, I forget, if I see, I remember, if I do, I know' illustrates the importance of learning. So health habits like other habits should be cultivated through will practice and by following certain rules rigidly. By repeatedly practicing healthy habits in the presence of health workers the general people learn the skill (e.g., handwashing) forever.

Known to Unknown

For imparting health education, one should proceed from the known to the unknown, one should start where the community people are and with what they understand and then proceed to new knowledge. The existing knowledge of the group should be used as pegs on which to hang new knowledge. In this way systematic knowledge is built-up. New knowledge will bring about a new enlarged understanding which can give. Rise to an insight into the problem participation. For example, before starting to ORS explain them regarding diarrhea.

Good Human Relations

Health educator should have a good human relation skill. Without good human relation skill he cannot develop trust among the people. He/She should have good personal qualities, should have a kind and sympathetic attitude and should be able to maintain friendly relations with people word of praise, love. Before starting any health education program developing good human relation is very important. A good human relation helps the health educator to address the needs of the people and can maintain a trust worthy relationship to own the confidence which is very essential success of the program.

Leaders

Community leaders can be used to reach people of the community and to convince them about the need for health education. The leaders may be political leader or social leader or leaders from any religious group, etc. In a community the people have well acceptance and trust on their leaders. So the health worker before starting any program have a meeting with community leaders and explain them the purpose of the program.

Methods and Approaches of Health Education

Health education is carried out at three main levels; individual, group and general public through mass media of communication. For effecting changes in "attitudes and behaviors", we rely on individual and group approach **(Fig. 4.2)**.

- Individual approach.
- Group approach.
- General approach/mass.

Individual Health Education

Health education at individual level is done to help individual to learn and assimilate health information to modify/change his/her attitude and behavior. There are many opportunities for individual health education. The methods mainly included:

- Personal interviews in the consultant room of the doctor.
- Health care center.
- The homes of the people.

The individual comes to the doctor or health care center because of illness. So opportunity is taken in educating regarding diet, nature of illness, causes of illness and its prevention, personal hygiene, environmental hygiene. The nursing staffs have also very important opportunities for undertaking health education.

Doctors and nurses, who are in direct contact with patients and their relatives, have opportunities for much individual health education. The community health nurse should not miss any opportunity during home visit to give a health message.

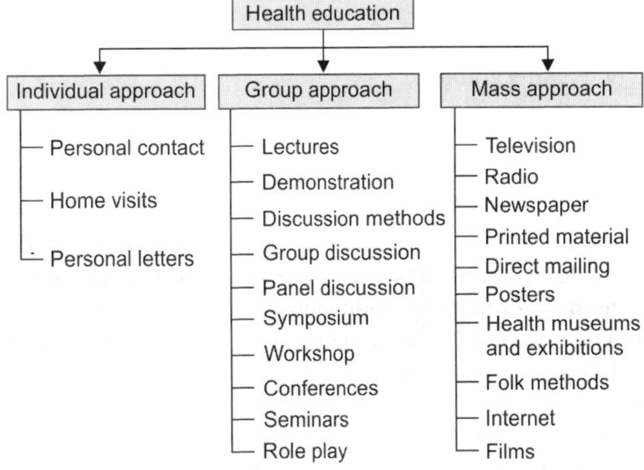

Fig. 4.2: Methods and approaches of health education.

The biggest advantage of individual health teaching is that we can discuss, argue and persuade the individual to change his behavior. The disadvantage is that the numbers we reach are small.

Group Health Education

The groups are many—mothers, school children, patients, industrial workers—to whom we can direct health teaching. The choice of subject in group health teaching is very important; it must relate directly to the interest of the group. For instance, mothers may be taught about baby care; school children about oral hygiene; a group of TB patients about tuberculosis, and industrial workers about accidents.

Group teaching is very effective way of educating a community. The choice of subject is very important in health teaching and subject must be the interest of the group. The methods of group teaching are given below:

Lectures

- A lecture may be defined as carefully prepared oral presentation of facts, organized thought and ideas by a qualified person.
- The chalk and talk communication has still a very important place in small group education.
- Lectures are the most widely used method of teaching, including health education.
- It is not a good method because communication mostly "one-way". There is no opportunity for the group to participate actively in learning. The lecture should be on a topic of current health interest, based on the needs of the group; it should not exceed 15 to 20 minutes; the subject matter should not deal with more than 5 or 6 points; the group should not be more than 30.
- The effect of the lecture depends upon the personality and performance of the speaker. Lecture may arouse interest in a subject. It may stimulate a group and give them basic information upon which to act.
- Used alone, the lecture method may fail to influence the health behavior of people. The lecture method can be made effective by combining with the following audio-visual aids.
    - Films and charts.
    - Flannel graphs.
    - Exhibits.
    - Flash cards.

Group Discussions

- Group discussion is considered a very effective method of health teaching. It is a "two way" communication; people learn by exchanging their views and experiences.
- This method is useful when the groups have common interests and similar problems.
- For an effective group discussion, the group should comprise not less than 6 and not more than 20 people. The participants are all seated in a circle, so that each is fully visible to all the others.
- There should be a group leader who initiates the subject, helps the discussion in the proper manner, prevents side-conversations, encourages everyone to participate and sums up the discussion in the end.
- If the discussion goes well, the group may arrive at decisions which no individual member would have been able to make alone. It is also desirable to have a person to record whatever is discussed. The "recorder" prepares a report on the issues discussed and agreements reached.
- In a group discussion, the members should observe the following rules:
    - Express ideas clearly and concisely.
    - Listen to what others say.
    - Do not interrupt when others are speaking.
    - Make only relevant remarks.
    - Accept criticism gratefully and
    - Help to reach conclusions.
- Group discussion is successful if the members know each other beforehand, when they can discuss freely. There is a good deal of evidence that group discussion is a very effective method of bringing about changes in the health behavior of people.
- Further, when a group of people decide collectively to accept an idea and act on it, the group acceptance strengthens and reinforces and gives the individual member courage to do the same. A well conducted group discussion is usually effective in reaching the right decisions and securing desirable action.

Panel Discussions

- In a panel discussion, 4 to 8 persons who are qualified to talk about the topic in front of a large group or audience.
- The panel comprises, a chairman or moderator. The chairman opens the meeting, welcomes the group and introduces the panel speakers. He introduces the topic briefly and invites the panel speakers to present their point of view. There is no specific agenda, no order of speaking and not set speeches.
- After the main aspects of the subject are explored by the panel speakers, the audience is invited to take part.
- The discussion should be spontaneous and natural. If members of the panel are unacquainted with this method, they may have a preliminary meeting, prepare the material on the subject and decide upon the method and plan of presentation.
- Panel discussion can be an extremely effective method of education, if it is properly planned and guided.

Symposium

- A symposium is a series of speeches on a selected subject.
- Each person or expert presents an aspect of the subject briefly. There is no discussion among the symposium members unlike in panel discussion. In the end, the audience may raise questions. The chairman makes a comprehensive summary at the end of entire session.

Workshop

The workshop is the name given to a novel experiment in education.

- It consists of a series of meetings, usually four or more, with emphasis on individual work, within the group, with the help of consultants and resource personnel. The total workshop may be divided into small groups and each group will choose a chairman and a recorder.
- The individuals work, solve a part of the problem through their personal effort with the help of consultants, contribute to group work and group discussion and leave the workshop with a plan of action on the problem.
- Learning takes place in a friendly, happy and democratic atmosphere, under expert guidance. The workshop provides each participant opportunities to improve his effectiveness as a professional worker.

Role Play

- Role playing or socio-drama is based on the assumption that many values in a situation cannot be expressed in words, and the communication can be more effective if the situation is dramatized by the group.
- The group members who take part in the socio-drama enact their roles as they have observed or experienced them. The audience is not passive but actively concerned with the drama.
- They are supposed to pay sympathetic attention to what is going on, suggest alternative solutions at the request of the leader and if requested come up and take an active part by demonstrating how they feel a particular role should be handled, or the like.
- The size of the group is thought to be best at about 25. Role playing is a useful technique to use in providing discussion of problems of human relationship.
- It is a particularly useful educational device for school children. Role playing is followed by a discussion of the problem.

Demonstrations

- It is a careful prepared presentation to show how to perform a skill or procedure.
- Practical demonstration is an important technique of health education.
- We show people how a particular thing is done–using a tooth brush, bathing a child, feeding of an infant, cooking, etc.
- A demonstration leaves a visual impression on the minds of the people and is more effective than the printed word.

Mass Level Approach

Mass level approaches in health education is for creating awareness in people at large, i.e., general public. The education is done using mass media of communication. These include radio, films, television, health exhibitions, posters, health magazines, newspapers, etc.

Mass Media

Mass Media denotes a section of the media specially designed to reach a large audience. Mass level approaches in health education is for creating awareness in people at large, i.e., general public. The term was coined in the 1920s with the advent of nationwide radio networks, mass-circulation newspapers and magazines. The education is done using mass media of communication. These include radio, films, television, health exhibitions, posters, health magazines, newspapers, etc.

Definitions

Mass media are media which can be used to communicate and interact with a large number of audiences.

Any channel carrying messages to a vast widespread general audience is called Mass Media, e.g., Newspaper, magazines, TV, Radio and Internet, etc. All are mass media communication.

Types

There are different types of mass media:

1. **Print media:** Newspaper, magazines
2. **Electronic media:** CD and DVD, movies, television.
3. **New age media:** Internet.

Each of these methods has its own advantages and disadvantages.

Radio

It is the most common, effective and easily available medium, even is rural and remote areas where other media are not reachable. This media is used for education of people. There are special health programs like World Health Day, World AIDS Day, Women's Day, Environmental Day, etc. Similarly through the radio, slogans and messages like small family, breastfeeding, immunization and other health programs can be broadcasted on radio regularly in different languages and areas.

But unawareness regarding broadcasting time, sound pollution, wrong and misleading messages, excessive use and forgetting the message are some disadvantages of this method.

Films

It is a very effective and extensive medium of not only health education, but even general education. Special documentary films are produced by films, division on specific topics for imparting information. But this medium is expensive and difficult to produce which is suitable for local audience.

Television

It is the most popular and effective media for the masses to create health consciousness among people at large. Television is no more expensive and is made available even in remote places.

The disadvantages of TV include receiving wrong messages, excessive advertising, disorders of eye-sight, publicity of wrong culture, consumerization.

Computer/Internet

Health education can be made available to individuals or groups by using internet system or instructional health programs. These will have an effective role in health education of the future. All telecast programs can be safely stored by feeding in a computer and these can be used as per requirement.

Health Exhibitions/Health Fairs

There are now becoming very popular to create public awareness. In these people who visit exhibitions/fairs directly come in contact with people who display their exhibits, interact with them and come to know variety of new ideas on health matters. It is very important that the exhibitions need to be organized properly to convey the messages of interest to people which would arouse their consciousness and motivation.

Posters

The main purpose of poster is to communicate the message to masses and to achieve this purpose an idea/message should be presented in a way to attract the attention of people. To send this message to the masses these are pasted at strategic points such as health centers, corners of the railway station, inter-state bus stop to seek attention of general public. The poster should be displayed for limited time otherwise it will lose its purpose. These should be used selectively to have its impact in imparting information.

Magazines and Journals

These are useful medium of imparting information to masses who are literate. But there are not many health magazines. Some of the magazines which are used to disseminate health information include Journal of Delhi Diabetic Forum, from Delhi, Swasth Hind from Central Health Education Bureau, Health Dialogue, published by Christian Medical Association of India, Center calling in English, Hamara Ghar in Hindi and Jana Swasth Rakshak by Mass Mailing unit of Family Welfare Division of Ministry of Health and Family Welfare.

Newspaper

Newspaper is one of the most widely used mass media which imparts information on health matters regularly and in accordance with the need of the time. Many newspapers have special health columns or supplementary health magazine to cover health aspects. This medium is used only for literate people.

Leaflets, Booklets and Pamphlets

Self-instruction material in the form of leaflets, booklets, pamphlets is frequently used by specialized clinics/health centers, etc. to impart information to specific groups and people in general to create awareness and consciousness on various aspects such as diabetes, HIV/AIDS, hypertension, heart disease, immunization, etc.

Folk Media

Folk media is the creative dissemination of information through cultural and performance arts. In many rural communities in India, oral traditions are very strong and people respond to communication through puppets, folk songs, drama, story-telling, folk dances. These methods have been found very successful in communicating health messages in various developing countries.

Folk theater, dance and music are still very popular in Indian states—there is Bhavai in Gujrat, Jatra in West Bengal, Burraktha in Andhra Pradesh, Therukootha in Tamil Nadu.

Other examples of theatre include—Tamasha, Jhanki and Nautanki—there are also traditional forms of dance include Kathakali, Bhangra, etc.

In traditional societies folk media have been popularly and successfully used to disseminate messages and even to pass on wisdom of older generation to the youth.

Folk media is prepared using local skilled people available in the community. Locally produced folk media is economical and very powerful. Cost involved is minimal, people get involved and the audience identifies with them because they are from the same community, speak the same language, have same social characteristics and values. The community people get encouragement and support from each other to solve their own health problems, promote and maintain health practices. The folk media is used as mass media through radio and television.

Objectives

- To coordinate the overall communication of the community.
- To convey the current messages to the community.
- To motivate the community development.
- To make more participation and cooperation for the community development.

Characteristics of Folk Media

- Its impact is much deeper.
- It is very useful for community development.
- No threat of cultural colonialism and foreign ideological domination.
- These media are comparatively cheap.
- Local talent and localized message would have more credibility than those centralized ones.
- Available to all and enjoyed by persons of different age groups at very low cost.

Advantages

- Being close to the people at the local level, these channels are potentially useful in the service of social concerns, as determined by local, provincial or national authorities themselves. They are more over abundantly present in areas where mass media technology has not been fully or effectively developed to capture sustained interest at local, provincial or national levels. Folk media personal forms of entertainment and communication. This is important because behavioral changes are most easily brought about by personal interaction.

- Another advantages of the traditional folk media is that they attract people who might not attend an educational meeting.

Approaches of Health Education

Regulatory Approach

Regulatory approaches require government agencies to restrict or direct the activities of regulated parties using terms and conditions within statutory and regulatory instruments, operating permits, licences, approvals or codes of practice. These may be specified for a whole sector or for an industrial process that is used across several sectors.

In this approach the society or the government seeks to protect health of the people through law and enforcement. Administrators make the rule and expect the community to accept and implement it. This approach is useful only in short-term or emergency situations. The impact is usually low in long term and thins out when the enforcement is withdrawn. The enforcement requires infrastructure and involves considerable cost.

Regulatory approaches range widely. Some are very restrictive tools that provide little flexibility, with government dictating the behavior for regulated parties to comply with environmental regulations. In contrast, innovative regulatory approaches allow parties more latitude in selecting the best means to comply with rules. Regulatory approaches are highly dependent on deterrents and, as a result, effective enforcement is essential to their success in achieving environmental goals.

Service Approach

Another form of "top down" approach is provision of health promotion services by the society or the government free of cost expecting the community to adopt and practice them. These approach aimed providing all types of health services needed by the people on their door steps based on the assumption that people would use them to improve their health status. Often these services initiated are not in tune with the "felt needs" of the people and thus never get accepted. For example when water sealed latrines provide by Government at free of cost but not used by people because they have not understood the importance of that. Hence it can be stated that, the service approach will be a failure when it is not based on the "felt needs" of the people.

Educational Approach

The educational approach is considered as one of the important means for bringing about changes in the health practices of people and helping them to recognize their health need. There are many problems which can be solved by proper education (example: Cessation of smoking, use of safe water and changing of habits, etc.) It involves proper communication and motivation of the community to make the right decision in order to attain health. Though it is a good method, it is a slow perseverance to have permanent and enduring results.

Primary Health Care Approach

This is new approach to health education starting from people with their full participation and active involvement in planning and delivering of health services based on the principle of primary health care, i.e., community involvement and intersectoral coordination. The underlying objective is to make the people about self-reliant of health.

INFORMATION EDUCATION AND COMMUNICATION

Information, education and communication (IEC) are interrelated. Education is obtained through information and communication; while education is a great source of information on the other hand, communication is a link for education and information. John M Last defines health education as "the process by which individuals and groups of people learn to behave in a manner conducive to the promotion, maintenance or restoration of health. This assumes that knowledge determines attitudes and attitudes in turn influences the behavior.

Education alone is not sufficient to initiate a behavior change because the target population requires access to proven preventive measures. In order to plug the existing gaps in health education, IEC came into practice in the early 1990s. IEC as stated by the World Health Organization "is an approach which attempts to change or reinforce a set of behaviors in a target audience regarding a specific problem in a predefined period of time". IEC activities were concerned with carrying out research on audiences to determine an effective way of delivering the appropriate information. It caters to the different needs of the people through various communication tools such as posters, brochures, radio broadcasts, and TV spots.

Definitions

IEC can be defined as an approach which attempts to change or reinforce a set of behaviors in a target audience regarding a specific problem in a predefined period of time.

IEC is the process learning that empowers people to make informed decisions and modify behaviors to attain a better standard of health.

An operational definition of 'IEC' refers to a public health approach aiming at changing or reinforcing health-related behaviors in a target audience, concerning a specific problem and within a predefined period of time, through communication methods and principles.

Aims of IEC

- To change the health behavior of individuals, family and community.
- To prepare background or basis for change in health behavior.
- To motivate or to adopt the health attitude.
- To change the norms of community.
- To facilitate education for audience about public health and to create awareness in public opinion.
- To obtain or garner social, political support for health activities.

The primary function of health communication is to provide scientific knowledge or information to people about health problems and how to maintain and promote health. People rarely seek such information although they have a right to know the facts about health and disease. Information should be easily accessible to the people. The Government, the media and health providers have an important social responsibility to provide factual and balanced health and health-related information to the people and awaken their interest on the basis of which they can make informed decisions. The cultural values, beliefs and norms of the people influence their acceptance of health information. Health information can be communicated through many channels to increase awareness and assess the knowledge of different population about various issues, products and behavior, channels might include interpersonal communication or mass media communication. Health information is an integral part of the national health system. It is a basic tool of management and a key input for the progress of any society.

The information gathered through the needs assessment provides the framework for the development of suitable IEC activities. Any activities and materials must always be culturally sensitive and appropriate.

Principles of Designing an IEC Program Activity

Activity to be based on Needs Assessment

When IEC program is planned, it should be planned based on their needs. To plan effective interventions, you must find out what are the needs of the people. What they know about various issues, including their ideas about: what causes sickness and disease and what maintains health, health care, traditional medicine, and reproductive health. It is important to build a relationship of trust and mutual respect in order to get accurate and complete information about sensitive issues. It is usually necessary to use multiple methods in undertaking a thorough needs assessment. Focus groups, individual interviews or Knowledge, Attitude, Behavior and Practice (KABP) surveys can be valuable ways to gather information. Only after there is an accurate picture of the individuals' knowledge, attitudes, behaviors, expectations and aspirations of health needs based on that you can determine the program to be best suited according to its needs.

Predetermine Clear Goals

There should be clear set of goals/objectives.

Goal

This is a broad statement of what you would like to see accomplished with the target audience in the end. Establish behavioral objectives that will contribute to achieving the goal. Objectives can be broadly defined as a general statement which attempts to give both shape and direction to set of more detailed intention for the future.

An Objectives must be SMART

S—Specific (What and Who)
M—Measurable (Something which can be measured)
A—Area Specific (Where)
R—Realistic (Achievable)
T—Time bound (When).

Assess the Influence of Underlying Social, Cultural, Environmental Condition

Underlying social, cultural, environmental condition can influence on the health status of the society because the culture has a strong impact on health belief and practices and it is very difficult to change it is. Influence of this must be considered. Before planning any program, i.e., in a program for prevention of malnutrition, we cannot force the people to take non-vegetarian items those are vegetarian people.

Proper Selection of Activities

Activities should have appropriate context. During the planning of any program there will be sufficient reason for selection of activities. There may be varieties of alternatives of any program during planning. During program planning there may be varieties of alternatives but the activities will be selected should have appropriate and sufficient background. All aspect of the activity must be coordinated and well-planned and focus should be on the target group. Activities must be linked with the availability of the support and resources.

Development of Appropriate Content of the Message

The content of the message and media must be complementary to each other. Training of the status on using the media may be considered. Always positive message should be emphasized and the content must reflect the nature and quality of the services available. Development and refinement of messages from time to time is necessary. Example of positive massage is 'Using condom You can prevent HIV, AIDS.' Negative massage having same meaning but we should never use it. 'Avoiding condom we can get HIV, AIDS.'

Participation of Target Group is Essential

During selection objectives the group will be selected for whom the massage will be develop. For example for MCH program the target groups are mothers and children.

Specially in any IEC program the target groups should be actively participated. If the target group is realized and participated then achievement is possible.

Provision for Periodic Evaluation should be Made

For any planned program, evaluation is essential to find out the effectiveness of the program. Periodic evaluation should be made to find out the behavior changes among the target group. Service provider must be respond to any demand that may be created by the people for effective IEC program.

The Essentials of IEC

Information, education and communication (IEC) combines strategies approaches and methods that enable individuals, families, groups, organizations and communities to play active roles in achieving, protecting and sustaining their own health. IEC activities not only need to have an appropriate context in which they are shaped, but it is crucial that health services providers be prepared to respond to any demand that may be created as a result of effective IEC activities. The influence of underlying social, cultural, economic and environmental conditions on health are also taken into consideration in the IEC processes. Identifying and promoting specific behaviors are desirable and usually the objectives of IEC efforts.

Steps in Developing IEC Activities

- The information gathered through the needs assessment provides the framework for the development of suitable IEC activities. Any activities and materials must always be culturally sensitive and appropriate. These are the major steps you should follow when designing an IEC activity.
- Conduct a need assessment
- Set goals and objectives in behavioral terms
- Establish behavioral objectives that will contribute to achieving the goal
  - Develop IEC materials and messages
    - Short, accurate, clear, relevant message
    - Repeated reinforcement to be done
    - Several version of same message
    - Suitable method and channel to selected.
  - Identify the potential barriers and ways to overcome
  - Identify the potential supports, resources and seek support as necessary
  - Establish an evaluation plan.

IEC Messages

- Develop IEC message. A good massage is short, accurate and relevant. It should be disseminated in the language of the target audience and should use vocabulary appropriated for that audience. The message tone may be humorous, deductive, authoritative, rational or emotionally appearing.
- Pretesting by trying out the materials with small groups from your larger target audience is an essential part of developing message and educational materials. It is through pretesting that you will ensure that people understand the message as intended, pretesting may need to be repeated frequently until you are sure your information is being conveyed as desired.

Determine suitable methods and channels of action and communication. Once the target audience is identified and researched and the key massage have been chosen. It is time to decide which media and combination of information channels will reach the target group. Both formal and informal groups can be targeted. Different channels to different jobs. Each has its own strengths and weakens, depending the role it will take in the communication program. The choice of messages and media will be influenced by many factors: cost, literacy levels, artistic style within the community, familiarity with and extent of penetrating of a particular medium for both service providers and users, and availability of the medium in the target populations community.

The development and reinforcement of messages and the choice of the communication channel or medium are inseparable. Very different messages will be developed for different media, for example radio, stories, poems, songs, posters or flip charts, for the nature of the medium affects what messages can be successfully used. The skills of those using the materials must also be considered. It may be necessary to provide training to those staff expected to use the material, for example it is important to recognize that placing a picture or poster on a clinic wall at which people may or may not look is quite different from using a series of pictures in the form of a flip chart as an educational tool in a group setting.

IEC Strategy

Any IEC strategy should be well planned, properly implemented, continuously monitored and timely evaluated for getting the best results.

Planning a Strategy

- Make comprehensive strategy. That means objectives should be clear, client centered and undertaking audience segmentation
- Know the community traditions
- Give emphasis on long-term capacity building
- Plan sufficient time, to foster changes in social and behavioral norms
- Link the IEC programs with healthcare service delivery program
- Plan for creation of such message that are salient, action oriented and attractive
- Focus IEC on most essential issues and their should be appropriate message for each audience
- Combine mass media with community, small group and individual activities for more effective campaign.
- Select appropriate timings for campaign

- Always emphasize positive behavior change
- Try to avoid information overloading especially when the umbrella campaign is to be carried out.

Implementing a Strategy

- Take support of community leaders. The use of opinion leaders and decision makers can enhance the success of an IEC project
- Involve the target audience actively in the design, implementation and monitoring of project, establish linkage with traditional healers, local NGOs and local support groups
- The interaction between health care provides at all levels and client is important element for successful IEC intervention
- A media campaign should use various broadcast and channels including TV, Radio, Print and traditional media in order to achieve maximum impact
- To spread message or for inaugural events, local holidays and festivals are more advantageous
- Logos and symbols should be pretested before launching. This is the outcome of IEC campaign that Red Ribbon symbolizes the international struggle around the HIV/AIDS
- In spite of expensive and elaborate products, simple, inexpensive, print materials can be more cost effective and useful
- IEC material should be distributed with distribution of relevant health commodities
- Along with the IEC team, non IEC professionals must be trained thoroughly for better implementation of IEC campaigns.

Monitoring and Evaluation of Strategy

- As a part of management information system (MIS) documentation of IEC programs inputs and experiences is important for knowing the success and failure
- Evaluation of IEC campaign should be considered from the very beginning
- Inexpensive methods like observation can be used for monitoring the campaign
- Carefully constructed and extreme specific questions should be asked for an evaluation. Both primary message and secondary message must be analyzed and distinguished properly
- The research and evaluation team should be well known about IEC project, for which they are engaged
- Evaluation framework should be responsive to program needs. It should provide information and feedback to program team to make corrections and adjustment in project during implementation phase and also in redesign it.

IEC activities were concerned with carrying out research on audiences to determine an effective way of delivering the appropriate information. It caters to the different needs of the people through various communication tools such as posters, brochures, radio broadcasts, and TV spots. It takes for granted that creating awareness will automatically leads to action and is made with the assumption that one size fits all. IEC gradually evolved to BCC and it is a part of BCC. IEC is substantially concerned with awareness generation while BCC goes one-step forward and its action-oriented.

BEHAVIOR CHANGE COMMUNICATION

Behavior means responses or reactions or acting in any situation. Change means act of changing or to become different or to modify. Behavior change can refer to any modification of human behavior. These days the most common term used in public health is Behavior Change Communication (BCC), a broad range of activities and approaches which focus on the individual, community, and environmental influences on behavior. Behavior is the range of actions and mannerisms made by humans or any organisms, systems, or artificial entities in conjunction with their environment, which includes the other systems or organisms around as well as the physical environment. It is controlled by a number of factors both internal and external. Sometime particular behavior can be injurious to health and lead to disorders.

Treatment of behavior-related diseases like HIV, non-communicable diseases is expensive but the cost of behavior change interventions is low. Change in behavior is emerging as an important strategy of prevention and control of many diseases specially non-communicable diseases and addictions. For example, in case of a diabetic disease, patient and their families have to access correct information about the disease, complications, treatment, advantages of lifestyle modification, available healthcare services. Information alone is insufficient to support behavior change. Influencing healthy behaviors and creating a supportive social environment is also important. It requires desire for learning and participation of patient, family and community. This type of behavior change communication will work when actions, messages and materials are planned with a goal in mind to educate people about diabetes and how to take care and where to go, etc.

Before individuals and communities change their behaviors, they must first understand basic facts about diabetes, change lifestyle, know importance of modifying diet, regular exercise and be given access to services. They must have social support of family and community for behavior change.

Behavior Change Communication (BCC) is an essential component of development. However, society-wide change is slow. Majority of researchers of health communication insist on behavior change programs that aims at increasing knowledge, stimulating dialogue, promoting attitude change, reducing stigma, improve skills etc. Scutchfield and Keck (2003) insist that the success of communication is determined by a variety of factors that may include: how much access the target audience has to information, whether the target audience has acquired sufficient knowledge and skills to perform the behavior among others. BCC is an effective communication approach which helps to promote changes in knowledge, attitudes, norms, beliefs and behaviors.

Definition

Behavior Change Communication (BCC) is an interactive process with communities to develop specific messages and methods using a variety of communication routes or pathways to develop positive behaviors; promote and maintain individual, community and societal behavior change.

Behavior Change Communication (BCC) is a communication strategy which encourages individual/community to change their behavior. It is a strategy that triggers people/society/communities to adopt healthy, beneficial and positive behavioral practices.

BCC is an interactive process with communities (as incorporated with a general program) to create custom-fitted messages and methodologies utilizing an assortment of correspondence channels to create positive practices; advance and support individual, network and cultural conduct change; and keep up suitable practices.

Importance of BCC

- **Increase knowledge:** BCC can ensure that people are given the basic facts about any disease condition or consequence of open field defecation when educator want to change the behavior of people in a language or visual medium which will increase their knowledge.
- **Community discussion:** BCC can encourage community discussions on the basic facts of disease conditions or any other factors which relate to it which will create more awareness among them.
- **Promote attitude change:** BCC can lead to appropriate attitudinal changes which we target for. For example, perceived complications of diabetes, prevention of communicable diseases like COVID-9, or use of toilet, etc.
- **Reduce stress of patient and family:** Provide information about the treatment, facilities, services in government and private health sector and self-help groups.
- **Create a demand for information and services:** BCC can urge individuals and communities to demand information on the area which information has been given for behavior change.
- **Promote services for prevention, care and support:** BCC can promote services for individuals and their family members; support groups for any type of diseases like HIV/AIDS, diabetics treatment and care and also any type of emerging diseases like COVID-19, etc.
- **Improve skills and make patient independent:** BCC programs can focus on teaching or reinforcing new skills and behaviors, such as regular exercise, modifying diet, taking insulin injection, precautions when alone or driving or traveling incase of DM or positive living, safe sex practice and prevention of opportunistic infections in case of HIV/AIDS. This will help in building confidence and taking decisions independently. BCC helps to trigger and stimulate people for adopting positive behavioral approaches.
- **More sustainable and acceptable:** BCC approaches are more sustainable and acceptable because it helps in modifying attitudes. By this approach message can be reach near the people by a variety of communication routes or pathways to develop positive behaviors; promote and maintain individual, community and societal behavior change which will be sustainable. It improve aptitudes and feeling of self-adequacy.

Human Behavior

In order to understand human behavior let us see how the perception of human being has changed from time to time. All organizations are composed of individuals, with different personality, attitudes, values, perception, motives, aspirations and abilities. The main reason to understand behavior is that individuals are different. No two individuals are similar. Before we proceed to understand human behavior, it is better to know what the term `behavior' means. Most people use the word 'behavior' means our conduct means behave in a particular way but behavior is anything that a person does. In psychology, behavior is regarded as any observable activity by human being. Most human behavior results from a combination of factors such as culture, attitudes, emotions, values, ethics, authority, rapport, persuasion, coercion and genetics. Behavior is the manner in which a person behaves, whether they can conform to the accepted social standards or not. Normal behavior means that which follows the rule or pattern or standard as set by the society; Word 'NORMAL' derived from the Latin word 'norma-' which means rule. When an individual is able to function adequately and performs daily living activities efficiently and feels satisfied with his lifestyle, he is said to have normal behavior. Human behavior is very much unpredictable. In behavior we cannot assume one set pattern of behavior. Lavitt classified behavior as: (i) Caused behavior, (ii) Motivated behavior, (iii) Goal oriented behavior. From these observations it can be understood that behavior is a dependent factor. By understanding behavior one can predict, direct, change and control behavior of individuals or group. There are generally four basic assumptions regarding nature of people: individual differences, a whole person, caused behavior (motivation) and value of the person (human dignity). Understanding past behavior is important for developing effective human skills, and it also provides a framework for predicting behavior. It also gives an idea to managers as to how behavior is similar in certain circumstances and changing in changing environmental condition. Behavior is the result of interaction between individual characteristics and the characteristics of the environment in which the behavior occurs. Each person has a unique combination of characteristics. Some of these characteristics are present from birth; others develop over time. These can be called as inherited and learned characteristics.

Characteristics of Normal Behavior

- A perception of reality.
- A positive attitude toward one's own self, accepting weaknesses and taking pride in strengths.
- Adequate in work, play and leisure.
- Willing to use problem solving approaches in life process.
- Capacity to adapt oneself to current situation.
- Capacity for withstanding anxiety and stress.

Principles of Human Behavior

- Almost all human behavior is learned.
- All behavior occur for a reason.
- No behavior occur "out of blue."
- Behavior continue to occur because they are effective.
- Behavior stop occurring when they are ineffective.

HEALTH BELIEF MODEL

The health belief model (HBM) is based on the understanding that a person will take a health-related action if that person feels that a negative health condition can be avoided and has a positive expectation that by taking a recommended action. The model defines the key factors that influence health behaviors as an individual's perceived threat to sickness or disease (perceived susceptibility), belief of consequence (perceived severity), potential positive benefits of action (perceived benefits), perceived barriers to action, exposure to factors that prompt action (cues to action), and confidence in ability to succeed (self-efficacy). When a health communicator want to change the behavior of the people he/she has to change the individual perception by giving importance on perceived benefits aspects to increase likelihood of taking positive action **(Fig. 4.3)**.

The HBM says a person will perform a health-related action if that person feels that a negative health condition can be avoided and has a positive outcome can achieved by accepting recommended action than he/she will avoid a negative health condition, i.e.,using condoms will be effective at preventing HIV, and believes that he/she can successfully take a recommended health action (i.e., he/she can use condoms comfortably and with confidence). People can vary greatly in regards to their perception of susceptibility. On one extreme are individuals who completely deny any possibility of acquiring the disease. In the middle are people who admit to the possibility of acquiring disease, but believe it will not likely happen to them. At the other end, people who are so fearful of acquiring the disease that they believe that they will in all probability acquire it. The more susceptible a person feels, the greater the likelihood they will take preventive measures. For example: In cancer control program for promotion of breast self-examination, the individual has to perceive herself for suspectable to breast cancer and the consequence/seriousness of it, then only she can practice it. In this program the Nurse has to teach them regarding breast self-examination, it's exact technique and benefits, ability to detect cancer an other diseases early. The health educator also can teach them on feeling good about oneself, feeling in control of one's health, and feeling more responsible toward oneself and one's family. In using this construct, health educators need to specify the exact action to be taken and specify the advantages or benefits that would result from that course of action. The health belief model is concerned with what people perceive, or believe, to be true about themselves in relation to their health.

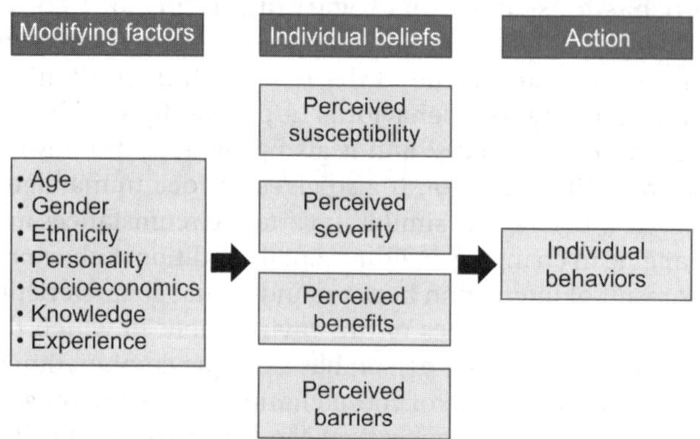

Fig. 4.3: Health belief model.

This model is based on components of individual perceptions of threat of a disease:

- **Perceived susceptibility to a disease:** It is the subjective belief that a person may acquire a disease or enter a harmful state as a result of a particular disease. It is the belief that one either may or may not contract a disease. The belief ranges from being afraid of contracting a disease to completely denying that certain behaviors will result in illness. For example, one person who smokes cigarettes may believe he or she is at danger for lung cancer and may stop smoking, while another person may believe smoking poses no serious threat and continues to smoke.
- **Perceived seriousness of a disease:** Belief in the extent of harm that can result from the acquired disease or harmful state of a particular behavior. This component is related to how much the person knows about the disease and can result in a change in health behavior.
  If a person who smokes believes that lung cancer can lead to physical disability or death and would, therefore, affect his or her ability to work and care for the family, the person is more likely to stop smoking.
- **Perceived benefits:** Perceived benefits is the belief in the advantages of the methods suggested for reducing the risk or seriousness of the disease of harmful state from a particular behavior is concerned with how effective the individual believes measures will be in preventing illness. This factor is influenced by:
  - The person's conviction that carrying out a recommended action will prevent or modify the disease.
  - The person's perception of the cost and unpleasant effects of performing the health behavior. For example, the person may believe that stopping smoking will prevent future breathing problems and that the initial withdrawal symptoms can be overcome; therefore, the person may stop smoking.

- **Perceived barriers:** Perceived barriers means the perceived impediments to taking action to improve a health condition. Barriers are mainly resources, previous believes and other resistances. Sometimes the new behavior will take too much time. The health educator should encourage the people and motivating them to overcome these barriers.
- **Cues to action:** Cues to Action are the causes or forces that would make a person feel the need to take action. Demographic variables (such as age and gender):
  - Sociopsychological variables (such as personality and peer group pressure).
  - Structural variables (such as knowledge and prior contact with the disease).

These factors interact to influence the perceived benefits of preventive action minus the perceived barriers to preventive action.

HBM has been adapted to explain and predict a variety of long- and short-term health behaviors:

1. Preventive behavior
2. Illness behavior
3. Sick role behavior.

BCC Ways to Influence Human Behavior

To influence behavior certain ways may be kept in mind as given:

- **Support:** The communicator should be act as a support system for the community people when changing their behavior. He/she should be always ready to solve the problem of the people and provide support specially in the form of service as per their needs along with appropriate information. The examples of services based on their needs are services like distribution of iron folic acid tablets or distributions of conventional contraceptives.
- **Inform:** Inform, advise or educate or otherwise build awareness, is very much important to adopt healthy behavior. Repeatedly by sharing health message a communicator can influence human behavior by repeatedly persuasion.
- **Legislation:** Legislation is the process or product of enrolling, enacting, or promulgating law by a legislature, parliament, or analogous governing body. Through legislation also the behavior can be changed some extends, e.g., Avoidance of smoking in public place or following traffic rules legislate, regulate, enforce with police will force people to adopt health promoting behavior.
- **Design:** Set environmental and physical context, design, engineer, availability, distribution of infrastructure in such a way that people are enabled to take action.

Steps of Behavior Change Through Behavior Change Communication

People proceed from lack of knowledge (unawareness) to gain in knowledge which is achieved with efforts on the part of health worker and the receiver of the message. There are some steps through which behavior changes takes places by BCC activities, these are as follows:

- **Knowledge:** Knowledge/Awareness means to know about health-related facts. It is the first step of behavior change process. In this step, one first learns about a new behavior and recalls messages and understands meaning of the messages.
- **Interests and approval:** It is the second step of behavior change process. In this stage when the clients will be well motivated then only, they will show the interest to know in details of health-related behavior. One then approves of the new behavior and responds favorably to messages. The person discusses the information with personal network (professional, colleagues, family and friends). Later he himself approves of the practices.
- **Intention:** One then believes this behavior is beneficial to them and intends to consult the provider. The person recognizes that the strategies can meet a personal need. The person intends to adopt these practices in future.
- **Practice:** The person goes to provider of information/supplies/services. One then attempts new behavior and continues to practice. This use to happen after analyzing the advantages and disadvantages of health messages.
- **Advocacy:** One can then promote the new behavior through their social or professional networks as a satisfied practitioner. He experiences and acknowledges personal benefits of adopting behavior and advocates it to others and supports the program in the community, e.g., A diabetic person develops habit of regular monitoring of blood sugar which helped him in diabetes control for himself, will tell other diabetic persons to do so. After practicing of health-related behavior the healthy habit will formed.

The Process of Behavior Changes within the Individual

Change within the individual might not come easily, but psychologists have developed effective ways to help people change their behavior. Therapists, physicians, and teachers use these techniques. Researchers have also proposed theories to explain how change occurs. Understanding the elements of change, the stages of change, and ways to work through each stage can help you achieve your goals.

- **The elements of change:** For changing our behavior everyone need to understand the three most important elements in changing a behavior.
- **Readiness to change:** Whether have the resources and knowledge to make a lasting change successfully?
- **Barriers to change:** Is there anything preventing you from changing?
- **Likelihood of relapse:** What might trigger a return to a former behavior?

Stages of Change Model

One of the best-known approaches to change is the Stages of Change or Transtheoretical Model, introduced in the late 1970s by researchers James Prochaska and Carlo

DiClemente. This model evolved through studies examining the experiences of smokers who quit on their own with those requiring further treatment to understand why some people were capable of quitting on their own. It was determined that people quit smoking if they were ready to do so. Thus, the Transtheoretical Model (TTM) focuses on the decision-making of the individual and is a model of intentional change. The TTM operates on the assumption that people do not change behaviors quickly and decisively. Rather, change in behavior, especially habitual behavior, occurs continuously through a cyclical process. The TTM is not a theory but a model; different behavioral theories and constructs can be applied to various stages of the model where they may be most effective.

The TTM posits that individuals move through six stages of change: precontemplation, contemplation, preparation, action, maintenance, and termination. Termination was not part of the original model and is less often used in application of stages of change for health-related behaviors. For each stage of change, different intervention strategies are most effective at moving the person to the next stage of change and subsequently through the model to maintenance, the ideal stage of behavior.

In this model, change occurs gradually and relapses are an inevitable part of the process. People are often unwilling or resistant to change during the early stages, but they eventually develop a proactive and committed approach to changing a behavior. This model demonstrates that change is rarely easy. It often requires a gradual progression of small steps toward a goal.

Stage 1: Precontemplation: In the precontemplation stage, people are not thinking seriously about changing and are not interested in any kind of help. People in this stage tend to defend their current bad habit(s) and do not feel it is a problem. They may be defensive in the face of other people's efforts to pressure them to quit. They do not focus their attention on quitting and tend not to discuss their bad habit with others. This stage is called "denial," but at Addiction Alternatives, we do not like to use that term. Rather, we like to think that in this stage people just do not yet see themselves as having a problem

Stage 2: Contemplation: In the contemplation stage people are more aware of the personal consequences of their bad habit and they spend time thinking about their problem. Although they are able to consider the possibility of changing, they tend to be ambivalent about it. In this stage, people are on a teeter-totter, weighing the pros and cons of quitting or modifying their behavior. Although they think about the negative aspects of their bad habit and the positives associated with giving it up (or reducing), they may doubt that the long-term benefits associated with quitting will outweigh the short-term costs. It might take as little as a couple weeks or as long as a lifetime to get through the contemplation stage. In fact, some people think about giving up their bad habit and may die never having gotten beyond this stage. On the plus side, people are more open to receiving information about their bad habit, and more likely to actually use educational interventions and reflect on their own feelings and thoughts concerning their bad habit.

Stage 3: Preparation/Determination: In the preparation/determination stage, people have made a commitment to make a change. Their motivation for changing is reflected by statements such as: "I have got to do something about this—this is serious. Something has to change. What can I do?" This is sort of a research phase: people are now taking small steps toward cessation. They are trying to gather information (sometimes by reading things like this) about what they will need to do to change their behavior. Or they will call a lot of clinics, trying to find out what strategies and resources are available to help them in their attempt. Too often, people skip this stage: they try to move directly from contemplation into action and fall flat on their faces because they have not adequately researched or accepted what it is going to take to make this major lifestyle change.

Stage 4: Action/Willpower: This is the stage where people believe they have the ability to change their behavior and are actively involved in taking steps to change their bad behavior by using a variety of different techniques. This is the shortest of all the stages. The amount of time people spend in action varies. It generally lasts about 6 months, but it can literally be as short as one hour! This is a stage when people most depend on their own willpower. They are making overt efforts to quit or change the behavior and are at greatest risk for relapse. Mentally, they review their commitment to themselves and develop plans to deal with both personal and external pressures that may lead to slips. They may use short-term rewards to sustain their motivation, and analyze their behavior change efforts in a way that enhances their self-confidence. People in this stage also tend to be open to receiving help and are also likely to seek support from others (a very important element).

Stage 5: Maintenance: Maintenance involves being able to successfully avoid any temptations to return to the bad habit. The goal of the maintenance stage is to maintain the new status quo. People in this stage tend to remind themselves of how much progress they have made. People in maintenance constantly reformulate the rules of their lives and are acquiring new skills to deal with life and avoid relapse. They are able to anticipate the situations in which a relapse could occur and prepare coping strategies in advance. They remain aware that what they are striving for is personally worthwhile and meaningful. They are patient with themselves and recognize that it often takes a while to let go of old behavior patterns and practice new ones until they are second nature to them. Even though they may have thoughts of returning to their old bad habits, they resist the temptation and stay on track. As you progress through your own stages of change, it can be helpful to re-evaluate your progress in moving up and down through these stages.

Stage 6: Relapse: In any behavior change, relapses are a common occurrence. When you go through a relapse, you might experience feelings of failure, disappointment, and frustration. The key to success is to not let these setbacks undermine your self-confidence. If you lapse back to an old behavior, take a hard look at why it happened. What triggered the relapse? What can you do to avoid these triggers in the future? While relapses can be difficult, the best solution is to start again with the preparation, action, or maintenance stages of behavior change. You might want to reassess your resources and techniques. Reaffirm your motivation, plan of action, and commitment to your goals. Also, make plans for how you will deal with any future temptations. Resolutions fail when the proper preparation and actions are not taken. By approaching a goal with an understanding of how to best prepare, act, and maintain a new behavior, you will be more likely to succeed.

Techniques of Behavior Change (Guiding Principles in Planning Behavior Change Communications Activity)

Behavior Change Communications (BCC) can be done through following techniques:

- **Dissemination of information:** The primary function of health communication is to provide scientific knowledge or information to people about health problems and how to maintain and promote health. People rarely seek such information although they have a right to know the facts about health and disease. Information should be easily accessible to the people. The Government, the media and health providers have an important social responsibility to provide factual and balanced health and health-related information to the people and awaken their interest on the basis of which they can make informed decisions. Dissemination of information is the first technique of BCC but this should be used where the audience having lack of information. The drawback is, it is source dominated and one way.
- **Providing education:** Education is a process, the chief goal of which is to bring about change in human behavior. Health education is the process of providing information, motivation and help to maintain and adopt healthy habits and lifestyles. Providing education means not only just passing of information, but also focuses on applying knowledge in skill building techniques by demonstrations, return demonstration like preparation of ORS, or any other skill practice. It build confidence and makes behaviors convenient.
- **Motivation:** It is the driving force to achieve something. In every person there is a fundamental desire to learn. Awakening of this desire is called motivation. It is used when information is established. Different appeals are instrumental for motivation, e.g., rationale appeal, emotional appeal, threat/fear appeal, joy/fun appeal.
- **Reinforcement:** Reinforcement is here repetition of messages and their at intervals which is extremely useful. It assists comprehension and understanding so health instruction needs reinforcement, It is used to sustain behavior change for repetitive types of behaviors. Need to be used with variations. Community based resources/ mechanisms should be established to reinforce the message.
- **Social pressure:** Social pressure is also a technique for Behavior Change Communications (BCC). When person in need of health services (for example, estimation of blood glucose) but not willing to avail health services or undergo treatment is encouraged by near and dear ones to avail health services.

Some of the guiding principles for making BCC effectives are as follows:

- BCC should be integrated with program goals from the start. BCC is an essential element of disease prevention, care and support programs, providing critical linkages to other program components, including policy initiatives.
- Formative BCC assessments must be conducted to improve understanding of the needs of target populations, as well as of the barriers to and supports for behavior change that their members face (along with other populations, such as stakeholders, service providers and community).
- The target population should participate in all phases of BCC development and in much of implementation.
- Stakeholders need to be involved from the design stage.
- Having a variety of linked communication channels is more effective than relying on one specific one.
- Pre-testing is essential for developing effective BCC materials.
- Planning for monitoring and evaluation should be part of the design of any BCC program.
- BCC strategies should be positive and action-oriented.

Steps of Organizing Behavior Change Communications Program

- **State program goals:** Identifying overall program goals is the first step in developing a BCC strategy. Specific program goals are established after reviewing existing data, epidemiological information and in-depth program situation assessments.
- **Involve stakeholders:** Key stakeholders need to be involved early on in every step of the process of developing programs and their BCC components. Stakeholders include policymakers, opinion leaders, community leaders, religious leaders and members of target populations.
- **Identify target populations:** To develop communication, it is important to identify the target populations as clearly as possible. Target populations are defined as primary or secondary. Primary populations are the main groups whose behavior the program is intended to influence. Secondary populations are those groups that influence the ability of the primary population to adopt or maintain appropriate behaviors.
- **Conduct formative BCC assessments:** A formative BCC assessment should start by seeking out all available studies, including data from in-depth assessments or

rapid ethnographic assessments, behavioral surveillance surveys and other related studies. After synthesizing this information, a formative BCC assessment protocol can be developed.

The formative BCC assessment should collect information on:
- Risk situations, showing in detail how decisions are made in different situations, including what influences the decisions and settings for risk
- Why individuals and groups practice the behaviors they do, and why they might be motivated to change (or unable to change) to the desired behaviors
- Perceptions of risk and risk behaviors
- Influences on behavior, such as barriers or benefits
- Insights of opinion leaders
- Patterns of service use and opinions about these services
- Perceptions of stigma and discrimination
- Future hopes, fears and goals
- Media and entertainment habits
- Health care-seeking behaviors
- Media resources.

- **Segment target populations:** Based on the formative BCC assessment, target populations can then be segmented. Population segments are often defined by psychosocial and demographic characteristics.
- **Define behavior change objectives:** What changes in behavior does the program intend to achieve? Observable changes in behavior, as specified in the behavior change objectives, are a final program outcome. Such changes include:
  - Knowledge change
  - Attitude change
  - Environmental change
- **Design BCC strategy and monitoring and evaluation (MandE) plan:** A plan for monitoring and evaluation needs to be drawn up during the initial stage of BCC strategy design. To monitor the course of a BCC strategy properly, it is necessary to establish effective information-gathering systems. These include reports, site visits and reviews of materials. Reporting tools and protocols must be standardized to ensure consistency.
- **Develop communication products and train providers:** It is important to develop an overall theme that will appeal to and attract target populations. The theme should stem from the BCC formative assessment and further consultation.
  - The theme should be positive.
  - Avoid blaming or stigmatizing.
  - Should call attention to the campaign and link its various elements together, functioning as a sort of umbrella.
  - It should be catchy and devised in such a way that all target populations can relate to it and identify with it.

  Steps to develop the overall theme and key messages:
  - Step 1. Develop a profile of the target population from formative BCC assessment.
  - Step 2. Identify desired behavior change.
  - Step 3. Understand and take into account the varying situations that could affect action and decision-making.
  - Step 4. Identify the information or data that you want to be understood by the target population.
  - Step 5. Develop key benefit statements that take the hopes and aspirations of the target population into account.
  - Step 6. Develop messages from key benefit statements. Messages should be simple, attractive and make clear the benefits of what is being promoted, through words or images.

  Choose channels: A channel is the way a message is disseminated. It is important to know which channels can most effectively reach particular target populations. Identifying the range of available channels should be part of every formative BCC assessment.
  - Mass media—for example, television or radio spots; articles in periodicals; or material in brochures, posters, flip charts, picture codes or comics.
  - In-person, by health workers, peer educators, counsellors, or other trained personnel.
  - Musical or dramatic performances and community events.
- **Conduct pre-testing:** It is important to pre-test at every stage with all audiences for whom the communication is intended, both primary and secondary. Pre-testing should be done of themes, messages, prototype materials, training packages, support tools and BCC formative assessment instruments. Pre-testing of media, messages and themes should evaluate:
  - Comprehension
  - Attraction
  - Persuasion
  - Acceptability
  - Audience members' degree of identification
- **Implement and monitor:** In the implementation phase, all elements of the strategy go into operation. All partners, programrs and channels of the BCC strategy must be closely coordinated. There must be links among critical program elements, such as supply and demand. It is also necessary during the implementation phase to review the preceding steps in the BCC process to ascertain whether the program has been addressing the target audiences' previously identified problems and needs. This can also help identify whether behavior change and communication goals are being achieved, and whether channels are being used as wisely as possible.
- **Evaluate:** Evaluation refers to the assessment of a project's implementation and its success in achieving predetermined objectives of behavior change. Various research designs are suitable for evaluating the impact of health communication programs:
  - Randomized control group design
  - Non-equivalent control group design
  - One-group, before after design
  - Interrupted time series design

- **Elicit feedback and modify the program:** As programs evolve, target populations acquire new knowledge and behaviors, and communication needs may change. The needs of target populations must be periodically reassessed to understand where they stand along the behavior change continuum. Monitoring and evaluation studies should lead directly to modifications of the overall program, as well as of the BCC strategies, messages and approaches.

SOCIAL AND BEHAVIOR CHANGE COMMUNICATION

Social and behavior change communication (SBCC) is the systematic application of interactive, theory-based, and research-driven communication processes and strategies to address tipping points for change at the individual, community, and social levels. A tipping point refers to the dynamics of social change, where trends rapidly evolve into permanent changes. It can be driven by a naturally occurring event or a strong determinant for change—such as political will that provides the final push to "tip over" barriers to change. Tipping points describe how momentum builds up to a point where change gains strength and becomes unstoppable **(Fig. 4.4)**.

Why the shift from Behavior Change Communication (BCC) to SBCC? Over the years, there has been a shift in how health education programs think about human behaviors. Approaches to behavior change have expanded beyond a focus on the individual in order to emphasize sustainable, social change. SBCC examine the problems from their multiplezides by analyzing personal, societal, and environmental factors to find the most effective leaning points for sustainable change. While BCC can achieve individual empowerment, SBCC is also using strategies that influence the physical, socioeconomic, and cultural environment to facilitate healthy norms and choices and remove barriers to them. In some situations, advocacy or social mobilization for policy change may support stronger and more immediate permanent change than campaigns that target individual behaviors. SBCC method aims to improve advocacy or mobilization for social action, along with BCC for personal change. BCC is thus part of SBCC, while SBCC builds on BCC.

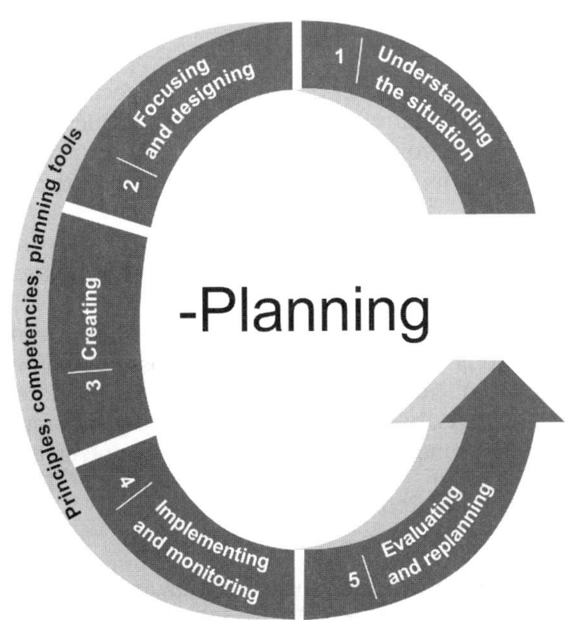

Fig. 4.4: Five steps process of SBCC.

Characteristics of SBCC

- **SBCC is a process:**
  - It is interactive, researched, planned, and strategic.
  - It aims to change social conditions and individual behaviors.
- **It uses a socioecological model:** SBCC applies a comprehensive, socioecological model to identify effective tipping points for change by examining: individual knowledge, motivation, and other behavior change communication concepts social, cultural, and gender norms, skills, physical and economic access, and legislation that contribute to an enabling environment.
- **SBCC uses three key strategies:**
  1. *Advocacy*—to raise resources as well as political and social leadership commitment to development actions and goals
  2. *Social mobilization*—for wider participation, coalition building, and ownership, including community mobilization
  3. *Behavior change communication*—for changes in knowledge, attitudes, and practices among specific audiences.

Process of SBCC

The SBCC process includes five steps shown **Figure 4.4**.

Understanding the Situation

- Identify what behavior(s) needs to be changed, who is performing the behavior(s), what are the motivating factors (drivers) and concerns* (barriers) regarding the current and desired behavior(s)
- **Identify and segment the Target Audience(s):** Target Audience(s) are the group of people whose behavior need to be changed. Identify and select the demographic characteristics of your Target Audience that differentiate them from the general population. This will help you focus on who to reach and how to reach them and engage them in your campaign.
- Identify drivers (motivating factors) and other influencing factors underlying behavior(s) you need to change
- **Create a Target Audience Profile:** To prepare the Target Audience Profile, select relevant demographic and psychographic information that will give you insights on how the Target Audience thinks, feels, and intends to act. It will help for monitoring their behavior change.

Focusing and Designing

There are three SBCC strategies to choose from:

1. **Behavior change communication:** Behavior change communication for changes in knowledge, attitudes, beliefs, and practices of specific target audiences. Behavior change communication reaches and engages the target audience through interpersonal communication (one-on-one and small group) and mass media.
2. **Social and community mobilization:** Social and community mobilization is required for wider participation, coalition building, and ownership. This can be achieved by engaging the target audience and creating an environment for the desired behavior(s) generally through commitment and participation of:
   - Professional or civic associations, groups, clubs
   - Social and business organizations or networks
   - Religious groups or associations
   - Community groups or associations
   - Political groups or associations
   - Crowdsourcing—petition or pledge website (e.g., Change.org)
3. **Advocacy:** Advocacy to raise resources and political and social leadership and commitment to actions and goals. Changes laws, policies, regulations (government and private) through support of:
   - Government decision makers, policymakers
   - Private sector decision makers
   - Donors and NGOs.

Creating

The intervention materials include key messages:

- **Develop the Key Message(s):** The Key Message is the information to be conveyed to the Target Audience to motivate them to accept the desired behavior. The Key Message addresses the key driver or motivating factors for the current behavior and communicate "Reason Why" we have to change our behavior. The key messages should communicate the consequences and risk of current behavior and the benefits that the desired behavior will which we can state as "call to action"
- **Develop the creative brief:** The creative brief is a document that will guide the creative design team or agency in designing the creative materials to communicate the Key Message.
  - A Creative Brief ensures that the materials are aligned with the campaign objectives, target audience profile, and Key Message. This is just like action plan of whole materials.
  - The creative brief has five sections:
    1. Goal and target audience
    2. Changes, barriers, and communication objectives
    3. Key message
    4. Manner and mood/tone of creative material(s)
    5. How the material(s) or activity fits into the media mix and other creative considerations.
- **Develop creative material(s):** Once the Creative Brief is prepared, the creative team or agency can now proceed with designing the creative materials. When the creative team or agency fully understands the Creative Brief, the next step will be for them to design the materials and present draft materials, e.g., storyboard of video, design of key visual, for your review and approval. The creative materials should have some criteria like command attention of publics, clarify the message, communicate a benefit (or a consequence), ensure that content within and among various materials have the same message and"look", create trust of publics and include a clear "Call to Action" in materials.
- **Pretest material(s):** Pretest messages/materials to ensure that the target audience finds the materials appealing, attractive, easily understandable, believable, relevant to their needs or situation and are motivated to act on the messages. The materials tested can be mockups of print materials or storyboards of video materials.
  A pretest will provide information on the following five elements:
  - *Appeal:* The materials and messages command attention and are attractive.
  - *Understandability:* The target audience readily understands what the material is saying without having someone else explain it.
  - *Believability:* The target audience accepts what the message/material is saying is correct and true.
  - *Relatability (resonance):* The target audience feels that the message/material is talking to them.
  - *Motivation to action:* The message/material moves the Target Audience to change their attitudes, beliefs, values and behaviors.
- **Prepare a media plan:** Prepare a media plan that will effectively reach the target audience. A media plan is the strategic use of media channels that will effectively reach and engage target audience to achieve objectives. The media plan is based on target audience and campaign budget.

Implementing and Monitoring

Implementation includes coordinates and executes planned activities and monitoring ensures that the activities are being conducted according to the time frame, using the planned inputs (quantity and quality), and producing the desired outputs.

- Inputs—items or resources needed for activities to be conducted, e.g., budget, staff, logistics, materials, expertise, and time
- Outputs—direct results of the activities, e.g., number of persons trained, number of groups oriented on the campaign, number and quality of creative materials (video, PSAs, billboards, print ads) produced, pretest of materials conducted, media placements implemented.

Evaluating and Replanning

Evaluation

- Determines whether the activities and outputs are producing desired results or outcomes based on the campaign's behavioral objectives

- Asks the question: Have we made progress against the campaign's behavioral and communication objectives?
- Can be conducted while the campaign is ongoing (mid-term evaluation) and at the end of the campaign (final evaluation) what to measure?

Behavioral objectives: Change in behaviors and practices of target audience before we can change behaviors, we need to change determinants, such as attitudes, beliefs, intentions to consume, and social norms/social acceptability etc. We also need to target and measure these changes in order to achieve our behavioral objectives based on our situation analysis and results of our baseline or pre-campaign research.

Replanning

Once the evaluation research (mid-term or end of campaign) is completed, you will have information on whether the campaign reached the right Target Audience (and how frequently), what the Target Audience recalled from the campaign, and whether those who recalled campaign messages have changed their attitudes, perception of social norms, intention to use, or self-reported use. The results from evaluation studies are generally compared between those who exposed messages or activities and those who did not recall any campaign message (not exposed to the campaign) to identify the effectiveness of the program. The data can be reviewed to determine changes to replan or strengthen the campaign.

Ten Principles of SBCC

1. Follow a systematic approach.
2. Use research (e.g., operations research), not assumptions, to drive your program.
3. Consider the social context.
4. Keep the focus on your audience(s).
5. Use theories and models to guide decisions.
6. Involve partners and communities throughout.
7. Set realistic objectives and consider cost effectiveness.
8. Use mutually reinforcing materials and activities at many levels.
9. Choose strategies that are motivational and action-oriented.
10. Ensure quality at every step.

INFORMATION SYSTEM

- The term "information system" usually refers to a computer-based system, one that is designed to support the operations, management, and decision functions of an organization.
- Information systems are "computer systems that collect, store, process, display, and communicate timely information needed in practice, education, administration and research". **—Malliarou, 2006; Malliarou et al. 2007**
- Information systems in organizations thus provide information support for decision makers. It encompasses transaction processing systems, management information systems, decision support systems, and strategic information systems.

Characteristics of Information System

- Information system cannot generate data by themselves, it can collect, record, store, process and retrieve data as per the needs of the users.
- These are designed for different levels of management.
- The information systems are facilitated with electronics equipment such as computers.
- The information systems should be integrated by the ways of databases.

Elements of an Information System

- **Hardware:** The equipment and devices for in putting, outputting secondary storage, processing as well as communication in the system.
- **Software:** The set of program to facilitate processing procedures. It includes systems software, application software and model base.
- **Database:** It is usually stored in the form of files and data bases on the physical storage media.
- **Procedures:** The operating procedures documented in the form of physical manuals constitute an information part of MIS.
- **Operating personnel:** The manpower operating these information system includes: system managers, system analysts, and data administrators, programers, and data entry and computer operators.

MANAGEMENT INFORMATION SYSTEM

A management information system (MIS) is defined as a combination of human attempts by computer to collect, store, recover information by using communication systems, it is used for improving management of organization activities. Management information systems, due to having advantages such as closer communication, more accurate control and more reliable data collection and faster processing of data and transforming them into information needed by managers are used in planning, organizing, leading and motivating, reporting and control. A MIS is an information system used for decision-making, and for the coordination, control, analysis, and visualization of information in an organization. The study of the management information systems involves people, processes and technology in an organizational context.

In a corporate setting, the ultimate goal of the use of a management information system is to increase the value and profits of the business. This is done by providing managers with timely and appropriate information allowing them to make effective decisions within a shorter period of time. Health Management Information Systems (HMIS) are one of the six building blocks essential for health system strengthening. HMIS is a data collection system specifically designed to support planning, management, and decision-making in health facilities and organizations.

'Management Information System is a system which provides management with the information it requires to monitor progress, measures performance, detect trends, evaluates alternatives, make decisions and to take corrective actions.'

—RR Durech

'Management Information System is defined as a formal system of gathering, integrating, comparing, analyzing and dispensing information internal and external to the enterprise in a timely, effective and efficient manner.'

—Koontz Harnold

'Management Information System is an integrated man machine system designed for providing information to support operational control, management control and decision-making functions in an organization.'

—Davis and Olson

Objectives of MIS

- To enhance communication among employees.
- To provide system for recording and aggregating information.
- To reduce the expenses related to employees manual activities.
- To support organization strategic goals and directions.

Purposes of MIS

- To provide management information to decision makers at various levels in the organization.
- To provide a basis to analyze warning signals that can originate both externally and internally.
- To automate routine operations thus avoiding human work in the processing tasks.
- To assist management in making routine decisions.
- To provide the information necessary to make non-routine decisions.

Uses of MIS

- To support decision-making and taking actions.
- To help to assess community needs, e.g., community needs assessment approach under RCH can make use of MIS for preparing subcentre action plans
- To prioritize the health needs
- To assess the performance of health workers or institutions like subcentre - PHC - CHC - district or state.
- To monitor program operations.
- To evaluate the program or it measure its success and failure.
- For better planning of services and programs at local level.
- To justify the resources spent (staff, money and material).
- For operational and epidemiological research purposes.
- MIS is useful for training of workers and medical officers and the supervisors.
- Helps to provide database or information to client or community whose livers it affects profoundly.

Classification of Management Information Systems

There are various types of management information systems. Mason and Swanson (1981) describe four categories of management information systems based on the level of support that the information system provides in the process of decision-making these are:

- Databank information system
- Predictive information system
- Decision-making information system
- Decision-taking information system.

Databank Information System

The responsibility of this information system is to observe, classify and store any item of data which might be potentially useful to the decision maker.

Predictive Information System

This system moves beyond pure data collection and the determination of trends over time. Predictive information systems provide for the drawing of inferences and predictions that are relevant to decision-making.

Decision-making Information System

This system goes one step further in the process of decision-making and incorporates the value system of the organization or its criteria for choosing among alternatives.

Decision-taking Information System

This is a decision system in which the information system and the decision maker are one and the same.

Implementation Method of MIS

It classify in 3 approaches, such as:

1. Direct approach
2. Parallel approach
3. Modular approach

Direct Approach

- Direct instillation of new system with immediate discontinuance of the old existing system is referred as "cold turnkey" approach. This approach becomes useful when these factors are considered.
- The new system does not replace the existing system.
- The old system is regarded absolutely no value.
- The new system is compact and simple.
- The design of new system is inexpensive with more advantages and less risk involved.

Parallel Approach

- The selected new system is installed and opened with current system. This method is expensive because of duplicating the facilities and personal maintain both systems.
- In this approach a target data is fixed when the operations of new one will operate on its own.

Modular Approach

This is generally recognized as "pilot approach" means the implementation of a system in the basis of organization on a piece-meal basis.

Advantages of MIS

- It supports and enhances the overall decision-making process.
- It enhances job performances throughout organization.
- It provides the means through which the activities can be monitored and information is distributed to the management, employees and clients.
- It provides the feedback on the effectiveness of risk control.

Disadvantages of MIS

- Unauthorized entries
- Backing
- Theft or corruption of data
- Incidence of sudden crash of the system.

Role of Nurse in Implementing MIS

- Ensure active cooperation of nurse and other allied health workers for the implementation of management information system.
- Allocate adequate resources for the implementation of management information system in the community and hospital.
- Appoint a nurse manager in each department of health to coordinate implementation of the system
- Form a team of coordinators from individual departments to encourage exchange of experience
- Provide sufficient staff in the community to assist with the implementation of MIS.
- Organize a kick-off meeting or a workshop for nurses and other health workers working in the community to provide them with information on new procedures, nurses' responsibilities in using the new system, and expected effects of the new system on nurses' work, patient care and the hospital and the community as a whole.
- Train nurse managers and other experienced nurses to assist with the training of other nursing staff.
- Adopt a unified methodological approach, prepare quality standardized documentation, develop a flexible system that can be readily modified, and actively involve the end user.
- Ensure continuous communication between system developers and users.
- The organizational changes that will occur with the implementation of the new system must be anticipated and presented to its users as a positive development and not as an additional task in their daily work.
- Ensure the participation of experts from all relevant fields in all phases of the project for the successful completion of the system.

INFORMATION TECHNOLOGY

Information technology (IT) is the use of computers to create, process, store, retrieve, and exchange all kinds of electronic data and information. IT is typically used within the context of business operations as opposed to personal or entertainment technologies, IT forms part of information and communications technology (ICT). An information technology system (IT system) is generally an information system, a communications system, or, more specifically speaking, a computer system—including all hardware, software, and peripheral equipment—operated by a limited group of IT users.

What does information technology encompass?

- The IT department ensures that the organization's systems, networks, data and applications all connect and function properly. The IT team handles three major areas:
  - Deploys and maintains business applications, services and infrastructure (servers, networks, storage);
  - Monitors, optimizes and troubleshoots the performance of applications, services and infrastructure; and
  - Oversees the security and governance of applications, services and infrastructure.

Most IT staff have different responsibilities within the team that break into several key areas including:

- **Administration:** Administrators handle the day-to-day deployment, operation and monitoring of an IT environment, including systems, networks and applications. Admins often perform a range of other duties such as software upgrades, user training, software license management, procurement, security, data management and observing adherence to business process and compliance requirements.
- **Support:** Help desk staff specialize in answering questions, gathering information and directing troubleshooting efforts for hardware and software. IT support often includes IT asset and change management, helping admins with procurement, handling backup and recovery of data and applications, monitoring and analyzing logs and other performance monitoring tools and following established support workflows and processes.
- **Applications:** Businesses rely on software to perform work. Some applications are procured and deployed from third parties, such as email server applications. But many organizations retain a staff of skilled developers that create the applications and interfaces—such as APIs—needed to deliver critical business capabilities and services. Applications might be coded in a wide array of popular languages and integrated with other applications to create smooth and seamless interactions between different applications. Developers might also be tasked with creating interactive business websites and building mobile applications. The trend toward agile or continuous development paradigms require developers to be increasingly involved with IT operations, such as deploying and monitoring applications.

- **Compliance:** Businesses are obligated to observe varied government- and industry-driven regulatory requirements. IT staff play a major role in securing and monitoring access to business data and applications to ensure that such resources are used according to established business governance policy that meets regulatory requirements. Such staff are deeply involved with security tasks and routinely interact with legal and business teams to prevent, detect, investigate and report possible breaches.

IT involves many things. Take, for instance, an IT department in a company. There are many people with many jobs and varied responsibilities. These responsibilities range from keeping systems and data secure to keeping networks up and running. There are people who input data, people who manage databases and people who do programming. There are also the decision makers, such as Chief Information Officers (CIOs), who decide how an IT department will operate and what components will be purchased.

IT also includes the management of data, whether it is in the form of text, voice, image, audio or some other form. It can also involve things related to the Internet. This gives IT a whole new meaning, since the Internet is its own realm. IT involves the transfer of data, so it makes sense that the Internet would be a part of IT. IT has become a part of our everyday lives and continues to proliferate into new realms.

TELEMEDICINE

Telemedicine is an upcoming field in health science arising out of the effective fusion of ICT with medical science having enormous potential in meeting the challenges of healthcare delivery to rural and remote areas. It is kind of system by the delivery of healthcare service done from a distance by all healthcare professionals using information communication technology for the exchange of different information. The term telemedicine has been derived from the Greek word 'tele' meaning at distance and medicine which is from the Latin word 'meden' meaning healing. Telemedicine is the used of modern telecommunications and information technology for the provision of clinic care to individuals at a distance and the transmission of information to provide that care, it includes the diagnosis, treatments, monitoring and education of patients using systems that allow ready access to expert advice and patients information no matter where the patient or relevant information is locate. Telemedicine relies on transfer of text, reports, voice, images and video, between geographically separated locations. Success relates to the efficiency and effectiveness of the transfer of information.

According to WHO

Telemedicine is the delivery of healthcare services where distance is a critical factors by all healthcare professional using information and communication technology for the exchange of valid information for diagnosis and treatment and prevention of disease and injuries, research and continuing education of healthcare providers all in the interest of advancing the health of individual and their community.

According to Williams

Telemedicine is defined as any health care provided to patient via technology across a distance. It also otherwise defined as the use of advance technologies to exchange health information and provide healthcare services across geographic area, time, social and cultural barriers.

The use of telecommunication is to provide medical information and services at may be as simple as to one health professional discussing a case over the telephone or as sophisticated as using satellite technology to broadcast or consultation between provides at two distant locations using video- conferencing equipment.

According to Americans Telemedicine Association

'Telemedicine is the use of medical information exchanged from one site to another via electronic communications for the health and education of the patient or healthcare provider and for the purpose of improving patient care'. In plain speak telemedicine is a process by which a patient is able to communicate his problems, (along with, if necessary details of medical investigations) to a doctor many miles away and receive necessary and relevant medical advice.

Objectives

- To provide quality care to the people who are residing in remotest areas.
- To reduce the cost of healthcare services.

Areas of Telemedicine Applications

- Cardiology
- Home care
- Radiology
- Emergency care
- Surgery
- Dermatology
- Psychiatry
- Oncology
- Pathology
- Ophthalmology
- Hematology
- ENT
- Nephrology
- Prehospital care

Applications

It can be also used for:
- Telehealth care
- Teleconsultation
- Telefollow-up
- Teleeducation
- Disease surveillance and program
- Disaster management can be tackle
- Telehome health care to elderly people

- Continuous medical education
- Public awareness
- Telementored or procedures or surgeries.

Evolution of Telemedicine in India

- **1996:** Deployment of First Indigenously Developed Hospital Information System Software by CDAC Noida at SGPGIMS, Lucknow, UP
- **1999:** Indigenous Development of Telemedicine Technology and Pilot Deployments by DeitY, MCIT, Government of India at AIIMS, New Delhi, PGIMER Chandigarh and SGPGIMS Lucknow
- **2000:** SATCOM based Telemedicine Deployment by ISRO at Apollo Hospitals, Aragonda
- **2001:** First telemedicine network between three institutions AIIMS-New Delhi, PGI Chandigarh and SGPGI-Lucknow, First National Conference on Telemedicine was held and a Scientific Body for promotion of Telemedicine in the Country Telemedicine Society of India, was formed
- **2001–2003:** Major Medical Institutions (Government and Corporate) initiated telemedicine activities and deployed hospital information system
- **2003–2004:** Deployment of SATCOM based TM nodes across the country by ISRO for Tele-education and Teleconsultation services
- **2005:** MoHFW constituted Indian Task Force for Telemedicine
- **2006:** Planning Commission approved budget for e-Health including Telemedicine in the 11th Five Year Plan School of Telemedicine and Biomedical Informatics (STBI) was set up at SGPGIMS, Lucknow by Government of UP. PHFI was awarded Grant-in-aid to have MoHFW 'Healthy India' Website for Health Education from 2007–08 to 2012–13
- **2007:** STBI at SGPGIMS, Lucknow was made National Resource Centre for Telemedicine and Biomedical Informatics by DeitY Government of India MoHFW, Government of India supported Teleophthalmology Project in many parts of the country MoHFW, Government of India supported Onco-NET Project.
- **2009:** MoHFW, supported National Rural TM Network with ₹25–50 Lakh to start the pilot projects on Telemedicine
- **2010:** National Medical College Network Project Conceived. SGPGIMS was made National Resource Centre for Telemedicine by MoHFW, MCTS launched by MoHFW, Government of India
- **2012:** EMR/EHR Standards by Expert Group of MoHFW establishment
- **2013:** Initiation of process of establishment of NMCN with Open Tender Basis. MCIT Initiative of National Optical Fibre Network (2011) to provide high speed bandwidth connectivity up to every Gram Panchayat wherein 2,50,000 shall have connectivity. As a Pilot Project of Teleconsultation three sites (PHC/CHC) as one Telemedicine Centre each block have been connected with one medical college in the states for Telemedicine activities.

Growth of TM Applications

Services can be Provided by Telemedicine

Sometimes telemedicine is best understood in terms of the services provided and the mechanisms used to provide those services. Here are some examples:

- **Primary care and specialist referral services** may involve a primary care or allied health professional providing a consultation with a patient or a specialist assisting the primary care physician in rendering a diagnosis. This may involve the use of live interactive video or the use of store and forward transmission of diagnostic images, vital signs and/or video clips along with patient data for later review.
- **Remote patient monitoring,** including home telehealth, uses devices to remotely collect and send data to a home health agency or a remote diagnostic testing facility (RDTF) for interpretation. Such applications might include a specific vital sign, such as blood glucose or heart ECG or a variety of indicators for homebound patients. Such services can be used to supplement the use of visiting nurses.
- **Consumer medical and health information** includes the use of the Internet and wireless devices for consumers to obtain specialized health information and on-line discussion groups to provide peer-to-peer support.
- **Medical education** provides continuing medical education credits for health professionals and special medical education seminars for targeted groups in remote locations.
    - *2001:* Teleradiology–still images
    - *2002:* Telecardiology–moving images, CME
    - *2003:* Telepathology, Teleophthalmology
    - *2004:* Teleoncology, Telesurgery
    - *2005:* Mobile Telehealth-augmentation
    - *2006:* Telemedicine for Primary healthcare.

What Delivery Mechanisms Can Be Used?

Networked programs link tertiary care hospitals and clinics with outlying clinics and community health centers in rural or suburban areas. The links may use dedicated high-speed lines or the Internet for telecommunication links between sites. ATA estimates the number of existing telemedicine networks in the United States at roughly 200 providing connectivity to over 3,000 sites.

- **Point-to-point connections** using private high speed networks are used by hospitals and clinics that deliver services directly or outsource specialty services to independent medical service providers. Such outsourced services include radiology, stroke assessment, mental health and intensive care services.
- **Monitoring center links** are used for cardiac, pulmonary or fetal monitoring, home care and related services that provide care to patients in the home. Often normal land-line or wireless connections are used to communicate directly between the patient and the center although some systems use the Internet.

- **Web-based e-health patient service sites** provide direct consumer outreach and services over the Internet. Under telemedicine, these include those sites that provide direct patient care.

Types of Telemedicine

Real Time (Synchronous)

Real time telemedicine could be as simple as a telephone call or as complex as robotic surgery. It requires the presence of both parties at the same time and a communication link between them that allows a real time interaction to take place. Video-conferencing equipment is one of the most common forms of technologies used in synchronous telemedicine. There are also peripheral devices which can attached to the computer or the video conferencing equipment which can aid in an interactive examination. For instant, a teleotoscope allows a remote physician to 'see' inside a patient's ear; a telestethoscope allows the consulting remote physician to hear the patient's heartbeat. Medical specialties conducive to this kind of consultation include psychiatry, family practice, internal medicine, rehabilitation, cardiology, pediatrics, obstetrics, genecology, neurology and pharmacy.

Store and Forward Telemedicine

Store and forward telemedicine involves acquiring medical data (like medical images, biosignals) and then transmitting this data to the doctor or medical specialist at convenient time for assessment offline. It does not require the presence of both parties at the same time. Dermatology (cf: teledermatology), radiology and pathology are the common specialties that are conductive to asynchronous telemedicine. A properly record Medical Record preferably in electronic form should be a component of this transfer. Telemedicine is most beneficial for population living in isolated communities and remote regions and is currently being applied in virtually all medical domains. Specialties that use telemedicine often use a 'tele' prefix; for example, telemedicine applied by radiologists is called Teleradiology. Similarly telemedicine as applied by cardiologists is termed as telecardiology, etc.

Categories of Services

Telemedicine can be provided three main categories of services. These are store-and-forward, remote monitoring and interactive services.

Store-and-forward

Store-and-forward is a telecommunications technique in which information is sent to an intermediate station where it is kept and sent at a later time to the final destination or to another intermediate station. The intermediate station, or node in a networking context, verifies the integrity of the message before forwarding it. Telemedicine can act as intermediate station involving acquiring medical data (like medical images, biosignals, etc.) and then transmitting this data to a doctor or medical specialist at a convenient time for assessment offline. It does not require the presence of both doctor and patient at the same time. A properly structured medical record preferably in electronic form should be a component of this transfer. The 'store-and-forward' process requires the clinician to rely on a history report and audio/video information in lieu of a physical examination.

Remote Monitoring

Remote monitoring also known as self-monitoring or testing, enables medical professionals to monitor a patient remotely using various technological devices. This method is primarily used for managing chronic diseases or specific conditions, such as heart disease, diabetes mellitus, or asthma. These services can provide comparable health outcomes to traditional in-person patient encounters, supply greater satisfaction to patients, and may be cost-effective.

Interactive Services

Interactive telemedicine services provide real-time interactions between patient and provider, to include phone conversations, online communication and home visits. Many activities such as history review, physical examination, psychiatric evaluations and ophthalmology assessments can be conducted comparably to those done in traditional face-to-face visits. In addition, 'clinician-interactive' telemedicine services may be less costly than in-person clinical visit.

Application of Telemedicine

- **Telehealth care:** The use of information and communication technology for prevention, promotion and to provide self-care facility across a distance. It includes:
  - Telecommunication
  - Telefollow up
- **Teleeducation:** Teleeducation should be understood as the development of the process of distance education based on use of information and telecommunication technology.
- **Disaster management:** Telemedicine can play an important role to provide healthcare facility to the victim of natural disaster such as Tsunami, earthquake *etc.*
- **Telephone health care:** Telemedicine technology can be applied to provide home health care to elderly people or patient with chronic illness.

Advantages of Telemedicine

Advantages for Patients

Telemedicine has been growing rapidly because it offers four fundamental benefits:

- **Improved access:** For over 40 years, telemedicine has been used to bring healthcare services to patients in distant locations. People at remote areas get top class medical facility from reputed hospital. Not only does telemedicine improve access to patients but it also allows physicians and health facilities to expand their reach, beyond their own offices. Hospital can spread their reach in remote villages and serve people without much investment or without the infrastructure. Given the provider shortages throughout the world—in both rural and urban areas—telemedicine has a unique capacity to increase service to millions of new patients.

- **Cost efficiencies:** Reducing or containing the cost of health care is one of the most important reasons for funding and adopting telehealth technologies. Telemedicine has been shown to reduce the cost of healthcare by Reducing travel cost and save time and increase efficiency through better management of chronic diseases, shared health professional staffing, reduced travel times, and fewer or shorter hospital stays.
- **Improved quality:** Studies have consistently shown that the quality of healthcare services delivered via telemedicine as good those given in traditional in-person consultations. In some specialties, particularly in mental health and ICU care, telemedicine delivers a superior product, with greater outcomes and patient satisfaction. Doctors can learn new technology by connecting foreign hospital.
- **Patient demand:** Consumers want telemedicine. The greatest impact of telemedicine is on the patient, their family and their community. Using telemedicine technologies reduces travel time and related stresses for the patient. Over the past 15 years, study after study has documented patient satisfaction and support for telemedical services. Such services offer patients the access to providers that might not be available otherwise, as well as medical services without the need to travel long distances.

Reduce Hospitalization and Save Time of Healthcare Provider

The patient can assess healthcare services at their residence. Generally the patient with minor illness and patient after care of postoperative condition need not came to hospital for minor consultation by which the time of healthcare provider can be saved.

Provide Patient Satisfaction

The patient used to like for treatment in their houses with presence of all relatives so this telemedicine helps in providing satisfaction to the patient by treating them in their own place.

Benefits for Doctors

- Excellent opportunity to share knowledge between physicians all over the world.
- Joint consultation with export physician and surgeons for better management of complicated cases.
- Local doctors can be updated at any time.
- Medical education in the form of teleconferencing.

Benefits for Government

- Reduces rush to medical facilities in cities.
- Improve monitoring facilities at rural centers.
- Increase reliance on Government Health care system.

Limitations of Telemedicine

- The overall cost of telecommunication system, especially data management apparatus and practical training of medical professionals is high.
- Virtual clinical treatment decreases human interaction among the healthcare professionals and patients that increases the risk of error in clinical services, if the service is delivered by inexperienced professional. Moreover, confidential medical information can be leaked through faulty electronic system.
- Telemedicine might take longer time for the difficulties in connecting virtual communication due to low internet speed or server problem. Moreover, this system cannot provide immediate treatment, such as, antibiotics.
- Low quality of health informatics records, like X-ray or other images, clinical progress reports, etc. run the risk of faulty clinical treatment.
- Telemedicine system requires tough legal regulation to prevent unauthorized and illegal service providers in this sector. Legal and ethical complications may arise.

Shortage of computer trained healthcare professionals and lack of training facility with lack of IEC.

- Privacy and security concern is also there. Evidence based practice is not practiced.
- The uneducated and poorly educated people cannot be assess this.
- All type of care cannot be provided in this method.

TELENURSING

Telenursing refers to the use of telecommunication and information technology for providing nursing services in health care whenever a large physical distance between patients and nurse or between a number of nurses. As a field it is a part of telehealth and has many points of contacts with other medical and nonmedical applications, such as telediagnosis, teleconsultation, telemonitoring, etc. The American Nurses Association has defined "telenursing as a subset of telehealth in which the focus is on the specific profession's practice (i.e., nursing)". Nurses' use technologies such as the Internet, computers, telephones, digital assessment tools and telemonitoring equipment in their practice to assess, plan, intervene and evaluate the outcomes of nursing care. This technique has expanded the scope of nursing practice across the states and international borders and it is also changing the face of standard nursing practice This is now a upcoming carrier option for the nurses of 21st century

Definition

Telenursing can be defined as using telecommunication devices to provide nursing care, utilizing the nursing process to care for individuals or specific patient populations, such as isolated groups of people. Telehealth focuses on delivery management and coordination of services and care.

Principles of Telenursing

- Engage in this practice to enhance their ability to provide safe, competent, compassionate and ethical care.
- Augment existing healthcare services. Enhance optimum access, where appropriate and necessary, provide immediate access to healthcare services.

JOURNALISM

The etymology of the word journalism, is outlined to the ancient Greek word hēmeroúsios or from the roots of the word diurnus which means 'daily', or from the Latin word diurnalis or diurnal. The word when traced historically had the meaning of either making a daily record (Swift) or the management and conduct of a journal or periodical work. A journalist was the person who is a writer of Journals or the Manager of a periodical work. Journalism is the activity of gathering, assessing, creating, and presenting news and information and also the product of these activities. Journalism can be notable from other activities and products by certain identifiable characteristics and practices. These characteristics not only separate journalism from other forms of communication, they are what make it indispensable to democratic societies. History reveals that in a democratic society, more news and information will be generated. Journalism is the collection, preparation, and distribution of news and related commentary and feature materials through such print and electronic media as newspapers, magazines, books, blogs, webcasts, podcasts, social networking and social media sites, and e-mail as well as through radio, motion pictures, and television. The word journalism was originally applied to the reportage of current events in printed form, specifically newspapers, but with the advent of radio, television, and the Internet in the 20th century the use of the term broadened to include all printed and electronic communication dealing with current affairs.

Definitions

- The Cambridge Advanced Learner's Dictionary and Thesaurus describes journalism as "The work of collecting, writing, and publishing news, stories and articles in newspapers and magazines or broadcasting them on the radio and television".
- The American Press Institute defines Journalism as 'the activity of gathering, assessing, creating, and presenting news and information. It is also the product of these activities'.
- Journalism can be defined as a searching, collecting, assessing, and editing of news or information which could be published or presented on a given media forum that could include press (newspaper or magazine or books), radio, television or the Internet.
- Journalism is the activity of gathering, writing, editing, and publishing or broadcasting news, as through newspapers and magazines or by radio and television.
- Journalism is the production and distribution of reports on the interaction of events, facts, ideas, and people that are the "news of the day" and that informs society to at least some degree. The word applies to the occupation (professional or not), the methods of gathering information, and the organizing literary styles. Journalistic media include: print, television, radio, Internet, and, in the past, newsreels.

An individual or individuals writing about things that have happened as in case of news reports, or an opinion generating piece called feature, or a feature on any given topic that informs people are called 'Journalists'. They work in Newspapers, Magazines, Radio or TV Channels and today they are also accomplished on the Internet. A journalist's work is called Journalism.

History

The earliest known journalistic product was a news sheet circulated in ancient Rome, the Acta Diurna, said to date from before 59 BC. The Acta Diurna recorded important daily events such as public speeches. It was published daily and hung in prominent places. In China during the Tang dynasty, a court circular called a bao, or "report," was issued to government officials. This gazette appeared in various forms and under various names more or less continually to the end of the Qing dynasty in 1911. The first regularly published newspapers appeared in German cities and in Antwerp about 1609. The first English newspaper, the Weekly News, was published in 1622. One of the first daily newspapers, The Daily Courant, appeared in 1702.

At first hindered by government-imposed censorship, taxes, and other restrictions, newspapers in the 18th century came to enjoy the reportorial freedom and indispensable function that they have retained to the present day. The growing demand for newspapers owing to the spread of literacy and the introduction of steam- and then electric-driven presses caused the daily circulation of newspapers to rise from the thousands to the hundreds of thousands and eventually to the millions.

Magazines, which had started in the 17th century as learned journals, began to feature opinion-forming articles on current affairs, such as those in the Tatler (1709–11) and the Spectator (1711–12). Appearing in the 1830s were cheap mass-circulation magazines aimed at a wider and less well-educated public, as well as illustrated and women's magazines. The cost of large-scale news gathering led to the formation of news agencies, organizations that sold their international journalistic reporting to many different individual newspapers and magazines. The invention of the telegraph and then radio and television brought about a great increase in the speed and timeliness of journalistic activity and, at the same time, provided massive new outlets and audiences for their electronically distributed products. In the late 20th century, satellites and later the Internet were used for the long-distance transmission of journalistic information.

The Profession

Journalism in the 20th century was marked by a growing sense of professionalism. There were four important factors in this trend: (1) the increasing organization of working journalists, (2) specialized education for journalism, (3) a growing literature dealing with the history, problems, and techniques of mass communication, and (4) an increasing sense of social responsibility on the part of journalists.

Before the latter part of the 19th century, most journalists learned their craft as apprentices, beginning as copyboys or cub reporters. The first university course in journalism was given at the University of Missouri (Columbia) in 1879–84. In 1912 Columbia University in New York City established the first graduate program in journalism, endowed by a grant from the New York City editor and publisher Joseph Pulitzer. It was recognized that the growing complexity of news reporting and newspaper operation required a great deal of specialized training. Editors also found that in-depth reporting of special types of news, such as political affairs, business, economics, and science, often demanded reporters with education in these areas. The advent of motion pictures, radio, and television as news media called for an ever-increasing battery of new skills and techniques in gathering and presenting the news. By the 1950s, courses in journalism or communications were commonly offered in colleges.

Concern for social responsibility in journalism was largely a product of the late 19th and 20th centuries.

By the late 20th century, studies showed that journalists as a group were generally idealistic about their role in bringing the facts to the public in an impartial manner. Various societies of journalists issued statements of ethics, of which that of the American Society of Newspaper Editors is perhaps best known.

In the second decade of the 21st century, social media platforms in particular facilitated the spread of politically oriented "fake news," a kind of disinformation produced by for-profit Websites posing as legitimate news organizations and designed to attract (and mislead) certain readers by exploiting entrenched partisan biases.

Different Forms of Journalism

- **News reporting:** A journalist gathers a news and either writes an article or reports about the same for a news channel either on Radio or a television or an internet forum. This could include an event, an occasion, a tragedy, a disaster or an investigative news piece.
- **Feature writing:** News or information can be transformed into a detailed style of writing or an opinion generating piece through feature writing. It could be a review of a movie or a book.
- **Discussion and debate boards:** The editorial page could carry articles with opinionated pieces of diverse opinions contrasted. Radio, internet and TV channels host debates and discussions moderated by renowned journalists.

Online Journalism

- **Blog writing:** News or information is also published in feature style writing on forums called blogs on the internet. The blog could also be made creative with videos, video links or pictures.
  - TV channels have recognized the power of the internet and have websites dedicated to the same. They run simultaneous news on these websites and provide reading matter.
  - Many journalists have turned to the internet for hosting their own shows, chat shows, reviews, humorous takes, interviews, opinionated pieces, etc.
  - Many citizens today report news and send videos and pictures thus giving a boost to the phenomenon of Citizen Journalism.
  - Wikis is another huge platform of information that is available for free. Many writers contribute to writing on this forum in order to benefit millions of people.
- **Mojo journalism:** The latest concept in journalism that basically means Mobile journalism. It is a kind of reporting wherein field reporting of events, stories or multimedia content occurs using smaller, connected mobile devices like smart phones, DSLR cameras, Laptops etc. This phenomenon has largely contributed to Citizen journalism too. Glen Mulcahy, Founder of Mojocon says, "Mobile Journalism is about empowering the individual storyteller to use whatever consumer technology they have available to them to make the best possible visual story that they can. I would like to think that Mobile Journalism definition can be extended to other mobile devices beyond smartphones, like DSLR cameras, laptops, GoPros."

Types of Journalism

Advocacy Journalism

Advocacy journalism is a genre of journalism that is fact-based, but supports a specific point of view on an issue.

Advocacy journalism is practiced by alternative media and special interest publications and programs, but might also apply to a single article in an otherwise-neutral publication.

In this type of journalism, the journalists can be openly biased about a particular person, or a group of people. Single-sided opinions are resented in this type of journalism.

Broadcast Journalism

Broadcast journalism is a type of news reporting presented to the public electronically or by radio instead of being published in newspapers.

Media in broadcast journalism include television, radio and the Internet.

Investigative Journalism

Investigative journalism is a form of journalism in which reporters deeply investigate a single topic of interest, such as serious crimes, political corruption, or corporate wrongdoing.

An investigative journalist may spend months or years researching and preparing a report. Investigative journalism is a primary source of information.

Most investigative journalism is conducted by newspapers, wire services, and freelance journalists.

Tabloid Journalism

Tabloid journalism is a style of journalism that emphasizes sensational crime stories, gossip columns about celebrities and sports stars, junk food news and astrology.

Although it is associated with tabloid-size newspapers, not all newspapers associated with tabloid journalism are tabloid size, and not all tabloid-size newspapers engage in tabloid journalism.

Tabloid journalism often concerns itself with rumors about the private lives of celebrities.

Yellow Journalism

Yellow journalism or the yellow press is a type of journalism that does not report much real news with facts.

It uses shocking headlines that catch people's attention to sell more newspapers.

Yellow press newspapers have several columns and front-page headlines about different types of news, such as sports and scandals.

CHAPTER 5 Nutrition

CONCEPT OF NUTRITION

Life cannot be sustained without adequate nourishment. Food is the basic necessity of life. Food that we eat is digested and assimilated in the body and used for its maintenance and growth. But if body does not meet its nutritional requirement, then it will give rise to many hazardous problems. From the nutritional point of view, the Indian society is actual society, consisting of a small group of well-fed and a very large group of undernourished. Nutritional problems are more prevalent among the poor sections due to the restrictions of diet imposed upon them by their poverty.

Nutrition is the selection of foods and preparation of foods and their ingestion to be assimilated by the body. By practicing a healthy diet, many of the known health issues can be avoided. The diet of an organism is what it eats, which is largely determined by the perceived palatability of foods.

Nutrition is the science of food values. It is relatively a new science, which was evolved from chemistry and physiology. The effect of food in our body is explained in nutrition. In other words, nutrition is defined as food at work in the body. In a broader sense nutrition is defined as 'the science of foods, the nutrients and other substances their action, interaction, and balance in relationship to health and diseases, the process by which the organism ingests, digests, absorbs, transport and utilizes nutrients and dispose off their end products, in addition nutrition must be concerned with the social, economic, cultural and psychological implication of food and eating.

Food is derived from plant or animal sources which may be solid, liquid or semisolid that provide energy and nutrients for maintenance, growth, and repair. It refers to anything, which nourishes the body, may be solids, semi-solids, and liquids which can be consumed and helps to sustain body and keep it healthy. It is a substance which after ingestion, digestion and absorption is capable being utilized by the body for its various functions. Food is an edible substance which contains one or more nutrients.

Diet: The foods one consumes. The quality of which affects health and the risk of chronic diseases. The word 'diet' is derived from the Greek word 'diatia' which means 'manner of living.'

The selection of food depends upon on number of factors like:

- Personal preference
- Positive and negative associations
- Habit
- Ethnic heritage/tradition
- Values
- Social pressure
- Emotional comfort
- Availability/convenience/economy
- Body weight and image
- Medical conditions
- Nutrition and health benefits.

Classification of Food

Food is classified in different ways. It can be classified by origin or source, classified by chemical composition or classified by predominant function.

Classification by origin: According to source or origin the food is classified as:

- Foods of animal origin
- Foods of vegetable origin.

Classification by chemical composition: According to chemical composition the food is classified as:

- Proteins
- Fats
- Carbohydrates
- Vitamins
- Minerals.

Classification by predominant function:

- **Body-building foods:** Meat, milk, poultry, fish, eggs, pulses, etc.
- **Energy-giving foods:** Cereals, sugars, fats, oils, etc.
- **Protective foods:** Vegetables, fruits, milk, etc.

Classification by nutritive value:

- Cereals and millets
- Pulses
- Vegetables
- Nuts and oil seeds
- Fruits
- Animal foods
- Fats and oils

- Sugar and jaggery
- Condiments and spices
- Miscellaneous food.

Functions of Food

Food is important for life. To be healthy and active, we should certainly have enough food. But the foods we eat should also be safe and rich in all the nutrients our body needs. Food does much more that satisfy your appetite. It provides nutrients that the body uses for growth and health. There are five types of nutrients that fall into two broad categories. Every nutrient have a wide variety of specific functions. Overall, the functions of food can be broadly classified into three main categories:

1. Physiological Functions of Food

The physiological functions of food can be further sub-divided as follow:

- **Energy giving food:** It acts as a fuel, the digested food releases energy at the cellular level in the presence of O_2 (combustion) and releases energy which is needed for various activities of the organism. The body needs a constant supply of energy to carry out the involuntary processes of which we are not even aware, like, respiration, circulation of blood, etc., which are essential for continuance of life which food provides.
- **Body building food:** It is needed for the growth and development of the organism. Food helps to produce new cells and tissues; repairs and replaces the old and worn out tissues. For the body building purposes, the major nutrients utilized are proteins and minerals.
- **Regulatory and protective functions of food:** It includes regulation of such varied activities as beating of the heart, maintenance of body temperature, muscle contraction, control of water balance, clotting of blood, removal of waste products from the body, etc. Food helps to keep our body healthy, increasing the immunity levels and fighting against the disease causing germs. For development of strong and healthy bones, muscles, healthy hair, nail and teeth.

2. Psychological Functions of Food

The second major function of food is the psychological function. Food must also satisfy certain emotional needs like sense of security, love and affection. People of different culture and cast have different food habits. The person begins to associate the food habits and foods commonly consumed by him, as it gives him a sense of security and satiety. The test of foods daily eaten by us, give us more mental satisfaction, then maintaining nutritional requirement. The food decorated properly gives more satisfaction to the individual.

3. Social Functions of Food

Food and eating has significant social meaning like any auspicious occasion like festivals. Share food with any other person implies social acceptance. Food is the common link between the individuals.

Refreshment served even at officials meeting creates a relaxed atmosphere, where people can exchange their views. The menu for such get-to-gather should bring the people together, rather than divide them. Foods help to strengthen mutual friendship.

Terminologies

Nutrition

The study of essential nutrients and the process by which nutrients are used by the body. It is a science that deals with all aspects of interaction between a living organism and the substances which help the organism to grow and sustain. It is concerned primarily with the part played by nutrients in body growth, development and maintenance. In short it is the process of ingestion, digestion, absorption and utilization of food. Nutrition is the process by which living organisms assimilate food to use for growth and health. Good nutrition happens when people get enough food and nutrients to be healthy and grow at a normal pace.

Dietetics

Dietetics is the practical application of the principles of nutrition; it includes the planning of meals for the well and the sick. Good nutrition means 'maintaining a nutritional status that enables us to grow well and enjoy good health'.

Nutrients

Nutrients are biochemical substances obtained from ingested food that allow the proper function of the body. If these nutrients are not present in our food in sufficient amount, the result is ill health. Important nutrients include carbohydrates, proteins, lipids, vitamins, minerals, and water. Food also contains many substances, which are non-nutrients, e.g., coloring and flavoring substances in food.

Classification of Nutrients

There are two types of nutrients: macronutrients (needed in relatively large amounts) or micronutrients (needed in smaller quantities).

Macronutrients

As 'macro' means large, macronutrients are nutrients needed in large amounts. It generally includes protein, fat, carbohydrate and water. The macronutrients (excluding fiber and water) provide structural material (amino acids from which proteins are built, and lipids from which cell membranes and some signaling molecules are built) and energy. Nutrients are substances needed for growth, metabolism, and for other body functions. There are three macronutrients: Proteins, carbohydrates, and fats.

Micronutrients

Micronutrients are the nutrients which named as such because they are needed only in minuscule amounts, these substances are the 'magic wands' that enable the body to produce enzymes, hormones and other substances essential for proper growth and development. As tiny as the amounts are, however, the consequences of their absence are severe. Iodine, vitamin A and iron are most important in global public health terms; their lack represents a major threat to the health and development of populations the world over, particularly children and pregnant women in low-income countries. The microminerals or trace elements include at least iron cobalt, chromium, copper iodine, manganese, selenium, zinc and molybdenum. Micronutrients also include vitamins which are organic compounds required as nutrients in tiny amounts by an organism.

TYPE I AND TYPE II NUTRIENTS

An alternative method of classifying nutrients as either type I or type II has recently been proposed (Golden, 1995). This classification is based on the way in which the body responds to a nutrient deficiency.

The type I and II classification is important because it emphasizes that poor growth is not caused solely by protein-energy malnutrition but can result from other nutrient deficiencies which may not be recognized and so appropriately treated. Furthermore, it demonstrates the importance of a wide range of nutrients in causing poor growth or weight loss, and therefore the need for a nutritionally balanced diet.

Over 40 nutrients are essential for better health. If even one is deficient then the person will not be healthy and less resistance to disease. But many are ignored by practitioners and their deficiency is not recognized. A type I response is characterized by specific physical signs of deficiency as a result of a reduced tissue concentration of the nutrient. For example, if the diet is deficient in a type I nutrient such as iron, there is an initial consumption of body stores followed by clinical signs characteristic of iron deficiency. The concentration of iron in the tissues is markedly reduced, but there is no effect on growth or body weight. In contrast, a type II response is characterized by reduced growth rate or weight loss in the absence of specific deficiency signs. For example, if the diet is deficient in a type II nutrient like zinc, growth stops, followed by weight loss. The concentration of zinc in the major tissues remains normal and there are no deficiency signs. Protein and energy (derived from carbohydrates and fat) are classified as type II nutrients.

They are divided into two groups in terms of the response to a deficiency.

Type I	*Type II*
• Iron • Iodine • Copper • Calcium • Selenium • Thiamin • Riboflavin • Pyridoxine • Niacin • Folate • Cobalamin • Vitamin A, D, E, K	• Nitrogen • Essential amino acid • Potassium • Magnesium • Phosphorous • Zinc • Sodium • Chloride

PROTEIN

The word protein means to 'take the first place'. In 1938 a Dutch Chemist Mulder, described that all living plants and animal contain certain substance without which life was not possible and this was identified as proteins. In constitution of body they stand next to the water.

Indeed proteins are of greatest importance in human nutrition. They are complex organic compounds containing the carbon, hydrogen, oxygen, nitrogen, and usually sulfur. Some proteins also contain phosphorus, iron, iodine, copper and other inorganic elements. Proteins are made up of much smaller units known as 'amino acids'.

There are 24 amino acids, which are stated to be needed by the human body, of which 9 are called 'essential', because the body cannot synthesize them. They must be obtaining from dietary proteins. The nine essential amino acids are Leucine, Isoleucine, Lysine, Methionine, Phenylalanine, Threonine Valine, Tryptophan and Histidine. Nonessential amino acids are Arginine, Asparagenic acid, Serine, Glutamic acid, Proline and Glycerine. Both essential and nonessential amino acids needed for synthesis for tissue protein. Nonessential amino acids can be synthesized by the body providing other building blocks are present. Animal proteins are rated superior to vegetables proteins because they are 'biologically complete', for example milk and egg proteins have a pattern of amino acids considered most suitable for human beings.

Protein is an important substance found in every cell in the human body. In fact, except for water, protein is the most abundant substance in your body. This protein is manufactured by your body utilizing the dietary protein you consume. It is used in many vital processes and thus needs to be consistently replaced. You can accomplish this by regularly consuming foods that contain protein.

Functions of Protein

Proteins are very essential for life processes, as there is hardly any important physiological function in which proteins do not participate. The important functions of proteins are:

Body-building, Repair and Maintenance

It is the most important function of protein. These are the major structural components of body tissues. In fact every living cell contains protein. The first need for proteins therefore is to supply the materials for the growth and development and the continuous replacement of the cell protein.

Protein is termed the building block of the body. It is called this because protein is vital in the maintenance of body tissue, including development and repair. Hair, skin, eyes, muscles and organs are all made from protein. This is why children need more protein per pound of body weight than adults; they are growing and developing new protein tissue.

Body Regulation

Many proteins have highly specialized functions in the regulation of body processes. All chemical reaction in the body are carried out by enzymes, which are protein in nature. Protein is a major element in transportation of certain molecules. For example, hemoglobin is a protein that transports oxygen throughout the body. Protein is also sometimes used to store certain molecules. Ferritin is an example of a protein that combines with iron for storage in the liver. Governing the body reaction are hormones, which are also proteins. Plasma protein has a fundamental role in the maintenance of water balance. Blood proteins also help in maintaining acid base balance of the body. The specific functions of hormones and enzymes are given below:

- **Hormones:** Protein is involved in the creation of some hormones. These substances help control body functions that involve the interaction of several organs. Insulin, a small protein, is an example of a hormone that regulates blood sugar. It involves the interaction of organs such as the pancreas and the liver. Secretin, is another example of a protein hormone. This substance assists in the digestive process by stimulating the pancreas and the intestine to create necessary digestive juices.
- **Enzymes:** Enzymes are proteins that increase the rate of chemical reactions in the body. In fact, most of the necessary chemical reactions in the body would not efficiently proceed without enzymes. For example, one type of enzyme functions as an aid in digesting large protein, carbohydrate and fat molecules into smaller molecules, while another assists the creation of DNA.

Body Protection

There is a protein called gamma globulin, which has a capacity to fight against invading organism. The body's resistance to disease is maintained in part by antibodies, which are protein in nature.

Energy-yielding

The energy needs of the body take priority over other needs, and if the diet does not furnish sufficient energy from carbohydrates and fats. The proteins of the diet as well as tissue protein will be used up for giving energy. One gram of protein gives 4 calories. If any body consume more protein than he need for body tissue maintenance and other necessary functions, his body will use it for energy. If it is not needed due to sufficient intake of other energy sources such as carbohydrates, the protein will be used to create fat and becomes part of fat cells.

Maintenance of Body Temperature

During the metabolism of proteins extra heat is liberated, which is used for maintaining the body temperature.

Formation of Antibodies

Protein forms antibodies that help prevent infection, illness and disease. These proteins identify and assist in destroying antigens such as bacteria and viruses. They often work in conjunction with the other immune system cells. For example, these antibodies identify and then surround antigens in order to keep them contained until they can be destroyed by white blood cells.

Food Sources

Protein can be found in a wide range of food. The best combination of protein sources depends on the region of the world, access, cost, amino acid types and nutrition balance, as well as acquired tastes. Some foods are high in certain amino acids, but their digestibility and the antinutritional factor present in these foods make them of limited value in human nutrition. Therefore, one must consider digestibility and secondary nutrition profile such as calories, cholesterol, vitamins and essential mineral density of the protein source.

On a worldwide basis, source of protein may be:

- **Plant source:** Proteins of plant origin include legumes, nuts, seeds and fruits. Foods contribute over 60% of the per capita supply of protein, on average.
- **Animal source:** Meat, products from milk, eggs and fish. In North America, animal-derived foods contribute about 70% of protein sources.

Whole grains and cereals are another source of proteins. However, these tend to be limiting in the amino acid lysine or threonine, which are available in other vegetarian sources and meats. Examples of food staples and cereal sources of protein, each with a concentration greater than 7%, are (in no particular order) buckwheat, oats, rye, millet, maize (corn), rice, wheat, bulgur, sorghum, amaranth, and quinoa.

Vegetarian sources of proteins in certain parts of the world, have higher concentrations of amino acids and are more complete sources of protein than whole grains and cereals. Examples of vegetarian foods with protein concentrations greater than 7% include soybeans, lentils, kidney beans, white beans, mung beans, chickpeas, cowpeas, lima beans, pigeon peas, lupines, wing beans, almonds, Brazil nuts, cashews, pecans, walnuts, cotton seeds, pumpkin seeds, sesame seeds, and sunflower seeds.

Protein Quality

It is not only the quantity of protein, which is important but also the quality. This depends mainly on the type and amount of particular amino acids present in the protein. Based on the quality of proteins, they can be classified into three classes.

Complete (First Class) Proteins

These contain all the nine essential amino acids in sufficient quantities so that a normal rate of growth can be maintained by the body. Mainly proteins from animal source belong to this class, i.e., milk, meat, eggs, fish, and poultry. Wheat germ and dried yeast have a biologic value approaching that of animal sources.

Partially Complete (Second Class) Proteins

They can maintain life, but they lack sufficient amount of some of the essential amino acids necessary for growth. Proteins from plant source like pulses, wheat and nuts belong to this class. By combining foods from two or more partially complete proteins, creates a complete protein. The amino acids that may be missing from one type of food can be compensated by adding a protein that contains that missing amino acid. When eaten in combination at the same meal, you are providing your body with all the essential amino acids it requires. These are considered complementary proteins when they are combined to compensate for each other's lack of amino acid. The example is the combination of all cereals, pulses, nuts, vegetables and fruits.

Incomplete (Third Class) Proteins

They can neither promote growth nor maintain life because they lack many of the amino acids or even if they contain, it is in very small amounts, Gelatin and zein which is found in corn are the examples which belongs to this class.

Recommended Daily Dietary Allowances

Recommended daily dietary allowances can determined on several factors including:
- Body weight and composition (increased muscle mass)
- Physical activity level
- Individual's energy and carbohydrate intake
- Overall energy intake
- Presence of illness or injury (e.g., Recovering from trauma or operation)
- Rate of growth in the individual (e.g., Greater during childhood)
- The body's need for nitrogen and essential amino acids.

The protein requirements vary from individual to individual. Apart from age and physiological conditions, factors like emotional disturbances infection and stress can affect a person's protein requirement. For proper utilization of protein, energy intakes should be adequate. Maximum amount of protein per kg of body weight is required during infancy, i.e., till one year of age. The requirement per kg of body weight slowly decreases as one reaches the adulthood and then it is stable, i.e., 1 g per kg of desirable body weight. During pregnancy and lactation the protein allowances for woman are increased over the basic level. The Indian Council of Medical Research (1990) has recommended the following standards in respect of protein requirement in India.

Estimated Requirements

US and Canadian Dietary Reference Intake guidelines:
- **Women aged 19 to 70 years old:** 46 g of protein per day (based on 57.5 kg individual).
- **Men aged 19 to 70 years of age:** 56 g of protein per day (based on 70 kg individual).

The recommended daily protein dietary allowance is based on a normal sedentary person.

Effects of Deficiency

- Abdominal enlargements
- Edema
- Depletion of plasma proteins
- Negative nitrogen balance
- Kwashiorkor
- Marasmus.

Table 5.1: Dietary reference intakes for protein.

DRI values (grams/kg/day)				
			RDA	
Age group	*Male*	*Female*	*Male*	*Female*
7 through 12 months	1	1	1.2 (11)	1.2 (11)
1 through 3 years	0.87	0.87	1.05 (13)	1.05 (13)
4 through 8 years	0.76	0.76	0.95 (19)	0.95 (19)
9 through 13 years	0.76	0.76	0.95 (34)	0.95 (34)
14 through 18 years	0.73	0.71	0.85 (52)	0.85 (46)
19 through 30 years	0.66	0.66	0.80 (56)	0.80 (46)
31 through 50 years	0.66	0.66	0.80 (56)	0.80 (46)
51 through 70 years	0.66	0.66	0.80 (56)	0.80 (46)
>70 years	0.66	0.66	0.80 (56)	0.80 (46)
Pregnancy: Increased protein requirements for 2nd half of pregnancy. 1st half use nonpregnant RDA.		0.88		1.1 (71)
Lactation		1.05		1.3 (71)

Estimated Average Requirement (EAR): The average daily nutrient intake level that is estimated to meet the requirements of half of the healthy individuals in a particular life stage and gender group.
Recommended Dietary Allowance (RDA): The average daily dietary nutrient intake level that is sufficient to meet the nutrient requirements of nearly all (97–98%) healthy individuals in a particular life stage and gender group.

Marasmus

Marasmus is a disease caused by a severe deficiency of protein and calories that affect infants and very young children, often resulting in weight loss and dehydration. Marasmus can develop into starvation and cause fatality caused by a lack of essential nutrients. People with marasmus appear bony with little muscle tissue.

Kwashiorkor

Kwashiorkor is a disease caused by a severe deficiency of protein in diets that contain calories mostly from carbohydrates such as yams, rice and bananas. It usually affects older children. People with kwashiorkor appear puffy in the abdomen area from retention of fluid, according to the University of Maryland Medical Center. Common symptoms of both marasmus and kwashiorkor include fatigue, irritability, diarrhea, stunted growth and impairment of cognition and mental health. Now Kwashiorkor and marasmus have been renamed as Severe Acute Malnutrition (SAM) is both a medical and social disorder and it is defined by weight for height. The details about SAM has described separately.

CARBOHYDRATES

Formerly the 'carbohydrate' is a simple sugars or substances, are composed of carbon, hydrogen, and oxygen, the last two being in the proportion to form water hence termed as 'Carbohydrate'. The general formula is $C_n H_{2n} O_n$. Carbohydrates are widely distributed in nature in the form of sugars, starches, celluloses and other substances. Carbohydrates are one of the main types of nutrients. They are the most important source of energy for our body. Our digestive system changes carbohydrates into glucose. This sugar is used for energy for the cells, tissues and organs. It stores any extra sugar in our liver and muscles for when it is needed.

Carbohydrates are called simple or complex, depending on their chemical structure. Simple carbohydrates include sugars found naturally in foods such as fruits, vegetables, milk, and milk products. They also include sugars added during food processing and refining. Complex carbohydrates include whole grain breads and cereals, starchy vegetables and legumes. Many of the complex carbohydrates are good sources of fiber.

Classification of Carbohydrates

The carbohydrates are classified into 3 groups:

1. **Monosaccharide:**
   - Glucose
   - Fructose
   - Galactose
2. **Disaccharides or compound sugar:**
   - Sucrose
   - Lactose
   - Maltose
3. **Polysaccharides:** Polysaccharides contain more than 2 sugars. They are pentose, hexoses and they present in all vegetables and bran's of cereals.

Functions of Carbohydrate

Providing Energy and Regulating Blood Glucose

Carbohydrates are the cheapest source of energy. One gram of carbohydrate gives 4 calories. Glucose is the main source of energy. So all types of carbohydrates are converted to glucose in body and then used for immediate tissue energy need. A small amount is stored as glycogen in the liver and muscles, and some is stored as fat in the adipose tissues. Glucose is the only sugar used by the body to provide energy for its tissues. Therefore, all digestible polysaccharides, disaccharides, and monosaccharide must eventually be converted into glucose or a metabolite of glucose by various liver enzymes. Because of its significant importance to proper cellular function, blood glucose levels must be kept relatively constant.

Sparing Protein and Preventing Ketosis

First of all, maintaining a regular intake of carbohydrates will prevent protein from being used as an energy source. Gluconeogenesis will slow down and amino acids will be free for the biosynthesis of enzymes, antibodies, receptors and other important proteins. Furthermore, an adequate amount of carbohydrates will prevent the degradation of skeletal muscle and other tissues such as the heart, liver, and kidneys. Ketosis will be prevented by taking proper amount of carbohydrate. Although the brain will adapt to using ketenes as a fuel, it preferentially uses carbohydrates and requires a minimum level of glucose circulating in the blood in order to function properly. Before the adaptation process occurs, lower blood glucose levels may cause headaches in some individuals. To prevent these ketotic symptoms, it is recommended that the average person consume at least 50 to 100 g of carbohydrates per day.

The first priority of metabolism during a prolonged fast is to provide enough glucose for the brain and other organs that dependent upon it for energy in order to spare proteins for other cellular functions. The next priority of the body is to shift the use of fuel from glucose to fatty acids and ketone bodies. From then on, ketones become more and more important as a source of fuel while fatty acids and glucose become less important.

Flavors and Sweeteners

One of the less important functions of carbohydrates is to provide sweetness to foods. Receptors located at the tip of the tongue bind to tiny bits of carbohydrates and send what humans perceive as a 'sweet' signal to the brain. However, different sugars vary in sweetness. For example, fructose is almost twice as sweet as sucrose and sucrose is approximately 30% sweeter than glucose.

Sweeteners can be classified as either nutritive or alternative. Nutritive sweeteners have all been mentioned before and include sucrose, glucose, fructose, high fructose corn syrup, and lactose. These types of sweeteners not only impart flavor to the food, but can also be metabolized for energy. In contrast, alternative sweeteners provide no food energy and include saccharin, cyclamate, aspartame, and acesulfame. Controversy over saccharin and cyclamate as artificial sweeteners still exists but aspartame and acesulfame are used extensively in many foods in the United States. Aspartame and acesulfame are both hundreds of times sweeter than sucrose but only acesulfame is able to be used in baked goods since it is much more stable than aspartame when heated.

Synthesis of B-complex

Being less soluble than other sugars remain in the intestine long enough to encourage the growth of desirable bacteria, which help in synthesis of B-complex vitamins. It also helps in better absorption and utilization of calcium.

Provide Bulk to the Diets

Cellulose, hemicelluloses and pectin's gives no nutrients to the body, but these fibers are very useful in providing bulk to the diets. These indigestible substances faceplate the elimination of intestinal wastes by stimulating the peristaltic movements of gastrointestinal tract and they also have the property of absorbing water thus giving bulk to the intestinal contents. Lack of adequate dietary fiber in diets containing refined foods, leads to constipation and colon cancer, also some of the dietary fibers like gum and mucilage's in our diets have been shown to lower blood cholesterol in hypercholesterolemia subjects and blood sugar in diabetes. Vegetables especially the leafy ones, fruits and unrefined cereals are rich in fiber and a generous inclusion of these provides a diet rich in fiber.

As Dietary Fiber

In general, the consumption of soluble and insoluble fiber makes the elimination of waste much easier. Since dietary fiber is both indigestible and an attractant of water, stools become large and soft. As a result, feces can be expelled with less pressure. However, not enough fiber consumption will change the constitution of the stool and increase the amount of force required during defecation. Excessive pressure during the elimination of waste can force places in the large intestine wall out from between bands of smooth muscle to produce small pouches called diverticula. Hemorrhoids may also result from unnecessary strain during defecation.

The disease of having many diverticula in the large intestine is known as 'diverticulosis'. Although diverticula is often asymptomatic, food particles become trapped in their folds and bacteria begin to metabolize the particles into acids and gases. Eventually, the diverticula may become inflamed, a condition known as 'diverticulitis'. To combat the disease, antibiotics are administered to the patient to destroy the bacteria while the intake of fiber in the diet is decreased until the inflammation has subsided. Once the inflammation has been reduced, a high fiber diet is begun to prevent a relapse.

Besides the prevention of intestinal disease, diets high in fiber have other health benefits. High fiber intake reduces the risk of developing obesity by increasing the bulk of a meal without yielding much energy. An expanded stomach leads to satisfaction despite the fact that the caloric intake has decreased.

Beyond dieters, diabetics can also benefit from consuming a regular amount of dietary fiber. Once in the intestine, it slows the absorption of glucose to prevent a sudden increase in blood glucose levels. A relatively high intake of fiber will also decrease the absorption of cholesterol, a compound that is thought to contribute to atherosclerosis or scarring of the arteries. Serum cholesterol may be further reduced by a reduction in the release of insulin after meals. Since insulin is known to promote cholesterol synthesis in the liver, a reduction in the absorption of glucose after meals through the consumption of fiber can help to control serum cholesterol levels. Furthermore, dietary fiber intake may help prevent colon cancer by diluting potential carcinogens through increased water retention, binding carcinogens to the fiber itself and speeding the passage of food through the intestinal tract so that cancer-causing agents have less time to act.

Source

Three main sources of carbohydrates are:

1. Starches
2. Sugar
3. Cellulose

Foods High in Starch

Starchy vegetables like peas, corn, lima beans and potatoes, dried beans, lentils and peas such as pinto beans, kidney beans, black eyed peas and split peas, grains like oats, barley and rice. (The majority of grain products in the US are made from wheat flour. These include pasta, bread and crackers but the variety is expanding to include other grains as well).

Sugar

Sugar is another type of carbohydrate which referred to as simple or fast-acting carbohydrate. Sugars are present in cane sugar, jaggery, honey, jam, jellies, dry fruits, sweets and fresh fruits, e.g., banana, sapota, grapes, mango.

Fibers

Dietary fibers such as cellulose, hemicellulose, pectin, gum and mucilage are important carbohydrates for several reasons. Soluble dietary fibers like pectin, gum and mucilage pass undigested through the small intestine and are degraded into fatty acids and gases by the large intestine. The fatty acids produced in this way can either be used as a fuel for the large intestine or be absorbed into the bloodstream. Therefore, dietary fiber is essential for proper intestinal health. Fiber comes from plant foods so there is no fiber in animal products such as milk, eggs, meat, poultry, and fish.

Fiber is the indigestible part of plant foods, including fruits, vegetables, whole grains, nuts and legumes. When you consume dietary fiber, most of it passes through the intestines and is not digested.

Good Sources of Dietary Fiber

Beans and legumes: Think black beans, kidney beans, pintos, chick peas (garbanzos), white beans, and lentils. Fruits and vegetables, especially those with edible skin (for example, apples, corn and beans) and those with edible seeds (for example, berries).

Whole grains: Whole wheat pasta, whole grain cereals (Look for those with three grams of dietary fiber or more per serving, including those made from whole wheat, wheat bran, and oats). Whole grain breads (To be a good source of fiber, one slice of bread should have at least three grams of fiber. Another good indication: look for breads where the first ingredient is a whole grain. For example, whole wheat or oats). Many grain products now have 'double fiber' with extra fiber added. Nuts—try different kinds. Peanuts, walnuts and almonds are a good source of fiber and healthy fat, but watch portion sizes, because they also contain a lot of calories in a small amount.

Recommended Daily Dietary Intakes

There is no fixed amount recommended for carbohydrates, but even then it should provide about 60–70% of the total energy. The daily diet of an adult should contain at least 40 g of dietary fiber.

Deficiency

The energy needs are not met if the diets are deficient in carbohydrates. The work efficiency is lowered. Also person becomes underweight. Growth will be slow in the case of children. Symptoms of ketosis may also develop. Lack of dietary fiber in the diet leads to constipation and colon cancer. If carbohydrates are consumed in excess they get accumulated as fat in the body leading to obesity and predisposes to diabetes and heart ailments.

FATS OR LIPIDS

Fat is an important component of our diets and serve a number of functions. These are also organic compound of carbon, hydrogen and oxygen. Fats are a wide group of compounds whose basis is in long-chain organic acids, called 'fatty acids'. More particularly, fats are *esters* of such organic acids formed with the alcohol glycerol. These differ from carbohydrates is that they have much smaller proportion of oxygen and much greater proportions of carbon and oxygen. Lipids are broadly classified into two groups, simple lipids and compound lipids. Simple lipids include fatty acids and waxes. All other lipids are included under compound lipids, e.g., carotenoids and phosphoglycerides.

The term 'fat' is generally applied to all triglycerides regardless of whether they are solid or liquid at room temperature. Triglycerides from animal sources contain a higher percentage of saturated fatty acids and are normally solids at room temperature and known as 'fats'. The plant triglycerides are rich in unsaturated fatty acids and are generally liquids at room temperature and called oils. Fats in the diets can be of two kinds, the visible and invisible fat. The visible fats are those which are derived from animal fats like butter, ghee and those derived from vegetables sources like mustard oil, groundnut oil, sunflower oil, etc. Apart from the added/visible fat, some amount of fat is present in other foods like cereals, pulses, oilseeds, milks, eggs and meats. The invisible fat is believed to contribute significance to the total fat and essential fatty acid content of the diet depending upon the foodstuffs present in the diet.

Types of Fat

- A *saturated fat* is a *fat* that consists of triglycerides containing only saturated fatty acids. Saturated fatty acids have no double bonds between the individual carbon atoms of the fatty acid chain. That is, the chain of carbon atoms is fully 'saturated' with hydrogen atoms. There are many kinds of naturally occurring saturated fatty acids, which differ mainly in number of carbon atoms, from 3 carbons (propionic acid to 36 (hexatriacontanoic acid). The nature of the fat depends upon the types of fatty acids which make up the triglycerides. All fats contain both saturated and unsaturated fatty acids but are usually described as 'saturated' or 'unsaturated' according to the proportions of fatty acids present. For example butter is often described as a 'saturated' fat because it has more saturated fatty acids than unsaturated fatty acids, while most vegetable oils are described as 'unsaturated' as they have more monounsaturated or polyunsaturated fatty acids.
- An *unsaturated fat* is a fat or fatty acid in which there is at least one double bond within the fatty acid chain. A fatty acid chain is monounsaturated if it contains one double bond, and polyunsaturated if it contains more than one double bond. Where double bonds are formed, hydrogen atoms are eliminated. Thus, a saturated fat has no double bonds, has the maximum number of hydrogens bonded to the carbons, and therefore is 'saturated' with hydrogen atoms. In cellular metabolism, unsaturated fat molecules contain somewhat less energy (i.e., fewer calories) than an equivalent amount of saturated fat.

Most 'unsaturated fats' are liquid at room temperature, are usually of vegetable origin and are commonly known as 'oils'. Vegetable and fish oils can be 'hardened' by a process which adds hydrogen atoms to some of the double bonds in the unsaturated fatty acids. This process is known as 'hydrogenation'. Hydrogenated vegetable oils are occasionally used in the manufacture of margarine and cooking fats, which may be used to produce cakes, biscuits and other bakery products.

Essential Fatty Acids

Certain fatty acids should be provided essentially in the diets, as they are not synthesized in the body. These are polyunsaturated fatty acids, namely linoleic, linolenic and arachidonic acids and are grouped as 'essential' fatty acids. They are required for metabolism and for maintenance of normal health of the skin. Therefore, proper type of fats which are rich in essential fatty acids, e.g., Peanut, cottonseed, corn, and sunflower oils, must be present in the diets. Animal fats are poor sources of essential fatty acids. However, it is only the linoleic acids which we really need as the other two can be synthesized in the body from the linoleic acid.

Food Sources

Dietary fats are derived from two main sources:

1. **Animal sources:** It includes butter, ghee, curd, whole milk, and its products meat, fish, poultry, and eggs.
2. **Plant sources:** They include all vegetables oils, e.g., groundnut, gingelly, mustard, cottonseed, sunflower, and coconut oil. Also it will include hydrogenated fats, margarine, nuts and oil seeds like cashewnut, peanuts, almonds, and mustard seeds.

Functions of Fat

- **Energy-yielding:** Fats are concentrated source of energy. One gram of fat gives 9 calories. Compared to carbohydrate it not only gives more amounts of energy but at a faster rate too.

- **Fats also perform the protein-sparing action** in the same way as carbohydrate does.
- **Storehouse of energy for the body's needs:** In fact not only amount of fats as such are stored in adipose tissue, but any amount of glucose, amino acids, not promptly utilized are also synthesized and stored in the body, thereby energy is continuously available from the stores in adipose tissues.
- **Insulation and padding:** The subcutaneous layer of fat is an effective insulator and reduces losses of body heat in cold weather, thus regulating the body temperature. The vital organs such as the kidneys are protected against physical injury by a padding of fat around the organs. Act like Cushion and protect the heart and other vital organs and Protect bones from injury.
- **Absorption of fat-soluble vitamins:** Fats help in absorption and transportation of fat-soluble vitamins in the body.
- **Provides essential fatty acids:** Fat is also the source of certain fatty acids which are essential for metabolism and for maintaining a normal skin.
- **Fats acts as a lubricant** for various body organs especially the organs of the gastrointestinal tract.
- **Gives satiety value:** Fat depresses the secretion of hydrochloric acid in the stomach, Thus the food stays in the gastrointestinal tract for a longer time and feeling of hunger is delayed.
- **Fat also increases the palatability** of the diet by adding flavor to many cooked preparations.
- Fats are also sources of essential fatty acids, an important dietary requirements.

Recommended Daily Dietary Intakes

The fat requirement mainly depends upon the energy needs of the individual. From physiological point of view there can be wide variation in fat intake and still good health can be maintained. On an average about 15–20% of the total energy should be supplied from fats. The dietary fats should be a good source of essential fatty acids and hence at least 50% of the dietary fat should be from vegetable oils rich in essential fatty acids.

Deficiency and Excess Intake of Fat

Deficiency

Just like carbohydrates deficiency, the energy needs will not be met if the diet is deficient in fat content. Hence leading to underweight, weakness and lowered work efficiency. In addition to this the deficiency of the essential fatty acids play a role in several metabolic reactions, a deficiency of these fatty acids is believed to lead to a skin condition known as 'phyrnoderma' (toad skin) in which the skin becomes rough and thick horny papules of the size of a pinhead irrupt in certain areas of the body, notably the thighs, buttocks and trunk. In addition to this, the deficiency of fat-soluble vitamins and essential fatty acids will also result. This will cause the ailments related to skin, eyes, bones, etc.

Excess

If excessive fat is consumed it will result in obesity gastro-intestinal disturbances, and predisposal to many other diseases like diabetes and cardiovascular ailments. In recent years there has been a revival of interest in the nutritional aspect of excessive intake of the fat in the diet in increasing the level of cholesterol.

MALNUTRITION

A pathological state resulting from a relative or absolute deficiency or excess of one or more essential nutrients; clinically manifested or detected only by biochemical, anthropometric or physiological tests. Malnutrition is caused by eating a diet in which nutrients are not enough or are too much such that it causes health problems. It is a category of diseases that includes under nutrition and over nutrition. Over nutrition can result in obesity and overweight. The World Health Organization (WHO) defines malnutrition as the cellular imbalance between the supply of nutrients and energy and the body's demand for them to ensure growth, maintenance, and specific functions **(Table 5.2)**.

Malnutrition generally implies under nutrition and refers to all deviations from adequate and optimal nutritional status in infants, children and in adults. In children, under nutrition manifests as underweight and stunting (short stature), while severely undernourished children present with the symptoms and signs that characterize conditions known as 'kwashiorkor', 'marasmus' or 'marasmic-kwashiorkor'.

Etiology

Figure 5.1 depicts the etiological factors of malnutrition.

Dietary Practices

A lack of adequate breastfeeding leads to malnutrition in infants and children, associated with the deaths of an estimated one million children annually. Illegal advertising of breast milk substitutes continues three decades after its 1981 prohibition under the WHO International Code of Marketing Breast Milk Substitutes.

Deriving too much of one's diet from a single source, such as eating almost exclusively corn or rice, can cause malnutrition. This may either be from a lack of education about proper nutrition, or from only having access to a single food source.

Diseases

Malnutrition can be a consequence of health issues such as gastroenteritis or chronic illness, especially the HIV/AIDS pandemic. Diarrhea and other infections can cause malnutrition through decreased nutrient absorption, decreased intake of food, increased metabolic requirements, and direct nutrient loss. Parasite infections can also lead to malnutrition.

Table 5.2: Classification of malnutrition.

Classification	*Definition*	*Grading*	
Gomez	Weight below % median WFA	Mild (grade 1) Moderate (grade 2) Severe (grade 3)	75–90% WFA 60–74% WFA <60% WFA
Waterlow	z-scores (SD) below median WFH	Mild Moderate Severe	80–90% WFH 70–80% WFH <70% WFH
WHO (wasting)	z-scores (SD) below median WFH	Moderate Severe	–3%</= z-score <–2 z-score <–3
WHO (stunting)	z-scores (SD) below median HFA	Moderate Severe	–3%</= z-score <–2 z-score <–3
Kanawati	MUAC divided by occipitofrontal head circumference	Mild Moderate Severe	<0.31 <0.28 <0.25
Cole	z-scores of BMI for age	Grade 1 Grade 2 Grade 3	BMI for age z-score <–1 BMI for age z-score <–2 BMI for age z-score <–3

(BMI: body mass index; HFA: height for age; MUAC: mid-upper arm circumference; SD: standard deviation; WFA: weight for age; WFH: weight for height; WHO: World Health Organization)

Poverty and Food Prices

Poor socioeconomic position was associated with chronic malnutrition since it inhibits purchase of nutritious foods such as milk, meat, poultry, and fruits. As much as food shortages may be a contributing factor to malnutrition in countries with lack of technology.

Agricultural Productivity

Local food shortages can be caused by a lack of arable land, adverse weather, lower farming skills such as crop rotation, or by a lack of technology or resources needed for the higher yields found in modern agriculture, such as fertilizers, pesticides, irrigation, machinery and storage facilities. As a result of widespread poverty, farmers cannot afford or governments cannot provide the resources necessary to improve local yields.

Climate Change

Climate change is of importance to food security, with 95% of all malnourished peoples living in the relatively stable climate region of the subtropics and tropics. According to the latest IPCC reports, temperature increases in these regions are 'very likely.' Even small changes in temperatures can lead to increased frequency of extreme weather conditions. Many of these have great impact on agricultural production and hence nutrition.

Mental Health Problems

Some patients with mental health conditions, such as depression, may develop eating habits which lead to malnutrition. Patients with anorexia nervosa or bulimia may develop malnutrition because they are ingesting too little food.

Improper Absorption

Some people may eat properly, but their bodies cannot absorb the nutrients they need for good health. Examples include patients with Crohn's disease or ulcerative colitis. Such patients may need to have part of the small intestine removed (ileostomy). Individuals who suffer from celiac disease have a genetic disorder that makes them intolerant to gluten. Patients with celiac disease have a higher risk of damage to the lining of their intestines, resulting in poorer food absorption. Patients who experience serious bouts of diarrhea and/or vomiting may lose vital nutrients and are at higher risk of suffering from malnutrition.

Alcoholism

This is a chronic (long-term) disease. Individuals who suffer from alcoholism can develop gastritis, or pancreas damage. These problems also seriously undermine the body's ability to digest food, absorb certain vitamins, and produce hormones which regulate metabolism. Alcohol contains calories, reducing the patient's feeling of hunger, so he/she consequently may not eat enough proper food to supply the body with essential nutrients.

In the poorer nations malnutrition is commonly caused by:

Food Prices and Food Distribution

It is ironic that approximately 80% of malnourished children live in developing nations that actually produce food surpluses (Food and Agriculture Organization). Some leading economists say that famine is closely linked to high food prices and problems with food distribution.

Lack of Breastfeeding

Experts say that lack of breastfeeding, especially in the developing world, leads to malnutrition in infants and

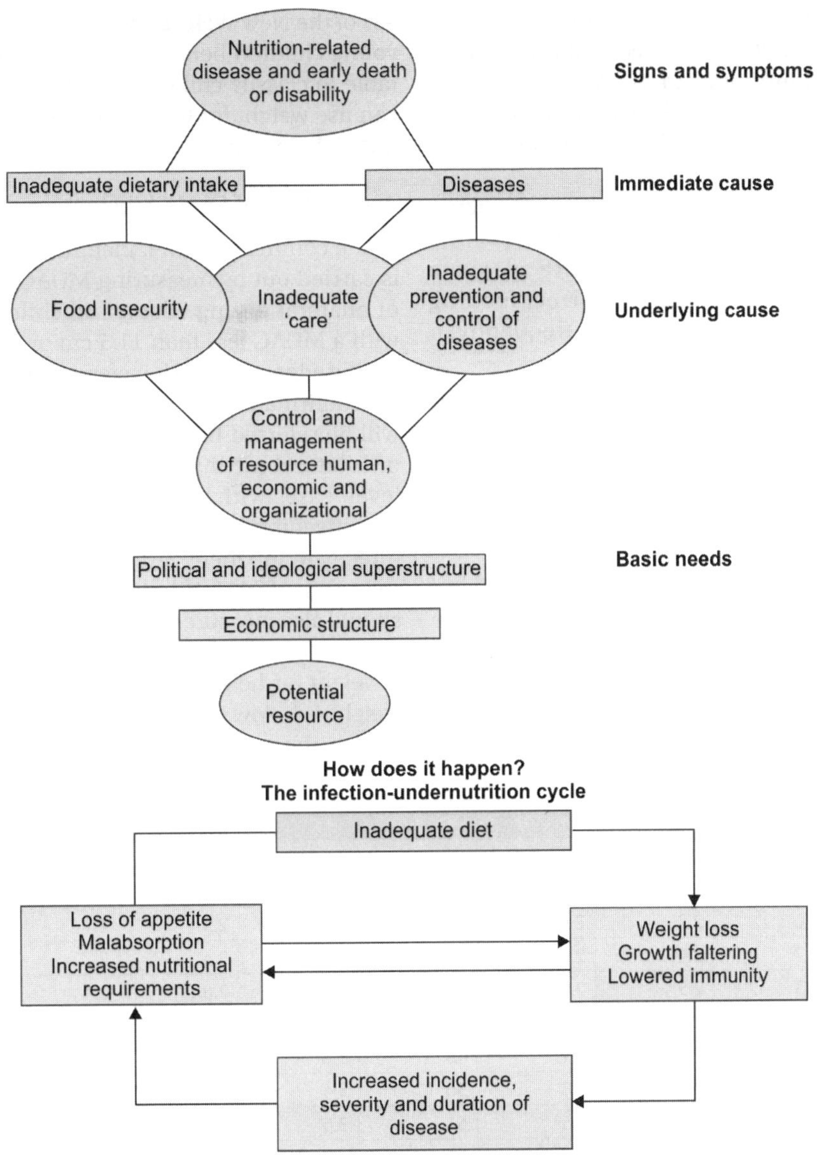

Fig. 5.1: Etiology of malnutrition.

children. In some parts of the world mothers still believe that bottle feeding is better for the child. Another reason for lack of breastfeeding, mainly in the developing world, is that mothers abandon it because they do not know how to get their baby to latch on properly, or suffer pain and discomfort.

Inadequate and inappropriate feeding practises, early or improper weaning practises, dietary taboos such as hot food, cold food, child food, etc., as well as eating habits and cultural practises connected to weaning and newborn feeding, are additional causes of malnutrition in children.

Though, there is a vast cause can relate to malnutrition all the cause can be categorized under two major heading. Those are deficiency of food in body and different disease conditions.

Classification of Undernutrition

The World Health Organization (WHO) defines malnutrition as the cellular imbalance between the supply of nutrients and energy and the body's demand for them to ensure growth, maintenance, and specific functions.

Underweight

Failure to achieve expected weight as compared to a healthy, well-nourished child of the same age is a sign of underweight and is recommended as a basic indicator of the status of a population's health. This condition can result from either chronic or acute malnutrition or both. Low weight for age (composite measure of acute and chronic malnutrition).

- **Stunting:** Stunting, or shortness, is an indicator of chronic (long-term) malnutrition. Failure to achieve expected length/height as compared to a healthy, well-nourished child of the same age is a sign of stunting. This is due to failure to receive adequate nutrition over a long period, frequent infection, sustained inappropriate feeding practices and poverty. Stunting is an important indicator of child growth and development. Stunting not only means stunted Bodies but also stunted Brains leading to stunted lives. India contributes to 31.2% of the stunted children population in the world which is the highest. The prevalence of stunting in India is 48% and the prevalence in Odisha is 45% (NHFS-3).

- **Wasting:** Wasting, or thinness, is an indicator of acute (short-term) malnutrition. Low weight for height.
- Wasting represents a recent failure to receive adequate nutrition, inadequate food intake, incorrect feeding practices, disease, and infection or more frequently, a combination of these factors.
- If a child fails to achieve expected weight for height, that is <-2 SD of the WHO Child Growth Standards median, then we will say the child is suffering from wasting.
- Severely wasted child is at 10 times the risk of Death.

Severe Acute Malnutrition

Severe acute malnutrition (SAM) is both a medical and social disorder and it is defined by weight for height (Z-score below -3 SD of the median WHO child growth standards), or Mid-upper arm circumference <115 mm/<11.5 cm, or Presence of bipedal nutritional edema. WHO and UNICEF recommend the use of a cut-off for weight for height below -3z of the New WHO growth standard to identify infants and young children being SAM. Use weight for height reference table to classify child as SAM if below -3z. A health worker can use weight for height reference table to classify child as SAM if below -3z.

Assessment of SAM Child

At the community level, identification of children with SAM is carried out by measuring MUAC and assessing presence of bilateral pitting edema. All children aged 6–59 months with a MUAC less than 11.5 cm or presenting with bilateral pitting edema should be referred to the nearest health facility for confirmation and treatment. Infants less than 6 months will be referred based on their weight for height indicator or bilateral pitting edema. If not possible at community level, cases with visible severe wasting and difficulties in breastfeeding should be referred. These infants will be sent directly to inpatient care for treatment. If the enrolment for treatment of SAM includes the weight for height criteria, staff should also measure the weight and the length or height of all children presenting and compare the child's weight against a weight for height look-up table to see whether the child's weight is below the -3 z-scores from the median. **Table 5.3** depicts the weight-for-length card.

Table 5.3: Weight-for-length reference card (below 87 cm).

Boys' weight (kg)					Length	*Boys' weight (kg)*				
–4 SD	–3 SD	–2 SD	–1 SD	Median	(cm)	Median	–1 SD	–2 SD	–3 SD	–4 SD
1.7	1.9	2.0	2.2	2.4	45	2.5	2.3	2.1	1.9	1.7
1.8	2.0	2.2	2.4	2.6	46	2.6	2.4	2.2	2.0	1.9
2.0	2.1	2.3	2.5	2.8	47	2.8	2.6	2.4	2.2	2.0
2.1	2.3	2.5	2.7	2.9	48	3.0	2.7	2.5	2.3	2.1
2.2	2.4	2.6	2.9	3.1	49	3.2	2.9	2.6	2.4	2.2
2.4	2.6	2.8	3.0	3.3	50	3.4	3.1	2.9	2.6	2.4
2.5	2.7	3.0	3.2	3.5	51	3.6	3.3	3.0	2.8	2.5
2.7	2.9	3.2	3.5	3.8	52	3.8	3.5	3.2	2.9	2.7
2.9	3.1	3.4	3.7	4.0	53	4.0	3.7	3.4	3.1	2.8
3.1	3.3	3.6	3.9	4.3	54	4.3	3.9	3.6	3.3	3.0
3.3	3.6	3.8	4.2	4.5	55	4.5	4.2	3.8	3.5	3.2
3.5	3.8	4.1	4.4	4.8	56	4.8	4.4	4.0	3.7	3.4
3.7	4.0	4.3	4.7	5.1	57	5.1	4.6	4.3	3.9	3.6
3.9	4.3	4.6	5.0	5.4	58	5.4	4.9	4.5	4.1	3.8
4.1	4.5	4.8	5.3	5.7	59	5.6	5.1	4.7	4.3	3.9
4.3	4.7	5.1	5.5	6.0	60	5.9	5.4	4.9	4.5	4.1
4.5	4.9	5.3	5.8	6.3	61	6.1	5.6	5.1	4.7	4.3
4.7	5.1	5.6	6.0	6.5	62	6.4	5.8	5.3	4.9	4.5
4.9	5.3	5.8	6.2	6.8	63	6.6	6.0	5.5	5.1	4.7
5.1	5.5	6.0	6.5	7.0	64	6.9	6.3	5.7	5.3	4.8
5.3	5.7	6.2	6.7	7.3	65	7.1	6.5	5.9	5.5	5.0
5.5	5.9	6.4	6.9	7.5	66	7.3	6.7	6.1	5.6	5.1
5.6	6.1	6.6	7.1	7.7	67	7.5	6.9	6.3	5.8	5.3
5.8	6.3	6.8	7.3	8.0	68	7.7	7.1	6.5	6.0	5.5
6.0	6.5	7.0	7.6	8.2	69	8.0	7.3	6.7	6.1	5.6

Contd..

Contd..

Boys' weight (kg)					*Length*	*Boys' weight (kg)*				
6.1	6.6	7.2	7.8	8.4	70	8.2	7.5	6.9	6.3	5.9
6.3	6.8	7.4	8.0	8.6	71	8.4	7.7	7.0	6.5	5.9
6.4	7.0	7.6	8.2	8.9	72	8.6	7.8	7.2	6.6	6.0
6.6	7.2	7.7	8.4	9.1	73	8.8	8.0	7.4	6.8	6.2
6.7	7.3	7.9	8.6	9.3	74	9.0	8.2	7.5	6.9	6.3
6.9	7.5	8.1	8.8	9.5	75	9.1	8.4	7.7	7.1	6.5
7.0	7.6	8.3	8.9	9.7	76	9.3	8.5	7.8	7.2	6.6
7.2	7.8	8.4	9.1	9.9	77	9.5	8.7	8.0	7.4	6.7
7.3	7.9	8.6	9.3	10.1	78	9.7	8.9	8.2	7.5	6.9
7.4	8.1	8.7	9.5	10.3	79	9.9	9.1	8.3	7.7	7.0
7.6	8.2	8.9	9.6	10.4	80	10.1	9.2	8.5	7.8	7.1
7.7	8.4	9.1	9.8	10.6	81	10.3	9.4	8.7	8.0	7.3
7.9	8.5	9.2	10.0	10.8	82	10.5	9.6	8.9	8.1	7.5
8.0	8.7	9.4	10.2	11.0	83	10.7	9.8	9.0	8.3	7.6
8.2	8.9	9.6	10.4	11.3	84	11.0	10.1	9.2	8.5	7.8
8.4	9.1	9.8	10.6	11.5	85	11.2	10.3	9.4	8.7	8.0
8.6	9.3	10.0	10.8	11.7	86	11.5	10.5	9.7	8.9	8.1
8.9	9.6	10.4	11.2	12.2	87	11.9	10.9	10.0	9.2	8.4
9.1	9.8	10.6	11.5	12.4	88	12.1	11.1	10.2	9.4	8.6
9.3	10.0	10.8	11.7	12.6	89	12.4	11.4	10.4	9.6	8.8
9.4	10.2	11.0	11.9	12.9	90	12.6	11.6	10.6	9.8	9.0
9.6	10.4	11.2	12.1	13.1	91	12.9	11.8	10.9	10.0	9.1
9.8	10.6	11.4	12.3	13.4	92	13.1	12.0	11.1	10.2	9.3
9.9	10.8	11.6	12.6	13.6	93	13.4	12.3	11.3	10.4	9.5
10.1	11.0	11.8	12.8	13.8	94	13.6	12.5	11.5	10.6	9.7
10.3	11.1	12.0	13.0	14.1	95	13.9	12.7	11.7	10.8	9.8
10.4	11.3	12.2	13.2	14.3	96	14.1	12.9	11.9	10.9	10.0
10.6	11.5	12.4	13.4	14.6	97	14.4	13.2	12.1	11.1	10.2
10.8	11.7	12.6	13.7	14.8	98	14.7	13.4	12.3	11.3	10.4
11.0	11.9	12.9	13.9	15.1	99	14.9	13.7	12.5	11.5	10.5
11.2	12.1	13.1	14.2	15.4	100	15.2	13.9	12.8	11.7	10.7
11.3	12.3	13.3	14.4	15.6	101	15.5	14.2	13.0	12.0	10.9
11.5	12.5	13.6	14.7	15.9	102	15.8	14.5	13.3	12.2	11.1
11.7	12.8	13.8	14.9	16.2	103	16.1	14.7	13.5	12.4	11.3
11.9	13.0	14.0	15.2	16.5	104	16.4	15.0	13.8	12.6	11.5
12.1	13.2	14.3	15.5	16.8	105	16.8	15.3	14.0	12.9	11.8
12.3	13.4	14.5	15.8	17.2	106	17.1	15.6	14.3	13.1	12.0
12.5	13.7	14.8	16.1	17.5	107	17.5	15.9	14.6	13.4	12.2
12.7	13.9	15.1	16.4	17.8	108	17.8	16.3	14.9	13.7	12.4
12.9	14.1	15.3	16.7	18.2	109	18.2	16.6	15.2	13.9	12.7
13.2	14.4	15.6	17.0	18.5	110	18.6	17.0	15.5	14.2	12.9
13.4	14.6	15.9	17.3	18.9	111	19.0	17.3	15.8	14.5	13.2
13.6	14.9	16.2	17.6	19.2	112	19.4	17.7	16.2	14.8	13.5
13.8	15.2	16.5	18.0	19.6	113	19.8	18.0	16.5	15.1	13.7
14.1	15.4	16.8	18.3	20.0	114	20.2	18.4	16.8	15.4	14.0
14.3	15.7	17.1	18.6	20.4	115	20.7	18.8	17.2	15.7	14.3
14.6	16.0	17.4	19.0	20.8	116	21.1	19.2	17.5	16.0	14.5
14.8	16.2	17.7	19.3	21.2	117	21.5	19.6	17.8	16.3	14.8
15.0	16.5	18.0	19.7	21.6	118	22.0	19.9	18.2	16.6	15.1
15.3	16.8	18.3	20.0	22.0	119	22.4	20.3	18.5	16.9	15.4
15.5	17.1	18.6	20.4	22.4	120	22.8	20.7	18.9	17.3	15.6

Gomez Classification

The child's weight is compared to that of a normal child (50th percentage) of the same age. It is useful for population screening and public health evaluations. Gomez classification of malnutrition in children is shown in **Table 5.4**.

Table 5.4: Gomez classification of malnutrition in children.

	Mild malnutrition	*Moderate malnutrition*	*Severe malnutrition*
Percent ideal body weight	80–90%	70–79%	<70%
Percent of usual body weight	90–95%	80–89%	<80%

- Percent of reference weight for age =

$$\frac{\text{Weight of patient}}{\text{Weight of a normal child of the same age}} \times 100$$

Wellcome Classification

Table 5.5 depicts the Wellcome classification.

Table 5.5: Wellcome classification: evaluates the child for edema and with the Gomez classification system.

Weight for age (Gomez)	*With edema*	*Without edema*
60–80%	Kwashiorkor	Undernutrition
<60%	Marasmic-kwashiorkor	Marasmus

Waterlow Classification

Chronic malnutrition results in stunting. Malnutrition also affects the child's body proportions eventually resulting in body wastage.

- Percent weight for height =

$$\frac{\text{Weight of patient}}{\text{Weight of a normal child of the same height}} \times 100$$

- Percent height for age =

$$\frac{\text{Height of patient}}{\text{Height of a normal child of the same age}} \times 100$$

Classification of Indian Academy of Pediatric

- Ist degree—weight between 80–70/of expected
- IInd degree—weight between 70–60/of expected
- IIIrd degree—weight between 60–50/of expected
- IVth degree—below 50/of expected assessment of SAM child must be added.

Marasmus

Marasmus is a severe form of malnutrition that consists of the chronic wasting away of fat, muscle, and other tissues in the body. Malnutrition occurs when your body does not get enough protein and calories. This lack of nutrition can range from a shortage of certain vitamins to complete starvation. Marasmus is one of the most serious forms of protein-energy malnutrition (PEM) in the world and it is common in the 1st year of life.

Etiology

- Balanced starvation
- Insufficient breast milk
- Dilute milk mixture or lack of hygiene.

Clinical Manifestations

Clinical manifestations includes wasting, muscle wasting, Growth retardation, Mental changes, No edema, Variable-subnormal temp, slow PR, good appetite, dizziness, fatigue often diarrhea, etc.

Kwashiorkor

Between 1–3 years old.

Etiology

- Very low protein but using calories from carbohydrate.
- In places where starchy foods are main staple.
- Never exclusively dietary.

Kwashiorkor is a form of severe *protein-energy malnutrition* characterized by edema, irritability, anorexia, ulcerating dermatoses, and an enlarged liver with fatty infiltrates. Sufficient calorie intake, but with insufficient protein consumption.

Clinical Manifestations

A. **Diagnostic signs:**
  - Edema
  - Muscle wasting
  - Psychomotor changes

B. **Common signs:**
  - Hair changes
  - Diffuse depigmentation of skin
  - Moonface
  - Anemia
  - Decreased muscle mass
  - Diarrhea
  - Failure to gain weight and grow
  - Fatigue
  - Large belly that sticks out (protrudes)
  - Lethargy or apathy
  - Loss of muscle mass

C. **Occasional signs:**
  - Flaky-paint rash
  - Coma
  - Hepatomegaly
  - Shock (late stage)

Treatment of PEM or SAM Child

Severe PEM is an emergency, hospitalization 1–3 months is desirable. On admission, treat vitamin deficiencies, dehydration and associated infections. In the acute phase, feeding started as soon as rehydrated and when edema is lost, full-strength feeds given with maintenance calories and protein; recovery after 2–3 weeks. Rehabilitation with high energy feeds (150–200 kcal/kg/day) started once full-strength feeds tolerated; recovery expected within 4-6 weeks on high energy feeds.

Organization of Management of SAM in Inpatient Services

SAM children with medical complications should be admitted in a health facility and NOT treated in an emergency ward or casualty department for the first 24–48 hours.

According to current WHO recommendations, hospital-based care for SAM is organized into phases:

- **Stabilization phase:** Treatment or prevention of hypoglycemia, hypothermia, dehydration, treatment of infections, correction of hydro-electrolytic balance, correction of micronutrient deficiencies, commencement of cautious feeding with F75 and stimulation of emotional and sensorial development.
- **Transition phase:** Appetite has returned, medical complications are under control and resolving, edema starts reducing, the child is given with feeds of F100 to foster child's weight gain.
- **Rehabilitation phase or catch up growth phase:** The child is given with feeds of F100 and also semi solid or solid home based diet for speedy recover.

Prognosis of PEM

Permanent impairment of physical and mental growth if severe and occurs early especially before 6 months old. First 48 hours critical, with poor treatment mortality may exceed 50%. Even with thorough treatment, 10% mortality may still occur. Some mortality causes are endocrine, cardiac or liver failure, electrolyte imbalance, hypoglycemia and hypothermia.

Prevention of Malnutrition

The most vulnerable group is mother and baby. For prevention of malnutrition some tips we have to remember for taking care of them.

- Starts breastfeeding within one hour of birth.
- Exclusive breastfeeding during the first six months of life with frequent, on-demand contribute to child spacing and lower fertility rates.
- Timely introduction of complementary foods at six months to ensure that the infant's energy and nutrient requirements are met.
- Age-appropriate complementary foods, adequate in terms of quality, quantity and frequency for children 6–23 months.
- Children are given iron and folic acid (IFA) supplements or IFA containing multiple micronutrient supplements to prevent anemia.
- Safe handling of complementary foods and hygienic complementary feeding practices.
- Full immunization and biannual vitamin A supplementation with deworming.
- Frequent, appropriate, and active feeding for children during and after illness, including oral rehydration with zinc supplements during diarrhea. Every child is fed, actively and frequently, with age-appropriate and nutrient dense foods, during and after illness, while frequent, on-demand breastfeeding continues to increase fluid and nutrient intake. Children with diarrhea receive appropriate rehydration therapy including a full course of zinc supplementation.
- Timely and quality therapeutic feeding and care for all children with severe acute malnutrition.
- Education and improved food and nutrient intake for adolescent girls particularly to prevent anemia. Dietary counseling, weekly iron and folic acid supplementation, twice yearly (six months apart) deworming.
- Improved food and nutrient intake for women, particularly during pregnancy and lactation.

CONCEPT OF FIRST 1,000 DAYS

The 1,000 days between a woman's pregnancy and her child's 2nd birthday (–9 to +24 months) offer a unique window of opportunity to shape healthier and more prosperous futures. The right nutrition during this 1,000 day window can have a profound impact on a child's ability to grow, learn, and rise out of poverty. It can also shape a society's long-term health, stability and prosperity. Mothers nutrition is of utmost importance to deliver a healthy child with optimal weight. During pregnancy, undernutrition can have a devastating impact on the healthy growth and development of a child. Babies who are malnourished in the womb have a higher risk of dying in infancy and are more likely to face lifelong cognitive and physical deficits and chronic health problems. For children under the age of two, undernutrition can be life-threatening. It can weaken a child's immune system and make him or her more susceptible to dying from common illnesses such as pneumonia, diarrhea and malaria.

Measures to Improve Nutrition in 1,000 Days

Solutions to improve nutrition in the 1,000 day window are readily available, affordable and cost-effective. They include:

- Ensuring that mothers and young children get the necessary macro and micronutrients they need during pregnancy, after birth until 2 years of age;
- Promoting good nutritional practices, including breastfeeding and appropriate, healthy foods for infants; and immunization as enlisted in the 10 essential nutrition interventions.
- Treating malnourished children with special, therapeutic foods.
- Feeding of children during illness.

OBESITY

An obese person has accumulated so much body fat that it might have a negative effect on their health. If a person's body weight is at least 20% higher than it should be, he or she is considered obese. If your Body Mass Index (BMI) is between 25 and 29.9 you are considered overweight. If your BMI is 30 or over you are considered Generalized, excessive accumulation of fat in subcutaneous and other tissues is known as 'obesity'.

Classification of Obesity

1. Classification according to 'desirable' weight standard: Overweight ~ ≥10% while Obese ~ ≥20%
2. The Centers for Disease Control (CDC) avoids using 'obesity' instead suggest two levels of overweight
3. The American Obesity Association uses: BMI of 25, overweight for adults and BMI of 30 is obesity because ~ BMI of 30, the marker for obesity in adults.

Obesity appears most frequently in the 1st year, 5–6 years and adolescence.

Etiology

- Excessive intake of food compared with utilization
- Genetic constitution
- Psychic disturbance
- Endocrine and metabolic disturbances rare
- Insufficient exercise or lack of activity.

Clinical Manifestations

- Fine facial features on a heavy-looking taller child
- Larger upper arms and thighs
- Genu valgum common
- Relatively small hands and fingers tapering
- Adiposity in mammary regions
- Pendulous abdomen with striae
- In boys, external genitalia appear small though actually average in size
- In girls, external genitalia normal and menarche not delayed
- Psychologic disturbances common
- Bone age advanced.

Treatment of Obesity

A. **1st principle:** Decrease energy intake:
   1. Initial med exam to R/O pathological causes
   2. 3-day food recall to itemize child's diet
   3. Plan the right diet
      a. Avoid all sweets, fried foods and fats
      b. Limit milk intake to not >2 glasses/day
      c. For 10–14 years, limit to 1,100–1300 cal diet for several months
   4. Child must be properly motivated and family involvement essential

B. **2nd principle:** Increase energy output:
   1. Obtain an activity history
   2. Increase physical activity
   3. Involve in hobbies to prevent boredom.

Complication of Obesity

Pickwickian Syndrome

- Rare complication of extreme exogenous obesity
- Severe cardiorespiratory distress and alveolar hypoventilation
- Includes, hypoxemia, cyanosis, CHF, etc.
- High O_2 concentration dangerous in cyanosis
- Weight reduction ASAP and quick.

VITAMINS

Concept of Vitamin

The term 'vitamin' is derived from the word 'vital amine' which means essential nitrogenous compounds. A **vitamin** is an organic compound and a vital nutrient that an organism requires in limited amounts. An organic chemical compound (or related set of compounds) is called a vitamin when the organism cannot synthesize. The term was coined by Polish Scientist, Funk, who gave the name 'vitamine' to anti-beriberi substance. Later on 'e' was dropped and thus the term 'vitamin' was coined. However with the discovery of more vitamins, it was soon realized that all the vitamins are not nitrogenous compounds; but all vitamins are essential for health. Vitamins are complex chemical substances, required by the body in very small amounts. They do not yield energy, but act as catalyst in various body process. Since vitamins cannot be manufactured in the body (atleast in sufficient amounts) they have to be supplied through the diet.

Vitamins are classified as either water-soluble or fat-soluble **(Fig. 5.2)**. In humans there are 13 vitamins: 4

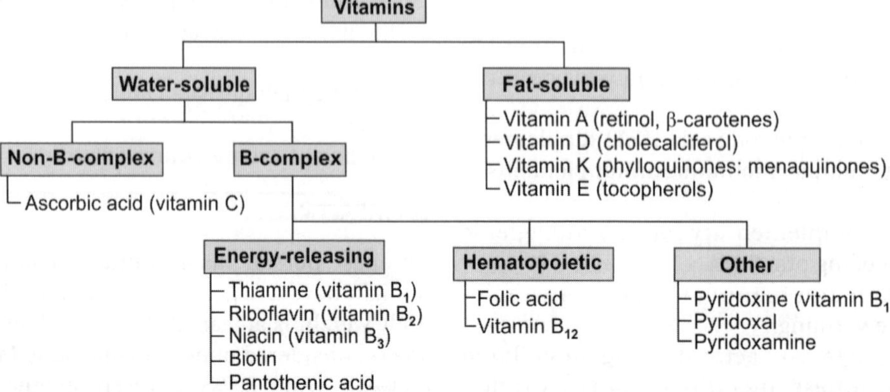

Fig. 5.2: Classification of vitamins.

fat-soluble (A, D, E, and K) and 9 water-soluble (8 B vitamins and vitamin C). Water-soluble vitamins dissolve easily in water and, in general, are readily excreted from the body, to the degree that urinary output is a strong predictor of vitamin consumption. Because they are not as readily stored, more consistent intake is important. Many types of water-soluble vitamins are synthesized by bacteria. Fat-soluble vitamins are absorbed through the intestinal tract with the help of lipids (fats). Because they are more likely to accumulate in the body, they are more likely to lead to hypervitaminosis than are water-soluble vitamins. Fat-soluble vitamin regulation is of particular significance in cystic fibrosis.

VITAMIN A

Vitamin A is a group of unsaturated nutritional organic compounds, that includes retinol, retinal, retinoic acid, and several provitamin A carotenoids, among which beta-carotene is the most important. Vitamin A has multiple functions: it is important for growth and development, for the maintenance of the immune system and good vision. Vitamin A is needed by the retina of the eye in the form of retinal, which combines with proteinopsin to form rhodopsin.

Vitamins A was discovered in the early nineteenth century by Dr McCollum and Davis. Dr McCollum carried out experiments on rats and found that when butter and egg yolk were added to the diet of group of rats, they were healthier, stronger as compared to the other group which were fed on lard and vegetables only. He came to the conclusion that butter and egg yolk contain some vital elements that were absent in lard and vegetables. In 1913, he isolated Vitamin A from butter and egg yolk.

Chemistry

Vitamin A occurs in several forms: as retinal, as an aldehyde and as retinoic acid. These several forms may be referred to as vitamin A. In its pure form, vitamin A is a pale yellow crystalline compound and occurs naturally in animals. It is soluble in fat solvents but insoluble in water, and is relatively stable to heat, acids and alkalis. It is easily oxidized and rapidly destroyed by ultraviolet radiation. The ultimate source of all vitamin A is in the carotenes which are synthesized by plants.

Animals, as well as man in turn convert a considerable portion of carotene of the foods they eat into vitamin A. Carotenes are dark-red crystalline compounds also known as 'Provitamin A' or precursors of vitamin A'. Alpha, Beta, Gamma, molecules of carotene are of significance in nutrition. Each molecule of beta-carotene yields two molecules of vitamin A. So it can conclude that vitamin A can be found in two principal forms in foods.

Retinol the form of vitamin A absorbed when eating animal food sources, is a yellow, fat-soluble substance. Since the pure alcohol form is unstable, the vitamin is found in tissues in a form of retinyl ester. It is also commercially produced and administered as esters such as retinyl acetate or palmitate.

The carotenes alpha-carotene, beta-carotene, gamma-carotene; and the *xanthophyl* beta-cryptoxanthin (all of which contain beta-ionone rings), but no other carotenoids, function as provitamin A.

Food Sources

Animal Source

Only animal foods contain vitamin A as such; fish-liver oil being the outstanding. Milk, butter, whole milk cheese, liver and egg-yolk contain good quantities of vitamin A. Vitamin A is not present in plant foods, but its precursor, carotene is present which is converted into vitamin A in the body.

Plant Source

Carotene is present in plants with green and yellow colorings. There is a direct correlation between the greenness of a leaf and its carotene content. Green leafy vegetables: spinach, turnip tops, beet greens, coriander leaves, curry leaves. Yellow vegetables: carrot, sweet potatoes, pumpkin. Yellow fruit: Papaya, mango, apricots, peaches.

Functions of Vitamin A

- Vitamin A is required for normal vision in dim light. The retina has two kinds of cells-rods and cones. Rods are sensitive to dim light, the cones respond to bright light. The rods contain a pigment called rhodopsin. Rhodospin is formed by the combination of a specific form of vitamin A with a protein. Rhodospin in the presence of bright light, breaks down into it components. In the dark these components, Vitamin A and protein again combine to regenerate rhodospin. This rhodospin helps us to see in dim light. This is called a visual cycle.
- Vitamin A is required to maintain the integrity of epithelium, especially the membranes that line eyes, the mouth and the gastrointestinal, respiratory and genitourinary tracts. These membranes offer resistance to bacterial invasion.
- Vitamin A is essential for normal skeletal and tooth development.
- It has a probable role in the immunological defense mechanism of the body.
- Vitamin A, in the retinoic acid form, plays an important role in gene transcription.

Embryonic Development and Reproduction

See **Table 5.6**.

Deficiency Diseases

Night blindness or Nictalopia is one of the earliest signals of vitamin A deficiency is impairment of dark adaptation. There should be continuous supply of retinol for normal visual function. Vitamin A deficiency depress the resynthesis of rhodopsin and interferes with the function of rods resulting in night blindness.

Table 5.6: Recommended dietary allowance of vitamin A.

Life stage group	*Adequate intakes (AI) μg/day*	*Upper limit μg/day*
Infants		
0–6 months	400	600
7–12 months	500	600
Children		
1–3 years	300	600
4–8 years	400	900
Males		
9–13 years	600	1700
14–18 years	900	2800
19 – >70 years	900	3000
Females		
9–13 years	600	1700
14–18 years	700	2800
19 – >70 years	700	3000
Pregnancy		
<19 years	750	2800
19 – >50 years	770	3000
Lactation		
<19 years	1200	2800
19 – >50 years	1300	3000

Dark Adaptation

More photons are required to excite already illuminated rod, whereas only a few photons are sufficient to excite rod cell in the dark. This property is called Dark adaptation. Bright light depletes stores of rhodopsin: When a person shifts suddenly from bright light to a dimly area there is difficult to see. A few minute later, rhodopsin is resynthesized and vision is improved. This period is called Dark adaptation time.

VITAMIN D

Vitamin D refers to a group of fat-soluble costeroids responsible for enhancing intestinal absorption of calcium, iron, magnesium, phosphate and zinc. Pure vitamin D was isolated in crystalline form in 1930 and was called 'calciferol'. It was also known as 'antiranchitic vitamin'.

Chemistry and Characteristic

Vitamin D is a group of sterol compounds possessing antirachitic properties, but only two are of nutritional interest. (i) Vitamin D_2 or ergocalciferol found in a plants and (ii) Vitamin D_3 or cholecalciferol which occurs in animal cells and activates in the skin on exposure to ultraviolet light. Pure vitamin D are white, crystalline compounds which are soluble in fats and fat solvents, but insoluble in water. They are stable to heat, alkalis and oxidation.

Functions

The functions of vitamin D especially works on bones and teeth, kidney and intestine.

Intestine

Promotes intestinal absorption of calcium and phosphorus and regulates the absorption of calcium and phosphorus from the intestinal tract. It renders the intestinal mucosa more permeable to calcium and phosphorus.

Kidney

Vitamin D regulates the enzyme 'alkaline phosphates' which regulates the release of phosphate organic compounds, thus it increases tubular reabsorption of phosphate in kidneys.

Bone

Stimulates normal mineralization, enhances bone reabsorption, affects collagen maturation. Thus vitamin D is required for normal bone and teeth development.

Food Sources

Sunlight

The sunlight is the major source of vitamin-D. Exposure to ultraviolet rays of the sunlight converts the precursor of vitamin D (7-dehydrocholestrol) present in the skin, to its active form.

Foods

Vitamin D occurs mainly in foods of animal origin. Fish liver oils are the richest natural source. Liver, eggs and butter contain useful amount. Small amounts are present in fresh milk and milk products. Fatty fish (such as tuna, salmon, and mackerel) are among the best sources of vitamin D. Beef liver, cheese, and egg yolks provide small amounts.

Mushrooms

Mushrooms provide some vitamin D. The vitamin D content is also being boosted by exposure to some commercially available mushrooms to ultraviolet light. Most milk in the United States is fortified with 400 IU vitamin D per quart.

Fortified Food

Vitamin D is added to many breakfast cereals and to some brands of soy beverages, orange juice, yogurt, and margarine. Check the nutrition fact panel on the food label.

Supplements

It can be very hard to get enough vitamin D from food sources alone. As a result, some people may need to take a vitamin D supplement. Vitamin D found in supplements and fortified foods comes in two different forms:

- D_2 (ergocalciferol)
- D_3 (cholecalciferol).

Daily Recommendations

Ten to fifteen minutes of sunshine three times weekly is enough to produce the body's requirement of vitamin D. The sun needs to shine on the skin of your face, arms, back, or legs (without sunscreen). The sunscreen should use after a few minutes in the sun.

People who do not live in sunny places may not make enough vitamin D. Skin that is exposed to sunshine indoors through a window will not produce vitamin D. Cloudy days, shade, and having dark-colored skin also cut down on the amount of vitamin D the skin makes.

The Recommended Dietary Allowance (RDA) for vitamins reflects how much of each vitamin most people should get on a daily basis. The RDA for vitamins may be used as goals for each person. How much of each vitamin you need depends on the age and gender. Other factors, such as pregnancy and your health, are also important.

Infants (Adequate Intake of Vitamin D)

- **0–6 months:** 400 IU [10 micrograms (mcg) per day]
- **7–12 months:** 400 IU (10 mcg/day).

Children

- **1–3 years:** 600 IU (15 mcg/day)
- **4–8 years:** 600 IU (15 mcg/day).

Older Children and Adults

- **9–70 years:** 600 IU (15 mcg/day)
- **Adults over 70 years:** 800 IU (20 mcg/day).

Pregnancy and Breastfeeding

600 IU (15 mcg/day).

In general, people over age 50 need higher amounts of vitamin D than younger people. Vitamin D toxicity almost always occurs from using too many supplements.

The safe upper limit for vitamin D is:

- 1,000 to 1,500 IU/day for infants
- 2,500 to 3,000 IU/day for children 1–8 years
- 4,000 IU/day for children 9 years and older, adults, and pregnant and breastfeeding teens and women.

One microgram of cholecalciferol (D_3) is the same as 40 IU of vitamin D.

Deficiency

Deficiency of vitamin D leads to Rickets in Children, a condition in which the level of calcium and phosphorus is always low. Bone growth cease and in more severe cases the bone which has already formed may be demineralized. This results in clinical changes which are observed by the swelling or bending of ribs. This condition is known as 'rachitie rosary'. The long bones increase at the ends and they may become curved instead of remaining straight. This leads to 'knock-knees', bowed legs, curvature of vertebral column and deformities of the pelvic bones. Softening of the skull, particularly in infants and the delayed closing of fontanelle is another feature of the deficiency of this vitamin. Deficiency in adults leads to Osteomalacia, a condition in which bones become fragile so that they are susceptible to fracture. In old age a deficiency of both vitamin D and calcium leads to osteoporosis, a condition in which bones become porous and break easily.

Side Effects

Too much vitamin D can make the intestines absorb too much calcium. This may cause high levels of calcium in the blood. High blood calcium can lead to:

- Calcium deposits in soft tissues such as the heart and lungs
- Confusion and disorientation
- Damage to the kidneys
- Kidney stones
- Nausea, vomiting, constipation, poor appetite, weakness, and weight loss.

VITAMIN E

Vitamin E refers to a group of ten lipid-soluble compounds that include both tocopherol and tocotrienols. It is key for strong immunity and healthy skin and eyes. In recent years, vitamin supplements have become popular as antioxidants. These are substances that protect cells from damage. However, the risks and benefits of taking vitamin E supplements are still unclear.

Chemistry and Characteristic

Vitamin E consists of a group of chemical substances called 'tocopherols'.

Alpha tocopherol is the compound possessing the greatest vitamin E activity. High temperature and acids do not affect the stability of this vitamin, but oxidation takes places in the presence of rancid fats or lead and iron salts. Decomposition occurs in ultraviolet light, alkalis and oxygen.

Functions

- The primary role of vitamin E is to act as an antioxidant. By accepting the oxygen, it helps to prevent the oxidation of vitamin A in the intestine, thereby sparing vitamin A.
- Though it is an antioxidant that protects body tissue from damage caused by substances called free radicals. Free radicals can harm cells, tissues, and organs. They are believed to play a role in certain conditions related to aging.
- Vitamin E reduces the oxidation of the polyunsaturated fatty acids, thereby helping to maintain the integrity of the cell membranes.
- It helps in releasing the energy from carbohydrates and fats, through the synthesis of a coenzyme. In some animals vitamin E is required to prevent the sterility.
- The body also needs vitamin E to help keep the immune system strong against viruses and bacteria.
- Vitamin E is also important in the formation of red blood cells and it helps the body use vitamin K. It also helps widen blood vessels and keep blood from clotting inside them.
- Cells use vitamin E to interact with each other and carry out many important functions.

Food Sources

- Vegetable oils (such as wheat germ, sunflower, safflower, corn, and soybean oils)
- Nuts (such as almonds, peanuts, and hazelnuts/filberts)
- Seeds (such as sunflower seeds)
- Green leafy vegetables (such as spinach and broccoli).

Although foods of animal origin are low in vitamin E, liver, heart, kidney milk and eggs are the animal sources of this vitamin. Human milk provides an adequate amount of vitamin E to infants, cow's milk is low in this vitamin.

Recommended Daily Allowances

The vitamin E requirement is linked to that of essential fatty acids. The requirement of vitamin E suggested is 0.8 mg/g of essential fatty acids.

Infants (Adequate Intake of Vitamin E)

- **0 to 6 months:** 4 mg/day
- **7 to 12 months:** 5 mg/day.

Children

- **1 to 3 years:** 6 mg/day
- **4 to 8 years:** 7 mg/day
- **9 to 13 years:** 11 mg/day.

Adolescents and Adults

- **14 and older:** 15 mg/day
- **Pregnant teens and women:** 15 mg/day
- **Breastfeeding teens and women:** 19 mg/day.

Deficiency

Vitamin E deficiency results in increased hemolysis (break down) of the red blood cells leading to anemia. Premature infants also shows a low level to tocopherol. In some species of animals, vitamin E deficiency is known to cause reproductive failure. In human beings vitamin E deficiency is not frequently reported.

VITAMIN K

Dr Dam (1935) found that a 'Koagulation Vitamin' was necessary to prevent fatal hemorrhages in chicks by promoting normal blood clotting. It is also known as the 'clotting vitamin', because without it blood would not clot. Some studies suggest that it helps maintain strong bones in the elderly. Vitamin K is actually a group of compounds. The most important of these compounds appears to be vitamin K_1 and vitamin K_2. Vitamin K_1 is obtained from leafy greens and some other vegetables. Vitamin K_2 is a group of compounds largely obtained from meats, cheeses, and eggs, and synthesized by bacteria.

Characteristics of Vitamin K

Vitamin K is found in nature in two forms: K_1 occurs in alfa-alfa and K_2 is produced by bacterial synthesis. These are soluble in fat. They are not destroyed by heat, but are unstable to alkalis, strong acids, oxidation and light.

Functions

- Vitamin K is essential for the formation of prothrombin and other clotting proteins by the liver.
- Vitamin K probably also participates in oxidative phosphorylation in the tissues.

Food Sources

The best way to get the daily requirement of vitamin K is by eating food sources. Vitamin K is found in the following foods:

- Green leafy vegetables, such as kale, spinach, turnip greens, collards, Swiss chard, mustard greens, parsley, romaine, and green leaf lettuce
- Vegetables such as Brussels sprouts, broccoli, cauliflower, and cabbage
- Fish, liver, meat, eggs, and cereals (contain smaller amounts).

Vitamin K is also made by the bacteria that line the gastrointestinal tract.

Recommended Daily Allowances

The variations in intestinal synthesis and in the diet have made it impossible to establish a daily allowance. Dietary deficiency is not believed to be a problem.

The Food and Nutrition Board at the Institute of Medicine recommended intakes for individuals—Adequate Intakes (AIs) for vitamin K.

Infants

- **0–6 months:** 2.0 micrograms per day (mcg/day)
- **7–12 months:** 2.5 mcg/day.

Children

- **1–3 years:** 30 mcg/day
- **4–8 years:** 55 mcg/day
- **9–13 years:** 60 mcg/day.

Adolescents and Adults

- **Males and females age 14–18:** 75 mcg/day
- **Males and females age 19 and older:** 90 mcg/day.

Deficiency

Deficiency usually occurs due to faulty absorption or due to liver disorders that affect the synthesis of prothrombin. Dietary deficiency is rather unusual.

A low level of prothrombin and other clotting factors leads to increased tendency to hemorrhages. Premature infants, anoxic infants and those whose mother have been taking anticoagulants are most susceptible to deficiency.

Vitamin B Complex

The vitamin B complex refers to all of the known essential water-soluble vitamins except for vitamin C. These include thiamine (vitamin B_1), riboflavin (vitamin B_2), niacin (vitamin B_3), pantothenic acid (vitamin B_5), pyridoxine (vitamin B_6), *biotin, folic acid* and the cobalamins (vitamin B_{12}). Each member of the B complex has a unique structure and performs unique functions in the human body. Vitamins B_1, B_2, B_3, and biotin participate in different aspects of energy production, vitamin B_6 is essential for amino acid metabolism, and vitamin B_{12} and folic acid facilitate steps required for cell division. Each of these vitamins has many additional functions. However, contrary to popular belief, no functions require all B complex vitamins simultaneously. Thiamine, Riboflavin, Niacin, Pyridoxine are cofactors to enzymes in energy metabolism, hence, deficiencies show up in quickly growing tissues such as epithelium. In general, supplements containing all eight are referred to as a **vitamin B complex**. Individual B vitamin supplements are referred to by the specific name of each vitamin. Thiamine, Riboflavin, Niacin, Pyridoxine are cofactors to enzymes in energy metabolism, hence, deficiencies show up in quickly growing tissues such as epithelium. Typical symptoms for the group include dermatitis, glossitis, cheilitis and diarrhea. Though nerve cells use lots of energy, so symptoms also show up in the nervous tissue are peripheral neuropathy, depression, mental confusion, lack of motor coordination and malaise.

THIAMINE OR VITAMIN B_1

Characteristics of Thiamine

Thiamine hydrochloride is a white crystalline substance. It has a faint yeast-like order and a salty, nut-like taste. It is readily soluble in water but not in fat solvents or fats. It is readily destroyed by heat in neutral or alkaline solution; in acidic medium it is resistant to heat up to 1200°C. Vitamin B_1, also known as 'thiamin,' is classified as a B complex vitamin. Very small amounts of vitamin B_1 are found in virtually all foods, and many commonly eaten foods contain substantial amounts.

Functions

Thiamine teams up with an enzyme to form a coenzyme. The latter acts as a catalyst in the oxidation processes:

- It is essential for the utilization of carbohydrates in the body; in deficiency there is accumulation of pyruvic acid and lactic acid in the tissues and body fluids.
- Thiamine is also essential for the maintenance of good appetite and normal digestion.
- It has a role in brain metabolism as the deficiency causes neurological and nervous disorders.

Food Sources

All the natural foods contain thiamine, even if in very small amounts. Important sources are dried yeast, whole grain cereals and pulses, oil seeds and nuts especially groundnuts, Meat, fish pork, eggs, vegetables and fruits are relatively poor sources.

Recommended Daily Allowances

Daily recommendations for dietary vitamin B_1 according to the National Academy of Sciences are listed below.

Pediatric

- **Newborns–6 months:** 0.2 mg (adequate intake)
- **Infants 7 months–1 year:** 0.3 mg (adequate intake)
- **Children 1–3 years:** 0.5 mg (RDA)
- **Children 4–8 years:** 0.6 mg (RDA)
- **Children 9–13 years:** 0.9 mg (RDA)
- **Men 14–18 years:** 1.2 mg (RDA)
- **Women 14–18 years:** 1 mg (RDA).

Adult

- **Men 19 years and older:** 1.2 mg (RDA)
- **Women 19 years and older:** 1.1 mg (RDA)
- **Pregnant or breastfeeding women:** 1.4 mg (RDA)

The recommended daily allowance is 0.5 mg/1000 Kcals.

Deficiency of Thiamine

Thiamine deficiency (Beriberi): The clinical manifestations of thiamine deficiency are beriberi and Wernick's encephalopathy. The pathology of beriberi is biochemically, there is accumulation of pyruvic and lactic acid in body fluids causing cardiac dysfunction such as cardiac enlargement especially right side, edema of interstitial tissue and fatty degeneration of myocardium, degeneration of myelin and of axon cylinders resulting in peripheral neuropathy and in chronic deficiency states, vascular dilatation and brain hemorrhages of Wernicke's Disease, resulting in weakness of eye movement, ataxia of gait and mental disturbance.

Beriberi exists in three forms, wet, dry and infantile beriberi:

1. **Wet beriberi:** Wet form of beriberi is characterized by heart involvement in which generalized edema, acute cardiac symptoms are present and it has a prompt response to thiamine administration
2. **Dry beriberi:** Dry form of beriberi is characterized by nerve involvement. The symptom includes edema not present, condition similar to peripheral neuritis or neurological disorders present
3. **Infantile beriberi:** Infantile beriberi is seen in breastfed infant of thiamine deficient mother which is also divided into:
   a. *Acute cardiac:* Ages 2–4 months; sudden onset of cardiac sign and symptoms such as cyanosis, dyspnea, systolic murmur and pulmonary edema with rales
   b. *Aphonic:* Ages 5–7 months; insidious onset of hoarseness, dysphonia or aphonia
   c. *Pseudomeningeal:* Ages 8–10 months; signs of meningeal irritation with apathy, drowsiness and even unconsciousness; occurs more often.

Prevention of Thiamine Deficiency

Beriberi can be prevented by consuming richest sources of thiamine are like pork, whole grain, enriched cereal grains and legumes. Improved milling system of rice to conserve thiamine avoiding excessive cooking of vegetables or polishing of cereals. In breastfed infants, prevention achieved by adding thiamine in maternal in diet in sufficient amounts.

Treatment

The drug of choice for treatment of beriberi is thiamine supplementation. Doses for conditions like beriberi and Wernicke-Korsakoff syndrome are determined by a doctor. For Wernicke-Korsakoff syndrome, thiamine is given intravenously. A daily dose of 50–100 mg is often taken as a supplement. In case of children, it is 10 mg daily for several weeks.

RIBOFLAVIN OR VITAMIN B_2

In its pure form this vitamin is bitter tasting, orange yellow, odorless compound in which crystals are needle-shaped. It dissolves sparingly in water to give a typical greenish yellow fluorescence. It is stable to boiling in acids, but in alkaline solutions it is readily decomposed by heat. It is also destroyed by exposure to light. Riboflavin is a B vitamin. It can be found in certain foods such as milk, meat, eggs, nuts, enriched flour, and green vegetables. Riboflavin is frequently used in combination with other B vitamins in vitamin B complex products.

Functions

- Riboflavin, like thiamine unites with the enzymes and helps in the tissue oxidation with the release of the energy, thus helping in protein, fat and carbohydrate metabolism and cellular respiration.
- Needed also by retinal eye pigments for light adaptation.

Food Sources

The richest source is dried yeast. Among the good sources are milk, liver, meat eggs, kidney and growing leafy vegetables. Cereals and fruits are not rich sources, but due to the large quantity consumed, they supply much of vitamin in the Indian diets.

Recommended Daily Allowances

The recommended daily allowances is 0.6 mg/1000 K cals. In case of infants and children less than 10 years, the recommended daily allowances 0.6–1.4 mg, for children more than 10 years 1.4–2 mg and it is depending on food intake of adults (0.025 mg/g dietary protein).

Deficiency of Riboflavin

Vitamin deficiency affects various metabolic and physiological activities in the body. Deficiency of vitamin B_2 directly affects the cellular processes running in the body. Vitamin B_2 deficiency is also known as 'vitamin B_2' riboflavin deficiency.

A vitamin B_2 deficiency affects the metabolism of carbohydrates, fats, ketone bodies, and proteins in the body. So it can be said that a vitamin deficiency directly affects a person's energy level. Another factor is that vitamin B_2 deficiency results in other vitamin deficiencies as well. It is easy to identify the signs of vitamin B_2 riboflavin deficiency. As riboflavin is regularly excreted from the urine, riboflavin deficiency symptoms become very common and easily identifiable. Riboflavin deficiency symptoms include:

- Bloodshot eyes
- Sore tongue and lips
- Infection in the mouth and throat
- Extreme and unusual sensitivity to light
- Irritability in the eyes
- Chapped lips.

The women need to take special care to ensure that they do not have a vitamin deficiency as riboflavin deficiency causes problems in the reproduction system, growth and repair of body tissues, as well as problems in the immune system.

NIACIN OR NICOTINIC ACID

It occurs in white needle-like bitter tasting crystals. It is moderately soluble in hot water, but only slightly soluble in cold water. It is stable to heat, alkalis, acids light and oxidation and unstable to reduction. If fact, it is one of the most stable of the vitamins. Niacin occurs in two form: Niacin and proniacin form, i.e., tryptophan. Human body can make 1 mg of vitamin from 50 to 60 mg of tryptophan. Thus if a diet contains large amount of tryptophan, it will provide enough niacin, even thought the diet might be low in its niacin content.

Functions

- Niacin is rapidly converted in the body to nicotinamide, which is a component of coenzymes which are essential for the metabolism of carbohydrates, fats and proteins.
- It is also essential for the normal functioning of skin, intestinal tract and the nervous system.

Food Sources

Poultry, meat and fish are the good sources, peanuts is also among good sources. Whole grains are fair sources of niacin. Potatoes, legumes and some green leafy vegetable contain fair amount of niacin but most fruits and vegetables are poor sources. Germination and fermentation enhances the value of niacin in the food.

Recommended Daily Allowances

The recommended daily allowances if 6.6 mg/1,000 Kcals, infants and children less than 10 years, the recommended daily allowances is 6–10 mg, for older individuals it is 10–20 mg.

Deficiency

Niacin deficiency results in pellagra. Pellagrazane involves the gastrointestinal tract, the skin and nervous system. Early signs include fatigue, headache, backache, loss of weight and loss of appetite, anorexia, weakness, irritability, numbness and dizziness, Nausea and vomiting are followed by diarrhea (i.e., loose motion is present). Classical triad of symptoms are dermatitis, diarrhea and dementia. Dermatitis may develop insidiously to sunlight or heat. The dermatitis first appears as symmetrical erythema followed by drying, scaling and pigmentation/vesicles and bullae at times, predilection for back of hands, wrists, forearms (pellagrous glove), neck (Casal's necklace) and lower legs (pellagrous boot). The GIT symptoms include are diarrhea, stomatitis or glossitis; feces pale, foul milky, soapy or at times steatorrheic. Mental changes include depression, irritability, disorientation, insomnia and delirium.

Treatment

- Niacin 50–300 mg daily which may be taken for a long time.
- Skin lesions may be covered with soothing lotions.

PYRIDOXINE OR VITAMIN B_6

Vitamin B_6 consists of a group of related pyridines: Pyridoxine, pyridoxal and pyridoxamine. Vitamin B_6 is soluble in water and relatively stable to heat and to acids. It is destroyed in alkaline solutions and is also sensitive to light.

Functions

Vitamin B_6 is the coenzymes for a large number of enzyme systems, most of which are:

- Vitamin B_6 is involved in the synthesis and catabolism of amino acids, synthesis of neurotransmitters, porphyrins and niacin.
- Plays important role in clinical conditions such as anemia, hyperemesis gravidarum, cardiac decompensation, radiation effects, skin grafting, INH therapy and seborrheic dermatitis.

Food Sources

Foods rich in pyridoxine are meat, poultry and fish, potatoes, sweet potatoes are fair sources. Yeast, whole wheat, corn, egg yolk, liver and lean meat are also good source.

Recommended Daily Allowances

Firm requirement not established but usually recommended: Infant: 0.1–0.5 mg, Child: 0.5–1.5 mg and Adult: 1.5–2 mg.

Deficiency

The deficiency of this vitamin causes convulsions, dizziness and vomiting. Other symptoms are cheilosis, glossitis and abdominal pain. According to their clinical manifestation the deficiency diseases is classified in three different types:

Neuropathic

The symptoms due to insufficient neurotransmitter synthesis, such as irritability, depression and somnolence.

Pellagrous

The symptoms due to low endogenous niacin synthesis, such as seborrheic dermatitis, intertrigo, angular stomatitis and glossitis.

Anemic

The symptoms due to low porphyrin synthesis, such as microcytic anemia and lymphopenia.

In genetic diseases involving pyridoxal phosphate enzymes also xanthurenic aciduria, cystathioninuria and homocystinuria.

Treatment for Pyridoxine Deficiency

- Pyridoxine 100 mg IM injection for seizures due to deficiency
- Children with pyridoxine dependency should be given 2–10 mg IM injection or 10–100 mg oral vitamin B_6.

FOLIC ACID GROUP

Folain is a generic term for folic acid (pteroylglutamic acid) and other compounds having the activity of folic acid. It consists of three linked components: a pteridine grouping, para-aminobenzoic acid, and glutamic acid, an amino acid. Pure folic acid occurs as a bright yellow. Crystalline compound, only slightly soluble in water. It is easily oxidized in an acid medium and is sensitive to light **(Table 5.7)**.

Functions

- Needed for RBC and DNA formation, cell multiplication especially GI cells
- Newly discovered functions:
  - Prevents neural tube defects
  - Prevents heart disease (reduces homocysteine levels)
  - Prevents colon cancer.

Food Sources

- It is present in the free form and in the conjugated form. Liver, kidney, deep green leafy vegetables are good sources of this vitamin. Wheat, cereals provide a fair amount.
- Dairy-foods, pork and light green vegetables are poor sources.

The ICMR expert committee, 1989 recommended the allowances of 'free' folic acid.

Deficiency

Folic acid deficiency results in megaloblastic anemia, glossitis and gastrointestinal disturbances. Services deficiency results

Table 5.7: Recommended daily allowances of folic acid.

Group folic acid	*Mcg/day*
Adults	1.0
Pregnancy	1.0
Lactation	1.5
Infants	0.2
Children	0.2–1.0

in infertility or even complete sterility. The anemia is the second most common cause of nutritional anemia in India.

Laboratory Findings

- Anemia macrocytic
- Serum folic acid <3 ng/mL, normal level = 5–20 ng/mL
- RBC folate levels indicator of chronic deficiency, normal level = 150–600 ng/mL
- Serum iron and vitamin B_{12} normal or elevated
- Formiminoglutamic acid in urine especially after oral histidine
- Serum LDH markedly high
- Bone marrow hypercellular.

Treatment

- Parenteral folic acid 2–5 mg/24 hours, response in 72 hours, same therapy will continue for 3–4 weeks.
- Blood transfusions only when anemia severe
- If pernicious anemia present, prolonged use of folic acid should be avoided.

CYANOCOBALAMIN OR VITAMIN B_{12}

This vitamin is the only cobalt containing substance essential for health. It occurs as deep red needle like crystals which are slightly soluble in water. This vitamin is absorbed from the ileum only. Its absorption depends on the presence of a mucoprotein enzyme produced by the gastric mucosa. The enzyme is called as intrinsic factor.

Functions

- It helps in the synthesis of nucleic acid and nucleoproteins.
- It is essential for the maturation of red blood cells in bone marrow.
- It is also required for the metabolism of nervous tissues.

Food Sources

It is present only in the foods of animal origin. Liver, meat, eggs and milk are goods sources. It is not found in the food of vegetable origin.

Recommended Daily Allowance

The RDA of vitamin B_{12} is 2.4 g for adult in all age groups. On the basis of a fetal deposition of 0.1 to 0.2 µg/day throughout pregnancy and evidence that maternal absorption of the vitamin becomes more efficient during pregnancy, the RDA is increased by 0.2 µg/day during pregnancy. So required RDA is 2.6. Similarly during lactation, RDA 2.8 µg/day of vitamin B_{12} is required.

Deficiency

Deficiency of this vitamin leads to pernicious anemia. This occurs only when there is a genetic deficiency which affects the formation of castle's intrinsic factors. Macrocytic anemia and degenerative changes of the nervous system may result after clinical manifestations include ataxia, paresthesias, hyporeflexia, Babinski responses, clonus and coma smooth, red and painful tongue, etc.

Treatment

- Prompt hematological response with parenteral vitamin B_{12} 1–5 mcg/24 hours.
- If there is neurological involvement 1 mg IM daily for at least 2 weeks.
- **Pernicious anemia:** Monthly vitamin B_{12} 1 mg IM necessary throughout patient's life.

ASCORBIC ACID OR VITAMIN C

Vitamin C is a white crystalline compound of relatively simple structure and closely related to monosaccharide sugars. It can be prepared synthetically at low cost from glucose. Of all the vitamins, vitamin C is the most easily destroyed. It highly soluble in water heat, light, alkalis, oxidative, enzymes and trace.

Functions

- Collagen is the major connective tissue in the body and hydroxyproline, found only in collagen, is formed from proline requiring ascorbic acid. Collagen is the cementing material that holds the cells of the body together. If there is defective collagen formation, endochondral bone formation stops.
- Vitamin C is necessary for the production of tissues for quick postoperative healing and for the maintenance of previously formed scar.
- It plays an important role in the normal metabolism of the amino acids.
- It helps in easy absorption of iron from gastrointestinal tract by the reduction of ferric iron to ferrous iron.
- Vitamin C is involved in hydroxylation reactions in the synthesis of steroids and epinephrine.

Food Sources

Fruits and vegetables are the main sources of this vitamin. Citrus fruits (amlas, oranges, grapes, fruits, lemons and limes) berries, melons, pineapples, guavas, pears, banana, apple, leafy vegetables, green pepper, tomatoes are good source of ascorbic acid. Milk, eggs, meat and poultry do not have any vitamin C. Human milk contains four to six times as much ascorbic acid than cow's milk to protect the infant from scurry. Dry legumes contain negligible amount which increase approximately seven times, during germination.

Deficiency

Deficiency of ascorbic acid results in defective formation of the intercellular cementing substance collagen. In the early stages are vague symptoms of irritability, digestive disturbances and anorexia. Mild vitamin C deficiency signs include ecchymoses, corkscrew hairs and the formation of petechiae due to increased capillary fragility resulting from weakened collagen fibrils. Severe deficiency results in decreased wound healing, osteoporosis, hemorrhaging, bleeding into the skin and friable bleeding gums with loosened teeth. A presenting feature is an infant with painful, immobile legs (pseudoparalysis), edematous in 'frog position' and occasionally with mass There is depression of sternum with 'rosary of scorbutic beads at the costochondral junction due to subluxation of the sternal plate. Orbital or subdural hemorrhages, melena and hematuria may be found. Low grade fever and anemia will usually present. Impairment of growth and development is common.

MINERAL ELEMENTS

Minerals are inorganic elements that originate in the earth and cannot be made in the body. They play important roles in various bodily functions and are necessary to sustain life and maintain optimal health, and thus are essential nutrients. Most of the minerals in the human diet come directly from plants and water, or indirectly from animal foods. However, the mineral content of water and plant foods varies geographically because of variations in the mineral content of soil from region to region. Minerals may be defined as those elements which remain largely as ash when plant and animal tissues are burnt. The human body contains more than 19 minerals, all of which must be derived from foods. A total of 4% of the body weight is made up of minerals. Some of the important minerals found in our body include calcium, phosphorus, iron, iodine, sodium, potassium, zinc and chloride. All these minerals are derived from the food we eat. Of these, calcium, phosphorus, sodium, potassium, chloride and magnesium are the minerals required in larger amounts by the body. Calcium and phosphorus account for three-fourth of the minerals present in the body, and five other elements account for most of the rest. Many of these elements are present in such minute amounts that they are referred to as a trace elements or micronutrients. Major minerals are those that our bodies need in quantities of 100 mg (milligrammes) or more per day, such as calcium, phosphorus, potassium, and chloride. Trace minerals, on the other hand, are needed in quantities less than 100 mg per day, such as iron, iodine, zinc, and copper, all of which are essential to our health. Minerals are important for the body in various ways. They are required to form such organic compounds like phosphoproteins, hemoglobin and thyroxin. Hard skeletal structures are formed with the help of elements like calcium, phosphorus and magnesium, whereas soft tissues contain a relatively high proportion of potassium. Mineral elements are also required in the constitution of enzymes; for maintaining osmotic pressure and water balance between intracellular and extracellular compartments; for proper functioning of the nervous system; for muscular contraction and so on. The amount of minerals present in the body, and their metabolic roles, varies considerably. Minerals provide structure to bones and teeth and participate in energy production, the building of protein, blood formation, and several other metabolic processes. Minerals are categorized into major and trace minerals, depending on the amount needed per day. The terms major and trace, however, do not reflect the importance of a mineral in maintaining health, as a deficiency of either can be harmful.

Table 5.8: Recommended daily dietary allowances of calcium.

Age group	*Recommended dietary allowance (RDA) per day*	*Tolerable upper intake level (UL) per day*
Infants 0–6 months	200 mg	1000 mg
Infants 7–12 months	260 mg	1500 mg
Children 1–3 years	700 mg	2500 mg
Children 4–8 years	1000 mg	2500 mg
Children 9–18 years	1300 mg	3000 mg
Adults 19–50 years	1000 mg	2500 mg
Adults 51–70 years Men Women	 1000 mg 1200 mg	 2000 mg 2000 mg
Adults >70 years	1200 mg	2000 mg
Pregnancy and lactation 14–18 years 19–50 years	 1300 mg 1000 mg	 3000 mg 2500 mg

CALCIUM

Calcium is the most important mineral required for human body for especially formation of bone and teeth. On the approximately 1,200 g of calcium present in the adult body, 99% is in the bones and teeth and remaining 1% is widely distributed in body fluids where it fulfils many functions **(Table 5.8)**.

Functions

- Calcium together with phosphorus and other elements gives rigidity to bones and teeth. This characteristic makes its possible for the bone to the support of the body. Bone forms protective cavities for vital organs—the heart and lungs in the chest cavity, the brain in cranial cavity.
- Calcium acts as a catalyst for the conversion of prothrombin to thrombin, this being one of the several steps in the clotting of blood.
- It activates the permeability of the cell membrane (regulating the passage of substances into and out of cells).
- It activates number of enzymes including lipase, adenosine; triphosphatase, and some proteolytic enzymes.
- It has a role in the transmission of nerve impulses (conveying message from one nerve cell to another).
- It is directly related to muscle contraction. In the absence of calcium, muscles lose their ability to contract.

Facilitates the actual process of contraction of the muscle cell. Assists the movement of sperm into an egg to fertilize the egg. It aids in the absorption of vitamin B_{12} from the ileum.

Food Sources

Dairy products such as milk, cheese, and yogurt are excellent sources of calcium. Certain green leafy vegetables such as mustard green, turnip greens, mint, spinach, carrot leaves rank next to dairy products in their calcium content. Citrus fruits, legumes, meats grains and nuts provide the least calcium. Fish with soft bones, canned sardines and salmon.

Deficiency

Deficiency of calcium in the diet results in retarded calcification of bones and teeth in the young. Due to the deficiency of calcium bones start bending and there is enlargement of ankle and wrists. In children, the deficiency disease is known as 'rickets' and in adults, as osteomalacia. Repeated pregnancies coupled with inadequate dietary intake can also given rise to the deficiency of calcium. The common symptoms of calcium deficiency includes Insomnia, anxiety, nervousness, depression, fatigue, muscle/joint pains, muscle spasms/cramps, high stomach acid, osteoporosis, seizures, birth defects, miscarriage, high blood pressure, irregular heart beat, cardiovascular disease, hemorrhagic stroke, aneurysms, PMS, dysmenorrhea (painful periods), etc.

PHOSPHORUS

Phosphorus is an essential macromineral. It is one of the most abundant minerals in the body. It normally makes up about 1% of total body weight. Phosphorus is required for normal functioning of every cell in the body but most of it, approximately 85%, is bound with calcium to form bones and teeth. Calcium phosphate is the major mineral component of bones. Phosphorus accounts for about 1% of body weight, or one-fourth of the total mineral elements in the body. About 85% of phosphorus is in combination with calcium in bones and teeth. Soft tissues contain much higher amounts of phosphorus than of calcium and most of it is in organic form **(Table 5.9)**.

Functions

- Main role is in binding with calcium to form healthy bones and teeth
- May be helpful in cases of vitamin D resistant rickets

Table 5.9: Phosphorus dosage/day.

Life stage/gender	*Phosphorus dosage/day*
Infants 0–6 months	100 mg
Infants 7–12 months	275 mg
Children 1–3 years	460 mg
Children 4–8 years	500 mg
Girls 9–13 years	1250 mg
Boys 9–13 years	1250 mg
Females 14–18 years	1250 mg
Males 14–18 years	1250 mg
Females 19–50 years	700 mg
Males 19–50 years	700 mg
Females older than 50 years	700 mg
Males older than 50 years	700 mg
Pregnant women 14–18 years	1250 mg
Pregnant women 19–50 years	700 mg
Lactating mothers 14–18 years	1250 mg
Lactating mothers 19–50 years	700 mg

- Needed for metabolism of carbohydrates and fats to produce energy
- Important for production of ATP (adenosine triphosphate), the molecule that the body uses to carry energy
- Required for synthesis of protein for growth and repair of cells and tissues, including nucleic acids (DNA and RNA)
- Needed to make phospholipids, such as phosphatidylcholine, that are structural components of cell membranes
- Helps the body utilize the B-complex vitamins
- Needed for heart muscle contraction and to regulate heartbeat
- May help alleviate multiple sclerosis
- Helps maintain normal acid-base (pH) balance in the body by acting as an important buffer
- Maintains calcium balance and helps prevent hypercalcemia (high blood calcium levels)
- Maintains kidney function
- Potassium and sodium phosphate taken orally are FDA-approved for use to help prevent or treat calcium-based kidney stones in people with hypercalciuria (high urine calcium levels) or those with calcium oxalate stones; avoid if stones are phosphate-based
- FDA-approved for treating occasional constipation, and to restore bowel function after surgery.

Food Sources

Milk and milk products are excellent sources of calcium. Certain green leafy vegetables such as mustard green, turnip greens, mint, spinach, carrot leaves rank next to dairy products in their calcium content. Citrus fruits, legumes, meats grains and nuts provide the least calcium.

Deficiency

Unusually low blood phosphate levels are called hypophosphatemia. Severe forms of it can result in death. However a deficiency of phosphorus is rare as it is present in most foods so deficiency of phosphorus is generally not seen in human beings.

MAGNESIUM

The amount of magnesium in the body is much smaller than that of calcium and phosphorus, i.e., about 20 to 35 g in the adult body. Of this about 60% are carbonates and phosphates at the surfaces of the bones. Most of the remaining magnesium is within the cells.

Functions

- It is required for numerous biological reactions involving the release of energy.
- It is a constituent of bone. It is involved in bone mineralization.
- It is also essential for normal metabolism of calcium and phosphorus.
- Its presence in the extracellular fluids regulates the transmission of nerve impulses.
- It activates the enzyme responsible for breakdown of glycogen.

Food Sources

Dairy products excluding butter provide enough magnesium. Flour and cereals products, dry beans soybeans, peas and nuts are good sources of magnesium. Green leafy vegetables are excellent sources because, magnesium is a part of chlorophyll.

Effect of Imbalances

Under normal conditions of health and food intake magnesium deficiency is not likely to occur. A deficiency of it may result from malabsorption syndrome, chronic alcoholism, toxemia of pregnancy or after intake of diuretics. Deficiency of magnesium results in neuromuscular irritability, tetanic convulsions, twitching, tremors, convulsions. In excess, it results in extreme thirst, excessive heat in the body, decrease in neuromuscular movements.

POTASSIUM

An adult body contains about 250 g of potassium of which about ninety seven% of the potassium in the body is in intracellular fluid (intracellular fluid refers to fluid inside the cells) while the remainder being in the extracellular fluid compartments (extracellular fluid refers to fluid outside the cells).

Functions

- Within the cell it maintains the osmotic pressure and fluids balance.
- It is required for the synthesis of proteins.
- It is required for enzymatic reactions taking place within the cell. Some potassium is bound to phosphate and is required for the conversion of glucose to glycogen.
- It is required for the transmission nerve impulse and for contraction of muscle fibers.

Food Sources

It is widely distributed in foods. Meat, poultry and fish are good sources. Fruits, vegetables and whole grain cereals are especially high in potassium. Banana, potatoes, tomatoes, carrots orange juice, grapefruit juice are rich sources.

Recommended Daily Allowance

The exact amount of potassium required is not known. A normal diet provides this mineral in sufficient amount.

Deficiency

Primarily the deficiency of potassium is not seen. Impaired appetite, severe malnutrition, chronic alcoholism and burn injuries can disturb the acid base balance and lower osmotic pressure.

SODIUM

An adult body contains approximately 120 g of sodium of which about 50% of the body's sodium is present in the extracellular fluid, 40% in bones and 10% or less in intracellular fluid. (Intracellular fluid refers to fluid inside the cell).

Functions

- It is required for maintenance of normal osmotic pressure and water balance.
- It is also required for maintaining the permeability of cell membrane.
- Sodium 'pump' helps to maintain the electrolyte difference between intracellular and extracellular fluid compartments.

Food Sources

Common salt or sodium chloride is the chief source of sodium in the diet. One tea spoon of salt provides almost 2000 mg sodium. It universally used to flavor the food we eat and is also used for preserving food for long periods. Numerous sodium compounds are used in food processing and preparation; baking soda, baking powder, sodium alginate, sodium propionate, sodium citrate.

Sodium is a naturally occurring constituent of animal's foods, including milk, egg, meat poultry and fish and in certain vegetables as spinach, celery, beet greens and fenugreek. Most vegetables, fruit, cereals, legumes are naturally low in sodium.

Recommended Daily Allowances

- 5–10 g of salt (sodium chloride) is sufficient for an average adult.
- An individual doing hard labor may need more.

Sodium Imbalance

- Osmotic pressure and the pH are seriously affected when there is a disturbance
- Concentrations of sodium in the extracellular fluid of the body tissues. When there is a retention of sodium in the tissue, edema occurs. In cardiac and renal failure sodium excretion gets reduced. Excess sodium losses occur during the hot weather causing muscular weakness, cramps, fatigue, vomiting and loss of appetite. In this case a small amount of salt may be added to liquid intake.
- With muscles and problems with the heart. Muscles in the body may cramp, feel weak or spasm. Muscle fibers may also begin to break down and release into the blood, causing damage to the kidneys. Eventually paralysis may occur and involve paralysis of the lungs, according to MedlinePlus. Abnormal heart rhythms are a potential side effect and are likely for people with heart disease. Fatigue and constipation are also possible complications of low potassium.

Complications of Low Sodium

Like potassium, having slightly low sodium levels may not cause any distinguishable symptoms. Chronic low sodium levels are much more likely to sneak by undetected than sudden drops in the electrolyte. Possible symptoms of low sodium levels include muscle spasms, nausea, fatigue, irritability and headache. Without proper treatment low sodium can cause a person to experience confusion, hallucinations and a decreased level of consciousness, according to MedlinePlus. The altered level of consciousness may include stupor and coma. These brain complications occur because the low sodium levels cause the cells in the brain to swell.

IODINE

About one-third of iodine present in an adult body variously estimated from 25 to 50 mg is found in the thyroid gland. The concentration in thyroid tissue is 2500 times as great as is any other tissue, all of which contain traces.

Functions

The only known function of iodine is as a constituent of thyroglobulin, a protein complex of several iodine-containing compounds. The thyroid hormone regulates the rate of oxidation within the cells and in doing so, regulates the physical and mental growth; the functioning of nervous and muscle tissues, circulating activity and the metabolism of all nutrients.

Food Sources

Iodine is supplied by food and water; the variations are wide depending upon the iodine content of the soils from which they come. People living in coastal areas and eating locally grown foods ingests enough iodine for their use. In hilly areas where there is a deficiency of iodine in food and drinking water—Iodinization of the salt is the only technique available to make good this deficiency in order to prevent goiter.

Recommended Daily Allowances

The daily requirement of iodine is 0.14 mg for an adult man and 0.10 mg for an adult woman. Growing children, pregnant and lactating women may need more.

Deficiency

Endemic goiter results in the parts of the world, where soil has a low iodine content.

Endemic goiter is a public health problem in sub-Himalayan region, Maharashtra and sub-Vindhya region, where 50% have goiter.

Goiter is characterized by the swelling of the thyroid gland.

IRON

Iron is chief among the trace elements required for the body. In an adult male it is approximately 3 to 5 g and in woman about 2 to 3 g. A major portion of the iron is in the red blood cells as hemoglobin. Muscle tissues contain about 3% of iron as myoglobin and the rest is stored as ferritin, hemosiderin, and siderophillin in liver, spleen, kidney and bone marrow **(Table 5.10)**.

Table 5.10: Recommended daily dietary allowance of iron.

Group	*Iron (mg)/day*
Adults male	28
Adult female	30
Pregnancy	38
Lactation	30
Infants	1.0 mg/kg body col
Children (1–9 years)	12–16
Adolescent boys (10–18 years)	34–50
Adolescent girls (10–19 years)	19–30

Functions

- Iron is a major constituent of a red-colored compound called hemoglobin presents in the blood. Iron is present in the hemoglobin (Hb). Hemoglobin is necessary for transport of oxygen to various parts of the body. Hb carries oxygen from the lings to the tissues and in turn helps in carrying carbon dioxide from the tissue to the lungs. From the lungs carbondioxide is then exhaled out.
- Iron is also present in the muscle in the form of myoglobin. Myoglobin has the capacity to store oxygen. This oxygen is used for muscle contraction and for other immediate needs of the muscle cells.
- Iron facilitates the complete oxidation of carbohydrate fats and proteins within the cell.
- Iron plays on important role in maintenance of specific brain.
- Iron forms a vital component of certain enzymes and substances that aid in metabolism.
- Iron has protective function. It helps in preventing infections.

Food Sources

Lean meats, deep green leafy vegetables and whole-grain cereals are good sources. Egg, yolk and organ meats are also among good sources. Liver is an excellent sources of iron. Other vegetable and fruits are fair source. Milk, cheese and ice cream are poor sources. Jaggery contain a good amount of iron.

Recommended Daily Allowances

The requirement of iron for the body is small, but due to poor absorption, much more is needed. From a vegetarian diet only 10% of the dietary iron is absorbed. For a mixed diet 15–20% absorption takes place.

Deficiency

Anemia results due to deficiency of iron. Usual symptoms are fatigue, giddiness, breathlessness on exertion, sleeplessness and loss of appetite. Paleness of the tongue, conjunctiva (white of eye) and nail bed is observed in an anemic person. In severe anemia, the nails of the fingers and toes becomes brittle and spoon shaped. Severe anemia can even lead to death.

FOOD GROUPS

A **food group** is a collection of foods that share similar nutritional properties or biological classifications. Nutrition guides typically divide foods into food groups and recommend daily servings of each group for a healthy diet to meet the nutrient requirements essential for good health, you need to eat a variety from each of the five food groups daily, in the recommended amounts.. It is often seen that most foodstuffs contain some nutrients in either more or lesser amounts than required. Thus, to be able to obtain all the nutrients and in adequate amounts, it is important to include different types of foodstuffs in our diet. On the other hand, it is also not possible to include, all the foodstuffs in our diet at one time. Therefore, to overcome this problem, food items providing same types of nutrients have been grouped together, termed as a 'Food Group'. It is not necessary to eat from each food group at every meal. In fact, in some instances, you only need to eat some of the foods in each food group a couple of times a week.

Food groups have been formed according to various methods from time to time. ICMR (1989) has classified the different foods items into five food groups as follow:

1. Cereal, roots and tubers
2. Pulses, nuts, and oil seeds
3. Milk, meat and their products
4. Fruits and vegetables
5. Fat and oils, sugar and jaggery.

In this classification, the foodstuffs providing similar nutrients have been grouped together.

CEREALS, ROOTS AND TUBERS

This group has been further subdivided into two:

Cereals and Cereals Products

The foodstuffs included in this group are rice, jowar, bajara, maize, bread, maida, etc. These food items are rich sources of energy and, thus provide energy to the body. Cereals are an important and economic source of energy. 100 g of cereals supply 340 kilocalories of energy. Cereals are also a significant source of proteins (8–11%) in the diets of people whose staple food is cereals. However, cereal protein is incomplete as it lacks an essential amino acid, lysine. When cereals are mixed with pulses in the same meal then the quality of protein improves through mutual supplementation. Cereals are also a good source of B-group vitamins, provided one consumes whole grain cereals, as most of B-group vitamins are present in the outer layer of the cereals. These vitamins are thus absent in refined cereals such as maida, etc. Whole grain cereal is also a good source of mineral iron, bajra, being the richest among all. Ragi is the only cereal, which contains appreciate amounts of calcium. Cereals are lacking in vitamin A and C. Both germination and fermentation of cereals significantly increase the B-group vitamins and vitamins C contents. Whole grain are a rich source of carbohydrates, protein, fiber, fats and oils and a wide range of vitamins and minerals including folate, thiamine, riboflavin, niacin and iron. However, when refined by the removal of the bran and germ, the remaining endosperm is mostly carbohydrate and lacks the majority of the other nutrients. Wheat flour contains glutelin and gliadin as proteins which are commonly known as 'gluten'. The strength of the wheat flour is based on the quality of gluten used. Whole grains chiefly furnish starch, proteins, minerals, B-vitamins and fiber. Refined cereals lose part of the protein, minerals, and B-complex vitamins in milling. They contain a little more starch than whole cereals. Whole grains contain more vitamins, minerals and fiber than refined grain and are valuable dietary sources of iron, phosphorus, thiamine and fiber.

Nutrient Content of Ragi, Maize and Jowar

Ragi

Ragi or finger millet is widely consumed without any refining by many people in rural areas. It contains B-vitamins but is poor in thiamine. Ragi is rich in minerals especially calcium. It is also rich in fiber and is a fair source of iron.

Maize or Corn

Maize, like any other cereal is rich in calories. It is deficient in amino acid lysine. It is a good source of carotene and contains thiamine and folic acid in appreciable amounts.

Jowar

Jowar or Sorghum is grown in Maharashtra, Karnataka, Madhya Pradesh, Gujarat, Uttar Pradesh and parts of Tamil Nadu. It is rich in carbohydrate, and B-complex vitamins. It is poor in vitamin A and rich in dietary fiber. Compared to rice, jowar is richer in protein but the quality is not as good as rice protein.

Starchy Roots and Tubers

Like potatoes, sweet potatoes, jam, colocasia, tapioca, etc., mainly provide carbohydrates and are thus grouped along with cereals under energy giving foods. These food items do not provide protein, as do cereals. Therefore it is not advisable to use them in place of cereals to provide energy for a very long time. These roots and tubers, can however, be used along with cereals in providing energy.

PULSES, NUTS AND OILSEEDS

This food groups include various pulses and legumes, like green gram, black gram beans, etc. Nuts and oilseeds like groundnuts, sesame are included in this group. The foodstuffs from this food group provide major portion of protein for vegetarians. The proteins from these sources are also second-class proteins. Pulse lack in essential amino acid, methionine and rich in lysine. On the other hand, cereals are lacking in essential amino and lystine and rich in methionine. Therefore when cereals and pulses are combined together, the quality of protein improves through mutual supplementation. Hence, cereal-pulse combination as in dosa, dal-roti, rice dal are good practice in Indian homes. Generally pulses give 340 calories per 100 g which is almost similar to cereal calorie. They are a rich source of protein containing about 18–25% protein. Soybean is an exception containing about 35 to 40% protein. All pulses contain sufficient amount lysine which is deficient in cereals and therefore they can supplement cereal protein. A mixture of cereals and pulses is superior to that of either one. Hence a combination of cereals and pulses is ideal for human consumption. Pulses contain 55–60% of carbohydrate including starch soluble sugar and fiber. They contain 1.5% lipids. Pulses also contain calcium, magnesium, zinc, iron, potassium and phosphorus. They are a poor source of carotene and vitamin C but fairly rich in niacin. Germination increases the vitamin C content of pulses. The thiamine content of pulses is equal to or exceeds that of cereals. Being rich in B-vitamins, they contribute significantly to B-vitamin intake.

Nuts and seeds have been valued for their oils as much as for a food in itself; their high content of energy, protein, vitamins, and minerals makes them a very nutritious food. Oilseeds like groundnuts, till, mustard, and sunflower seeds, etc. also have good amounts of proteins. The oil cake or meal left after the extraction of oils is rather a very good source of proteins. This oil cake should be incorporated in the diets in combination with other protein food to improve protein. Apart from proteins, nuts also contain a high amount of fat; therefore they are good sources of energy also.

MILK, MEAT AND THEIR PRODUCTS

The foodstuffs included in this food groups are:

- Milk and its products.
- Eggs, meat, fish, poultry, etc.

All these foodstuffs provide us with first class proteins, i.e., their protein contain all the essential amino acids, in adequate amounts. The food items from this group thus help in body building and maintenance processes.

Milk and its Products

Milk is a complex fluid containing protein, fat, carbohydrate, vitamins and minerals. The main protein in milk is casein and it constitutes 3.0–3.5% of milk. The fat content of milk varies from 3.5% in cow's milk to about 8.0% in buffalo's milk. Fat is present in the form of fine globules varying in diameter from 1 to 10 mm (micrometers). Milk also contains phospholipids and cholesterol. Lactose is the sugar present in milk. The important minerals in milk are calcium, phosphorus, sodium and potassium. Milk is an excellent source of riboflavin and a good source of vitamin A. However, milk is a poor source of iron and ascorbic acid. The small amount of iron present is bioavailable. There are different types of processed milk. Raw milk is processed into the following types of milk.

- **Skimmed milk:** Skim milk is whole milk from which fat has been removed by a cream separator. The quantity of fat is usually 0.05 to 0.1%. It contains all other milk nutrients, except vitamin A and D, but can be fortified by the addition of these vitamins.
- **Toned milk:** Toned milk is prepared by using milk reconstituted from skim milk powder. Skimmed milk is prepared by removing fat from milk in a cream separator. The skimmed milk is then mechanically dried to give skim milk powder. It is mixed with buffalo milk containing 7% fat. The fat content of toned milk should be less than 3%.
- **Standardized milk:** In standardized milk the fat content is maintained at 4.5% and soluble non-fat is 8.5%. It is prepared from a mixture of buffalo milk and skim milk.
- **Homogenized milk:** Homogenization is a mechanical process that reduces the size of fat globules by forcing milk through small apertures under pressure and velocity. When milk is homogenized, the average size of the globule will be 2 micrometers. The decrease in the size of fat globules increases their number and surface area. The newly formed fat droplets brings about stabilization of the milk emulsion and thus prevents rising of the cream. Homogenized milk has a creamier texture, bland flavor and whiter appearance.
- **Evaporated milk:** It is made by evaporating more than half the water from milk under vacuum, at a temperature of 74°–77°C. It is then fortified with vitamin D, homogenized and filled into cans 56 and sterilized at a temperature of 118°C for 15 minutes and cooled. The treatment employed lends a brown color and characteristic flavor owing to the reaction between sugar and protein.
- **Condensed milk:** It is obtained when whole milk is concentrated to about one-third of its original volume and has about 15% sugar added to it. The preparation of condensed milk involves: (i) filtration and pasteurization of milk, (ii) preheating and evaporation, (iii) addition of sterilized sugar syrup, (iv) homogenization.
- **Flavored milk:** It is the milk prepared by the addition of flavor such as rose, pista, badam, cardamom, etc., to pasteurized whole milk.
- **Milk powder:** Milk powder is prepared by dehydrating whole milk in drum driers or spray driers. In the case of drum or roller drying, the milk is filtered, pasteurized, homogenized and then fed into roller driers which are internally heated with steam. The dried milk is obtained as a thin sheet and is powdered. In spray drying, the homogenized milk is blown as a fine spray into a preheated vacuum chamber resulting in fine dry powder. The milk powder is collected, cooled and packed.

Milk Products

- **Khoa:** Khoa is prepared by evaporating whole milk in an open cast iron pan with continuous stirring until it is semisolid. It is used extensively in the preparation of Indian sweets.
- **Cream:** Cream is the fat of milk and is used in the preparation of sweets. It is made by simmering large quantities of milk until a thick layer of milk fat and coagulated protein

form on the surface. It can be consumed with or without the addition of sugar.

- **Butter:** Butter is obtained from cream by churning. When cream is churned, the fat globules are destabilized and coalesce until the milk separates into two phases—viz. the butter and the aqueous phase. Butter is removed and washed. Butter is used as a cooking medium in many Indian recipes. It is one of the main ingredients in cakes, biscuits, icing and bread.
- **Ghee:** Ghee is butter oil. It is prepared by melting butter and separating the moisture from butter by heating. It is used in preparing Indian sweets, savories, curries and variety rice like pulav and biriyani.
- **Paneer:** Paneer is a soft cheese prepared by addition of lemon juice or citric acid to hot milk and precipitating the casein. The liquid released in this process is known as 'whey' and the resultant curd is tied in a muslin cloth and hung for a day to squeeze any liquid present in it. The soft cheese (paneer) that is obtained is used in Indian gravies and pulavs. It is a very good source of protein.
- **Cheese:** It involves the curdling of milk with enzyme rennet under microbially controlled condition. Milk is held at about 27°C in vats and a lactic acid culture is added. When the milk gets acidic, rennet is added to it and the milk is allowed to coagulate. The curd formed is cut and heated to about 37°C with constant stirring to remove the whey. The whey is drained. Salt is mixed with the curd and it is pressed to remove further amount of whey. The cheese formed is coated with paraffin to prevent loss of moisture. The paraffined cheese is allowed to ripen for three to six months at temperatures between 45° to 60°C. Cheese is a concentrated source of protein.
- **Curd:** Curd is prepared by heating milk to about 50°C. A teaspoon of curd (starter) from an earlier batch of curd is added and is mixed thoroughly. The lactic acid bacteria present in the starter curdles the milk. The bacteria breaks down lactose to lactic acid thereby increasing the acidity of milk. When the pH reaches 4.6, the milk protein casein coagulates as curd. The optimum temperature for the formation of curd is 35°–40°C and the time needed for curd formation is 8–12 hours depending on the atmospheric temperature. Curd is used as a dressing on salads made from fresh vegetables and combines well with plain cooked rice.
- **Yoghurt:** This is a coagulated milk product with curd like consistency. It is made from partially skimmed or whole milk and it has a slightly acidic flavor. In the production of yoghurt, a mixed culture of *Lactobacillus bulgaricus, Streptococcus thermophilus and Lactobacillus acidophilus* is added to pasteurized milk and incubated at 42°C to 46°C.

All the dairy products are the best sources of calcium. They supply protein, riboflavin, and vitamins A and D (if fortified). This group helps promote strong bones and healthy teeth. Milk is a very important food for growing children, as it provides them with good quality proteins and they are also able to digest it. For small infants this is the only food, which is easily digested and assimilated in the body.

Eggs, Meat, Fish and Chicken

Meat is a very good source of protein. The average protein content of meat varies from 16–25%. The amino acid pattern of meat protein is of outstanding nutritive value. The fat content of meat varies from 5–40%. Depending on the type, breed and age of the animal, fat is distributed throughout meat in small particles of large masses. Fat deposited uniformly in small sheets in the connective tissue within the muscle is called 'marbling'. This contributes tenderness and flavor to the meat. Meat fats are rich in saturated fatty acids. The cholesterol content of meat is 75 mg/100 g. Carbohydrate is found in small quantities and present in the form of glycogen and glucose. Meat is a good source of iron, zinc and phosphorus. It also contains sodium and potassium. It is an excellent source of B-complex vitamin particularly B_{12} which is absent in plant foods. Liver is an excellent source of iron and vitamin A.

Poultry: The term poultry refers to domestic fowls reared for their flesh and egg. It includes chicken, duck, geese, turkey, pigeon, etc. Poultry meat has a high protein content varying from 18–25%. It contains all the essential amino acids required for body building. Fat content of poultry is influenced by age and species of the bird. Young birds have little fat content. Chicken fat is unsaturated and is therefore better than the fat of red meat. Poultry flesh is a good source of B-vitamin and minerals. Egg: The term egg mainly refers to the egg of hen and duck. An average egg weighs 50 g. approximately and is composed of the shell, egg white and yolk. The weight is distributed in the different parts as follows **(Table 5.11)**.

These are also excellent sources of first class protein, which can be totally utilized in our body for building the body. They also contain B-group vitamins in good amounts. Among this liver is very good source of vitamin A and vitamin B_{12}. Eggs contain nearly all the nutrients, but are particularly good source of protein, fats, vitamin A, iron, calcium and phosphorus **(Table 5.12)**.

Table 5.11: Percentage composition of an egg.

Part	*Weight %*
Shell	9-12
Egg white	58–60
Egg yolk	31–33

Table 5.12: Nutrients in an egg.

Calories	*70 Cal/292.88 kJ*
Fat	5 g
Cholesterol	195 mg
Sodium	65 mg
Carbohydrate	1 g
Protein	6 g

FRUITS AND VEGETABLES

Fruits and vegetables provide vitamins and minerals required for growth and maintenance of health and are thus termed as protective foods. This food includes fresh vegetables and fruits which provide protective nutrients to our body, i.e., vitamins and minerals. The foodstuffs included in this group are spinach, methi, cabbage, cauliflower, carrot, papaya, mango, apple, tomato, lemon, orange, guava, amla, etc. A fruit is a mature ovary of a flower. The fleshy portion of the pericarp makes up the chief edible portion of the fruit. Fruits can be classified as follows:

- **Berries:** Gooseberry, grapes, strawberry.
- **Citrus:** Lemon, lime, orange, sweet lime.
- **Drupes:** Peach, plums, apricot.
- **Melons:** Water melon, musk melon
- **Pomes:** Apple, pear.

Green leafy vegetables, orange, yellow-colored fruits and vegetables provide us mainly with carotenes (precursor of vitamin A) vitamin C is found in citrus fresh fruits. Vitamin B group is also present in green leafy vegetables. Some fruits like peaches, pineapple and vegetables like fenugreek, mustard leaves, horse gram leaves are exceptionally good sources of iron. **Green leafy vegetables** are an inexpensive rich source of many nutrients such as carotene, ascorbic acid, folic acid, calcium, iron and fiber. They are a poor source of protein. Calcium is basically furnished by green leafy vegetables. Fruits and vegetables also provide dietary fiber to our meals. The fibrous tissues, which are not digested, help to move the food through the digestive tract and regulate excretion of body wastes. Vegetables are low in fat and can be used liberally in low calorie diets for weight reduction. Besides providing nutrients they add variety to the diet. They make the diet attractive by their texture, flavor and colorphyto chemicals refers to the wide variety of plant compounds naturally produced by plants. They include plant pigments and flavoring substances. Fruits and vegetables with bright colors, viz. yellow, orange, red, green, blue, purple contain phytochemicals. Beta-carotene, vitamin C and vitamin E are nutrients that function as antioxidants. An antioxidant is a substance that significantly reduces or prevents oxidation of fatty acids and protein thus preventing cell and tissue damage caused by free radicals in the body. Free radicals are unstable molecules resulting from normal metabolic processes. During these processes oxygen molecules lose an electron, which creates an unstable (molecule) thereby causing oxidative stress. These free radicals attack healthy cells in the body in the hope of finding another electron to stabilize themselves. This process can cause damage to healthy cells.

FATS AND OILS, SUGAR AND JAGGERY

Fats and oils like vegetables oils; hydrogenated fats and pure ghee are very concentrated sources of energy providing 9 Kcal/g. They are mainly used as the cooking medium and hence do form a necessary part of the diet. Fats and oils help to increase the palatability of our food. Sugar, jaggery and honey supplies energy in the form of carbohydrates. These food items provide about 4 Kcal/g. Sugar is the main source of energy in the form of carbohydrate. Apart from providing carbohydrates, jaggery is also a good source of iron. Although, most of the food items are covered under these five food groups, but still some widely used food items are uncovered. Condiments and spices are also used in our diet which are mainly added to make the food tasty and appealing. Though they contain significant amounts of certain nutrients, but since these are used in very small quantities, they do not contribute much to the nutritive value of the diet.

The ICMR classification is based on grouping foodstuffs according to the similarity in nutrients found in them. To incorporate the goodness of all the food groups in one's diet, one most choose some foodstuffs out of the two energy giving food groups, i.e., cereals, roots, and tubers, and fat, oil and sugar and some food items out of either pulses or meats for body building purpose. The fruits and vegetables however are a must in every meal. Thus, some items from the energy giving food groups, bodybuilding food groups and protective food group must be incorporated in every meal. For case in planning diets and for the sack of simplicity and remembrance, the food groups have also been divided according to their functions. Thus on the basis of three physiological functions of food, food items have been grouped into three food groups as follows:

Energy-giving Food Groups

The food stuffs included in this food groups are cereals, like wheat, rice, bajra, jawar, etc. roots and tubers like potato, colocasia, and sugar, jaggery, ghee oil, butter, etc. All these foodstuffs are either rich sources of carbohydrates of fats and provide us with energy. These foodstuffs give the strength to carry on the various day-to-day activities.

Body-building Food Groups

The food items included in this food group are milk and its products, meat, fish, pulses, nuts, soybeans, etc. The food from this group mainly provide us with proteins and some vitamins and minerals to aid in the growth of the body and for the maintenance of the body by repair of worn out tissues.

Body-protective and Regulatory Food Groups

The food items included in this group are fruits, green vegetables and other vegetables. The nutrients derived from these foodstuffs are vitamins and minerals. These nutrients help us to fight against disease and infections. Vitamins and minerals also aid in the regulation of various body processes. If some food items from the three functional food groups are included in each meal, then our meal becomes a complete meal. To make our meals complete, it is not necessary to go in for elaborate menus, but by simple and judicious selection of menus, we can achieve a complete and balanced meal, e.g., incorporation of any vegetable in parathas and having them with curds.

BALANCED DIET

A balanced diet is one that gives your body the nutrition it needs to function properly. In order to get truly balanced nutrition, one should obtain the majority of his/her daily calories from fresh fruits and vegetables, whole grains, and lean proteins.

Definition

Balanced diet can be defined as 'the one which contains different types of foods in such quantities and proportions that the need for all the nutrients are adequately met and a small extra provision is made for nutrients as a margin of safety'.

Thus, our meals will only be said to be adequate and balanced when the quantity of food consumed is sufficient to meet our daily requirements, plus there is an allowance to be stored in the body to be used in conditions of stress. When a person due to some reasons, is not able to consume the required amount of nutrients, like in fevers or fasting, then the body stores of these nutrients are utilized. The quantity of our meals can be improved or is said to be optimum when our diets are complete. Every meal should have foodstuffs providing energy, protein, and vitamins, and minerals.

The component of a balanced diet will, however differ according to age, sex, physical activity, economic status and physical state of human being, which shall be discussed in detail in the next chapter. However, as an example a day's diet for an adult man belonging to middle income group is given below. Meal planning means planning diets which will provide all nutrients in required amounts and proportions, i.e., adequate nutrition. As the family's well-being and health are depended on how well they are fed. It is a challenge to every meal-planner to meet it and when well done, it proves to be a satisfying and rewarding experience. Besides others factors such as digestibility, palatability, economy, family customs, related to religion, food fads, etc. It also determines whether the food can be actually supplied and utilized by the individual. What are the characteristics of a well-planned meal? First of all it should be remembered that food has to be palatable before it can become nutritious, as majority of people will not eat something they do not like, even if it has excellent nutritive value. We should remember that appetite is the pleasurable anticipation of foods and depends not only on hunger but also on taste, texture, appearance and attractiveness of the foods, pleasantness of the surrounding and a cheerful frame of mind. Meal planning thus, is both an art and a science: an art in the skillful blending of colors, texture and flavor: and a science in the wise choice of food for optimum nutrition and digestion.

MEAL PLANNING

The meal planning helps to make the best use of the material, time and financial resources.

To obtain meals that meet the physical, social and psychological needs of the individual and families. It is very important to plan family meals in order to fulfill the nutritional requirement of the family members. This is essential to keep them strong, healthy, and free from any disease and deficiency of any kind. Meal planning is of utmost importance because it economizes on time, labor and fuel.

While planning meals, the methods of working can be carefully throughout, so that there is maximum retention of nutrients and minimum losses.

Meals can be planned according to the budget of the family. There can then be maximum utilization of money, if it is spent in the best possible way. Once can have a rich diet without buying expensive foods. Meal planning, therefore, encourages one to plan within the family means.

Meal planning allows one to select different foods from the same food group and avoid monotony. Besides, use of variety of foodstuffs is important from nutritional points also.

Meal planning determines the adequacy of the diet, the kinds of foods purchased, its quality and cost, the way it is stored, prepared and served.

Objectives of Meal Planning

- To satisfy the nutritional needs of the family members.
- To keep expenditure within family food budget.
- To take into account the food preference of individual members.
- Using methods of cooking to retain maximum nutrients.
- To economize on time, fuel and energy.
- To serve attractive and appetizing meals.

Factors Affecting Meal Planning

Meal planning whether for the simplest family meal or for an elaborate company dinner, involve consideration of a number of factors. These are:

Nutritional Adequacy

Meal pattern must fulfill the family needs, so that the nutrition requirement of each individual in the family are met. These requirements differ from person to person according to age, sex, activity and physiological condition, therefore, due consideration should be given to each member of the family. The best way to ensure nutritional adequacy of a diet is to select the food from all the five food groups. The different requirements for different family members does not mean that separate cooking is to be done for all of them. But the diet can be planned in such a way that while cooking the same food the nutritional requirements of all the members can be catered, e.g., by increasing or decreasing the amount of certain foodstuff by including some extra protein food for growth periods. For instance, the same salad can be used for both the overweight and the underweight members of the family if the dressing is omitted for the former.

Economy

The amount of money available, depending upon the socioeconomic status also effects the meal planning.

The major part of the income is spent on food. Therefore, one should spend economically to get maximum utilization. Although the budget of a family of moderate-income group may not provide for foods of the luxury class, it can still offer variety and opportunity for choice. Food budgets in lower income families permit even more limited choice and it may become increasingly necessary to depend on cereal foods for the main or substantial part of the meal. Then the problem faced is the supplementation of these cereal with foods necessary for a balanced diet. Although it may become difficult to plan, it is nevertheless possible. Thereby, it is very important to know the less expensive alternative for the more expensive recommended foods, having high nutritive value. Such recipes and foods should be included in meal preparation like using cereal pulse combination, e.g., khichri, paushtik roti, seasonal vegetables; butter milk; jaggery, pickle and chutney.

The Facilities and Help Available

The time spent in cooking depends on other facilities and other help availability of servant, using readymade foods, using labor saving devices. However, time like money needs to be budgeted for its best use. Time management in the preparation of foods is essential for the home maker who is also employed outside the home.

Satiety Value

Any individual meal should provide enough satiety value, so that one does not feel hungry till it is time for the next meal. Proteins and fats have greater satiety value as compared to carbohydrates, e.g., a breakfast of just tea and toast will not provide enough satiety value till lunch, whereas, a breakfast of milk, cereal, eggs and fruit will provide enough satiety value till lunch.

Personal Likes and Dislikes

Although the recommended dietary allowances for each of the classes of food should be followed, there is room for individual preference amongst the foods in each class. Some people make personal likes and dislikes the only basis for the inclusion or exclusion of certain foods in their meals—the failure to include milk is a common practice. It is always better to change the form of the food rather than to completely omit it. For example, milk can be given in the form of curd, cheese, custard or other sweet dish, soyabeans in the form of soya flour chapatis mixed with wheat flour.

Religion, Traditions and Customs

They are important in determining the food included in the diet, type of meal and the dishes served to the individual of family. For instance, Muslims do not eat pork, whereas Hindus do not eat beef. Rice is considered an auspicious dish at festivals and marriages. Widows are generally not served fish in Bengal. Therefore, religion, traditions and customs should be kept in view while planning meals for a family.

Variety

It is very important, because nobody likes to eat even his favorite food stuff over and over again. Therefore, to introduce variety, do not repeat same food items during daymeal. Also variety in meal planning is the sum total of many kinds and classes of food served in pleasing color combinations, with judicious mixture of soft and crisp foods, blunt and sharp flavors, hot and cold dishes. It ensures better nutrition and also result in more interesting meals with an attractive variety of texture, color, taste and appearance which in turn stimulates appetite and please the palate. Various methods of working can also introduce a variety—a meal consisting of tandoori roti, dal and seasonal green vegetable also with a crisp salad.

Schedules of Family Members

When planning meals, one needs to think of the schedules (time table) of the family members—meal times and the number of meals eaten at home and those that are eaten away from home. If packed lunches are made, the menus need to be modified to ensure that the items can be packed and the menu is appetizing even when cold.

Family Size and Composition

The family size affects the foods that can be served. It is known that the money spent for food per person decreases as the family size increases, when the family income remains constant. Staples such as wheat and rice are bought in larger amounts but quantity of milk, vegetables and fruits is lowered. Thus, the quality of the diet is affected. Family composition affects the kind and amounts of mood needed and pattern of meals served. For example, when children are below 5 years of age, more milk is required, the numbers of meals are more, as the child cannot take large amount at a time. As the child grows the meal pattern changes to accommodate the school hours and the need to pack lunch or snack may arise. Older members of the family may require change in consistency of food due to faulty teeth.

Meal Times

It is also an important factor in meal planning. The meals should be planned according to the time for meal, i.e., whether it is breakfast, lunch or dinner. Normally while planning the meal for whole day, it is seen that 1/3rd of days requirement are met by lunch 1/3rd by dinner and 1/3rd by breakfast and evening tea. But this is not a rigid schedule and can be changed according to individual requirement. But as long as the total nutritional requirements are being met.

Occasion

For daily meals the first importance is given to nutritive value. However, for special occasion, special importance has to be given to color, appearance, number of dishes to be included, but at the same time nutritive value can not be ignored. Similarly each festival has its specific food item which should always be given importance, e.g., preparing Sweets for Deepawali, Cake for X'mas, Sevian for Eid, etc.

Meal Planning for Different Meals in a Day

Breakfast

It is very important meal as taken after 10–12 hours long gap between dinner and breakfast the next day. It should be well planned, nutritious attractive and should provide 1/3rd to 1/4th of the day's requirements, but do not make it very heavy which would lead to lethargy. The school children usually miss breakfast and as a result, they cannot concentrate on studies after some time.

Breakfast should include cereal preparation—Paratha, puri, toast, porridge.

- Protein food—eggs, sausages, milk.

Low-cost Menu

1. Banana (any seasonal fruit)
2. Cereal and protein food—'missi' roti
3. Tea/butter milk/milk.

Middle-cost Menu

1. Apple or orange
2. Paratha (stuffed) with curds or toast and butter, milk/tea and pickle, or puri, vegetable preparation and a glass of milk lassi.

Western Menu/High Cost Menu

1. Fruit juice (orange, pineapple).
2. Porridge (cornflakes, rice, flakes, oatmeal, etc.) with milk.
3. Fried eggs with sausages/poached egg/panner-sabzi.
4. Buttered toast.
5. Coffee/tea.

Lunch

It is the main meal, hence an important meal. About 1/3rd of the total day's requirements should be provided. The members who are not at home for the lunch, should be given packed lunch, which should be nutritious, easy to carry, attractive and with some variety.

Packed Lunch Menu (for School Children)

- Dal/paneer-stuffed paratha.
- Fruit, e.g., orange.
- Piece of cake.

Or

- Sandwiches (paneer/egg/beans)
- Sweet (peanut chikki/besan ladoo/halwa/burfi).

For children food stuff should have variety, but it has to be handy too.

Packed Lunch Menu (for Adults)

- Parathas/chapatis
- Dry vegetable
- Dry dal.

However, on holidays when everyone is at home, menu with difference is prepared.

Normal Lunch Menu (on Holidays)

- Soup
- Cereal preparation—rice/pulao/chapati/puri/paratha
- Meat curry/egg curry/kabuli channas, pulse preparation, etc.
- Vegetable preparation, carrot, pea, sabzi/koftas
- Curd preparation.
- Salad.
- Desert/fruit: Custard/kheer/carrot-halwa/soufflé/pudding/fruit salad.

The selection of food items and number of dishes can vary according to the socioeconomic status.

On the other hand, where normally lunch is eaten at home, the menu should be simpler. Also dishes like curries, rice, curd, etc., can be included which are otherwise difficult to carry, some of the examples are:

- Moong whole, brinjal bharta, rice/chapati, curd fruit.
- Stuffed tandoori paranthe, curd, potato-pea curry, fruit.
- Chapati, pea-paneer curry, pumkin sabzi, curd fruit.
- Rice, sambhar, sweet curd mixed with fruits.

Evening Tea

It is generally light and usually includes snacks, sweets, pakoras, cutlets, mathri and tea/coffee/juice.

For children something heavy should be given like sandwiches, ladoos, burfi, cakes, etc.

If tea time is special occasion, 3–4 snacks and beverage can be served.

Normal Evening Tea Menu

- Pakoras, tea
- Tomato sandwich, tea
- Mathri, ladoo, tea
- Biscuit, vadas, tea
- Jalebi, wafers, tea.

Evening Tea Menu (for Special Occasions)

- Rainbow sandwich, coconut rolls, cashewnuts fried, tea.
- Cutlets, rasgullas, chirwa, biscuit, tea.
- Chocolate burfi, samosa, pastry, wafers, tea.
- Coconut burfi, khandwi, gulabjamun, dal-month, tea.
- Cashewnut burfi, peanut cutlets, chocolate cake, chirwa, tea.

Dinner

It is also the main meal and should provide 1/3rd of day's requirements and should make up for all deficiencies in person's meal, e.g., if curd has not been taken in the morning, include it in the dinner. Menu has to be elaborate when someone is invited. Otherwise, menu is like lunch.

For festivals, prepare particular food according to sanity of festivals, e.g., various sweets on Deepawali, cake on Christmas, Sevian on Eid, Gujiya on Holi, etc.

Tips for Menu Planning

- Consider whole day as a unit rather than individual meals.
- Try to distribute carbohydrates, fats and proteins throughout the day, so that no meal has predominance of any kind of food stuff.
- Use seasonal foods because they are best in flavor and cheap, however, avoid giving the same food stuff and especially in the same meal, e.g., do not give tomato soup, tomato macroni and tomato salad for the same meal. But, during the day things like cereals, butter, milk have to be repeated.
- Take care of color, flavor and texture by giving contrast in each meal, e.g., keep the color combination of dishes in mind while planning the meal. The dishes can be garnished to bring about more color in diet. Flavor of food should be blended with each other. There should also be some contrast in texture, e.g., some dishes can be soft and some dishes can be crisp, like with the soup we can given toasted bread, etc.
- There should be a balance between the dishes like some dishes should be light and some should be heavy, e.g., filling soup can be served with light main meal and vice versa.
- Include the favorite foods of the family at different meals, but at the same time do not be limited to only these foods and try to introduce new dishes, so that food habits can be expanded.
- Money can be saved on food by following methods:
  a. Buying bigger packs.
  b. Compare the prices before buying.
  c. Wholesale markets are cheaper than retail ones.
  d. Cook just the required amounts: if food is left over then make use of it by converting to another dish, etc.
  e. Use seasonal fruits and vegetables.
  f. Keep accounts.

Time can also be saved by following methods:

- Plan meal for several days at a time.
- Buy dry ingredients together at least for a month.
- Avoid going market during crowded hours.
- Arrange things properly in kitchen so as to save the time while working.
- Use pressure cooker.
- Plan your time while working.
- Use labor saving devices, e.g., mixer, but possible only in case the money is available to purchase them.

How to Plan a Diet

Keeping in mind, all the points discussed above for meal planning, the diet is planned as a day's menu with suitable meal pattern for particular individual. Further, to judge the adequacy of diet in terms of various nutrients, it is treated for detailed calculations. For this purpose, food composition tables (Nutritive Value of Indian Foods, NIN, ICMR) are used which give the nutritive value of several food stuffs per 100 gram of the edible portion. Generally detailed calculations are done for three important nutrients—1st for energy, then 2nd is for protein and the 3rd important nutrients is variable depending upon the requirements for the individual for whom the diet is planned.

The following example illustrates the planning of diet along with the detailed calculations.

Aim: To plan a day's diet for an adult man aged 28 years, who is a moderate worker belonging to middle income group.

General Information

- **Age:** 28 years
- **Sex:** Male
- **SES:** Middle income group
- **Activity:** Moderate worker

Recommended Daily Dietary Allowances

- **Energy:** 2875 K. cals
- **Thiamine:** 1.4 mg
- **Protein:** 60 g.

General Considerations

- The subject is a moderate worker, so his RDA is taken accordingly and the diet should be nutritionally balanced.
- His traditions, customs and beliefs should be kept in mind.
- His likes and dislikes should be kept in mind.
- The third important nutrient for the subject is thiamine, as thiamine's allowances are related energy intake, i.e., to carbohydrate utilization.
- Variety in the menu is essential and it should be provided in forms of color, texture and flavor.
- Food items included should be of moderate cost with the inclusion of seasonal fruits and vegetable, etc., hereby economic factor is also kept in mind.
- The planned meal should be able to provide enough satiety value. Planned diet should be according to the climate and availability of food should be kept in mind.
- The meal should be served in a pleasant atmosphere.

Menu

Breakfast

- Besan paratha
- Curds
- Coffee

Lunch

- Chapati
- Palak-Paneer
- Banana

Evening Tea

- Potato chops with chutney
- Tea

Dinner

- Rice (fried)
- Chapati
- Pineapple and lemon ice cream.

DIET PLAN FOR DIFFERENT AGE GROUPS

Infants

Infancy is a period of rapid growth. The average birth weight of newborn is 3 kg In first few days the newborn loses about 10% of body weight. Infant usually doubles the weight at 6 months and triples at the age of 1 year and 4 times at the age of 2 years. The baby measures 50 cm at birth, 60 cm at 3 months, 70 cm at 9 months and 75 cm at 1 year.

A diet lacking essential calories, minerals, vitamins, or fluids is considered inadequate. Breast milk provides the best nutrition for these vital first months of growth when compared to infant formula. For example, breastfeeding aids in preventing anemia, obesity, and sudden infant death syndrome; and it promotes digestive health, immunity, intelligence, and dental development.

After 6 months there is gradually introducing foods other than breast milk in the child's feeding schedule which is known as complementary feeding. Breast milk is sufficient till 6 months and after that complementary feeding is required to meet the excess demand of the body.

Age (months)	*Energy (Kcal)*	*Protein(g)*	*Calcium mg/dL*
0–6	108/kg	2.05/kg	500
6–12	98/kg	1.65/kg	450

Nutritional requirement for infants have largely been based on breast milk intake combine with supplementary diet. Documented evidences shows that infants grow well on exclusive breast-feeding for first 6 months of life.

Nutrition Contents of Breastfeeding

See **Table 5.13**.

Table 5.13: Nutrition contents of breastfeeding.

Nutrient	*Content/100 mL*
Calories	67 kcal
Proteins	1.1 g
Fat	3.5 g
Lactose	7.0 g
Sodium	0.9 mEq
Potassium	1.4 mEq
Calcium	35 mg
Phosphorus	15 mg
Iron	30–50 µg
Zinc	120 µg
Vitamin A	60 µg
Vitamin C	5.2 mg

Nutritional Requirement for Toddler and Preschool Going Children

During second year of life the weight gain is about 2 to 2.5 kg from the period of infancy. During 3 to 5 years of age the weight gain for the baby is 1.5 kg to 2 kg. Length of the newborn is approximately 50 cm (20") at birth which increases to 75 cm (29") at the age of one year. During the second year, the increase in height is about 10 cm and during 3–5 years height gain is 6–7 cm. As growth proceeds during childhood, there are changes in proportion of water, muscle tissues, fat deposition and the skeletal structure. During the second year of life, the child start developing a sense of individuality which is distinct from his mother. Preschool age is age of imitation and sex identification.

Item-wise Requirements Diet for Toddler and Preschool Children (In Grams)

See **Table 5.14**.

A Day's Sample Diet for a 5-year-old Child

See **Table 5.15**.

Nutritional Requirement for School Going Children

By school going age most of the children establish a particular pattern of food intake relative their peers. At school, he is exposed to food patterns which may be different from those

Table 5.14: Item-wise requirements diet for toddler and preschool children (in grams).

Food items	*1–3 years*	*4–6 years*
Cereals	175	270
Pulses	35	35
Leafy vegetables	40	50
Other vegetables	20	30
Roots and tubers	10	20
Milk	300	250
Oil and fats	15	25
Sugar and jaggery	30	40

Table 5.15: A day's sample diet for a 5 year old child.

Meal	*Food*	*Amount*
Early morning	Milk with sugar	200 mL
Breakfast	Paratha with curd or egg and bread	1 paratha 1 egg, 2 slice of bread
Mid morning	Fruit or fruit juice	1 fruit/1 glass fruit juice
Lunch	Rice, mixed vegetables, curd chapati	Rice small plate Mixed vegetables Small katori, curd ½ katori Chapati 1–2
Evening	Milk + biscuit	150 mL, 4–6 biscuit
Dinner	Dal, Chapati, Salad	1 katori dal, chapathi 2
Bed time	Fruit custard	1 katori

at homes and want to accept them. Behavior at meal times may be a problem as children are usually at hurry. They may rush to their breakfast due to early school timing and with their evening meals due to play and other activities. The adequacy of children's food depends not only on food available to them but also on food environment. Advertising and TV have a strong influence on the type of food chosen by children. So it is essential for parents to take special care when meal planning for them.

Balanced Diet Requirements for School Going Children

See **Table 5.16**.

A Day Sample Diet Plan for 8-year-old Child

See **Table 5.17**.

Nutritional Requirement for Adolescence

During this period growth and development take place at all level namely physiological, psychological and social. During this period rapid growth take place accomplished by hormonal changes, sexual maturation and often emotional bouts. This stage is called as second growth spurt. The growth spurt in girls occurs at 11–14 years and boys at 13–16 years. Changes in body composition occur due to hormonal influence which regulates the development of sex characteristics. At this stage of life adolescent girls and boys develop sexual maturity. At this stage child develops his identity and decision-making ability.

Balanced Diet Requirements for Adolescents (in grams)

See **Table 5.18**.

A Sample Menu Plan for a 14-year Boy

See **Table 5.19**.

Nutrition for Adulthood

By this stage, the body growth particularly in terms of height and weight stops to a certain extent but the breakdown and repair of body tissues goes on. Proper nutrition in adulthood ensures good health in old age. Various factors like age, sex, climate, activity, body growth, stress affect our body need for different nutrients.

Balanced Diet Requirements for Adult (in grams)

See **Table 5.20**.

One Day Menu for an Adult (Sedentary Work)

- **Energy:** 2875 kcal
- **Protein:** 60 g (60 kg wt.)

See **Table 5.21**.

Nutrition for Aged People

Adequate nutrition and balanced diet is important even in old age to prevent and control the common hazards of aging. The changes are associated with aging are loss of teeth, decrease neuromuscular coordination, impaired hearing and failing vision, diminished sense of taste and smell,

Table 5.16: Balanced diet requirements for school going children.

Food items	*Quantity (in grams)*
Cereals	300–400
Pulses	45
Leafy vegetables	50
Other vegetables	50
Roots and tubers	30
Milk	250
Fat and oil	40
Sugar and jaggery	45

Table 5.17: A day sample diet plan for 8-year-old child.

Meal	*Food*	*Quantity*
Breakfast	Sandwich and milk or omlet bread	Sandwich 2, milk 1 cup, egg, two slicebread
Midmorning	Stuffed paratha paneer and one fruit	Paratha 1 and one fruit
Lunch	Rice, curd, mixed vegetables	Rice 1 small plate, curd 1 small katori, mixed vegetables ½ katori
Evening snacks	Milk or cold coffee biscuits	Milk or cold coffee 1 cup biscuits 4–6
Dinner	Dal/meat, vegetables chapati	Dal/meat, small katori ½ katori 2 night Friut custard/ice cream 1 katori

Table 5.18: Balanced diet requirements for adolescents (in grams).

	Girls		
Food stuffs	*13–15 years*	*16–18 years*	*Boys 13–18 years*
Cereals	400	420	320
Pulses	70	70	70
Leafy vegetables	100	100	150
Other vegetables	150	175	150
Milk	600	600	600
Fat and oil	30	40	30
Sugar and jaggery	30	30	30

Table 5.19: A sample menu plan for a 14 years boy.

Meal	*Food*	*Quantity*
Early morning	Milk with sugar	200 mL
Breakfast	Boiled egg/omlet, bread or paratha with	1 egg, 2 slice bread or paratha 1, ½ katori curd
Mid-morning	Fruit salad or fruit juice 200 mL	Fruit juice 200 mL
Lunch	Fried rice, vegetables, curd chapati, salad	One plate, one katori 1–2 chapaties
Dinner	Dal/channa/chicken curry, vegetables, chapaties	1 katori/1 katori, 2 chapaties
At night	Ice cream/kheer/fruit custard	1 katori

Table 5.20: Balanced diet requirements for adult (in grams).

	Adult man			*Adult woman*		
Food stuffs	***Sedentary workers***	***Moderate workers***	***Heavy workers***	***Sedentary workers***	***Moderate workers***	***Heavy workers***
Cereals	460	520	670	410	440	575`
Pulses	40	50	60	40	45	50
Leafy vegetable	40	40	40	100	100	150
Other vegetable	60	70	80	40	40	100
Roots and tubers	50	60	80	50	50	60
Milk	150	200	250	100	150	200
Oil and fats	40	45	65	20	25	40

Table 5.21: One day menu for an adult (sedentary work).

Meal	*Food*	*Quantity*
Early morning	Milk with sugar or tea	1 cup
Breakfast	Egg with bread or paratha with curd, coffee	1 egg, 2 breads, 2 parathas,1 cup
Mid-day	Fruit salad or fruit juice or tea with biscuits	1 cup tea, 4–6 biscuits
Lunch	Vegetables Chapati Rice, curd, mixed salad	1 katori 2 1 plate, curd 1 katori
Evening tea	Tea with snacks	1 cup tea
Night dinner	Dal/rajama Vegetables Chapati	1 katori 1 katori 3
Bed time	Kheer/fruit	1 katori/1 fruit

Table 5.22: General diet plan for elderly.

Day	*Breakfast (8:00–9:00 AM)*	*Mid-morning (11:00–11:30 AM)*	*Lunch (1:30–2:00 PM)*	*Evening (4:30–5:30 PM)*	*Dinner (8:00–9:00 PM)*
Monday	Boiled egg or low fat paneer multigrain sandwich + 1 glass fresh fruit juice/tea/ coffee (with less sugar)	1 bowl boiled sprouts	1 bowl rice,1 bowl dal/rajma/ chana/beans, 1 small bowl curd,1 bowl cucumber salad, 1 bowl green vegetable Non-veg: Less oil-less spicy chicken/fish/egg curry	Unsweetened green tea + Mixed nuts and seeds (almond, chia, walnut)	Green pea-potato curry (potato to be less) + 2 plain chapati 1 glass warm milk (before bed)
Tuesday	1 bowl vegetable poha + 1 apple and ½ bowl curd	1 bowl vegetable salad	2 chapati + 1 bowl paneer curry OR 1 bowl fish curry (100 g) + 1 cup buttermilk	1 cup tea + 2 digestive biscuits Seasonal fruits (seasonal, orange, apple, pear, guava)	1 bowl vegetable soup, 2 plain roti/ chapati,1 bowl soy bean curry
Wednesday	1 bowl oatmeal/oats upma + 1 glass green and fruit smoothie (best to add apple, carrot and beet)	1 fistful of dry fruits	2 multigrain atta chapati + 1 bowl rice + 1 bowl chana curry + ½ bowl bottle guard curry + 1 cup buttermilk	1 small bowl roasted chana + 1 cup light tea	2 chapati + 1 bowl mixed vegetable
Thursday	2 slice brown bread + 1 slice low fat cheese + 1 small bowl sprouts	1 bowl of mixed fruits	1.5 bowl veg pulav rice + 1 bowl moong dal tadka + 1 small bowl low fat curd + 1 plate green raw salad	1 cup light tea + 2 wheat rusk	2 chapati + 1 bowl mixed dal
Friday	2 idli with sambar/2 plain dosa + 1 fruit	1 bowl plain puffed rice with cucumber and boiled chana	1 cup rice + 1 bowl chicken curry (150 g) OR low fat paneer/tofu curry + 1 glass buttermilk	1 fistful dry fruits	2 plain rice dosa + 1 bowl mixed veg masur dal
Saturday	2 plain utthapam + 1 tablespoon green chutney	1 bowl boiled sprouts	2 chapati + 1 bowl cabbage curry + 1 bowl moong dal + 1 small bowl curd/yogurt	1 bowl of mixed fruits	2 chapati + 1 bowl any mixed vegetable curry

anorexia, physical discomfort, incomplete digestion, etc. The rate of blood flow through kidneys decrease. Loneliness, depression, anxiety, fragile and weak bones are the features of aging people **(Table 5.22)**.

FOOD ADULTERATION

Dictionary says: Being mixed with extraneous material; the product of adulterating or the act of adulterating (especially the illicit substitution of one substance for another). Food adulteration is subtle murder practiced in the community and is gravest of socioeconomic crime. It has direct impact on economy, health, character and progress of a Country.

Definition

Food adulteration is defined as the intentional addition of non-permitted foreign matter.

The Federal Food, Drug and Cosmetic (FD and C) Act (1938) provides that food is 'adulterated' if it meets any one of the following criteria:

- It bears or contains any 'poisonous or deleterious substance' which may render it injurious to health.
- It bears or contains any added poisonous or added deleterious substance (other than a pesticide residue, food additive, color additive, or new animal drug, which are covered by separate provisions) that is unsafe.
- Its container is composed in whole or in part of any poisonous or deleterious substance which may render the contents injurious to health.
- It bears or contains a pesticide chemical residue that is unsafe.
- It is, or it bears or contains, an unsafe new animal drug.
- It is, or it bears or contains, an unsafe color additive.
- It consists, in whole or in part, of 'any filthy, putrid, or decomposed substance' or is otherwise unfit for food.
- It has been prepared, packed, or held under unsanitary conditions (insect, rodent, or bird infestation) whereby it may have become contaminated with filth or rendered injurious to health.
- It has been irradiated and the irradiation processing was not done in conformity with a regulation permitting irradiation of the food in question.
  Note: FDA has approved irradiation of a number of foods, including refrigerated or frozen uncooked meat, fresh or frozen uncooked poultry, and seeds for sprouting.
- It contains a dietary ingredient that presents a significant or unreasonable risk of illness or injury under the conditions of use recommended in labeling (for example, foods or dietary supplements containing aristolochic acids, which have been linked to kidney failure, have been banned).
- A valuable constituent has been omitted in whole or in part or replaced with another substance; damage or inferiority has been concealed in any manner; or a substance has been added to increase the product's bulk or weight, reduce its quality or strength, or make it appear of greater value than it is (this is 'economic adulteration'); it is offered for import into the United States and is a food that has previously been refused admission, unless the person reoffering the food establishes that it is in compliance with US law [21 USC § 342].
- The Federal Meat Inspection Act and the Poultry Products Inspection Act contain similar provisions for meat and poultry products.

Adulterant

Any material which is or could be employed for the purposes of adulteration.

An article of food shall be deemed to be adulterated: An adulterant is a chemical substance which should not be contained within other substances (e.g., food, beverages, and fuels) for legal or other reasons. The addition of adulterants is called adulteration.

Common Adulterants

Pulses such as moong or channa: Here adulterant is Metanil Yellow and Kesari Dal (Added to enhance the yellow color of a food substance). Its harmful effect is that it is highly carcinogenic and if consumed over a continuous period of time it can also cause stomach disorders.

Green Chilies, Green Peas and Other Vegetables

Here adulterant is Malachite Green (To accentuate the bright, glowing green color of the vegetable). Argemone seeds (used to add bulk and weight) that it is a colored dye that has proven to be carcinogenic for humans if consumed over a long period of time.

Mustard Seeds and Mustard Oil

Here adulterant is Argemone seeds (used to add bulk and weight). Papaya seeds (used to add bulk) that the consumption of these could cause epidemic dropsy and severe glaucoma. Young children and senior citizens with poor immunity are more susceptible to this.

Paneer, Khoya, Condensed Milk and Milk

Here adulterant is starch (used to give it thick, rich texture). Its harmful effect is that it is unhygienic, unprocessed water and starch can cause stomach disorders. Starch greatly reduces the nutritional value of the ingredient.

Icecream

Here adulterant is pepperonil, ethylacetate, butraldehyde, emilacetate, nitrate, washing powder, etc., are not less than poison. Pepper oil is used as a pesticide and ethyl acetate causes terrible diseases affecting lungs, kidneys and heart. Ice cream is manufactured in extremely cold chamber where fat is hardened and several harmful substances are added. Also a kind of gum is added which is sticky and slow melting. This gum is obtained by boiling animal parts like tail, the nose, the udder, etc.

Black Pepper

Here adulterant is Papaya seeds (used to add bulk). Its harmful effect is that Papaya seed can cause serious liver problems and stomach disorders.

Coffee Powder

For coffee powder adulterant is Tamarind seeds, chicory powder (used to add bulk and color). It is harmful effect is that it can cause diarrhea, stomach disorders, giddiness and severe joint pains. Some other adulterants: The starch in rice powder or wheat flour, often added to thicken cream, could be identified by the blue color produced by a dilute solution of iodine in aqueous potassium iodide.

Red Wine

Adulterated with the juice of bilberries or elderberries produced a deep blue precipitate with lead acetate.

Of all forms of adulteration the most reprehensible was the use of poisonous coloring matters in the manufacture of jellies and sweets. The bright colors used to attract children often contained lead, copper or mercury salts. Food-preservatives have a very extensive use, which often constitutes adulteration. Salt is the classic preservative, but is seldom classified as an adulterant. Salicylic, benzoic, and boric acids, and their sodium salts, formaldehyde, ammonium fluoride, sulfurous acid and its salts are among the principal preservatives. Many of these appear to be innocuous, but there is danger that the continued use of food preserved by these agents may be injurious. Some preservatives have been conclusively shown to be injurious when used for long period.

Coal tar colors are employed a great deal, pickles and canned vegetables are sometimes colored green with copper salts.

Turmeric is used in mustard and some cereal preparations. Any jellies, which are colored so as to simulate finer ones. In confectionery, dangerous colors, such as chrome yellow, Prussian blue, copper and arsenic compounds are employed.

Cream is adulterated with gelatin, and formaldehyde is employed as a preservative for it.

Butter is adulterated to an enormous extent with oleomargarine, a product of beef fat.

Brick dust in chili powder, colored chalk powder in turmeric.

Contaminants Use for Adulteration

There is a wide variety of contaminants use for adulteration which are injurious for health. Physical contaminants like bone, rock, grit and metal; Chemical contaminants like pesticides, insecticides, herbicides, Other chemical-contaminants PBB, PCB, arsenic, tin also make us to prone for some life-threatening diseases other than this other Food adulterants are non-permitted colors like Rhodamine B, Rhodamine G Auramine Orange I/Orange II/Orange G, Bismark Brown. Non-permitted sweeteners Cyclamate, Dulcin Artificial Sweeteners like, Acesulfame K (300 ppm), Saccharin (100 ppm) Aspertame (700 ppm), Sucralose (300 ppm). Neotame (33 ppm) makes the food dangerous for health.

Impact of Food Adulteration

The impact of food adulteration affecting not only the consumer but also it affects the country as a whole consumer pays more money for the foodstuffs of lower quality. Some forms of adulteration are harmful. Injurious to health, even may result in death, the common adulterant and their effects are listed in **Table 5.23**.

Table 5.23: Adverse effects of adulterants.

Adulterant	*Adverse effects*
Argemone oil	Epidemic dropsy
Mineral oil	Hepatic damage/carcinoma
Kesari dhal	Lathyrism
PBB, PCB	Endocrinological dysfunction, neurotoxicity
Metanil yellow	Anemia, blindness, convulsions

Codex Alimentarius Commission

A Joint FAO/WHO Food Standards Program was established in 1962, and a joint subsidiary body was created, the Codex Alimentarius Commission (CAC). The CAC aims to promote harmonization of standards and facilitate International trade. Food standards in India are based on CAC.

Laws in India

In India, as early as 1860, the adulteration of foodstuffs was prohibited under the Penal Code (Sec 272, 273). 'Adulteration of food-stuffs and other goods' was later included in the Concurrent List (III) of the Constitution of India. It then, became possible for the Central Government to enact an All India legislation on this subject.

Prevailing Food Standards in India:
- The PFA standards
- The AGMARK
- The ISI (Bureau of Indian Standards).

The PFA Standards

The PFA standards are based on the Prevention of Food Adulteration Act, 1954.

Prevention of Food Adulteration Act, 1954

The Prevention of Food Adulteration Act, (PFA) 1954 operated by the Directorate General of Health Services, Ministry of Health was designed for the following purposes:
- It formulates and monitors the standard of quality and purity of foods with emphasis on prevention of adulteration of foods.
- It is the basic structure intended to protect the common consumer against the supply of adulterated foods.
- It makes provision for prevention of adulteration of food and lays down the rule that no person shall manufacture for sale, store, sell or distribute any adulterated or misbranded food or food which contravenes the provision of act or rules.

- It has set the yardstick to ascertain adulteration. According to this act, a food is deemed to be adulterated, if:
  - It is not of the nature, substance and quality, which the food ought to be.
  - It contains any other substance which affects, or if the article is so processed so as to affect injuriously the nature, substance and quality of the food.
  - It contains added inferior or cheaper substance that affects the nature and quality of the food.
  - Any constituent of the food is removed so as to affect injuriously the nature, quality and substance of the food.
  - It is prepared, packed and stored under unsanitary conditions.
  - It contains any filthy, disgusting, rotten, decomposed substance of a diseased animal or vegetable substance or is insect-infested or otherwise unfit for human consumption.
  - The article is obtained from a diseased animal.
  - The article contains a poisonous ingredient or any other ingredient injurious to health.
  - The container renders the food injurious to health.
  - It contains excessive or prohibited colors.
  - It contains excessive or prohibited preservatives.
  - It does not satisfy the standards prescribed by the authorities.

Under the provision of the PFA Act, the Government of India has promulgated PFA rules which specifies the following details:

- Qualification, duties and functions of food analysts, food inspectors and central food laboratory.
- Procedure for drawing test samples and sending them to the analyst and laboratory.
- Specification for the identity and purity of food.
- Tolerance for contaminants, preservatives, emulsifiers and other additives.

AGMARK Standard

The word Agmark is derived from the words' Agricultural Marketing'. It is a standard of quality based on the physical and chemical characteristics of food, both the natural and those acquired during processing. Products graded under AGMARK include vegetable oils, ghee, butter, rice, groundnut, pulses and spices. These standards ensure accurate weight and correct selling price.

Bureau of Indian Standards

The Bureau of Indian Standards lays down criteria for standardization of vegetables and fruit products, spices and condiments, animal products and processed food. Manufacturers are allowed to use the BIS label on each unit of their product, if their products conform with the standards laid down by BIS. The products are checked for quality by laboratories certified by BIS. BIS is also known as 'ISI' (Indian Standard Institution). Some of the items which require compulsory BIS certification under PFA Act include artificial food colors, natural food colors, food additives, infant formula, milk-cereal based weaning foods, milk powder and condensed milk.

Revised from Time to Time by 'Central Committee for Food Standards'

It is a centrally sponsored Act but implementation is largely carried out by state and local govt. bodie in the respective areas. Center plays vital role in proper coordination, monitoring and surveillance of the program throughout the country. A chain of food laboratories and 4 Regional Central food appellate Central Food Laboratories (Kolkata, Mysore, Ghaziabad, Pune) DGHS organizes the in-service training program for different functionaries like Food Inspectors, Analysts, Senior officers, etc., responsible for implementation of PFA Act. FPA Act, 1954 amended in 1964, 1976, 1986 to make it more stringent.

Minimum 6 months imprisonment with a minimum of ₹1,000 fine for proven cases and the punishment may extend up to Life imprisonment and a fine not less than ₹5,000 if it comes under IPC-Section 320.

FOODBORNE ILLNESS OR DISEASE

Foodborne illness or disease (colloquially referred to as food poisoning) is any illness resulting from the spoilage of contaminated food by pathogenic bacteria, viruses, or parasites that contaminate food, as well as prions (the agents of mad cow disease), and toxins such as aflatoxins in peanuts, poisonous mushrooms, and various species of beans that have not been boiled for at least 10 minutes. Food poisoning can caused by the infection of food with microorganisms or ingestion of toxins product.

Over 200 diseases are caused by eating food contaminated with bacteria, viruses, parasites or chemical substances such as heavy metals. This growing public health problem causes considerable socioeconomic impact though strains on healthcare systems lost productivity, and harming tourism and trade. These diseases contribute significantly to the global burden of disease and mortality.

Foodborne diseases are those which are caused by contamination of food and occur at any stage of the food production, delivery and consumption chain. They can result from several forms of environmental contamination including pollution in water, soil or air, as well as unsafe food storage and processing.

Foodborne diseases encompass a wide range of illnesses from diarrhea to cancers. Most present as gastrointestinal issues, though they can also produce neurological, gynecological and immunological symptoms. Diseases causing diarrhea are a major problem in all countries of the world, though the burden is carried disproportionately by low- and middle-income countries and by children under 5 years of age.

Causes and Types of Foodborne Illness

Foodborne illness is caused by consuming contaminated foods or beverages. Many different disease-causing microbes or pathogens can contaminate foods, so there are many different types of foodborne illnesses.

Most foodborne diseases are infections caused by a variety of bacteria, viruses, and parasites. Other diseases are poisonings caused by harmful toxins or chemicals that have contaminated food.

Foodborne diseases are classified into:

1. **Foodborne infections:** Foodborne infection is caused by the ingestion of food containing live bacteria which grow and establish themselves in the human intestinal tract. These can either be bacterial, viral or parasitic. Body reacts by raising temperature. Foodborne infection tend to have long incubation periods in comparison to foodborne intoxication.
2. **Foodborne intoxications:** Foodborne intoxication is caused by ingesting food containing toxins formed by bacteria which resulted from the bacterial growth in the food item. These diseases caused by consumption of food containing biotoxicants, metabolic products and poisonous substance.

Milk-borne Infections

Salmonella Poisoning

Salmonellosis is a disease resulting from the ingestion of salmonella along with contaminated food. This is mainly a foodborne illness and milk and milk products appear to be commonly involved. There are about 2000 closely related biotypes of salmonella that can cause food poisoning in humans. It is during the mishandling of milk that the causative microorganism may enter these foods and their subsequent growth during holding may lead to salmonellosis.

Causative Microorganism

- Salmonella typhi cause typhoid
- Salmonella paratyphi A, B, C cause Paratyphoid
- Salmonella enteritidis leads to food poisoning.

Sources

- Water is one of the most important source of salmonella, as it frequently gets contaminated through fecal matter. If polluted water is used for washing of utensils and equipment it can also lead to contamination of milk. Silage is another source of salmonella.
- Handlers are the carriers in active cases.
- External agents like flies also acts as a source of contamination.
- Animals suffering from salmonellosis, under certain conditions, excrete viable microorganisms in their milk.

Symptoms

- **Typhoid fever:** Characterized by continuous fever, inflammation of intestines, formation of intestinal ulcers, enlargement of spleen, characteristic raised spot eruptions on the abdomen and toxemia.
- **Paratyphoid fever:** Resembling typhoid fever but it is milder than typhoid. Approximately 10^5 to 10^7 microorganisms per mL are required to cause infection.
- **Salmonellosis:** Nausea, vomiting, abdominal pain, diarrhea, chills, headache, prostration, muscular weakness, drowsiness, moderate fever, restlessness, etc.

Incubation Period

About 7–14 days for typhoid and 1 to 7 days for paratyphoid.

Diagnosis

Microorganism may be present in feces; urine and blood are identified by microscopic, cultural, fermentative and serological tests. Widal test is used for typhoid.

Prevention and Control

- Adequate treatment of water
- Infected individuals, who had infection should not handle milk
- Follow hygienic conditions during production, processing and storage
- Educating the people about food and personal hygiene
- Periodic examination of individuals who handle foods for public consumption
- Pasteurization and other adequate heat treatment of milk and milk products
- Control of flies
- Treatment of affected individuals.

Bacillary Dysentery (Shigellosis)

This is one of the common foodborne infection and outbreaks are associated with consumption of unpasteurized milk.

Causative Microorganism

- *Shigella dysenteriae*
- *Shigella sonnei*
- *Shigella flexneri*

Source

- Milk contaminated with water, flies and utensils
- Milk handlers.

Symptoms

Shigellosis is an acute intestinal disease characterized by diarrhea with blood, pus or mucous, fever, vomiting, abdominal cramps and tenesmus.

Diagnosis

Isolation of microorganism by taking rectal swabs and plating on desoxycholate citrate agar, incubation period is 1–4 days.

Prevention and Control

- Strict sanitary condition should be enforced in dairy workers particularly in pasteurization plants and retail outlets dispensing milk in bulk
- Attendants looking after the patients should be prohibited from contact with milk or utensils
- Take precautions to exclude flies.

Streptococcal Infection

Streptococcal infections like septic sore throat, scarlet fever and food poisoning are treated to the consumption of milk and its products. Humans and animals both can contaminate milk with streptococci. Although streptococcal food poisoning through milk and milk products is not well established, yet a few strains of Group D Streptococci or enterococci have produced toxic metabolites in milk and their toxigenic potentials is ascertained in animal models.

Causative Microorganism

- *Streptococcus pyogenes:* Scarlet fever, septic sore throat, tonsillitis and septicaemia
- *Streptococcus agalactiae:* Mastitis in animals.

Sources

- Animals infected with *Streptococcus agalactiae* may harbor microorganisms in udder and acts as a source of pathogens
- Personnel directly connected with the care and milking of animals in a dairy herd may act as vectors of mastitis and cause mastitis in other animals as these carry the pathogens on skin of hands, etc.
- Enterococci are chiefly of fecal origin and fecal contamination of milk and milk products may introduce lot of enterococci in these products
- Milking machines may help in the transfer of pathogens to milk and also to other animals with the help of infected teat cups
- Human carriers of *Streptococcus pyogenes* contaminate milk during handling and processing
- Human carriers disseminating pathogenic *Streptococcus pyogenes* may also infect animals that develop clinical or subclinical udder infections, and in turn pass out these microorganism into milk
- Milk products may get contaminated from raw milk infected with streptococci.

Symptoms

- **Septic sore throat:** Characterized by high and irregular fever, sudden onset of fever, inflammation and swelling of lymph glands of throat and sometimes involving the formation of abscess around tonsils and in cervical lymph glands.
- **Scarlet fever:** It is an acute febrile disease of throat, accompanied by a scarlet rash. Invasion of other parts of body may occur by microorganisms resulting in infection of middle ear, kidney. Scarlet rash is due to elaboration of a toxin.
- **Food poisoning:** The symptoms resembles staphylococcal food poisoning, however, these are of mild type. Incubation period is 1–3 days.

Diagnosis

For septic sore throat, throat swabs should be taken and observed for the presence of hemolytic streptococci of lancefield group A. Dick test is used to detect scarlet fever. Food poisoning can be diagnosed by the isolation of causative microorganisms their enterotoxin typing and toxigenicity.

Prevention and Control

- Adequate heat treatment of milk
- Holding milk at lower temperature
- Rejection of milk from the suspected quarters
- Milk showing abnormal changes should not be pooled
- Regular checking of the health of dairy workers
- Fecal contamination of milk should be avoided.

Milk-borne Intoxications

Staphylococcal Poisoning

Infection of milk by some strains of *Staphylococcus aureus* leads to the elaboration of enterotoxins by these that cause gastroenteritis in humans.

Toxins

Staphylococci produce different metabolic end products such as:

- Hemolysin/staphylolysin (α, β, γ and δ)
- Leukocidin
- Necrotizing factor
- Lethal factor
- Enterotoxin
- Coagulase.

Among different toxins, enterotoxin is responsible for major food poisoning outbreaks. *Staphylococcus aureus* is capable of growing and producing enterotoxins in raw milk at a concentration of 10^6 microorganisms per mL. However, not all the strains of microorganisms are capable of producing enterotoxins. The toxin production is faster in milk with low count. In poor quality milk, competition with other microorganisms and changes brought about by these, e.g., acidity, depletion of nutrients inhibit toxin production.

Sources

Human handlers are the main source as the microorganisms and present in nose, skin, wounds, pimples and boils. Animals affected with mastitis are the other sources.

Symptoms

Nausea, vomiting, abdominal cramps, diarrhea, sweating, headache, prostration, etc. Mortality is low, incubation period is 1–16 hours, and symptoms last for 24–48 hours.

Diagnosis

Biological methods, serological methods, coagulase test and thermo nuclease test.

Prevention and Control

- Adequate heating destroys staphylococci but not the enterotoxin. So, heating within few hours of production

would inhibit the multiplication of staphylococci and hence, no toxin production
- Adequate cooling immediately after producing milk also inhibits multiplication of staphylococci.
- Postpasteurization contamination should be avoided
- Infected handlers should not be allowed to handle milk
- Animals having mastitis should be isolated.

Botulism

Botulism poisoning is the severest of all the food poisonings, as it affects the nervous system and is often extremely fatal. However, milk is rarely involved in the causation of botulism as fluid milk is not a suitable medium for the growth of causative agent being an anaerobe. In sour milk *Clostridium botulinum* cannot survive due to low pH. But it is quite prevalent in canned products like condensed milk and processed cheese in view of the existing anaerobic conditions favorable for its growth.

Toxins

Although, the microorganism is heat resistant, it produces a variety of heat labile toxins that can be destroyed at 100°C within few minutes. Different types of toxins A to G are produced by the microorganism and out of these at least four A, B, E and F are known to affect human. These toxins are lethal in small doses. It is estimated that 0.1 µg of toxin may cause death of person and 1 mg of purified toxin is sufficient to kill a population of million people.

Sources

Soil and water

Symptoms

Nausea, vomiting, fatigue, dizziness, headache, and dryness of skin, mouth, and throat. As it acts on central nervous system (CNS), it leads to paralysis of muscles, double vision and respiratory failure, resulting in to death. Incubation period is 12–96 hours.

Diagnosis

Microscopic examination, animal inoculation and cultural identification.

Prevention and Control

- Adequate heating of product destroys toxin (1000°C per 10–20 minute)
- Hygienic conditions is adopted during production of milk
- Chilling after production should be essential
- Acidity inhibits the causative microorganism
- Reject bulged cans and spoiled foods.

E. coli Poisoning

E. coli is known to be associated with enteritis in infants and adults as well as with traveler's diarrhea and food poisoning. Milk and milk products like icecream, kulfi, dried milks, cheese, etc., can be contaminated with toxigenic *E. coli* that can produce the enterotoxins under favorable conditions. A minimum of 10^5 to 10^7 cells per gram are required to produce enterotoxins sufficient to cause food poisoning.

Toxins

E. coli can produce two types of enterotoxins named as heat labile and heat stable toxins. The labile toxin can be inactivated at 65°C per 30 min.

Sources

- Water supplies contaminated with fecal matter
- Unhygienic practices by handlers may introduce the microorganism in to milk chain
- Infected animal may also excrete the microorganisms.

Symptoms

Children are more susceptible. Symptoms due to heat labile toxins are almost similar to symptoms of cholera. Massive watery diarrhea occurs due to accumulation of fluid in the intestines. In case of heat stable toxin, the symptoms include diarrhea with or without vomit that is not bloody and without inflammatory exudates in stool. Fever may be present in children but not in adults. Incubation period is 8–24 hour.

Prevention and Control

- Fecal contamination of water supply should be avoided
- Handlers should follow strict hygiene practices
- Cross contamination from infected animals should be avoided.

Cholera

Cholera is one of the acute diarrheal diseases caused by *Vibreo cholerae*. It frequently occurs in the form of massive epidemics. Unhygienic practices are mainly responsible for outbreak. Although, cholera is mainly water-borne disease, the involvement of milk may also transmit the disease. The causative microorganism adheres to the epithelial lining of mucosa in the small intestines, where it produces enterotoxin that causes loss of fluid and electrolytes from the body followed by dehydration.
- Milk infected by soiled hands of a patient
- Use of infected water for dairy purpose
- Adulteration of milk with contaminated water.

Symptoms

In mild cases of cholera, diarrhea appears to be the only symptom. In severe cases, diarrhea, vomiting, rice water stools, abdominal pain, thirst, dehydration are major symptoms. The disease runs a short course terminating in death, sometimes within 12 hours after the appearance of first symptoms. Incubation period is few hours to 5 days, usually 3 days.

Diagnosis

Intraperitoneal inoculation of Guinea pigs with pure culture results in the death of the animal within 24 hours.

Prevention and Control

- Proper pasteurization of milk and its products.
- Sanitary disposal of human excreta
- Protection of water by boiling
- Sanitary preparation and handling of products
- Control or destruction of house flies
- Public health education
- Isolation of patients and carriers
- Disinfection of stools and vomit and articles soiled by the patients
- Food left by the patients should be burnt
- Room of patient should be thoroughly cleaned and disinfected
- Use of cholera vaccine in exposed population group.

Fungal Intoxications

The common types of fungal intoxications that result through milk are those caused by *Asperigillus* and other molds like *Pencillium, Fusarium* etc.

Aflatoxicosis

Aflatoxicosis is a common type of fungal intoxication caused by the common molds, *Aspergillus flavus* and *Aspergillus parasiticus* by virtue of their ability to produce aflatoxin. Aflatoxin can be present in milk as preformed toxin or it can be secreted in milk by the milch animal that has been fed with aflatoxin containing feed. Therefore, even with satisfactory sanitation and hygiene during production and processing of milk, the mycotoxins can be transferred to consumer. Upon ingestion, the aspergillus toxins are metabolized by milch animals and are secreted into milk in form of M1 and M2 that are also toxic to the consumers.

- **Types of aflatoxins:** *Aspergillus flavus* produces B1, B2, B2a. B1 is the most abundant and most toxic of the aflatoxin. G1, G2 and G2a toxins (produced by *Aspergillus flavus* only) are extremely heat stable, potent and exhibit very strong toxicity apart from being highly carcinogenic. The recommended upper permissible limit of aflatoxin in foods is 0.5–15 μg/kg.
- **Source:** Aerial contamination and soil contaminated foods introduce mold spores in milk and milk products.
- **Symptoms:** Liver hyperplasia, tissue hemorrhage, anorexia, hepatitis and finally death in animals. The vital organs like spleen, pancreas and kidney may also be involved in aflatoxicosis.
- **Prevention and control:**
  - Prevent contamination of milk and milk products
  - Prevent fungal growth by storing the product under proper conditions and by use of fungi-static agents
  - Detoxification of aflatoxins by physical, chemical or biological agents. However, this is relatively impractical in dairy products.

Milk-borne Toxifications

Bacillus cereus Poisoning

It occurs due to ingestion of contaminated food with *Bacillus cereus* or its spores and produces three types of toxins:

1. Hemolysin
2. Lecithinase
3. Enterotoxin.

Sources

- From mastitis udder
- Spores from animal's teat and skin equipment's
- Soil; directly or indirectly.

Symptoms

Two major classifications of symptoms:

1. **Diarrhea:** Abdominal pain and cramps, profuse watery diarrhea, rectal tenesmus. Moderate nausea with rare vomiting. Lecithin's releases phosphoryl choline, a toxic substance from lecithin.
2. **Vomiting:** Acute attack of nausea and vomiting, diarrhea is not common.

Prevention and Control

- Proper cooling of milk
- Maintenance of environmental hygiene and air quality

Clostridium perfringens Poisoning

Clostridium perfringens: It causes gas gangrene. The anaerobic conditions inside canned foods are favorable for growth of *C. perfringens.* Five different enterotoxins—A, B, C, D and E are produced, where A and C causes food poisoning.

Sources

- From soil and feces
- Dust, fodder, milk
- Fecal contamination of water.

Symptoms

Diarrhea, vomiting, abdominal pain; incubation period is 8–22 hours. Sometimes it is fatal.

Prevention and Control

- Proper cooling of milk
- Maintenance of environmental hygiene and air quality
- Hygiene during production, processing, etc.

FOOD HYGIENE/FOOD SAFETY

Food is a potential source of infection and is liable to contamination by microbes, at any point during its journey from the producer to the consumer. Food hygiene, which refers to the many practices needed to safeguard the quality of food from production to consumption. This is sometimes referred to as 'from farm to fork' or 'from farm to table', because it includes every stage in the process from growing on the farm, through storage and distribution, to finally eating the food. It also includes the collection and disposal of food wastes. Throughout this chain of events there are many points where, directly or indirectly, knowingly or unknowingly, unwanted chemicals and microorganisms may contaminate the food. Everyone who works with food is responsible for ensuring that consumers are protected from contaminated food and the risk of food poisoning, which causes extreme discomfort, absence from work or school and, in some cases, death. People get sick from food poisoning because the food they have eaten has contained bacteria, viruses or chemicals. It can take from an hour to a few days to develop food poisoning, depending on the cause, and the best way of preventing food poisoning is to use safe food handling practices. Bacteria are the biggest problem, because they are so common, and are found in soil, on animals, people and even clothes. In the kitchen, bacteria often come from vegetables and raw meat. Sometimes these bacteria can move from raw ingredients to cooked food, in a process called cross contamination.

Food safety, nutrition and food security are closely linked. Unsafe food creates a vicious cycle of disease and malnutrition, particularly affecting infants, young children, elderly and the sick. In addition to contributing to food and nutrition security, a safe food supply also supports national economies, trade and tourism, stimulating sustainable development. The globalization of food trade, a growing world population, climate change and rapidly changing food systems have an impact on the safety of food. WHO aims to enhance at a global and country-level the capacity to prevent, detect and respond to public health threats associated with unsafe food. Food hygiene are the conditions and measures necessary to ensure the safety of food from production to consumption (Food Chain Sequence). Handling, preparing and storing food or drink in a way that best reduces the risk of consumers becoming sick from the foodborne disease. Food hygiene falls under the umbrella term 'food safety'. Food hygiene itself does not include all the other key areas of food safety.

Food safety refers to an entire system of managing risks. Meanwhile, food hygiene refers to an individual set of practices for controlling only one aspect.

Concept of Food Safety and Food Hygiene

Food safety refers to the management systems that establishments must have in place if they sell food. It ensures that the food in any establishment - from restaurants and supermarkets to delis, food trucks, and cafés - is safe to eat and as advertised. There are various pieces of legislation in place for food safety, but the Food Safety Act 1990 is the main framework for all food safety laws.

Under food safety law, the key elements of food safety are:

- Ensuring everyone follows good food hygiene practices. This includes personal hygiene, safe handling of food, preventing cross-contamination, cleaning procedures, allergen control, safe storage of food, and cooking temperatures.
- Implementing appropriate food management systems. This refers to the overarching system that keeps food and the premises safe and hygienic. The main aspect is HACCP, but it also refers to recordkeeping, labeling, traceability, supply and delivery, and staff training.
- Maintaining hygienic premises. The maintenance of the building is another key aspect of risk prevention. This includes the general cleanliness and upkeep of the building, having an appropriate layout, suitable lighting, ventilation, pest control, and waste management.
- *Food hygiene* is an essential aspect of food safety. It refers to the processes that directly involve food—including storage, preparation, and cooking. Good practices in these areas ensure that customers receive food that is safe and as described.
- Food hygiene may be defined as the sanitary science which aims to produce food which is safe for the consumer and of good keeping quality. It covers a wide field and includes the rearing, feeding, marketing and slaughter of animals as well as the sanitation procedures designed to prevent bacteria of human origin reaching food stuff. Food hygiene in its widest sense, implies hygiene in the production, handling, distribution and serving.
- WHO (1984) has defined food hygiene as all conditions and measures that are necessary during production, processing, storage, distribution and preparation of food to ensure that it is safe, wholesome and fit for human consumption. The primary aim of food hygiene is to prevent food poisoning and other foodborne illness.

The key elements of food hygiene are:

- **Personal hygiene:** This includes handwashing, protective clothing, illness procedures, and other duties (such as avoiding smoking).
- **Preventing cross-contamination:** This includes preventing bacterial, physical, chemical, and allergenic contamination, particularly by having appropriate equipment in place (such as separate cutting boards).
- **Cleaning procedures:** Thorough cleaning of the kitchen, equipment, and kitchenware (including plates and cutlery) is vital.
- **Allergen control:** All businesses must clearly explain which foods are allergenic and must prevent allergens from cross-contaminating other food.
- **Safe storage of food:** This includes storage locations and containers, a FIFO system, labeling, and temperature control.
- **Cooking temperatures:** Businesses must ensure they cook and hold food at appropriate temperatures to prevent bacterial risks.

FIVE KEYS TO SAFER FOOD

The core messages of the five keys to safer food are: (1) keep clean; (2) separate raw and cooked; (3) cook thoroughly; (4) keep food at safe temperatures; and (5) use safe water and raw materials.

Keep Clean

While most microorganisms do not cause disease, dangerous microorganisms are widely found in soil, water, animals and people. These microorganisms are carried on hands, wiping cloths and utensils, especially cutting boards, and the slightest contact can transfer them to food and cause foodborne diseases. So keeping clean is an important aspect of food safety.

Wash Hands

- Wash your hands before handling food and often during food preparation, before taking food and during serving also.
- Wash your hands after going to the toilet, after toileting baby or changing any diaper
- Wash and sanitize all surfaces and equipment used for food preparation
  - After playing with pet animal
  - Whenever hands are soiled
  - After changing a diaper, blowing your nose
  - Handling rubbish, handling chemicals
  - Playing with pets, smoking.

How to Wash Hands?

- Wet your hands with warm running water
- Add soap, then rub your hands together for at least 20 seconds—making a soapy lather on both the front and back of your hands, as well as between your fingers and under your nails
- Rinse your hands well under warm running water—dry hands thoroughly with a clean towel.
- Then turn off the water with a clean paper towel and dispose in a proper receptacle.

Cleanliness of Slaughtering House

If slaughtering of animals at home then:

- Keep the area clean and separate from food preparation areas.
- Change clothes and wash hands and equipment after slaughtering.
- Do not slaughter sick animals.
- Wash hands to prevent contamination with fecal material.
- Keep domestic and other live animals away from the food growing, preparation and storage areas (e.g., pets, poultry, animals raised in the home).

Separate Raw and Cooked Food

Cross-contamination is a term used to describe the transfer of microorganisms from raw to cooked food. Separation must occur at all phases of food preparation including slaughter plates used for raw food should not be used for cooked food. Store raw foods below cooked foods to avoid cross-contamination. Cross-contamination of foods occurs when the microorganisms from raw food are transferred to cooked foods. Cross-contamination can occur at any time from slaughter until consumption. Separation of raw and cooked foods must occur throughout all phases of food preparation including slaughter to prevent dangerous microorganisms on raw foods from transferring to cooked foods. It is important to remember that when a plate that has been used for raw food, it should not be used again for cooked foods until it is washed with soap and water. For example, if you place raw meat onto a plate that same plate should not be used again for the cooked meat because the cooked meat will become contaminated with the juices of the raw meat.

To prevent the transfer of disease-causing microorganisms from raw foods to cook foods during storage, raw foods should be stored below cooked foods. The juices from the raw food can drip onto and contaminate the cooked food. So separate of raw meat, poultry and seafood from other foods by using separate equipment and utensils such as knives and cutting boards for handling raw foods.

Cook Thoroughly

Cook food thoroughly, especially meat, poultry, eggs, and seafood. Since bacteria are found on the outer surface of meat, the centre of an intact piece of meat is usually sterile and safe from bacteria. However, when meat is minced or ground, the bacteria on the outside are mixed into the meat and thus are present throughout the meat. It is important to cook these food until the centre reaches a temperature of 70°C. Cooking foods to a temperature above 70°C kills microorganisms on foods within 30 seconds. When food must be prepared at lower temperatures, a longer cooking time is needed because the microorganisms are being killed at a slower rate and more time is needed to ensure they are killed. When reheating already cooked foods, they should be reheated until piping hot (70°C) throughout the entire food. The middle of the food should not still be cool. For meat and poultry, make sure that juices are clear, not pink. Ideally, use a thermometer to measure the temperature. Proper cooking can kill almost all dangerous microorganisms. Studies have shown that cooking food to a temperature of 70°C can help ensure it is safe for consumption. Foods that require special attention include minced meats, rolled roasts, large joints of meat and whole poultry.

- Be aware of on-going diseases in your area such as Avian influenza. Human health risks from these diseases
- May require additional controls such as using personal protective gear. Contact the local government authority for further information.
- Remove feces from the home and keep it separate from food growing, preparation and storage areas.

Storing and Handling Food

- Keep food covered to protect it from dust, insects, sneezes, etc. Always use a clean cover—never re-use plastic or aluminium wrap.
- Keep raw meat and seafood, eggs, ready-to-eat food (such as fruit and vegetables) and cooked meals separated in the fridge. Always wrap and store cooked foods above raw foods in the fridge.
- Keep perishable foods hot (above 60°C) or cold (below 5°C). Check the temperature of your fridge regularly—in hot weather it may need adjusting to keep food cold.

- Arrange food in your fridge so cold air can easily circulate around it. Never overstock your fridge. Fridges work better and are cheaper to run if they are defrosted regularly.
- Bacteria that cause food poisoning can grow easily on high-risk foods such as dairy products, meat (including poultry), fish and seafood. Given time and the right temperature conditions, bacteria can multiply quickly to dangerous levels. Bacteria grow best at temperatures between 5°C and 60°C. This temperature range is known as the 'temperature danger zone'. To keep high-risk foods out of the temperature danger zone.

Always keep high-risk foods at the following temperatures:

- Above 60°C for foods such as roasts, stews, casseroles, soups and curries
- Below 5°C for foods including sliced meats, desserts, dairy products, sandwiches and salads.
- Always defrost frozen food in the fridge or in a microwave oven set on 'defrost'. Defrosting food on the bench top can be unsafe, and increase bacteria growth in foods as they defrost.
- Make sure food is cooked thoroughly. Joints of meat and poultry should reach at least 75°C in their center—this will kill most harmful bacteria. Make sure meat and poultry juices are clear, not pink.
- Cook and serve food immediately—never leave high-risk food out at room temperature. Any food left out for more than four hours should be thrown away.
- Refrigerate promptly all cooked and perishable food at or below 5°C. Portion food before cooling, for example slice meats and cut large poultry into smaller portions. Place liquid foods such as casseroles in shallow containers (no more than 5 cm deep) to allow for rapid cooling and place in the fridge as soon as it stops steaming.
- If reheating food, make sure it is reheated until steaming hot.
- Do not store food too long, even in the fridge. Keep for a maximum of 3 days.

Handling of Food

- Always wash your hands thoroughly with soap and hot water:
  - Before handling food, especially cooked food
  - After going to the toilet
  - Between handling raw and cooked foods.
- Avoid using bare hands to touch food. Use tongs, forks and spoons whenever possible.
- Always clean and sanitize work surfaces and utensils. Sanitizers kill bacteria, while detergents only remove dirt and grease.
- Wash fruits and vegetables, especially if eaten raw.
- Use safe, treated water when preparing food and cleaning.
- Use separate cutting boards and knives for each type of food, for example raw meat, fish, vegetables and cooked foods.
- Use paper towels whenever possible. Dishcloths and towels can carry bacteria.
- Protect food preparation areas and food from pests, insects and pets.

For proper hygiene, a number of food handling rules must be followed. A common guideline for all types of food is that when cooking or handling any food, you should first make sure that the work area and utensils and tools are well cleaned and disinfected.

DIFFERENT BRANCHES OF FOOD HYGIENE

- Milk hygiene
- Meat hygiene
- Fish hygiene
- Egg hygiene
- Hygiene of vegetables and fruits
- Food handlers hygiene
- Sanitation of eating place.

Milk Hygiene

Milk may be defined as the whole lacteal secretion of mammary glands of the mammals obtained by the process of milking of one or more individuals (animals) during the period following at least 72 hours after calving or until the milk is free from colostrum containing not less than 3.5% fat and 8.5% SNF (Solids Not Fat). It is a white opaque fluid with few exceptions where it is tinge (coloring spot yellowish-color particularly within a breed. Milk is an efficient vehicle for a great variety of disease agents. It can get contaminated by various sources like udder, utensils, personal hygiene of the handlers, storage environment, water, etc. A joint FAOWHO expert committee (1970) on milk hygiene classified milk-borne disease as under:

- Infections of animals that can be transmitted to man.
  - Tuberculosis
  - Streptococcal infections
  - Anthrax
- Infections primary to man that can be transmitted through milk:
  - Typhoid and paratyphoid fevers
  - Cholera
  - Enteropathogenic *Escherichia coli.*

Clean and Safe Milk

- First essential is a healthy and clean animal.
- Secondly, the premises where the animal is housed and milked should be sanitary.
- Milk vessels must be sterile and kept covered.
- Water supply should be bacteriologically safe.
- Milk handlers must be free from communicable diseases.
- Milk should be cooled immediately to 10°C after it is drawn to retard bacterial growth.

Methylene Blue Reduction Test

- It is indirect method for detection of microorganisms in milk.
- Test is carried out on the milk accepted for pasteurization

- Definite quantity of methylene blue is added to 10 mL of milk and sample is held at a uniform temperature of 37°C until the blue color is disappeared.
- This test serves as confirmation of heavy contamination and compared with direct counts of bacteria, it saves time and money.

Pasteurization of Milk

Pasteurization is the process of heating something up quickly then cooling it back down. Pasteurizing milk destroys 99.9% of disease-causing microorganisms and extends the shelf-life to 16–21 days from the time it was packaged.

High Temperature Short Time

In the United States, the most common method of pasteurization is High Temperature Short Time (HTST). This method involves using metal plates and hot water to raise the temperature of the milk to at least 161°F (71°C) for no less than 15 seconds, or 145°F (62°C) for 30 minutes, followed by rapid cooling.

Higher Heat Shorter Time

Similar to HTST pasteurization, Higher Heat Shorter Time (HHST) uses slightly different equipment and higher temperatures for a shorter time. Using HHST, milk can be heated anywhere from 191°F (89°C) - 212°F (100°C) for its specified time.

Ultra High Temperature

Another popular method of pasteurization is Ultra High Temperature (UHT). This process involves heating the milk using commercially sterile equipment and filling it under aseptic conditions into hermetically sealed packaging. The milk must be heated to 280°F (138°C) for at least two seconds, then rapidly cooling it down. UHT kills more bacteria (good and bad) and gives it a much longer shelf-life. UHT milk does not need refrigeration, until opened, and is shelf-stable for at least six months.

Ultra Pasteurized

Not to be confused with UHT, Ultra Pasteurized (UP) milk is heated using commercially sterile equipment, but it is not considered sterile because it is not hermetically sealed. Milk is heated to 280°F (138°C) for at least two seconds, then rapidly cooling it down. Since the milk is not hermetically sealed, it must be refrigerated with an average shelf-life of 30–90 days.

Meat Hygiene

In meat hygiene following points are important

Meat Inspection

Animal intended for slaughter are subjected to proper antemortem and postmortem inspection by qualified veterinary staff. Meat inspection is a very important process before being accepted or rejected. Antimortem inspection should be carried out for every animal before slaughtering. The term antemortem "before death". It is the inspection of live animals and birds prior to being slaughtered to ensure that animals are properly rested and that proper clinical information, which will assist in the disease diagnosis and to identify sick animals.

Like antemortem inspection routine postmortem examination of a carcass should be carried out as soon as possible after the completion of dressing. It helps to detect abnormalities, so that products only conditionally fit for human consumption are passed as food. Signs of generalized disease are inflammation of joints and lesions in different organs. Postmortem rejection is based on following diseases like *Cysticercus bovis*, liver fluke, abscesses, *Sarcocystis* species, hydatidosis, septicemia, parasitic and nodular infections of liver and lungs, tuberculosis, *Cysticercus cellulose*. Good meat qualities should be neither pale pink nor a deep purple tint and should be firm elastic to touch, should not be slimy and have an agreeable odor. Animals or meat found unfit for human consumption should be destroyed or denatured.

Slaughter House Hygiene

Hygiene of slaughter house is important to prevent contamination of meat during the process of dressing. There is a Model Public Health Act (1955) in India, which standardizes on the location, structure, disposal of wastes, water supply, examination of animals, storage of meat, transportation of meat and miscellaneous other activities connected with meat processing.

Slaughter houses should be preferably away from residential areas. Floors and walls up to 3 feet should be impervious and easy to clean. Blood, offal, etc., should not be discharged into public sewers but should be collected separately. Water supply should be independent, adequate and continuous. Animals other than those to be slaughtered should not be allowed inside the shed.

Storage of Meat

Meat should be stored in fly-proof and rat-proof rooms; for overnight storage, the temperature of the room shall be maintained below 5°C. If required meat shall be transported in fly-proof covered vans.

Fish Hygiene

Fish deteriorates or loses its freshness because of autolysis which sets in after death and because of the bacteria with which they become infected. Before cutting or cooking, make sure that it is kept in a fit condition. To do this, make sure that the scales are firm, the gills are reddish and the eyes are bulging, 'shiny clear and prominent'. Stale fish should be condemned. Fish deteriorates or loses its freshness because of autolysis which sets in after death and because of the bacteria with which they become infected. Cooking at a minimum temperature of 65°C is recommended for fish.

For tinned fish inspection also required. The tin must be new and clean without leakages or rusting. There should be no evidence of having been tampered with such as sealed openings. On opening the tin, the contents should not blown out which indicates decomposition.

Egg Hygiene

Egg is considered among the most nutritious and healthiest foods on the planet. Egg is an excellent source of protein, with all the essential amino acids that body needs to maintain good health. In addition, it also contains several minerals and vitamins, which are required for healthy living. Eggs are accepted by all communities without restriction to any religion, and are consumed globally by children, adults, and old people.

Although the majority of freshly laid eggs are sterile inside, the shells become contaminated by fecal matter from the hen. Microorganisms including pathogenic Salmonella can penetrate a cracked shell and enter the egg yolk leading to spoilage. Eggs can also be pasteurized to increase the shelf-life.

Testing of Freshness of Eggs

Floating Test

To test freshness of the eggs first fill the bowl with enough cold water to completely cover the egg, then gently drop the egg into the bowl of water. If it sinks to the bottom, turns on its side, and stays there, it is very fresh. If the egg sinks but floats at an angle or stands on end, the egg is a bit older (a week to two weeks old) but still okay to eat. If the egg floats, it is too old and should be discarded as shown in **Figure 5.3**.

The Egg White Test/Breaking Test

This test is a good choice when you plan on cracking the egg before cooking it or adding to a baked good recipe. Crack the egg onto a plate or other flat surface and look closely at the consistency of the egg white—it should be slightly opaque, not spread out too much, and appear thick and somewhat sticky. If it is watery, clear, and runny, the egg has lost its freshness. This is due to the fact that as eggs age, the white turns liquidy and breaks down. You will also notice the yolk will be slightly flat on top instead of rounded as shown in **Figure 5.4**.

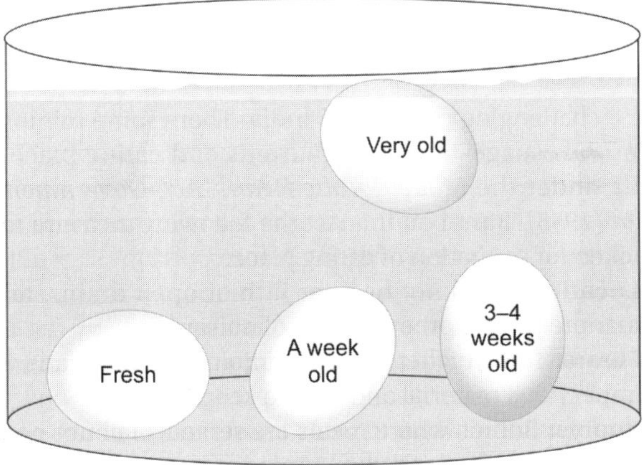

Fig. 5.3: Floating test of egg.

The Sniff Test

Often when there is a sulfur odor—whether it has to do with eggs or not—it is described as "rotten eggs." That is because eggs that have gone bad emit a strong sulfur smell. If the egg is really past its prime, you may smell it through the shell; but if not and you are concerned about freshness, take a whiff after you crack it.

Fruits and Vegetables Hygiene

Vegetables and fruits host many pathogens like bacteria, fungal, protozoan which can enter the plant material during or after harvesting. Generally proper washing and sanitization are employed to increase shelf-life and product safety. Freshly harvested products are routinely washed to remove soils, pesticide residues, insects, plant debris, and microbes.

The following measures can be taken to reduce the risks from microbiological contamination:

- When shopping, select fruits and vegetables that look fresh and are in good condition; avoid items with an off-odor, or that are obviously damaged or mouldy. Do not buy packaged vegetables that have liquid in the bag, though some condensation in packs of prepared salad is normal.
- Handle produce carefully: Buy fruits and vegetables only what you need. Some fruits and vegetables, such as apples and carrots, can be stored, but most items should be used within a few days.
- Put products into a clean, cold (5°) refrigerator promptly. Bananas, tomatoes, or fruits that need further ripening can be kept at room temperature.
- Read and follow label instructions for packaged fruit and vegetables, such as "keep refrigerated" or "use by " or "best before". Throw away anything you have kept for too long, or that looks or smells spoiled.
- Wash fruits and vegetables in lots of clean running water before eating. Peel and discard outer leaves or rinds. Thoroughly scrub vegetables if you want to eat the skin. Use a vegetable brush and water to scrub items with tough skin, such as melons, apples, or carrots, before cutting and serving raw. Smaller, more delicate fruits, such as berries, are easily rinsed in a colander thus limiting the potential damage. Thorough washing removes harmful bacteria, viruses, and residues left on the surface.
- Cover dishes made with cut fruits and vegetables. Leave prepared fruit salads and other cut produce in the refrigerator until serving. Discard these items if they have been out of the refrigerator for more than four hours.
- Fresh fruit and vegetables are tasty and satisfying to eat and are essential in providing the necessary vitamins, minerals and fiber in our diet. Let us enjoy their wide variety everyday as part of a healthy diet.

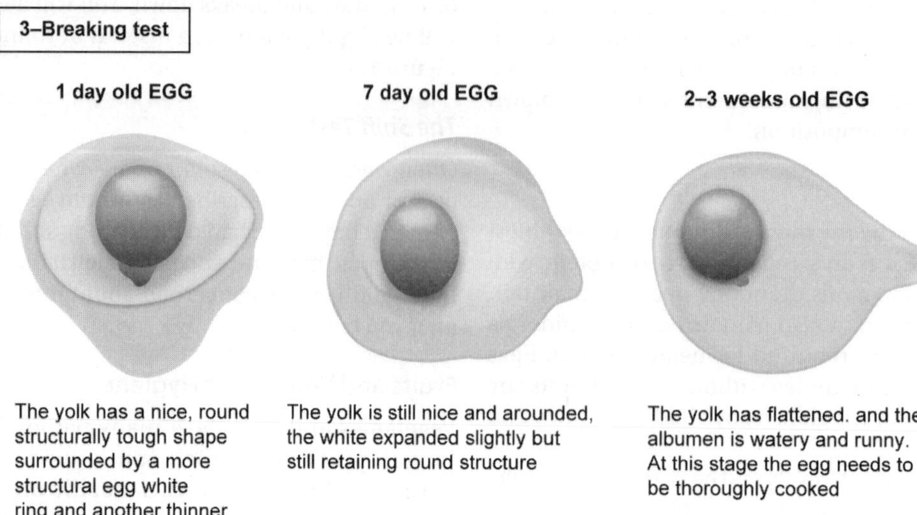

Fig. 5.4: Breaking test of egg to test freshness.

Hygiene for Food Handlers

Food sanitation rests directly upon the state of personal hygiene and habits of the person working in food industries. The infections which are likely to be transmitted by the food handlers are diarrhea, dysenteries, typhoid and paratyphoid fevers, enteroviruses, viral hepatitis, protozoa cysts, eggs of helminths, streptococcal and staphylococcal infections and salmonellosis. Medical examination carried out of all food handlers at the time of employment. Any person with a history of typhoid fever, diphtheria, chronic dysentery, tuberculosis or any other communicable disease should not be employed. Persons with wounds, skin infections should not be permitted to handle food or utensils. The day to day health appraisal of the food handlers is also equally important; those who are ill should be excluded from food handling. Any illness which occurs in a food handler's family should at once be notified.

Education of food handlers in matters of personal hygiene, food handling, utensils, dishwashing, and insect and rodent control is the best means of promoting food hygiene. Personnel hygiene to be promoted: (a) Hands: The hands should be clean at all times. Scrubbed and washed with soap and water immediately after visiting a lavatory. Nails to be kept trimmed and free from dirt. A checklist can be used by food handler for personal hygiene practices.

Checklist for Food Handler

The checklist for hygienic practice used by food handler should contain following points:

- Uniforms, aprons (or clothes) should be clean at the beginning of a work shift
- Wear a hair restraint (hat or hairnet)
- Keep fingernails short and clean
- Avoid touching nose, mouth, hair and skin during food preparation
- Do not smoke in food premises
- Do not cough or sneeze directly onto food. Wash hands after coughing or sneezing
- Wash your hands after blowing your nose
- Avoid wearing jewellery while handling and preparing food
- Avoid using strong perfumes/after shaves
- Do not wear uniforms or aprons outside the food preparation area
- Cover all wounds or cuts on hands or arms completely with bright-colored waterproof wound strip
- Wear disposable gloves if there is a wound on the hand. Change both gloves and wound strip regularly
- Food handlers to be free from any illnesses such as gastro or the flu
- Cease work and report to the manager while ill
- Hands must be washed before: Working Handling food and utensils
- Hands must be washed after: Using the toilet handling raw food coughing, sneezing, eating, drinking or smoking, licking fingers, handling waste, changing soiled clothes, touching ears, nose, hair, mouth, or other bare body parts, handling animals or any other unhygienic practice.

Sanitation of Eating Places

It is a challenging problem in India. There some minimum standards suggested for restaurants and eating places in India under the *Model Public Health Act, Government of India (1955).* Based on this Act the following measure must be taken for sanitation of eating place:

- **Location:** Shall not be near filth or open drain, stable, manure pit and other sources of nuisances.
- **Floors:** To be higher than the adjoining land, made with impervious material and easy to keep clean.
- **Rooms:** Rooms where meals are served shall not be less than 100 sq. feet and shall provide accommodation for a maximum of 10 persons.

- Walls up to 3 feet should be smooth, corners to be rounded; should be impervious and easily washable
- Lighting and ventilation—ample natural lighting facilities aided by artificial lighting with good circulation of air are necessary.
- **Kitchen:** It should be ample floor space, window opening, proper flooring and ventilation.

ASSESSMENT OF NUTRITIONAL STATUS

Introduction

Nutritional assessment is the interpretation of anthropometric, biochemical (laboratory), clinical and dietary data to determine whether a person or groups of people are well nourished or malnourished (over-nourished or undernourished. Assessment of Nutritional Status is the current body status, of a person or a population group, related to their state of nourishment (the consumption and utilization of nutrients). The nutritional status is determined by a complex interaction between internal/constitutional factors and external environmental factors: Internal or constitutional factors like: age, sex, nutrition, behavior, physical activity and diseases. External environmental factors like: food safety, cultural, social and economic circumstances. The complex interaction between internal or constitutional factors and external environmental factors. An ideal nutritional status occurs when the supply of nutrients conforms to the nutritional requirements or needs. It is also influenced by food intake, quantity and quality, and physical health. The spectrum of nutritional status spread from obesity to severe malnutrition.

Purposes of Nutritional Assessment

The purpose of nutritional assessment is to:

- Identify individuals or population groups at risk of becoming malnourished
- Identify individuals or population groups who are malnourished
- To develop health care programs that meet the community needs which are defined by the assessment
- To measure the effectiveness of the nutritional programs and intervention once initiated Iodine.

Methods of Nutritional Assessment

Nutritional status is assessed by two types of methods; direct and indirect. The direct methods deal with the individual and measure objective criteria, while indirect methods use community indices that reflect the community nutritional status/needs. Indirect Methods of Nutritional Assessment: Ecological variables including agricultural crops production, economic factors, e.g., household income, per capita income, population density, food availability and prices, cultural and social habits, vital health statistics: morbidity, mortality and other health indicators, e.g., infant and under-five mortality, utilization of maternal and child health care services, fertility indices and sanitary conditions.

Direct Methods of Nutritional Assessment

Direct methods are summarized as ABCD:

- Anthropometric methods
- Biochemical, laboratory methods
- Clinical methods
- Dietary evaluation methods.

Indirect Methods of Nutritional Assessment

These are again categorized in three categories:

1. Ecological variables including crop production
2. Economic factors, e.g., per capita income, population density and social habits.
3. Vital health statistics particularly infant and under 5 mortality and fertility index.

Direct Method

Anthropometry

The word anthropometry comes from two words: Anthropo means 'human' and metry means 'measurement'. Nutritional Anthropometry is concerned with the measurements of the variations of physical dimensions and body composition at stages of life cycle and different planes of nutrition. Anthropometry is the measurement of body height, weight and proportions. It is an essential component of clinical examination of infants, children and pregnant women. It is used to evaluate both under and over nutrition. The measured values reflects the current nutritional status and do not differentiate between acute and chronic changes. Other anthropometric Measurements are midarm circumference, skin fold thickness, head circumference, head/chest ratio, hip/waist ratio.

Anthropometry for Children

Anthropometry for children include accurate measurement of height and weight is midarm circumference, head circumference, chest circumference, etc. The results can then be used to evaluate the physical growth of the child. For growth monitoring the data are plotted on growth charts over a period of time that is enough to calculate growth velocity, which can then be compared to international standards.

Height

The height of the individual is the sum of four components: leg, pelvis, spine and skull or measuring height, the subject stands erect and bare footed on a stadiometer with a movable head piece. The head piece is leveled with skull vault and height is recorded to the nearest 0.5 cm.

Weight Measurement

Weight gain is an indicator of growth in children. It is measured with the help of the weighing scale. Body weight should be determined after the first void and before ingestion of food. The weight for age can be compared with the standards of ICMR and the nutritional status can be interpreted. Use a regularly calibrated electronic or balanced-beam scale for taking weight. Spring scales are less reliable. The subject should weigh in light clothes, no shoes. Read to the nearest 100 g (0.1 kg) for accurate measurement.

Head Circumference

The measurement of head circumference is a standard procedure to detect pathological condition in children. Head circumference is related mainly to brain size. At birth the circumference of head is greater than that of the chest.

Chest Circumference

The circumference of the head and the chest are about the same at six months of age. After this the skull grows slowly and the chest more rapidly. Therefore between the ages of six months and five years the chest/head circumference ratio of less than one may be due to failure to develop or due to wasting of muscle and fat of chest. In nutritional anthropomertry the chest/head circumference ratio is of value in detecting under nutrition in early childhood.

Midupper Arm Circumference

Midupper arm circumference (MUAC) at birth in a healthy child is between 10–11 cm. Over the first year the increment in MUAC is 3 to 4 cm as the muscles of the arms start to develop. In the preschool age the increase in MUAC is only one cm. Hence there is not much difference between the MUAC of a 3 year old from that of a 5 year old. So MUAC is an age independent index. The field workers in nutrition in our country have fixed the desirable value for MUAC as 12 cm for Indian preschool children. The WHO has recommended 14 centimeter as a desirable value for MUAC for preschool children. Hence in screening malnourished children in a community, this method is used with ease. When the value of MUAC is less than 12 cm among 1–5 year old children, they are designated as malnourished. In the field condition a bangle with a diameter of 4 centimeter can be used as a tool to detect malnutrition. When the bangle moves smoothly over the midupper arm of the child, it indicates malnutrition. The bangle test can be conducted with ease in field condition to screen malnourished children.

Nutritional Indices in Adults

The international standard for assessing body size in adults is the body mass index (BMI).

BMI is computed using the following formula:

- BMI = Weight (kg)/Height (m^2)

BMI (WHO: Classification)

- BMI <18.5 = Underweight
- BMI 18.5–24.5 = Healthy weight range
- BMI 25–30 = Overweight (grade 1 obesity)
- BMI >30–40 = Obese (grade 2 obesity)
- BMI >40 = Very obese (morbid or grade 3 obesity)

Evidence shows that high BMI (obesity level) is associated with type 2 diabetes and high-risk of cardiovascular morbidity and mortality. For assessing obesity other assessment tools are waist circumference, hip circumference and waist and hip ratio.

Waist Circumference

Waist circumference is measured at the level of the umbilicus to the nearest 0.5 cm. The subject stands erect with relaxed abdominal muscles, arms at the side, and feet together. The measurement should be taken at the end of a normal expiration. Waist circumference predicts mortality better than any other anthropometric measurement. It has been proposed that waist measurement alone can be used to assess obesity, and two levels of risk have been identified:

	Males	Female
Level 1	>94 cm	>80 cm
Level 2	>102 cm	>88 cm

Level 1 is the maximum acceptable waist circumference irrespective of the adult age and there should be no further weight gain but level 2 denotes obesity and requires weight management to reduce the risk of type 2 diabetes and CVS complications.

Hip Circumference

Hip circumference is also an important anthropometric measurement use to assess obesity. It is measured at the point of greatest circumference around hips and buttocks to the nearest 0.5 cm.

For measuring the hip circumference the subject should be standing and the measurer should squat beside him. Both of the measurement should taken with a flexible, non-stretchable tape in close contact with the skin, but without indenting the soft tissue.

Interpretation of WHR (Waist and Hip Ratio)

Waist and hip ratio can be calculated. High-risk waist and hip ratio = >0.80 for females and >0.95 for males. A WHR below these cut-off levels is considered as generally low risk of obesity.

Advantages of Anthropometry Method

- Objective with high specificity and sensitivity
- Measures many variables of nutritional significance (Ht, Wt, MAC, HC, skin fold thickness, waist and hip ratio and BMI).
- Readings are numerical and gradable on standard growth charts
- Readings are reproducible.
- Inexpensive and need minimal training

Limitations of Anthropometry

- Interobservers errors in measurement
- Limited nutritional diagnosis
- Problems with reference standards, i.e., local versus international standards.
- Arbitrary statistical cut-off levels for what considered as abnormal values.

Biochemical, Laboratory Methods

Biochemical tests can be used to detect the deficiencies by analyzing blood, urine, stools and phlem. For example, estimation of hemoglobin in blood to detect iron deficiency. Hemoglobin estimation is the most important test, and useful index of the overall state of nutrition. Beside anemia it also tells about protein and trace element nutrition. Other investigation can include:

- Stool examination for the presence of ova and/or intestinal parasites
- Urine dipstick and microscopy for albumin, sugar and blood
- Specific lab tests like measurement of individual nutrient in body fluids (e.g., serum retinol, serum iron, urinary iodine, vitamin D) and detection of abnormal amount of metabolites in the urine (e.g., urinary creatinine/ hydroxyproline ratio)
- Analysis of hair, nails and skin for micronutrients.

Advantages of Biochemical Method

- It is useful in detecting early changes in body metabolism and nutrition before the appearance of overt clinical signs.
- It is precise, accurate and reproducible.
- Useful to validate data obtained from dietary methods, e.g., comparing salt intake with 24-hour urinary excretion.

Limitations of Biochemical Method

- Time consuming
- Expensive
- They cannot be applied on large scale
- Needs trained personnel and facilities.

Clinical Assessment

Clinical examination is an important practical method for assessing the nutritional status of a community. Essentially, the method is based on examination for changes of skin, eyes, hair and buccal mucosa or in organs near the surface of the body such as the parotid and thyroid glands. Clinical assessment must always be carried out by individuals with adequate training. It is the simplest and most practical method of ascertaining the nutritional status of a group of individuals which utilizes a number of physical signs, (specific and non specific), that are known to be associated with malnutrition and deficiency of vitamins and micronutrients.

Steps of Clinical Assessment

- Good nutritional history should be obtained
- General clinical examination, with special attention to organs like hair, angles of the mouth, gums, nails, skin, eyes, tongue, muscles, bones, and thyroid gland for observance of any deviation
- Detection of relevant signs helps in establishing the nutritional diagnosis like pallor (on the palm of the hand or the conjunctiva of the eye), Bitot's spots on the eyes, pitting edema, goiter and severe visible wasting, angular stomatitis, cheilosis, spongy and bleeding gum, any sign can be detected.

By this method from sign and symptoms nutritional deficiency disease can be assessed.

Advantages

- Fast and Easy to perform
- Inexpensive
- Noninvasive.

Limitations

Did not detect early cases.

Dietary Assessment

Nutritional intake of humans is assessed by five different methods. These are:

1. 24 hours dietary recall
2. Food inventory method
3. Food expenditure pattern method
4. Diet history
5. Weighment method.

24 Hours Dietary Recall Dietary methods of assessment include looking at past or current intakes of nutrients from food by individuals or a group to determine their nutritional status. You can ask what the family or the mother and the child have eaten over the past 24 hours and use this data to calculate the dietary diversity score. In this method a set of standardized cups suited to local conditions are used. The standard cups help the respondent to recall the quantities of the food prepared and fed to individual members on the previous day. This is usually done for three consecutive days. The advantage of this method is that the intake of each food item by the specific individual in the family such as pre-school child, adolescent, pregnant women can be assessed using the cups.

Dietary Diversity

Dietary diversity is a measure of the number of food groups consumed over a reference period, usually 24 hours. Generally, there are six food groups that our body needs to have everyday. These can be represented in the food guide pyramid which is reproduced in **Figure 5.5**.

Food Inventory Method

This method is usually employed in Institutions where homogenous group of people take their meals in a common kitchen, e.g., Hostels, orphanages. In this method the amount of food stuff issued to the kitchen as per the issue register is taken into consideration. No direct measurement or weighing is done. A study period of one week is desirable.

Food Expenditure Pattern Method

In this method information on the amount spent on food and non-food items during the previous month or week is collected using a questionnaire. This method avoids actual weighing of foods.

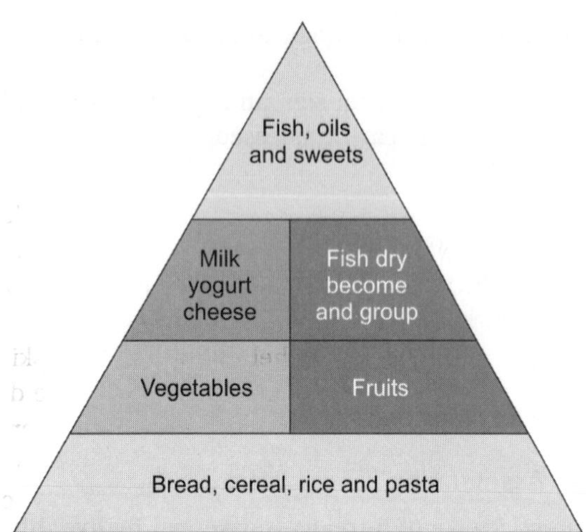

Fig. 5.5: Food pyramid including three groups of food.

Diet History

This method is useful for obtaining qualitative details of diet and studying patterns of food consumption at household and industrial level. The procedure includes assessment of the frequency of consumption, different foods, daily or number of times in a week or fortnight or occasionally. This method is used to study meal pattern, dietary habits, food preferences, and avoidances during sickness.

Weighment Method

In this method, the food either raw or cooked is actually weighed using an accurate balance. It is ideal to conduct the survey for seven consecutive days. Every day food is weighed in the morning and evening before actual cooking. The age, sex, physiological status of the family members should be noted down. Nutrient intake is then calculated using the ICMR food composition tables. Though this method is accurate as the foods are directly weighed, it requires extreme cooperation of the house wives. The information on food and nutrient consumption is compared with the recommended allowances of the ICMR and the adequacy is determined. A combination of dietary, clinical and biochemical assessment is desirable for assessment of nutrition status of individuals or communities.

Indirect Methods

Vital Statistics

Malnutrition influences morbidity, mortality, life expectancy and other health statistics. Hence vital statistics may therefore be considered as indirect indication of the nutritional status of the community. Infant mortality rate, maternal mortality rate and morbidity rate are the vital statistics that can be used to assess the nutritional status of the community.

Assessment of Socioeconomic Status

Less per capita income, high population density, poor social habits, low food availability, increased family size, unsanitary living conditions, inadequate knowledge of nutritional needs, inappropriate weaning practices are powerful social cultural and economic factors, which influence nutritional status.

Ecological Variables

Ecological variables like assessment of crop production is also an indicator for assessing nutritional status. Poor crop production can leads to unavailability.

METHODS OF COOKING

Heat is transferred to the food during cooking by conduction, convection, radiation or microwave energy. Cooking takes place by moist and dry heat. Moist heat involves water and steam. Air or fat are used in dry heat.

Moist Heat Methods

Boiling

Boiling is a method of cooking foods by just immersing the food in water at 100°C and maintaining the water at that temperature till the food become tender. Rice, egg, dhal, meat, roots and tubers are cooked by boiling.

Merits

- Simple method—It does not require special skill and equipment.
- Uniform cooking can be achieved.

Demerits

- Continuous excessive boiling leads to damage in the structure and texture of food.
- Loss of heat labile nutrients such as B and C vitamins if the water is discarded.
- Time consuming—Boiling takes more time to cook food and fuel may be wasted.
- Loss of color—water soluble pigments may be lost.

Stewing

It refers to the simmering of food in a pan with a tight fitting lid using small quantities of liquid to cover only half the food. This is a slow method of cooking. The liquid is brought to boiling point and the heat is reduced to maintain simmering temperatures (82°C–90°C). The food above the liquid is cooked by the steam generated within the pan. Apple, meat, especially tougher meats suitable for slow-cooking, such as beef. Poultry, sausages, seafood, vegetables and legumes are usually stewed.

Merits

- Stewing is used to prepare various types of gravy-based dishes
- Loss of nutrients is avoided as water used for cooking is not discarded.
- Highly enhances and the natural flavor is retained.

Demerits

The process is time consuming and there is wastage of fuel.

Steaming

It is a method of cooking food in steam generated from vigorously boiling water in a pan. The food to be steamed is placed in a container and is not in direct contact with the water or liquid. Idli, custard and idiappam are made by steaming. Vegetables can also be steamed.

Merits

- Less chance of burning and scorching.
- Texture of food is better as it becomes light and fluffy, e.g., Idli.
- Cooking time is less and fuel wastage is less.
- Steamed foods like idli and idiappam contain less fat and are easily digested and are good for children, aged and for therapeutic diets.
- Nutrient loss is minimized.

Demerits

- Steaming equipment is required.
- This method is limited to the preparation of selected foods.

Pressure Cooking

When steam under pressure is used the method is known as 'pressure cooking' and the equipment used is the pressure cooker. In this method the temperature of boiling water can be raised above 100°C. Rice, dhal, meat, roots and tubers are usually pressure cooked.

Merits

- Cooking time is less compared to other methods.
- Nutrient and flavor loss is minimized.
- Conserves fuel and time as different items can be cooked at the same time.
- Less chance for burning and scorching.
- Constant attention is not necessary.

Demerits

- The initial investment may not be affordable to everybody.
- Knowledge of the usage, care and maintenance of cooker is required to prevent accidents.
- Careful watch on the cooking time is required to prevent over cooking.

Poaching

This involves cooking in the minimum amount of liquid at temperatures of 80–85°C that is below the boiling point. Egg and fish can be poached.

Merits

- No special equipment is needed.
- Quick method of cooking and therefore saves fuel.
- Poached foods are easily digested since no fat is added.

Demerits

- Poached foods may not appeal to everybody as they are bland in taste.
- Food can be scorched if water evaporates due to careless monitoring.
- Water soluble nutrients may be leached into the water.

Blanching

In meal preparation, it is often necessary only to peel off the skin of fruits and vegetables without making them tender. This can be achieved by blanching. In this method, food is dipped in boiling water for 5 seconds to 2 minutes depending on the texture of the food. This helps to remove the skin or peel without softening food. Blanching can also be done by pouring enough boiling water on the food to immerse it for some time or subjecting foods to boiling temperatures for short periods and then immediately immersing in cold water. The process causes the skin to become loose and can be peeled off easily.

Merits

- Peels can easily be removed to improve digestibility.
- Destroys enzymes that bring about spoilage.
- Texture can be maintained while improving the color and flavor of food.

Demerits

Loss of nutrients if cooking water is discarded.

Dry Heat Methods

Roasting

In this method food is cooked in a heated metal or frying pan without covering it, e.g., Groundnut.

Merits

- Quick method of cooking.
- It improves the appearance, flavor and texture of the food.
- Spices are easily powdered if they are first roasted.

Demerits

- Food can be scorched due to carelessness.
- Roasting denatures proteins reducing their availability.

Grilling

Grilling or broiling refers to the cooking of food by exposing it to direct heat. In this method food is placed above or in between a red hot surface. Papads, corn, phulkas, chicken can be prepared by this method.

Merits

- Enhances flavor, appearance and taste of the product.
- It requires less time to cook.
- Minimum fat is used.

Demerits

Constant attention is required to prevent charring.

Toasting

This is a method where food is kept between two heated elements to facilitate browning on both sides. Bread slices are cooked by toasting.

Merits

1. Easy and quick method.
2. Flavor improved.

Demerits

- Special equipment required.
- Careful monitoring is needed to prevent charring.

Baking

In this method, the food gets cooked in an oven or ovenlike appliance by dry heat. The temperature range maintained in an oven is 120–260°C. The food is usually kept uncovered in a container greased with a fat coated paper. Bread, cake, biscuits, pastries and meat are prepared by this method.

Merits

- Baking leads a unique baked flavor to foods.
- Foods become light and fluffy—cakes, custards, bread.
- Certain foods can be prepared only by this method—bread, cakes.
- Uniform and bulk cooking can be achieved, e.g., bun, bread.
- Flavor and texture are improved.
- Variety of dishes can be made.

Demerits

- Special equipment like oven is required.
- Baking skills are necessary to obtain a product with ideal texture, flavor and color characteristics.
- Careful monitoring needed to prevent scorching.

Sauteing

Sauteing is a method in which food is lightly tossed in little oil just enough to cover the base of the pan. The pan is covered with a lid and the flame or intensity of heat is reduced. The food is allowed to cook till tender in its own steam. The food is tossed occasionally, or turned with a spatula to enable all the pieces to come in contact with the oil and get cooked evenly. The product obtained by this method is slightly moist and tender but without any liquid or gravy. Foods cooked by sauteing are generally vegetables which are used as side dishes in a menu. Sauteing can be combined with other methods to produce variety in meals.

Merits

- Takes less time.
- Simple technique.
- Minimum oil is used.

Demerits

Constant attention is needed as there is chance of scorching or burning.

Frying

In this method, the food to be cooked is brought into contact with larger amount of hot fat. When food is totally immersed in hot oil, it is called deep fat frying. Samosa, chips, pakoda are examples of deep fat fried foods. In shallow fat frying, only a little fat is used and the food is turned in order that both sides are browned. For example, omelette, cutlets, parathas.

Merits

- Very quick method of cooking.
- The calorific values of food is increased since fat is used as the cooking media.
- Frying lends a delicious flavor and attractive appearance to foods.
- Taste and texture are improved.

Demerits

- Careful monitoring is required as food easily gets charred when the smoking temperature is not properly maintained.
- The food may become soggy due to too much oil absorption.
- Fried foods are not easily digested.
- Repeated use of heated oils will have ill effects on health.

COMBINATION OF COOKING METHODS

Braising

Braising is a combined method of roasting and stewing in a pan with a tight fitting lid. Flavors and seasonings are added and food is allowed to cook gently. Food preparations prepared by combination methods are: Uppuma—roasting and boiling. Cutlet—boiling and deep frying. Vermicilli payasam—roasting and simmering.

Microwave Cooking

Microwaves are electromagnetic waves of radiant energy with wavelengths in the range of 250×10^6 to 7.5×10^9 Angstroms. The most commonly used type of microwave generator is an electronic device called a magnetron which generates radiant energy of high frequency. A simple microwave oven consists of a metal cabinet into which the magnetron is inserted. The cabinet is equipped with a metal fan that distributes the microwave throughout the cabinet. Food placed in the oven is heated by microwaves from all directions.

Moist foods and liquid foods can be rapidly heated in such ovens. Food should be kept in containers made of plastic, glass or china ware which do not contain metallic substances. These containers are used because they transmit the microwaves but do not absorb or reflect them.

Merits

- Quick method—10 times faster than conventional method. So loss of nutrients can be minimized.
- Only the food gets heated and the oven does not get heated.

- Food gets cooked uniformly.
- Leftovers can be reheated without changing the flavor and texture of the product.
- Microwave cooking enhances the flavor of food because it cooks quickly with little or no water.

Demerits

- Baked products do not get a brown surface.
- Microwave cooking cannot be used for simmering, stewing or deep frying.
- Flavor of all ingredients do not blend well as the cooking time is too short.

Solar Cooking

Solar cooking is a very simple technique that makes use of sunlight or solar energy which is a nonconventional source of energy. Solar cooker consists of a well insulated box which is painted black on the inside and covered with one or more transparent covers. The purpose of these transparent covers is to trap heat inside the solar cooker. These covers allow the radiation from the sun to come inside the box but do not allow the heat from the hot black absorbing plate to come out of the box. Because of this, temperature up to 140°C can be obtained which is adequate for cooking.

Merits

- Simple technique—requires no special skill.
- Cost effective as natural sunlight is the form of energy.
- Original flavor of food is retained.
- There is no danger of scorching or burning.
- Loss of nutrients is minimum as only little amounts of water is used in cooking.

Demerits

- Special equipment is needed.
- Slow cooking process.
- Cannot be used in the absence of sunlight—rainy season, late evening and night.

FOOD PRESERVATION

Food is the basic necessity of man and is invaluable for healthy existence. However, most foods fit for consumption undergo deterioration and spoilage. In order to combat this problem foods have to be preserved. Food preservation can be defined as the science that deals with the process of prevention of decay or spoilage of food thus allowing it to be stored in a fit condition for future use. Preservation of food increases the shelf-life of foods and thus ultimately ensures its supply during times of scarcity and natural drought.

Principles of Food Preservation

- Prevention or delay of microbial decomposition:
  - By keeping out microorganisms (asepsis)
  - By removal of microorganisms (e.g., filtration)
  - By hindering the growth and activity of microorganisms, e.g., refrigeration, dehydration, addition of chemical preservatives.
  - By killing microorganisms, e.g., boiling.
  - Irradiation.
- Prevention or delay of self-decomposition of food.
  - By destruction or inactivation of enzymes, e.g., by blanching. The steaming or boiling of fruits or vegetables in water for few minutes to inactivate natural enzymes and facilitates removal of skin is known as 'blanching'.
  - By prevention or delay of purely chemical reactions, e.g., prevention of oxidation by the use of antioxidants.
- Prevention of damage caused by insects, animals and mechanical causes.

Methods of Food Preservation

A perusal of the history of food preservation reveals that food preservation had its beginning from time immemorial and could be traced to nearly a thousand years ago. Salting of meat, fish, and vegetables was the oldest method of preservation and could be traced back to the ancient Egypt and Greek civilizations. Pickling in salt and vinegar, sun-drying and preservation of fruits and vegetables in sugar and honey were among the other methods used. Storage of food in frozen conditions was also practiced for centuries in places where freezing temperatures were recorded.

Use of Low and High Temperatures

Use of Low Temperatures

Microbial growth and enzyme reaction are retarded in foods stored at low temperatures. The lower the temperature, the greater the retardation. The low temperatures employed can be:

- Cellar storage temperature (about 15°C)
- Refrigerator or chilling temperature (0°C to 5°C).
- Freezing temperature (–18°C to – 40°C).

Cellar Storage Temperatures (About 15°C)

Temperatures in cellars (under ground rooms) where surplus food is stored in many villages are usually not much below that of the outside air and is seldom lower than 15°C of many spoilage organisms or of the plant enzymes. Decomposition is however, slowed down considerably.

Root crops, potatoes, onions, apples and similar foods can be stored for limited periods during the winter months.

Refrigerator or Chilling Temperature (0°C to 5°C)

Chilling (refrigerator), temperatures are obtained and maintained by means of ice or mechanical refrigeration. Fruits and vegetables, meats, poultry, fresh milk and milk products, fish and eggs can be preserved from two days to a week when held at this temperature. In addition to the foods mentioned above, foods prepared for serving or left-overs may also be stored in the household refrigerator. The best storage temperature for many foods, eggs, for example, is slightly above 0°C. The optimum temperature of storage varies with the product and is fairly specific for any given food. Besides temperature, the relative humidity and the composition of the atmosphere can affect the preservation of the food. Commercial cold storages with proper ventilation and automatic control of temperatures are now used throughout the country (mostly in cities) for the storage of semi perishable products such as potatoes and apples. This has made such foods available throughout the year and has also stabilized their prices in these cities. Low temperatures chiefly inhibit the growth of microorganisms although freezing may result in the destruction of some microorganisms.

Freezing Temperature

Freezing may preserve foods for long periods of time provided the quality of the food is good to begin with and the temperature of storage is far below the actual freezing temperature of food.

Some microorganisms are destroyed during freezing preservation. The chief preservative effect of freezing temperatures lies in the inability of microorganisms to grow at freezing temperature. In vegetables, enzyme action may still produce undesirable effects on flavor and texture during freezing. The enzymes therefore must be destroyed by heating before the vegetables are frozen.

Slow Freezing Process

It is also known as 'sharp freezing'. In this method, the foods are placed in refrigerated cabinets at temperatures ranging from –4°C to –29°C. This method is adopted in home-freezers. Freezing may require from 3 to 72 hours under such conditions.

Quick Freezing Process

The lower temperatures used –32°C to –40°C freeze foods so rapidly that fine crystals are formed and the time of freezing is greatly reduced over that required in sharp freezing. The fine crystals formed by quick freezing have a lesser effect on breaking up plant and animal cells than do methods of slow freezing that produce coarser ice crystals. In quick freezing, large quantity of food can be frozen in a short period of time.

Dehydro Freezing

Dehydro freezing of fruits and vegetables consists of drying the food to about 50% of its original weight and volume and then freezing the food to preserve it. The quality of dehydro frozen fruits and vegetables is equal to that of fruits and vegetables frozen without preliminary drying. The cost in packing, freezing, storing and shipping of such foods is less because of the reduction in weight and volume of foods during dehydro freezing.

Use of Heat or High Temperatures

The destruction of microorganisms by heat is due to the coagulation of the protoplasm. The temperature and time used in heat processing a food depend upon the nature of the food and what other methods are combined with heat. The various degrees of heating used in preservation of food can be classified into three: (a) Pasteurization, (b) Heating up to 100°C or 212°F and (c) Heating above 100°C.

Pasteurization

The time and temperature used in the pasteurization process depend upon the product treated and the method used. In pasteurization, most of the spoilage organisms are killed but a few survive and hence must be inhibited by low temperatures or some other method, if spoilage is to be prevented. There are two methods of pasteurization—flash method and holder method. In flash method, otherwise called high temperature short time method, a high temperature for a short time is used, while in the holder method or low-temperature long-time method, a lower temperature for a longer time is used. There are slight variations in the time and temperature used for pasteurizing different foods, like milk, cream, ice cream mix and wines.

Heating up to a Temperature of About 100°C

Most methods of cooking come under this. This temperature can be obtained by boiling any liquid food, by immersing a container in boiling water or by exposure to steam. Before the use of pressure cookers and autoclaves, canning was done at 100°C and this killed all bacteria except spores.

Heating above 100°C (212°F)

Temperatures above 100°C are obtained by means of steam under pressure as in a pressure cooker or autoclave. Sterilization of foods can be brought about at 121°C for 15 minutes under moist conditions.

CANNING PROCEDURE

The details of canning procedures vary with the nature of the food to be canned, but there are certain important operations common to canning of all foods. (1) Cleaning (2) Blanching (3) Exhausting, (4) Sealing the container (5) Sterilizing the sealed container and (6) Cooling the container.

Cleaning

The first step in canning, whether done in the home or on a large scale in factories, is the thorough cleaning of the raw food to be preserved. By this means most of spoilage organisms are removed. On a large scale, cleaning is done with the help of various kinds of washers. The raw materials may be subjected to high pressure sprays or strong flowing streams of water, while passing along a moving belt.

Blanching

Blanching consists of the immersion of raw food materials, especially vegetables and fruits, into hot water or exposure to live steam. Blanching serves as an additional hot water wash.

It softens fibrous plant tissues, inhibits the action of enzymes and fixes the natural color of certain products making them more attractive in appearance.

Exhausting

Gases are expelled by passing the open can containing the food through an exhaust box in which hot water or steam is used to expand.

NUTRITION EDUCATION

Good nutrition prolongs independence by maintaining physical strength, mobility, endurance, hearing, vision, and cognitive abilities. Eighty-seven% of older Americans have one or more chronic diseases that can be improved by nutrition therapy, including cancer, chronic lung disease, heart disease, dementia, diabetes mellitus, high blood cholesterol, high blood pressure, osteoporosis, obesity and overweight, and failure to thrive (Draft Nutrition Screening Initiative Policy Statement: Nutrition: Proven Effective in Managing Chronic Disease in Older Americans).

Nutrition education can be defined as any set of learning experiences designed to facilitate the voluntary adoption of eating and other nutrition-related behaviors conducive to health and well-being. It is an integral part of providing nutrition services to older persons.

Nutrition services providers must conduct nutrition education activities, consistent with the goals and content described below, at a minimum of two times per calendar year at each site. Nutrition education presents general information related to health and nutrition, often to groups in clinic waiting rooms or community settings. Educators may be trained counsellors or health volunteers who deliver prepared talks on specific topics, often using visual aids. They should encourage clients to ask questions and direct them to additional information as needed.

Nutrition education should include information on physical activity in addition to nutrition. In recognition of the importance of physical activity on health and the prevention of disease, the Dietary Guidelines for Americans recommend being physically active each day. Regular physical activity sustains the ability of older adults to live independently, and benefits individuals with arthritis and those with depression and anxiety. It may reduce the risk of cognitive decline in older adults, and is effective in helping to manage many chronic diseases.

Nutrition Education Goals

To create positive attitudes toward good nutrition and physical activity and provide motivation for improved nutrition and lifestyle practices conducive to promoting and maintaining the best attainable level of wellness for an individual.

To provide adequate knowledge and skills necessary for critical thinking regarding diet and health so the individual can make healthy food choices from an increasingly complex food supply.

To assist the individual to identify resources for continuing access to sound food and nutrition information.

Nutrition Education Content

The Dietary Guidelines, which include maintenance of a healthy weight, daily physical activity, food safety, and moderation of alcohol intake should serve as the framework for all nutrition education activities. The Dietary Guidelines can be found here.

A nutrition education program makes available information and guidance pertaining to:

- **Food,** including the kinds and amounts of food that are required to meet one's daily nutritional needs.
- **Nutrition,** including the combination of processes by which the body receives substances necessary for maintenance of its functions and for growth and renewal of its components, i.e., ingestion, digestion, absorption, metabolism, and elimination.
- **Behavioral practices,** including the factors which influence one's eating and food preparation habits.
- Consumer issues, including the management of food purchasing power to obtain maximum food value for the money spent.
- **Information on physical activity:** Information on the roles of nutrition and physical activity in maintaining health and independence, and preventing or managing chronic diseases such as diabetes, heart disease, high blood pressure, osteoporosis, and arthritis.

Nutrition Education Activities

Nutrition education consists of activities which provide visual and verbal information and instruction to participants or participants and caregivers in a group or individual setting. The presentations or activities may be led by an RD or ICE, or someone else overseen by an RD or individual with comparable expertise. The minimum length of one nutrition education presentation is five minutes.

Examples of nutrition education activities include: presentations, cooking classes, food preparation demonstrations, field trips, plays, panel discussions, planning and/or evaluating menus, food tasting sessions, question and answer sessions, gardening, physical fitness programs, videos, etc. For home-delivered participants, activities can include the distribution of educational materials.

When nutrition education is being provided by the nutrition program service provider, all costs associated with the delivery of nutrition education services must be budgeted and charged appropriately to that service.

Principles of Nutrition Education Program

An effective nutrition intervention program will integrate good instructional design and learning principles and use media that facilitate a high degree of individualization.

The effect of an intervention on the target population's knowledge and behavior depends on the intervention's application of 6 basic educational principles.

1. **Consonance:** Degree of fit between program activities with its objective, or degree to which communication is directed toward accomplishing the intended outcome. Here before planning a health education program the organizer should check the objectives should be met by the activities planned.
   Example: In a health education program for losing weight of obese people, if exercise is not included, this show the program lacked consonance or in a program to teach glucose self-monitoring, teaching the benefits of glucose monitoring without showing how to monitor would be insufficient.
2. **Relevance:** Take into account client's knowledge, beliefs, circumstances, prior experience and reading level before selecting topic method of education and other activities of health education. The degree to which the intervention is geared to clients.
3. **Individualization:** Allows clients to have personal questions answered or instructions paced according to individual learning progress. Client learn in different way and different rates a program is more effective when it targets to an individual.
4. **Feedback:** Feedback helps clients learn by providing a measuring stick to determine how much progress they are making. By evaluation of clients knowledge or by measuring the achievement of objectives, feedback can be given to the clients which help him/her to learn more.
5. **Reinforcement:** Reinforcement is designed to reward for the desired behavior. It is the process of encouraging or establishing a belief or pattern of behavior. In behavioral psychology, reinforcement is a consequence applied that will strengthen an organism's future behavior whenever that behavior is preceded by a specific antecedent stimulus. "Positive feedback leads to reinforcement." Praise and congratulations are very effective in rewarding change behavior.
6. **Facilitation:** Facilitation is the action of facilitating something. A facilitator is a person who helps a group of people to work together better, understand their common objectives, and plan how to achieve these objectives, during meetings or discussions. Measures taken to accomplish desired actions or eliminate obstacles.

Principles of adult learning will be followed in nutrition education program.

Adult learners will learn best when subject matter is directly tied to their own realm of experience. Their learning is facilitated when they can make connections between their past experiences and their current concern. They are motivated to learn by the relevance of the topic to their lives. Adult learners will retain new information best when they are actively involved in problem-solving exercises and hands-on learning. An effective nutrition education program takes into account the learning styles and motivations of the target population. So for effective educational program:

- Make learning problem-centered.
- Make information concrete and define all abstract terms.
- Make learning collaborative between the educator and the learner.
- Encourage participatory approaches to learning.
- Ask open-ended questions to draw out what adults already know about the topic.
- Seize the "teachable moments" which are life transitions.
- Increase the adult learners' sense of self-worth by validating their experiences.
- Establish a positive learning environment.

The importance of nutrition education as a means for improving nutrition of the community in the developing countries has increased rapidly during the recent past.

Importance of Nutrition Education

- Lack of awareness about the dietary requirements and nutritive value of different food is the main cause for prevailing malnutrition among school children, pregnant women, lactating mother and other vulnerable sections of the community.
- Nutrition education should be practical and should be easily adaptable to the socioeconomic status, food habits and the available local food resources generally needed for the purpose of demonstration and feeding of the locally available audience. Nutrition education program should become a part of the community.
- Enhancing people's motivation towards a healthy lifestyle for prevention of obesity
- Facilitating the people's ability to take corrective action
- Improving environmental supports.

Objectives of Nutrition Education

The main objectives are as follows:

- To develop nutrition advisory services and nutrition education programs for the public.
- To participate and coordinate in community nutrition programs with the cooperation of people working in other disciplines like social workers, village health workers and nurses, etc., and also with the help of social welfare agencies.
- To help in developing supplementary nutrition program where ever necessary.
- To improve the nutritional levels of the community by the available means.

Methods of Nutrition Education of the Community

The various important methods of nutrition education are:

- Lectures and demonstrations
- Workshops
- Group discussion
- Panel discussion
- Workshop
- Mass approach.

Lectures and Demonstration

The lecture on nutrition should be simple and easily understandable. It should be easily adoptable by the people attending the program. The group should not be more than 25. To make the method more effective AV aids can be used such as flipchart, flannel graph, exhibits, etc. The demonstrations should be simple and these should make good use of locally available resources with the help of which it can be easily adopted by the community. The combination of lecture and demonstration is more effective especially when demonstrating any food preparation.

- **Group discussion:** Group discussion is a very effective method of health communication in which people interact in a face to face manner. The group should not be less than 6 and more than 12 members. The participants should be sited in a circle so that each is fully visible to other. Nutrition education will be more effective if this method will be combine with method
- **Panel discussion:** In a panel discussion there are 4 to 8 person who are qualified to talk about the topic (e.g., nutritional problems and their management) in front of a large group of audience. There is no specific agenda, no order of speaking and no set speaker. After starting of the discussion, the main aspect of the subject are explored by the panel speaker. The audience is invited to take part and their doubts are cleared by the speakers.
- **Workshop:** The workshop is the name given to a noble experiment in education. It consist of a series of meetings usually four or more with emphasis on individual work, within the group, with the help of a consultant and it is divided into two groups and each group will choose a chairman and a recorder. The nutrition work should discuss the prevailing nutritional problem in the community in simplest form and the solution for it.
- **Mass approach:** Mass approach like film and slide shows, poster, charts and exhibition, books, pamphlets, bulletins and newspaper, radio and television are also effective methods of nutrition education.

Posters, Charts and Exhibition

Posters should be simple and should immediately catch the attention of the viewers and should be written in the regional language. The letters should be clearly and easily visible at a distance too. Charts also should be in a position to stimulate the interest of the people. The charts should be well-balanced with the use appropriate colors and should not be crowded. Exhibitions having posters and charts are the best mode for educating the community. It should be set up keeping in mind the educational level of the people the education program is catering to.

Books, Pamphlets, Bulletins and Newspaper Articles

Printed matter for nutrition education is suitable for educating students, teachers and other professionals. These materials should be made available in regional languages and should give sufficient information.

Radio and Television

Radio and television programs reach a large number of audience within no time. Jokes, stories, dramas, etc., involving the nutritional problem help to create large scale awareness. These are the methods which can be useable for both educated and illiterate people also. Not only this role play, strict play and sociodrama can be used as effective methods of nutrition education.

NUTRITIONAL REHABILITATION

Nutritional rehabilitation is the practical training to mothers of children with malnutrition in selecting, preparing food from locally available cheap sources and feeding them back to health.

Child under nutrition encompasses stunting (chronic malnutrition), wasting (acute malnutrition) and deficiencies of micronutrients (essential vitamins and minerals). It significantly contributes to under-five mortality as undernourished children have increased susceptibility to infections and hence frequent episodes of diarrhea, acute respiratory infections, malaria and measles. It also leads to growth retardation and impaired psychosocial and cognitive development. This has impact on education attainment. The degree of cognitive impairment is directly related to the severity of stunting and iron deficiency anemia. Children who are affected by moderate/sever acute malnutrition during the critical stage of life between conception and age two, if not provided with timely and quality care, will find it difficult to achieve their full potential. Scientific evidence has shown that beyond the age to two to three years, many effects of chronic under nutrition are irreversible. This means that to break the intergenerational transmission of poverty and under nutrition, children at risk must be reached during their first two years of life.

This may due to lack of knowledge on selection and preparation of foods, its quality, quantity and maintenance of hygiene. So, it is the role of a community health nurse to teach community people regarding prevention of malnutrition and correction of malnutrition by demonstrating different food preparation procedures. Sometimes the child with acute malnutrition will be transferred to NRC for intensive feeding to recover lost weight, development of emotional and physical stimulation, capacity building of the primary caregivers of the child with acute malnutrition through sustained counseling and continuous behavioral change activities. Thus, NRC will be intended to function as a bridge between hospital and home care. Hence, NRC will be a short stay home for children with acute malnutrition along with the primary caregivers.

NATIONAL NUTRITION POLICY

In spite of the significant improvement of the food production and advancement of science since independence, under nutrition continues to be a widespread problem in India. In the year 1993, Govt. of India announced National Nutrition Policy 1993. As nutrition is a multisectorial issues, it needs to be tackle at various levels through direct nutrition interventions for especially vulnerable groups as well as through various development policy instruments which will create condition for improved nutrition.

Goals

Eradication of malnutrition.

Important Strategy

The important strategies of NNP are as follows:

- Direct measures or short-term measures are:
  - Nutrition interventions for especially vulnerable groups.
    - Expanding the safety net—The universal immunization program, oral rehydration therapy, and the integrated child development services have a considerable impact on child survival and forms of malnutrition.
    - Improving growth monitoring between age group 0 to 3 years, with closer involvement of the mothers.
    - Reaching the adolescent girls through ICDS so as to make them ready for safe motherhood.
    - Ensuring better coverage of expectant women in order to reduce the incidence of low birthweight babies.
  - To control and eliminate micronutritional deficiencies.
  - Popularize of low cost nutritious food.
  - Fortification of essential food.
  - To prevent vitamin A deficiency and making available iodine deficiency disorders control programs to all.
- Indirect policy measurements or long-term institutional and structural changes:
  - Food security: In order to ensure aggregate food security, a per capita availability of 215/kg/person/year of food grain needs to be attained.
  - Improvement of dietary pattern through production and demonstration.
  - Improving the purchasing power of the urban and rural poor and improving the public food distribution system.
  - Land reforms.
  - Better coverage of health and family welfare service.
  - Basic health and nutrition knowledge.
  - Prevention of food adulteration.
  - Nutrition surveillance.
  - Monitoring of nutrition program.
  - Research into various aspects of nutrition, both on the consumption side and the supply side.
  - Equal remuneration for women.
  - Information, education and communication regarding nutrition.
  - Minimum wage administration.
  - Community participation.
  - Education and literacy particularly that of women.

THE VILLAGE HEALTH, SANITATION AND NUTRITION COMMITTEE

One of the key elements of the National Rural Health Mission is the Village Health, Sanitation and Nutrition Committee (VHSNC). The committee has been formed to take collective actions on issues related to health and its social determinants at the village level. They are particularly envisaged as being central to 'local level community action' under NRHM, which would develop to support the process of Decentralised Health Planning. Thus the committee is envisaged to take leadership in providing a platform for improving health awareness and access of community for health services, address specific local needs and serve as a mechanism for community-based planning and monitoring.

The committee is formed at the revenue village level and it should act as a subcommittee of the Gram Panchayat. It should have a minimum of 15 members which should comprise of elected member of the Panchayat who shall lead the committee, all those working for health and health-related services should participate, community members/beneficiaries and representation from all community sub-groups especially the vulnerable sections and hamlets/habitations. ASHA residing in the village shall be the member secretary and convener of the committee.

Objective of VHSNCs is to:

- Inform the community about the health programs and government initiatives.
- Enable community to participate in the planning and implementation of the programs, and take collective action for attainment of better health status in the village.
- Take action on social determinants and all public services that directly or indirectly affect health and health outcomes.
- Facilitate the community to voice health needs, experiences and issues related to—access of health services such that the institutions of local government and public health service providers can take note and undertake appropriate action.
- Equip Panchayats with the understanding and mechanisms required for them to play their role in governance of health and other public services and provide leadership to the community for collective action to improve health status.
- Provide support and facilitate the work of community health workers like ASHA and other frontline health care providers, who form a crucial interface between the community and health institute VHSNC is to be formed at the level of revenue village.

Composition of the VHSNC

The VHSNC should have at least 15 members. It may have more members.

Key Principles Governing the Composition of the VHSNC

- Elected members, especially women members of the panchayat resident in the village should be enabled to lead.
- All those working for health or health-related services should be able to participate.
- The voices of service users of health services—especially of mothers should find place.

- There should be representation from all community subgroups, especially from poorer and more vulnerable sections.
- All habitations/hamlets should have representation.

Members of VHSNC

- **Elected gram panchayat members:** Those members who are residents of the village are to be preferred, like the women Ward Panch. In areas where there are no elected panchayats, members of tribal councils, could be considered. Though more than one elected member of a panchayat can be included in the VHSNC, their numbers should be limited to one-third of the total number of members, and preference should be given to women panchayat members. Members of the permanent standing committees of the gram panchayat who are usually elected members should also be preferably included.
- **ASHAs:** All ASHAs of the village should be on the committee. In small villages there would be only one ASHA per VHSNC.
- **Frontline staff of government health-related services:** The ANM of the health department, the anganwadi worker of the ICDS, and the school teacher should be included as regular members only if they are resident in that particular village. Otherwise they qualify to be special invitees. Volunteers/village level workers of other government departments, e.g., The hand pump mechanic of Public Health and Engineering Department (PHED) or the field coordinators of the MNREGA program, should also be considered if they are resident in the village.
- **Community-based organizations:** Representatives of existing community-based organizations like Self-Help Groups, Forest Management Committees, Youth Committees, etc.
- **Pre-existing committees:** If there are separate committees on School Education, Water and Sanitation or Nutrition, the first effort should be to integrate these committees with VHSNC. If that is not possible or till the time it has not been done, key functionaries of each of these bodies should be included as a member in the VHSNC and chairperson of the VHSNC should also become a member of these committees.
- **Service-users:** Pregnant women, lactating mothers, mothers with children of up to 3 years of age, and patients with chronic diseases who are using the public services should also find place.

  Note: At least 50% should be women members and SCs, STs and minorities should be well-represented.
- **Special invitees:** Other than members a more general category of special invitees can be included. They can attend the meeting and indeed their presence and interaction with the committee is essential. They are generally not residents of the village. This includes Medical Officer of the local PHC, Facilitator of the ASHA program, Supervisors in health and ICDS departments, Panchayat secretary and Block Development Officer, Zilla and block panchayat member.

  Ideally the medical officer and block development officer should participate in every VHSNC meeting at least once or twice a year. ASHA Facilitators who are also facilitators for other community processes including the VHSNC itself should attend the VHSNC meetings more regularly.

Chairperson

The Chairperson of the VHSNC is a woman elected member of the gram panchayat (panch) preferably from among the SC/ST communities, who is a resident of that village. If there is no woman panch from that village, then preference should be given to any panch from the SC/ST. But this is a decision arrived at between the gram panchayat and VHSNC with the ANM and ASHA playing a facilitating role.

Member Secretary and Convener

The ASHA will be the Member Secretary and Convener of VHSNC. She can play a very important role in providing a more organized support mechanism and more sustained building of capacity of the VHSNC. She also has better community ownership and acceptance.

She has been involved in health-related issues over the past few years. For successful achievement of her objectives especially as related to health promotion, prevention and community mobilization, the ASHA also requires an active VHSNC.

Joint Bank Account

- Once the VHSNC has been constituted, an account in the nearest bank should be opened. It is to this bank that the fund of the VHSNC shall be credited.
- The joint signatories of the VHSNC account would be the Chairperson of the VHSNC (female panchayat member) and the Member Secretary (ASHA).
- If any other persons, for example ANM, AWW are amongst the joint signatories of the account they should be replaced as per the above guideline.
- All withdrawals from VHSNC account must be done by signature of both the signatories (if the account is operated by two signatories) or by two of the three signatories (if the account is operated by three signatories). The decision on expenditure of untied fund will only be done through a written approved proposal of the VHSNC with signatures of its members.

Roles and Responsibilities of Key VHSNC Members

Chairperson of the Committee

The Chairperson will:

- Be responsible for ensuring that meetings are held on monthly basis.
- Lead the monthly meetings of the committee and ensure smooth coordination amongst members for effective decision-making.

- Represent the VHSNC in the Standing Committee of the Panchayat on health and share details of work undertaken by VHSNC at the village level.
- Helps the VHSNC to undertake village health planning and take responsibilities for necessary actions and follow-ups.
- Help the VHSNC to formulate annual plan.
- Ensure that the issues/plans emerging from village health monitoring and planning are reflected in the Gram Sabha and Gram Panchayat proceedings.
- Ensure that the records are adequately maintained.

Member Secretary and Convener of the Meeting

- ASHA acts as the member secretary and convener of the committee. She will fix the schedule and venue for monthly meetings of the committee.
- Ensure that meetings are conducted regularly with participation of all members.
- Draw attention of the committee on specific constraints and achievements related to health status of the village community and enable appropriate planning.
- Facilitate collection of information for village level planning-related to total population of the village, number of maternal and infant deaths, JSY/JSSK beneficiaries, children immunized, malnourished children and those referred to Nutrition Rehabilitation Centre (NRC), number of households and details of families falling under marginalized groups such as—those below poverty line, SC/ST category, women headed households, landless families working as daily wage laborers, families living in distant hamlets, migrant labors and individuals with disability.
- Maintain records on gaps identified in health or other related sectors. This includes identifying the cause of the gap, recording the decision on collective action as needed by the village to address the gap, and designating the persons responsible for leading the collective action, the specified timeframe to undertake the action, and recording follow-up action.
- Undertake regular update of the cashbook and maintain other necessary records related to the funds.
- Provide information on activity-wise fund utilization to the committee every month and with bills and vouchers/documents on a quarterly basis.
- Work with Chairperson for the annual presentation of the activities and expenditures in the annual Gram Sabha, its social audit and getting the approval of the Statement of Expenditure (SOE) by the Gram Panchayat, and timely submission of the SOE to the ASHA Facilitators or at the block level.

The Anganwadi Worker

She is an important member of the VHSNC. She has a critical role in enabling VHSNC to take action on addressing malnutrition.

She will:

- Provide information on hamlet-wise malnutrition status of children (less than six years of age) and presenting before the committee any specific challenges related to the functioning of AWC or help she needs for improving her effectiveness.
- Help in mapping the marginalized households needing nutrition services and extends support in forming and implementing nutrition component of the village health plan.
- Be accountable for ensuring the provision of take home ration for children of less than three age group, pregnant/lactating mothers, and supplementary food for children 3–6 years, and bringing the issues related to nonavailability of supplementary nutrition before the committee.
- Inform VHSNC of any difficulties she faces in providing Anganwadi services.
- Be held accountable by the VHSNC for providing hot cooked meals in accordance with norms.

Auxiliary Nursing Midwife

She will:

- Provide information to VHSNC regarding available services, schemes, and services for maternity and child health.
- Share details on marginalized groups or those unreached through health services and seek the support of the VHSNC to reach these populations.
- Inform the VHSNC on the deaths in the village, especially maternal and child death and their probable causes.
- Facilitate or support the committee in preparing a village action plan to address the issue of reaching the marginalized and unreached groups with health services.
- Inform VHSNC of any difficulties she faces in providing health services.
- Be made accountable by the committee for smooth functioning of subcenter and provision of quality services and regular conduct of VHND.

Role of Representatives from other Departments Like Education, Water and Sanitation, and Department of Woman and Child Development

- The mandate of the VHSNC encompasses health, sanitation, drinking water and nutrition as well as the education, particularly in the context of the programs like Mid-day meal, and other programs implemented by Department of Woman and Child Development. Accordingly the VHSNC has the role of providing oversight and monitoring of their services to ensure convergent action on wider determinants of health such as drinking water, sanitation, female literacy, nutrition and women and child health.
- These representatives will—inform VHSNC on various developments, enable VHSNC to monitor and take action

on challenges faced in implementing the respective programs. This will ensure action on improving social determinants of health. This also allows VHSNC to ensure local level accountability in delivery of social sector programs.

Accredited Social Health Activist Facilitator

The ASHA Facilitator is instrumental in facilitating the VHSNC meeting. She is also responsible for collecting utilization certificates and other records for submitting to the BMO.

If there is more than one ASHA in the VHSNC village, then one of them is to be selected by consensus as Member-Secretary and convener. This could also be by rotation amongst the ASHAs after a two or three year period but that is a local decision.

ASHA Facilitator (or Block Mobilizer) should organize a meeting of all ASHAs of the village in the presence of the Panch. Selection of the ASHA who would become the Member Secretary would be as per consensus in the meeting.

Activities of VHSNC

- Monthly meetings
- Accounting for the United Village Fund
- Community monitoring of health care facilities
- Facilitating service delivery in the village
- Management of United Village Health Fund
- Record maintenance
- Organizing local collective action for health promotion
- Monitoring and facilitating access to essential public services
- Village health planning.

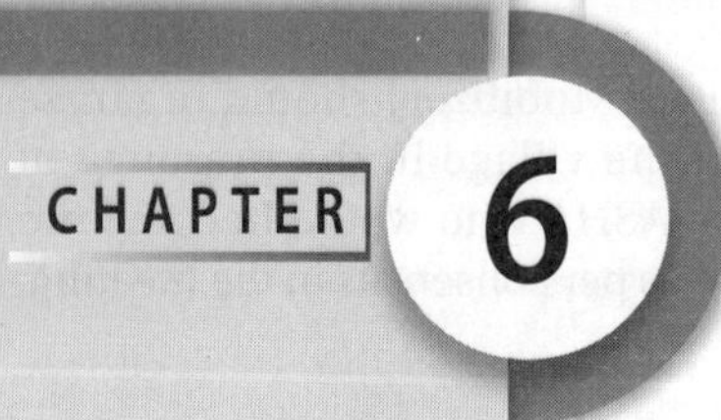

Environment and Health

CONCEPT OF ENVIRONMENT AND ENVIRONMENTAL HEALTH

The term 'environment' has been derived from the French word 'Environia', which means 'to surround'. It refers to both abiotic (physical or nonliving) and biotic (living) environment. The word 'environment' means surroundings in which organisms live. Environment and the organisms are two dynamic and complex components of nature. Environment regulates the life of the organisms, including human beings. Human beings interact with the environment more vigorously than other living beings. We can also define it as 'environment is the combination of all the physical and organic factors that act on a living being. The environment encompasses all living and nonliving things occurring naturally on earth or it encompasses the interaction of all living species with the climate, weather, and natural resource'.

Definition

Webster's Dictionary defines the environment as 'the circumstances, objects, conditions by which one is surrounded, the complex of physical, chemical and biotic factors that act upon an organism or an ecological community and determine its form and survival, the aggregate of social, cultural factors that influence the life of an individual or community'.

Environmental Health

Environmental health is determined by the changes that are taking place in the biosphere comprising of number of ecosystem (ecology as a science and branch of biology helps in understanding the changes that are taking places and the balance which can be maintained in the biosphere) for wholesome environmental health. So, it is very important for a nurse to understand the concept of ecology, ecosystem, basic principles of ecology/ecosystems and ecological balance.

Many factors combine together to affect the health of individuals and communities. Whether people are healthy or not is determined by their circumstances and environment. To a large extent, factors such as where we live, the state of our environment, genetics, our income and education level, and our relationships with friends and family, all have considerable impacts on health, whereas the more commonly considered factors such as access and use of health care services often have the less of an impact.

Components of Environment

There are mainly three components of environment:

Physical Component

The physical component of environment is also known as 'abiotic component' or 'natural component'. The meaning of 'abiotic' or 'physical' is nonliving; so, abiotic environment includes nonliving things, like, land water and air conditions, atmosphere and climatic factors, such as sunbeams, rainwater, precipitation, moisture, pressure and wind speed, etc. The physical or abiotic components of environment have a greater effect on living beings. The biotic and abiotic components both are interdependent with each other.

Importance

- Physical environment is responsible for the residential facilities of living beings.
- Soil, water and air are the necessary nutrient element providers for the living beings.
- All the living beings are surrounded by atmosphere in the combination of different types of gases. The living beings take oxygen and other gases from the atmosphere for their survival.
- It also controls the climatic factors like weather.
- Soil is responsible for the works and food crops for the living beings. It also provides different types of minerals which are very necessary for the growth of life.
- Water is one of the most necessary things for the living beings.

Biological Component

Biological component is the living component of an ecosystem comprising of plants, animals, and microorganisms (bacteria and fungi). They carry out different functions and based on their role, they are classified into three main groups. These are: (1) Producers; (2) Consumers; (3) Decomposers.

Importance

They carry out different functions based on their roles as producers, consumers and decomposers. **Producers (plants) produce foods** by photosynthesis process using chlorophyll in the presence of sunlight, which is consumed by primary consumers or herbivores. Then secondary consumers or primary carnivores eat herbivores and lastly, all are discomposed by decomposers like microorganisms but all depend upon each other.

Sociocultural Component of Environment

Sociocultural component of environment involves the culture and lifestyle of the human beings which is created by the man through his different social and cultural activities and thinking. The historical, cultural, political, moral, economic aspects of human life constitute to the social or cultural environment.

Importance

- Culture involves the religion of the human, relations with each other, etc. In a society, there are different types of people, they have different religion, different thinking, which has culture of its own and same culture group people having their own lifestyle.
- The social or cultural environment affects the behavior of human beings and, hence, it has a great importance.
- The development of a child highly depends upon culture and society.
- Some sociocultural belief has also negative impact on health.

Though environments is having different components, in simple words, environment is the sum total of conditions in which an organism has to survive or maintain its life process. It influences the growth and development of living forms. In other words, environment refers to those surroundings that surround living beings from all sides and affect their lives. It consists of atmosphere, hydrosphere, lithosphere and biosphere. Its chief components are soil, water, air, organisms and solar energy.

NATURAL RESOURCES

Our environment provides us with a variety of goods and services necessary for our day to day lives. These natural resources include, air, water, soil, minerals, along with the climate and solar energy, which form the nonliving or 'abiotic' part of nature. The 'biotic' or living parts of nature consists of plants and animals, including microbes. Plants and animals can only survive as communities of different organisms, all closely linked to each in their own habitat, and requiring specific abiotic conditions. Thus, forests, grasslands, deserts, mountains, rivers, lakes and the marine environment all form habitats for specialized communities of plants and animals to live in. Interactions between the abiotic aspects of nature and specific living organisms together form ecosystems of various types. Natural resources can be defined as the resources that exist (on the planet) independent of human actions. This includes all valued characteristics such as commercial and industrial use, aesthetic value, scientific interest and cultural value. These are the resources that are found in the environment and are developed without the intervention of humans. Common examples of natural resources include air, sunlight, water, soil, stone, plants, animals and fossil fuels.

Natural resources are naturally occurring materials that are useful to man or could be useful under conceivable technological, economic or social circumstances or supplies drawn from the earth, supplies such as food, building and clothing materials, fertilizers, metals, water and geothermal power. For a long time, natural resources were the domain of the natural sciences. Based on the availability are two types of natural resources:

Renewable

Renewable resource, also known as a flow resource is a natural resource which will replenish to replace the portion depleted by usage and consumption, either through natural reproduction or other recurring processes in a finite amount of time in a human time scale. When the recovery rate of resources is unlikely to ever exceed a human time scale, these are called perpetual resources. Renewable resources are a part of earth's natural environment and the largest components of its ecosphere. A positive life-cycle assessment is a key indicator of a resource's sustainability. The examples of renewable resources are air, water, soil, sunlight, forests, etc.

- **Air:** Air is a renewable resource. All living organisms need oxygen, nitrogen (directly or indirectly), carbon (directly or indirectly) and many other gases in small quantities for their survival.
- **Water:** Water is a natural resource which is not only found on the surface of the earth in rivers, oceans, lakes, and streams but also underground. Water is renewable because it is recycled in reasonably short periods of time. To simplify the water cycle, fresh water is found in streams, reservoirs and underground. When people use this resource, waste water will flow into the ocean.
- **Sunlight:** Other examples of renewable resources are sunlight, which is consumed as solar energy. Sunlight replenishes instantaneously.
- **Forests:** Forests are renewable natural resource capable of providing several major and minor forest products and contribute substantially to economic development. The forests consist of and conserve a variety of flora and fauna, which form a rich biodiversity and play a vital role in the environmental stability and ecological balance. Forests, once destroyed take thousands of years to regrow into fully developed natural ecosystems with their full complement of species. Forests thus can be said to be—have like nonrenewable resources if over-used
- **Soil:** Soil is renewable and is constantly forming and eroding. Mountains are eroded by wind, rain and frost breaking them down to rocks then sand and silt. Exposed soil gets washed out to sea then settles to be compressed

into rocks that in turn gets pushed back up due to plate tectonics. From there the cycle repeats in self and gets expanded by plant material mixing in to give the rich topsoil we like to grow our crops in.

- **Agricultural food:** Though agriculture is a renewable source, recent times to produce more and more food by the addition of extra chemicals and modern agriculture system like irrigation, which leads to the development of saline soil, and the use of artificial fertilizers eventually ruin soil quality, and pesticides, which are a health hazard for humans as well as destroying components vital to the long-term health of agricultural ecosystems, creates a variety of environmental problems, which ultimately lead to the formation of unproductive land.
- **Nonagricultural food:** Though most food has its origin in renewable resources but still overuse can create problems. Fish are today being over-harvested until the catch has become a fraction of the original resource and the fish are incapable of breeding successfully to replenish the population. When the population of a species of plant or animal is reduced by human activities, until it cannot reproduce fast enough to maintain a viable number, the species becomes extinct. Many species are probably becoming extinct without us even knowing, and other linked species are affected by their loss.

Nonrenewable

Nonrenewable resources are nonrenewable in nature because once these resources are used up, they cannot be replaced, which is a major problem for humanity as we are currently dependent on them. There are four major types of nonrenewable resources: oil, natural gas, coal, and nuclear energy. Oil, natural gas, and coal are collectively called fossil fuels. Fossil fuels were formed within the earth from dead plants and animals over millions of years—hence the name "fossil" fuels. They are found in underground layers of rock and sediment. Pressure and heat worked together to transform the plant and animal remains into crude oil (also known as petroleum), coal, and natural gas.

The plants and animals that became fossil fuels lived in a time called Carboniferous Period, around 300-360 million years ago. The energy in the plant and animal remains originally came from the sun; through the process of photosynthesis, solar energy is stored in plant tissues, which animals then consume, adding the energy to their own bodies. When fossil fuels are burned, this trapped energy is released.

Crude Oil

Crude oil is a liquid fuel fossil that is used mostly to produce gasoline and diesel fuel for vehicles, and for the manufacturing of plastics. It is found in rocks below earth's surface and is pumped out through wells.

Natural Gas

Natural gas is widely used for cooking and for heating homes. It consists mostly of methane and is found near oil deposits below earth's surface. Natural gas can be pumped out through the same wells used for extracting crude oil.

Coal

Coal is a solid fossil fuel that is used for heating homes and generating power plants. It is found in fossilized swamps that have been buried beneath layers of sediment. Since coal is solid, it cannot be extracted in the same manner as crude oil or natural gas; it must be dug up from the ground.

Nuclear Energy (Uranium)

Apart from fossil fuels, the other category of nonrenewable resources is nuclear fuels. It is primarily obtained through the mining and refining of uranium ore, a naturally occurring radioactive element below the earth's surface. Nuclear energy comes from radioactive elements, mainly uranium, which is extracted from mined ore and then refined into fuel. Uranium is found in small quantities, and miners often gather the uranium deposits for refining and purification. The mineral generates power through a process known as nuclear fusion, which creates enough pressure to run turbines and generate nuclear power.

Approximately 80% of the total amount of energy used globally each year comes from fossil fuels. We depend on fossil fuels because they are energy-rich and relatively cheap to process. But a major problem with fossil fuels, aside from their being in limited supply and by burning them, carbon dioxide releases into the atmosphere. Rising levels of heat-trapping carbon dioxide in the atmosphere is the main cause of global warming.

Alternative energy sources, such as wind and solar energy, are a possible solution to the depletion of nonrenewable sources. Both of these clean energy sources are available in unlimited supply.

NATURAL RESOURCES AND ASSOCIATED PROBLEMS

Associated Problems: Renewable Resources

Global livestock and fisheries resources can also not be expanded beyond certain limits. Only up to a limited extent resources of biosphere can be safely exploited. Though an enormous quantity of water is present, for fresh water life depends largely on precipitation, which to is available only in a finite quantity. Its uneven distribution over earth' surface has caused large area to become infertile deserts.

Water Pollution or Scarcity

Water sources can be overused or wasted to such an extent that they locally run dry. Water sources can be so heavily polluted by sewage and toxic substances that it becomes impossible to use the water. Water pollution truly harms biodiversity and aquatic ecosystems. The toxic chemicals can change the color of water and increase the amount of minerals—also known as eutrophication—which has a bad impact on life in water. Thermal pollution, defined by a rise in the temperature of water bodies, contributes to global warming and causes serious hazard to water organisms. Water pollution has very negative effects on public health. A lot of diseases result from drinking or being in contact with contaminated water, such as diarrhea, cholera, typhoid, dysentery or skin infections. In zones where there is no available drinking water, the main risk is dehydration obviously.

Sunlight

Sunlight having a lots of positive effects on health however manufactured chemicals, especially manufactured halocarbon refrigerants, solvents, propellants, and foam-blowing agents (chlorofluorocarbons (CFCs), HCFCs, halons) create hole in ozone layer. Ozone layer depletion increases the amount of UVB that reaches the earth's surface. Laboratory and epidemiological studies demonstrate that UVB causes non-melanoma skin cancer and plays a major role in malignant melanoma development. In addition, UVB has been linked to the development of cataracts, a clouding of the eye's lens.

Effects of Deforestation Loss of Species

Seventy percent of the world's plants and animals live in forests and are losing their habitats due to deforestation, according to National Geographic. Loss of habitat can lead to species extinction. It also has negative consequences for medicinal research and local populations who rely on the animals and plants in the forests for hunting and medicine. The loss of trees and other vegetation can cause climate change, desertification, soil erosion, fewer crops, flooding, increased greenhouse gases in the atmosphere, and a host of problems for indigenous people. By destroying the forests, human activities are putting entire ecosystems in danger, creating natural imbalances, and putting life at threat. Scientists estimate that India should ideally have 33% of its land under forests. Today we have only about 12%. Thus we need not only to protect existing forests but also to increase our forest cover.

Soil Erosion

Soil erosion is the displacement of the upper layer of soil; it is a form of soil degradation. This natural process is caused by the dynamic activity of erosive agents, that is, water, ice (glaciers), snow, air (wind), plants, animals, and humans. In accordance with these agents, erosion is sometimes divided into water erosion, glacial erosion, snow erosion, wind (aeolian) erosion. Some human activities that increase soil erosion are deforestation, agricultural practices and urbanization. Tree roots anchor the soil. Without trees, the soil is free to wash or blow away can also lead to silt entering the lakes, streams and other water sources. This can decrease local water quality and contribute to poor health in populations in the area.

Air

Air is a renewable source but due to deforestation, industries and burning of chemicals and fossil fuels which produce gaseous pollutants and pollute the air. Air pollution can also cause headaches, dizziness, and nausea. Long-term health effects from air pollution include heart disease, lung cancer, and respiratory diseases such as emphysema. Air pollution can also cause long-term damage to people's nerves, brain, kidneys, liver, and other organs. Air pollution can damage crops and trees in a variety of ways. Ground-level ozone can lead to reductions in agricultural crop and commercial forest yields, reduced growth and survivability of tree seedlings, and increased plant susceptibility to disease, pests and other environmental stresses. Air pollution can harm us when it accumulates in the air in high enough concentrations. Air pollution can leads to a variety of air-borne disease

Associated Problems: Nonrenewable Resources

Greenhouse Gas Emissions

Though nonrenewable resources, such as coal and oil, are the primary source of power in the world, and they are used to power vehicles, factories, and homes. Although affordable, they can be harmful to the environment and are one of the notable contributors to global warming. Most nonrenewable energy resources produce carbon dioxide as a byproduct. The CO_2 gets trapped in the atmosphere and is the main cause of climate change, according to most climatologists. Different types of nonrenewable energy fuels emit different levels of greenhouse gases. For example, coal is considered the worst emitter of carbon dioxide while for example natural gas produced around 28% of carbon dioxide emissions. The concerns about greenhouse gas emissions and climate change are cross-cutting. It is not just about direct impacts of rising temperatures and changing weather patterns as floods or dry seasons proliferate that impact human livelihoods.

Air Pollution

Nonrenewable energy sources are not just altering our earth's atmosphere by increasing the amount of greenhouse gas emissions. They also emit a variety of pollutants that affect people's health and the environment. For example, coal-fired power plants are the single largest source of mercury emissions in the US. When mercury is emitted into the air, it deposits on the ground or in water. This way it can accumulate in organisms of species that inhabit the area (such as fish), passing through the food chain. This has profound effects on our biodiversity but also creates real risks for people, as studies have found that exposure to mercury can lead to neurological and neuro-behavioral effects in embryos and young children. Other air pollutants emitted due to fossil fuel combustion include sulfur dioxide, nitrogen oxides and particulate matter.

Acid Rain and Water Pollution

It is not just the air that we breathe which gets polluted. Dangerous pollutants that are emitted into the air can take a part in the water cycle cause acid rain which forms when sulfur and other chemicals are introduced into the atmosphere from industrial processes. Chemicals suspended in the air then turn the rain mildly acidic.

Acid rain is corrosive to machinery and disrupts local ecosystems. In terms of the environment, acid rain changes the acidity of lakes and streams which can be very harmful to fish and other aquatic organisms; it is also damaging to trees thereby weakening forest ecosystems.

Thermal Pollution

Both fossil fuel plants and nuclear power plants require water to run and help cool the power plant. The water they use is also needed for other purposes, such as maintaining local ecosystem functions or agriculture. When the plants release that water back into the environment, its temperature is changed and as a result its quality has been degraded. Heated water that is reintroduced to the environment contains lower levels of dissolved oxygen which can stress native wildlife, for example increasing the heart rate of fish or decreasing fertility.

Land Pollution and Waste Generation

It is also important not to forget environmental impacts that come about as a result of the extraction of nonrenewable resources or the disposal of the waste they generate. There is very clear evidence illustrating the impact of surface mining both in the short and long-term. For instance, huge volumes of excess rock or soil are dumped in other locations such as nearby valleys affecting those ecosystems.

When it comes to the land that is being mined, in the long-term these sites are left with poor soil quality and sometimes due to the chemicals used the lands ends up being polluted as well as any nearby water reserves. In case of uranium and waste disposal create some very critical issues for which no long-term solution has been found due to the radioactive nature of the ore being mined.

Oil Spills and Other Accidents

Lastly, there is something to be said about unintended consequences or rather unforeseen and accidental effects. Oil spills are extremely damaging to nearby shores and ecosystems.

Over Consumption of Natural Resources

Now a days a major part of natural resources consumed in the technologically advanced or 'developed' world, usually termed 'the North'. The 'developing nations' of 'the South', including India and China, also overuse many resources because of their greater human population. However, the consumption of resources per capita (per individual) of the developed countries is up to 50 times greater than in most developing countries. Advanced countries produce over 75% of global industrial waste and greenhouse gases. Energy from fossil fuels is consumed in relatively much greater quantities in developed countries. Their per capita consumption of food too is much greater as well as their waste of enormous quantities of food and other products, such as packaging material, used in the food industry. The USA for example with just 4% of the world's population consumes about 25% of the world's resources. Producing animal food for human consumption requires more land than growing crops. Thus countries that are highly dependent on nonvegetarian diets need much larger areas for pastureland than those where the people are mainly vegetarian.

Unplanned Land Use

Land as a resource is now under serious pressure due to an increasing 'land hunger' to produce sufficient quantities of food for an exploding human population. It is also affected by degradation due to misuse. Land and water resources are polluted by industrial waste and rural and urban sewage. They are increasingly being diverted for short-term economic gains to agriculture and industry. Natural wetlands of great value are being drained for agriculture and other purposes. Semi-arid land is being irrigated and overused. Land itself is a major resource, needed for food production, animal husbandry, industry, and for our growing human settlements. The different forms of intensive land use are frequently extended at the cost of 'wild lands', our remaining forests, grasslands, wetlands and deserts.

Thus, it is essential to evolve a rational land-use policy that examines how much land must be made available for different purposes and where it must be situated. For instance, there are usually alternate sites at which industrial complexes or dams can be built, but a natural wilderness cannot be recreated artificially. Scientists today believe that at least 10% of land and water bodies of each ecosystem must be kept as wilderness for the long-term needs of protecting nature and natural resources.

ROLE OF INDIVIDUAL IN CONSERVATION OF NATURAL RESOURCES

Individuals role in energy conservation and saving energy

- Switch off light, fan and other appliances when not in use.
- Use solar heater for cooking.
- Dry the cloth in the sunlight instead of driers.
- Use always pressure cookers.
- Grow trees near the house to get cool breeze instead of using AC and AI cooler.
- Ride bicycle or just walk instead of using scooter for short distance.
- Replacing tube lights with CFLs and LEDs.
- Construct buildings in such a way that maximum amount of sunlight can be obtained.
- Try to dry cloths in sunlight instead of drier of washing machine.
- Using solar cookers for cooking food.
- Buying energy efficient appliances, always checking energy consumption figure.
- Minimize use of automobiles by using bicycles, public transport, carpooling, etc.
- Trying to reside near the place of work, if possible.
- Keeping vehicles tuned for low consumption of fuel.

- Checking fuel consumption data while buying a new vehicle.
- Following the advice given by Petroleum Conservation Research Association.
- Wearing adequate woolen clothes during winter instead of using heat convector.
- Growing deciduous trees at proper place outside the house. They will cut off intense heat during the summers, cut off electricity consumption and will provide a cool breeze.
- Observe December 14 as world energy conservation day.

Individuals role in conservation of water:

- Not keeping water taps running.
- Use minimum water for all domestic purposes.
- Check the water leaks in pipes and repair them properly.
- Reuse the soapy water, after washing clothes for washing courtyard, carpets, etc.
- Use drip irrigation.
- Rainwater harvesting system should be installed in all the houses.
- Sewage treatment plant may be installed in all industries and institution.
- Continuous running of water taps should be avoided.
- Watering of plants should be done in the evening to minimize evaporation losses and not watering them in the mid-day.
- Installing water saving toilets that use optimum water per flush.

Individual's role in sustainable agriculture and soil protection: Some of the measures in sustainable agriculture and soil protection are:

- Reducing use of chemicals such as fertilizers and pesticides to check soil pollution.
- Using biofertilizers
- Using biological control measures for pest control.
- Avoid over irrigation without proper irrigation to prevent water logging.
- Discouraging monoculture practice in agriculture.
- Adopting mix cropping
- Grow different type plants, i.e., trees, herbs and shrubs.
- In the irrigation process, using strong flow of water should be avoided.
- Adopting drip irrigation/sprinkling irrigation to avoid washing out soil nutrients. Observing December 23 as world farmers day.
- Observing June 17 as a day to combat desertification and deserts.
- Observe November 21–27 as national land resource conservation week.

Individuals role in food security or conservation of food resources: Some of the measures to achieve food security are:

- Sustainable use of food by cooking proper amount and not wasting it.
- Eating only as much as required for sustenance of life.
- Consuming local and seasonable vegetables and so as to save energy on their transportation.
- Buy only organically grown food
- Discourage packed, canned and preserved food
- Shift from nonvegetarian to vegetarian
- Observe October 16 as world food day and November 21 as world fishery day.
- Do not store large amount of food grains and protect them from damaging insects.

Individual's role in conservation of minerals: Some of the measures to conserve minerals are:

- Minimize the use of minerals which are likely to be depleted or exhausted.
- Minimize use of jewelry to conserve scarce minerals.
- Recycle and reuse minerals and glasses
- Buy durable products that lasts long
- Buy efficient vehicles
- Repair and reuse bicycles
- Use recyclable utensils.

Individual's role in conservation of forests: Individual's role in conservation of forests are:

- Use nontimber product.
- Planting ornamentals, herbs, shrubs, or suitable trees in and around the house.
- Grassing must be controlled
- Minimize the use of paper and fuel.
- Avoid the construction of dam, road in the forest areas.
- Not uprooting the existing trees while constructing a house but planting fast growing plant species in open area of the house.
- Maintain lawn and garden in open place in your house, if possible participating in community plantation programs.
- Encourage mass scale tree plantation programs and cooperate with NGOs engaged in saving trees.
- Plant trees generously in barren fields and tag tree plantation with year ceremonies such as birth day, marriage anniversary, etc.
- Observe and encourage to observe July 1–7 as Van Mahotsav Week.

EQUITABLE USE OF RESOURCES FOR SUSTAINABLE LIFE-STYLE

Scarcity of resources is the burning problem of modern technology. The twenty-first century will see growing human needs for resources since many parts of the world are using natural resources at a rate faster than the natural processes can replenish it. Natural resources are limited. For example, the existing water sources are being subjected to heavy pollution. Global climatic changes are altering the quality of fresh water sources as a consequence of unknown effects on the hydrological cycle. Sustainable development is currently being discussed as a focal theme in the field of development, planning and other associated aspects. In the light of self-defeating current mode of development and recurrent natural calamities, people are urged to ponder over the faults, shortcomings, lacunae, discrepancies and limitations of the ongoing developmental process and production system.

It is essential to sustain the natural resources. We should conserve natural resources so that it may yield sustainable benefit to the present generation while maintaining its potential to meet the needs of the future generation. There are three specific objectives to conserve living resources:

1. To ensure that any utilization of the ecosystem is sustainable.
2. To preserve biodiversity and
3. To maintain essential ecological processes.

Resource management should be less energy-intensive, suitable to local ecology and needs of the people, less cost-intensive and more viable in terms of economy, ecology and culture.

There is a big divide in the world as North and South, the more developed countries (MDCs) and less developed countries (LDCs), the haves and the have nots. The MDCs have only 22% of world's population, but they use 88% of its natural resources, 73% of its energy and command 85% of its income. As the rich nations continue to grow, they will reach a limit.

If they have a growth rate of 10% every year, they will show 1024 times increase in the next 70 years. Will this much of growth be sustainable? The answer is 'No' because many of our earth's resources are limited and even the renewable resources will become unsustainable if their use exceeds their regeneration.

Thus, the solution to this problem is to have more equitable distribution of resources and wealth. We cannot expect the poor countries to stop growth in order to check pollution because development brings employment and the main problem of these countries is to tackle poverty.

The poor in the LDCs are at least able to sustain their life. Unless they are provided with such basic resources, we cannot think of rooting out the problems related to dirty, unhygienic, polluted, disease infested settlements of these people, which contribute to unsustainability.

Thus, the two basic causes of unsustainability are over population in poor countries who have under consumption of resources and over consumption of resources by the rich countries, which generate wastes. In order to achieve sustainable lifestyles it is desirable to achieve a more balanced and equitable distribution of global resources and income to meet everyone's basic needs. The rich countries will have to lower down their consumption levels while the bare minimum needs of the poor have to be fulfilled by providing them resources. A fairer sharing of resources will narrow down the gap between the rich and the poor and will lead to sustainable development for all and not just for a privileged group.

ECOLOGY

The word 'ecology', derived from the Greek word 'Oikos' meaning habitation, and 'logos' meaning discourse or study, implies a study of the habitations of organisms. Ecology was first described as a separate field of knowledge in 1866 by the German Zoologist Ernst Haeckel, who invented the word 'ecology' for 'the relation of the animal to its organic as well as its inorganic environment'.

Definitions

- Ecology is the science of study of all the relations of every organism to all its environment. **—Taylor, 1936**
- Ecology is the study of structure and functions of nature. **—Odum, 1963**
- Ecology is the study of environmental interaction which controls the welfare of living things regarding their distribution. Ecology is the branch of biological science and is concerned with the study of interrelationship of living and nonliving things.

Ecology has been variously defined by other investigators as 'scientific natural history', 'the study of biotic communities', or 'the science of community population'. Probably the most comprehensive definition of ecology, which is the simple one and which is most often given is 'a study of animals and plants in their relations to each other and to their environment'.

Meaning

According to above definition, 'ecology' is explained as a 'science study'.

- The components of nature which include different forms of life and their physical and chemical environment.
- The process of interaction among different forms of life and nonliving things (physical and chemical environment)
- How different forms of life can live in harmonious relations to their surroundings.
- How different forms of life and their surroundings can be controlled and regulated to maintain their health and welfare.

Areas of Ecological Concern

Ecological concern comprises of four areas—population, community, ecosystem and biosphere. These are included in biological spectrum which starts from protoplasm, cells, tissues, organs, organ system, organism, population, ecosystems and biosphere.

Biological spectrum shows successive organization from cell to biosphere. Out of this spectrum, ecology is concerned with the last four areas.

Population

From the ecological point of view, population refers to the group of individuals of any one kind of organism living together in a particular place.

Community

In ecological sense, 'community' refers to the association of various populations in a particular locality. This is also known as 'biotic community'.

Ecosystem

An ecosystem is formed when the community (various types of population) and nonliving environment interact and function together. It is the unit of study in ecology.

Biosphere

Biosphere refers to the world of living and nonliving things and is comprised of the part of earth (the lithosphere), the thin layer of air above the surface of earth (atmosphere) and water (hydrosphere). The biosphere extends vertically into the atmosphere to about 10 kms, downwards into the ocean about 35,000 feet and into the earth's surface about 23,000 feet. The sun remains the chief source of energy and supports the life within the biosphere. The nutrients necessary or life are drawn from air, water and soil. Recycling of nutrient takes place by virtue of various cycles in the biosphere for life to continue and balance to be maintained.

The biosphere is compared to a number of ecosystems on the land, in the air and in water which helps in maintaining life from the highest peak of mountain to deep down below the sea level. The ecosystems in the biosphere interact delicately in controlled and orderly manner to assure the survival and growth of biotic community.

There are four ecological levels, which include population, communities, ecosystem and biosphere.

ECOSYSTEM

The term 'ecosystem' was proposed in 1935 by a British botanist Professor Arthur Tansley. An ecosystem includes all the living things (plants, animals and organisms) in a given area, interacting with each other, and also with their nonliving environments (weather, earth, sun, soil, climate, and atmosphere). An ecosystem is formed when the community (various types of population) and nonliving environment interact and function together. A small puddle at the back of the home is the best example where all sorts of living things, from microorganisms to insects and plants, may be available. These may depend on nonliving things, like water, sunlight, turbulence in the puddle, temperature, atmospheric pressure and even nutrients in the water for life.

Size

The size of an ecosystem can vary. It can exist in a small area, such as underneath a rock, a decaying tree-trunk, small aquarium or it can exist in large forms, such as entire rain-forest or an ocean. Technically, the earth can be called a 'huge ecosystem.' As long as both the living organisms and nonliving things are present and interact together, life is sustained and it is considered as an ecosystem. An ecosystem can be created artificially in a test tube in the laboratory. The biosphere is made of a number of ecosystems, such as ponds, lakes, streams, rivers, seas and seashore, grasslands, deserts, forests, etc.

To make things simple, ecosystems can be categorized into three main scales:

- **Micro:** A small-scale ecosystem, such as a pond, puddle, tree trunk, under a rock, etc.
- **Messo:** A medium-scale ecosystem, such as a forest or a large lake.
- **Biome:** A very large ecosystem or collection of ecosystems with similar biotic and abiotic factors, such as an entire rainforest with millions of animals and trees, with many different water bodies running through them.

Ecosystem boundaries are not marked (separated) by rigid lines. They are often separated by geographical barriers, such as deserts, mountains, oceans, lakes and rivers. As these borders are never rigid, ecosystems tend to blend into each other. This is why a lake can have many small ecosystems with their own unique characteristics. Scientists call this blending 'ecotone.'

Components

There are two major components of an ecosystem:

1. **Living organisms:** The living organisms refer to the biotic community which includes plants, animals and microbes. Plants in the presence of sunlight convert carbon dioxide and water into carbohydrate, and thus manufacture their own food. So, they are called 'producers.' Animals, on the other hand, consume the product of plants and animals. So, they are also called 'consumers.' Microbes including bacteria, fungi and insects break down the dead organic matter, consume some of the decomposed products and release simple substances which are used by the plants to manufacture their food. They are called 'decomposers.'
2. **Nonliving things:** The nonliving things are called 'abiotic components.' These are comprised of physical and chemical substances, which include sunlight, water, oxygen, carbon dioxide, minerals, dead plants and animal matter and other factors, such as temperature, light, heat, wind and rainfall, etc. All these help in growth of plants and animals. There are a number of cycles, such as carbon cycle, nitrogen which helps in ecosystem's maintenance.

Environment and health hydrogen cycle, energy cycle, etc. which help in manufacturing of food by plants, maintenance of composition of air, formulation of moisture and rain, maintenance of healthy soil, temperature, weather conditions and agricultural aspects, etc.

Ecosystems can be put into two groups. If the ecosystem exists in a water body, like an ocean, fresh water or puddle, it is called an 'aquatic ecosystem.' Those that exist outside the water bodies are called 'terrestrial ecosystems.'

Levels of Organization

To understand the levels of belonging in an ecosystem, let us discuss the following terminology **Figure 6.1**.

Individual, Species, Organism

An individual is any living thing or organism. Individuals do not breed with individuals from other groups. Animals,

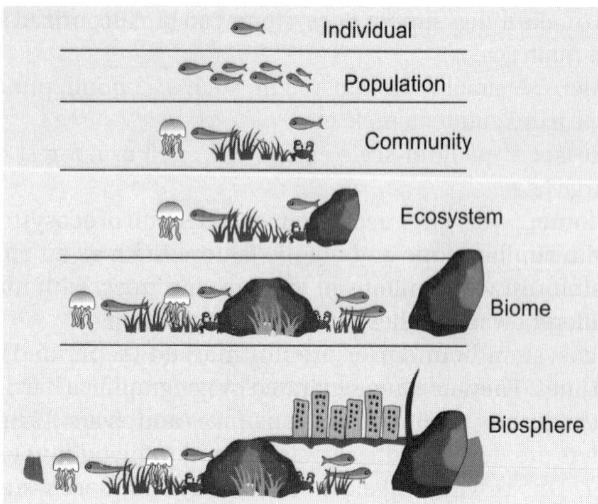

Fig. 6.1: Levels of organization.

unlike plants, tend to be very definite with this term because some plants can cross-breed with other fertile plants.

In the diagram above, the goldfish is interacting with its environment, and will only cross-breed with other gold fishes just like her.

Population

It refers to a group of individuals of a given species that live in a specific geographic area at a given period of time. For example, Gill and his family and friends and other fishes of Gill's species. Note that populations include individuals of the same species, but may have different genetic make-up such as hair/eye/skin color and size between themselves and other populations.

This includes all the populations in a specific area at a given point of time. A community includes populations of organisms of different species. In the diagram above, note how populations of goldfishes, salmons, crabs and herrings coexist in a defined location. A great community usually includes biodiversity.

Ecosystem

As explained in the pages earlier, ecosystems include more than a community of living organisms (abiotic) interacting with the environment (abiotic). At this level, note how they depend on other abiotic factors, such as rocks, water, air and temperature.

Biome

A biome, in simple terms, is a set of ecosystems sharing similar characteristics with their abiotic factors adapted to their environments. Biomes are very large ecological areas on the earth's surface, with fauna and flora (animals and plants) adapting to their environment. Biomes are often defined by abiotic factors, such as climate, relief, geology, soils and vegetation. A biome is not an ecosystem, although, in a way, it can look like a massive ecosystem. There are five major categories of biomes on earth—desert biomes, aquatic biomes, forest biomes, grassland biomes and tundra biomes.

Biosphere

When we consider all the different biomes, each blending into the other, with all the human beings living in many different geographic areas, we form a huge community of humans, animals and plants, in their defined habitats. A biosphere is the sum of all the ecosystems established on earth.

Food Chain and Food Web

The living organisms of the ecosystems of biosphere have feeding relationship with one another to sustain life and maintain balance in these. In this feeding relationship, one organism becomes the food for another, which, in turn, becomes food for the third organism, third for fourth—this goes on to form a chain. Food chains are usually in a sequence, with an arrow used to show the flow of energy. Below are some living things that can fit into a food chain. All the food chains begin from a plant (the producer) and end at a microorganisms (the decomposer). In this way, there is a flow of solar energy in the form of food energy from the plant to a series of organisms. A food chain is not the same as a food web. A food web is a network of many food chains and is more complex.

The sun is the source of all the energy in food chains. Green plants, usually the first level of any food chain, absorb the sun's light energy to make their own food by the process of photosynthesis. Green plants (autotrophs) are, therefore, known as 'Producers' in a food chain.

The second level of the food chains is called the 'Primary Consumer'. These consume the green plants. Animals in this group are usually herbivores. Examples include insects, sheep, caterpillars and even cows.

The third in the chain are 'Secondary Consumers'. These usually eat up the primary consumers and other animal matter. They are commonly called 'carnivores' and examples include lions, snakes and cats.

The fourth level is called 'Tertiary Consumers'. These are animals that eat secondary consumers.

Quaternary Consumers Eat Tertiary Consumers

At the top of the levels are predators. They are animals that have little or no natural enemies. They are the 'bosses' of their ecosystems. Predators feed on preys. A prey is an animal that predators hunt to kill and feed on. Predators include owls, snakes, wild cats, crocodiles and sharks. Humans can also be called 'predators'.

When any organism dies, detritivores (like vultures, worms and crabs) eat it up. The rest are broken down by decomposers (mostly bacteria and fungi), and the exchange of energy continues. Decomposers start the cycle again.

Principles

The laws of ecosystem/ecology help to explain the status of a man's health as well as environmental health. In simple and informal forms, these are as under everything is related to everything else.

It means all living organism and nonliving things in an ecosystem are interconnected. It implies that any change or manipulation in any one of the living or nonliving component may have a very harmful effect on the environment, e.g., use of pesticides on crops especially which are eaten raw cause harmful effects like gastrointestinal disturbances and neurological problems, etc. Pesticides can also palate the soil and the pollutant can affects successive crops.

Everything Must Go Somewhere

It means the organisms excretion or waste is taken by other organisms as food. This helps in removal of waste excreted by various forms of life from the environment to quite an extent.

Nature Knows Best

It means the changes brought about by human beings in any natural system do not always improve the system. It may cause harmful effect, e.g., conditioning of air temperature and humidity by air conditioner, treatment of soil with insecticide, use of fertilizer in agriculture may improve certain aspect of life but may cause many harmful effects on living organism and disturb nature.

Preservation of Nature

In order to preserve the nature (biosphere), anything which is removed must be added and anything which is added must be removed. For example, trees must be planted, if these are removed, poisonous gases and substances must be removed from the air and water, which is added through automobiles. Oxygen and water which are used must be replaced. In this way, it helps in maintaining a balance in the environment.

To what extent these laws are obeyed or disobeyed by people will determine the health of our biosphere. This will depend upon their knowledge, skill, attitude and behavior.

Ecological Balance

The ability of nature to remain unchanged is called 'balance of nature' or 'ecological balance'. The whole biosphere is an ecosystem, a system of 'give-and-take' among the plants, animals and their physical surroundings. In theory, it is a close cycle and remains in balance, but, in practice, it is seldom in a state of balance. The process of interaction to sustain life on earth and maintain balance in this biosphere goes on. In an environment, we find many organisms which are harmful to man and also many conditions, which are difficult to live in, e.g., very hot (humid conditions) or very cold (dry conditions) **(Fig. 6.2)**.

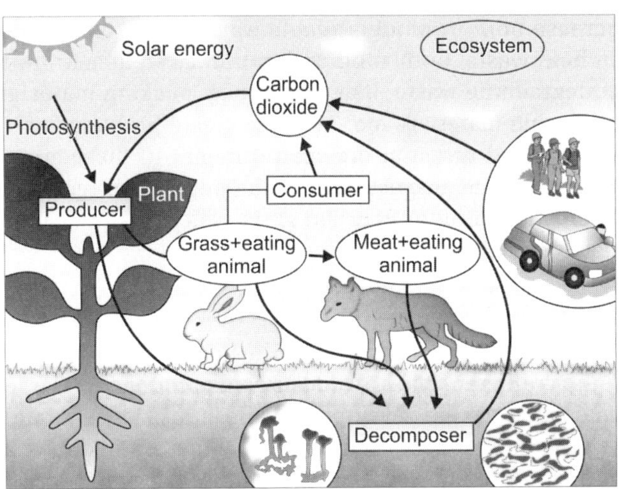

Fig. 6.2: Ecological balance.

In order to sustain life, live healthy and comfortably, man has to make lots of adjustments to his environment. In this process of adjustment, he has devised various artificial ways to modify his environment. Many chemicals and medicines have been manufactured to kill the harmful organisms. Many man-made resources have been developed to make life comfortable, fast, healthy and lengthy. All man-made resources have been useful in improving the living conditions in many ways but have been found to pollute the environment and affect the ecological balance. It causes many health problems, like occupational hazards and diseases, cardiovascular and neuromuscular diseases, cancer, etc.

Factors Affecting Ecosystem

The changes which are taking place in the environment in the various ecosystems of our biosphere affect the ecosystem. Some changes are cyclic and are transient because of seasonal variation and changes (e.g., flood, droughts, etc.). Whereas some others are irreversible and permanent, e.g., geological transformation, continental drifts, etc. The changes done by human beings become more prominent, making the environment unwholesome. The air we breathe every moment is not fresh. The man-made factors affecting the ecosystem are as follows:

Population Explosion

According to the Census 2011, the population is 1.21 billion in India with 20 million added every year. However, most of the growth is taking place in the developing countries. However, at present, some developing countries have very low rates of population growth, whereas some high-income countries have high rates because of immigration. Population and economic growth in urban centers have been increasing pressure on ecosystems. However, dense urban settlement is considered to be a lesser burden on the environment than the urban and suburban sprawl. Moreover, pressures on some ecosystems have been significantly lowered by the movement of people to urban areas. This population explosion, especially in the specific urban areas (urban slums) is creating problems due to overcrowding, depletion/natural resources and development of man-made resources by industrialization, green revolution, etc. The rapid increase in our population is creating the problem of waste management. There is an increase both in biodegradable waste, like excrements, kitchen, waste, both solid and liquid, as well as in non-biodegradable waste, like plastic bag, packing material, disposable materials, etc. All these create problems of its disposal and threat to the environment. All these create problems of its disposal. Increasing population results in the creation of slums in urban areas, which, in turn, causes an adverse effect on the environment.

Industrialization

By developing industrial revolution in the twentieth century, different types of industries, like cottage and large-scale industries are developed. All the industries generate a lot of waste products, such as gases, effluents, solid matter, thermal waste, etc. These waste materials are often released directly into the air, rivers, streams, drains on the land which deteriorate our environment and cause harmful effects not only to human beings but also other animals, plants, and also destroy the nonliving things, like buildings and monuments. Industrialization also increases the number of daily wagers.

Urbanization

There has been an increase in urbanization of our population. It is due to industrial revolution, poverty and lack of resources and services in the villages. People from the villages migrate to the towns and cities for employment, education, etc., resulting in overcrowding and slums most often on the unauthorized land. Usually, in these areas, there is a lack of the basic amenities, like water, electricity, drainage, toilet facilities, etc. Often the slum-dwellers try to attain the electricity and water connections through foul means. This situation not only creates administrative problems but also causes adverse effects on the environment and results in many physical, mental and social health problems for the slum-dwellers and city people.

Automobiles

Automobiles save time, efforts and labor of all the people in their transportation. But the exhaust from the automobiles is composed of carbon monoxide, hydrocarbon, lead, and nitrogen oxide, which crate a great havoc in the atmosphere.

It also causes traffic jams with long halting time at the signals. This increases the emission of exhaust in the air leading to air pollution. Vehicles are also the cause of noise pollution in the environment.

Modern Agricultural Practices

Irrigational activities in rural areas often lead to logging of water which promotes breeding of mosquitoes. At times, in certain areas, due to excessive irrigation from canal water, the land becomes marshy and useless for cultivation. Chemical fertilizers and insecticides are used in order to maintain high productivity. The insecticides and chemical fertilizers have lasting effects on agriculture products and passed to various animals through food chain or food webs and cause harmful effects on the organisms.

Change in Economic Activity

Global economic activity has increased nearly sevenfold in the last 50 years. As per capita income grows, demand for many ecosystem services increases and the structure of consumption also changes. The share of income devoted to food, for example, decreases in favor of industrial goods and services.

Socio-political Factors

These factors include decision-making processes and the extent of public participation in them. The trend toward democratic institutions over the past 50 years has helped empower local communities. There has also been an increase in multilateral environmental agreements.

Cultural and Religious Factors

In this context, culture can be defined as the values, beliefs, and norms that a group of people share. It conditions individuals' perceptions of the world, and suggests the courses of action, which can have an important impact on the environment.

Deforestation

Deforestation refers to the reducing forest area due to demand of wood for constructing houses, buildings, industries, dams, roads and also wood for fire as required by human beings. These have been in demand since the time a human being has lived in the biosphere, but, at present, due to increase in population and modernization, these activities have increased. Because of deforestation, there is reduced vegetation and also soil erosion on the hills. Thus, water is not held and flows along with soil into the river, thus resulting in floods. Deforestation also reduces the amount of water being transferred from the ground to the air because of reduced number of trees causing change in climate and also causing adverse effects on the environment.

Radioactive Substances

Radioactive substances, like radium, uranium, etc. emit radiations and pollute the environment, causing cancers to the human beings. These substances are used in laboratories, hospitals and power plants where nuclear bombs are manufactured. These radioactive wastes require special methods of disposal. If not followed properly, these can pollute water and also air, etc.

Natural Calamities

Natural calamities are grave disasters or misfortune of great magnitudes, which occur by nature and cause disruption on the environment. These calamities include floods, earthquakes, draughts, cyclones, volcanoes, landslides, avalanches and tidal waves in the seas. In floods, due to the excessive overflow of water from the river to nearby villages and towns, the entire life and environment get disrupted. Earthquakes are tremors of the earth's surface. These can range from mild to severe and can cause widespread destruction of the environment. Drought is mainly caused due to lack of rainfall, which results in the lack of vegetation of any form and makes it difficult for the people to survive. Cyclone erupts with violent disturbances in the atmosphere with high-speed wind, and frequent rainfall and thunderstorm, which disrupts the environment. During landslide, falling of large mass of earth along the slope of mountain on to the area down the mountain causes a lot of damage. Usually, heavy rainfall and deforestation cause landslide. Similarly, volcanoes and tidal waves can harm the environment. Volcanoes refer to the ejection of various gases, ashes and molten rock (lava) with tremendous heat from within the earth through weak surface of a mountain. Similarly, tidal there is an occurrence of exceptionally large waves in the ocean when earthquake occurs deep inside the bottom. These waves destroy the towns, cities, etc.

BIODIVERSITY

Variation is the law of nature. It occurs every moment and everywhere. The variations take place at micro levels which may be linear or cyclic. The variety and variability of organisms and ecosystems is referred to as biological diversity or biodiversity. Biodiversity is the term used to describe the variety of life found on earth and all the natural processes. The World Commission on Environment and Development (WCED) constituted by the UN General Assembly published a report in 1987 which provided a boost and endorsement to the need for conserving the world's rich biodiversity. Biodiversity includes ecosystem, genetic and cultural diversity, and the connections between these and all the other species.

The different aspects of biodiversity all have a very strong influence on each other.

Definitions

The Canadian Biodiversity Strategy defines biodiversity as 'the variety of species and ecosystems on earth and the ecological processes of which they are a part, including ecosystem, species, and genetic diversity. In short, the term is used to refer to life in all its forms and the natural processes that support and connect all forms.

Biodiversity is not easily defined because it is more than just the sum of its parts, as all of its elements are integral to maintaining functioning, evolving resilient ecosystems.

The variety of life at every hierarchical level and spatial scale of biological organizations: genes within populations, populations within species, species within communities, communities within landscapes, landscapes within biomes, and biomes within the biosphere.

The levels of organization of biodiversity include ecosystems, species and gene components.

The United Nations Convention on Biological Diversity provides a similar definition for biodiversity: 'the variability among the living organisms from all sources including, inter alia (among other things), terrestrial, marine and other aquatic ecosystems and the ecological complexes of which they are part; this includes the diversity within the:

- Species are a complete, self-generating, unique ensemble of genetic variation, capable of interbreeding and producing fertile offspring. They (and their subspecies and populations) are generally considered to be the only self-replicating units of genetic diversity that can function independently.
- Genes are the working units of heredity; each gene is a segment of the DNA molecule that encodes a single enzyme or structural protein unit. Genetic diversity is the foundation of all biodiversity's. Genetic variation permits populations to adapt to the changing environment and continue to participate in life's processes.

The three primary attributes of biodiversity are:

1. **Composition:** Composition is the identity and variety of an ecological system. Descriptors of composition are typically lists of the species resident in an area or an ecosystem and measures of composition include richness and diversity of species.
2. **Structure:** Structure is the physical organization or pattern of a system, from habitat complexity as measured within the communities to the pattern of habitats (or patches) and other elements at a landscape scale.
3. **Functions:** Functions are the result of one or more ecological and evolutionary processes, including predation, gene flow, natural disturbances and mycorrhizal associations as well as abiotic processes, such as soil development and hydrological cycles. Examples of functions include predator-prey systems, water purifications and nutrient cycle.

Appropriate conservation and sustainable development strategies attempt to recognize this as being integral to any approach to preserving biodiversity. Almost all cultures have their roots in our biological diversity in some way or the other. Biodiversity boosts the ecosystem's productivity where each species, no matter how small, has an important role to play.

Types of Biodiversity

There are three essential types of biodiversity, which are shown in **Figure 6.3**:

1. Species biodiversity
2. Genetic biodiversity
3. Ecological biodiversity

Genetic Diversity

It refers to differences between the genetic resources of organisms. Each individual of a particular species differs from the other in its genetic constitution. That is why every human is different from another. Similarly, the species of rice, wheat, maize, barley, etc., have different varieties.

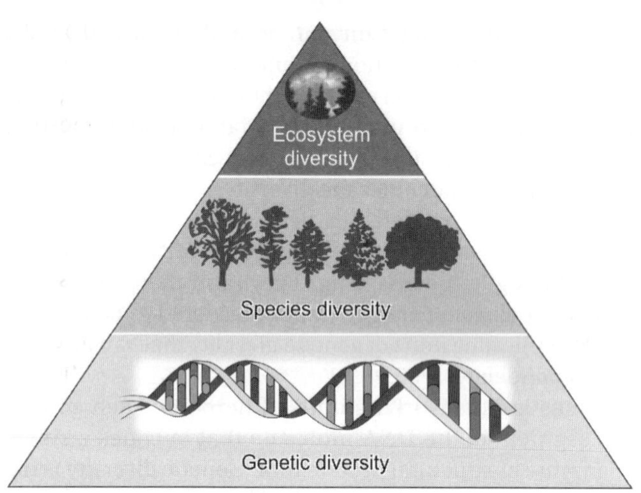

Fig. 6.3: Types of biodiversity.

Each member of any animal or plant species differs widely from other individuals in its genetic makeup because many combinations of genes are possible that give specific characteristics to each individual. This genetic variability is essential for the healthy reproduction of a species.

Today, the diversity of nature is being exploited more by using wild relatives of crop plants to create new varieties of more productive crops and breed better domestic animals. Modern biotechnology manipulates genes to develop better types of drugs and a variety of industrial products. Although all species have come from a single or common ancestor, species diverge and produce new unique characteristics over time, thus contributing to biodiversity.

Species Diversity

The species' diversity refers to a group of similar organisms that typically mate to produce offspring. They commonly share the same ancestry. It is the number of different species that are represented in a given community. Species diversity is the most basic classification unit and includes all species ranging from plants to various microorganisms. Additionally, two different individuals from the same species group are also not exactly similar; they have diversity. For instance, two other human beings are not the same. Apart from this, people situated in entirely different regions have a significant level of diversity. The total numbers of different species of plants and animals located in an area form this type of diversity. It is believed that there are about 5–10 million species in the world; however, only 1.75 million of those species have been named scientifically so far on earth.

There are two constituents of species diversity:

1. **Species richness:** Number of different species present in an ecosystem. Tropical areas have greater species richness as the environment is conducive for a large number of species.
2. **Species evenness:** Relative abundance of individuals of each of those species. If the number of individuals within a species is fairly constant across communities, it is said to have a high evenness and if the number of individuals varies from species to species, it is said to have low evenness. High evenness leads to greater specific diversity.

Ecological Diversity

Ecological diversity is the complex network of different species present in local ecosystems and the dynamic interactions. An ecosystem consists of organisms of many several species living in a region and their connections through the flow of energy, nutrients, and matter. Those relationships occur as organisms of different species interact with each other. The primary source of energy in almost every ecosystem is the sun. The radiant energy of the sun is converted into chemical energy by plants. This energy flows from those systems when animals eat plants and are then consumed by other animals in return. Fungi get energy by decomposing organisms, which release nutrients back into the soil.

Thus, an ecosystem comprises living components (microbes, plants, animals, and fungi) and nonliving components (climate and chemicals) connected by energy flow and interact with each other. Ecological biodiversity is associated with plant and animal species living together and connected by the food chain and food webs. Diversity in various ecosystems, such as deserts, rainforests, mangroves, etc., also includes ecological diversity. It is generally observed between different ecosystems in a region.

Ecological diversity has three major perspectives. The diversity of different species in a landscape is typically measured in three distinct scales. They are termed alpha diversity, beta diversity, and gamma diversity.

Alpha Diversity

Alpha diversity is the type of ecological diversity found within a specific region, community, or ecosystem. More specifically, alpha diversity refers to the species diversity within a community at a local scale or small scale, most often the size of one ecosystem, comprises two components, i.e., species richness and evenness. Generally, it is represented by the total number of different species (or species richness) in that particular region. This is often measured by the total number of taxa or distinct organism groups within the corresponding ecosystem (species, genera, and families). In particular, if we think of diversity in an area, we refer to the alpha diversity more often than not.

Beta (β) Diversity

Beta diversity is the inter-community diversity expressing the rate of species turnover per unit change in habitat. Beta diversity refers to the type of ecological diversity measured by distinguishing the species diversity between different ecosystems or along with environmental gradients. The measurement of beta diversity typically involves comparing the number counts of taxa unique to each ecosystem. In simple words, it is the measure of species diversity between two separate entities at a larger scale, usually separated by a specific geographical barrier such as the mountain ridge or the river. It is the rate of change in species composition across habitats or among communities. Furthermore, beta diversity determines a quantitative measure of the diversity of communities that experience the changing environments.

Gamma (γ) Diversity

Gamma diversity is the overall diversity at landscape level includes both α and β. Gamma diversity typically refers to all species richness over a large region (at a vast scale). It is the measure of the complete diversity for various distinct ecosystems within a region. In simple words, it is often studied as a biome where the species diversity is observed between several ecosystems. This usually ranges over the areas such as the whole mountain slope or the complete littoral zone of a seashore.

Let us understand these three perspectives with the help of an example. Suppose an area of mountain slope is the landscape. The mountain slope usually contains various patches of grasslands and forests. Here, alpha diversity refers to all such species diversity situated within every single grassland or forest patch of the slope. Beta diversity refers to all such species diversity located between any two patches and their corresponding communities. Lastly, the given landscape's gamma diversity refers to all those species diversity present along with the entire range of the slope.

Value of Biodiversity

Biodiversity provides a variety of environmental services from its species and ecosystems that are essential at the global, regional and local levels. It is essential for preserving ecological processes, such as fixing and recycling of nutrients, soil formation, circulation and cleansing of air and water, global life support, maintaining the water balance within ecosystems, watershed protection, maintaining stream and river flows throughout the year, erosion control and local flood reduction. Food, clothing, housing, energy, medicines are all resources that are directly or indirectly linked to the biological variety present in the biosphere.

- **Consumptive use value:** A straight consumptive use is the direct utilization of timber, food, fuelwood and fodder by local communities. The diversity of organisms provide food, clothing, shelter, medicines, proteins, enzymes, papers, sports goods, musical instruments, beverages, narcotics, pets, zoo specimens, tourism and raw material for business prospects, etc.
- **Productive use value:** This category comprises of marketable goods. The biotechnologist uses bio-rich areas to prospect and search for potential genetic properties in plants or animals that can be used to develop better varieties of crops for use in farming and plantation programs or to develop better livestock. To the pharmacist, biological diversity is the raw material from which new drugs can be identified from plant or animal products. To industrialists, biodiversity is rich storehouse from which to develop new products. For the agricultural scientist, the biodiversity is the basis for developing better crops. A variety of industries, like pharmaceuticals are highly dependent on identifying compounds of great economic value from the wide variety of wild species of plants located in undisturbed natural forests called "biological prospecting".
- **Social values:** Social value of biodiversity prospecting motivated habitat conservation in some areas, as traditional societies valued it as a resource. Ecosystem people value biodiversity as a part of their livelihood as well as through cultural and religious sentiments. A great variety of crops have been cultivated in traditional agricultural systems and permitted a wide range of produce to be grown and marketed throughout the year and acted as an insurance against the failure of one crop. In recent years, farmers have begun to receive economic incentives to grow cash crops for national or international markets, rather than to supply local needs. This has resulted in local food shortages, unemployment, landlessness, and increased vulnerability to drought and floods.
- **Ethical and moral values:** Ethical values related to biodiversity conservation are based on the importance of protecting all forms of life against illegal activities like cloning of animals, smuggling of valuable biodiversity instances, bio-piracy, illicit trade etc. In India, several generations have preserved nature through local traditions. However, immediate benefit rather than ethics appears to be modern man's objective.
- **Aesthetic value:** Biodiversity is a direct source of pleasure and aesthetic satisfaction—its contribution to quality of life, outdoor recreation and scenic enjoyment. They provide opportunities for recreational activities such as hiking, canoeing, bird watching, river rafting, rock climbing, trekking, parasailing, and nature photography. The designing of thousands of new horticultural species, wildlife conservation, landscape luxury, national parks, zoological and botanical gardens, snake, crocodile, butterfly parks, and biotechnologically manipulated novel curios species added to the existing aesthetics.
- **Option value:** Keeping future possibilities open for their use is called 'option value'. It is impossible to predict which of our species or traditional varieties of crops and domestic animals will be of greatest use in the future. Important ecosystem services and uses for plants and animals are still unknown and await discovery. It becomes valuable if targets are based on policy of obtaining wealth from wastes.

Threats to Biodiversity

The diversity in India, i.e., forests, grasslands, wetlands, mountains, deserts and marine ecosystems face many pressures. One of the major causes for the loss of biological diversity in India has been the depletion of vegetative cover in order to expand agriculture. Since most of the biodiversity rich forests also contain the maximum mineral wealth and also the best sites for water impoundment, mining and development projects in such areas have often led to destruction of habitats. Poaching and illegal trade of wildlife products too have adversely affected biological diversity. The threats to Biodiversity change can be natural or man-made. Man-made threats are developmental pressure like construction, forest-based industries, hydel/irrigation projects, mining, oil drilling, pollution, resource extraction, etc., road and transport, etc. The common threats to biodiversity are described below.

Climate Change

Long-term and irreversible change that occurs in the earth's climate can increase or decrease the temperature of the atmosphere which has major effects on the environment such as rising of the sea levels, and glacial retreats. The biodiversity of organisms are affected due to such change regarding their population, distribution, level of the ecosystem, and even the individuals' morphology and function. Due to increase in temperature, organisms have already adapted by expanding their ranges in latitudes many species population have declined because of this behavior. Aside from this, many animals have exhibited changes in the timings of their physiological functions. These include the birds and insects migrating and mating earlier than usual, which then result in some failure in breeding and production of young.

Regarding ecosystems, studies revealed that climate change has brought the expansion of many desert ecosystems and thus have effects on the function and services that the ecosystem can provide.

For humans, the rapidly increasing rate in climate change imposes great threats for human security as the natural resources are becoming more and more limited. At present, global warming and climate change already have irreversible impacts on biodiversity. And these effects, if not mitigated, can lead to more significant threats in the future.

Habitat Loss and Degradation

Habitat loss refers to changes in the environment that result to the rendering of a specific habitat to be functionally valuable. The habitat can no longer accommodate and support the life of the organisms present, thereby declining their population.

Habitat loss may either be caused by natural events like natural calamities and geological events or anthropogenic activities like deforestation and man-induced climate change.

In the process the organisms that were once living in a particular area or region are displaced and are forced to relocate which resulting in biodiversity reduction. Man-made efforts like the practice of clearing out ecosystems for agriculture conversion, industrial expansion, logging and mining, continues to displace organisms of their natural habitat.

Pollution

All forms of pollution like water, air, or land pollution, appear to be a threat to all life forms on earth and plays a major threat to biodiversity when it comes to the nutrient loading of the elements nitrogen and phosphorus. In Europe, atmospheric nitrogen is the only pollutant that has not decreased in concentration since the implementation of legislation. Its mere presence poses huge challenges to the conservation measures intended to natural habitats and species living there. Furthermore, the presence of nitrogen compounds in water systems can cause eutrophication (excessive plant and algal growth).

The presence and accumulation of phosphorus in water systems can alter the way food webs function. Excessive phosphorus, like nitrogen can result to the uncontrolled growth of planktonic algae thus increasing organic matter deposition in the seabed.

Another form of pollution that can damage and kill living organisms is acid rain. Acid rain, as its name suggests, is rain that is composed of harmful acids (i.e., nitric and sulfuric acid). This rain is usually a result of pollution coming from the excessive burning of fossil fuels.

Some types of pollution, like the depletion of the ozone layer, can be reversible. However, this shall only happen when humans stop or limit the use of various chemicals that contribute to its destruction.

Invasive Species

An exotic or unnatural species can be any kind of organism that has been introduced to a foreign habitat. This introduction can cause major threats to the native species as they often become subjected to great competition for resources, disease, and predation. When these species have successfully colonized the area, they are already called "invasive" ones.

The greatest threat that invasive species can bring is their capability to change an entire habitat. These species are highly adaptable and can easily dominate a certain area. Because many natural species survive only in a particular environment, they tend to be displaced, or worse, perish.

Overexploitation: Overexploitation refers to the act of overharvesting species and natural resources at rates faster than they can actually sustain themselves in the wild. Because of this, species population is put into great risk of reduction. Overharvesting, overfishing, and overhunting are some examples of overexploitation. Additionally, some species of living organisms find it hard to reproduce when their number is too small. So as a population or ecosystem continues to suffer from low species diversity, the probability of getting wiped out completely when a natural disaster or other forces increases.

Other Potential Threats

Aside from the five aforementioned threats, there are still a lot of drivers that may either directly or indirectly contribute to the loss of biodiversity. One good example of this are the epidemics and infectious diseases of wildlife such as Ebola virus disease, infectious bursal disease, and flu. This phenomenon does not only affect wildlife but also human health as well.

Biodiversity Conservation

Biodiversity conservation is the protection and management of biodiversity to obtain resources for sustainable development. Biodiversity conservation has three main objectives:

1. To preserve the diversity of species.
2. Sustainable utilization of species and ecosystem.
3. To maintain life-supporting systems and essential ecological processes.

Biodiversity and its Conservation Methods

Biodiversity refers to the variability of life on earth. It can be conserved in the following ways:

- In-situ Conservation
- Ex-situ Conservation

In-situ Conservation

In-situ conservation of biodiversity is the conservation of species within their natural habitat. In this method, the natural ecosystem is maintained and protected. The in-situ conservation has several advantages which are described bellow:

- It is a cost-effective and convenient method of conserving biodiversity.
- A large number of living organisms can be conserved simultaneously.
- Since the organisms are in a natural ecosystem, they can evolve better and can easily adjust to different environmental conditions.

Certain protected areas where in-situ conservation takes place include national parks, wildlife sanctuaries and biosphere reserves.

National Parks

These are small reserves maintained by the government. Its boundaries are well demarcated and human activities such as grazing, forestry, habitat and cultivation are prohibited, e.g., Kanha National Park, Bandipur National Park.

Wildlife Sanctuaries

These are the regions where only wild animals are found. Human activities such as timber harvesting, cultivation, collection of woods and other forest products are allowed here as long as they do not interfere with the conservation project. Also, tourists visit these places for recreation.

Biosphere Reserves

Biosphere reserves are multi-purpose protected areas where the wildlife, traditional lifestyle of the inhabitants and domesticated plants and animals are protected. Tourist and research activities are permitted here.

Ex-situ Conservation

Ex-situ conservation of biodiversity involves the breeding and maintenance of endangered species in artificial ecosystems such as zoos, nurseries, botanical gardens, gene banks, etc. There is less competition for food, water and space among the organisms.

Advantages of Ex-situ conservation:

- The animals are provided with a longer time and breeding activity.
- The species bred in captivity can be reintroduced in the wild.
- Genetic techniques can be used for the preservation of endangered species.

Strategies for Biodiversity Conservation

Following are the important strategies for biodiversity conservation:

- All the varieties of food, timber plants, livestock, microbes and agricultural animals should be conserved.
- All the economically important organisms should be identified and conserved.
- Unique ecosystems should be preserved first.
- The resources should be utilized efficiently.
- Poaching and hunting of wild animals should be prevented.
- The reserves and protected areas should be developed carefully.
- The levels of pollutants should be reduced in the environment.
- Deforestation should be strictly prohibited.
- Environmental laws should be followed strictly.
- The useful and endangered species of plants and animals should be conserved in their nature as well as artificial habitats.
- Public awareness should be created regarding biodiversity conservation and its importance.

WATER

Introduction

Water is one of the most vital natural resources for all lives on earth. The availability and quality of water always have played an important part in determining not only where people can live, but also their quality of life. Even though there always has been plenty of fresh water on earth, water has not always been available when and where it is needed.

Water covers 71% of the earth's surface. It is vital for all known forms of life. On earth, 96.5% of the planet's water is found in seas and oceans, 1.7% in groundwater, 1.7% in glaciers and the ice caps of Antarctica and Greenland, a small fraction in other large water bodies, and 0.001% in the air as vapor, clouds (formed of solid and liquid water particles suspended in air), and precipitation. Only 2.5% of the earth's water is freshwater, and 98.8% of that water is in ice and groundwater. Less than 0.3% of all freshwater is in rivers, lakes, and the atmosphere, and an even smaller amount of the earth's freshwater (0.003%) is contained within biological bodies and manufactured products. Water on earth moves continually through the water cycle of evaporation and transpiration (evapotranspiration), condensation, precipitation, and runoff usually reaching the sea. Evaporation and transpiration contribute to the precipitation over land. Safe drinking water is essential to humans and other life forms even though it provides no calories or organic nutrients. Access to safe drinking water has improved over the last decades in almost every part of the world, but approximately one billion people still lack access to safe water. Safe wholesome water is essential for every individual for a healthy life.

Safe Wholesome Water

Definition

Potable water is free from harmful microorganisms and substances, even if it may have color, odor, or taste problem due to dissolved minerals. 'Wholesome' water is fit to use for drinking, cooking, food preparation or washing without any potential danger to human health by meeting the requirements of regulations made under Section 67 (Standards of Wholesomeness) of the Water Act, 1991. These stipulate the criteria that the water must meet in order to protect the lifelong health of the population. These parameters include limits on:

- Biological quality (including levels of bacteria and oocysts)
- Chemical quality (including levels of metals, solvents, pesticides and hydrocarbons)
- Physical qualities (including color, taste and odor)
- However, wholesome water to be suitable for washing (i.e., washbasins, baths, showers and bidets).

If an alternative water source is being considered, its reliability to provide the necessary quantity of water should also be assessed. Where the quantity cannot be guaranteed (excluding exceptional events, as even water mains can burst and cause cuts), a back-up supply will be needed. If the back-up supply is from a wholesome water source, there must be no possibility of contamination of the wholesome water supply by non wholesome water (by strict compliance with the water regulations).

Water Resources

Water resources are divisible into three distinct categories:

The surface-water resources, the groundwater resources and rainwater resources. Each of these categories is a part of the earth's water circulatory system, called the 'hydrologic cycle', and is derived from precipitation, which is rainfall plus snow.

Surface water resource: Sea, river, stream, tanks, lake, pond, etc.

Groundwater resources: Shallow well, deep well, tube well, boreholes and spring, etc.

Rainwater: Generally collected and stored, referred to as 'harvested rainwater'.

Uses of Water

Water can be used in a community in various ways.

Domestic Purposes

For domestic purpose, the water can be used in cooking, bathing, drinking, washing, flushing the toilets and gardening, etc. It is estimated that 8% of worldwide water use is for household purposes. Basic household water requirements have been estimated by Peter Gleick at around 50 liters per person per day, excluding water for gardens.

Public Amenities

For public amenities, water is used in cleaning streets, recreational purposes, like swimming pools, public fountains, fire protection and public parks. Recreational water use is usually a very small but growing percentage of total water use. Recreational water use is mostly tied to reservoirs. Commercial water use includes fresh water for motels, hotels, restaurants, office buildings, other commercial facilities, and civilian and military institutions. Domestic water use is probably the most important daily use of water for most people.

Industrial Purposes

Industrial water use is a valuable resource to the nation's industries for such purposes, as processing, cleaning, transportation, dilution, and cooling in manufacturing facilities. Major water-using industries include steel, chemical, paper, and petroleum refining. Industries often reuse the same water over and over for more than one purpose.

Agricultural Purposes

Irrigation water use is water artificially applied to farm, orchard, pasture, and horticultural crops, as well as water used to irrigate pastures, for frost and freeze protection, chemical application, crop cooling, harvesting, and for the leaching of salts from the crop root zone. Nonagricultural activities include self-supplied water to irrigate public and private golf courses, parks.

Animal Husbandry

Livestock water use includes water for stock animals, feed lots, dairies, fish farms, and other nonfarm needs. Water is needed for the production of red meat, poultry, eggs, milk, and wool, and for horses, rabbits, and pets. Livestock water use only includes fresh water.

Mining

Mining water use includes water for the extraction of naturally occurring minerals; solids, such as coal and ores; liquids, such as crude petroleum; and gases, such as natural gas. The category includes quarrying, milling (such as crushing, screening, washing, and flotation), and other operations as part of mining activity. A significant portion of the water used for mining, about 32%, is saline.

Thermoelectric Power

Thermoelectric power water use is the amount of water used in the production of electric power generated with heat. The source of the heat may be from fossil fuels, nuclear fission, or geothermal. Fossil fuel power plants typically reuse water. They generate electricity by turning a turbine using steam power. After the steam is used to turn the turbines, it is condensed back to water by cooling it. The condensed water is then routed back to the boiler, where the cycle begins again.

HARDNESS OF WATER

Water that does not form an immediate lather with soap is called 'hard water'. Hardness of water is due to the presence of soluble calcium, magnesium or iron compounds. The most common compounds are calcium bicarbonate $Ca(HCO_3)_2$, magnesium bicarbonate $Mg(HCO_3)_2$, calcium sulfate $CaSO_4$ and magnesium sulfate $MgSO_4$. The addition of soap forms an insoluble scum. The scum consists of insoluble salts of these metals.

Water that forms an immediate lather with soap is called 'soft water'. Such water does not have dissolved salts of calcium, magnesium and iron.

Types of Hardness

Depending upon the behavior of water towards soap, hardness is divided into two types.

Temporary Hardness

Hardness of water due to the presence of soluble bicarbonates of calcium and magnesium is called 'temporary hardness'. When water containing dissolved carbon dioxide passes over solid carbonates (chalk or limestone deposits, etc.), these compounds get dissolved in water. Rainwater and distilled water are always soft because they do not have dissolved (soluble) salts.

Temporary hardness is removed in the following ways:

- **By boiling the water:** Boiling promotes the formation of carbonate from the bicarbonate and precipitates calcium carbonate out of solution, leaving water that is softer upon cooling.
- Chemical methods.
- By adding slaked lime $[Ca(OH)_2]$ to hard water, insoluble carbonates are formed. The insoluble calcium carbonate is the 'fur' (or scale) formed in kettles, boilers, pipes, etc.

Permanent Hardness

This is due to the presence of chlorides and sulfates of calcium and magnesium. Permanent hardness is hardness (mineral content) that cannot be removed by boiling. When this is the case, it is usually caused by the presence of calcium sulfate and/or magnesium sulfates in the water, which do not precipitate out as the temperature increases. Such hardness can be removed by the addition of washing soda. This removes both the temporary and the permanent hardness of water.

Effects of Hard Water

- With hard water, soap solutions form a white precipitate (soap scum) instead of producing lather, because the 2+ ions destroy the surfactant properties of the soap by forming a solid precipitate (the soap scum). A major component of such scum is calcium stearate, which arises from sodium stearate, the main component of soap.
- Hard water also forms deposits that clog plumbing. These deposits, called 'scale', are composed mainly of calcium carbonate ($CaCO_3$), magnesium hydroxide ($Mg(OH)_2$), and calcium sulfate ($CaSO_4$). Calcium and magnesium carbonates tend to be deposited as off-white solids on the inside surfaces of pipes and heat exchangers. The resulting build-up of scale restricts the flow of water in pipes. In boilers, the deposits impair the flow of heat into water, reducing the heating efficiency and allowing the metal boiler components to overheat. In a pressurized system, this overheating can lead to failure of the boiler.
- The presence of ions in an electrolyte, in this case, hard water, can also lead to galvanic corrosion, in which one metal will preferentially corrode when in contact with another type of metal, when both are in contact with an electrolyte.
- In swimming pools, hard water is manifested by a turbid, or cloudy (milky), appearance to the water. Calcium and magnesium hydroxides are both soluble in water. The solubility of the hydroxides of the alkaline-earth metals to which calcium and magnesium belong (group 2 of the periodic table) increases moving down the column. Aqueous solutions of these metal hydroxides absorb carbon dioxide from the air, forming the insoluble carbonates, giving rise to the turbidity.

WATER POLLUTION

Water pollution is a major global problem which requires ongoing evaluation and revision of water resource policy at all levels (international down to individual aquifers and wells). It has been suggested that it is the leading worldwide cause of deaths and diseases, and that it accounts for the deaths of more than 14,000 people daily. An estimated 580 people in India die of water pollution-related illness everyday. Around 90% water in the cities of China is polluted and as of 2007, half a billion Chinese had no access to safe drinking water. In addition to the acute problems of water pollution in developing countries, developed countries continue to struggle with pollution problems as well.

Water pollution is defined as something that adversely impairs the beneficial use of water. It is the contamination of water bodies (e.g., lakes, rivers, oceans, aquifers and groundwater). Water pollution occurs when pollutants are directly or indirectly discharged into water bodies without adequate treatment to remove harmful compounds.

Classification and Sources

Physical Pollution

Physical pollution is the introduction of discarded materials into the environment. Physical pollution might be referred to as trash and is the direct result of human actions. Physical pollutants, such as discarded water bottles and plastic bags along with waste materials from industrial or manufacturing processes, do not naturally degrade and can accumulate or leach chemicals into the ground or water supplies as they break down.

Chemical Pollution

Chemical pollution is another type of pollution. It is defined as the introduction of chemicals into the environment. Agricultural practices are one example of a chemical pollution source. Chemical water pollutants are generally atoms or molecules, which have been discharged into natural water bodies, usually by activities of humans. Common examples of such chemical water pollutants are mercury emanating from mining activity, certain nitrogen compounds used in agriculture, chlorinated organic molecules arising from sewage or water treatment plants or various acids which are the externalities of various manufacturing activities.

Radioactive Pollution

Radioactive substances are really merely a special sub-class of chemical pollutants, and by mass represent the smallest of the contributors to water pollution; however, their potential for harm allows recognition as a separate class. In fact, most discharge of radioactivity is not from the negligible escape from nuclear power plants, but rather it arises from agricultural practices, such as tobacco farming, where radioactive contamination of phosphate fertilizer is a common method of introduction of radioactive materials into the environment.

Biological Pollution

Common pathogenic microbes introduced into natural water bodies are pathogens from untreated sewage or surface run-off from intensive livestock grazing. One of the most common disease agents is *Giardia lamblia*, a parasitic protozoan common in fecal material of many fauna including humans. This and other protozoans and bacteria are important causes of illness and mortality in developing countries where population density, water scarcity and inadequate sewage treatment combine to occasion widespread parasitic and bacterial disease.

Thermal Pollution

Thermal pollution is the rise or fall in the temperature of a natural body of water caused by human influence. Thermal pollution, results in a change in the physical properties of water. A common cause of thermal pollution is the use of water as a coolant by power plants and industrial manufacturers. Elevated water temperatures decrease oxygen levels, which can kill fish, and can alter food chain composition, reduce species biodiversity, and foster invasion by new thermophilic species. Thermal pollution can also be caused by the release of very cold water from the base of reservoirs into warmer rivers.

Causes

Industrial Waste

Industries produce huge amount of waste, which contains toxic chemicals and pollutants. Industries do not have proper waste management system and drain the waste in the fresh water which goes into rivers, canals, and later, into the sea.

Mining Activities

Mining is the process of crushing the rock and extracting coal and other minerals from underground. These elements when extracted in the raw form contain harmful chemicals and increase the amount of toxic elements when mixed up with water, which may result in health problems.

Marine Dumping

The garbage produced by each household in the form of paper, aluminum, rubber, glass, plastic, food is collected and deposited into the sea in some countries. These items take from 2 weeks to 200 years to decompose. When such items enter the sea, they not only cause water pollution but also harm animals in the sea.

Accidental Oil Leakage

Oil spills pose a huge concern as large amount of oil enters into the sea and does not dissolve with water, thereby causing problems for local marine wildlife, such as fish, birds and sea otters.

Agriculture

The use of fertilizers and pesticides in agriculture can cause chemical pollution in water.

WATER PURIFICATION

Water purification is the process of removing undesirable chemicals, biological contaminants, suspended solids and gases from contaminated water. There are a wide variety of methods for water purification. The common methods used include physical processes, such as filtration, sedimentation, and distillation; biological processes, such as slow sand filters or biologically active carbon; chemical processes, such as flocculation and chlorination and the use of electromagnetic radiation, such as ultraviolet light. Water-borne diseases depicts in **Table 6.1.**

Purification on Small Scale

Household Treatment

Straining: Straining water is an important first step of water purification. Pouring muddy or dirty-looking water through

Table 6.1: Water-borne diseases.

Disease	*Pathogen*	*Causes*
Adenovirus infection	Adenoviridae virus	Drinking contaminated water
Amebiasis	*Entamoeba histolytica* parasite	Fecal matter of an infected person (usually ingested from infected water supply)
Campylobacteriosis	*Campylobacter jejuni* bacteria	Chicken, unpasteurized milk, water
Cryptosporidiosis	*Cryptosporidium* parasite	Fecal matter of an infected person (can survive for days in chlorinated pools)
Cholera	*Vibrio cholerae* bacteria	Contaminated drinking water, rivers and coastal waters
E coli 0157:H7	*Escherichia coli* bacteria	Undercooked ground beef, imported cheese, unpasteurized milk or juice, cider, alfalfa sprouts
Giardiasis	*Giardia lamblia* parasite	Swallowing recreational water contaminated with *Giardia*
Hepatitis A	Hepatitis A virus	Ready-to-eat foods, fruit and juice, milk products, shellfish, salads, vegetables, sandwiches, water
Legionellosis	*Legionella pneumophila* bacteria	Contaminated water
Salmonellosis	*Salmonella* bacteria	Poultry, eggs, meat, meat products, milk, smoked fish, protein foods, juice
Vibrio infection	*Vibrio parahemolyticus, Vibrio vulnificus* bacteria	Raw shellfish, oysters
Viral gastroenteritis	*Calicivirus*	Water, ready-to-eat foods (salad, sandwiches, bread), shellfish

a piece of fine, clean cotton cloth will often remove a certain amount of the suspended solids and insect larvae contained in the water. The cloth selected should be clean and adequate as it is to be used for filtering the water. If the dirt does not pass through the cloth, then removal of dirt is not possible. A cotton cloth can works best for straining. The cloth should not be so thick that it takes a very long time to filter.

Washing the cloth between usages will make straining more effective. Straining alone is unlikely to make water from a contaminated source completely safe to drink. But it makes household water treatment easier.

Boiling: Boiling water is the safest method of purification. Boiling water kills germs and parasites. The water undergoes to a full, rolling boil for at least five minutes to be safe, with some experts recommending an even longer time. The downside of boiling your drinking water is that it removes the oxygen and the water ends up tasting flat. You can improve its quality by pouring it back and forth between two containers to put oxygen back in, or simply shake it up.

Chemical disinfection: 'Water disinfection' means the removal, deactivation or killing of pathogenic microorganisms. Microorganisms are destroyed or deactivated, resulting in termination of growth and reproduction. When microorganisms are not removed from drinking water, drinking water usage will cause people to fall ill. Bleaching powder, chlorine solution, high test hypochlorite (HTH) can be used for disinfection purposes, chlorine may be used in gas, liquid or solid form to disinfect water. Because chlorine gas is highly toxic and can be dangerous if released into the atmosphere, the danger is avoided by the use of chlorine in liquid form (sodium hypochlorite) or solid form (calcium hypochlorite). Household bleach is made up of 3–6% sodium hypochlorite and the EPA recommends using it to disinfect water in emergency situations. Calcium hypochlorite water purification tablets are readily available for emergency situations as well. While chlorine is a highly effective and widely used method of water disinfection, it reacts with organic compounds in water, forming trihalomethanes (THMs) and haloacetic acids, which are carcinogenic in large quantities. The best way to avoid this is to remove as many organics as possible, prior to disinfection. Iodine, like chlorine, is available in liquid and tablet forms. Iodine is recommended for emergency use only, in limited quantities. Iodine water purification is not recommended for people who are pregnant, have thyroid disease, or iodine allergy.

Ceramic filters: Ceramic filters are an inexpensive and effective type of water filters, that rely on the small pore size of ceramic material to filter dirt, debris, and bacteria out of water. Water is carefully introduced to one side of the filter, which acts to block the passage of anything larger than the pore size. Typically bacteria, protozoa, and microbial cysts are removed but the filters are not effective against viruses since they are small enough to pass through to the other 'clean' side of the filter. Ceramic water filters (CWF) may be treated with silver in a form that will not leach away. The silver helps to kill or incapacitate bacteria and prevent the growth of mold and algae in the body of the filter.

Disinfection of Well

Well disinfection can eliminate or reduce many different kinds of harmful bacteria and viruses as well as harmless bacteria which can cause unpleasant taste and odor. However, disinfection will not correct water problems caused by chemical contamination from nitrate, fuels, pesticides, or other substances.

Step 1. Determine the depth of water in the well: The company that constructed the well should be able to provide the measurements of well depth and water level. The depth

Table 6.2: Volume of water per foot of well depth based on the diameter of the well.

Well-casing diameter (inches)	*Water volume per foot of water depth (gallons)*[1]
4	0.65
6	1.47
8	2.61
10	4.08
12	5.88
18	13.22
24	23.50
30	36.72
36	52.87

[1]Volume of water calculated as the volume of a cylinder multiplied by 7.48 gallons/cubic foot.

Table 6.3: Amount of chemical required to create a chlorine concentration of 200 ppm.

Chemical name	*Amount per 100 gallons of water*
Liquid laundry bleach (5.25% NaOCl)	3 pints
Commercial strength bleach (12–17% NaOCl)	1 pint
Chlorinated lime (25% $CaOCl_2$)	11 ounces
Dairy sanitizer (30% $CaOCl_2$)	9 ounces
High-test calcium hypochlorite (65–75% $Ca(OCl)_2$)	4 ounces

of the water is calculated by subtracting the water level from the depth of the well. For example, depth of the well is 50 feet and the water level is at 40 feet. The well contains 10 feet of water (50 – 40 = 10 feet).

Step 2. Determine the volume of water in the well: For determining the volume of water inside, diameter of the well measurement is essential. The measured inside diameter of the well was assumed 30 inches. The next step is to find the gallons per foot of depth for a 30-inch well. For above example, we would multiply the depth of the water in the well (10 feet) by 36.7 gallons of water per foot of water depth **Table 6.2** to get 367 gallons of well water (10 × 36.7 = 367 gallons of water in the well).

Step 3. Estimate the volume of water in the distribution system: If there is distribution system, total up the water storage in the system (including the water heater, pressure tank, etc.) and add 50 gallons for the pipeline. If there is a 30-gallon hot water heater and a 30-gallon pressure tank, you need to add 110 gallons for the distribution system.

Step 4. Determine the water contained in the entire system: Add the water volume in the well to the water contained in the distribution system to get 477 gallons (367 gallons in the well plus 110 gallons in the distribution system).

Step 5. Determine the amount of chlorine product required for a 200 ppm solution: There are varieties of products available in the market. Based on the product of chlorine, the amount will be calculated **Table 6.3**.

Introduce the chlorine material into the well and distribution system: The best way to introduce chlorine material into the well is to dissolve the chlorine in a 5-gallon bucket of fresh water. Be sure the bucket is made of plastic and has been thoroughly washed. Then pour the chlorine solution into the well. Try to splash the solution on the sidewalls of the well-casing as much as possible. Attach a hose to the water hydrant or faucet nearest to the well and run water through the hydrant and back into the well. This will thoroughly mix the chlorine solution and well water.

As an alternative to bleach, one can purchase well safe sanitizer kit.

Another method of shock chlorinating a large-diameter well is to place tablets or powder in a weighted porous sack (tightly woven burlap works well). Raise and lower the sack in the well water. Remember that only the portions of the well coming in contact with the chlorine will be disinfected. Be sure to allow the sack to touch the bottom of the well during this process.

For small-diameter wells (4–6-inch diameter), there is not enough room in the well-casing to use a sack. Instead, dissolve the tablets or powder in a bucket of water and introduce into the well-casing as described for using liquid chlorine sources. Again, use a nearby hydrant and hose to circulate water through a portion of the distribution system to assure that the chlorine material is thoroughly mixed with well water.

If a strong chlorine odor is not detected at each site, add more chlorine to the well. This may be an indication that your well contains iron, hydrogen sulfide or organic materials. The reason for the lack of odor is caused by the reaction between chlorine and another ionic particle.

Disinfection in Large Scale

The components of a typical water purification system comprise one or more of the following measures:

- Storage
- Filtration
- Disinfection

Storage

Storage provides a reserve for water where further contamination can be prevented. As a result of storage, a very considerable purification takes place. By storage, the impurities settle down in 24 hours by gravity, the water becomes clear and allows to pass the light and reduces the work of filter. Certain chemical changes like the aerobic bacteria oxidizes the organic matter present in the water with aid of dissolved oxygen. As a result, the content of free ammonia is reduced and a rise of nitrate occurs. The biological changes in storage system are 90% of the pathogenic organisms die in 5–7 days' storage.

Filtration

It is an important purification system as it provides 98 to 99% purification. There are two types of sand filtration. It can be either rapid or slow. The difference between the two is not simply a matter of the speed of filtration, but also the underlying concept of the treatment process. Slow sand filtration is essentially a biological process, whereas rapid sand filtration is a physical treatment process. Slow sand filters have an advantage over rapid sand filters in that they produce microbiologically 'clean' water which should not require disinfection to inactivate any bacteria, although the addition of a disinfectant to provide a residual for the distribution system is still advisable. However, because of their slow flow rate, slow sand filters require large tracts of land if they are to supply large populations and can be relatively labor-intensive to operate and easy to maintain.

Slow Sand Filtration

Slow Sand Filters

The first use of sand filters to purify the water supply dates back to 1804 in Paisley, Scotland by John Gibb, then by James Simpson for the Chelsea Waterworks Company in London in 1829.

The elements of slow sand filters are:

- Supernatant (raw) water
- Sand bed of filter medium
- Underdrainage sytem
- Filter control

Supernatant (raw) water: The supernatant water layer provides the driving force for raw water to pass through the bed of filter medium and creates a detention time of several hours for the raw water to be treated, during which period particle may settle and/or agglomerate or be subjected to other physical or (bio)chemical processes.

Sand bed of filter medium: The most important part of the filter is the sand bed. The thickness of the sand bed is about 1 meter. It consists of a bed of graded sand like filter sand, coarse sand, fine gravel and course gravel. The sand should be free from clay, loam and organic matter.

The sand bed presents a large surface area; 1 cubic meter of filter sand presents some 15,000 sq meters of surface area. Water percolates through the sand very slowly (a process taking 2 hours or more) and as it does so, it is subjected to a number of purification processes—mechanical staining, sedimentation, absorption, oxidation and bacterial action, all playing their part. The designed rate of filtration of water normally lies between 0.1 and 0.4 m^3/hour per sq. meter of sand bed surface.

Vital layer: Slow sand filters work through the formation of a gelatinous layer (or biofilm) called the hypogeal layer or Schmutzdecke in the top few millimetres of the fine sand layer. The Schmutzdecke is formed in the first 10–20 days of operation. This is also called 'vital layer', or 'biological layer'. This layer consists of thread-like algae and numerous forms of life including plankton, diatoms and bacteria. The formation of vital layer is known as 'ripening of the filter'. When it is fully formed, it extends for 2–3 cm into the top portion of the sand bed. The vital layer is called as the heart of the slow sand filter. It removes organic matter, holds back bacteria and oxidizes ammoniacal nitrogen into nitrate and helps in making bacteria-free water. As the reestablishment of the schmutzdecke takes several days, the plant has to have sufficient capacity to supply the water demand.

Underdrainage system: The underdrainage system serves two purposes—it provides an unobstructed passage for the filtered water and supports the bed of filter medium. It usually consists of main and lateral drains made of perforated or nonjointed pipes, concrete blocks, or well-burnt bricks. The underdrains are covered by layers of graded gravel. The gravel, laid with large-sized pieces at the bottom and progressively reducing in size to the top, prevents sand grains from entering into the drainage system.

Filter control: The filter is equipped with certain valves and devices which are incorporated in the outlet pipe system. The purpose of this is to maintain a constant rate of filtration. An important component of the regulation system is the 'venturi meter' which measures the bed resistance or loss of 'head' when the resistance builds up. The operator opens the regulating valve so as to maintain a steady rate of filtration. When the loss of head exceeds 1.3 m, it is uneconomical to run the filter.

Slow sand filters may be used where there is sufficient land and space, as the water must be passed very slowly through the filters. These filters rely on biological treatment processes for their action rather than physical filtration. The filters are carefully constructed using graded layers of sand, with the coarsest sand, along with some gravel at the bottom and finest sand at the top. Drains at the base carry treated water away for disinfection. Filtration depends on the development of a thin biological layer called the 'zoogleal layer' or *Schmutzdecke*, on the surface of the filter.

Process of Purification

The purification starts in the supernatant raw water layer where large particles will settle into the filter bed and smaller particles may agglomerate to settleable flocs due to physical or bio(chemical) interactions. Under the influence of sunlight, algae will grow, producing oxygen which helps the biological processes. The number of bacteria will decrease and there will be reduction of organic matter due to biochemical oxidation.

Major part of the removal of impurities and considerable improvement of the physical, chemical and bacteriological quality of raw water takes place in the filter bed and especially in the Schmutzdecke. In this top layer abound micro-organisms, such as algae, plankton, diatoms and bacteria, which, through their tremendous biological activity, break down organic matter.

As the water passes through the bed, it is constantly changing direction so that particles carried by the water come into contact with the filter grains by various transport mechanisms. The grains become covered with a sticky layer of mainly organic material which, in turn, absorbs these particles by various attachment mechanisms. At the same time, the active micro-organisms (bacteria, protozoa, bacteriophages) in the sticky layer around the grain feed on the impurities caught as well as on each other. In this way, degradable organic matter, including bacteria and viruses of fecal origin, is gradually broken down and converted into water, carbon dioxide and harmless inorganic salts. The life-filled zone where these purification mechanisms take place extends to about 0.4–0.5 m down from the surface of the filter bed, but it gradually decreases in activity downwards as the water is purified and contains less organic matter and nutrients. At greater depth in the filter bed, the products of the biological processes are further removed by physical processes (adsorption) and chemical action (oxidation).

The transport, attachment and purification mechanisms described will only function effectively if a sufficient detention time in the filter bed is allowed for the water to be treated. Especially, when slow sand filtration is the main treatment process, the rate of filtration should be kept low (0.1 and 0.2 m/h) or 0.1–0.2 m^3/m^2 bed area per hour. Another important parameter for the purification process is the oxygen content of water. The activity of the biomass will decrease considerably if the oxygen content of water into the filter medium falls below 0.5 mg/L. If the anaerobic conditions occur, obnoxious impurities may be released to the water by the biomass. Such occurrences may be prevented by aeration of the raw water presedimentation of the raw water or recycling part of the aerated effluent to the supernatant water reservoir. For additional aeration of filtered water, the outlet weir chamber should be provided with suitable ventilation.

Rapid Sand Filter

Rapid sand filtration is now commonly used worldwide and is far more popular than slow sand filtration. The principal factor in this decision has been the smaller land requirement for rapid sand filters and lower labor costs. However, rapid sand filters do not produce water of the same quality as slow sand filters and a far greater reliance is placed on disinfection to inactivate bacteria. It is also worth noting that rapid sand filters are not effective in removing viruses. It is commonly used in municipal drinking water facilities as part of a multiple-stage treatment system.

Rapid sand filtration is a physical drinking water purification method. As freshwater flows through a sand-and-gravel bed, the majority of suspended particles are removed. Rapid sand filters provide rapid and efficient removal of relatively large suspended particles but they cannot provide safe drinking water unless pretreatment (i.e., coagulation-flocculation) and post-treatment (e.g., chlorine disinfection) is applied.

Rapid sand filters evolved at the end of the 19th century in the United States. By the 1920s, they were widely used as a major water purification method, since necessary facilities required less land area compared to *slow sand filters.*

Treatment Process and Basic Design Principles

The major parts of a gravity rapid sand filter are:

- Chamber: Filter tank or filter box
- Filter media (sand)
- Gravel support
- Underdrainage system
- Wash water troughs.

The filter chamber is usually made out of reinforced concrete, filled with sand and gravel to the height of 1.5–2 meters. The water is supplied to the top of the sand-bed and filtered as it flows through the layers of graded sand and gravel. A system of perforated pipes on the bottom drains the chamber (WHO 1996). The filter chamber can be constructed as open tanks (rapid gravity filters) or closed tanks (pressure filters).

The filtering is carried out by the following steps:

Mechanical Straining

First, relatively large suspended particles get stuck between the sand grains as they pass the filter medium.

Adsorption

It is the process by which molecules of a substance, such as a gas or a liquid, collect on the surface of another substance, such as a solid. The molecules are attracted to the surface but do not enter the solid's minute spaces as in absorption. The smaller particles adhere to the surface of the sand grains caused by the effect of the van der Waals forces.

Coagulation-Flocculation

Coagulation-flocculation is a chemical water treatment technique typically applied prior to sedimentation and filtration (e.g., rapid sand filtration) to enhance the ability of a treatment process to remove particles. Coagulation is a process used to neutralize charges and form a gelatinous mass to trap (or bridge) particles thus forming a mass large enough to settle or be trapped in the filter. Flocculation is gentle stirring or agitation to encourage the particles thus formed to agglomerate into masses large enough to settle or be filtered from solution.

Sedimentation

Sedimentation means gravity settling of particles in a liquid such that they accumulate. It is one of the most basic water treatments for both drinking water and wastewater. It is a simple, physical pretreatment of water prior to application of other purification treatments such as filtration and disinfection. It removes undesirable small particulate suspended matter (sand, silt and clay) and some biological contaminants from water under the influence of gravity. The longer the water is held undisturbed, the more the suspended solids and pathogens will settle to the bottom of the container. Adding coagulants can accelerate the sedimentation process. Three common chemicals used for this purpose are aluminum sulfate, poly aluminum chloride (also known as 'PAC' or 'liquid alum' and 'ferric sulfate').

Filtration

This filtering process is determined by two basic physical principles. First, relatively large suspended particles get stuck between the sand grains as they pass the filter medium (mechanical straining). Second, smaller particles adhere to the surface of the sand grains caused by the effect of the van der Waals forces (physical adsorption). A chemical filter-aid (i.e., coagulant or flocculant) might be added to promote additional adhesion. In the course of these processes, more and more particles accumulate in the filter medium, increasingly causing clogged filters and decreased performance. Initial filtering performance can be re-achieved through cleaning of the filter bed. This is usually conducted through backwashing.

Backwashing: The flow of water is reversed, so that treated water flows backwards through the filter. The sand is resuspended and the solid matter is separated in the surface water. Often, air is injected additionally to support the cleaning process (WHO 1996). As soon as most particles are washed out and the backward flowing water is clear, the filter is put back to operation. Clearly, relatively large quantities of sludge are generated through backwashing and require some form of treatment before discharge into the environment.

Rapid sand filtration is a highly effective method to remove turbidity, if it is correctly applied (Brikke and Bredero 2003).

WATER QUALITY STANDARDS

Drinking water quality standards describe the quality parameters set for drinking water. Despite the truism that every human on this planet needs drinking water to survive and that water may contain many harmful constituents, there are not universally recognized and accepted international standards for drinking water. Even where standards do exist, and are applied, the permitted concentration of individual constituents may vary by as much as ten times from one set of standards to another.

The guidelines for drinking water quality recommended by WHO (1993 and 1996) relate to the following variables:

- Acceptability aspects
- Microbiological aspects
- Chemical aspects
- Radiological aspects.

Acceptability Aspects

The provision of drinking-water that is not only safe but also acceptable in appearance, taste and odor is of high priority. Water that is aesthetically unacceptable will undermine the confidence of consumers, will lead to complaints and, more importantly, could lead to the use of water from sources that are less safe. To a large extent, consumers have no means of judging the safety of their drinking-water themselves, but their attitude towards their drinking-water supply and their drinking-water suppliers will be affected to a considerable extent by the aspects of water quality that they are able to perceive with their own senses. It is natural for consumers to regard with suspicion water that appears dirty or discolored or that has an unpleasant taste or smell, even though these characteristics may not in themselves be of direct consequence to health. The appearance, taste and odor of drinking-water should be acceptable to the consumer. Water that is aesthetically unacceptable can lead to the use of water from sources that are aesthetically more acceptable, but potentially less safe.

Turbid and Color

Turbidity (the cloudiness caused by fine suspended matter in the water). On aesthetic ground, the drinking water should be free from turbidity. Turbidity is sometimes due to the inorganic material present in the ground water which interferes with the disinfection and microbiological determination. The drinking water must be colorless. Turbidity and color of the water is mainly due to organic substances, biological activity and industrial pollution.

Taste and Odor

Taste and odor can enter water in a variety of ways. Surface water sources can become contaminated through algal blooms or through industrial wastes or domestic sewage introducing taste- and odor-causing chemicals into the water. Groundwater supplies can be afflicted with dissolved minerals, such as iron and manganese, which enter the water when it passes through rocks underground. Tastes and odors can also enter either type of water in the raw water transmission system and in the treatment plant due to algal growths, accumulated debris and sludge, or disinfection byproducts. The distribution system can have many of the same causes of taste and odor mentioned above, with the addition of problems resulting from cross-connections and low-flow zones.

The best way to treat taste and odor problems is prevention. Algal blooms in reservoirs can be prevented by using copper sulfate while algae growing on walls of the treatment plant basins can be removed through shock treatment with chlorine. Since hydrogen sulfide is produced during anaerobic conditions, preventing these conditions in the reservoir, the distribution system, and in sludge in the sedimentation basin will prevent hydrogen sulfide formation. In the distribution system, periodic flushing and maintaining an adequate chlorine residual will keep the pipes clean and odor-free.

Temperature

Cool water is generally more pleasant but it tends to decrease the efficiency of treatment process, including disinfection and it may have a deleterious effect on quality of water. However, high temperature enhances the growth of microorganism and other problems like taste and odor, color, etc. So, no guideline value is recommended for temperature and also it is impractical.

Total Dissolved Solids

Total dissolved solids (TDS) in drinking-water consist mainly of chloride, sulfate, carbonates, sodium, magnesium and calcium. Excessive dissolved solids in drinking-water may lead to objectionable taste, and corrosion or encrustation in water distribution system. At concentrations greater than approximately 1,000 mg/L, the taste of water becomes increasingly unpalatable. As far as health aspects are concerned, there is no evidence of adverse physiological reactions at TDS levels greater than 1,000 mg/L. On the contrary, there are vague indications from epidemiological studies that high levels of certain salts (calcium and magnesium) may have beneficial health effects.

Fluoride levels between 0.5 and 1 mg/L provide substantial protection against dental caries. However, for fluoride, the margin between beneficial and toxic effects is rather small. Excessive exposure may lead to adverse health effects varying from mottling of teeth to crippling of skeletal fluorosis. The guidelines recommend a GV of 1.5 mg/L on the assumption that the daily per capita consumption of drinking-water is about 2 liters. At this level, dental fluorosis may occur in a certain proportion of the population. Nitrate and nitrite in drinking-water may be of natural origin, or can be leached from septic tanks, pig farms and feed lots. Use of fertilizers (too much and at the wrong time of the year) can also result in nitrate pollution. High concentration of nitrate, and especially nitrite, in drinking-water may cause methemoglobinemia. Groups especially susceptible to methemoglobin formation are young infants, children and pregnant women. Epidemiological studies indicate that at levels of nitrates less than 50 mg/L (as nitrate), there does not seem to be any problem with methemoglobinemia. There are considerable uncertainties as to the level of nitrite which may cause such clinical effects. On the assumption that nitrite was ten times more potent than nitrate (on a molar basis) with respect to methemoglobin formation, the guidelines recommend a provisional GV of 3 mg/L (as nitrite). In addition, since nitrite and nitrate exert similar toxicological effect and may occur simultaneously, the following condition was also specified.

The most significant health effect from lead is the association of lead exposure with reduced cognitive development and intellectual performance in children. Results of studies on children with blood lead concentrations below 25 µg/dL indicate that, on an average, the intelligence quotient (IQ) is reduced by 1–3 points for each 10 µg/dL increment in the blood lead concentration. Existing epidemiological studies do not provide evidence of a threshold. Steps are now being taken to reduce all sources of lead exposure of children with some apparent success in various countries. In countries where lead has been removed from petrol, and where there is no specific source of excess lead exposure, blood lead concentrations in children are decreasing and are now approximately 4–6 µg/dL. The almost complete elimination of lead-soldered side-seams in canned foods in a number of countries has also contributed to the reduction in lead exposure. Corrosion control measures are being implemented to reduce hardness (the reduced ability to get lather using soap).

pH Value

Basically, the pH value is a good indicator of whether water is hard or soft. The pH of pure water is 7. In general, water with a pH lower than 7 is considered acidic, and with a pH greater than 7 is considered basic. The normal range for pH in surface water systems is 6.5 to 8.5, and the pH range for groundwater systems is between 6 and 8.5 in general, water with a pH < 6.5 could be acidic, soft, and corrosive. Acidic water could contain metal ions, such as iron, manganese, copper, lead, and zinc. In other words, acidic water contains elevated levels of toxic metals. Water with a pH > 8.5 could indicate that the water is hard. Hard water does not pose a health risk, but can also cause aesthetic problems. These problems include an alkali taste to the water (making that morning coffee taste bitter!), formation of scale deposits on dishes, utensils, and laundry basins, difficulty in getting soaps and detergents to lather, and the formation of insoluble precipitates on clothing.

Hardness

Hard water requires more soap and synthetic detergents for home laundry and washing, and contributes to scaling in boilers and industrial equipment. Hardness is caused by compounds of calcium and magnesium, and by a variety of other metals. Water is an excellent solvent and readily dissolves minerals it comes in contact with. As water moves through soil and rock, it dissolves very small amounts of minerals and holds them in solution. Calcium and magnesium dissolved in water are the two most common minerals that make water 'hard.'

Microbial Aspects

Securing the microbial safety of drinking-water supplies is based on the use of multiple barriers, from catchment to consumer, to prevent the contamination of drinking water or to reduce contamination to levels not injurious to health. Safety is increased if multiple barriers are in place, including protection of water resources, proper selection and operation of a series of treatment steps and management of distribution systems (piped or otherwise) to maintain and protect treated water quality. The preferred strategy is a management approach that places the primary emphasis on preventing or reducing the entry of pathogens into water sources and reducing reliance on treatment processes for removal of pathogens. In general terms, the greatest microbial risks are associated with ingestion of water that is contaminated with feces from humans or animals (including birds). Feces can be a source of pathogenic bacteria, viruses, protozoa and helminths. Faecally derived pathogens are the principal concerns in setting health-based targets for microbial safety. Microbial water quality often varies rapidly and over a wide range.

Short-term peaks in pathogen concentration may increase disease risks considerably and may trigger outbreaks of waterborne diseases. Furthermore, by the time microbial contamination is detected, many people may have been exposed. For these reasons, reliance cannot be placed solely on end-product testing, even when frequent, to determine the microbial safety of drinking-water.

Particular attention should be directed to a water safety framework and implementing comprehensive water safety plans to consistently ensure drinking-water safety and thereby protect public health. Failure to ensure drinking-water safety may expose the community to the risk of outbreaks of intestinal and other infectious diseases. Outbreaks of waterborne diseases are particularly to be avoided because of their capacity to result in the simultaneous infection of a large number of persons and potentially a high proportion of the community.

AIR

INTRODUCTION

The immediate environment of man comprises of air on which depend all forms of life. Apart from supplying the life-giving oxygen, air and atmospheric conditions serve several functions. The human body cooled by the air contact; the special senses of hearing and smell function through air-transmitted stimuli; disease agents may be conveyed by air. Pollution of air by dust, smoke, toxic gases and chemical vapors has resulted in sickness and death. Human beings need a continuous supply of air to exist.

Generally, dry air contains:
- 78.09% nitrogen
- 20.95% oxygen
- 0.93% argon
- 0.039% carbon dioxide
- And small amounts of other gases too.

Air also contains a variable amount of water vapor, on an average around 1% at sea level, and 0.4% over the entire atmosphere. Although air content and atmospheric pressure vary at different layers, air suitable for the survival of terrestrial plants and terrestrial animals currently is only known to be found in earth's troposphere and artificial atmospheres **(Fig. 6.4)**.

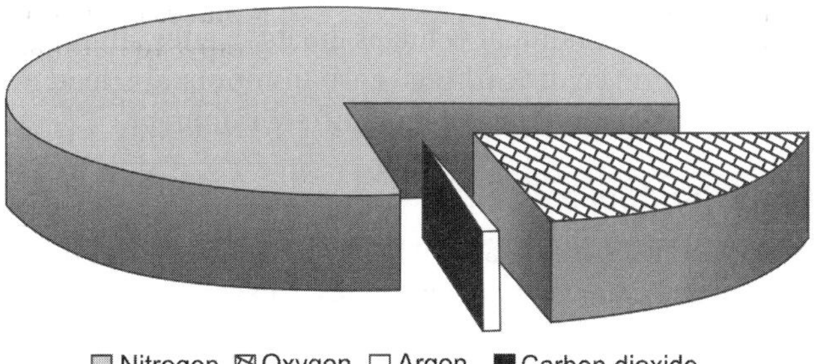

Fig. 6.4: Composition of air.

Changes in Air of Occupied Room

Human occupancy and activity vitiate air in occupied rooms and give a sense of discomfort to the occupants. The changes in air that take place in confined places are both chemical and physical.

a. **Chemical changes:** The air becomes progressively contaminated by carbon dioxide and the oxygen content decreases due to metabolic processes. An average person at rest gives off 0.7 c.ft. of carbon dioxide per hour; this may increase up to 2 c.ft. during physical activity. In a mixed gathering comprising all age groups, the per capita output of carbon dioxide is taken as 0.6 c.ft. per hour.
b. **Physical changes:** The most important changes that occur due to human occupancy are the physical changes. There are:
   - **Rise in temperature:** The indoor temperature tends to rise as a result of the emanation of body heat. A man at rest gives off approximately 400 Btu per hour. One Btu (British Thermal Unit) is the quantity of heat required to raise the temperature of one pound of water by 1 degree. Under the condition of physical exertion, the heat output may go up to 4,000 Btu.
   - **Increase in humidity:** There is an increase in the relative humidity due to moisture evaporated from the skin and lungs. The expired air contains about 6% of water vapor per 24 hours in the form of perspiration. It has been calculated that a human being releases 18.4 g of water vapor per hour when sleeping and up to 175 g of water vapor when engaged in really vigorous exercises.
   - **Decrease in air movement:** In crowded places, the natural movement of air is impeded.
   - **Body odors:** Unpleasant odors arise from foul breath, perspiration, bad oral hygiene, dirty clothes and other sources.
   - **Bacterial pollution:** The exhaled air contains microorganisms in suspension and saprophytic bacteria and may include pathogenic bacteria.

Comfort Zone

The **comfort zone** is a psychological state in which a person feels familiar, at ease, in control and experiences low anxiety and stress. In the zone, the majority of adults feel comfortable and a steady level of performance is possible. There is no unanimous decision on a single zone of comfort for all the people because comfort is quite a complex subjective experience, which depends not only on physical, physiological factors but also on psychological factors, which are difficult to determine. Considering only the environmental factors, comfortable thermal conditions are those under which a person can maintain normal balance between production and loss of heat, at normal body temperature and sweating. The level at which one functions with ease and familiarity, i.e., the temperature range (between 28 and 30°C) at which the naked human body is able to maintain a heat balance without shivering or sweating is considered as comfort zone.

Comfort conditions may be defined as the human environment that must provide light, air, and thermal comfort. Comfort is best defined as the absence of discomfort. People feel uncomfortable when they are too hot or too cold, or when the air is odorous and stale. Positive comfort conditions are those that do not distract by causing unpleasant sensations of temperature, drafts, humidity, or other aspects of the environment. Considering only environmental factors, comfortable thermal conditions are those under which a person can maintain normal balance between the production and loss of heat.

Comfort zones evaluated in India are as given below:

Corrected effective temperature in degree celcius	
Pleasant and cool	20
Comfortable and cool	20–25
Comfortable	25–27
Hot and comfortable	27–28
Extremely hot	28+
Intolerably hot	30+

Indices of Thermal Comfort

Thermal comfort refers to the subjective feeling of temperature in an environment. It is a complex entity. Much work was done to determine what constitutes 'thermal comfort'. Optimum levels of thermal comfort help in maximizing productivity. Measurement of thermal comfort levels is complex and several indices have been put forward from time to time to express thermal comfort and heat stress. These are:

- **Air temperature** was used for a long time as an index of thermal comfort, but it was realized that air temperature alone was not an adequate index. Initially, the air temperature as measured from a dry bulb thermometer was taken as the indicator of thermal comfort. But it was found to be a unsatisfactory measure as comfort levels depended on other factors too.
- **Air temperature and humidity:** Air temperature and humidity were considered together to express thermal comfort; even this was found to be unsatisfactory.
- **Cooling power:** Still later, air temperature, humidity and air movement were considered together and expressed as 'cooling power' of the air. An instrument was devised by Hill called the 'kata thermometer' to measure the cooling water. These indices plus mean radiant heat are used by the Bulgarian standards to evaluate the thermal comfort.

Effective Temperature

The different factors determining thermal comfort—air temperature, humidity and air movements are combined together into a single index called 'effective temperature'. Effective temperature is the temperature in an environment with 100% humidity and no air movements which will induce the same level of thermal comfort as in the present situation. For example, if the effective temperature is said to be 30°C, it means that the thermal comfort is equivalent to one in an environment with temperature 30°C, 100% humidity and no air movements. But effective temperature does not take into consideration the effect of radiant heat energy.

Corrected Effective Temperature

This index is an improvement over the effective temperature index. Instead of the dry bulb temperature, the reading of the globe thermometer is used to allow for radiant heat. That is, the CET scales deal with all the four factors, namely air, temperature, velocity, humidity and mean radiant heat. Corrected effective temperature is measured using a combination of:

- Globe thermometer—to measure air temperature adjusted for radiant heat
- Wet bulb thermometer—to measure humidity
- Air speed measurement.

AIR POLLUTION

Air pollution is an atmospheric condition in which certain substances, like gases, particulate matter, radioactive substances, etc., are present in concentrations which can cause undesirable effects on human environment. It occurs in many forms. The **pollutants** include sulfur dioxide (SO_2), nitrogen oxides (NO_x), ozone (O_3), carbon monoxide (CO), volatile organic compounds (VOC), hydrogen sulfide (H_2S), hydrogen fluoride (HF), and various gaseous forms of metals. They are corrosive to various materials which cause damage to cultural resources, can cause injury to ecosystems and organisms, aggravate respiratory diseases, and reduce visibility.

Sources of Air Pollution

The major sources of air pollution include industries, automobiles, chemical fertilizers, combustion of coal, fuel oil and natural gas, and tobacco smoking, and dust of drugs produced during milling and sieving. Large stationary sources, such as fossil fuel-fired power plants, smelters, industrial boilers, petroleum refineries, and manufacturing facilities as well as farm area and other mobile sources are the sources of air pollution.

Automobiles

Automobiles include on-road transportation, like vehicles, such as cars, sports utility vehicles, and buses. In addition, there is also a 'non-road' or 'off-road' category that includes gas-powered lawn tools and mowers, farm and construction equipment, recreational vehicles, boats, planes, and trains, etc. They emit hydrocarbons, carbon monoxide, lead and nitrogenous oxide which pollute the environment.

Agricultural Sources

Agricultural sources may be due to hoist animals and grow crops, which can generate emissions of gases and particulate matter. For example, animals in a barn or restricted area (rather than field grazing), produce large amounts of manure. Manure emits various gases, particularly ammonia into the air. This ammonia can be emitted from the animal houses, manure storage areas, or from the land after the manure is applied. In crop production, the misapplication of fertilizers, herbicides, and pesticides can potentially result in air pollution. The chemical fertilizers which are used to increase agriculture production produce pollutants, like nitrogen oxide, sulfur dioxide, ammonia and urea dust, which pollute the air in the community and neighborhood.

Industries

Industries include factories, power plants, dry cleaners and degreasing operation. Manufacturing industries release large amount of carbon monoxide, hydrocarbons, organic compounds, and chemicals into the air, thereby depleting the quality of air. Some of the examples of important industrial sources are: (a) thermal power plants which produce sulfur-dioxide, nitrogen-oxide and ash particles; (b) cement factories which produce cement dust, carbon-monoxide and sulfur-dioxide; (c) steel plants which produce sulfur-dioxide, carbon-monoxide and other particles. Petroleum refineries also release hydrocarbons and various other chemicals that pollute the air and also cause land pollution.

Mining operations: Mining is a process wherein minerals below the earth are extracted using large equipment. During the process, dust and chemicals are released in the air causing massive air pollution. This is one of the reasons which is responsible for the deteriorating health conditions of workers and nearby residents.

Indoor or domestic sources of air pollution: Household cleaning products, painting supplies emit toxic chemicals in the air and cause air pollution. Domestic combustion of coal, wood or oil is a major source of smoke, dust sulfur dioxide and nitrogen oxide in house. The **combustion of coal, fuel oil and natural gas** can be used in factories, power plants, in some other places also. These produce carbon-dioxide, carbon-monoxide, sulfur dioxide, ash particles and, thus, pollute air.

Tobacco Smoke

Tobacco smoke emitted by smokers in the households and public places pollute the air of the houses and public places. The tobacco smoke emits nicotine which is very injurious to health of other people too.

Natural Sources

Although much air pollution results from some type of human activities, naturally occurring elements, such as pollen grains from plants and flowers, ash from volcanic eruptions, dust from fields, airborne microorganisms, etc., also pollute the air.

Other Sources

Other sources include burning of refuse, incinerator, nuclear energy programs activity also contribute gases and particulates to our atmosphere.

Types of Air Pollutants

More than 100 types of air pollutants have been identified. The major types of pollutants are carbon monoxide gas from motor vehicle exhaustion, or the sulfur dioxide released from factories, nitrogen oxides, particularly nitrogen dioxide, are expelled from high temperature combustion sulfuric acid, nitric acid, carbonic acid, etc. An air pollutant is a substance in the air that can have adverse effects on humans and the ecosystem. The substance can be solid particles, liquid droplets or gases. A pollutant can be of natural origin or man-made. Pollutants are classified as ***primary*** or ***secondary***.

- **Primary pollutants:** These are usually produced from a process, such as ash from a volcanic eruption. Other examples include carbon monoxide gas from motor vehicle exhaustion, or the sulfur dioxide released from factories. Nitrogen oxides, particularly nitrogen dioxide, are expelled from high-temperature combustion, and are also produced during thunderstorms by electric discharge. Volatile organic compounds (VOCs) those are highly reactive organic compounds release through incomplete combustion and industrial source are also primary pollutants.
- **Secondary pollutants:** These are not emitted directly. Rather, they form in the air when primary pollutants react or interact. Sulfuric acid, nitric acid, carbonic acid are the examples of secondary pollutants. Ground level ozone is a prominent example of a secondary pollutant. Some pollutants may be both primary and secondary; they are both emitted directly and formed from other primary pollutants.
- **Carbon monoxide (CO):** It is produced when fuels, such as gas, oil, coal or wood do not burn fully. When fire burns in an enclosed space, such as a room, the oxygen is gradually used up and replaced with carbon dioxide. When the fuel is unable to burn fully it releases carbon monoxide or sometimes burning of fuel from automobiles, trucks, heavy-construction equipment, farming equipment and residential heating can produce carbon monoxide. After breathing in carbon monoxide, it enters your bloodstream and mixes with hemoglobin (the part of red blood cells that carries oxygen around your body), to form carboxyhemoglobin. When this happens, the blood is no longer able to carry oxygen, and this lack of oxygen causes the body's cells and tissues to die. Other symptoms include chest pain in heart patients, headaches, reduced mental alertness control, motor vehicle and industrial emissions. Use oxygenated gasoline during winter months.
- **Nitrogen dioxide (NO_2):** It is an important air pollutant because it contributes to the formation of photochemical smog, which can have significant impact on human health.

The major source of nitrogen dioxide is the burning of fossil fuels—coal, oil and gas. Most of the nitrogen dioxide in cities comes from motor vehicle exhaustion (about 80%).

Other sources of nitrogen dioxide are petrol and metal refining, electricity generation from coal-fired power stations, other manufacturing industries and food processing. The main effect of breathing in raised levels of nitrogen dioxide is the increased likelihood of respiratory problems. Nitrogen dioxide inflames the lining of the lungs, and it can reduce immunity to lung infections. This can cause problems, such as wheezing, coughing, colds, flu, bronchitis, lung irritation and damage. Reacts in the atmosphere to form ozone and acid rain. Controls motor vehicle and industrial combustion emissions.

- **Lead (Pb):** It is a metal found naturally in the environment as well as in manufactured products. The major sources of lead emissions have historically been from fuels in on-road motor vehicles (such as cars and trucks) and industrial sources, metal smelters, resource recovery, leaded gasoline, etc. Lead poisoning is a type of metal poisoning and a medical condition in humans and other vertebrates caused by increased levels of the heavy metal lead in the body. Lead interferes with a variety of body processes and is toxic to many organs and tissues including the heart, bones, intestines, kidneys, and reproductive and nervous systems. It interferes with the development of the nervous system and is therefore particularly toxic to children, causing potentially permanent learning and behavior disorders. Symptoms include abdominal pain, confusion, headache, anemia, irritability, and in severe cases seizures, coma, and death. Replace leaded paint with nonlead substitutes. As a result of EPA's regulatory efforts to remove lead from on-road motor vehicle gasoline, emissions of lead from the transportation sector dramatically declined by 95% between 1980 and 1999, and levels of lead in the air decreased by 94% between 1980 and 1999. Today, the highest levels of lead in air are usually found near lead smelters. The major sources of lead emissions to the air today are ore and metals processing and piston-engine aircraft operating on leaded aviation gasoline.
- **Sulfur dioxide (SO_2):** Coal or oil burning power plants and industries, refineries, diesel engines increases lung disease and breathing problems for asthmatics. Reacts in the atmosphere to form acid rain. Reduces the use of high-sulfur fuels (e.g., use low-sulfur reformulated diesel or natural gas). Sulfur dioxide is generally formed when reactive organic gases (ROGs) and nitrogen oxides react in the presence of sunlight. ROG sources include any source that burns fuels (e.g., gasoline, natural gas, wood, oil), solvents, petroleum processing and storage and pesticide. The three effects of sulfur dioxide are: breathing difficulties, lung tissue damage, damage to rubber and some plastics.
- **Prevention:** Reduce motor vehicle ROG and nitrogen oxide emissions through emission standards, reformulated fuels, inspection programs and reduced vehicle use. People with asthma or chronic lung or heart disease are the most sensitive to SO_2. It also damages trees and crops. SO_2, along with nitrogen oxides, is the main precursor of acid rain. This contributes to the acidification of lakes and streams, accelerated corrosion of buildings and reduced visibility.
- **Hydrogen sulfide:** It is heavier than air and may travel along the ground. It collects in low-lying and enclosed, poorly ventilated areas, such as basements, manholes, sewer lines, underground telephone vaults and manure pits. Hydrogen sulfide is both an irritant and a chemical asphyxiant with effects on both oxygen utilization and the central nervous system. Its health effects can vary depending on the level and duration of exposure. Repeated exposure can result in health effects occurring at levels that were previously tolerated without any effect. Low concentrations irritate the eyes, nose, throat and respiratory system (e.g., burning/tearing of eyes, cough, shortness of breath). Asthmatics may experience breathing difficulties. The sources are geothermal power plants, petroleum production and refining, sewer gas.

Other Classifications of Pollutants

The pollutants present in the air should be identified and categorized so that appropriate measures can be adopted to combat pollution. Solid matter: light, fine and coarse particles, hydrocarbons, aromatics. Liquid substances: smoke, soot, fly-ash, dust, mist, fumes, organic acids, inorganic acids. Gases: sulfur dioxide, nitrogen oxide, carbon dioxide.

EFFECTS OF AIR POLLUTION

Air pollution has many injurious effects not only on the health of people but also on all other animals. It also has adverse effects on soil, plants, monuments, buildings and climate, etc.

Effects on Human Health

Air pollution is very injurious to human health. It can cause various problems ranging from minor ailments to blindness, respiratory distress and deaths as it happened during Bhopal Gas Tragedy on 3rd December, 1984. The severity and nature of problems depend upon the type of concentration of pollutants in the air. The air pollution can cause the following disorders in the human beings:

- **Respiratory disorders:** Generally, the air pollution causes irritation of nose and throat, respiratory damage which includes bronchitis, asthma, emphysema, etc. It also increases susceptibility to infection of respiratory tract. These problems are due to pollution of air with chlorine, nitrogen, oxide, sulfur dioxide, ozone, suspended particles, fluorides and aldehydes.
- **Heart problems:** Air pollution with carbon monoxide is the main cause of heart disorders. Carbon monoxide when inhaled reduces oxygen in the blood, which increases the risk of heart attacks. Burning charcoal in the closed rooms at nights in winters have resulted in deaths in sleep due to choking because of carbon monoxide. Other pollutants, such as sulfur dioxide, ozone and particulate matter can also cause heart diseases.

- **Brain damage and nervous breakdown:** Hydrogen sulfide in the air can cause brain damage and affect the nervous system. Lead can cause permanent brain damage and reduce ability to concentrate, irritation and hyperactivity in children below five years of age. Children may become below average in growth and development. The main source of lead is exhaust from automobiles. It has a cumulative effect.
- **Cancer:** Inhalation of diesel and petrol exhaust can cause lung cancer because of carbon particles and benzene. Some of the hydrocarbons can cause anemia and blood cancer.
- **Eye problems:** Air polluted with nitrogen oxide, sulfur dioxide, ozone, etc. can cause irritation, conjunctivitis and even blindness like in Bhopal Gas Tragedy mentioned earlier.
- **Birth defects and stunted growth in children:** Particulate matter, vitiated air, tobacco smoke and vehicle exhaust which contain carbon monoxide and benzene can produce low birthweight babies with stunted growth. Chances of abnormal babies are high in mothers who smoke during pregnancy.

Effects on Soil

Air pollution abrades, corrodes and tarnishes soil. These effects reduce the fertility of soil.

Effects on Plants

Air pollutants cause disappearance of chlorophyll, the green-coloring matter which is responsible for photosynthesis; breakdown of plant cells and premature leaf fall. Ozone mainly affects field crops, fruits and fruit trees.

Effects on Monuments and Buildings

Monuments like Taj Mahal are facing grave danger from air pollution. The black soot released from Mathura oil refineries is causing blackening of Taj Mahal. Similarly, other buildings and monuments are getting affected by polluted air.

Other Effects of Air Pollution

- **Smog:** Smoke mixed with fog is called 'smog'. This usually happens during winter from December to January in places where there is accumulation of smoke due to heavy traffic jam on roads and industries.

  Smog can be very injurious to health if it contains sulfur dioxide, carbon monoxide and nitrous oxide in sufficient quantity. Incident of injurious smog happened in London in 1952 when 4,000 people died and in Tokyo in 1972, when 8,000 people died.
- **The greenhouse effect:** Normally, the solar energy from the sun reaches the earth to be utilized by plants and animals. Heat is produced in this process which gets radiated in the space and the temperature of the earth's surface is maintained.

  But due to burning of fuel, carbon dioxide and water vapors are released in the air and form a layer along with ozone layer in the atmosphere. This layer allows the solar energy from the sun to pass through on to earth's surface but traps the heat back in the earth's atmosphere which results in gradual warming of earth's atmosphere. This is affecting change in weather leading to natural calamities and many related health problems.
- **Acid rain:** The pollutants like sulfur dioxide, oxides of nitrogen, unburnt hydrocarbons which are released from motor vehicles, thermal plants, oil refineries by burning of coal and petroleum products combine with moisture in the air and rainwater and produce sulfuric acid and nitric acid which fall along with the rain called 'acid rain'. The acid rain pollutes soil, water and reduces the growth of crops and fishes in river, streams, canals and ponds. It also stops the growth of plants and destroys the buildings made of marble and stone and statues made up of metals. Acid rain can cause respiratory problems, such as asthma, bronchitis and emphysema. Acid rain was first detected by Robert Angus Smith in 1872. The biggest effect of acid rain was detected in 1981 in USA when it was found that almost all fishes had disappeared in the spirit lake in New York due to acid rain.
- **Ozone depletion:** Though the presence of ozone in the atmosphere within 10 kms of earth's surface is harmful but its presence at a height of 25–40 kms above the surface of the earth protects plants and animals from the harmful effects of ultraviolet (UV) rays from the sun.

  The ozone layer acts as a shield on the earth. It absorbs 99% of the UV radiations from the sun which are harmful to life on the earth. But, it allows infrared rays of the sun to pass through, which are useful for warming the earth. The presence of ozone layer in the atmosphere within 25–40 kms of height from earth protects people from having skin cancer and eye problems. It also helps in maintaining the climatic conditions of the earth.

  But, the ozone layer is getting depleted by the aerosols used by jet airplanes; fluorocarbons, hydrocarbons, etc., released from refrigerators, air conditioners, etc. By now, about 5–10% of ozone layer has got depleted.

  Air pollution is, therefore, very harmful to animals, plants and nonliving things in the biosphere. It causes various disorders, many of which are fatal. The sudden air pollution as happened in Bhopal Gas Tragedy led to severe respiratory distress and suffocations and deaths in large number of people at a time.

Monitoring, Prevention and Control of Air Pollution

Monitoring

The indicators for monitoring air pollution include sulfur dioxide, smoke and suspended particles. These are monitored daily over a number of areas. The results are then collected by a central agency and interpreted. Sulfur dioxide is measured in urban and industrial areas. Smoke concentration is measured with the help of filter paper by photoelectric meter and expressed as micrograms/cubic meter as an average level over a period of time. Grit and dust particles are measured and interpreted once in a month. Air pollution index takes into consideration more than one indicators to analyze the severity of pollution.

Air pollution monitoring in India is done by Central Pollution Control Board since 1990 in major cities which include: Ahmedabad, Mumbai, Kolkata, Delhi, Hyderabad, Jaipur, Kanpur, Kochi, Chennai and Nagpur. Long-term air quality trends are evaluated on the basis of dust, sulfur dioxide, nitrogen dioxide, lead, hydrogen sulfide and ammonia. The findings demonstrated the presence of suspended particulate matter in coastal cities and industrial sites. It also indicates the possibility of acid rain in the urban atmosphere.

Prevention and Control

Air pollution can cause many health disorders in man related to respiratory system, cardiovascular system, nervous system, eyes, etc. Usually these problems occur gradually due to long exposure to polluted air and become very serious by the time the problems are diagnosed. But these problems can be prevented and controlled by taking appropriate measures of prevention and control of air pollution which are briefly described in this section. These include:

- **Containment method:** In this method the pollutants are prevented to escape from their source into the surrounding air. This is done by various mechanical devices, e.g., in factories exhaust fans, suction apparatus, air-cleaning devices, etc., are installed to effect ventilation and cleaning of air before discharge into the atmosphere, in automobiles, filters are used in the exhaust pipes to prevent the escape of toxic substances, air is injected into the exhaust pipe to convert exhaust compounds into less toxic, abatement equipment are installed in the existing engines to improve combustion, etc.
- **Replacement method:** In this method, pollution, producing substances and processes are replaced by nonpolluting substances and processes, e.g., use of CNG instead of diesel in automobiles, use of nonleaded petrol instead of leaded petrol, use of solar cooker, gobar gas/natural gas instead of firewood, coal, etc. for cooking; replacement of coal-based electricity production plants by hydroelectric power or wind-powered generators, etc.
- **Dilution:** Dilution refers to reducing of pollutants in the air which can be done by extensive planting of trees and vegetation around the industrial and residential areas. This is usually called 'establishing the green belt'. It is also done by discharging the gases/smoke through long chimney high up to the atmosphere where it gets dispersed and diluted.
- **Disinfection of air:** In the recent years, disinfection of air has received much attention. The method includes mechanical ventilation which helps in reducing vitiated air and bacterial density, ultraviolet radiation for disinfecting operation theaters and infectious disease wards, etc., chemical mists (Triethylene glycol vapors) control bacteria, application of oil on floor to reduce infection.
- **Legislative method:** It refers to establishing of an Act (Law) which can set some norms for precautionary measures to be implemented by the factories, automobiles, etc. The Government of India has enacted Air (Prevention and control of Pollution) Act, 1981. Usually, difficulties are experienced in the implementation of the Act.
- **International action:** Air pollution is considered a global problem. Therefore, WHO has established regional centers at London, Washington, Moscow, Nagpur and Tokyo and 20 other laboratories in various parts of the world. These laboratories and centers are set up to study the air pollution level and issue warning of air pollution where and when necessary.
- **Mechanical ventilation:** Mechanical ventilation, especially in houses, public places. Health centers and hospital wards help in removing used air (vitiated air) and replacing it with fresh air. It also reduces the bacterial content.
- **Dust control:** Dust control can be done by frequent wet dusting and wet cleaning of floors of health centers, hospital wards, houses, roads, etc. This not only reduces dust but also the bacterial content.
- **Management of transport and road traffic:** It includes having good public transport system so that people travel by this system and not by individual car, car pooling or which will discourage using individual cars, better traffic management, which will help in reducing congestion on roads. All these measures reduce air pollution.

No single method is good enough in the prevention and control of air pollution. It requires the implementation of all these methods to have good effects.

AIR POLLUTION CONTROL

Air pollution can be controlled by two fundamental ways:

1. **Preventive technique:** It includes use of devices for removal of pollutants from exhaust gases, e.g., scrubbers, dry and wet collectors, filters, electrostatic precipitators, etc., building of higher stake facility for discharging of pollution into the air.
2. **Effluent control:** Substitution of raw materials causing more pollution with that of less pollution-causing materials. Use of nonconventional fuels, like Gobar gas, Biogas, CNG and LPG must be prepared and encouraged for.

Nurses' Contribution in Prevention and Control of Air Pollution

- Identifying air pollutants in the house, neighborhood, villages and towns. This may include smoke from various sources, exhaust from automobiles, vapor and gases from chemicals and pesticides, etc.
- Creating awareness among families, community leaders and people at large about these pollutants and their adverse effects on human health, animals and plants.
- Educating and motivating families, community leaders and people at large about:

- Prevention of smoke from various sources in homes, neighborhoods and community.
- Importance of cross-ventilation, wet sweeping and moping.
- Avoidance of cigarette smoking in homes and public places.
- Safe and proper storing of chemical fertilizers, DDT and bleaching powder.
- Surveillance of the occurrence of airborne diseases.
- Using a fuel-efficient vehicle and maintaining it properly.
- Resort to alternative energy sources, like solar power and wind power, whenever possible.

- Encourage the people to use technologically advanced air pollution-control equipment, like fabric filters and wet scrubbers. While fabric filters will help to remove the dust particles in a process referred to as 'bag filtration', wet scrubbers will help to remove acid gases, like sulfur dioxide, present in the atmosphere.

LIGHTING

Good lighting is required for good vision. It can be possible by arranging some factors that help effectively to reading process. If lighting is not in a good pattern, it leads to headache, stress and other fatigue, etc., requirement of good lighting is surely needed to run our daily workout without losing efficiency. For effective vision, some light factors are essential that are sufficiency, distribution, absence of glare, absence of sharp shadows, steadiness, color of light, surroundings and angle of light, etc.

FACTORS ESSENTIAL FOR GOOD LIGHTING

- **Sufficiency:** Sufficiency of lighting enables the eye to discern the details of the object as well as the surroundings without eye strain. Insufficient lighting causes eye strain. Sufficient lighting is termed as about an illumination that comes out from a 15–20 candles which is accepted as a basic minimum satisfactory vision. The illumination requirements vary from as little as 5-feet candles in stairways and corridors to 100-feet candles in some industries.
- **Distribution:** The efficient vision without any eye stress occurs by uniformity in light distribution. Light distribution should be proper by establishing the source of light generally from the left side. Two or three sources of light from any side with same intensity can be used, i.e., the source of light is needed to be with same voltage. If there are contrast differences in light, it will strain the eyes and affect the visual accuracy adversely. Proper dispersal of light, without the production of shadow therefore, necessary for efficient vision.
- **Absence of glare:** Glare is excessive contrast. There should be excessive light and high intensity of light causes glare, e.g., torch lights. These lights are pointed and cause to glare. Another best example of glare is the automobile headlights at night, the same light during daylight would not cause glare owing to the absence of excessive contrast. Glare may be directly from a light source or reflected glare from sources, such as tabletops of a polished furniture. Glare causes annoyance. It is not possible for our eye to effectively read in glared light because glare causes acute discomfort and reduction in critical vision.
- **Absence of sharp shadows:** Shadows occur when any object takes place between the light source and field of vision. Shadows create stress and need to be clear for proper reading process. Slight shadows are inevitable, but sharp and contrasting shadows are disturbing. Like glare, shadows cause confusion to the eye and therefore, should not be present in the field of vision. In incandescent bulbs, it always creates shadiness but fluorescent bulbs are proper to avoid shadows and for effective reading.
- **Steadiness:** The term refers to stable condition of light. Light must be constant with constant contrast and intensity. Flickering lights create eyestrain and headache.
- **Color of light:** The color of light is not very important so long as the intensity is adequate. Since natural light has a soothing effect on eyes, the artificial light should be as possible as the daylight color. By using red or violet lights, the effective reading will not take place, because the intensity of these lights is higher than normal.
- **Surrounding:** As a requirement to good lighting background has a major role to play because when a black object is viewed against a dark background, recognition is difficult. High levels of illumination will be required where there is little color contrast. For efficient vision, color schemes in rooms are important. The walls in the rooms and ceilings create reflection and it is essential for accumulation of light. Ceilings and roofs should have a reflection factor of 80%; walls 50–60%; and furniture 30–40%. There should not be much reflection from the floor, not more than 15–20%. Contrasting colors are often used to prevent accidents, e.g., culverts, bridges, etc.
- The glass walls or black backgrounds lose the efficiency of light because glass walls emit the light outside and black background absorbs the light and there is probably no reflection. So, surroundings should be in a normal condition by using proper materials causing reflection.
- **Angle of lighting:** Light source should be established in a proper way that leads to effective lighting by reflection. If the light is established in an improper condition, there will not be any reflection and the efficiency will be lost. For effective reading, light source would be better to be established on the left side of the wall rather than on the ceiling and other sides.

Measurement of Light

What we perceive as light is a narrow wavelength band of electromagnetic radiation from about 380–780 nm (nanometer). Light containing all visible waves is perceived as white. There is considerable confusion about units of light measurement. There are four measures of importance. For each of these four measures again, there are a number of terms and also a great variety of names. The four measures are: (1) Luminous intensity, which is the 'power' of a light source considered as a point radiating in all directions; this is measured as candles or candle power; (2) Luminous flus, which is the flow of light related to a unit of solid angle measured in lumens; (3) Illumination or illuminance, which is the amount of light reaching a surface measured in lux per unit area; and (4) Brightness or luminance which is the amount of light reflected from a surface measured in lamberts.

Lumens: 'Lumen' is the unit of total light output from a light source. If a lamp or fixture is surrounded by a transparent bubble, the total rate of light flow through the bubble is measured in lumens. Lumens indicate a rate of energy flow. Thus, it is a power unit, like the watt or horsepower. Typical indoor lamps have light outputs ranging from 50 to 10,000 lumens. Lumen is used in most types of lamps to compare lamp outputs, and to calculate lamp energy efficiencies (which are expressed as lumens per watt). Lumen output is not related to the light distribution pattern of the lamp. A large fraction of a lamp's lumen output may be useless if it goes in the wrong directions.

Footcandles and lux: 'Footcandles' and 'lux' are units that indicate the density of light that falls on a surface. This is what light meters measure. For example, average indoor lighting ranges from 100 to 1,000 lux, and average outdoor sunlight is about 50,000 lux. The footcandle is an older unit based on English measurements. It is equal to one lumen per square foot. It is being replaced by lux, a metric unit equal to one lumen per square meter. One footcandle is 10.76 lux. Although footcandles are now officially obsolete, they probably will continue to be used.

A lamp produces a certain amount of light measured in lumens. This light falls on surfaces with a density that is measured in footcandles or lux. A person looking at the scene sees different areas of his visual field in terms of levels of brightness, or luminance, measured in candelas per square meter. Many characteristics other than light intensity are important in selecting light sources. These include color, operating temperature, starting time, etc.

Daylight factor: Since the intensity of daylight illumination is liable to change from one moment to another, it is not measured in terms of foot candles. Reliance is placed on a factor called the 'daylight factor (DF)'. It is the ratio of illumination at a given point to illumination at a point exposed simultaneously to the whole hemisphere of the sky (taken as 500 foot-candles) excluding direct sunlight. The daylight factor may be summarized as follows:

$$DF = \frac{\text{Instantaneous illumination indoors}}{\text{Simultaneously occurring illumination outdoors}} \times 100$$

The daylight factor in a building may be rapidly determined by a modified photo-electric meter known as a 'daylight factor meter'. It is recommended that in living rooms, the daylight factor should be at least 8% and in kitchens about 10%.

Natural Lighting

Natural lighting is derived partly from the visible sky and partly from reflection. In fact, much light comes to the rooms by reflection from light-colored objects. Efficient utilization of natural light calls for careful design, location and orientation of buildings and relationship between buildings (town planning). Natural lighting also depends upon the time of the day, season, weather and atmospheric pollution. Since natural light is accompanied by radiant heat, all attempts should be made to exclude radiant heat while admitting daylight.

SUGGESTIONS FOR IMPROVING DAYLIGHT ILLUMINATION

The following general principles are taken into consideration in planning for the best utilization of daylight.

Orientation

The brightness of the sky is not constant on the east and west and 'therefore' the illumination is subject to variation in buildings facing east or west. Further, the direct penetration of sunlight from the east or west may heat up the rooms unduly in the tropics, especially during summers. Buildings are, therefore, oriented, wherever possible, towards north or south for uniform illumination. This is particularly essential for schools, factories and laboratories, where uniform lighting is required. When a building faces east and west, window shades are used to protect against direct penetration of sunlight.

Removal of Obstructions

Removal of obstructive items either wholly or partially is likely to give the most effective improvement in lighting.

Windows

Windows should be properly planned, as the actual lighting of any room is influenced by the amount of visible sky, the size, shape and arrangement of window openings. A tall window gives better penetration of light. Broad window gives better diffraction of light.

Interior of the Room

In order to obtain the full benefit of the natural illumination, the ceiling should be white, the upper portion of the walls light and tinted, and lower portions dark so as to give a perfect contrast to eyes.

ARTIFICIAL LIGHTING

Daylight may not meet the requirements of illumination during all hours, and especially during cloudy days. It should be supplemented by artificial illumination for adequate illumination. Artificial lighting should be as close as possible to daylight in composition. There are five systems of artificial lighting—direct, semi-direct, indirect, semi-indirect and direct-indirect.

Direct Lighting

In direct lighting, 99–100% of the light is projected directly towards the working area. Direct lighting is efficient, economical, but tends to cast sharp shadows. It should not fall into the eyes.

Semi-Direct

Here 10–40% of the light is projected upwards so that it is reflected back on the object by the ceiling.

Indirect

Light does not strike a surface directly, because 90–100% of the light is projected towards the ceiling and walls. This gives a general illumination of the whole room but not of any object.

Semi-Indirect

Here, 60–90% of the light is directed upwards, and the rest downwards.

Direct-Indirect

Here, light is distributed equally. No one system can be recommended to the exclusion of others.

Methods of Artificial Illumination

Filament Lamps

These are widely used. The electric current heats up the tungsten filament and the light emitted depends upon the temperature. The hotter filaments produce the bluer light. Accumulation of dust on the bulbs reduces illumination by 30–40%. The bulbs and shades, therefore, should be cleaned frequently.

Fluorescent Lamps

Fluorescent lamps are economical in the use of electric current; they are cool and efficient; the light emitted simulates natural light. The lamps consist of a glass tube filled with mercury vapor and an electrode fitted at each end. The inside of the tube is coated with fluorescent chemicals, which absorb practically all the ultraviolet radiation and remit the radiation in the visible range.

The total emission of energy from the two lamps is as follows:

	Light	*Heat*
Filament	5%	95%
Fluorescent	21%	79%

Lighting Standards

The eye responds to illumination ranging from 0.1 lux (full moonlight night) to 1,10,000 lux (bright sunshine). There is considerable confusion about standards because of the adaptability of the eye. Many standards have been published but these standards are arbitrary. The visual efficiency increases with the increase of illumination, but the curve flattens out at higher levels. The law of diminishing returns applies. A useful rule of thumb is that the illumination level should be 30 times higher than the level at which the task can just be done. It is worth repeating there are no exact lighting standards and it is usually better to err on the side of too much light, provided glare can be avoided.

Biologic Effects of Light

Considerable attention has recently been focused on the biologic effects of light. The observation that daylight could cause the in vitro degradation of bilirubin is now being used as a therapeutic measure in premature infants with hyperbilirubinemia. Other biologic effects of light include effect on biologic rhythms of body temperature, physical activity, the stimulation of melanin synthesis, the activation of precursors of vitamin D, adrenocortical secretion and food consumption.

LAND AND ITS POLLUTION

Land is the solid part of earth's surface while soil is the upper layer of the earth in which plants are grown. About 40% of the land is covered by desert. The rest of the land is used for making houses and buildings for various service organizations and institutions for agriculture and forests, for industrialization, urbanization, roads and highways, railways for mining, etc.

Definition

Land pollution is defined as the addiction of chemicals and organic substances in the soil which reduce its productive capacity and addition of all other unwanted substances in an indefinite proportion which deteriorates environment.

Land pollution is the degradation of earth's land surfaces often caused by human activities and their misuse of land resources. It occurs when:

- Waste is not disposed properly.
- Hazardous disposal of urban and industrial wastes.
- Exploitation of minerals.
- Improper use of soil by inadequate agriculture practices.

Land Pollutants

The various unwanted chemicals, organic and other substances which get added in an indefinite proportion in the soil and on land and destroy the soil, cause soil erosion and deteriorate environment.

The major land pollutants include pollutants which are washed out of the atmosphere with rain; pesticides and biocides; artificial fertilizers; household refuse, garbage, old papers, trash, industrial waste, construction debris, improper landfills, etc. Plastic has become a major land pollutant. Plastic bags, papers and wrappers stay undecayed for a long period on the land and create nuisance in the environment and become sources of health hazards.

Soil Erosion

Soil erosion refers to removal of upper fertile layer of the earth by wind and water. Soil erosion is due to overgrazing, deforestation and defective agricultural practices. Soil erosion can be prevented by controlling overgrazing and deforestation, by proper agricultural practices and by planting trees. The presence of trees and forests does not allow the wind or water to carry away with it a layer of soil.

Sources of Land Pollutants

There are a number of sources of land pollutants. These are presented below:

- **Waste matter from living habitat:** The waste matter from living habitat includes kitchen waste, refuse and sewage from household; solid and liquid waste from stables and butcher houses; dry and wet refuse from roads and streets, etc. The solid waste matter from household, stables and butcher houses, roads and streets, etc. is disposed of by burial in trenches using different methods of disposal. The problem arises when the burial of the trenches is not done properly and improper waste disposal system causes waste accumulation and improper sanitation system.

  The sewage from living habitats is disposed of by mechanical and biological treatment of the sewage. The effluents and sludge which are the byproducts of sewage disposal can contaminate soil if these are thrown on the surface of earth or used for cultivation without proper disposal. In some places, sewage may be directly thrown on the surface of earth which contaminates the soil or improper sanitation system causes sludge to leak at surrounding soil, which serves breeding ground for flies, rats, microorganisms which can contaminate soil and cause various problems.
- **Waste matter from agriculture:** With growing human population, demand for food has increased considerably. Farmers often use highly toxic fertilizers and pesticides to get rid of insects, fungi and bacteria from their crops. However with the overuse of these chemicals, they result in contamination and poisoning of soil. The waste matter, which is released from modern agricultural practices, includes different types of fertilizers, biocides, i.e., pesticides, herbicides, weedicides, etc. Pesticides which are persistent in nature are chlorinated hydrocarbon insecticides, e.g., DDT, HCH, endrin, lindane, heptachlor, endosulfan, etc. Residues of these pesticides in soils have long-term effects especially under the temperate conditions. These get washed away by wind and water into soil. This leads to chemical and biological contamination of soil.
- **Increase in urbanization and population:** Construction uses up forest land leading to increase in demand for raw materials, like timber. This leads to the exploitation and destruction of forests. On the other side, large quantities of sewage and solid wastes are produced because of increasing population and growth of cities and towns. But facilities for their safe and efficient collection, removal and disposal are inadequate which result in contamination of soil and deterioration of environment.
- **Waste matter from industries:** Industrial activities also are a contributing factor to land pollution. Industrial wastes are the effluents discharged from chemical industries, paper and pulp mills, tanneries, textile mills, steel industries, distilleries, refineries, pesticides and fertilizer industries, pharmaceutical industries, food processing industries, cement industries, thermal and nuclear power plants, mining industries, etc. may produce variety of toxic substances which are harmful for health. Thermal power plants generate a large quantity of 'fly ash.' Huge quantities of these wastes are dumped on land which cause land pollution. Often the waste water from industries is discharged either in the streams and river or in the drainage system. But in some places, it is thrown directly on the land either surrounding the industries or at some distance which contaminates the land. The solid waste from the industries is also left on the land surface for short or long duration, which pollutes the soil and environment.
- **Sociocultural practices:** In rural areas, open field defecation is a socio culturally accepted practice and is in vogue in almost all the villages throughout the country. Open field defection is also practiced in urban slums out of necessity and convenience. This practice pollutes and contaminates the soil with some microorganisms and worms which get transmitted to people and cause gastrointestinal diseases, especially hookworm infestation which enter the body through bare feet.
- **Construction activities:** Due to urbanization, large amount of construction activities are taking place, which has resulted in large waste articles, like wood, metal, bricks, plastic that can be seen by naked eyes outside any building or office which is under construction.
- **Mining activities:** During extraction and mining activities, several land spaces are created beneath the surface. We constantly hear about land caving in; this is nothing but nature's way of filling the spaces left out after mining or extraction activity.
- **Deforestation and soil erosion:** Deforestation carried out to create dry lands is one of the major concerns. Land, that is once converted into a dry or barren land, can never be made fertile again, whatever the magnitude of measures to redeem it. Land conversion, meaning the alteration or modification of the original properties of the land to make it usable for a specific purpose, is another major cause. This hampers the land immensely. Also there is a constant waste of land. Unused available land over the years turns barren; this land then cannot be used. So, in search of

more land, potent land is hunted and its indigenous state is compromised with.

Effects of Land Pollution

Land pollution contaminates the soil and water with microorganisms and helminths which can cause some gastrointestinal diseases, especially by drinking contaminated water, eating raw vegetables and by walking barefoot and swimming in contaminated swimming pools.

The diseases include diarrheal diseases, typhoid, hepatitis A and E, poliomyelitis, dysentery, work infestation, especially hookworm and guinea work. *Clostridium tetani* are usually present in the soil which get transmitted to human beings through deep skin injuries and by using contaminated hands and articles at the time of delivery and abortion. The land when contaminated with toxic chemicals and pesticides leads to problem of skin cancer and human respiratory system and also pesticides can damage crops, kill vegetation, and poison birds, animals, and fish. Most pesticides kill or damage life forms other than those intended. The toxic chemicals can reach our body through foods and vegetables that we eat as they are grown in polluted soil.

In addition, land pollution can contaminate air and water and can cause various harmful effects to plants and animals. The effects of land pollution are very hazardous and can lead to the loss of ecosystems. When land is polluted, it directly or indirectly affects the climatic pattern.

Land pollution with waste matter from household, stables, butcher houses, etc., when not collected, removed and disposed of properly, deteriorates the environment and causes sanitation problems. This creates health problems due to breeding of flies, mosquitoes, rats, etc. Soil polluted with various toxic chemicals is injurious to plants and vegetations. Sometimes, it can seriously disrupt the balance of nature, and, in extreme cases, can cause human fatalities.

Prevention and Control of Land Pollution

It is very important to preserve and maintain the quality of land to prevent harmful effects on men, animals and plants. Some of the measures which are followed and need to be followed are as under:

- Safe disposal of excreta and sewage, both in rural and urban areas as discussed in this chapter under prevention and control of water pollution.
- Use of garbage (animal and plant waste) for producing manure, bio-gas, etc., especially in the rural areas.
- Controlled use of artificial fertilizers and biocides.
- Avoid using the material which cannot be reused or recycled.
- Recycling of wastes and used metals. Waste metals, like iron, copper, aluminum, etc., can be melted and used to make useful products. Waste paper, gases, rubber and plastics can also be recycled.
- Improvement of slums.
- Encourage use of biodegradable materials to reduce soil pollution.
- Stopping the use of open spaces, fields, banks of rivers, ponds, etc., as toilets. Proper latrines should be provided in rural and slum areas.

Nurses' Contribution in Prevention and Control of Land Pollution

- Identifying and helping families and community people identify the land pollution at the neighborhood and community level, e.g., wet and dry garbage/refuse from household, stables, streets, etc., trash, building material, etc.
- Creating awareness among families, leaders and people at large regarding safe collection, removal and disposal of dry and wet refuse and waste water from household, neighborhood and community.
- Educating and motivating families, leaders and people at large regarding:
  - Maintenance of environment sanitation.
  - Association of increasing community's population with sanitation problems and acceptance of small family norms.

NOISE AND ITS POLLUTION

Noise means 'wrong sound, in the wrong place, at the wrong time'. Man is living in an increasingly noisy environment. The 20th century has been described as the 'century of noise'. Noise has become a very important 'stress factor' in the environment of man.

It is another hazardous pollutant present in our environment. It threatens not only the health of human beings but also the health of all other living organisms. It is a serious hazard in all big cities, such as Delhi, Mumbai, Chennai, Kolkata, Bengaluru, etc. Sound is a form of energy that causes sensation of hearing.

Sound forms the basis for speech which is the main mode of communication in human beings. Sound travels through the air or any other substance in the form of longitudinal waves. These waves are produced by the vibrations of the sound-producing sources. The sound waves reach the ear and through its vibrating mechanisms, the nerve message travels from the inner ear to the brain and the sound is heard. Thus, there are three conditions necessary for the production and hearing of sound, i.e., sound-producing vibrating body, a medium for the sound waves to travel and an ear to detect the sound waves.

Properties of Noise

Noise has two important properties: loudness or intensity, and frequency.

Loudness

Loudness or intensity depends upon the amplitude of the vibrations which initiated the noise. The loudness of noise is measured in decibels (dB). When we say that sound is 60 dB, it means that it is 60 dB more intense than the smallest distinguishable noise or the 'reference' sound pressure, which is understood to be 0.0002 microbars or dynes/cm^2. A dyne is 1/10,00,000th of atmospheric pressure. Normal conversation produces a noise of 60–65 dB; whispering 20–30 dB; heavy street traffic, 60–80 dB; and boiler factories, about 120 dB. A daily exposure up to 85 dB is about the limit people can tolerate without substantial damage to their hearing.

Frequency

The frequency of the sound waves is denoted by Hertz (Hz). One Hz is equal to one wave per second. Human ears can detect frequencies between 20 and 20,000 Hz. This range is known as 'audible range'. This range gets reduced with age and other factors. Frequencies above 20,000 Hz are known as 'ultrasonic waves' while below 20 Hz are known as 'infrasonic waves'. These are inaudible to man, but audible to animals, like dogs, bats, etc.

The intensities of the sound can be measured in decibels. Sound up to 80 decibels (db) is safe for human beings. The sound level of normal talking is usually 60 db and that of whispering is between 30 and 35 db.

Terminology

The sounds we hear can be musical sounds and noises. These are defined as under:

- **Musical sounds:** These are defined as the sounds which have regular and periodic vibrations. These sounds are pleasant to the ears. Musical sounds stimulate brain activities and cause relaxation.
- **Noises:** Noises are defined as the sounds which have irregular and nonperiodic vibrations. These sounds produce jarring and unpleasant sensations on the ears. It is the high intensity sound which causes pollution and is harmful. Noise thus can also be defined as any unwanted sound that produces undesired psychological or physiological effects on an individual. Sound becomes unwanted when it either interferes with normal activities, such as sleeping, conversation, or disrupts or diminishes one's quality of life. Not all noise can be called 'noise pollution'. If it does not happen regularly, it may be termed as 'nuisance'.
- **Noise pollution:** It refers to the pollution of environment with high intensity of sound produced from various sources and which can cause harmful effects on human beings, other animals and plants. A noise of 90 db can produce temporary hearing loss but a noise of 160 db sound can cause complete deafness, e.g., the sound from the jet aircraft during take-off at close range can cause total deafness due to rupturing of eardrum.

Sources of Noise Pollution

There are various sources of noises which pollute our environment and differ at various places which are presented underneath.

- **Sources at domestic sites:** These include various types of electronic sound and video systems, e.g., radio, loudspeaker, television, record player, etc. and other electronic machines, such as mixers and grinders, coolers, air-conditioners, Tullu pumps, generators and grass-cutter machines, etc. Others include loudspeakers of sound systems and TVs, ipods and earphones. Another example may be your neighbor's dog barking all night everyday at every shadow it sees, disturbing everyone else in the apartment.
- **Sources at roadside:** These include bulldozers, concrete mixers, cutting and crushing machines, hammer strikes, etc. All these produce thundering and roaring sounds which cause noise pollution which are very harmful to workers as well as people living in and around the areas.
- **Sources at factory sites:** These include various types of noise-producing machines, e.g., drilling and milling machines, rollers, cranes, etc., and produce very high-intensity sounds which are deafening and harmful otherwise to workers and people in the surrounding areas.
- **Other sources:** These include loudspeakers, drum-beating, rock music, airplanes, trains, crackers and fireworks, etc. Use of loudspeakers during various cultural and religious functions, especially till late nights/whole night, which is very disturbing, especially for children, elders, sick, etc.

Effects of Noise Pollution

As per WHO, the prescribed optimum noise level is 45 db during the day and 35 db during the night and anything above 80 db is hazardous. Noise pollution can cause several harmful effects to human beings. These are as under:

- **Auditory fatigue:** Auditory fatigue is characterized by whistling and buzzing of ears and occurs in places where sound intensity is of 90 db.
- **Deafness (hearing loss):** The noise can cause temporary and permanent deafness. Usually, a noise of 90 db can produce a temporary hearing loss, which disappears after 24 hours of exposure to noise. If the ears do not get chance to recover due to repeated or continuous exposure to noise, the deafness can become permanent. A sound of 160 db, such as the sound from the jet aircraft and noise from some factories can cause complete deafness either due to rupture of eardrum or damage of the inner ear or both. It can cause pain in the middle ear, loss of equilibrium and dizziness.
- **Changes in psychosocial behavior:** It is observed that repeated or continuous exposure to noise causes annoyance, tension, nervousness and anxiety, temper tantrums, etc. It also causes fatigue, insomnia, inefficiency at work, impairs concentration, etc.
- **Physiological changes:** Exposure to noise is found to affect cardiovascular system. It increases heart rate and blood pressure, decreases peripheral circulation. It also increases intracranial pressure and sweat. It is said to affect digestive system and cause peptic ulcer. General

symptoms, such as giddiness, nausea and fatigue may also occur. Noise interferes with sleep. Noise is also said to cause visual disturbance. It is said to cause a narrowing of pupils, affect color perception and reduce night vision.

Other Effects

- **Interference with speech:** Noise interferes with speech communication. In everyday life, the frequencies causing most disturbance to speech communication lie in the 300–500 Hz range. Such frequencies are commonly present in noise produced by road and air traffic. For good speech intelligibility, it is considered that the speech sound level must exceed the speech interference level (SIL) by approximately 12 db.
- **Efficiency:** A low level of noise is always desired in work environment. Reduction in noise has been found to increase work output by increasing concentration.
- **Economic losses:** Besides affecting health, noise is also a significant factor in economic losses. The potential cost of noise-induced hearing loss to industry is quite huge.

Prevention and Control of Noise Pollution

There are various ways of prevention and control of noise pollution. Some of these are listed as under:

- The noise source can be reduced by use of good-quality silencers and muffin in the vehicles, use of insulating material at places where noise is produced, e.g., planting of trees and hedges along the roads and streets, reducing the volume of musical devices, such as radios, televisions, record players, loudspeakers, etc.
- Hearing protection is recommended for all workers who are consistently exposed to noise louder than 85 db in the frequency bands above 150 Hz. Workers must be regularly rotated from noisy areas to comparatively quiet posts in factories. Periodical audiogram check-ups and use of earplugs, earmuffs are also essential as the situation demands.
- Noise-producing activities should be limited to specified hours of the day and night, e.g., air flights, construction work, etc.
- Proper planning of city like division of the city into zones with separation of areas concerned with industry and transport is essential. Railway yards, aerodromes, industries, etc., should be installed away from residential areas. Wherever such provisions are not possible, green belts should be laid down around these installations. House fronts should lie not less than 15 meters from the road and the intervening space should be thickly planted with trees and bushes, widening of main streets to reduce the level of noise penetration into dwellings can be done.
- The use of pressure horns and loudspeakers should be banned in the residential areas.
- The workers should be exposed for limited hours to high-intensity sounds in the industries. There should be frequent changes from high-intensity zones to quiet zones.
- Proper maintenance of motors and machines should be done.
- Education of people regarding noise pollution is very important and should be done.
- Many countries have enacted specific legislation to control noise pollution from various sources. In India, making loud noise is punishable by law with imprisonment up to 5 years or fine up to 1 lac or both. In case it continues, an additional fine may be extended to ₹5,000 per day. If the above contravention continues beyond a period of 1 year after the date of conviction, imprisonment may be extended to 7 years.

Nurses' Contribution in Prevention and Control of Noise Pollution

- **Identify sources of noise:** The nurse can help the family members and community people identify the sources of noise pollution in their houses, neighborhood and community and also help them in reducing noise at their source by using good-quality silencers and muffin in the vehicles, using of insulating material at places where noise is produced as like planting of trees.
- **Creating awareness:** Creating awareness among families, leaders and people at large regarding the harmful auditory and nonauditory effects of noise on human health by which the individuals can protect themselves from the noise. This is especially applicable for industrial workers, traffic police, people working in railway stations, etc. Educating and motivating people regarding prevention and control of noise pollution at their household, neighborhood and community level are also important.

RADIOACTIVE POLLUTION

The radioactive pollution of environment is due to advanced technology and modernization of man's activities. It includes radioactive pollution of atmosphere, water, soil, and food. The radioactive substances are very hazardous to all living organisms. It is becoming very important to understand about it as it will help in creating awareness among the community people taking precautionary measures.

Definitions

- **Radioactive substances:** The substances (elements) which emit invisible ionizing radiations due to nuclear disintegration are called 'radioactive substances'. For example: uranium, radium, thorium and polonium, etc.
- **Radioactivity:** The emission of invisible ionizing radiations from radioactive substances is known as 'radioactivity'.
- **Radioactive pollution:** The presence of invisible ionizing radiations produced from radioactive substances in the atmosphere, water, food, etc., which are harmful, refers to radioactive pollution.

Types of Radiation

There are three different types of ionizing radiations, which are emitted from the nucleus of radioactive substances, such as thorium, uranium, radium, etc. The radiation includes α (alpha) particles, β (beta) particles and γ (gamma) rays:

- **α particles:** α particles are positively charged. These are very harmful (10 times more harmful than X-rays), when taken internally either by ingestion or inhaled through air. But fortunately a particles have little penetrating powers in the body.
- **β particles:** β particles are negatively charged. These can penetrate the skin but generally do not reach deep-seated organs when delivered externally. These can damage the skin and affect eyes.
- **γ rays:** γ-rays are electromagnetic radiations. These are of short wavelength. These have high penetrating power and are more dangerous than α and β rays.

In addition to these rays, there are X-rays which are man-made electromagnetic radiations and are in great use in medical field. Like γ rays, X-rays are also of short wavelength and have penetrating power. These are also highly hazardous when used frequently.

All these rays are ionizing radiations which have high energy value to penetrate inside the body tissue and get deposited there. Roentgen is the unit of measurement of radioactivity of radioactive substance. This unit of measurement is named after a great scientist William Roentgen, who discovered X-rays. The safest limit of radioactivity for human beings is 0.25 roentgen per week.

There are a number of nonionizing electromagnetic radiations which have long wavelength, less energy value and less penetrating power than the radiations mentioned above. These radiations include ultraviolet, visible light, infrared, microwave and radiofrequency radiations.

Sources of Radiation Pollution

There are two major categories of sources of radioactive pollution. These are natural and man-made sources.

Natural Sources

The natural sources of radioactive radiation mainly include radiation from the environment and cosmic radiation. The cosmic rays which originate in outer space are weakened as they pass through the atmosphere. At ordinary living altitudes, their impact is about 35 mrad a year. At altitudes above 20 km, cosmic radiation becomes important. The radioactive substances, such as radium, uranium, thorium, etc., are present in the soil, rocks and radioactive gases, such as radon and thoron are present in the air. It is estimated that man derives about 50 mrad per year from terrestrial radiation. It is estimated that, man derives about 50 mrad per year from terrestrial radiation. These substances and gases release radioactive radiation and contaminate air, water, soil and food. Similarly, cosmic rays from sun, stars, etc. also release radioactive radiation in the atmosphere.

All these natural sources of radiation in the environment expose human beings at the risk of radiation.

Man-made Sources

The man-made sources of radioactive radiation include: X-rays, radioactive substances which are used in the field of medicines, nuclear power plants, nuclear explosions, nuclear weapons, industries using radioactive substances, satellites, rockets, mining and refining processes, etc.

- **X-rays:** The greatest man-made sources of radiation exposure to the general population at the present time are medical and dental X-rays. Two distinct groups involved in these are patients and radiologists, and medical technician. Experimental and epidemiological data currently do not support the proposition that there is a threshold dose of radiation below which there is no increased risk of cancer. However, this is under increasing doubt. It is estimated that the additional radiation will increase a person's cumulative risk of getting cancer by age 75 by 0.6–1.8%. The amount of absorbed radiation depends upon the type of X-ray test and the body part involved. CT and fluoroscopy entail higher doses of radiation than do plain X-rays.
- **Radioactive fallout:** Nuclear explosions release a tremendous amount of energy in the form of heat, light, ionizing radiation and many radioactive substances, the important being the isotopes of carbon (C14) iodine (I131), cesium (Cs137) and strontium (Sr90). Cs137 and Sr90 are considered most important because they are liberated in large amounts and remain radioactive for many years. The 'half-life' of Sr90 is about 28 years and that of Cs137 30 years. These radioactive particles released into the atmosphere float down to earth for some years afterwards. Because of air currents, the particles are distributed fairly evenly over the whole human race. A country where there had been no explosions, showed that a dose of 33 mrems per person was received from this source.
- **Miscellaneous:** Some everyday appliances (e.g., TV sets, luminous wrist watches) are radioactive. But radiation from these sources at present is too small to be important.

All these sources produce radioactive gases which pollute the atmosphere and radioactive waste which may contaminate water and soil if not disposed of properly. Radioactive waste can be dangerous for millions of years. Radioactive pollution can also be due to electronic devices, such as color TVs, computers, radium watches, cellular phones, etc.

Effects of Radioactive Pollution

Though radioactive substances have been responsible for advancement in medicine, informatics, communication, agriculture, industries, space technologies, etc. but have many harmful effects on human health.

Chronic exposure to low level of radiation can cause many somatic and genetic problems. In early stages, it can cause depigmentation of skin and loss of hair. In the long run, it can cause diseases like blood cancer, cancer of various parts of the body, like thyroid, lungs, bones, etc., genetic changes in future generation, etc. Thus, it reduces life expectancy of people.

Because of radioactive pollution of atmosphere, food, water, soil, etc., there are increasing incidences of these diseases. Acute exposure to radiation causes radiation sickness which is characterized by vomiting, sore throat, diarrhea, bleeding under the skin and other organs, etc.

One of the examples of devastating effects of radiation in the 20th century was the use of nuclear bomb on Hiroshima and Nagasaki (cities in Japan) in 1945. Thousands (15–20%) of people died of radiation, 20–30% died of fire of the explosion. Even after years, people kept suffering from cancer of lungs, breast, thyroid, bones, cataract, etc. Babies born today still have many genetic problems.

Prevention and Control of Radiation

It is the man-made sources which increase the risk of exposure to radioactive radiations and so also exposure to X-rays constitute the greatest risk. The following measures are advocated and implemented:

- Safe disposal of radioactive waste from nuclear plants, hospitals, laboratories, industries, etc. The methods used are: releasing of radioactive gases high up in the air where these get diluted and disposed; storing of radioactive waste until its radioactivity is reduced; and chemical treatment of waste before its final disposal.
- Initiating efforts to stop nuclear explosion.
- Underground testing of nuclear explosion.
- Use of radiation therapy within prescribed limits and when absolutely required.
- Avoidance of unnecessary X-ray examinations especially in case of children and pregnant women.
- Thorough monitoring and surveillance of X-ray plants, workers and handling of X-ray machines and procedures.
- Application of protective measures while carrying any diagnostic or therapeutic procedure involving use of radioactive substances, etc.
- Controlled exposure of workers in the industries, labs, and nuclear medicine departments of hospitals.
- Monitoring of level of concentration in the industries, labs and nuclear medicine departments, etc.
- Creating awareness among people regarding radioactive radiations and use of such electronic devices at homes.

Protection from radiation is the concern of international organizations like the International Atomic Energy Agency (IAEA), World Health Organization (WHO) and the International Commission of Radiological Protection (ICRP). Their main concern is to promote peaceful use of atomic energy. These organizations are working towards developing guidelines for radiation protection, code of practice for safe operation of nuclear power plants and international safety standards.

Nurses' Contribution in Prevention and Control of Radioactive Pollution

a. Identifying and helping families and community people identify sources of radioactive pollution in their homes and community, e.g., electronic gadgets, radium watches, cellular phones, etc.
b. Creating awareness among families and community people at large about the harmful effects of radioactive pollution on health.
c. Educating families and community people at large regarding:
   - The controlled use of electronic devices in their homes.
   - Lobbying for peaceful use of atomic energy.

In general, it can be seen that community health nurses, while dealing with families and community people at large, make use of nursing process to assess this quality and safety of environment, plan and implement actions to improve their living environment. The major nursing intervention includes education of people in the community in its various settings. Education is both formal and informal, planned and incidental. The nurses act as motivators and change agents.

Nurses are directly not responsible for environmental health. This is the responsibility of other authorities. They act as an advocate and report to these agencies and involve them if necessary to deal with any such environmental situation along with community people.

HOUSING

'Housing' in the modern concept includes not only the 'physical structure' providing shelter, but also the immediate surroundings, and the related community services and facilities. It has become part of the concept of 'human settlement', which is defined as 'all places in which a group of people reside and pursue their life goals; the size of the settlement may vary from a single family to millions of people.'

Goals of Housing

The generally accepted goals of housing are:

- **Shelter:** The house should provide a sanitary shelter which is a basic need for security and a sense of connection within communities.
- **Family life:** That the house should provide adequate space for family life and related activities, viz. preparation and storage of good, meeting, sleeping individual activities and other basic activities. The adequacy of housing at this level has been found to have a direct impact on such things as worker productivity and family stability.
- **Access to community facilities:** A third element of housing is accessibility to community services and facilities, such as health services, schools, shopping areas, places of worship, etc. The availability of a suitable range of housing contributes to a community's ability to function in efficient, equitable, prosperous and sustainable ways. Adequate and appropriate housing is, thus, fundamental to vital, and livable conditions.
- **Family participation in community life:** Family is part of the wider community. Community is important to family in many ways. It can offer help in times of need; it is an important source of making friends. Communities are able to prove their efforts and improve their living conditions.

- **Economic stability:** Housing is a form of investment of personal saving. It provides for economic stability and well-being of the family.
- **Improve health:** Stable, affordable and accessible housing linked to health, justice and community support services is critical to helping people live independently and improve life opportunities related to family, work, education, recreation or other pursuits. Objectives for housing need to be seen in this context.

The implementation of social goals in housing requires that the Government should:

- Introduce social housing scheme
- Establish both minimum and maximum standards
- Create financial and fiscal institutions geared up to helping the low-income people obtain credit for building or renovating their houses.

CRITERIA FOR HEALTHFUL HOUSING

An expert committee of the WHO recommended the following criteria for healthful housing similar to the Basic Principles of Healthful Housing published by the American Public Health Association:

- Healthful housing provides physical protection and shelter;
- It provides adequate means for cooking, eating, washing and excretory functions;
- It is designed, constructed, maintained and used in a manner such as to prevent the spread of communicable diseases;
- It provides for protection from hazards of exposure to noise and pollution;
- It is free from unsafe physical arrangements due to construction or maintenance, and from toxic and harmful materials; and
- It encourages personal and community development, promotes social relationships, reflects as regards the ecological principles, and by these means, promotes mental health.

The minimum standards are still maintained by building regulations, the aim being improvement of housing and environmental conditions for the majority of families within the limits set by the available resources and objectives. The standards in India are those recommended by the EHC (1947). These are mentioned as follows:

Site

(a) The site should be elevated from its surroundings that it is not subject to flooding during rains; (b) It should have an independent access to a street of adequate width; (c) It should be away from the breeding places of mosquitoes and flies; (d) It should be away from the nuisance, such as dust, smoke, smell, excessive noise and traffic; (e) It should be in pleasing surroundings; (f) The soil should be dry and safe in founding the structure and should be well-drained. 'Made-soil', i.e., ground that is leveled by dumping refuse is very unsuitable for building purposes for at least 20–25 years. The subsoil water level should be below 10 feet (3 meters).

Setback

For proper lighting and ventilation, there should be an open space all around the house. This is called 'setback'. In the rural areas, it is recommended that the built-up area should not exceed one-third of the total area; in the urban areas, where land is costly, the built-up area may be up to two-thirds. The setback should be such that there is no obstruction to proper lighting and ventilation.

Floor

The floor should be pucca and satisfy the criteria, like it should be impermeable so that it can be easily washed and kept clean and dry. (a) Mud floors tend to peak up and cause dust, so these are not recommended; (b) The floor must be smooth and free from cracks and crevices to prevent the breeding of insects and harborage of dust; (c) The floors should be damp-proof; (d) The height of the plinth should be 2–3 feet (0.6– meter).

Walls

(a) The walls should be reasonably strong; (b) These should have a low heat capacity, i.e., these should not absorb heat and conduct the same; (c) These should be weather-resistant; (d) These should be unsuitable for harborage of rats and vermin; (e) These should not be easily damaged and smooth. These standards can be attained by 9-inch bricks—all plastered smooth and colored cream or white.

Roof

The height of the roof should not be less than 9 feet (3 meters) in the absence of air-conditioning for comfort. The roof should have a low heat transmittance coefficient.

Rooms

The number of living rooms should not be less than two, at least one of which can be closed for security. The rooms may be open on one side if that side lies a private courtyard. The number and area of rooms should be increased according to size of family, so that the recommended floor space per person may be made available.

Floor Area

The floor area of a living room should be at least 120 sq ft (12 sq m) for occupancy by more than one person and at least 100 sq ft (10 sq m) for occupancy by a single person. The floor area available in living rooms per person should not be less than 50 sq ft; the optimum size is 100 sq ft.

Cubic Space

Unless means are provided for mechanical placement of air, the height of rooms should be such as to move an air space of at least 500 cubic feet per capita, preferably 1,000 cubic feet.

Windows

- Unless mechanical ventilation and artificial lighting are provided, every living room should be provided with at least two windows, and at least one of them should open directly on to an open space.
- The windows should be placed at a height of no more than 3 feet (1 m) over the ground in living rooms.
- Window area should be 1/5th of the floor area. Doors and windows combined should have 2/5th of the floor area.

Lighting

The daylight factor should exceed 1% per half the floor area.

Kitchen

Every dwelling house must have a separate kitchen. The kitchen must be protected against dust and smoke, adequately lighted, provided with arrangements for bring food, fuel and provisions, provided with water supply, and a sink for washing utensils, and fitted with arrangements for proper drainage. The floor of the kitchen must be impervious.

Privy

A sanitary privy is a must in every house, belonging exclusively to it and readily accessible. In the more developed areas of the world, the majority of dwelling units are equipped with water-carriage systems.

Garbage and Refuse

The house should have facilities for bathing and washing belonging exclusively to it and providing adequate privacy.

Water Supply

The house should have a safe and adequate water supply available at all times.

Housing and Health

Housing is part of the total environment of man and, being a part, it is, to some extent, responsible for the status of a man's health and well-being. It is difficult, however, to demonstrate the specific cause-and-effect relationship because housing embraces so many facets of environment. By deductive reasoning, a strong relationship can be established between poor housing and the following conditions:

- **Respiratory infections:** Common cold, tuberculosis, influenza, diphtheria, bronchitis, measles, whooping cough, etc.
- **Skin infections:** Scabies, ringworm, impetigo, leprosy.
- **Rat infestation:** Plague.
- **Arthropods:** Houseflies, mosquitoes, fleas and bugs.
- **Accidents:** A substantial proportion of house accidents is caused by some defect in the home and its environment.
- **Morbidity and mortality:** High morbidity and mortality rates are observed where housing conditions are substandard.
- **Psychosocial effects:** These effects must not be overlooked. The sense of isolation felt by persons living in the upper floors of high buildings is now well known to have harmful effects. Often, also, people living in densely populated urban areas feel a similar sense of isolation, which may lead to neurosis and behavior disorders.

If the definition of health given by WHO is applied, we have also to take into consideration the broader aspects of mental and social well-being of individuals and families, i.e., factors related to satisfaction of physiological, psychological and social needs.

Overcrowding is a health problem in human dwellings. It may promote the spread of respiratory infections, such as tuberculosis, influenza and diphtheria. High morbidity and mortality rates are observed where housing conditions are substandard.

The accepted standards with respect to overcrowding are as follows:

Standards with Respect to Overcrowding

Persons per Room

The degree of overcrowding can best be expressed as the number of persons per room, i.e., number of persons in the household divided by the number of rooms in the dwelling **Table 6.4**. The room standard is contravened when the number of persons sleeping in a dwelling and the number of rooms available as sleeping accommodation is such that two persons of opposite sexes, who are not living together as husband and wife, must sleep in the same room. For this purpose, children under the age of ten shall be left out of account, and a room is available as sleeping accommodation if it is of a type normally used in the locality either as a bedroom or as a living room.

The WHO-accepted standards for floor space are as follows:

- A baby under 12 months is not counted, and children from 1 to 10 years are counted as half-a-unit.
- Overcrowding is considered to exist if two persons over 9 years of age, not husband and wife, of opposite sexes are obliged to sleep in the same room.

(A baby under 12 months is not counted; children from 1–10 are counted as half-a-unit).

Table 6.4: Number of persons per square meter.

Area (in square meter)	*No. of person(s)*
11 or more	2
9–10	1.5
7–9	1
5–7	0.5
Under 5	Nil

Sex Separation

Overcrowding is considered to exist if 2 persons over 9 years of age, not husband and wife, of opposite sexes are obliged to sleep in the same room.

Indicators of Housing

- **Physical indicators:** These are based on floor space, cubic space, room height, persons per room, rooms per dwelling, environmental quality (e.g., air, light, water, noise, sewage disposal, etc.).
- **Economic indicators:** These are cost of the building, rental levels, taxes, expenditure on housing, etc.
- **Social indicators:** The following were proposed at an inter-regional seminar on the Social Aspects of Housing, organized by the UN in 1975.
  - Indicators related to prevention of illness:
    - Frequency of illness due to inadequate sewage and garbage collection
    - Frequency of illness associated with contaminated water source
    - Frequency of insect-borne diseases
    - Frequency of illness due to overcrowding
    - Frequency of illness due to accidents
    - Frequency of illness due to proximity to animals
    - Access to medical facility.
  - Indicators related to comfort:
    - Thermal comfort
    - Acoustic comfort
    - Visual comfort
    - Spatial comfort
  - Indicators related to mental health and social well-being:
    - Frequency of suicides in the neighborhood
    - Neglected and abandoned youth in the neighborhood
    - Drug abuse (including alcohol) in the neighborhood.

House Site and Construction Assistance

The scheme was included in the State Sector as a part of Minimum Needs Programme and formed the core of the rural housing program during the seventh and subsequent five year plan. This scheme has two components—provision of free house sites and construction assistance with varying proportions of subsidy and loan in different states. Construction assistance planned to benefit 3.5 million families directly as part of Minimum Needs Programme. This is exclusive of other special rural housing programs intended for specific beneficiary groups.

Indira Awas Yojana

The Indira Awas Yojana (IAY) was introduced in the Central Sector in 1985–1986 as part of the Rural Landless Employment Guarantee Programme (RLEGP). These types of houses have one room, one kitchen attached with latrine, bathroom and a smokeless chulha.

DISPOSAL OF WASTES

Disposal of wastes is now largely the domain of sanitarians and public health engineers. However, health professionals need to have a basic knowledge of the subject since improper disposal of wastes constitutes a health hazard. Further the health professional may be called upon to give advice in some special situations, such as camp sanitation or coping with waste disposal problems when there is a disruption or breakdown of community health services in natural disasters. These aspects are considered in this section.

The term 'solid wastes' includes garbage (food waste), rubbish (paper, plastic, wood, metal, throw-away containers, brass), demolition products (bricks, masonry, pipes), sewage treatment residue (sludge and solids from the coarse screening domestic sewage), dead animals, manure and other discarded material. Strictly speaking, it should not contain night soil. In India and in other countries as well, it is not uncommon to find night soil in collection of refuse. The output of daily waste depends upon the dietary habits, lifestyles, living standards and the degree of urbanization and industrialization. The per capita daily solid waste produced ranges between 0.25 and 2.5 kg in different countries.

Effects of Accumulation of Solid Waste

- It decomposes and favors fly-breeding
- It attracts rodents and vermins
- The pathogens which may be present in the solid waste may be conveyed back to man's food through flies and dust
- There is a possibility of water and soil pollution
- Heaps of refuse present an unsightly appearance and nuisance from bad odors
- Increased incidence of vector-borne diseases.

Sources of Refuse

- Refuse that is collected by the street-cleansing service of avenging is called 'street refuse'. It consists of leaves, straw, paper, animal droppings and litter of all kinds.
- Refuse that is collected from markets is called 'market refuse'. It contains a large proportion of putrid vegetable and animal matter.
- Refuse that is collected from stables is called 'stable litter'. It contains mainly animal droppings and left-over animal feeds.
- Industrial refuse comprises a wide variety of wastes ranging from completely inert materials, such as calcium carbonate to highly toxic and explosive compounds.
- The domestic refuse consists of ash, rubbish and garbage. Ash is the residue from fire used for cooking and heating. Rubbish comprises paper, clothing, bits of wood, metal, glass, dust and dirt.
- Garbage is waste matter arising from the preparation, cooking and consumption of food. It consists of waste food, vegetable peelings and other organic matter.

Garbage needs quick removal and disposal because it ferments on storage.

Storage

The first consideration should be given to the proper storage of refuse, while awaiting collection.

- **Galvanized steel dustbin:** The galvanized steel dust bin with close fitting cover is a suitable receptacle for storing refuse. The capacity of a bin will depend upon the number of users and frequency of collection. The output of refuse per capita per day in India is estimated to vary from 1/10 to 1/20 c. ft. For a family of 5 members, a bin having a capacity of 5/10 or 1/2 c. ft. would be needed. If collection is done once in three days, a bin having a capacity of 1-1/2 or 2 c. ft. would be adequate. A recent innovation in the western countries is the 'paper sack'. Refuse is stored in the paper sack, and the sack itself is removed with the contents for disposal and a new sack is substituted.
- **Public bins:** Public bins cater for a larger number of people. They are usually without cover in India because people do not like to touch them. They are kept on a concrete platform raised 2–3 inches above the ground level to prevent flood water entering the bins. In bigger municipalities, the bins are handled and emptied mechanically by lorries fitted with cranes.

Collection

The method of collection depends upon the funds available. House-to-house collection is by far the best method of collecting refuse. In India, there is no house-to-house collection system. People are expected to dump the refuse in the nearest public bin, which is usually not done. Refuse is dispersed all along the street, and some of it is thrown out in front and around the house. As a result, an army of sweepers is required for sweeping the streets in addition to the gang for collecting the refuse from public bins. The refuse is then transported in refuse collection vehicles to the place of ultimate disposal. Dead animals are directly transported to the place of disposal.

The collection methods normally practiced in this country need drastic revision and improvement in the interest of better hygiene. The Environmental Hygiene Committee (1949) recommended that municipalities and other local bodies should arrange for the collection of refuse not only from the public bins but also from individual houses. A house-to-house collection will result in a simultaneous reduction in the number of public bins. The open refuse cart should be abandoned and replaced by enclosed vans. Mechanical transport should be used wherever possible as it is more practical and economical than the 19th-century methods. There is a wide variety of refuse collection vehicles of all shapes and sizes. The latest arrival in the western countries is the 'Dustless Refuse Collector' which has a totally enclosed body.

Methods of Disposal

There is no single method of refuse disposal which is equally suitable in all circumstances. The choice of a particular method is governed by local factors, such as cost and availability of land and labor. The principal methods of refuse disposal are as follows:

Dumping

Refuse is dumped in low-lying areas partly as a method of reclamation of land but mainly as an easy method of disposal of dry refuse. As a result of bacterial action, refuse decreases considerably in volume and is converted gradually into humus. Kolkata disposes of its refuse by dumping and the reclaimed land is leased out for cultivation. The drawbacks of open dumping are: (i) the refuse is exposed to flies and rodents; (ii) it is a source of nuisance due to the smell and unsightly appearance; (iii) the loose refuse is dispersed by the action of the wind; and (iv) the drainage from dumps contributes to the pollution of surface and ground water. A WHO Expert Committee (1967) condemned dumping as 'the most insanitary method that creates public health hazards, nuisance, and severe pollution of the environment'. Dumping should be outlawed and replaced by sound procedures.

Controlled Tipping

Controlled tipping or sanitary landfill is the most suitable method of refuse disposal where suitable land is available. It differs from ordinary dumping in that the material is placed in a trench or other prepared area, adequately compacted, and covered with earth at the end of the working day. The term 'modified sanitary landfill' has been applied to those operations where compaction and covering are accomplished once or twice a week.

Three methods are used in this operation—the trench method, the ramp method and the area method.

1. **Trench method:** Where leveled ground is available, the trench method is usually chosen. A long trench is dug out 2–3 m (6–10 feet) deep and 4–12 m (12–36 feet) wide, depending upon the local conditions. The refuse is compacted and covered with excavated earth. Where compacted refuse is placed in the fill to a depth of 2 m (6 feet), it is estimated that one acre of land per year will be required for 10,000 population.
2. **Ramp method:** This method is well suited where the terrain is moderately sloping. Some excavation is done to secure the covering material.
3. **Area method:** This method is used for filling land depressions, disused quarries and clay pits. The refuse is deposited, packed and consolidated in uniform layers up to 2–2.5 m. (6–8 feet) deep. Each layer is sealed on its exposed surface with a mud cover at least 30 cm (12 inches) thick. Such sealing prevents infestation by flies and rodents and suppresses the nuisance of smell and dust. This method often has the disadvantage of requiring supplemental earth from the outside sources.

Chemical, bacteriological and physical changes occur in buried refuse. The temperature rises to over 60°C within 7 days and kills all the pathogens and hastens the decomposition process. Then it takes 2–3 weeks to cool down. Normally, it takes 4–6 months for complete decomposition of organic matter into an innocuous mass. The tipping of refuse in water should not be done as it creates a nuisance from odors given off by the decomposition of organic matter. The method of controlled tipping has been revolutionized by mechanization. The bulldozer achieves the tasks of spreading trimming and also spreading top soil.

Incineration

Refuse can be disposed of hygienically by burning incineration. It is the method of choice where suitable land is not available. Hospital refuse which is particularly dangerous is best disposed of by incineration. Incineration is practiced by several industrialized countries, particularly in large cities due to lack of suitable land. Incineration is not a popular method in India because the refuse contains a fair proportion of fine ash which makes the burning difficult. A preliminary separation of dust or ash is needed. All this involves head outlay and expenditure, besides manipulative difficulties in the incinerator. Further, disposal of refuse by burning is a loss to the community in terms of the much-needed manure. Burning, therefore, has a limited application in refuse disposal in India.

Composting

Composting is a method of combined disposal of refuse at night soil or sludge. It is a process of nature whereby organized matter breaks down under bacterial action, resulting in the formation of relatively stable humus-like material called the 'compost' which has considerable manurial value for the soil. The principal byproducts are carbon dioxide, water and heat. The heat produced during composting, 60°C or high over a period of several days, destroys eggs and larvae, flies, weed seeds and pathogenic agents. The end-product called 'compost' contains a few or no disease-producing organisms and is a good soil-builder, containing small amounts of the major plant nutrients, such as nitrates and phosphates.

Mechanical composting: Another method of composting known as 'mechanical composting' is becoming popular. In this, compost is literally manufactured on a large scale by processing raw materials and burning out a finished product. The refuse is first cleared of salvageable materials, such as rags, bones, metal, glass, etc. which are likely to interfere with the grinding operation. It is then pulverized in pulverizing equipment in order to reduce the size of particles to less than 2 inches. The pulverized refuse is then mixed with sewage. The factors which are controlled in the operation are a certain carbon-nitrogen ratio, temperature, moisture, pH and aeration. The entire process of composting is complete in 4 : 6 weeks. This method of composting is in vogue in some of the developed countries, e.g., Holland, Germany, Switzerland, and Israel. The Government of India is considering the installation of mechanical composting plants in selected cities. Cities such as Delhi, Nagpur, Mumbai, Chennai, Pune, Allahabad, Hyderabad, Lucknow and Kanpur have offered to join the government for setting up pilot plants for mechanical composting.

Manure Pits

In the rural areas in India, there is no system for the collection and disposal of refuse. Refuse is thrown around the houses discriminately, resulting in gross pollution of the soil. The problem of refuse disposal in rural areas can be solved by digging manure pits and covered with earth after each day's dumping. Two such pits will be needed; when one is closed, the other one will be in use. In 5–6 months' time, the refuse is converted into manure, which can be returned to the field. This method of refuse disposal is effective and relatively ample in rural communities.

Burial

This method is suitable for small camps. A trench 1.5 m wide and 2 m deep is excavated, and at the end of each day, the refuse is covered with 20–30 cm of earth. When the level of the trench is 40 cm from ground level, the trench is filled with earth and compacted, and a new trench is dug out. The contents may be taken out after 4–6 months and used on the fields. If the trench is 1 m in length for every 200 persons, it will be filled in about one week.

Public Education

Refuse disposal cannot be solved without public education. People have very little interest in cleanliness outside their homes. Many municipalities and corporations usually look for the cheapest solution, especially in regard to refuse disposal. What is needed is public education on these matters, by all town methods of health education, viz. pamphlets, newspapers, broadcasting programs, films, etc. Police enforcement of the news may also be needed at times.

Economics and Finance

If refuse disposal is to be carried out efficiently, hygienically and economically, heavy capital outlay will be needed, whatever system of disposal is adopted. In the highly industrialized units, up to 20% of municipal budgets are spent on the collection and disposal of solid wastes, and even more will be required if the job is to be done adequately.

International Cooperation

An organization named the International Solid Wastes and Public Cleansing Association (ISWA) was formed in 1970 to assist countries in the general endeavor to improve sanitary services. A WHO International Reference Centre has also been set up in Switzerland to collect, evaluate and disseminate information on waste-disposal practices and to foster research.

EXCRETA DISPOSAL

Public Health Importance

Human excreta is a source of infection. It is an important cause of environmental pollution. Every society has a responsibility for its safe removal and disposal so that it does not constitute a threat to public health. Improper excreta disposal are caused soil pollution, water pollution, contamination of food, and propagation of flies and spread of food-borne and water-borne diseases, like dysentery, diarrhea, cholera, hookworm disease, ascariasis, typhoid and paratyphoid fever, viral hepatitis and similar other intestinal infections and parasitic infestations. These diseases are not only a burden on the community in terms of sickness, mortality and a low expectation of life, but a basic deterrent to social and economic progress. Proper disposal of human excreta, therefore, is a fundamental environmental health service without which there cannot be any improvement in the state of community health.

Extent of the Problem in India

In many areas of the world, including India, excreta disposal is a problem of grave importance. Nearly 74% of India's population lives in rural areas and the majority of the people 'go to the fields' for defection and thereby pollute the environment with human excrement. The situation is in no way better in the urban areas too. The Health Survey and Planning Committee (1962) reported that not more than 15% of the urban population in India had the amenity of a sewerage system.

Statistics indicate that the intestinal group of diseases claims about 5 million lives every year while another 50 million people suffer from these infections. Surveys carried out in the community development block areas in Andhra Pradesh, Assam, Bihar, Madhya Pradesh, Manipur, Odisha, Rajasthan and West Bengal show that the enteric group of fevers is very common in the rural areas—the annual incidence varying from 102–2119 per 1,00,000 of population. Hookworm disease is also known to be highly prevalent. About 45 million people are estimated to be infested with hookworms. The solution to the problem is only through hygienic disposal of human excreta which is the cornerstone of all public health services.

How Disease is Carried from Excreta

Let us consider how the fecal-borne diseases are transmitted to a new host. The human excreta of a sick person or a carrier of disease is the main focus of infection. It contains the disease agent, which is transmitted to a new host through various channels:

- Water
- Fingers
- Flies
- Soil and
- Food.

Fecal-oral transmission of organisms causing the diseases occurs mostly through fecal contamination of food, water, and hands, which is not at all apparent. Very small amounts of feces can carry enough organisms to cause the diseases.

Community medicine aims at breaking the disease cycle at vulnerable points. The disease cycle may be broken at various levels—segregation of feces, protection of water supplies, protection of food, personal hygiene and control of flies. Of these, the most effective step would be to segregate the feces and arrange for its proper disposal so that the disease agent cannot reach the new host, directly or indirectly. In simple terms, this barrier can be provided by a 'sanitary latrine' and a disposal pit. The more elaborate schemes envisage installation of a sewerage system and sewage treatment plants.

Methods of Excreta Disposal

These are a number of methods of excreta disposal. Some are applicable to unsewered areas, and some to sewered areas. Classification and description of the various methods of excreta disposal are given below.

Service-type Latrines (Conservancy System)

Shallow trench latrines: A simple improvement on open defecation fields is to provide shallow trenches in which people can defecate. This allows users to cover feces and improves the overall hygiene and convenience of an open defecation system. Trenches need only be 200–300 mm wide and 150 mm deep. Their length depends on the number of users to 3–3.5 m (10–12 feet) and necessary for 100 people and shovels may be provided to allow each user to cover their excreta with soil. Separate trenches should be provided for men and women. The earth from the trench should be piled up at the side. People should be instructed to cover feces with each time they use the latrine. The shallow trench is a rudimentary arrangement for a short period (up to one week). When the trench is filled to 30 cm (12 inches) below the ground level, it must be covered with earth, heaped above the ground level and compacted; if necessary, a new trench must be dug.

Deep trench latrines: This type of latrine is intended for camps of longer duration from a few weeks to a few months. The trench is 1.8–2.5 m (6–8 feet) deep and 75–90 cm (30–35 inches) wide. Depending upon the local customs, a seat or a squatting plate is provided. A superstructure is built for privacy and protection. Deep trench latrines involve the sitting of several cubicles above a single trench, which is used to collect excreta. However, care should be taken not to provide too many latrines side by side. The recommended maximum length of trench is 6 meters, providing six cubicles. Other requirements are the same as for shallow trench latrines.

Bucket latrines: In the situations where there is limited space, it may be appropriate to provide buckets or containers in which people can defecate. These should have tight-fitting lids and should be emptied at least once a day. Disinfectants may be added to reduce contamination risks and odor. Containers can be emptied into a sewerage system, a landfill site or waste-stabilization ponds. This measure will only be appropriate where there are no other immediate action options and users find the method acceptable. It is, therefore, not used in most situations.

Water seal latrines: A further improvement in the designing of sanitary latrines for rural families is the hand-flushed 'water seal' type of latrine. Here the squatting plate is fitted with a water seal. The water seal performs two important functions:

- It prevents access by flies. That is, the night soil is sealed off from flies by a small depth of water contained in a bent pipe called the 'trap'.
- It prevents escape of odors and foul gases and, thereby, eliminates the nuisance from smell. Once the latrine is flushed, night soil is no longer visible.

These merits have rendered the water seal type of latrine more acceptable to rural people than the borehole or pit privy without water seal. Several designs of water seal latrines have been tested in the field, and two types have gained recognition for wide use. These are the PRAI type, evolved by the Planning Research and Action Institute, Lucknow (Uttar Pradesh, India) and the RCA type, designed by the Research-cum-Action Projects in Environmental Sanitation of the Ministry of Health, Government of India. Of these two types, the RCA latrine has been accepted as a suitable design for side adoption in different parts of the country. The parts of a water-sealed latrine, whether RCA type or PRAI type, are essentially the same. The differences are in matters of minor engineering detail.

The essential features of the RCA latrine and its installation are described below:

Location: The safe distance between the latrine and a source of water supply will depend upon the porosity of the soil, level of ground water, its slope and direction of flow. In general, it may be stated that latrines of any kind should not be located within 15 m (50 feet) from a source of water supply, and should be at a lower elevation to prevent the possibility of bacterial contamination of the water supply. Where possible, latrines should not be located in areas usually subject to flooding.

Squatting plate: The squatting plate or slab is an important part of a latrine. It should be made of an impervious material so that it can be washed and kept clean and dry. If kept dry, it will not facilitate the survival of hookworm larvae. In recommending squatting plates, due consideration should be paid to the habits of the Indian people who defecate in the squatting position and use water for anal washing. The slab of the RCA latrine has been designed to meet the above needs. It is made of cement concrete with minimum dimensions of 90 cm (3 feet) square and 5 cm (2 inches) thickness at the outer edge. There is a slope 1/2-inch towards the pan. This allows drainage into the latrine of the water used for ablution or cleansing purposes. A circular squatting plate of 90 cm (3 feet) diameter and of 5 cm (2 inches) uniform thickness has also been found satisfactory. For the convenience of the users, raised footrests are included in the squatting plate.

The pan receives the night soil, urine and wash water. The length of the pan is 42.5 cm (17 inches). The width of the front portion of the pan has a minimum of 12.5 cm (5 inches) and the width at its widest portion in 20 cm (8 inches). There is a uniform slope from front to back of the pan. The pan is given a smooth finish.

Trap: The trap is a bent pipe, about 7.5 cm (3 inches) in diameter and is connected with the pan. It holds water and provides the necessary 'water seal'. The water seal is the distance between the level of water in the trap and the lowest point in the concave upper surface of the trap. The depth of the water seal (AB) in the RCA latrine is 2 cm (3/4 inches). The water seal prevents the access by flies and suppresses the nuisance from smell.

Connecting pipe: When the pit is dug away from the squat plate, the trap is connected to the pit by a short length of connecting pipe 7.5 cm (3 inches) in diameter and at least 1 m (3 feet) in length with a bend at the end.

A latrine of this type is called the 'indirect type' because the pit is sited away from the squatting plate. In the direct type, there is no need for a connecting pipe. The direct type is best suited for areas where the ground is hard and does not easily cave in. The direct type is cheaper and easier to construct and occupies less space. An advantage with the indirect type is that when the pit fills up, a second pit can be put into operation by merely changing the direction of the connecting pipe. Therefore, the indirect type is usually preferred.

Dug well: The dug well or pit is usually 75 cm (30 inches) in diameter and 3–3.5 m (10–12 feet) deep and is covered. In loose soil and where the water-table is high, a lining of earthenware ring or bamboo matting can be used to prevent caving in of the pipe. When the pit fills up, a second pit is dug nearby and the direction of the connecting pipe is changed into the second pit. When the second pit fills up, the first one may be emptied and reused.

Superstructure: The desired type of superstructure may be provided for privacy and shelter. An attractive superstructure with a neat finish is desirable as this will be generally well maintained.

The life of a latrine will depend upon several factors, such as care in usage and maintenance. The latrine should be used only for the purpose intended and not for disposal of refuse or other debris. The squatting plate should be washed frequently and kept clean and dry. People should learn to flush the pan after use with adequate quantity of water. One to two liters of water are sufficient to flush the RCA latrine. Thus, proper maintenance involves health education of the people which is very necessary for the success of any latrine program.

SEPTIC TANK

The septic tank is a watertight masonry tank into which household sewage is admitted for treatment. It is a satisfactory means of disposing excreta and liquid wastes from individual dwellings, small groups of houses and institutions, which have adequate water supplies but do not have access to public sewerage system.

Design Features

There are various designs in septic tanks. Some are double-chambered and some single-chambered. A single-chambered septic tank has been found satisfactory for small installations. Tanks with more than two compartments are expensive and have shown little advantage over the two- or multiple-chambered septic tanks.

The main design features of a septic tank are as follows:

- **Capacity:** The capacity of a septic tank will depend upon the number of users. A capacity of 20–30 gallons of 2-1/2-5 c. ft. per person is recommended for household septic tanks. The minimum capacity of a septic tank should be at least 500 gallons. Septic tanks are not recommended for large communities.
- **Length:** The length is usually twice the breadth.
- **Depth:** The depth of a septic tank is from 1.5–2 m (5–7 feet).
- **Liquid depth:** The recommended liquid depth is only 1.2 m (4 feet)
- **Air space:** There should be a minimum air space of 30 cm (12 inches) between the level of liquid in the tank and the undersurface of the cover.
- **Bottom:** In some septic tanks, the bottom is slopping towards the inlet end. This facilitates retention of solids.
- **Inlet and outlet:** There is an inlet and outlet pipe, which are submerged.
- **Cover:** The septic tank is covered by a concrete slab of suitable thickness and provided with a manhole.
- **Retention period:** Septic tanks are designed in this country to allow a retention period of 24 hours. Too long a retention period will result in undue septicity of the effluent, whereas too short a period gives insufficient treatment.

Working of a Septic Tank

The solids settle down in the tank, to form 'sludge', while the lighter solids including grease and fat rise to the surface to form 'scum'. The solids are attacked by the anerobic bacteria and fungi and are broken down into simpler chemical compounds. This is the first stage of purification, called 'anerobic digestion'. The sludge is much reduced in volume as a result of anerobic digestion, and is rendered stable and inoffensive. A portion of the solids is transferred into liquids and gases (principally methane) which rises to the surface in the form of bubbles.

The liquid which passes out of the outlet pipe from time to time is called the 'effluent'. It contains numerous bacterial, cysts, helminthic ova and organic matter in solution or fine suspension. The effluent is allowed to percolate into the subsoil. It is dispersed by means of perforated or open-jointed pipes laid in trenches 90 cm (3 feet) deep and the trenches are then covered with soil. The effluent percolates into the surrounding soil. There are millions of aerobic bacteria in the upper layers of the soil, which attack the organic matter present in the effluent. As a result, the organic matter is oxidized into stable end-products, i.e., nitrates, carbon dioxide and water. This stage of purification is called 'aerobic oxidation'.

To sum up, two stages are involved in the purification of sewage. The first stage, anerobic digestion takes place in the septic tank proper, and the second stage, aerobic oxidation takes place outside the septic tank, in the subsoil. Together, these two stages complete the purification of sewage.

Operation and Maintenance

The use of soap water and disinfectants, such as phenol should be avoided as they are injurious to the bacterial flora in the septic tank. Undue accumulation of sludge reduces the capacity of the septic tank and interferes with proper working. Therefore, the contents of the septic tank should be bailed out at least once a year. This operation is called 'desludging'. The bailed out sludge is disposed of by trenching. Newly built septic tanks are first filled with water up to the outlet level and then seeded with ripe sludge drawn from another septic tank, to provide the right type of bacteria to carry out the decomposition process.

Aqua Privy

The aqua privy functions like a septic tank and has been used in different regions in the country. The privy consists of a water-tight chamber filled with water. A short length of a drop pipe from the latrine floor dips into the water. The shape of the tank may be circular or rectangular. The size of the tank depends upon the number of users. A capacity of one cubic meter (35 cubic feet) is recommended for a small family, allowing 6 years or more for the cleansing purposes. Aqua privies are designed for public use also.

Night soil undergoes purification by anerobic digestion. Since there is evolution of gases, a vent should be provided for the escape of gases into the atmosphere. The vent should be open above the roof of dwellings. The effluent is far from innocuous. It contains finely divided fecal matter in suspension and may carry parasitic and infective agents. It should be treated in the same manner as the effluent from a septic tank by subsoil irrigation or absorption. The digested sludge which accumulates in the tank should be removed at regular intervals.

SULABH SHAUCHALAYA

The 'Sulabh Shauchalaya' model, the invention of a Patna-based firm, is a low-cost pour-flush, water-seal type of latrine, which is not being used in many parts of India. Basically, it is an improved version of the standard hand-flush latrine (e.g., RCA type). It consists of a specially designed pan and a water-seal trap. It is connected to a pit 3 feet square and as deep. The excreta undergoes bacterial decomposition and is converted to manure (compost). The method requires very little water.

Through Sulabh International, the investors not only build but also maintain the system of Sulabh Community

Latrines. Their usual structure is a lavatory block of several dozen seats, with a bathing block adjoining. The system is to charge ₹2 per user (who is given soap powder by the sulabh attendant after use). Recently, Delhi has opted for this system in all its slums. This system has drawn praise among the ecologists and planners.

It has very limited use under Indian conditions. It consists of a metal tank containing a disinfectant fluid. The active ingredients of the fluid are formaldehyde and quaternary ammonium compounds. In addition, a harmless water dye and a deodorizing substance are usually incorporated. A seat with a cover is placed directly over the tank. Nothing except the toilet paper should be thrown into the chemical closely.

WATER CARRIAGE SYSTEM

The water carriage system or sewerage system implies collecting and transporting of human excreta and waste water from residential, commercial and industrial areas, by a network of underground pipes, called sewers to the place of ultimate disposal. It is the method of choice for collecting and transporting sewage from cities and towns where population density is high. There are two types of water carriage system—the combined sewer system and the separate sewer system. In the combined system, the sewers carry both the sewage and surface water. In the separate system, surface water is not admitted into sewers. The separate system is considered the system of choice today. Although the first sewers were laid in 1867 in Calcutta (now Kolkata), the Mudaliar Committee (1962) reported that not more than 15% of the urban population in India had the amenity of a sewerage system. The problem is heavy investment—a heavy outlay of capital is needed to install a water-carriage system. Since water is needed for flushing the toilets and for conveying the human wastes, there can be no sewerage system without a piped water supply.

A water carriage system consists of the following elements:

Household Sanitary Fittings

Where sewers exist, every house is expected to be connected to the nearest sewer. The usual household sanitary fittings are: (i) water closet; (ii) urinal; and (iii) washbasin. Water closets may be broadly divided into two types—Indian squatting type and the western commode type, which is an ideal water closet bowl (western type). It is recommended that for efficient performance: (a) the water seal area should not be more than 7.5 cm; (b) there should not be any sharp corners in the trap design; (c) the volume of water in the trap should be as little as possible, preferably not exceeding 1.75 liters to maintain a minimum of 50 mm deep water seal; and (d) the interior of the bowl should be vertical, at least 50–75 mm just above the surface of water seal. The water closets are provided with a 'flushing rim'. Human excreta are directly received into the water in the closet without soiling the sides. The flushing removes all traces of excreta from the side and keeps the closet clean. The closet is connected to a small cistern by a pipe 2.5–3.75 cm (1–1.5 inches) in diameter. The flushing cistern normally holds 15 liters (3 gallons) of water and works by symphonic action. The flushing cisterns can be classified as high level, low level and integrated depending upon the height of location above the water closet bowel or pan. The Indian squatting type WC pans are used with high-level flushing cisterns.

House Drain

The house drain is usually 10 cm (4 inches) in diameter and is laid in the courtyard about 15 cm (6 inches) below the ground level on a bed of cement concrete with a sufficient gradient towards the main drain. The house drain empties the sewage into the main sewer or public drain.

Public Sewer

The trunk sewers are not less than 22.5 cm (9 inches) in diameter; bigger ones may be 2–3 m (8–10 feet) in diameter. They are laid on a bed of cement concrete, about 3 m (10 feet) below the ground level, with sufficient gradient to ensure what is known as 'self-cleansing' velocity. This varies from 2–3 feet per second. The trunk sewers collect sewage from several houses and transport to the main outfall or place of final disposal.

Sewer Appurtenances

These are (a) manholes, and (b) traps which are installed in the sewerage system. Manholes are openings built into the sewerage system. They are placed (a) whenever there is a change in the direction of sewers, (b) at the meeting point of two or more sewers, and (c) at distances of 100 meters in long straight runs. These openings permit a man to enter the sewer for inspection, repairs and cleansing. Workers entering the manholes are liable to gas-poisoning and asphyxiation. Due precautions should be taken to ensure their safety. TRAPS are of various kinds. These are the devices designed to prevent foul gases entering the houses and to remove sand, grit and grease from the sewage. Traps are placed in three situations: (a) under the basins of water closets; (b) where the house drain joins the public drain (intercepting trap); and (c) where surface waste water enters the drains.

The installation of a sewerage system is a huge engineering problem. It involves considerable planning, designing, construction, operation, maintenance and administration, each calling for specialized skills. Sewer systems are designed, like water supplies, for the service for one generation (30 years). Social aspects of excreta disposal will be added here.

Social Aspects of Excreta Disposal in India

India is a land of villages and about 74% of its population lives in villages. The problem of sanitation, therefore, is one of 'rural sanitation'. Surveys have shown that 90% of the population 'go to the open fields' for defection. This habit of indiscriminate fouling of the surroundings with human excrement is generations-old, and rooted firmly in the cultural behavior of the Indian village people.

In urban areas, the latrine is considered a necessary part of house. In rural areas, by and large, people have not accepted latrines with any enthusiasm, and even when installed, only a few used them regularly. The problem in rural sanitation is how to overcome the resistance of the village people, and induce them to use sanitary latrines. Research studies have indicated that there is only one way to solve the problem, i.e., through health education.

The reasons found by the social scientists are listed as follows: (1) latrines are associated with bad smell; (2) they are the breeding places of flies; (3) they are something foul and dirty so that one should not have them close to his/her house; (4) latrines are costly and beyond their means to install; and (5) they do not know how fecal-borne diseases are spread. In short, people have a bad image of latrines in their minds. Secondly, using a latrine goes against a daily habit pattern of going to the fields. The use of latrines involves a drastic change in the day-to-day behavior of a large number of people.

The solution to the problem lies in teaching the people first the reasons why latrines are important. The teaching should be undertaken by all the known methods of health education, like direct discussion, group discussion, latrine demonstration, and use of visual aids and, above all, service facilities. The ultimate goal of health education will be to motivate the rural people towards acceptance and use of sanitary latrines.

Surface Water Drainage in Urban Areas

Many low-income communities in the developing countries consider storm-water drainage to be their most urgent need as far as urban infrastructure is concerned. It is the coastal regions of the world that have the highest average rainfall, but the flat estuarine terrain and often impermeable alluvial soil make drainage difficult. Even in the arid areas where average rainfall is low, tropical rainfall—when it comes—is more intense than in temperate climates, and the lack of vegetation and of adequate drainage means that torrents of water can form in minutes, causing damage to homes and property, which will take years to repair. The lack of drainage is especially serious where the ground is either steeply sloping, as in Hong Kong or very flat as in Kolkata, Bangkok and Manila.

Deaths due to drowning in floods or burial beneath landslides or collapsing homes are perhaps the most dramatic signs of the suffering that drainage can help to alleviate. Less noticeable to an outsider, but of greater impact on the residents living in a poor community is the steady toll of disease, disability and death by standing water.

First in the public health importance are the many 'fecal-oral' infections acquired by consumption of contaminated food and drink. Children are particularly exposed to infection when playing or bathing in surface water. Surface water becomes contaminated with pathogens from blocked sewers and overflowing septic tanks. This contaminated surface water can infect people in many ways.

Another important group of diseases related to poor drainage is transmitted by mosquitoes, and malaria is the best example. Transmission can be particularly intense in urban areas, where there are relatively few animals to divert the vector species of mosquito from human blood meals. Drainage construction is an effective mosquito control measure. It is cheaper than application of insecticides and does not have to be repeated regularly. Unlike insecticides, it can have no detrimental effect on the environment; on the contrary, it constitutes an environmental improvement.

Urban poor may often build on land with drainage problems, but good urban planning can help to avoid making these problems worse. One of the simplest planning measures is to set out regular plots before house-building starts in an area, leaving space for well-aligned roads. Adequate road width and alignment will make it much easier to build drains when they are needed later.

SEWAGE

Sewage is a major carrier of disease (from human wastes) and toxins (from industrial wastes).

The safe treatment of sewage is thus crucial to the health of any community. It is waste water from a community, containing solid and liquid excreta, derived from houses, street and yard washings, factories and industries. It resembles dirty water with an unpleasant smell. The term 'sullage' means the waste water which does not contain human excreta, e.g., waste water from kitchens and bathrooms. The amount of sewage that flows in the sewers depends upon:

- **Habits of the people:** If people use more water, there will be more sewage
- **Time of the day:** Sewage does not flow uniformly throughout the day. It is subject to different seasons. In the morning, when people tend to use more water, there is greater quantity and flow; in mid-day, the flow is less, and again there is a slight increase in the evening. The average amount of sewage which flows through the sewerage system in 24 hours is called the 'dry weather flow'.

Health Aspects

Unless prompt measures are taken to provide proper means of sewage disposal, the following environmental problems may be created:

- Creation of nuisance, unsightliness and unpleasant odors
- Breeding of flies and mosquitoes
- Pollution of soil and water supplies
- Contamination of food
- Increase in the incidence of disease, especially enteric and helminthic diseases.

Composition

Sewage contains 99.9% of water. The solids which comprise barely 0.1% are partly organic and partly inorganic; they are partly in suspension and partly in solution. The offensive nature of the sewage is mainly due to the organic matter which it contains. The organic matter decomposes according to the laws of nature, during which process, it gives off offensive odors. In addition, sewage is charged with numerous living organisms derived from feces, some of which may be agents to disease. It is estimated that one gram of feces may contain about 1,000 million of *E. coli*, 10–100 million of fecal streptococci, and 1–10 million spores of Cl. perfringens besides several others. An average adult excretes daily some 100 grams of feces.

Aim of Sewage Purification

Raw sewage or inadequately treated sewage should not be discharged into rivers, sea or other sources of water supply. This is because the oxygen in the water supply is used up by the numerous aerobic bacteria found in the sewage. Depletion of oxygen may lead to the death of the plant and animal in water. Furthermore, the water may yield an offensive smell because of the release of hydrogen sulfide.

The main aim of sewage treatment is to 'stabilize' the organic matter so that it can be disposed of safely; and, to convert the sewage water into an effluent of an acceptable standard of purity which can be disposed of into the land, rivers or sea.

A standard test which is an indicator of the organic content of the sewage is biochemical oxygen demand (BOD).

The 'strength' of the sewage is expressed in terms of:

- **Biochemical oxygen demand (BOD):** It is the most important test done on sewage. It is defined as the amount of oxygen absorbed by a sample of sewage during a specified period, generally 5 days, at a specified temperature, generally 20°C for the aerobic destruction or use of organic matter by the living organisms. BOD values range from about 1 mg/L for natural waters to about 300 mg/L for untreated domestic sewage. If the BOD is 300 mg/L and above, sewage is said to be 'strong'; if it is 100 mg/L, it is said to be 'weak'.
- **Chemical oxygen demand (COD):** The COD test measures the oxygen equivalent of that portion of the organic matter in a sample which is susceptible to oxidation by a strong chemical oxidizer. If wastes contain toxic substances, this test may be the only practical method for determining the organic load.
- **Suspended solids:** The suspended solids are yet another indicator of the 'strength' of sewage. The amount of suspended solids in domestic sewage may vary from 100–500 ppm (mg/L). If the amount of suspended solids is 100 mg/L, the sewage is said to be weak; if the amount is 500 mg/L, the sewage is said to be strong.

Decomposition of Organic Matter

The decomposition of organic matter in sewage takes place by the following two processes:

- **Aerobic process:** It is the most efficient method of reducing the organic matter in sewage. The process requires a continuous supply of free dissolved oxygen. The organic matter is broken down into simpler compounds, namely CO_2, water, ammonia, nitrites, nitrates and sulfates by the action of bacterial organisms including fungi and protozoa.
- **Anerobic process:** Where the sewage is highly concentrated and contains plenty of solids, the anerobic process is highly effective. The end-products of decomposition are methane, ammonia, CO_2, and H_2. In anerobic decomposition, the reactions are slower and the mechanism of decomposition extremely complex.

MODERN SEWAGE TREATMENT

Modern sewage treatment plants are based on biological principles of sewage purification, where the purification is brought about by the action of anerobic and aerobic bacteria. The treatment of sewage may be divided into two stages—primary treatment and secondary treatment.

In primary treatment, the solids are separated from the sewage partly by screening and partly by sedimentation and subjected to anerobic digestion which is the first stage in purification. In secondary treatment, the effluent is subjected to aerobic oxidation, which is the second stage in purification.

Primary Treatment

Screening

Sewage arriving at a disposal work is first passed through a metal screen which intercepts large floating objects, such as pieces of wood, rags, masses of garbage and dead animals. Their removal is necessary to prevent clogging of the treatment plant. These are removed by screens consisting of metal bars spaced at 19 mm intervals, which are placed across the influent channels. Tines (metal combs) rake the collected matter off these, and heavy objects such as rocks (which would otherwise damage the equipment) are allowed to sink into a hopper. The remaining solids are dewatered using a compacting screw and then collected for landfilling off- site. About 6 m of large solid matter is collected this way each day. The screen consists of vertical or inclined steel bars usually set 5 cm (2 inches) apart. In some plants, the screens are of the fixed type while in others, the screens are of the moving type. The screenings are removed from time to time either manually or mechanically, and disposed of by trenching or burial.

Grit Chamber

Sewage is then passed through a long narrow chamber called the grit chamber or detritus chamber. In this chamber, the waste water is aerated by air pumped through perforated pipes near the floor of the tanks. This aeration makes the water less dense, causing the grit to settle out. As the air jets are positioned such that the water is swirling as it moves down the tanks, the suspended solids are prevented from settling out. This chamber is approximately 10–20 meters in length; it is so designed as to maintain a constant velocity of about 1 foot per second, with a detention period of 30 seconds to 1 minute. The function of the grit chamber is to allow the settlement of heavier solids, such as sand and gravel, while permitting the organic matter to pass through. The grit which collects at the bottom of the chamber is removed periodically or continuously, and disposed of by plain dumping or trenching.

Primary Sedimentation

Sewage is now admitted into a huge tank called the 'primary sedimentation tank'. It is a very large tank, holding from 1/4 to 1/3 the dry weather flow. There are various designs in primary sedimentation tank. By far, the most common is the rectangular tank. Sewage is made to flow very slowly across the tank at a velocity of 1–2 feet per minute. The sewage spends about 6–8 hours in the tank. During this long period of relatively still conditions in the tank, a very considerable amount of purification takes place mainly through sedimentation of suspended matter. Nearly 50–70% of the solids settle down under the influence of gravity. A reduction of between 30 and 40% in the number of coliform organisms is obtained. The organic matter which settles down is called 'sludge' and is removed by mechanically operated devices, without disturbing the operation in the tank. While this is going on, a small amount of biological action also takes place in which the micro-organisms present in the sewage attack complex organic solids and break them down into simpler soluble substances and ammonia. A certain amount of fat and grease rises to the surface to form scrum, which is removed from time to time and disposed of. When the sewage contains organic trade wastes, it is treated with sulfate. Addition of one of these chemicals precipitates the animal protein material quickly.

Secondary Treatment

The effluent from the primary sedimentation tank still contains a proportion of organic matter in solution or colloidal state, and numerous living organisms. It has a high demand for oxygen and can cause pollution of soil or water. It is subjected to further treatment, aerobic oxidation, by one of the following methods:

Trickling Filter Method

The trickling filter or percolating filter is a bed of crushed stones or canker, 1–2 m (4–8 feet) deep and 2–30 m (6–100 feet) in diameter, depending upon the size of the population. The effluent from the primary sedimentation tank is sprinkled uniformly on the surface of the bed by a revolving device. The device consists of hollow pipes, each of which has a row of holes. The pipes keep rotating, sprinkling the effluent in a thin film on the surface of the filter. Over the surface and down through the filter, a very complex biological growth consisting of algae, fungi, protozoa and bacteria of many kinds occurs. This is known as the 'zoogleal layer'. As the effluent percolates through the filter bed, it gets oxidized by the bacterial flora in the zoogleal layer. The action of the filter is thus purely a biological one, and not one of filtration as the name suggests. The term 'filter' is a misnomer. The trickling filters are very efficient in purifying the sewage. They do not need rest pauses because wind blows freely through the beds supplying the oxygen needed by the zoogleal flora. The biological growth or zoogleal layer lives, grows and dies. The dead matter sloughs off, breaks away and is washed down the filter. It is a light green, flocculent material and is called 'humus'. The oxidized sewage is now led into the secondary sedimentation tanks or humus tanks.

Activated Sludge Processing

Activated sludge processing is the modern method of purifying the sewage in place of the trickling filter. The 'heart' of the activated sludge process is the aeration tank. The effluent from the primary sedimentation tank is mixed with sludge drawn from the final settling tank (also known as 'activated sludge' or 'return sludge'; this sludge is a rich culture of aerobic bacteria). The proportion of activated sludge to the incoming effluent is of the order of 20–0%. The mixture is subjected to aeration in the aeration chamber for about 6–8 hours. The aeration is accomplished either by mechanical agitation or by forcing compressed air continuously from the bottom of the aeration tank. This latter method, also known as 'diffuse aeration', is considered a better method of aeration. During the process of aeration, the organic matter of the sewage gets oxidized into carbon dioxide, nitrates and water with the help of the aerobic bacteria in the activated sludge. The typhoid and cholera organisms are definitely destroyed, and the coliforms greatly reduced. Activated sludge plants occupy less space, and require skilled operations. One acre of activated sludge plant does the work of 10 acres of percolating filter. Activated sludge process is, therefore, best suited for larger cities and the percolating filter for smaller towns because they are cheaper to install and easier to operate.

Secondary Sedimentation

The oxidized sewage from the trickling filter or aeration chamber is led into the secondary sedimentation tank where it is detained for 2–3 hours. The sludge that collects in the secondary sedimentation tank is called 'aerated sludge' or 'activated sludge' because it is fully aerated. It differs from the sludge in the primary sedimentation tank in that it is practically inoffensive and is rich in bacteria, nitrogen and phosphates. It is valuable manure if dehydrated. Part of the activated sludge is pumped back into the 'aeration tanks' in the activated sludge process and the rest pumped into the sludge digestion tanks for treatment and disposal.

Sludge digestion: One of the greatest problems associated with sewage treatment is the treatment and disposal of the resulting sludge. One million gallons of sewage produce 15–20 tons of sludge. The sludge is a thick, black mass containing 95% of water, and it has a revolting odor. There are a number of methods of sludge disposal:

- **Digestion:** Modern sewage treatment plants employ digestion of sludge as the method of treatment. If sludge is incubated under favorable conditions of temperature and pH, it undergoes anerobic autodigestion in which complex solids are broken down into water, carbon dioxide, methane and ammonia. The volume of sludge is also considerably reduced. It takes 3–4 weeks or longer for complete sludge digestion. The residue is inoffensive, sticky and tarry mud which will readily form excellent manure. Sludge digestion is carried out in special tanks known as 'sludge digestion tanks'. Methane gas, which is a byproduct of sludge digestion, can be used for heating and lighting purposes.

- **Sea disposal:** The coastal towns and cities can dispose of sludge by pumping it into the sea.
- **Land:** Sludge can be disposed of by composting with town refuse.

Disposal of Effluent

- **Disposal by dilution:** Disposal into water courses such as rivers and streams is called 'disposal by dilution'. The effluent is diluted in the body of water and the impurities are oxidized by the dissolved oxygen in water. The diluting capacity of the river or the receiving body of water and its dissolved oxygen contents are important considerations before discharging the effluent into a river or any body of water. Since people use river water for drinking purpose, the effluent must be rendered free from pathogenic organisms by adequate chlorination. The Royal Commission in England in its Fifth Report (1908) recommended that an effluent from a sewage treatment plant should not have more than 30 mg/L of suspended solids and the 5-day BOD of the effluent, including the suspended matter, should not exceed 20 mg/L. These standards assumed that the river or body of water into which the effluent passed would provide an 8:1 dilution. These standards have been the backbone of subsequent work on the purity of sewage effluent. During the past few years, the industry has developed hundreds of new chemicals which are released into the sewerage system. Some of these chemicals are not removed by biological treatment. Consequently, the effluent may contain substances toxic to man, or substances that can kill fish, damage agriculture or interfere with the normal functioning of a stream. In many places in the UK, the effluent standards have been raised from the original Royal Commission values of 30 mg/L of suspended solids and 20 mg/L of BOD to 10 mg/L of each. The WHO is seized with this problem, and is fostering research in 'tertiary' methods of treatment or 'polishing' the effluent further.
- **Disposal on land:** If suitable land is available, the effluent can be used for irrigation purposes (e.g., the Okhla Sewage Treatment Plant in Delhi).

Other Methods of Sewage Disposal

The following are the other methods of sewage disposal:

Sea Outfall

Coastal towns and cities may dispose of their sewage by discharging it into the sea. For instance, nearly two-thirds of untreated sewage of Greater Mumbai are discharged everyday into the Arabian Sea. Purification takes place by dilution in the large body of sea water, and the solids get oxidized slowly. The drawback of this method is that the offensive solid matter may be washed back to the shore and create public nuisance. In order to prevent this, the sewage outfall is designed to discharge the sewage into deep water at many points.

River Outfall

Raw sewage should never be discharged into rivers. The present-day practice is to purify the sewage before it is discharged into rivers. How far the sewage should be purified depends upon the dilution the river provides to carry on aeration and self-purification.

Land Treatment (Sewage Farming)

If sufficient and suitable land (porous soil) is available, sewage may be applied to the land after grit removal, screening and a short period of settlement. This type of treatment is practiced in some Indian towns and cities and is known as 'Sewage Farming or Broad Irrigation'. An acre of land would be required to treat the sewage of 100–300 persons. The land is first laid into ridges and furrows. Sewage is fed into the furrows intermittently and crops are grown on the ridges. The crops that are found suitable to grow are those which do not come in contact with sewage and are likely to be eaten raw. Fodder grass and potatoes seem to be the most paying crops. Fruit trees, whose fruits are high above the ground (e.g., plantain), can be grown. But sugarcane, coriander, cucumber, tomato, onion, etc. should not be grown. The farm should be under the direction of a competent agricultural expert. During the rainy season, it may not be possible to operate the sewage farms. Badly managed farms stink, a condition described as 'sewage sickness' because of the lack of sufficient aeration and rest pauses to the land. Alternate methods of disposal may have to be provided during the rainy season.

Oxidation Pond

A cheap method of sewage treatment is the oxidation pond which has been referred to by many different names, such as waste stabilization pond, redox pond, sewage lagoons, etc. The term 'waste stabilization pond' is more appropriate. The term 'waste' includes both sewage and industrial wastes. Although an old method of purifying sewage, oxidation pond has attracted the attention of public health engineers only recently. Over 50 ponds are working at present in India. The first large-scale installation was the one at Bhilai, where it serves a population of 1,00,000.

The oxidation pond is an open, shallow pool 1–1.5 m (3–5 feet) deep with an inlet and outlet. To qualify as an oxidation pond, there must be the presence of: (a) algae;

(b) certain types of bacteria which feed on decaying organic matter; and (c) sunlight. The organic matter contained in the sewage is oxidized by bacteria (hence oxidation pond) to simple chemical compounds, such as carbon dioxide, ammonia and water. The algae, with the help of sunlight, utilize the carbon dioxide, water and inorganic minerals for their growth. Thus, there is a mutually beneficial biological balance between the algae and bacteria in oxidation ponds. Oxygen that is needed for oxidation is derived to a small extent from the atmosphere but mostly from the algae which liberates oxygen under the influence of sunlight. Consequently, sunlight is an important factor in the proper functioning of oxidation ponds. Cloudy weather definitely lowers the efficiency of the process.

The oxidation ponds are predominantly aerobic during sunshine hours as well as some hours of the night. In the remaining hours of the night, the bottom layers are generally anerobic. Thus, the sewage purification in oxidation ponds is brought about by a combination of aerobic and anerobic types of bacteria. The effluent may be used for growing vegetable crops (land irrigation) or may be discharged into a river or other water courses after appropriate treatment. Mosquito nuisance is avoided by keeping weed growth in the neighborhood of oxidation ponds to a minimum and the water-line free from marginal vegetation. There is no odor nuisance associated with these ponds when they are properly maintained. Oxidation ponds have become an established method of purifying sewage for small communities.

Oxidation Ditches

Other methods recommended are oxidation ditches and aerated lagoons. These methods make use of mechanical rotors for extended aeration. For treatment of the wastes of a population between 5,000 and 20,000, an oxidation ditch requires an area of one acre as compared to 22 acres for an oxidation of pond and 2.5 acres for an aerated lagoon. These are low-cost treatment methods for the purification of sewage.

THERMAL POLLUTION

Thermal pollution is defined as the presence of waste heat in the water which can cause undesirable changes in the natural environment.

Sources of Thermal Pollution

Certain processes, like evaporation, convection, radiation, and use of equipment, such as dryers, evaporators, etc. may sometimes lead to thermal pollution.

Effects of Thermal Pollution

Thermal pollution, in turn, decreases the oxygen content in the atmosphere and, thus, leads to ill effects on human beings' health.

Control of Thermal Pollution

- **Cooling ponds:** The pond receives thermal energy in the water from the plant's condensers and the energy is dissipated mainly through evaporation. Once the water has cooled in the pond, it is reused by the plant. New water is added to the system ('make-up' water) to replace the water lost through evaporation.

  Many such ponds have secondary outdoor recreational purposes that include fishing, swimming, boating, camping and picnicking. One example is Lake Anna in Virginia, which provides cooling water for the North Anna Nuclear Generating Station.
- **Spray ponds:** Here the water is sprayed through nozzles where fine droplets are formed.
- **Cooling towers:** (a) Wet cooling tower: cool air entering from sides takes away the heat and cools the water. Large amount of water is lost through evaporation; (b) Dry cooling tower: There is no water loss in this method but installation and operation cost of dry cooling tower is many times higher than the wet cooling tower.

CLIMATE CHANGE

Climate change affects the social and environmental determinants of health—clean air, safe drinking water, sufficient food and secure shelter. Between 2030 and 2050, climate change is expected to cause approximately 2,50,000 additional deaths per year, from malnutrition, malaria, diarrhea and heat stress. The direct damage costs to health (i.e., excluding costs in health-determining sectors such as agriculture and water and sanitation), is estimated to be between USD 2–4 billion/year by 2030. Areas with weak health infrastructure—mostly in developing countries—will be the least able to cope without assistance to prepare and respond. Reducing emissions of greenhouse gases through better transport, food and energy-use choices can result in improved health, particularly through reduced air pollution.

Climate change is caused by increases in the amount of greenhouse gases (such as carbon dioxide, methane and nitrous oxide) in the atmosphere, which cause the earth's average temperature to rise.

Greenhouse gases trap heat in the atmosphere, raising air and sea temperatures. They are primarily produced through the burning of fossil fuels (like coal) for electricity generation, as well as through agricultural, mining, land management and transport practices.

Impacts of Climate Change

Rising Sea Levels

Climate change impacts rising sea levels. Average sea level around the world rose about 8 inches (20 cm) in the past 100 years; climate scientists expect it to rise more and more rapidly in the next 100 years as part of climate change impacts.

Melting Ice

Projections suggest climate change impacts within the next 100 years, if not sooner, the world's glaciers will have disappeared, as will the Polar ice cap, and the huge Antarctic ice shelf, Greenland may be green again, and snow will have become a rare phenomenon at what are now the world's most popular ski resorts.

Torrential Downpours and More Powerful Storms

While the specific conditions that produce rainfall will not change, climate change impacts the amount of water in the atmosphere and will increase producing violent downpours instead of steady showers when it does rain. Hurricanes and typhoons will increase in power, and flooding will become more common.

Heatwaves and Droughts

Despite downpours in some places, droughts and prolonged heatwaves will become common. Heating disturbs the entire global weather system and can shift cold upper air currents as well as hot dry ones. Single snowballs and snowstorms do not make climate change refutations. Increasingly, however, hot, dry places will get hotter and drier, and places that were once temperate and had regular rainfall will become much hotter and much drier.

Human societies will be seriously affected by extremes of climate such as droughts and floods. A changing climate would bring about changes in the frequency and/or intensity of these extremes. This is a major concern for human health. A warming climate can contribute to the intensity of heat waves by increasing the chances of very hot days and nights. Climate warming also increases evaporation on land, which can worsen drought and create conditions more prone to wildfire and a longer wildfire season.

Changing Ecosystems

As the world warms, entire ecosystems will move. Already rising temperatures at the equator have pushed such staple crops as rice north into once cooler areas, many fish species have migrated long distances to stay in waters that are the proper temperature for them. Farmers in temperate zones are finding drier conditions difficult for crops such as corn and wheat, and once prime growing zones are now threatened. Some areas may see complete ecological change.

Reduced Food Security

One of the most striking impacts of rising temperatures is felt in global agriculture, although these impacts are felt very differently in the largely temperate developed world and in the more tropical developing world. Different crops grow best at quite specific temperatures and when those temperatures change, their productivity changes significantly. In North America, for example, rising temperatures may reduce corn and wheat productivity in the US mid-west. The productivity of rice, the staple food of more than one third of the world's population, declines 10% with every 1°C increase in temperature.

Pests and Disease

Rising temperatures favor agricultural pests, diseases and disease vectors. Pest populations are on the rise and illnesses once found only in limited, tropical areas are now becoming endemic in much wider zones. In Southeast Asia, for example, where malaria had been reduced to a wet season only disease in most areas, it is again endemic almost everywhere year around. Likewise, dengue fever, once largely confined to tropical areas, has become endemic to the entire region. Increased temperatures also increase the reproduction rates of microbes and insects, speeding up the rate at which they develop resistance to control measures and drugs.

GLOBAL WARMING

Global warming is a phenomenon of climate change characterized by a general increase in average temperatures of the earth, which modifies the weather balances and ecosystems for a long time. It is directly linked to the increase of greenhouse gases in our atmosphere, worsening the greenhouse effect.

In fact, the average temperature of the planet has increased by 0.8°C (33.4°F) compared to the end of the 19th century. Each of the last three decades has been warmer than all previous decades since the beginning of the statistical surveys in 1850.

At the pace of current CO_2 emissions, scientists expect an increase of between 1.5° and 5.3°C (34.7°–41.5°F) in average temperature by 2,100. If no action is taken, it would have harmful consequences to humanity and the biosphere.

Causes

The greenhouse effect is a natural phenomenon. However, the increase in greenhouse gases is linked to human activities. It is thus no surprise that the world's leading climate scientists believe that human activities are very likely the main cause of global warming since the mid-twentieth century. The human activities like:

Fossil Fuels

The massive use of fossil fuels is obviously the first source of global warming, as burning coal, oil and gas produces carbon dioxide—the most important greenhouse gas in the atmosphere—as well as nitrous oxide.

Deforestation

The exploitation of forests has a major role in climate change. Trees help regulate the climate by absorbing CO_2 from the atmosphere. When they are cut down, this positive effect is lost and the carbon stored in the trees is released into the atmosphere.

Intensive Farming

Another cause of global warming is intensive farming, not only with the ever-increasing livestock, but also with plant protection products and fertilizers. In fact, cattle and sheep produce large amounts of methane when digesting their food, while fertilizers produce nitrous oxide emissions.

Waste Disposal

Waste management methods like landfills and incineration emit greenhouse and toxic gases—including methane—that are released into the atmosphere, soil and waterways, contributing to the increase of the greenhouse effect.

Mining

Modern life is highly dependent on the mining and metallurgical industry. Metals and minerals are the raw materials used in the construction, transportation and manufacturing of goods. From extraction to delivery, this market accounts for 5% of all greenhouse gas emissions.

Overconsumption

Finally, overconsumption also plays a major role in climate change. In fact, it is responsible for the overexploitation of natural resources and emissions from international freight transport, which both contribute to global warming.

Global Warming Effects

Here are some consequences that are documented in the Intergovernmental Panel on Climate Change Special Report on Global Warming:

On Biodiversity

The increase of temperatures and the climate upheavals disturb the ecosystems, modify the conditions and cycles of plant reproduction. The scarcity of resources and climate change are changing life habits and migratory cycles of animals. We are already witnessing the disappearance of many species—including endemic species—or, conversely, the intrusion of invasive species that threaten crops and other animals.

Global warming therefore impacts biodiversity. It is the balance of biodiversity that is modified and threatened. According to the IPCC, a 1.5°C (34.7°F) average rise might put 20–30% of species at risk of extinction. If the planet warms by more than 2°C, most ecosystems will struggle.

On Oceans (Ice Melting)

Because of global warming, permafrost and ice are melting massively at the poles, increasing the sea level at a rate never known before. In a century, the increase reached 18 cm (including 6 cm in the last 20 years). The worst case scenario is a rise of up to 1 m by 2,100.

The acidification of the oceans is also of great concern. In fact, the large amount of CO_2 captured by the oceans makes them more acidic, arousing serious questions about the adaptability of seashells or coral reefs.

On Humans

Human beings are not spared by these upheavals. Climate change is affecting the global economy. It is already shaking up social, health and geopolitical balances in many parts of the world. The scarcity of resources like food and energy gives rise to new conflicts.

Rising sea levels and floods are causing population migration. Small island states are in the front line. The estimated number of climate refugees by 2050 is 250 million people.

On the Weather

For decades now, meteorologists and climatologists around the world have been watching the effects of global warming on the weather phenomena. And the impact is huge: more droughts and heatwaves, more precipitations, more natural disasters like floods, hurricanes, storms and wildfires, frost-free season, etc.

Prevention of Global Warming

Renewable Energies

The first way to prevent climate change is to move away from fossil fuels. We have to choose the alternative renewable energies like solar, wind, biomass and geothermal.

Energy and Water Efficiency

Producing clean energy is essential, but reducing our consumption of energy and water by using more efficient devices (e.g., LED light bulbs, innovative shower systems) is less costly and equally important.

Sustainable Transportation

Promoting públic transportation, carpooling, but also electric and hydrogen mobility, can definitely help reduce CO_2 emissions and thus fight against global warming.

Sustainable Infrastructure

In order to reduce the CO_2 emissions from buildings caused by heating, air conditioning, hot water or lighting, it is necessary to build new low energy buildings, and to renovate the existing constructions.

Sustainable Agriculture and Forest Management

Encouraging better use of natural resources, stopping massive deforestation as well as making agriculture greener and more efficient should also be a priority.

Responsible Consumption and Recycling

Adopting responsible consumption habits is crucial, be it regarding food (particularly meat), clothing, cosmetics or cleaning products. Last but not least, recycling is an absolute necessity for dealing with waste.

Global warming is the slow increase in the average temperature of the earth's atmosphere because an increased amount of the energy (heat) striking the earth from the sun is being trapped in the atmosphere and not radiated out into space.

The earth's atmosphere has always acted like a greenhouse to capture the sun's heat, ensuring that the earth has enjoyed temperatures that permitted the emergence of life forms as we know them, including humans. Without our atmospheric greenhouse the earth would be very cold. Global warming, however, is the equivalent of a greenhouse with high efficiency reflective glass installed the wrong way around.

HEAT WAVE

Across the globe, hot days are getting hotter and more frequent, while we are experiencing fewer cold days. Over the past decade, daily record high temperatures have occurred twice as often as record lows across the continental United States, up from a near 1:1 ratio in the 1950s. Heat waves are becoming more common, and intense heat waves are more frequent in the US. West, although in some parts of the country the 1930s still holds the record for number of heat waves.

If greenhouse gas emissions are not significantly curtailed, daily high and low temperatures will increase by at least 5°F in most areas by mid-century, rising to 10°F by late century. The National Climate Assessment estimates 20–30 more days over 90°F in most areas by mid-century.

Heat waves are more dangerous when combined with high humidity. The combination of temperature and humidity is measured by the heat index. A recent study projects that the annual number of days with a heat index above 100°F will double, and days with a heat index above 105°F will triple, nationwide, when compared to the end of the 20th century.

Effects of Heat Waves

Extreme heat can increase the risk of other types of disasters. Heat can exacerbate drought, and hot, dry conditions can in turn create wildfire conditions. Buildings, roads, and infrastructure absorb heat, leading to temperatures that can be 1–7°F hotter in urban areas than outlying areas. A phenomenon known as the urban heat island effect. This impact is most intense during the day, but the slow release of heat from the infrastructure (or an atmospheric heat island) overnight can keep cities much hotter than surrounding areas. Rising temperatures across the country pose a threat to people, ecosystems, and the economy.

Extreme heat is one of the leading causes of weather-related deaths in the United States, killing an average of more than 600 people per year from 1999–2009.

Heat stress occurs in humans when the Acid rain dissolves body is unable to cool itself effectively. Normally, the body can cool itself through sweating, but when humidity is high, sweat will not evaporate as quickly, potentially leading to heat stroke.

Hot days are also associated with increases in heat-related illnesses, including cardiovascular and respiratory complications and kidney disease. In extreme temperatures, air quality is also affected. Hot and sunny days can increase the production of ground-level ozone, a harmful pollutant that is the main component of smog, which can damage the respiratory system and is particularly harmful for those with asthma.

Greater use of air conditioning requires more electricity which, depending on the electricity source, emits other types of pollution, including particulates that have an impact on air quality too. These increases in ozone and particulate matter can pose serious risks to people, particularly the same vulnerable groups directly impacted by heat mentioned above.

High temperatures can be damaging to agriculture. Plant growth is negatively impacted by high daytime temperatures and some crops require cool night temperatures. Heat waves also increase the chances of livestock experiencing heat stress, especially when night time temperatures remain high and animals are unable to cool off. Heat-stressed cattle can experience declines in milk production, slower growth, and reduced conception rates.

Warmer temperatures affect many aspects of the US energy system, including production, transmission, and demand. While higher summer temperatures increase electricity demand for cooling, at the same time, they can lower the ability of transmission lines to carry power, possibly leading to electricity reliability issues like rolling blackouts during heat waves.

Resilience Strategies for Extreme Heat

- Identifying vulnerable populations and creating heat preparedness plans with all residents in mind, that may include steps like opening cooling centers during periods of extreme heat and adopting workplace heat stress standards.
- Installing cool and green roofs and cool pavement to reduce the urban heat island effect.
- Planting trees to provide shade and to cool the air through evapotranspiration.
- Pursuing energy efficiency to reduce demand on the electricity grid, especially during heat waves.

ACID RAIN

When fossil fuels such as coal, oil and natural gas are burned, the chemicals like sulfur dioxide and nitrogen oxides are produced. When these chemicals react with water and other chemicals in the air to form sulfuric acid, nitric acid and other harmful pollutants like sulphates and nitrates and spread upwards into the atmosphere, and are carried by air currents, to finally return to the ground in the form of acid rain, fog or snow. Acid rain, or acid deposition, is a broad term that includes any form of precipitation with acidic components, such as sulfuric or nitric acid that fall to the ground from the atmosphere in wet or dry forms.

Causes

- Burning of fossil fuels to generate electricity. Two thirds of SO_2 and one fourth of NOX in the atmosphere come from electric power generators.
- In the US coal burning power plants contribute to about 70% of sulfur dioxide. In Canada oil refining, metal smelting and other industrial activities account for 61% of sulfur dioxide pollution.
- **Vehicles and heavy equipment:** Motor vehicle exhaust fumes are the main source of nitrogen oxides.
- Manufacturing, oil refineries and other industries.
- Acid pollutants also occur as dry particles and gases, which when washed from the ground by rain, add to the acids in the rain to form a more corrosive solution. This is called acid deposition.

Winds can blow SO_2 and NOX over long distances and across borders making acid rain a problem for everyone and not just those who live close to these sources.

Effects

- The corrosive nature of acid rain causes many forms of environmental damage.
- The acids in acid rain chemically react with any object they come in contact with. Acids react with other chemicals by giving up hydrogen atoms.
- Acid rain dissolves and washes away nutrients in the soil which are needed by plants. It can also dissolve naturally occurring toxic substances like aluminum and mercury, freeing them to pollute water or poison plants.
- Acid rain indirectly affects plants by removing nutrients from the soil in which they grow. It affects trees more directly by creating holes in the waxy coating of leaves, causing brown dead spots which affect the plant's photosynthesis. Such trees are also more vulnerable to insect infestations, drought and cold.
- Acid rain that falls or flows as ground water to reach rivers, lakes and wetlands, causes the water in them to become acidic. This affects plant and animal life in aquatic ecosystems.
- Acid rain also has far reaching effects on wildlife. By adversely affecting one species, the entire food chain is disrupted, ultimately endangering the entire ecosystem. Different aquatic species can tolerate different levels of acidity. For instance clams and mayflies have a high mortality when water has a pH of 6.0, while frogs can tolerate more acidic water, although with the decline in supply of mayflies, frog populations may also decline. Land animals that are dependent on aquatic organisms are also affected.
- Acid rain and dry acid deposition damages buildings, automobiles, and other structures made of stone or metal. The acid corrodes the materials causing extensive damage and ruins historic buildings. For instance the Parthenon in Greece and the Taj Mahal in India have been affected by acid rain.
- Although surface water polluted by acid rain does not directly harm people, the toxic substances leached from soil can pollute water supply. Fish caught in these waters may be harmful for human consumption. Acid, along with other chemicals in the air, produces urban smog, which causes respiratory problems.

Solutions

- The best way to stop the formation of acid rain is to reduce the emissions of sulfur dioxide and nitrogen oxides into the atmosphere. This can be achieved by using less energy from fossil fuels in power plants, vehicles and industry.
- Switching to cleaner burning fuels is also a way out. For instance using natural gas which is cleaner than coal, using coal with lower sulfur content, and developing more efficient vehicles.
- If the pollutants have already been formed by burning fossil fuels, they can be prevented from entering the atmosphere by using scrubbers in smokestacks in industry.
- These spray a mixture of water and limestone into the polluting gases, recapturing the sulfur.
- In catalytic converters, the gases are passed over metal coated beads that convert harmful chemicals into less harmful ones. These are used in cars to reduce the effects of exhaust fumes on the atmosphere. Once acid rain has affected soil, powdered limestone can be added to the soil by a process known as liming to neutralize the acidity of the soil.

OZONE LAYER DEPLETION

Ozone is formed by the action of sunlight on oxygen. It forms a layer 20–50 kms above the surface of the earth. This action takes place naturally in the atmosphere, but is very slow.

Ozone is a highly poisonous gas with a strong odor. It is considered a pollutant at ground level and constitutes a health hazard by causing respiratory ailments like asthma and bronchitis. It also causes harm to vegetation and leads to a deterioration of certain materials like plastic and rubber. Ozone in the upper atmosphere however, is vital to all life as it protects the earth from the sun's harmful ultraviolet radiation. In the 1970s, scientists discovered that chemicals called chlorofluorocarbons or CFCs, which were used as refrigerants and aerosol spray propellants, posed a threat to the ozone layer. Not only this other chemicals and industrial compounds such as bromine, halocarbons and nitrous oxides from fertilizers may also attack the ozone layer. Since the early 1980s, scientists detected a thinning of the ozone layer in the atmosphere above Antarctica. This phenomenon is now being detected in other places as well including Australia.

Ozone layer depletion is the gradual thinning of the earth's ozone layer present in the upper atmosphere. Ozone depletion also consists of a much larger springtime decrease in stratospheric ozone around earth's polar regions, which is referred to as the ozone hole.

Effects of Ozone Layer Depletion

- The depletion of the ozone layer has harmful effects on the human health, animals, environment and marine life.
- Studies demonstrate that an increase in UV-B rays causes a higher risk of skin cancer, plays a major role in malignant melanoma development, sunburns, quick ageing, eye cataracts, blindness and weekend immune system.
- Direct exposure to ultraviolet radiations also leads to skin and eye cancer in animals.
- UV-B rays negatively affect plants, crops. It may lead to minimal plant growth, smaller leaf size, flowering and photosynthesis in plants, lower quality crops for humans. And decline in plant productivity would in turn affect soil erosion and the carbon cycle.
- Planktons and zooplankton are greatly affected by the exposure to UV-B rays. These are higher in the aquatic food chain. If the planktons declines, it would likely have wide-reaching effects for all marine life in the lower food chain.

Solutions to Ozone Layer Depletion

- Montreal Protocol was proposed in 1987 to unite the world to cut out production and import of ozone-depleting substances. The Montreal Protocol phases down the consumption and production of the different ozone depleting substances (ODS) in a step-wise manner, with different timetables for developed and developing countries.
- Every individual should also take steps to prevent the depletion of the ozone layer. One should avoid using pesticides and shift to natural methods to get rid of pests instead of using chemicals.
- The vehicles emit a large amount of greenhouse gases that lead to global warming as well as ozone depletion. Therefore, the use of vehicles should be minimized as much as possible.
- Most of the cleaning products have chemicals that affect the ozone layer. We should substitute that with eco-friendly products.
- Maintain air conditioners, as their malfunctions cause CFC to escape into the atmosphere.

WASTELAND RECLAMATION

Loss of vegetation cover leads to loss of soil through erosion, which ultimately creates wastelands. This is one of the pressing problems of the country. Loss of soil has already ruined a large amount of cultivable land in our country. If it remains unchecked, it will affect the remaining land. Unless we adequately safeguard our 'good' lands, we may eventually face a serious shortage of food grains, vegetables, fruit, fodder and fuel wood. Hence, conservation of soil, protecting the existing cultivable land and reclaiming the already depleted wastelands figures prominently among the priority tasks of planning for the future.

Wasteland reclamation is the concept of ecological restoration. Examples include the rehabilitation of land that has been degraded by soil erosion, by salinization and waterlogging or by chemical contamination. Land reclamation involves a wide range of disciplines from the physical (e.g., engineering, pedology, geomorphology, and biology) and the social sciences.

Methods of Wasteland Reclamation

Wasteland can be classified into three forms: (1) Easily reclaimable, (2) Reclaimable with some difficulty, (3) Reclaimable with extreme difficulty. Easily reclaimable wastelands can be used for agricultural purposes. Those which can be reclaimed with some difficulty can be utilized for agro-forestry. Wastelands that are reclaimed with extreme difficulty can be used for forestry or to recreate natural ecosystems.

Agriculture: Wasteland can be reclaimed for agriculture by reducing the salt content which can be done by leaching and flushing. Gypsum, urea, potash and compost are added before planting crops in such areas.

Agro forestry: This involves putting land to multiple uses. Its main purpose is to have trees and crops inter- and/or under planted to form an integrated system of biological production within a certain area. Thus, agro forestry implies integration of trees with agricultural crops or livestock management simultaneously.

Forestry: Attempts to grow trees in highly nonalkaline saline soils have been largely unsuccessful. Field experiments have shown that species like Eucalyptus, Prosopis and Acacia Nilotica could not be grown in highly alkaline soil. Studies have shown that if tree seedlings are planted with a mixture of original soil, gypsum, and manure, better growth can be achieved. It is however important to use indigenous species of trees so that the program recreates the local ecosystem with all its species.

Need for Wasteland Development

Wasteland development provides a source of income for the rural poor. It ensures a constant supply of fuel, fodder and timber for local use. It makes the soil fertile by preventing soil erosion and conserving moisture. The program helps maintain an ecological balance in the area. The increasing forest cover helps in maintaining local climatic conditions. Regenerated vegetation cover helps in attracting birds which feed on pests in the surrounding fields and function as natural pest controllers. The trees help in holding back moisture and reduce surface runoff rates thus helping in the control of soil erosion.

SOCIAL ISSUES AND ENVIRONMENT

Social aspects, development and environment have a strong relation. Development aims at improving global economy and standard of living yet leads to environmental degradation. Major factor is unsustainable resource use and unsustainable growth practices environmental issues may present themselves as temporary or permanent changes to the atmosphere, water, and land due to human activities, which can result in impacts that may be either reversible or irreversible which are also responsible for social issues.

SUSTAINABLE DEVELOPMENT

By the 1970s most development specialists began to appreciate the fact that economic growth alone could not bring about a better way of life for people unless environmental conditions were improved. Development strategies in which only economic considerations were used, had begun to suffer from serious environmental problems due to air and water pollution, waste management, deforestation and a variety of other ill effects that seriously affected peoples' well-being and health. There were also serious equity issues between the "haves and the have nots" in society, at the global and national levels. The disparity in the lifestyles between the rich and the poor was made worse by these unsustainable development strategies.

Thus increasingly the world began to see the need for a more equitable use of earth resources. "The control over natural resources and the wealth that it produces also begins to create tensions between people that can eventually lead to both strife within a country and wars between nations". Development has to be visualized in a holistic manner, where it brings benefits to all, not only for the present generation but also for future generation. There is an urgent need to interlink the social aspects with development and environment. According to GH Brundtland (Norwegian Prime Minister and Director of WHO) Sustainable development is defined as *"meeting the needs of the present without compromising the ability of future generation to meet their own needs".*

Key aspects for sustainable development:

- **Inter-generational equity:**
  - We should minimize any adverse impacts on resources and environment for future generations
  - We should handover a safe, healthy, and resourceful environment to our future generations
  - This is possible only if we stop over exploitation of resources, reduce waste discharge and emissions and maintain ecological balance.
- **Intra-generational equity:**
  - The development process should seek to minimize the wealth gaps within and between nations
  - The technology should address to the problems of developing countries, producing drought tolerant varieties for uncertain climates, vaccines for infectious diseases, clean fuel for domestic and industrial use
  - This will support the economic growth of poor countries, narrowing the wealth gap and lead to sustainability.

Measures for sustainable development:

- **Using appropriate technology:**
  - Appropriate technology is the one which is locally adoptable, eco-friendly, resource efficient, and culturally suitable (involves local resources and labor).
  - Using indigenous technologies are more useful, cost effective, and sustainable.
  - The technology should use less resources and produce minimum waste
- **Adopting 3R's (reduce, reuse, recycle)**
  - 3R approach reduces the pressure on resources and reduces waste generation and pollution
  - **Minimizing the resource use:** Reduced demand for any metallic product will decrease the mining of their metal and cause less production of waste
  - **Using them again and again:** The refillable containers which are discarded after use can be reused, e.g., discarded rubber tubes can be used as rubber bands
  - **Recycling the material:** Recycling is the reprocessing of discarded materials into new useful products, e.g., recycling of paper
- **Promoting environmental education and awareness:**
  - This will help in changing the thinking and attitude of people towards our earth and the environment
  - Introducing the subject right from school stage will inculcate a feeling of belongingness to the earth in the small children
  - Earth thinking will help to transform our lifestyles to sustainable ones
- **Resources utilization as per carrying capacity:**
  - *Carrying capacity:* Any system can sustain limited number of organisms on sustainable basis.
  - If the carrying capacity of a system is crossed, environmental degradation starts.
  - Carrying capacity has the two basic components:
    1. Supporting capacity: The capacity to regenerate
    2. Assimilative capacity: The capacity to tolerate different stresses
  - If the resources are utilized based on the above two properties then sustainability can be achieved.

URBAN PROBLEMS RELATED TO ENERGY

Now a days huge quantities of energy has been consumed by urban population or in urban areas however in the past, urban housing required relatively smaller amounts of energy than we use at present. Traditional housing system in India required very little temperature adjustments as the materials used, such as wood and bricks handled temperature changes better than the current concrete, glass and steel of ultra-modern buildings.

Until the 1950s many urban kitchens were based on fuelwood or charcoal. This was possible and practical when homes had chimneys and kitchens were isolated from the rest of the house but smoke became a problem when housing changed to apartment blocks. Kerosene thus became a popular urban fuel. This changed to electrical energy and increasingly to natural gas by the 1970s in most parts of urban India.

Urban hubs in hot climates need energy for cooling. The early systems of fans changed into air-conditioning, which consumes enormous quantities of energy. New buildings in our country have taken to using large areas covered by glass. While in cold climates this uses the greenhouse effect to trap the warmth of the sun inside, in our hot climate this adds several degree to the temperature inside. Thus it requires even more energy to run large central air conditioning units. High rise buildings in urban centers also depend on energy to operate lifts and an enormous number of lights.

Urban transport depends on energy mainly from fossil fuels. Most urban people use their own individual transport rather than public transport systems for a variety of reasons. Urban transport in different cities and even different parts of a city are either inefficient or overcrowded. Thus even middle income groups tend to use their own private vehicles. This means more and more vehicles on the road which leads to traffic congestion, waste of time for all the travelers, and a great load of particulate matter and carbon monoxide from the exhaust of vehicles. This causes a rise in the number of people having serious respiratory diseases. Thus there is a need to develop a more efficient public transport system and discourage the use of individual vehicles in all our urban areas.

Each of us as an ecologically conscious or ecofriendly individual must reduce our use of energy. An unnecessary light left on carelessly adds to energy use. Imagine the amount of energy wasted by thousands of careless people. If we learned to save electricity, we would begin to have a more sustainable lifestyle.

WATER CONSERVATION

Conserving water has become a prime environmental concern. Clean water is becoming increasingly scarce globally. With deforestation surface runoff increases and the sub-soil water table drops as water has no time to seep slowly into the ground once vegetation is cleared. As many areas depend on wells, it has become necessary to go on making deeper and deeper wells. This adds to the cost and further depletes underground stores of water. This could take years to recharge even if the present rate of extraction is reduced which seems hardly possible in most situations. Water being one of the most precious and indispensable resources needs to be conserved. The following strategies can be adopted for conservation for water.

Decreasing runoff losses: This can be achieved by:

- Contour cultivation on small furrows and ridges across the slopes trap rainwater and allow more time for infiltration.
- Conservation bench terracing involves construction of a series of benches for catching the runoff water.
- Water spreading is done by channeling or lagoon travelling. Channeling means a series of diversions with vertical intervals and lagoon travelling means small depressions are dug in the area so that there is temporary storage of water.
- Chemical wetting agents or conditioners like gypsum when applied to sodic soils improves soil permeability and reduce runoff.
- Surface crop residues tillage, mulch, animal residues.
- Water storage structures like farm ponds, dug wells.

Reducing evaporation losses:

- Horizontal barrier of asphalt placed below the soil surface increases water availability.
- A co-polymer of starch and acrylonitrile called super slurper absorbs water 4,000 times its weight.
- By keeping free water surface area minimum as reservoirs and lakes are the water bodies with large surface area which is possible by adopting following measures:
  - The reservoir site may be selected in such a way that area to storage ratio is minimum.
  - To avoid water loss water could be stored below ground.
  - When there are number of reservoirs on one river the water may be stored in one large reservoir when possible rather than in several small reservoir.

Storing water in soil:

- Soil should be wetted to field capacity. Field capacity (Cc) corresponds to the superior limit of available water and represents the moisture of the soil after drainage of the water contained in the macropores by gravity action. This moisture condition favors higher absorption of water and nutrients by the plants.
- Leaving the soil fallow for one season water can be made available for the next season for crop growth.

Reducing irrigation losses: Technological measures to reduce seepage, leakage and percolation losses in irrigation include the lining of canals and watercourses, and promoting modern irrigation technologies such as pipe, sprinkler and drip systems. Irrigation in early morning or late evening can helps in reducing water losses.

Reuse of water:

- Water reuse generally refers to the process of using treated wastewater (reclaimed water) for beneficial purposes such as agricultural and landscape irrigation, industrial processes, nonpotable urban applications (such as toilet flushing, street washing, and fire protection), groundwater recharge, recreation, and direct or undirected water supply. Treated waste water can be used for ferti irrigation
- Using grey water from washings, bath tubs for watering gardens washing cars.

Preventing wastage of water at household level:

- Closing taps when not in use
- Repairing any leakage from pipes.

Increasing block pricing: The consumer has to pay a proportionately higher bill with higher use of water. Water and wastewater tariffs determine the level of revenues that service providers receive from users in centralized or semi-centralized systems for the appropriate catchment, purification and distribution of freshwater, and the subsequent collection, treatment and discharge of wastewater.

RAINWATER HARVESTING

Rainwater harvesting (RWH) is the collection and storage of rain, rather than allowing it to runoff. Rainwater is collected from a roof-like surface and redirected to a tank, cistern, deep pit (well, shaft, or borehole), aquifer, or a reservoir with percolation, so that it seeps down and restores the ground water. Rainwater harvesting is one of the simplest and oldest methods of self-supply of water for households, and residential and household-scale projects, usually financed by the user.

In present age, concrete houses, well-built roads, footpaths and well concreted courtyards have left few open grounds.

With the decrease in natural forest cover, increase in concrete jungles and decrease in exposed earth very little open ground is left for water to soak in and thereby increasing the ground water table.

- So, artificial recharging of groundwater is extremely essential.
- Rainwater harvesting is a technique of increasing the recharge of ground water by capturing and storing water which is done by constructing special water harvesting structures like dug wells, percolation pits, lagoons, check dams, etc.

Objectives

- To reduce runoff loss
- To avoid flooding of roads
- To meet the increasing demands of water
- To raise the water table by recharging ground water.

Rainwater harvesting techniques: There are two major techniques of rainwater harvesting.

1. **Surface runoff harvesting:** In this method, rainwater flows away as surface runoff and can be stored for future use. Surface water can be stored by diverting the flow of small creeks and streams into reservoirs on the surface or underground. It can provide water for farming, for cattle and also for general domestic use. Surface runoff harvesting is most suitable in urban areas.

   Rooftop rainwater/storm runoff can be harvested in urban areas through:
   - Recharge pit
   - Recharge trench
   - Tubewell
   - Recharge well
2. **Groundwater recharge:** Groundwater recharge is a hydrologic process where water moves downward from surface water to groundwater. Recharge is the primary method through which water enters an aquifer. The aquifer also serves as a distribution system. The surplus rainwater can then be used to recharge groundwater aquifer through artificial recharge techniques.

   Rainwater in rural areas can be harvested through:
   - Gully plug
   - Contour bund
   - Dug Well recharge
   - Percolation tank
   - Check dam/Cement plug/Nala bund
   - Recharge shaft.

Although rainwater harvesting measure is deemed to be a desirable concept since the last few years, it is rarely being implemented in rural India. Different regions of the country practiced a variety of rainwater harvesting and artificial recharge methods. Some ancient rainwater harvesting methods followed in India which includes Madakas, Ahar Pynes, Surangas, Tankas, etc.

The Mewar region of Rajasthan has a rich legacy of traditional water harvesting systems to share the available water for cultivation. There are various types of rainwater harvesting systems.

- **Medhbandi:** Medhbandi means resistance, counteraction, opposition or obstruction. This is a stone embankment built on a hill slope to help create a level field for cultivation. It controls erosion and conserves moisture by providing obstruction in warer flow.
- **Naada/bandha:** These are stone check dams across streams or gullies that are constructed to capture runoff on a stretch of fertile land that is submerged in water during the monsoon. The land not only becomes more fertile after trapping silt, but also retains substantial quantities of water in the soil. These dams are constructed in phases over several years. The height is slowly increased up to the right height of the check dam which determines the size of the naada.
- **Hembar:** These are small temporary dams constructed with stones, twigs and mud over a seasonal stream when water flows in it is reduced to a point that it cannot be taken directly to the fields for irrigation.
- **Chak:** Chak is a big plot of land, usually a carnot or village pasture land, enclosed by a stone boundary wall called kot. Tree plantations, seeding of grass for fodder, contour bunds with trenches and loose stone check dams are developed in the chak. The chak is used for fodder and fuel wood. It reduces soil erosion and enhances recharge of ground water.
- **Talab:** The Mewar region is well-known for its built reservoirs (talabs). Udaipur City is famous for its large number of talabs, and is called the lake city. A small reservoir of less than five bighas is called talai, a medium sized lake is called bandh or talab and a bigger lake is called sagar or samand.
- **Sazakuva:** This is an open dug well which has several owners. In Mewari language, saza means partner. This is an important method for irrigation in the Aravalli hills. About 70,000 wells in the Udaipur District provide water for 80% of the area under irrigation and provide water for their owners. These are considered common property resources.

Applications/Uses of Rainwater Harvesting Systems

Domestic Use

Rooftop rainwater harvesting is used to provide drinking water, domestic water, water for livestock, water for small irrigation, and a way to replenish groundwater levels. Kenya has already been successfully harvesting rainwater for toilets, laundry, and irrigation and Australia use harvested rainwater for cooking and drinking.

Agriculture

In regards to urban agriculture, rainwater harvesting in urban areas reduces the impact of runoff and flooding. The combination of urban 'green' rooftops with rainwater catchments have been found to reduce building temperatures by more than 1.3°C. Rainwater harvesting in conjunction with urban agriculture would be a viable way to help meet the United Nations Sustainable Development Goals for cleaner and sustainable cities, health and wellbeing, and food and water security.

Industry

Frankfurt Airport has the biggest rainwater harvesting system in Germany. The system helps save approximately 1 million cubic meters of water per year. The cost of the system was 1.5 million dm (US$63,000) in 1993. This system collects water from the roofs of the new terminal which has an area of 26,800 square meters. The water is collected in the basement of the airport in six tanks with a storage capacity of 100 cubic meters. The water is mainly used for toilet flushing, watering plants and cleaning the air conditioning system.

Rainwater harvesting was adopted at the Velodrome—the London Olympic Park—in order to increase the sustainability of the facility. A 73% decrease in potable water demand by the park was estimated. Despite this, it was deemed that rainwater harvesting was a less efficient use of financial resources to increase sustainability than the park's blackwater recycling program.

Advantages of Rainwater Harvesting

The benefits of rainwater harvesting system are listed below:

- Less cost.
- Helps in reducing the water bill.
- Decreases the demand for water.
- Reduces the need for imported water.
- Promotes both water and energy conservation.
- Improves the quality and quantity of groundwater.
- Does not require a filtration system for landscape irrigation.
- This technology is relatively simple, easy to install and operate.
- It reduces soil erosion, stormwater runoff, flooding, and pollution of surface water with fertilizers, pesticides, metals and other sediments.
- It is an excellent source of water for landscape irrigation with no chemicals and dissolved salts and free from all minerals.

Disadvantages of Rainwater Harvesting

In addition to the great advantages, the rainwater harvesting system has a few disadvantages like unpredictable rainfall, unavailability of the proper storage system, etc.

Listed below are few more disadvantages of the rainwater harvesting process:

- Regular maintenance is required.
- Requires some technical skills for installation.
- Limited and no rainfall can limit the supply of rainwater.
- If not installed correctly, it may attract mosquitoes and other waterborne diseases.
- One of the significant drawbacks of the rainwater harvesting system is storage limits.

WATERSHED MANAGEMENT

The word "watershed" introduced in 1920 was used for the "water parting boundaries". Watershed is that land area which drains or contributes runoff to a common outlet. It is a geographic unit (a piece of land) that collects, stores, and releases water. Collected water comes from rain, snow melt and fog. The water is stored in lakes, ponds, sub-surface soil etc. The stored water is released through rivers, streams and ground water flow. The watershed is defined as the land area from which water drains under gravity to a common drainage channel like streams, rivers, lake, estuary, and even the ocean. A watershed ranges from few square kilometers to few thousand square kilometers in size. The water shed comprises complex interactions of soil, land, vegetation, land use activities and water. Rivers originate in streams that flow down mountains and hill slopes. A group of small streams flow down hillsides to meet larger streams in the valley which forms the tributaries of major rivers.

Watershed management implies an effective conservation of soil and water resources for sustainable production with minimum nonpoint resources (NFS) pollutant losses. It involves management of land surface and vegetation so as to conserve the soil and water for immediate and long-term benefits to the farmers, community and society as a whole.

The management of a single unit of land with its water drainage system is called watershed management. It is a technique that has several components. This includes soil and water management and developing vegetative cover and prevention of watershed degradation etc. The natural drainage pattern of a watershed unit if managed appropriately can bring about local prosperity by a year round abundance of water that improves the quality of human life in the area.

Types of Watershed

The watershed is a natural hydrological entity that covers a specific aerial expanse of land surface from which the rainfall runoff flows to a defined drain, channel, stream or river at any particular point. The watersheds are classified based on their size as macro, micro and mini watershed. The macro watershed size is 1,000 to 10,000 ha. The small micro hydrologic unit in the hierarchal system is termed as Micro watershed having size of 500–1,000 hectares (ha) and smallest mini watershed size is 10–100 ha.

Causes of watershed degradation:

- Overgrazing
- Deforestation
- Mining
- Construction activities
- Industrialization

- Soil erosion
- Shifting cultivation.

Watershed management: Rational utilization of land and water resources for optimum production causing minimum damage to the natural resources is known as watershed management.

Objectives of watershed management:
- To promote sustainable economic development through optimum use of land, water and vegetation
- To restore ecological balance through sustainable development of natural resources
- Minimizing soil erosion and moisture retention
- To minimize the risk of floods, droughts, and landslides
- To manage watershed for the beneficial developmental activities like domestic water supply, irrigation, hydro-power generation, etc.

Watershed management practices:
- **Water harvesting:**
  - Proper storage of water is done for use in dry seasons in low rain fall areas.
  - It also helps in moderation of floods
  - This is carried out by construction of percolation tanks, dug wells, check dams, etc., at the base of hill/mountain such that the rainwater will not runoff and thus gets stored.
  - Giving enough time for water to percolate in to sub-soil and enhance the ground water table.
- **Afforestation and agro forestry:**
  - In watershed development, afforestation and crop plantation play very important role.
  - They help to prevent soil erosion and retention of moisture.
  - In high rain fall areas woody trees are grown in between crops to reduce runoff and loss of fertile soil.
  - In Dehradun, trees like Eucalyptus, grasses like Chrysopogon are grown along with maize or wheat.
  - Woody trees include Sheesham, Teak, etc.
- **Mechanical measures to reduce runoff loses and soil erosion:** Several mechanical measures are followed to reduce runoff loses and soil erosion
  - Terracing
  - Bunding
  - Bench terracing
  - No-till farming
  - Contour cropping
  - Strip cropping

  Bunding has proved to be a very useful method in reducing runoff, peak discharge and soil loss in Dehradun.
- **Scientific mining and quarrying:** Due to improper mining, the hills lose stability and get disturbed resulting in landslides, rapid erosion, etc.
  - Contour trenching at an interval of 1 m on overburden dump
  - Planting some soil binding plants like Ipomoea, Vitex
  - Draining of water courses in the mined area are recommended for minimizing the destructive effects of mining.
- **Public participation:**
  - People's involvement including the farmers and tribals is a key to success any watershed management program, particularly the soil and water conservation
  - The communities are to be motivated for protecting a freshly planted area
  - Maintaining water harvesting structures implemented by Government or NGOs
  - Properly education the people
- Successful watershed management has been done at Haryana state through active participation of the local people.

ENVIRONMENTAL ETHICS

Environmental ethics deals with issues related to the rights of individuals that are fundamental to life and wellbeing. This concerns not only the needs of each person today, but also those who will come after us. It also deals with the rights of other living creatures that inhabit our earth. There is an urgent need to inculcate sensitivity towards environmental degradation among people by fostering environmental ethical values. Environmental ethics attempts to define what is right and what is wrong regardless of cultural differences. We human beings have a fundamental duty towards nature to respect and care for the earth, protect life-support systems, biodiversity and ensure sustainable development. The following are the environmental ethical values to be inculcated:

Environmental consciousness: Environmental consciousness, a multi-dimensional construct, represents a mental state of an individual. It is found distinct from its antecedents and associated behaviors varying from low general level to high product-specific level. Environmental consciousness is a question of values or general (primitive) beliefs on the relationship between human beings and the environment. Environmental consciousness includes environmental concern like willingness to make financial sacrifices for environmental amelioration, attitude towards environmentally destructive acts and self-report of involvement in proenvironmental behavior.

Humility and reverence: The difference between reverence and humility is that reverence is veneration; profound awe and respect, normally in a sacred context while humility is the characteristic of being humble; humbleness in character and behavior. Generally people having humbling in nature for environment while we are enjoying the beauties of nature. In such moments, we become aware of ourselves as one among many—one person in an enormous world, one species among millions. Environmentalists may remind us here that the nature in which such experiences occur is vanishing, that biodiversity is in a moment of decline (a sixth mass extinction) for which humans bear some, perhaps a great, burden of guilt. For the environmentally conscious this is perhaps a humiliating rather than a humbling reminder.

The word "revere" can be defined as having a deep respect or admiration for something. Reverence for life is a fundamental experience of being human—to be in awe of life and all its forms of expression. When we hold our environment and natural world with reverence, we are often inspired toward conscious, ethical, and moral decision-making about how to live on our planet. This could include a commitment to do no harm, to live sustainably, and to take action towards protecting the planet's oceans, forests, and species.

Responsibility and commitment: Responsibility is the state of being responsible, accountable, or answerable while commitment is the act or an instance of committing, putting in charge, keeping, or trust, especially. Commitment is defined to be a kind of promise or pledge to do something in future. But responsibility means you have to finish the work with or without commitment. IBM's corporate environmental programs date back to the 1960s. In 1971, Thomas J. Watson, Jr., IBM's CEO at the time, formalized the company's commitment to environmental protection with our Corporate Policy on IBM's Environmental Responsibilities. Updated a number of times over the years, the policy and the environmental programs supporting it have defined and driven IBM's longstanding commitment to environmental leadership across all of our business activities.

Respect for all forms of life and landscape: Respect for all forms of life is an essential value. Increasing human population interacts with local and global environments to deplete biodiversity and resources humans depend on, thus challenging societal values centered on growth and relying on technology to mitigate environmental stress. Although the need to address the environmental crisis, central to conservation science, generated greener versions of the growth paradigm, we need fundamental shifts in values that ensure transition from a growth-centered society to one acknowledging biophysical limits and centered on human well-being and biodiversity conservation.

Global environmental citizenship: Environmental citizenship is the idea that we all should take responsibility for how we interact with the environment. We should adopt a green lifestyle to keep the air clean. Since air pollution is damaging to the environment and human health, we all need to play our part in reducing the level of air pollution in our neighborhoods. Environmental protection acts should be followed by every citizen of India. Everyone can get involved in the local consultation process on the sustainable community strategy for their area. Industries and businesses have a tremendous impact on the environment. Help them to act responsibly as you make your consumer choices on goods or services. Think green before you buy. If you intend to buy a new electronic or electrical appliance, find out from your retailer about their take back schemes for an old equivalent appliance. Refuse to buy products with excessive packaging. In this way we can fulfil our environmental citizenship role.

Self-reliance: Self-reliance on one's own powers and resources rather than those of others. Self-reliance is the ability to depend on yourself to get things done and to meet your own needs. An example of self-reliance is growing your own food. The capacity to rely on one's own capabilities, and to manage one's own affairs; independence not to be dependent. We can make self-reliance to a commitment to preserve natural resources for the benefit of present and future generation, follow appropriate standards for exploration of natural resources based upon use and share with each other and care for the earth.

Adoption of eco-friendly culture: We have to develop eco-friendly culture by adopting eco-friendly lifestyle. This can be achieved by:

- Consume organic produce and try growing your own food. Try and consume food that is produced locally or available in local market.
- Use more public transport and walk wherever possible.
- Recycle and reduce the amount of waste.
- Adopt modern technology by paying your bills online, screenshot your travel documents and access your bank statements online to adopt a paper-free lifestyle.
- Encourage composting of plant and kitchen waste and turns it into food for plants.
- Stop littering by educating public about the health hazards and inculcate the habit of disposing of your trash in a dustbin.

Preservation of Diversity on The Planet

Biodiversity is more than simply the collection of plants and animals on earth; it is about local ecosystems and promoting healthy conditions for organisms to thrive. While protecting the rainforests sounds like a daunting task, there is a lot we can do to promote and preserve local biodiversity at home like support local farms, save the bees and plant local flowers, fruits and vegetables, etc.

The spectrum of common environmental activities for inculcating environmental ethical values are:

- Using recycled paper for notes and circulars
- Diverting wastes from kitchen to the garden
- Switching off unnecessary lights
- Using bicycles or walking
- Using public transport systems
- Collecting rainwater
- Avoiding usage of freshwater for gardening
- Using cloth towels instead of paper towels
- Avoiding unnecessary outdoor lighting
- Organizing tree-plantation campaigns
- Reducing volume of radio and television to reasonable levels
- Listening to radio programs on environment and its problems
- Organizing eco-clubs
- Placing trash cans and dustbins around the college premises
- Observing Environment Day on 5th June and Earth Day on 22nd April
- Planting trees in and around the campus
- Encouraging healthy lifestyles through balanced nutrition, exercise and helping enforce environment protection laws

- Staging short plays on environmental crisis to create environmental awareness
- Conserving energy resources by avoiding unnecessary wastage of energy
- Cutting and displaying pictures and newspaper cuttings depicting environmental crisis.

THE ENVIRONMENTAL PROTECTION ACT

Environmental Act means the Act that regulate the impact of human activities on the environment. Environmental Act covers a broad range of activities that affect air, water, flora or fauna. It includes acts that relate to protection of animals and plants.

The Central Government is empowered to take measures necessary to protect and improve the quality of the environment by setting standards.

The Environment Protection Act (1986)

Environment Protection Act, 1986 Act of the Parliament of India. This Act was passed to protect the environment, as there was a growing concern over the deteriorating state of the environment. The decline in the environmental quality, was evidenced by increasing pollution, loss of forest cover and an increasing threat to biodiversity. In the wake of the Bhopal gas Tragedy or Bhopal Disaster, the (Government of India) enacted the Environment Protection Act of 1986 under Article 253 of the Constitution. Passed in May 1986, it came into force on 19 November 1986. It has 26 sections and 4 chapters. The purpose of the Act is to implement the decisions of the United Nations Conference on the Human Environment. They relate to the protection and improvement of the human environment and the prevention of hazards to human beings, other living creatures, plants and property.

Although there were several existing laws that dealt directly or indirectly with environmental issues, it was necessary to have a general legislation for environmental protection because the existing laws focused on very specific types of pollution, or specific categories of hazardous substances or were indirectly related to the environment through laws that control land use, protect our National Parks and Sanctuaries and our wildlife. However, there were no overarching legislation and certain areas of environmental hazards were not covered. There were also gaps in areas that were potential environmental hazards and there were several inadequate linkages in handling matters of industrial and environmental safety. This was essentially related to the multiplicity of regulatory agencies. Thus there was a need for an authority which could assume the lead role for studying, planning and implementing long-term requirements of environmental safety and give directions to, as well as coordinate a system of speedy and adequate response to emergency situations threatening the environment.

This Act was thus passed to protect the environment, as there was a growing concern over the deteriorating state of the environment. As impacts grew considerably environmental protection became a national priority in the 1970s. The decline in the environmental quality, was evidenced by increasing pollution, loss of forest cover and an increasing threat to biodiversity.

The presence of excessive concentrations of harmful chemicals in the atmosphere and aquatic ecosystems leads to the disruption of food chains and a loss of species. These are symptoms of a rapidly deteriorating environment. The growing risks of environmental accidents and threats to life support systems now looms threateningly over our civilization. The decision taken at the conference in Stockholm strongly voiced these environmental concerns and several measures were made possible for environmental protection. While the need for a wider general legislation to protect our environment is now in place, it has become increasingly evident that our environmental situation continues to deteriorate.

Public concern and support is crucial for implementing the EPA. This must be supported by an enlightened media, good administrators, highly aware policy makers, informed judiciary and trained technocrats who together can influence and prevent further degradation of our environment. Each of us has a responsibility to make this happen.

The Act is an "umbrella" legislation designed to provide a framework for central government coordination of the activities of various central and state authorities established under previous laws, such as the Water Act and the Air Act.

The Environment (Protection) Act, 1986 not only has important constitutional implications but also an international background. The spirit of the proclamation adopted by the United Nations Conference on Human Environment which took place in Stockholm in June 1972, was implemented by the Government of India by creating this Act.

THE AIR POLLUTION PREVENTION AND CONTROL ACT

Government passed this Act in 1981 to clean up our air by controlling pollution. Sources of air pollution such as industry, vehicles, power plants, etc. are not permitted to release particulate matter, lead, carbon monoxide, sulfur dioxide, nitrogen oxide, volatile organic compounds (VOCs) or other toxic substances beyond a prescribed level. To ensure this, Pollution Control Boards (PCBs) have been set up by government to measure pollution levels in the atmosphere and at certain sources by testing the air. This is measured in parts per million or in milligrams or micrograms per cubic meter.

The particulate matter and gases that are released by industry and by cars, buses and two wheelers is measured by using air sampling equipment.

The main objectives of the Act are as follows:

- To provide for the prevention, control and abatement of air pollution.
- To provide for the establishment of Central and State Boards with a view to implement the Act.

- To confer on the Boards the powers to implement the provisions of the Act and assign to the Boards functions relating to pollution.

Air pollution is more acute in heavily industrialized and urbanized areas, which are also densely populated. The presence of pollution beyond certain limits due to various pollutants discharged through industrial emission are monitored by the Pollution Control Boards.

Powers and functions of the Boards Central Board: The main function of the Central Board is to implement legislation created to improve the quality of air and to prevent and control air pollution in the country. The Board advises the Central Government on matters concerning the improvement of air quality and also coordinates activities, provides technical assistance and guidance to State Boards and lays down standards for the quality of air. It collects and disseminates information in respect of matters relating to air pollution and performs functions as prescribed in the Act.

State Pollution Control Boards: The State Boards have the power to advice the State Government on any matter concerning the prevention and control of air pollution. They have the right to inspect at all reasonable times any control equipment, industrial plant, or manufacturing process and give orders to take the necessary steps to control pollution. They are expected to inspect air pollution control areas at intervals or whenever necessary. They are empowered to provide standards for emissions to be laid down for different industrial plants with regard to quantity and composition of emission of air pollutants into the atmosphere. A State Board may establish or recognize a laboratory to perform this function.

The State Governments have been given powers to declare air pollution control areas after consulting with the State Board and also give instructions for ensuring standards of emission from automobiles and restriction on use of certain industrial plants.

Penalties: Persons managing industry are to be penalized if they produce emissions of air pollutants in excess of the standards laid down by the State Board. The Board also makes applications to the court for restraining persons causing air pollution in every State. Whoever contravenes any of the provision of the Act or any order or direction issued is punishable with imprisonment for a term which may extend to three months or with a fine of ₹10,000 or with both, and in case of continuing offence with an additional fine which may extend to ₹5,000 for every day during which such contravention continues after conviction for the first contravention.

What can an individual do to control air pollution?

- When you see a polluting vehicle take down the number and send a letter to the Road Transport Office (RTO) and the Pollution Control Board (PCB).
- If you observe an industry polluting air, inform the PCB in writing and ascertain if action is taken.
- Use cars only when absolutely necessary. Walk or cycle as much as possible instead of using fossil fuel powered vehicles.
- Use public transport as far as possible, as more people can travel in a single large vehicle rather than using multiple small vehicles which add to pollution.
- Share a vehicle space with relatives and friends. Carpools minimize the use of fossil fuels.
- Do not use air fresheners and other aerosols and sprays which contain CFCs that deplete the ozone layer.
- Do not smoke in a public place. It is illegal and endangers not only your own health but also that of others.
- Coughing can spread bacteria and viruses. Use a handkerchief to prevent droplet infection which is air-borne. It endangers the health of other people.

THE WATER POLLUTION PREVENTION AND CONTROL ACT

The Government has formulated this Act in 1974 to be able to prevent pollution of water by industrial, agricultural and household wastewater that can contaminate our water sources. Wastewater with high levels of pollutants that enter wetlands, rivers, lakes, wells as well as the sea are serious health hazards. Controlling the point sources by monitoring levels of different pollutants is one way to prevent pollution by giving a punishment to a polluter. However, it is also the responsibility of people in general to inform the relevant authority when they see a likely source of pollution. Individuals can also do several things to reduce water pollution such as using biodegradable chemicals for household use, reducing use of pesticides in gardens, and identifying polluting sources at workplaces and in industrial units where oil or other petroleum products and heavy metals are used. Excessive organic matter, sediments and infecting organisms from hospital wastes can also pollute our water. Citizens need to develop a watchdog force to inform authorities to take appropriate actions against different types of water pollution. A polluter must pay for his actions. However, preventing pollution is better than trying to cure the problems it has created, or punishing offenders.

Objectives

The main objectives of the Water Act are to provide for prevention, control and abatement of water pollution and the maintenance or restoration of the wholesomeness of water.

It is designed to assess pollution levels and punish polluters. The Central Government and State Governments have set up Pollution Control Boards that monitor water pollution.

Functions of the Pollution Control Boards

The Government has given the necessary powers to the Pollution Control Boards to deal with the problems of water pollution in the country. The Government has also suggested penalties for violation of the provisions of the Act.

Central and State water testing laboratories have been set up to enable the Boards to assess the extent of water pollution and standards have been laid down to establish guilt and default.

The Central and State Boards are entitled to certain powers and functions which are as follows:

Central Board: It has the power to advise the Central Government on any matters concerning the prevention and control of water pollution. The Board coordinates the activities of the State Boards and also resolves disputes. The Central Board can provide technical assistance and guidelines to State Boards to carry out investigations and research relating to water pollution, and organizes training for people involved in the process. The Board organizes a comprehensive awareness program on water pollution through mass media and also publishes data regarding water pollution. The Board lays down or modifies the rules in consultation with the State Boards on standards of disposal of waste. The main function of the Central Board is to promote the cleanliness of rivers, lakes, streams and wells in the country.

State Boards: They have the power to advise the State Government on any matters concerning water pollution.

- It plans a comprehensive program for the prevention of water pollution by collecting and disseminates information on water pollution and participates in research in collaboration with the Central Board in organizing training of people involved in the process.
- The Board inspects sewage or trade effluents, treatment plants, purification plants and the systems of disposal and also evolves economical and reliable methods of treatment of sewage and other effluents and plan the utilization of sewage water for agriculture.
- The State Board advises State Governments with respect to location of industries. Laboratories have been established to enable the Board to perform its functions.
- The State Boards have the power to obtain information from officers empowered by it who make surveys, keep records of flow, volume, and other characteristics of the water.
- They are given the power to take samples of effluents and suggest the procedures to be followed in connection with the samples. The concerned board analyst is expected to analyze the sample sent to him and submit a report of the result to the concerned Board. The Board is required to send a copy of the result to the respective industry. The Board also has the power of inspecting any plant record, register, document or any material object, and can conduct a search in any place in which there is reason to believe that an offence has been conducted under the Act.

Penalties are charged for acts that have caused pollution. This includes failing to furnish information required by the Board, or failing to inform the occurrence of any accident or other unforeseen act. An individual or organization that fails to comply with the directions given in the subsections of the law can be convicted or punished with imprisonment for a term of three months or with a fine of ₹10,000 or both and in case failure continues an additional fine of ₹5,000 every day. If a person who has already been convicted for any offence is found guilty of the same offence again, he/she after the second and every subsequent conviction, would be punishable with imprisonment for a term not less than two years but which may extend to seven years with fine.

What can individuals do to prevent water pollution?

- Inform the Pollution Control Board of any offender who is polluting water and ensure that appropriate action is taken. One can also write to the press.
- Do not dump wastes into a household or industrial drain which can directly enter any water body, such as a stream, river, pond, lake or the sea.
- Do not use toilets for flushing down waste items as they do not disappear but reappear at other places and cause water pollution.
- Use compost instead of chemical fertilizers in gardens.
- Avoid use of pesticides at home like DDT, Malathion, Aldrin, and use alternative methods like paste of boric acid mixed with gram flour to kill cockroaches and other insects. Use dried neem leaves to help keep away insects.

THE WILDLIFE PROTECTION ACT

This Act passed in 1972, deals with the declaration of National Parks and Wildlife Sanctuaries and their notification. It establishes the structure of the State's wildlife management and the posts designated for Wildlife Management. Before 1972, India had only five designated national parks. Among other reforms, the Act established schedules of protected plant and animal species; hunting or harvesting these species was largely outlawed. The Act provides for the protection of wild animals, birds and plants; and for matters connected therewith or ancillary or incidental thereto. It extends to the whole of India. It provides for setting up Wildlife Advisory Boards and prohibits hunting of all animals specified in Schedules I to IV of the Act. Plants that are protected are included in schedule VI.

In 2002 The Amendment to the Wildlife Protection Act become more stringent for preventing the commercial use of resources by local people. It has brought in new concepts such as the creation of Community Reserves.

Penalties

- A person who breaks any of the conditions of any license or permit granted under this Act shall be guilty of an offence against this Act. The offence is punishable with imprisonment for a term which may extend to three years or with a fine of ₹25,000 or with both.
- An offence committed in relation to any animal specified in Schedule I, or Part II of Schedule II, like the use of meat of any such animal, or animal articles like a trophy, shall be punishable with imprisonment for a term not less

than one year and may extend to six years and a fine of ₹25,000.

- In the case of a second or subsequent offence of the same nature mentioned in this sub-section, the term of imprisonment may extend to six years and not less than two years with a penalty of ₹10,000.

What can an individual do?

- If you observe an act of poaching, or see a poached animal, inform the local forest department official at the highest possible level. One can also report the event through the press. Follow-up to check that action is taken by the concerned authority. If no action is taken, one must take it up to the chief wildlife warden of the state.
- Say 'no' to the use of wildlife products and also try to convince other people not to buy them.
- Reduce the use of wood and wood products wherever possible.
- Avoid misuse of paper because it is made from bamboo and wood, which destroys wildlife habitat. Paper and envelopes can always be reused.
- Create a pressure group and ask government to ensure that the biodiversity of our country is conserved.
- Do not harm animals. Stop others from inflicting cruelty to animals.
- Do not disturb birds' nests and fledglings.
- When you visit the zoo do not tease the animals by throwing stones or feeding them, and prevent others from doing so.
- If you come across an injured animal do what you can to help it.
- If the animal needs medical care and expert attention contact the Society for the Prevention of Cruelty to Animals in your city.
- Create awareness about biodiversity conservation in your own way to family and friends.
- Join organizations, which are concerned with protection of biodiversity, such as Worldwide Fund For Nature -India (WWFI), Bombay Natural History Society (BNHS), or a local conservation NGO.

FOREST CONSERVATION ACT

To appreciate the importance of the Forest Conservation Act of 1980, which was amended in 1988, it is essential to understand its historical background. The Indian Forest Act of 1927 consolidated all the previous laws regarding forests that were passed before the 1920's. The Act gave the government and forest department the power to create reserved forests, and the right to use reserved forests for government use alone. It also created protected forests, in which the use of resources by local people was controlled. Some forests were also to be controlled by a village community, and these were called village forests.

The Act remained in force till the 1980s when it was realized that protecting forests for timber production alone was not acceptable. The other values of protecting the services that forests provide and its valuable assets such as biodiversity began to overshadow the importance of their revenue earnings from timber. Thus a new Act was essential. This led to the Forest Conservation Act of 1980 and its amendment in 1988.

This act establishes three categories of forests:

1. Reserve forest
2. Protected forest
3. Village forest

Reserved forest constituted by the State Government on any forest land on which the Government has proprietary rights, in which local people are prohibited. Protected forest, which comes under government protection in order to check the deforestation, as well as ensures need of forest products for commercial use. Village forest is a forest in which the villagers guards the forest and cutting and transportation of trees.

What can an individual do to support the Act?

- Be alert to destructive activities in your local green areas such as reserved forests and protected forests, and in protected areas (national parks and wildlife sanctuaries). Report any such act to the forest department as well as the press. Report of violations can be made to the conservator of forest, district forest officer, range forest officer, forest guard or the district commissioner, or local civic body.
- Acquaint yourself with the laws, detailed rules and orders issued by the government.
- Be in touch with concerned local NGOs and associations. Organize one with other like minded people if none exist in your area.
- Create awareness about the existence and value of national parks and sanctuaries and build up a public opinion against illegal activities in the forest or disturbance to wildlife.
- Pressurize the authorities to implement the forest and wildlife laws and rules to protect green areas.
- Take legal action if necessary and if possible through a public interest litigation (PIL) against the offending party. Use the help of NGOs who can undertake legal action.
- Help to create public pressure to change rules laws and procedures when necessary.
- Use better, ecologically sensitive public transport and bicycle tracks. Do not litter in a forest area.
- Participate in preservation of greenery, by planting, watering and caring for plants.

Whom should forest offences be reported to?

If you as a citizen come across anyone felling trees, encroaching on forest land, dumping garbage, cutting green wood, lighting a fire, or creating a clearing in reserved forests, protected forests, national park, sanctuary or other forest areas, you must report it to the forest/wildlife officers concerned. For urgent action one can contact the police. In fact you should file an FIR in any case because it serves as an important proof that you have made the report.

ISSUES INVOLVED IN ENFORCEMENT OF ENVIRONMENTAL LEGISLATION

- Environmental legislation is evolved to protect our environment as a whole, our health, and the earth's resources. The presence of a legislation to protect air, water, soil, etc. does not necessarily mean that the problem is addressed.
- Once a legislation is made at the global, National or State level, it has to be implemented.
- For a successful environmental legislation to be implemented, there has to be an effective agency to collect relevant data, process it and pass it on to a law enforcement agency. If the law or rule is broken by an individual or institution, this has to be punished through the legal process. Information to law enforcement officials must also come from concerned individuals.
- In most situations, if no cognizance is given, the interested concerned individual must file a PIL for the protection of the environment.
- There are several NGOs in the country such as WWF-I, BEAG and the BNHS which take these matters to court in the interest of conservation. Anyone can request them to help in such matters. There are also legal experts such as MC Mehta who have successfully fought cases in the courts to support environmental causes.

Environment impact assessment (EIA): For all development projects, whether government or private, the Ministry of Environment and Forests (MoEF) requires an impact assessment done by a competent organization.

- The EIA must look into physical, biological and social parameters. EIAs are expected to indicate what the likely impacts could be if the project is passed.
- The MoEF has identified a large number of projects that need clearance on environmental grounds. The EIA must define what impact it would have on water, soil and air. It also requires that a list of flora and fauna identified in the region is documented and to specify if there are any endangered species whose habitat or life could be adversely affected.
- New projects are called 'green field projects' where no development has been done. Projects that already exist but require expansion must also apply for clearance. These are called 'brown field projects'.
- After the Environmental Protection Act of 1986 was passed, an EIA to get an environmental clearance for a project became mandatory.
- An EIA is not intended to stop all types of development. The siting of an industry can be selected carefully and if it is likely to damage a fragile area an alternate less sensitive area must be selected.

Using an environmental calendar of activities:

- **February 2:** World Wetland Day is celebrated to create awareness about wetlands and their value to mankind. On February 2nd 1971, the Ramsar Convention on Wetlands of International importance was signed at Ramsar in Iran.
- **March 21:** World Forestry Day can be used to initiate a public awareness campaign about the extremely rapid disappearance of our forests. The program must be action oriented and become an ongoing process with activities such as tree plantation
- **April 7:** World Health Day—The World Health Organization (WHO) came into existence on this day in 1948. A campaign for personal sanitation and hygiene to understanding issues of public health, occupational health, etc. can be carried out.
- **April 18:** World Heritage Day can be used to arrange a visit to a local fort or museum. Environment also includes our cultural monuments. Students could use this opportunity to create awareness among the local people about their very valuable heritage sites.
- **April 22:** Earth Day was first celebrated in 1970 by a group of people in the USA to draw attention to increasing environmental problems caused by humans on earth. This day is now celebrated all over the world with rallies, festivals, clean-ups, special shows and lectures.
- **June 5:** World Environment Day marks the anniversary of the Stockholm Conference on Human Environment in Sweden in 1972, where nations of the world gathered to share their concern over human progress at the expense of the environment.
- **June 11:** World Population Day is a day when the vital link between population and environment could be discussed in seminars held at college and other NGOs.
- **August 6:** Hiroshima Day could be used to discuss our own Bhopal Gas Tragedy and the Chernobyl disaster.
- **September 16:** World Ozone Day was proclaimed by the United Nations as the International Day for the preservation of the ozone layer. This is a good occasion for students to find out more about the threats to this layer and initiate discussion on what they can do to help mitigate this global threat. The day marks the Montreal Protocol signed in 1987 to control production and consumption of ozone depleting substances.
- **September 28:** Green Consumer Day could be used to create an awareness in consumers about various products. Students could talk to shopkeepers and consumers about excess packaging and a campaign to use articles which are not heavily packaged could be carried out.
- **October 1–7:** Wildlife Week can consist of seminars on conserving our species and threatened ecosystems. The State Forest Departments organize various activities in which every student should take part. A poster display, a street play to highlight India's rich biodiversity can be planned. Wildlife does not only mean animals, but includes plants as well.

COMMONLY USED INSECTICIDES AND PESTICIDES

Insecticides are substances used to kill insects. They include ovicides and larvicides used against insect eggs and larvae, respectively. Insecticides are used in agriculture, medicine, industry and by consumers. Insecticides are claimed to be a major factor behind the increase in the 20th-century's agriculture.

Insecticides are substances used to kill insects. They include ovicides and larvicides used against insect eggs and larvae, respectively. Insecticides are used in agriculture, medicine, industry and by consumers. Insecticides are claimed to be a major factor behind the increase in the 20th-century's agricultural productivity. Nearly all insecticides have the potential to significantly alter ecosystems; many are toxic to humans and/or animals; some become concentrated as they spread along the food chain.

PESTICIDES

Pesticides include insecticides, herbicides and fungicides. Pesticide is any substance or mixture of substances intended for preventing, destroying, repelling, or mitigating any pest. Pest means any organism that damages crops, injures or irritates livestock or man, or reduces the fertility of land. Pesticide derived from Latin words pestis means "deadly contagious disease." During the late middle ages, when the bubonic plague killed a third of all humans, it was commonly known as "the pest and cide means to kill. There are several thousand different types in use and almost all of them are possible causes of water pollution. For example, DDT, malathion, parathion, deltamethrin and others have been sprayed in the environment for long periods of time for the control of disease vectors such as mosquitoes, and to control the growth of weeds and other pests. The pollution by chemicals such as pesticides may have long-term consequences, such as groundwater pollution. Most of the water supplies in India are found contaminated due to the pesticide discharge.

According to a study conducted in India by ICMR, 85% of milk samples found to have pesticides level above the acceptable limits. The most common pesticides found were organochlorines and organophosphorus. Among the organochlorines, HCH and DDT were frequently detected and among organophosphorus, endosulfan. Malathion and chlorpyrifos pesticides were also most frequently detected. Once the pesticide is released in the environment, they have different distribution and persistence patterns in air, water and soil. Many pesticides which are used in homes have been found in house dust for many days to weeks after the application. Climatic characteristics also play a role in persistence. Studies in the Arctic have shown that insecticides and herbicides persist 3–8 times longer in cold climates than in temperate zones. The most persistent pesticides are termed "persistent organic pollutants" (POPs) and may represent long-term dangers.

Insecticides: Insecticides are the sub-class of pesticides. It means a substance used to kill or destroy insects. Insects are small air-breathing arthropod of the class insecta, having a body divided into head, thorax, and abdomen, three pairs of legs, and (in most species) two pairs of wings. Insecticide derived from Latin insectum means (animal that has been) cut into sections and cide. The pesticide is a broad term that means any chemical that kills the pest, i.e., weed, insect, bacterial fungus, etc. whereas, insecticides only kill the insects **(Fig. 6.5)**.

Classification of Pesticides

Pesticides are classified on the basis of various criteria such as toxicity (hazardous effects), pest organism they kill and pesticide function, chemical composition, mode of entry, mode of action, how or when they work, formulations and sources of origin **(Table 6.5)**.

Classification of Pesticides on the Basis of Toxicity

Toxicity of pesticide mainly depends on two factors namely dose and time. Hence, how much of the substance is involved (dose) and how often the exposure to the substance occurs (time) give rise to two different types of toxicity—acute and chronic toxicity.

Acute toxicity: Acute toxicity refers to how poisonous a pesticide is to a human, animal or plant after a single short-term exposure. A pesticide with a high acute toxicity

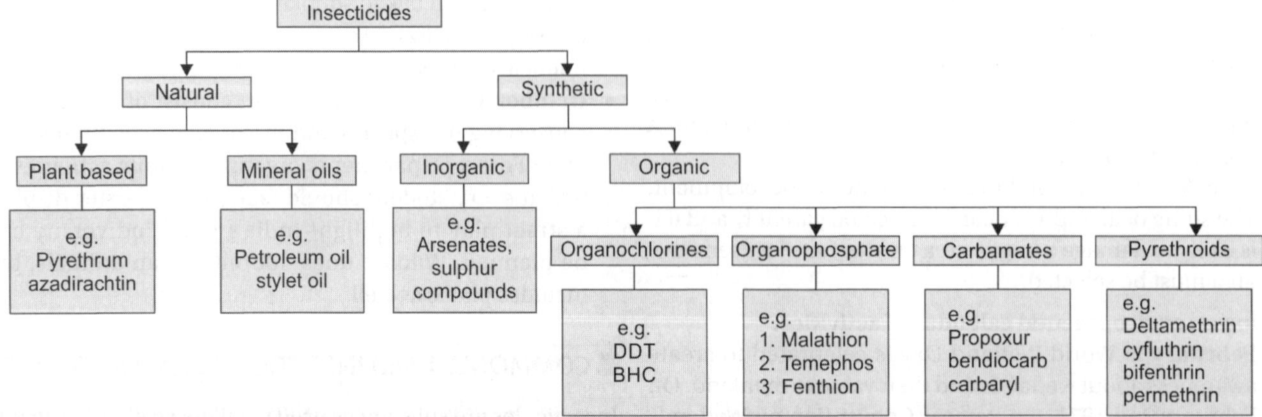

Fig. 6.5: Overall classification of insecticides.

Table 6.5: Pesticides types on the basis of pest organism they kill.

Sl No.	Type of pesticide	Target pests/functions	Examples
1.	Acaricides	Substances that are used to kill mites and ticks or to disrupt their growth or development	DDT, dicofol, chlorpyrifos, permethrin, etc.
2.	Algicide	Substances that used to kill or inhibit algae	Copper sulphate, diuron, oxyfluorfen, etc.
3.	Antifeedants	Chemicals which prevent an insect or other pest from feeding	Chlordimeform, azadirachtin, etc.
4.	Avicides	Chemicals that are used to kill birds	Strychnine, fenthion, etc.
5.	Bactericides	Compounds that isolated from or produced by a microorganism or a related chemical that is produced artificially, which are used to kill or inhibit bacteria in plants or soil	Streptomycin, tetracycline, etc.
6.	Bird repellents	Chemicals which repel the birds	Diazinon, methiocarb, etc.
7.	Chemosterillant	Chemicals that renders an insect infertile and thus prevent it from reproducing	Diflubenzuron
8.	Desiccants	Act on plants by drying their tissues	Boric acid
9.	Fungicides	Chemicals which are used to prevent, cure eradicate the fungi	Cymoxanil, thiabendazole, Bordeaux mixture
10.	Herbicide softener	A chemical that protect crops from injury by herbicides, but does not prevent the herbicides from killing weeds	Benoxacor, cyometrinil
11.	Herbicides	Substances that are used to kill the plants, or to inhibit their growth or development	Alachlor, paraquat, 2,4-D
12.	Insect attractant	A chemical that lures pests to trap, thereby removing them from crops animals and stored products	Gossyplure, gyplure
13.	Insect growth regulator	A substance that works by disrupting the growth or development of an insect	Diflubenzuron
14.	Insecticides	A pesticide that is used to kill insects or to disrupt their growth or development	Azadirachtin, DDT, chlorpyrifos, malathion, etc.
15.	Larvicides	Inhibit the growth of larvae	Methoprene

is deadly even when a very small amount is absorbed. Acute toxicity may be measured as acute oral toxicity, acute dermal toxicity and acute inhalation toxicity.

Chronic toxicity: Chronic toxicity is delayed poisonous effect from exposure to a pesticide. Chronic toxicity of pesticides concerns the general public as well as those working directly with pesticides because of potential exposure to pesticides on/in food products, water and the air.

Pesticides are Classified Based on their Mode of Action

- **Insecticides:** Compounds which kill or repel insects and related species, e.g., organophosphates, organochlorine, carbamates, etc.
- **Herbicides:** Compounds which kill weeds/prevent growth of undesirable herbs or weeds in the field, e.g., parquet, atrazine, etc.
- **Fungicides:** Compounds which kill fungi and moulds, e.g., Captan, Captafol, etc.
- **Rodenticides:** Compounds which kill rats, mice, moles and other rodents, e.g., anticoagulants, arsenic, strychnine, etc.
- **Acaricides:** Compounds which kill mites, ticks and spiders, e.g., azobenzene, chlorobenzilate, etc.
- **Nematicides:** Compounds which kill nematodes, e.g., ethylene bromide
- **Molluscicides:** Compounds which kill the molluscs such as snails and slugs, e.g., metaldehyde.
- **Miscellaneous pesticides:** Compounds of lead, copper, mercury, nicotine, etc.

Classification Based on Sources of Origin

Pesticide are natural or biological agents that are used to kill unwanted plants or animal pests. Based on the source of origin, pesticide may be classified into biopesticides and chemical pesticides.

- **Biopesticides:** These act on the target pests and strongly linked organisms. Biopesticides include microbial pesticides (containing a live bacterium, fungus, virus, protozoan or alga as active ingredient), and chemicals that are derived from animals, bacteria, fungi and plants. They are less toxic, decomposed easily and required in small quantities. There are three major classes of Biopesticides.
  - **Microbial pesticides:** The active ingredient is microorganism such as bacteria or fungi, e.g., bacterial toxins produced by *Bacillus thuringiensis*, and *Bacillus sphaericus* acts on mosquito larvae, black fly larvae.

- **Plant incorporated protectants:** Pesticides produced by plant naturally and genetic material introduced together is termed as plant incorporated protectants.
- **Biochemical pesticides:** Pesticides which include natural material that have nontoxic mechanism to controls pests, e.g., insect sex pheromones.
- **Chemical pesticides:** These are of wide range which affect large group of nontarget organisms. Chemical pesticides are quite toxic and not always biodegradable. Chemical pesticides are further divided into organochlorine, organophosphate, carbamates and pyrethroids.

MEDICAL ENTOMOLOGY

Arthropods comprise the most numerous varieties of living things in the environment of men. Some of them are man's allies, helping in the fertilization of flowers, but the majority of arthropods, in general, are either of no use to man or are his most dangerous enemies. A study of the arthropods of medical importance is known as medical entomology, which is an important branch of preventive medicine. It is the branch of science that deals with insects that cause diseases, or that serve as vectors of organisms that cause diseases in human beings. In medical entomology, for example, research may pertain to the interactions of the arboviruses and their hosts and involve physiology, genetics, biology, and ecology.

Arthropods of Medical Importance

See **Tables 6.6 and 6.7**.

Arthropods and Transmission of Disease

Arthropods transmit the disease in the following ways:

- **Transmission through direct contact:** Arthropods get transferred from one person to another, either through direct contact or due to proximity and, thus, spread the disease.

Table 6.6: Classes of arthropods.

Class: Insects	*Class: Arachnida*	*Class: Crustacea*
• Mosquitoes: Anophelines, culicines	• Ticks: ▪ Hard ticks ▪ Soft ticks	• Cyclops
• Flies	• Mites (chiggers):	
▪ Houseflies	*Leptotrombidium* and trombiculid mites	
▪ Sandflies	Itch mite	
▪ Tsetse flies		
▪ Black flies		
• Human lice:		
▪ Head and body lice		
▪ Crab lice		
• Fleas:		
▪ Rat fleas		
▪ Sand fleas		
• Reduviid bugs		

Table 6.7: Arthropod-borne diseases.

Arthropod	*Diseases transmitted*
1. Mosquito	Malaria, filarial, viral encephalitis (e.g., Japanese encephalitis) Hemorrhagic fevers (e.g., yellow fever, dengue)
2. Housefly	Typhoid and paratyphoid fever, diarrhea, dysentery, cholera, gastroenteritis, amoebiasis, helminths' infestations, poliomyelitis, conjunctivitis, trachoma, anthrax, yawn, etc.
3. Sand fly	Kala-azar, oriental sore, sand fly fever, oroya fever
4. Tsetse fly	Sleeping sickness
5. Louse	Epidemic typhus, relapsing fever, trench fever, pediculosis
6. Rat flea	Bubonic plague, endemic typhus, chiggerosis, hymenolepis diminuta
7. Black fly	Onchocerciasis
8. Reduviid bug	Chagas disease
9. Hard tick	Tick typhus, viral encephalitis, viral fevers, viral hemorrhagic fever (e.g., Kyasanur forest disease, tularemia, tick paralysis, human babesiosis)
10. Soft tick	Q fever, relapsing fever
11. Trombiculid mite	Scrub typhus, rickettsial pore
12. Itch mite	Scabies
13. Cyclops	Guinea worm disease, fish tapeworm (*Desulfobacter latus*)
14. Cockroaches	Enteric pathogens

- **Mechanical transmission:** Here the disease is transferred from one place to the other by carrier arthropods. Insects and parasites, mechanically carrying the infection with them, sit at a place and, thus, spread the disease.
- **Biological transmission:** Malaria, filarial, and plague, etc., are transmitted through biological transmission only. In this case, the pathogens grow in the insect or the arthropod or part of their lifecycle is completed in the insect host and then the disease is transmitted.

Principles of Arthropod control

The general principles of arthropod control are explained as follows:

- **Environmental control:** This offers the last approach to the control of arthropods, because the results are likely to be permanent. For example, environmental manipulations are elimination of breeding places (source reduction), filling and drainage operation.
- **Chemical control:** A wide range of insecticides belonging to the organ chlorine, organophosphorus and carbonate groups of compounds are available for vector control.
- **Biological control:** To minimize environmental pollution with toxic chemicals, great emphasis is now being placed on biological control.
- **Genetic control:** Much progress has taken place in the recent years in theoretical and applied aspects of genetic control of arthropods.

MOSQUITOES

Mosquitoes are found all over the world but, in tropical countries, they are found in large numbers. Human blood-sucking mosquitoes are more dangerous.

Mosquito-borne diseases:

- Anopheles: Malaria
- Culicine: Filaria, encephalitis
- Arêtes: Dengue fever, hemorrhagic fever
- Mansuria: Malayan filariasis

Body Structure

A mosquito's body structure has three parts. Head is semicircular in shape with a pair of eyes. There are needle-like structures in front of head called 'proboscis'. Mosquitoes use it for biting. These are large and round. It has a pair of wings on its back and three pairs of legs on its front or abdomen. Abdomen is long and narrow with ten segments. Last two of these segments form the sex organs of a mosquito.

Life Cycle

There are four stages in the life cycle of a mosquito. These are eggs, larvae, pupa and adult.

1. **Eggs:** A female mosquito lays 100–250 eggs at a time. A newborn mosquito remains in egg stage for 1–2 days and then it enters the next stage of life cycle **(Fig. 6.6)**. Mosquito's eggs are laid in slow-moving or stagnant pools of fresh water to provide suitable habitat for the larvae once they hatch. Different species of mosquitoes prefer different water conditions; some prefer shaded areas, whereas some prefer direct sunlight. However, some species will lay mosquito eggs on moist, often-flooded soil in anticipation of the next rise in water. Those eggs can survive winter, waiting for spring or summer rains to cover them over.

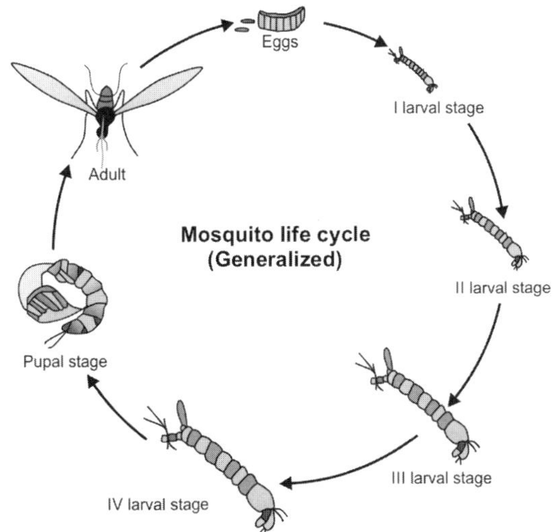

Fig. 6.6: Life cycle of a mosquito.

Note: Each larval stage is larger than the previous one. Molting occurs between each larval and pupal stage. Larval and pupal stages are aquatic.

2. **Larvae:** It lives in dirty and stagnant water and it floats freely in it. It feeds in bacteria and small plants like algae. This stage continues for 5–7 days. These larvae are predatory, feeding on other aquatic insects and organisms, but they themselves can also be eaten by fish, copepods and other creatures. Most larvae lay at an angle to the water surface and breathe through a specialized tube-like organ, known as a 'siphon', but Anopheles larvae lack the siphon and so lay parallel to the water's surface in order to breathe. Each larva must shed its skin (molt) four times before reaching the stage where it forms a pupa.
3. **Pupa:** The pupa is just like a butterfly pupa. This is of colon or comma shape. This is actually the rest period. At this stage, it does not eat anything and continues to float on the surface of the water. It goes under water on sensing danger. This stage is of 1–2 days, after which the pupa splits and the adult emerges. The length of the full cycle is dependent on whether the conditions were optimal for that species of mosquito, and specifically based on temperature.
4. **Adult:** An adult mosquito comes but by bursting the outer layer of pupa. The male mosquito has a shorter life as compared to the female mosquito. Under normal circumstances, a mosquito lives for 2 weeks. The male adult mosquitoes usually live for about a week, feeding on nectar—they also possess very bushy antennae for seeking out females to mate with. Female mosquitoes have specialized mouthparts that allow them to feed on blood.

Other Facts About Mosquitoes

- Generally, mosquitoes are found in dark places, corners, stagnant water, coolers, kitchen cabinets, bathrooms and toilets and also more in the rainy season.
- Male mosquitoes do not bite, only female mosquitoes bite because they require blood to lay eggs.
- After biting or sucking blood, mosquitoes rest on the walls; therefore, DDT, etc. are sprayed on the walls.
- Mosquitoes can fly up to 3 miles.

Methods of Controlling the Mosquitoes

A number of methods are used to control mosquitoes. These methods can be classified into two types:

1. Methods of protection against mosquito bites
2. Methods of eradication of mosquitoes, which also include the anti-larval and anti-adult measures.

Protection Against Mosquito Bites

- Fixing the mosquito nails or wire mesh in the windows and doors.
- Use of mosquito nets while sleeping.
- **Smoke:** Mosquitoes can be repelled or made inactive by burning dry neem leaves, mosquito repellent coils, etc.
- **Use of repellents:** These substances (insulin, odomos, diethyltoluamide, etc.) are rubbed on the skin, due to which mosquitoes do not perch on the skin.

- Weaning gown or full sleeves shirt and pyjama is also effective to cover the body in case of unavailability of mosquito net.
- Using fogging machine can reset mosquitoes.

Eradication of Mosquitoes

Both adult as well as larvae are attacked to eradicate mosquitoes:

- Eradicate mosquitoes
- Controlling the environment
- Use of larvicides
- Use of insecticides
- Genetic control.

LOUSE

Louse is a wingless parasite, which lives on the bodies of mammals and birds. Louise is directly related to the poor standards of cleanliness. Women and children are more infected with them than men **(Fig. 6.7)**.

Kinds of Louse

- **Head louse (Pediculus capitis):** Head lice are wingless insects spending their entire life on the human scalp and feeding exclusively on human blood. Unlike body lice, head lice are not the vectors of any known diseases. Except for rare secondary infections that result from scratching at bites, head lice are harmless, and they have been regarded by some as essentially a cosmetic rather than a medical problem.
- **Body louse (Pediculus corporis):** Body lice are hard to find on the skin because, when not feeding, they hide and plant their eggs in the folds or seams of clothing. Body lice live in the seams and linings of clothing, blankets, and sheets and move to the body when feeding.
- **Pubic/crab louse (Pthirus pubis or crab louse):** As per their names, head lice are found in head, body louse in the body and pubic louse (crab louse) in the pubic region. The head and body louse have almost the same physical size and shape, but the crab louse has a rounder body and its second and third pairs of legs are larger than the first pair near its head. Pubic lice are found among coarse hairs around the rectal area and sex organs, but occasionally, migrate to the eyebrows, eyelashes, head or over the body if the person is unusually hairy. Crab lice live on the hairy parts of the body, usually in the pubic and perinatal regions. Since prepubertal children have no hair in these areas, crab lice are uncommon before adolescence. It is difficult to remove them manually.

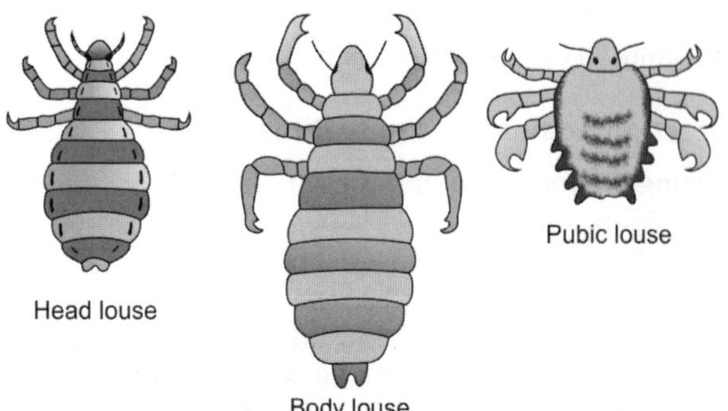

Fig. 6.7: Types of louse.

Structure and Lifestyle

Body of louse is flat and is composed of three parts—head, throat and abdomen. Louse uses its mouth to suck the blood. It has a pointed head with five antennae. In distinguishing three kinds of louse, head lice and body lice are morphologically indistinguishable. However, body lice are slightly larger. These lice have abdomens longer than their breadth and their six legs are equal in size. In contrast, the abdomen of the crab louse is about as wide as or even slightly wider than its length, and the second and third pairs of legs are thicker than the first pair. Crab lice are much smaller than head lice and body lice. Head lice and pubic lice are highly dependent upon human body warmth and will die if separated from their host for 24 hours. Body lice are harder since they live on clothing and can survive if separated from human contact for up to a week without feeding.

Life cycle of louse passes through the following stages **(Fig. 6.8)**.

Eggs

A female lays up to 300 eggs at the rate of 4–9 eggs per day. These are firmly attached to the root of hair. Their common name is 'nits'. This stage continues for 6–9 days.

Larvae

The larva is similar to an adult louse; the only difference is that it is smaller in size. It remains in this stage for 10–15 days.

Adult

Under favorable conditions, an adult louse lives for 30–50 days.

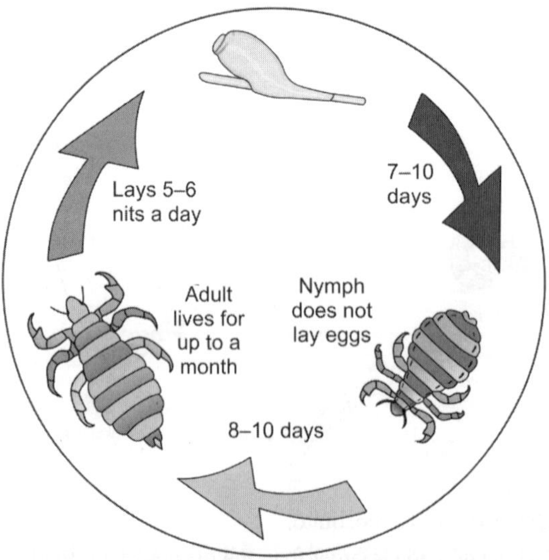

Fig. 6.8: Life cycle of a louse.

Transmission of Disease

Except for rare secondary infections that result from scratching of bites, head lice are harmless but body lice transmit a number of diseases through bites or infected excreta. The diseases are typhoid, trench and relapsing fever, all serious diseases. The body louse, which is generally limited to those who do not bathe frequently, can transmit certain diseases. Among the three kinds of human lice, only the body louse has been implicated as vector, a carrier of louse-borne disease, like relapsing fever and epidemic typhus. In past times, typhus epidemic, relapsing fever, trench fever, dermatitis, itching, etc., are major diseases caused by it.

Modes of Transmission

Direct Contact

- Sleeping together
- Contact in crowded places
- Students sharing a bench in the school.

Indirect Contact

- Spread through used clothes, bed, sharing combs, and towels, etc.
- Infected items of hotels, dharamshalas, inns, etc. and clothes and combs of schools.

Control of Louse

Protection Against Louse

It includes various aspects of personal hygiene:
- Daily bath
- Clothes, especially undergarments, should be changes everyday
- Special care of a female child's and a woman's hair
- Proper cleaning of bed, towels, bed linen and bed sheets, etc.
- Hot water to be used for washing clothes. Clothes to be dried in sunlight, hot iron to be used on those clothes
- Combs, hair brushes, hair pins and clips, etc. should be clean and separate for individual use.

Use of Insecticides for Killing the Lice

- Apply 10% DDT on hair and head, and cover it for 24 hours with a cloth. Wash it off after the specified time period. This process should be repeated after every 7–10 days, so that all the nits and lice, etc. are destroyed completely.
- 1% malathion should be sprayed on the inner surface of the undergarments. This destroys the body lice.
- Mixture of coconut oil and kerosene also effectively destroys the lice. Many medicines are also available in the market to kill lice.

FLIES

Housefly

Houseflies are a symbol of filth and poor sanitation. Flies are of many types. In India, flies can be seen all around the year.

Body Structure

Musca domestica is the most common species of a housefly. It is 6–7 mm long with hairy-brown color. Its body has three parts—head, thorax and abdomen. Head has a pair of eyes, two antennae and proboscis. It has two wings and three pairs of legs which are attached to thorax. Its body and legs are covered with innumerable fine hair, which secrete sticky fluid that helps in transmission of diseases.

Life Cycle (Fig. 6.9)

- **Eggs:** The female fly lays eggs in the human excreta, manure heaps or garbage and vegetables refuse. It lays 120–150 eggs at a time, which are shiny and resemble grains of rice. Eggs take 8–24 hours to hatch.
- **Larvae:** Eggs hatch into larvae or maggots. These are buried under manure heaps. They crawl to reach to their food larvae, also known as maggots. Maggots are legless, white insects that feed from the egg-laying site for 3–5 days. During this time, maggots molt several times. This stage continues of 2–9 days.
- **Pupa:** Larvae grow into pupa. It is barrel-shaped and brown in color. This stage is also known as the rest period of the life cycle. Its duration can be of 3–6 days. Fly pupae are similar in function to butterfly cocoons. Their hard, brown shells protect the inactive, developing flies. Over the course of 3–6 days, the pupae develop legs and wings, ultimately emerging as full-grown houseflies.
- **Adult life:** Generally, it takes 5–6 days to reach this stage. During summer, this stage may last for 8–20 days. The adult female houseflies are capable of reproduction within 2–3 days.

Other Facts About Flies

- Flies grow in manure, human and animal excreta, garbage, environment with poor sanitation and heaps of refuse.
- Phlegm, saliva, feces, pars and other fluids excreted from the body attract them more.
- Flies do not consume solid substances. They vomit on them and suck the food in liquid state.
- They can fly up to 6.5 kms. Generally, they continue to fly in circles.

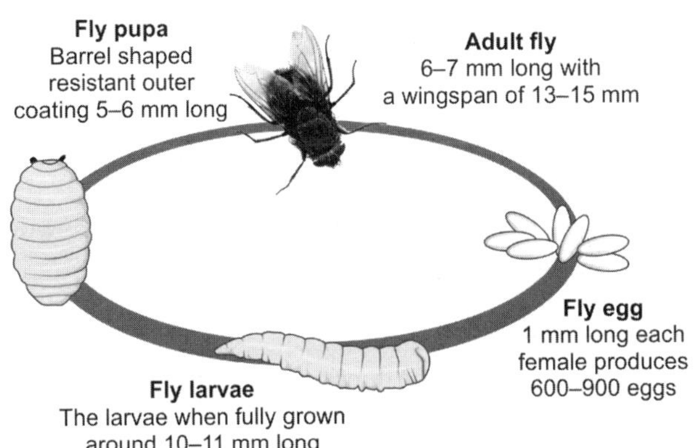

Fig. 6.9: Life cycle of a housefly.

- Flies are always covering around the garbage and always remain close to breeding places.
- Generally, flies live for 15 days in summers and 25 days in winters.

Transmission of Disease by Flies

- Mechanical transmission
- Food pipe transmission: Bacteria are stored safely in the food pipe of flies.

Fly-borne Diseases

Flies are of many types which are responsible for different diseases. Given below are the types of flies and the diseases which they spread.

- **Houseflies:** Diarrhea, cholera, dysentery, gastroenteritis, typhoid, amebiasis, trachoma, conjunctivitis
- **Sandflies:** Sand fly fever, kala-azar
- **Tsetse flies:** Sleeping sickness
- **Black flies:** Dermatitis/skin diseases.

Methods to Control Flies

Flies control program is undertaken with the following objectives:

- To control the breeding of flies
- To destroy flies
- To protect the edible substances from being infected by flies
- Educating people about the maintenance of cleanliness through health education.

Following methods are used to achieve these objectives:

Environmental Control

Breeding grounds of flies can be destroyed through the following methods of cleanliness:

- Proper collection and disposal of garbage and refuse
- Being careful about cleanliness in the kitchen
- Changing the habits of defecation, stopping open-air/field defecation and using sanitary latrines
- Building sanitary latrines in camps and conferences
- Improving the level of personal hygiene and domestic and environmental cleanliness.

Destruction of Flies

- Flies can be destroyed by using insecticides as DDT, BHC, Lindane, etc.
- Using fly paper to attract, trap and kill the flies. Similarly, fly swatter, tube light, etc. can also be used.
- Flies can be controlled by dusting some special powders on tablecloth, furniture, etc.

Preventive Measures

- Using wire mesh on the doors and windows of the houses, hospitals, hotels and restaurants.
- Food and the other edible substances should always be kept covered.
- Cut fruits, left-over vegetables, milk, tea and glasses and cups used for consuming liquids should be immediately cleaned and kept at the proper place.
- Toilets and urinals should always be closed.
- Developing the habit of frequent washing of hands and arranging for sink in the kitchen.
- Proper cleaning of food-serving and kitchen utensils.
- Health education.

Flies are a symbol of insanitation. This further under-lines the importance of personal and environmental hygiene. Thus, health education plays an important role in controlling the flies.

Sand Fly

Sand fly is the second most harmful fly after housefly. It is associated with a number of diseases. It is light or dark brown in color and the shape of its body is similar to that of a mosquito.

The body has three parts—head, thorax and abdomen. It cannot fly but can jump to a certain distance. It lives for almost 2 weeks.

Head

The head bears a pair of long and hairy antenna. Palpi and proboscis and one pair of prominent black eyes are present.

Thorax

The thorax bears a pair of wings and three pair of legs. The wings are upright in shape and hairy. The second longitudinal vein is branched twice. The legs are long and slender and out of proportion to the size of the body.

Abdomen

The abdomen has ten segments and is covered with hair. In the female, the tip of abdomen is rounded, while in the male, claspers are attached to the last abdominal segment.

Life Cycle of a Sand Fly

The life cycle of a sand fly is characterized by complete metamorphosis, having four developmental stages as shown in **Figure 6.10**:

- **Egg:** The female generally lays eggs in the damp dark places in the cattle sheds and poultry. The eggs vary from 40–60 in number, brownish in color. The eggs measure about 0.4 mm in length. Eggs hatch in 1–2 weeks' time.
- **Larva:** The larva is maggot-like structure, having large head, thorax and abdomen and two long bristles on the last abdominal segment. It feeds on the decaying organic matter and becomes a pupa in about 2 weeks' time.
- **Pupa:** Pupae are found in cracks and crevices in the wall. The pupa stage lasts for about one week.
- **Adult:** The average life of a sand fly is about 2 weeks.

Control Measures

Sand flies are easily controlled because they do not move long distance from their breeding places.

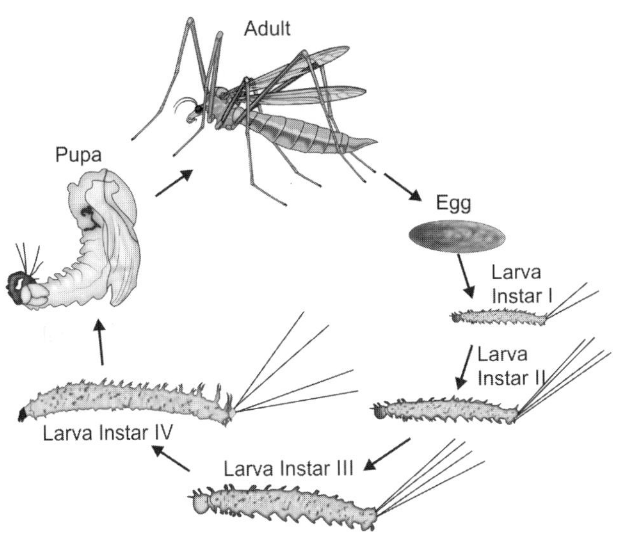

Fig 6.10: Life cycle of sand fly.

Insecticide

Spray of DDT 1-2 g/sq m or lindane 0.2 g/sq m is useful in effective controlling of the sandflies. Spraying should be done in the human dwellings, cattle sheds and poultry. Its residue may remain effective for a period of 3 months.

Sanitation

Removal of shrubs and vegetation, filling of cracks and crevices in the wall, and floor and distance of cattle sheds and poultry from human habitations are some of the important points to be taken care of. Paying attention to cleanliness of animal sheds, homes and healthy eating habits within the premises can also reduce their number.

Tsetse Fly

Tsetse fly is found in Africa. It is very similar to a housefly. Its life cycle is unusual and it lives for almost 100 days. It attacks on men, animals, birds, snakes, etc. It produces sleeping sickness. It is essential to use insecticides and maintain the cleanliness of vegetation to control its menace. Its total eradication is possible through genetic control techniques.

FLEAS

Fleas are brown-colored. These are wingless insects with hard external skin and stout body. Fleas are for the main cause of plague.

The body of flea is made up of three parts—head, thorax and abdomen. It sucks blood with its mouth. Thorax has three segments with three pairs of legs attached to them. Abdomen is also divided into ten segments. Male flea has a coiled structure in its abdomen called 'penis' **(Fig. 6.11)**.

It has four stages in this life cycle, namely eggs, larva, pupa and adult flea. Fleas lay their eggs in the hair and holes of mice. Generally, they live for a month. Female fleas require a blood meal prior to laying eggs. Eggs are laid on the host animal, and typically drop into the bedding or nest of the host. Larvae then feed on organic material present in the nest/bedding. Once the cocoon is created, flea pupae can survive for several months without feeding.

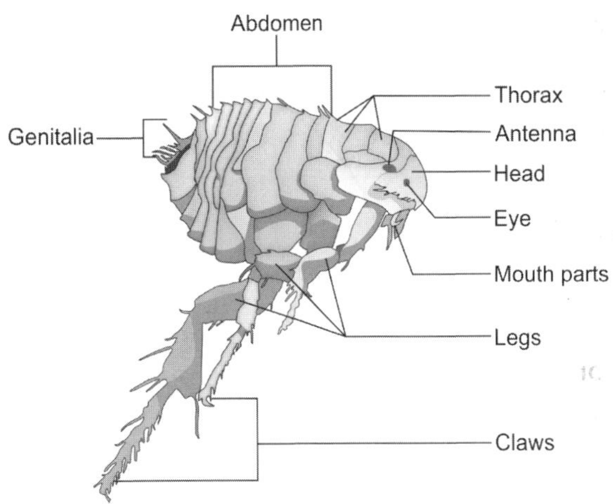

Fig. 6.11: Structure of fleas.

LIFE CYCLE

Eggs

The flea life cycle begins when the female lays after feeding. Eggs are laid in batches of up to 20 or so, usually on the host itself, which means that the eggs can easily roll onto the ground. Because of this, areas where the host rests and sleeps become one of the primary habitats of eggs and developing fleas. The eggs take around 2 days to 2 weeks to hatch as shown in **Figure 6.12**.

Larvae

Flea larvae emerge from the eggs to feed on any available organic material such as dead insects, feces, and vegetable matter. In laboratory studies, some dietary diversity seems necessary for proper larval development. Blood-only diets allow only 12% of larvae to mature, whereas blood and yeast or dog chow diets allow almost all larvae to mature. They are blind and avoid sunlight, keeping to dark places such as sand, cracks and crevices, and bedding.

Pupae

Given an adequate supply of food, larvae pupate and weave silken cocoons within 1–2 weeks after three larval stages. After another week or two, the adult fleas are fully developed and ready to emerge. They may remain resting during this period until they receive a signal that a host is near-vibrations (including sound), heat, and carbon dioxide are all stimuli indicating the probable presence of a host. Fleas are known to overwinter in the larval or pupal stages.

Adult Flea

Once the flea reaches adulthood, its primary goal is to find blood and then to reproduce. Its total life span can be as short as 1 year, but may be several years in ideal conditions. Female fleas can lay 5,000 or more eggs over their life, allowing for phenomenal growth rates, average 30–90 days.

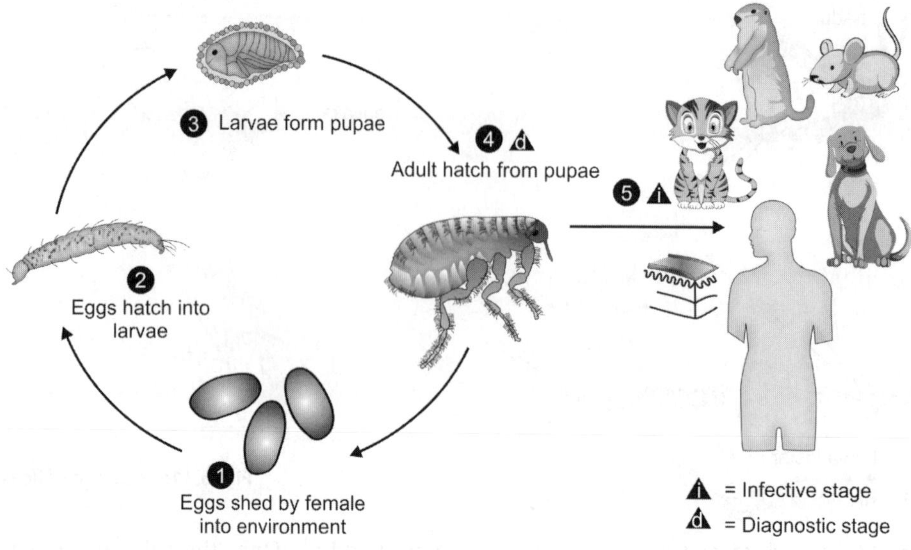

Fig. 6.12: Life cycle of fleas.

A flea might live a year and a half under ideal conditions. These include the right temperature, food supply, and humidity. Generally speaking, an adult flea only lives for 2 or 3 months. Without a host for food a flea's life might be as short as a few days. With ample food supply, the adult flea will often live up to 100 days.

Kinds of Fleas

There are three major kinds of fleas:
1. Rat fleas
2. Dog and cat fleas
3. Human fleas

Fleas are also found in other mammals.

Transmission of Disease

Fleas transmit the disease in the following ways:
- Mechanical transmission
- Biting and through human excreta.

Both male as well as female fleas bite. They spread through grains, cotton, gunny bags (jute), etc.

Fleas and Plague

Rat fleas are responsible for plague. The number of fleas found on rats help in judging their density and spread. This is also known as 'flea index'. Bites of fleas inject the plague bacilli in the body of the prey. Rat fleas are responsible for endemic typhus and bubonic plague while sucking the blood. These deposit the refuse which has the disease-causing bacilli. In such conditions, infection is caused due to scratching of the area bitten by fleas.

Methods of Control

- Rat eradication
- Spraying insecticides (especially in the mice holes)
- Use of flea repellents (such as benzyl benzoate).

BUGS

Bugs are the common problem for the rural as well as urban areas. These are generated mainly due to improper sanitation. They are found in beds and mattresses of homes, bus stations, hospitals, inns, railway stations, dharamshalas, community homes, and old furniture, books, cracks and creeks, and boxes, etc.

Bugs are brown-colored, flat insects. They have three pairs of legs, eyes, two antennae and a head. It has a proboscis-like structure below its head. A bug uses it to suck blood. Bugs are the cause of disturbed sleep, dermatitis, itching, etc. and become a carrier of diseases. Insecticides like DDT, BHC, gammaxene, benzene, etc. are sprayed at their resting and hiding places to control them. Maintaining the sanitation and cleanliness of public and community places and exposing clothes to sunlight from time to time are also essential.

TICKS

Ticks are oval in shape and there is no clear division of their body. Both male and female ticks bite. Their life cycle passes through four stages. These are external parasites of vertebrate animals. They are responsible for the transmission of typhus, encephalitis, hemorrhagic fever and relapsing fever. These can be controlled by maintaining cleanliness, filling cracks and holes and spraying insecticides, like DDT, lindane, etc.

MITES

This is an extremely small round arthropod that lives as a parasite in the human skin. It is known as the 'itch mite'. It lays eggs under the upper layers of skin. When the larvae begin to hatch out of the eggs and crawl on the skin, they produce itching. Scratching leads to bacterial and fungal infections. A person suffering from the itch may transmit it to other people as well.

The four stages in the life cycle of mite are egg, larvae, nymph and adult, which get completed in 10–15 days. A mite lives for 1–2 months.

Mite and Scabies

Scabies is a disease that is produced by mites. Fingers and the place in between the wrist, underarms, hips, lower abdomen, feet and palms are the places where terrible itching is felt, especially in the night. Many family members might be affected by it. In acute cases, papules, boils and lesions might also be present.

Control

- Using insecticides to destroy mites
- Environmental control: This includes filling the cracks of the walls and enhancing the level of cleanliness in the house
- Paying proper attention to personal hygiene
- Using intimate formulations (repellents) on the skin
- The following can also be used for the treatment of scabies: benzyl benzoate 25%, emulsion, sulfur ointment 10%, titmouse and benzene hexachloride
- For effective control of scabies, all the members of the family should be treated together.

RODENTS

Rodents are such a part of human environment which damage the walls of a house, papers, clothes, priceless articles and edible substances. They also pose a threat to the health and are responsible for the transmission of many fetal diseases.

Types of Rodents

- **Domestic rodents:** Black rats, Norway rats and house mice are included in this. Black rats are founding shops and ships. This is a very agile rat.
- **Wild rodents:** There are many species of wild rodents. One of its species named *Tatera indica* is the natural and ample source of epidemic plague in India.

Transmission of Disease

Rodents transmit the disease by:

- Directly baling the human body
- Contaminating food and water, and
- Through rat fleas.

Rodents are responsible for diseases, like plague, typhus, trichinosis, rat-bite fever and amebic dysentery.

Methods of Rodent Control

The following are the important methods of rodent control:

- Maintaining the cleanliness:
  - Foodstuff must be covered
  - Constructions of rat-proof buildings, shops, kitchen, etc.
  - Proper waste disposal
  - Filling the cracks and holes of the walls and floor
  - Roofs should not become their shelters.
- **Trapping:** Rats can be trapped using rat-traps and their numbers can be reduced
- Use of rodenticides or rat poison
- **Other methods:** Cyanogas is pumped into the barrows and holes, etc.

Community Health Nurse and Pest Control

Community health nurse has the following responsibilities related to pest control:

- Informing the society about the diseases and dangers of insects.
- Explaining them the reasons behind the origin of insects/pests and the utility of the methods of controlling them.
- Exhibiting the availability and use of pest control techniques.
- Educating people about pest control and the timely evaluation of techniques used in it.

CHAPTER 7

Maternal and Child Health Care

INTRODUCTION TO THE CONCEPT OF MATERNAL AND CHILD HEALTH CARE

Maternal and child health care (MCH) is a very important component of family welfare services, which not only contributes to improving community health status but also helps in promoting small family norms and population stabilization. The maternal and child health care services are rendered as a comprehensive mother-baby package because mother and baby are one entity. Mother and baby package interventions are strategic interventions and are the pillars of child survival and safe maternal and child health aims to improve the global state of health of women and men looking to have a child. The term 'maternal and child health' refers to the promotive, preventive, curative and rehabilitative health care for mothers and children. It includes the subareas of maternal health, child health, family planning, school health, handicapped children, adolescence and health aspects of care of children in special settings, such as day care. It is a planned examination, observation and guidance given to the pregnant women from conception till the time of labor.

Maternal health is now referred to as 'reproductive health (RH)'. According to the World Health Organization (WHO), it is defined as a state of complete physical, mental and social well-being and not merely the absence of disease or infirmity in all matters relating to the reproductive system and its functions and processes. It implies that people are able to have a satisfying and safe sex life; are informed about and to have access to safe, effective, affordable and acceptable methods of family planning as well as other methods of their choice for the regulation of fertility, which are not against the law; are able to have access to appropriate health care services that will enable women to go safely through pregnancy and childbirth and provide the couples with the best chance of having healthy babies.

MCH care is the health service provided to mothers (women in their child-bearing age) and children. The targets for MCH are all women in their reproductive age groups, i.e., 15–49 years of age, children, school-age population and adolescents.

Burden of Mother and Child

In many countries, mother and children constitute a priority group. In India, women in the child-bearing age (15–44 years) constitute 22.2% and children <15 years of age about 35.3% of the total population. Together they constitute nearly 57.5% of the total population. By virtue of their numbers, mother and children are the major consumers of health services. They not only constitute a large group but also a 'vulnerable' or special risk group. The risk is connected with child-bearing in the case of women; and growth and development and survival in the case of infants and children.

Mother and child must be considered as one unit. It is because, during the antenatal period, the fetus is the part of the mother. The period of development of fetus in the mother is about 280 days. During this period, the fetus obtains all the building material and oxygen from the mother's blood. Child health is closely related to maternal health. A healthy mother brings forth a healthy baby. There is less chance of premature birth, still birth or abortion.

Definition

The term 'maternal and child health' refers to the promotive, preventive, curative and rehabilitative health care for mother and children. It includes the subareas of maternal health, child health, family planning, school health, handicapped children, adolescence, and health aspects of care of children in special settings, such as day care.

Appropriate care during pregnancy, delivery and postnatal period substantially reduces perinatal and neonatal death.

Objectives

- Reduction of maternal, perinatal, infant and childhood mortality and morbidity
- Promotion of reproductive health
- Promotion of the physical and psychological development of the child and adolescent within the family
- Every child receives adequate care and proper nourishment
- Every child is immunized and protected from diseases
- Their growth and development are monitored and deviation is identified and treated on time
- Care is rendered by the trained personnel

- Mother and family members are educated and trained to give proper care to their children to promote their health
- Prevent malnutrition
- Prevent communicable diseases
- Early diagnosis and treatment of the health problems
- Health education and family planning service.

Goals and Strategy

Goals of Maternal Health

- To reduce the risk of death to 1 in 500 or more pregnancies or <2 per 1,000 live births
- To have 100% deliveries conducted by trained personnel
- To have minimum 90% institutional deliveries.

Strategies of Maternal Health Care

The strategies of maternal health care are as follows:

- **Accessibility of maternal health care:** The basic maternal care which includes quality of antenatal care, clean and safe delivery and postpartum care available to all pregnant women.
- Information, education and communication to all women, families and communities regarding:
  - Special needs of pregnant and lactating mothers
  - High-risk factors
  - Signs and symptoms of complications
  - Arrangement for transport during emergency
  - Prepare for confinement
  - Timely referral.
- **Technical competency of healthcare providers:** The health personnel at all levels, i.e., community health center and hospital be knowledgeable, skillful in management of normal pregnancies and deliveries and detection and management of high-risk cases and complications and their timely referral
- Availability of appropriate and well-equipped referral facility at first level, and secondary and tertiary levels
- Availability of transport facility at the village level for transporting and mothers during emergencies
- Monitoring of performance in hospital, primary health center and other health facilities with labor rooms to increase proportion of institutional deliveries
- Improving newborn care.

Targets of Maternal and Child Health Services

According to National Health Policy, 2002, the goals to be achieved by 2015 are:

- Reduced maternal mortality rate—100/1 lakh
- Reduced infant mortality rate—30/1,000
- Death rate of 1 to 4 years old age-group—below 10/1,000
- Size of family—2 to 3 members
- Birth weight of child—minimum 2.5 kg
- Weight of minimum 90% of total children—according to height-weight chart.

Recent Trends in MCH Care

Mother and child care have become the foremost priority of primary health care in every country. This indicates the transformation in thinking about mother and child health care. A description of modern and latest nature of this care is explained below:

- **Integration of care:** Earlier maternal and child health care services were divided into antenatal, child care and family planning. Different agencies were working independently in these areas but, in its present form, all these services are provided at one place in a unified form. Naturally, it is comfortable for the mothers and children and is helpful in increasing the capability and effectiveness of services.
- **Risk approach:** The risk among mothers and infants is identified and special care is given to them immediately. Along with it, the normal group is provided the required maternal and infant health services.
- **Manpower changes:** According to the new concept, maternal and child health services should not be left to traditional health workers (ANM, TBA, health visitors), rather MPW, TBA, Anganwadi workers, ASHA. Specialists of the field and child volunteers (Bal Sevikas) and workers of NGO should also be involved, so that the best-level care and targets and maternal and child health care can be achieved.
- **Primary health care:** Achieving 'health for all' is possible only through primary health care.
  - It makes available the information about protection and resources for mother and child health care.
  - Primary healthcare is family-centered health system; therefore, maternal and child health services are its main and essential constituents.
- **Reproductive and child health:** As per the decision taken in World Women Conference, Beijing (1995), maternal and child health services have been included in reproductive and child health services. In our country, a number of programs and services are underway which are related to MCH care.

Components of MCH Services

Services to the Mother

- Preconception care
- Antenatal care
- Intranatal care
- Postnatal care
- Family planning services.

Services to the Children

- Essential and immediate newborn care
- Care of 'at risk' newborn
- Continuing care of the client
- Care of the toddlers (preschool children)
- Care of school children
- Care of the children of employed mothers

- Care of the handicapped children
- Placement of the children.

PRECONCEPTIONAL CARE

Preconceptional care is the service to the woman before she conceives. Ideally it should start (for a potential mother) much before marriage. The components of preconceptional care are the preventive aspects of antenatal care that are educational, informal and genetic counseling.

Educational: The high school and college girl students are given knowledge about anatomy and physiology of reproductive system, pathology of STDs including HIV/AIDS. They are also given education about planned parenthood, family welfare and mother craft.

Informal: They are informed about the benefits of medical supervision during pregnancy and the facilities available for the same. They are also informed about the Medical Termination of Pregnancy Act (MTP-Act).

Genetic counseling: This means improvement in the genetic constitution in the individual family by counseling the individual or the couple. Here the measures are directed to the individual family level. This is of two types—prospective counseling and retrospective counseling.

1. **Prospective counseling:** This is true prevention. A heterozygous individual with recessive traits should not marry another heterozygous individual. Diseases like thalassemia, sickle cell anemia, G6PD deficiency are prevented.
2. **Retrospective counseling:** This is done, when a hereditary disorder has already occurred in the family. The different methods adopted are contraception, termination of pregnancy, in the event of diagnosing a defective fetus by sonography, sterilization of person with harmful trait, *in vitro* fertilization and embryo transfer, avoiding exposure to X-rays, ionizing radiations, etc., treatment of hemophilia with antihemophilic globulin, etc.

ANTENATAL CARE

Antenatal period starts from the time of conception to the onset of labor. In the rural areas, antenatal care is provided by health worker female.

Objectives

- To promote the health of the mother and to maintain it.
- To protect her health.
- To preserve the physiological aspects of pregnancy.
- To detect the 'high-risk' mothers and to give them special attention.
- To prevent complications of pregnancy.
- To prepare her physically fit and mentally alert to cope up with pregnancy.
- To prepare her for breastfeeding.
- To teach her the mother craft.
- To sensitize her the need of family planning.
- To reduce MMR and IMR.

Goals of Antenatal Care

- To reduce maternal and perinatal mortality and morbidity rates
- To improve the physical and mental health of women and children
- To prepare the woman for labor, lactation, and care of her infant
- To detect early and treat properly complicated conditions that could endanger the life or impair the health of the mother or the fetus
- To prevent, identify, and ameliorate maternal and fetal abnormalities that can adversely affect the pregnancy outcome
- To decrease financial barriers for the care of mothers.

Antenatal Care

- Support and encourage psychological adjustment to pregnancy, childbirth, breastfeeding and parenthood
- Promote awareness of the social and psychological components of child-bearing and their influences on the family
- Monitor the progress of pregnancy to ensure the health and well-being of mother and fetus
- Monitor all women for signs of obstetric difficulties through close personal attention and diagnostic tests, where essential and indicated
- Recognize deviations from the normal, and treat or refer as required
- Recognize that women who develop warning signs may return to normal following treatment and might not necessarily be continued to be regarded or treated as at risk
- Build a trustworthy relationship between the woman and her caregivers
- Provide the woman with information with which she can make suitable decisions
- Actively involve relevant members of the woman's family or friends in the experience of pregnancy, encouraging the supportive role that they might play and recognizing that they too might need support.

Components of Antenatal Care

Components of antenatal care are:
- Antenatal registration and maintenance card
- Antenatal history
- Antenatal examinations
- Antenatal visits
- Antenatal investigations
- Antenatal advice
- Antenatal services.

Antenatal Registration and Maintenance of Antenatal Card

Registration of the mother is done in the antenatal register after confirming the pregnancy clinically in the hospital and after 12 weeks of missing the period in the rural areas by the female health worker. An antenatal card is prepared by writing the registration number, identifying data and details of previous and present history, including family history and chief complaints if any.

Antenatal history, antenatal examination and investigations can be carried during antenatal visit and also antenatal advice can be provided. So it is explained details under antenatal visits.

- **Antenatal services:** These services are rendered by Government of India. These are:
  - *Nutritional services:* Under the National Programme of Integrated Child Development Services Scheme (ICDS) all rural, expectant, malnourished mothers are given a 'supplementary food' daily, which provides 600 kcals of energy including 20 gm of protein to prevent malnutrition in mothers.
- **Immunization services:** Every mother should be immunized against tetanus. First dose should be given to the mother in the first antenatal visit and second dose should be given after 1 month of 1st dose. If she has conceived within the 5 years of previous complete immunization, one booster dose of tetanus is enough. Immunization against erythroblastosis fetalis. If the mother is Rh -ve and the fetus is Rh +ve, mother is given Rh anti-D-immunoglobulin during 28th week and 34th week to prevent erythroblastosis fetalis.
- **Medicinal services:** If the woman is registered within the first trimester of pregnancy, she should be given folic acid supplementation for improving the growth of the fetal neural tissue. It is recommended that the woman be given 5 mg of folic acid once a day, till 12 weeks of pregnancy. After that, she is to be advised a combination of iron and folic acid (IFA). All pregnant women need to be given one tablet of IFA (100 mg elemental iron and 0.5 mg folic acid) every day for at least 100 days, starting after the first trimester at 14–16 weeks of gestation. This is the dose of IFA given to prevent anemia (prophylactic dose). If a woman is anaemic (Hb <11 g/dL) or she has pallor, give her two IFA tablets per day for three months. This means a woman with anemia in pregnancy needs to take at least 200 tablets of IFA. This is the dose of IFA needed to correct anemia (therapeutic dose). Women with severe anemia (Hb <7 g/dL) or those who have breathlessness and tachycardia due to anemia, should be started on the therapeutic dose of IFA and also referred to the MO in the PHC for further management. Anthelmintic drugs should be given once during the second trimester to deworm her.
- **Family welfare services:** If the mother is primigravida, she is sensitized about different contraceptive methods and if she wants to have a second child, she is motivated for spacing with a IUD after delivery.
- **Educational services:** As and when the mother develops any health problems, she is educate about that to take treatment correctly and completely. She is also educated about child rearing practices.

Number and Timing of Visits

It must ensure that every pregnant woman makes at least four visits for antenatal care, including the first visit/registration. These visits recommended only for the pregnancies without complications, studies have shown that additional visits do not improve the maternal or perinatal outcome.

The first visit is recommended as soon as the pregnancy is suspected. This is meant for registration of pregnancy and the first antenatal check-up.

The second visit should be scheduled between the 4th and 6th months (around 26 weeks). The third one should be planned in the 8th month (32 weeks), and the fourth one in the 9th month (36 weeks).

Early Timing of the First Visit/Registration

The first visit or registration of a pregnant woman for ANC should take place as soon as the pregnancy is suspected. Every married woman in the reproductive age-group should be encouraged to visit her health provider or inform you if she believes herself to be pregnant. Ideally, the first visit should take place in the first trimester (first 3 months of pregnancy), before or at the 12th week of pregnancy. However, even if a woman comes late in her pregnancy for registration, she should be registered, and care given to her according to the gestational age.

Importance of Early Registration

Early registration is required to:

- Assess the health status of the mother and to obtain baseline information on blood pressure (BP), weight, etc.
- Screen for complications early and manage them appropriately by referral as and where required.
- Help the woman recall the date of her last menstrual period (LMP).
- Give the woman the first dose of tetanus toxoid injection (Inj. TT) well within time (after 12 weeks of pregnancy). Help the woman access facilities for an early and safe abortion, if she does not want to continue with her pregnancy. Be alert to the possibility that the abortion might be an attempt at female feticide. [Refer to the Government of India (GoI) Ministry of Health and Family Welfare (MoHFW), Guidelines for the Medical Termination of Pregnancy (MTP)]. Build a good rapport with the pregnant woman. You, as the provider of care during pregnancy, must give plenty of time to counsel the woman and her family. Start the woman on a regular dose of folic acid during the first trimester.

Antenatal Visit

- WHO recommends a minimum of four ANC visits. A pregnant woman should visit health center/hospital at care at least 4 times during pregnancy for antenatal check-up. Registration and 1st ANC check-up: As soon as the period is missed or within the first 3 months of the missing period

- 2nd ANC check-up: In the 4th to 6th months of pregnancy
- 3rd ANC check-up: In the 7th to 8th months of pregnancy.
- 4th ANC check-up: In the 9th month of pregnancy.

Activities During the First Antenatal Care Visit

After the diagnosis of pregnancy, the initial assessment interview can establish the trusting relationship between the nurse and the pregnant woman—establishing a rapport, getting information about the woman's physical and psychological health, and obtaining a basis for anticipatory guidance for pregnancy.

History Taking

History-taking includes the following components:

Personal and Social History

This includes the woman's name, age, occupation, address, and phone number, marital status, duration of marriage, religion, nationality and language, housing and finance.

Menstrual History

A compete menstrual history is important to establish the estimated date of delivery. It includes the LMP, age of menarche, regularity and frequency of menstrual cycle, and the contraception method. Any previous treatment of menstrual expected date of delivery (EDD) is calculated as follows: first day of LMP – 3 months + 7 days and change the year. Example: calculate EDD if LMP was August 30, 2007 = June 6, 2008.

Obstetrical History

Obstetrical history includes history of previous pregnancies that may alert the care provider to possible problems in the present pregnancy, which includes gravida, para, abortion, and living children, weight of infant at birth and length of gestation, labor experience, type of delivery, location of birth, and type of anesthesia, maternal or infant complications, previous operations, such as cesarean section and genital repair, and cervical, etc.

History of Present Complaints

Ask the patient if she has any current problems, such as nausea and vomiting, abdominal pain, headache, urinary complaints, vaginal bleeding, edema, backache, heartburn, and constipation.

Medical and Surgical History

Chronic conditions, such as diabetes mellitus, hypertension, and renal disease can affect the outcome of pregnancy and must be investigated.

Family History

Family history provides valuable information about the general health of the family, and it may reveal information about patterns of genetic or congenital anomalies, including DM, hypertension, heart disease, cancer and anemia.

Physical Examination

Physical examination is important to detect the previously undiagnosed physical problems that may affect the pregnancy outcome and to establish baseline levels that will guide the treatment of the expectant mother and fetus throughout pregnancy.

In every antenatal visit, the physical examination should be carried out as follows:

General Examination

It includes general appearance, body-build and gait. Body mechanics and changes in posture and gait should be addressed. Body mechanics during pregnancy may produce strain on the muscles of the lower back and legs. The face is observed for skin color as pallor and pigmentation as chloasma. Observe the eyes for edema of the eyelids and color of conjunctiva. Healthy eyes are bright and clear. Edema of the extremities or face necessitates further assessment for signs of pregnancy-induced hypertension.

Vital Signs

Blood Pressure

It is taken to ascertain normality and provide a baseline reading for a comparison throughout pregnancy. In late pregnancy, raised systolic pressure of 30 mm Hg or raised diastolic pressure of 15 mm Hg above the baseline values on at least two occasions of 6 or more hours apart indicates toxemia.

Pulse

The normal pulse rate is 60–90 BPM. Tachycardia is associated with anxiety, hyperthyroidism, or infection.

Respiratory Rate

The normal respiratory rate is 16–24 BPM. Tachypnea may indicate respiratory infection or cardiac disease.

Temperature

Normal temperature during pregnancy is from 36.2–37.6°C. Increased temperature suggests infection.

Cardiovascular System

Venous congestion can develop into varicosities. It is most commonly noted in the legs, vulva, and rectum, as edema.

Height and Weight

An initial weight is needed to establish a baseline for weight gain throughout pregnancy. Recommendations for weight gain during pregnancy are often made based on the woman's body mass index.

Breast

Assess breast size, symmetry, condition of nipple, and the presence of colostrum.

Gastrointestinal Systems

Mouth

The gum may be red, tender, and edematous as a result of the effects of increased estrogen. Observe the mouth for dryness or cyanosis of the lips, gingivitis of the gums, septic focus or caries of the teeth.

Intestine

Assess for the bowel sound, constipation or diarrhea.

Vaginal Discharge

Ask the woman if she is having any type of vaginal discharge.

Observe the neck for enlarged thyroid gland and scars of the previous operations.

Abdomen

The size of the abdomen is inspected for the height of the fundus, which determines the period of the gestation, multiple pregnancies.

The shape of the abdomen is inspected for fetal lie. The position of the abdomen is longer if the fetal lie is longitudinal as occurring in 99.5% of the cases. The abdomen is lower and broad if the lie is transverse. Fetal movement is inspected as an evidence of fetal life and position. The fetal heartbeat can be heard by stethoscope after the 20th week or doppler after 8th week. Normal fetal heart rate is 120–160 beats/min.

Neurological System

Deep tendon reflexes should be evaluated because hyperreflexia is associated with complications of pregnancy.

Skin

- Pallor of the skin may indicate anemia
- Jaundice may indicate hepatic disease
- Chloasma and linea nigra related to pregnancy
- Striae gravidarum should be noted
- Nail beds should be pink with instant capillary return.

Legs

Legs should be noted for edema.

Following ANC visits: In every antenatal subsequent visit complete physical examination with checking of blood pressure, weight gain to be measure by the health worker. She inquires about physical changes that are related directly to the pregnancy, such as the woman's perception of fetal movement, any exposure to contagious illness, medical treatment and therapy prescribed for nonpregnancy problems since the last visit; tetanus toxoid and other examinations as indicated. The urine examination is necessary for measuring the sugar and albumin levels.

Follow-up

Advise the mother to follow-up according to the schedule of antenatal care that is mentioned before, advise the mother to follow-up immediately if any danger sings appear, describe the importance of follow-up to the mother.

Health Teaching During Pregnancy

Hygiene

Daily wash is necessary all over because it is stimulating, refreshing, and relaxing. Warm shower or sponge bath is better than tub bath. Hot bath should be avoided because it may cause fatigue and fainting. Regular washing of the genital area, axilla, and breast is necessary in case of increased discharge and sweating. Vaginal douches should be avoided except in case of excessive secretion or infection.

Breast Care

Wear firm, supportive bra with wide straps to spread weight across the shoulder. Wash the breasts with clean tap water (no soap, because that could have a drying effect) daily to remove the colostrum and to reduce the risk of infection. It is not recommended to massage the breast. This may stimulate oxytocin hormone secretion and possibly lead to contraction. Advise the woman to be mentally prepared for breastfeeding. Advise the pregnant woman to express colostrum during the last trimester of pregnancy to prevent congestion.

Dental Care

The teeth should be brushed carefully in the morning and after every meal. Encourage the woman to visit her dentist regularly for routine examination and cleaning. Encourage the woman to snack on nutritious foods, such as fresh fruit and vegetables to avoid sugar coming in contact with the teeth. A tooth can be extracted during pregnancy, but local anesthesia is recommended.

Dressing

The woman should avoid wearing tight cloths, such as belt or constriction bands on the legs because these could impede lower extremity circulation. Suggest wearing shoes with a moderate to low heel to minimize pelvic tilt and possible backache. Loose and light clothes are the most comfortable.

Travel

Many women have questions about travel during pregnancy. Early in normal pregnancy, there are no restrictions. Late in pregnancy, travel plans should take into consideration the possibility of early labor. Traveling should be avoided in case of abortion history.

Sexual Activity

Sexual intercourse is allowed with moderation, is absolutely safe and normal unless specific problems exist, such as vaginal bleeding or ruptured membrane. If a woman has a history of abortion, she should avoid sexual intercourse in the early months of pregnancy.

Exercises

Exercises should be simple. Walking is ideal, but long periods of walking should be avoided. The pregnant woman should avoid lifting heavy weights, such as mattresses or furniture, as it may lead to abortion. She should avoid long periods of standing because it predisposes her to varicose veins. She should avoid setting with legs crossed because it will impede circulation. Exercises help in developing a good posture, reducing constipation and insomnia, alleviating uncomfortable, postural backache and fatigue. Ensure good muscle tone and strong pelvic support, developing good breathing habits, ensure good oxygen supply to the fetus, preventing circulatory stasis in the lower extremities, promoting circulation, and lessen the possibility of venous thrombosis. During exercises, jerking or bouncing should always be avoided.

Contraindications

Some of the contraindications of exercises are vaginal bleeding, severe anemia, and history of preterm labor, extreme over- or underweight, hypertension, and heart, lung and thyroid diseases.

Sleep

The pregnant woman should lie down to relax or sleep for 1 or 2 hours during the afternoon. At least 8 hours' sleep should be obtained every night and increased towards term, because the highest level of growth hormone secretion occurs at sleep. Advise the woman to use natural sedatives, such as warm bath and a glass of warm milk. A good sleeping position is Sims' position. This puts the weight of the fetus on the bed, not on the woman, and allows good circulation in the lower extremities. Avoid resting in supine position, as supine hypotension syndrome can develop.

Hazards

The pregnant woman should avoid the following hazards:

- **Occupational hazards:** Lead, mercury, X-rays and ethylene oxide
- **Infection:** Rubella, toxoplasmosis, syphilis
- **Smoking and alcohol** increase risk for pregnancy, prematurity, fetal death, mental retardation and congenital anomalies.
- **Drugs:** As sedative and analysis, anticoagulant, antithyroidism, hormones and antibiotics.

Diet

The daily requirement of nutrients in pregnancy is extra 300 calories, 20 grams protein in addition to more iron and calcium. Women should be advised to eat more vegetables, fruits, proteins, and vitamins and minimize their intake of fats.

Managing the Minor Disorders of Pregnancy

Nausea and Vomiting

Nausea and vomiting generally occur between 4 and 6 weeks of gestation, which may be due to hormonal influences—hCG, progesterone, estrogen; emotional factors like tension, etc. Advise the antenatal mother for adequate rest and relaxation, eating small six meals a day rather than three large meals. Explain them regarding solid food which is tolerated better than liquid food, like crackers or pieces of dry toast, carbohydrate snacks at bedtime can prevent hypoglycemia, which cause nausea and vomiting. Food should not have a strong odor, should not be either very hot or very cold, and fried or greasy foods should be avoided.

Heartburn

Heartburn is a common minor disorder. Progesterone hormone relaxes the cardiac sphincter of the stomach and allows reflex or bubbling back of gastric contents into the esophagus and the pressure of the growing uterus on the stomach from about 30–40 weeks.

The woman should take precautions like avoid lying flat, sleeping with more pillows and lying on the right side, take small frequent meals, take antacids. Taking baking soda in a glass of water is contraindicated because of the possibility of retention of sodium and subsequent edema, avoid fried, spicy, and fatty food and avoid citrus juices, etc.

Backache

Backache may be due to muscular fatigue and strain that accompany poor body balance. It may be due to increased lordosis during pregnancy in an effort to balance the body.

The pregnancy hormones sometimes soften the ligaments to such a degree that some support is needed. Regular exercises like sitting with knees slightly higher than the hips can help.

The pregnant woman should be reassured that once delivery of the baby is done, the ligaments will return to their prepregnant strength.

Urinary Frequency

Urinary frequency may occur due to the pressure of the growing uterus on the bladder. The problem will get resolved when the uterus rises into the abdomen after the 12th week. Kegel exercises are sometimes recommended to help maintain the bladder.

Varicosities

Progesterone relaxes the smooth muscles of the veins and results in sluggish circulation. The valves of the dilated veins become inefficient and varicose veins result. Weight of the uterus partially compresses the veins returning blood from the legs.

For the prevention of this condition, lying flat on the bed with the feet elevated, and moving the legs above is better than standing still can help.

Constipation

Intestinal motility decreases during pregnancy as a result of progesterone and iron supplementation. Management of this condition includes the food to have an ample amount of fruit and green vegetables which contain fibers, drinking a lot of water, exercise and walking. Laxatives could be prescribed by the physicians.

Danger Signs of Pregnancy

The danger signs of pregnancy are:
- Vaginal bleeding including spotting
- Persistent abdominal pain
- Severe and persistent vomiting
- Sudden gush of fluid from vagina
- Absence or decrease in fetal movement
- Severe headache
- Edema of hands, face, legs and feet
- Fever above 100°F (>37.7°C)
- Dizziness, blurred vision, double vision and spots before eyes
- Painful urination.

Risk Approach in Maternal Care

Risk approach is a managerial tool for health services to identify people at risk as early as possible and intervene in order to reduce the risk. The basic concept behind this approach is that all the women in reproductive age-group are vulnerable to disease, death and disability. However, all women are not equally vulnerable and this approach helps to identify mothers who are at a higher risk than others with a lesser risk.

Purpose

The main objective of the at-risk approach is the optimal use of the existing resources for the benefit of the majority. It attempts to ensure a minimum of care for all while providing guidelines for the diversion of limited resources to those who most need them. That means:
- To care for all but to pay special attention to those in greatest need.
- The diversion of limited resources to those who most need them.
- Detection of risk factors requires knowledge of the characteristics associated with poor outcomes and the ability to recognize and measure them.

High-risk Pregnancy

Definition

A pregnancy is defined as high-risk when there is likelihood of an advance outcome to the woman and her baby that is >the incidence than the outcome in general publication.

Identification of High-risk in a Pregnant Woman

One of the main aims of antenatal care is identification of woman at risk and to provide appropriate management. The identification is made from women's history, examinations and investigations carried prior to pregnancy. In practice, identification of risk pregnancy can be carried out in two ways:

General Risk Scoring

According to general risk scoring system the women are classified into different categories for which different and appropriate management system or strategies can be implemented.

Following are the ways of calculating risk:
- The number of risk factors present
- By the asthmatic sum of all factors
- Weighted risk for each individual factors present
- By collecting weighted risk by further mathematical process.

Specific Risk Recognition

In practice, this is by far the most commonly used method of risk recognition. In this, a woman is identified having a risk factor for specific advance outcomes and, as a consequence, she receives additional management to treat the disease.

General Risk Factors

- **Age <18 years (young prime):** There is a grave risk to both mother and child because the teenaged mother (i) is still growing and not adequately equipped to cope with the pregnancy and labor, low birth-weight baby, poor breastfeeding due to incomplete development of breast; (ii) is not psychologically prepared for the responsibilities of marriage, pregnancy and recurring of children; (iii) has increasing nutritional requirement by virtue of her own growth and the growing fetus, thus, has a greater risk for anemia. Domiciliary visit, proper guidance and counseling may be helpful to prevent these problems.
- **Elderly prime, i.e., 30 years and over:** Having the baby in too late in life leads to increased risk of complications in pregnancy and labor, which include: (i) heavy bleeding before and after birth; (ii) malpresentation resulting in difficult labor; (iii) induced aggravated blood pressure; (iv) delay in explosion of placenta; (v) low birthweight baby; (vi) Forceps delivery or cesarean operation; (vii) chromosomal abnormalities. Regular vigilance for the raised blood pressure and fetal assessment is very essential.
- **Parity >4 (having >four pregnancies):** Due to repeated pregnancy, the problems include malnutrition, antepartum and postpartum hemorrhages; (iii) difficult and obstructed labor resulting in perineal tear and uterine rupture; (iv) prolapsed uterus; (v) stillbirth; (vi) neonatal death; (vii) premature delivery; (viii) low birthweight baby, etc. This is due to weakening of tissues, depletion of nutrients and overall physical health of the mother.

Table 7.1: Risk factors management by past obstetric history.

Risk factors	*Nature*	*Management*
Previous history of ectopic pregnancy	Chance of recurrence of maternal anxiety	Early USG to confirm abnormalities
Previous stillbirth or neonatal death	Risk depends on causes, not all recurrent	Try and find out the cause, and establish management according to the cause
Previous congenital anomalies	Possible recurrence	Prenatal detailed diagnosis as early as possible. Proper counseling
Baby weight is –2 SD (–2 SD is two standard less than normal deviation)	IUGR	Grade-II fetal check
Baby weight +2 SD (+2 SD is more than two standard deviations)	Gestational diabetes	May be diabetes mellitus. Random glucose should behave in 28–32 weeks
Antibodies	Hemolytic disease	Specific protocol. Assess renal functions, blood pressure and grade II fetal check
Proteinuria (PET)	Recurrence	Assess renal function, BP, grade-II fetal check—specific plan depending on the case
Preterm delivery	Recurrence	Careful observation for pain—advice for bed rest
Uterine scar	Uterine rupture/previous cesarean section	Review of mode of delivery at 36 weeks
Short labor	Recurrence and neonatal risk	Specific management plan at 36 weeks
PPH	Recurrence	Specific plan at 36 weeks
Problem with baby	Recurrence and maternal anxiety	Obtain detailed and specific plan

- **Having too close pregnancies:** When the interval between the two pregnancies is <three years, it can create problems during pregnancy. It is because the mother did not get enough time to recover completely or fully from the stress and strain of the previous pregnancies. She also suffers from nutritional deficiency anemia, and low birth weight baby. Other children in the family get neglected as the mother cannot give attention to them.
- **Non-caucasian:** It denotes a race which indicates the black or dark skin race. These people having seen the risk of hemoglobinopathy (i.e., the risk of a group of inherited diseases including thalassemia and sickle cell diseases) or Africans are suspected to be infected with HIV. So, investigations should be done properly.
- **Single parent (financial and social):** This is also a general factor. If one parent is absent (maybe he or she is dead or divorced), there may be poor antenatal attendance due to lack of education. So, domiciliary visits are needed. If necessary, discuss the plan for labor and delivery, and consider engaging into other social works as well.

Specific Risk Factors Management by Past Obstetric History

See **Table 7.1**.

Risk Factors (Past Medical Surgical History)

Risk factors	*Nature*	*Management*
Smoker	IUGR	Advise to reduce and stop smoking; Grade-I fetal check
Excess alcohol	IUGR, fetal alcohol syndrome	Grade-II fetal check—alert the pediatrician
Chronic disease and the prescribed drugs	Possible adverse effect of disease on pregnancy	Obstetrician and pediatrician
Hemoglobin-opathy	Sickle or thalassemia traits, have risk or affected fetus. Sickle disease: (i) IUGR; (ii) IUGR	Test partner should offer prenatal diagnosis. Encourage hydration. Check renal function regulation test of midstream urine
Drug abuse	IUGR, neonatal withdrawal	Serological testing, Grade-II fetal check
Anesthetic problem, A-H diabetes	Recurrence	Alert the pediatrician, consult an anesthetician, random glucose at 28 and 32 weeks
FH congenital anomaly	Possible recurrence	Obtain detailed diagnosis
Subfertility	Anxiety, multiple pregnancy, hypertension or gestational diabetes	Reassure vigilance for hypertension

Schematic risk factors from examination see **Table 7.2.** Schematic risk factor arising in pregnancy see **Table 7.3.**

NATAL CARE

Concept

Natal care refers to care during confinement/delivery/birth of a child. The birth of a child is a normal physiological process but, at any time, any difficulty may arise and complications can occur. About 1% of deliveries tend to be abnormal and another 4% tend to be difficult.

Table 7.2: Schematic risk factors from examination.

Risk factors	*Nature*	*Management*
Weight >85 kg	Hypertension, gestational diabetes	Vigilance advised for raised blood pressure, random glucose at 28–32 weeks
Weight <45 kg	IUGR	Grade-I fetal check
Primigravida and height <152 cm	Cephalopelvic disproportion	Plan for labor if fetal head unengaged at 40 weeks
Cardiac murmur	A symptomatic heart disease	Consider cardiological opinion

Table 7.3: Schematic risk factor arising in pregnancy.

Risk factors	*Nature*	*Management*
Vaginal bleeding	<20 weeks' miscarriage	Acute referral to hospital, early hospitalization and complete rest
BP >140/90	Preeclampsia IUGR	IP BP >160/100 and proteinuria, hospital admission and care using preagreed protocol
Multiple pregnancy	Anemia, hypertension, IUGR, preterm delivery, congenital abnormalities	Iron/folate supplement, vigilance for raised blood pressure, preterm uterine activity, Grade-II fetal check, more frequent visits
SDF	IUGR	Fetal assessment using preagreed protocol
LFD	Big baby and compilations, gestational diabetes, hydramnios, multiple pregnancy	Fetal assessment using preagreed protocol, random glucose
Polyhydramnios	Big baby and compilations, abnormal fetus	Fetal assessment using preagreed protocol, random glucose
Malpresentation after 35 weeks	Delivery problem	Look for cause and make plan for labor
Reduce fetal movement	Poor maternal perception, fetal disease	Immediate nonstress test and fetal assessment
Preterm ROM	Preterm labor amnionitis, pyelonephritis	Hospital admission and, managed with protocols, treat (5 days) monthly midstream urinal

Objectives

- To prevent infection
- To prevent injury to both mother and baby
- To detect and deal with any complications
- To resuscitate the baby and to provide immediate care to it.

General Principles

- The deliveries must be conducted by trained and skillful health personnel under clean surroundings by clean and correct method.
- The use of five cleans is advocated. It includes the use of clean hands with clean finger nails, clean surface and surroundings, clean blade, clean cord-tie. Keeping the birth canal clean by avoiding unsafe practices, clean cutting of cord and its care.
- The cord should be ligated at two places 6 cm and 9 cm from the umbilicus and cut between these two points.
- Family should not be allowed to apply any ointment, oil, ash or cow dung on the cord since such practices are dangerous and may cause tetanus infection.

Conditions for Referrals

The trained dais and health workers (females) should be watchful to identify any problem and emergency and must refer the mother to the first referral unit (FRU) hospital immediately to avail timely medical help when necessary. The mother should be watched for the following symptoms/conditions during labor:

- Prolonged labor beyond 12 hours with not much progress
- Continuous and excessive bleeding during the process of delivery
- Fits and unconsciousness
- High fever or dehydration
- Malpresentation
- Difficulty in breathing or in passing urine, etc.
- Sluggish or no pains after rupture of membranes
- Good pains for an hour or so after rupture of membranes but with no progress
- Meconium-stained liquor or slow (<120/m), irregular or excessive (>160/m) fetal heart rate
- Nonseparation of placenta within half-an-hour of childbirth
- Incomplete separation of placenta
- Postpartum hemorrhage or collapse.

These deliveries can be conducted at home and in the health institutions. All high-risk mothers and where home conditions are not safe should be delivered in the health centers and hospitals. The ratio may vary in different states, e.g., 90% of the deliveries in Kerala are conducted in health institutions, while in most of the northern states, majority of the deliveries are conducted at home.

POSTNATAL CARE

Concepts and Objectives

It refers to care which is rendered to both mother and baby after delivery. It starts soon after birth of baby and continues for 6 weeks. The first 48 hours following delivery are the most critical in the entire postpartum period. Most of the important complications of the postpartum period, which can lead to maternal death, occur during these 48 hours. Hence, a woman who has just delivered needs to be closely monitored during the first 48 hours. The next most critical period is the first week following the delivery. A substantial number of complications can occur during this period, both for the mother as well as for the baby. Hence, another visit has to be paid to the mother (and the baby) in the first 7–10 days. The objectives of postnatal care are:

- To restore, promote and maintain health of the mother and baby
- To promote breastfeeding
- To prevent complications
- To establish good nutrition for the baby
- To prevent infection and identify any health problem/ disorder in the baby
- To support and strengthen the parents' confidence, and their role within their family and cultural environment.
- To motivate for planned and small family norms
- To educate mother and family on various aspects of mother and child care.

Immediate Care of a Newborn

Care of the baby soon after birth is very important. The aim of immediate care is to help the newborn baby to adjust to the new environment, which is quite harsh for the baby. The objectives of the care are:

- To establish and maintain breathing of the baby (i.e., cardiopulmonary function)
- To maintain body temperature
- To prevent infections
- To detect any congenital abnormalities.

Cleaning of the Airway

Immediately after birth, the baby should cry and breathe. If the baby is crying and the breathing is normal, then there is no need for resuscitation. In order to promote breathing, the airway needs to be cleared of mucus and any other secretions. The secretions can be drained by lowering the head and gentle patting at the back. If necessary, gentle suction of mucus should be done. If the baby does not cry and breathe within a minute, resuscitation must be done using various alternative measures, such as suction, ventilation by mouth-to-mouth breathing or bag and mask administration of oxygen, etc. Resuscitation is required in babies who are subjected to hypoxia in labor.

Maintenance of Body Temperature

As soon as the baby is born, he is exposed to an environment which is colder in winter and hotter in summer. The newborn baby has the risk of hypothermia or hyperthermia because of immature heat-regulating system. The hypothermia also results because of evaporation of amniotic fluid from the body surface. The mortality rate in hypothermic babies is twice high as that of babies without hypothermia.

The risk of hypothermia is greatly reduced by placing the baby near a source of warmth after immediately and carefully dried with towel or clean cloth, wrapped in a clean cloth, kept close to the mother for skin-to-skin contact and breastfed as soon as possible, preferably within an hour of birth. A normal baby, who is crying well after birth, can be placed in skin-to-skin contact with the mother's abdomen and covered with a dry cloth. The maternal body heat will provide the extra warmth required. It is also an additional assurance to the mother of the baby's well-being. In case of severe hypothermia, the child should be referred immediately to the FRU/hospital, as the case may be. In any case, the child should be protected from draughts. Extra care must be taken for preterm/low birthweight babies. In a PHC setting, additional heat can be provided by placing the baby under a source of heat, such as a lamp with a 200-watt bulb or under a radiant warmer.

Ensure that during and after the delivery, no fans are running in the delivery room, and no windows are open through which air currents blow into the room.

Care of the Eyes

It is very important to take care of the eyes as the child is born to prevent ophthalmia neonatorum due to variety of infections especially, Neisseria gonorrhoeae, and chlamydia trachomatis in mothers. Ophthalmia neonatorum can cause severe disability.

The care of eyes includes wiping of each eye from inside to outside with boiled and then cooled swabs, one for each eye as the child is born before he opens the eyes. A single application of either 1% freshly prepared silver nitrate or 1% tetracycline ointment is applied within 1 hour of delivery. Also treat the mother and her husband for gonorrhea. The eyes should be cleaned at birth and once everyday using sterile cotton swabs soaked in sterile water or normal saline. Each eye should be cleaned using a separate swab.

Care of the Umbilical Cord

The umbilical cord should be cut after it stops pulsating so that the child has the benefit of getting blood. The cord should be ligated in two places, 6 cm and 9 cm from the umbilicus and cut in between with sterilized scissors/ blade and tied with sterilized cord to prevent from tetanus. Nothing needs to be applied to the cord. The cord should be kept dry. Special instructions should be given to the mother and family not to apply anything, e.g., any oil, ash or cow dung on the cord. Such customs increase the danger of the tetanus infection. The mother should be instructed to prevent the cord from getting soiled with the newborn's urine or feces.

The cord dries, shrinks and falls off within 5–8 days by aseptic necrosis.

APGAR Scoring

APGAR scoring is a device to monitor the physical condition of the baby. It is determined by immediate observation of the heart rate, respiration, muscle tone, reflex response and color of the infant. Graded score is given to each of the signs on three-point scale. The observation is done at 1 minute and again at 5 minutes after birth.

A total score ranges from 0–10. A score ranging from 0–3 indicates severe depression, from 4 to 6 mild depression and from 7–10 no depression. A score below 6 needs immediate care. Low APGAR score at 5 minutes after birth is a very serious indicator. The baby can develop complications and has high-risk of mortality during the neonatal period.

Care of the Skin

The care of the skin is very important to protect the child from any infection and keep the baby clean and warm. The vernix on the baby's body is protective in nature. Therefore, if culturally acceptable, the bathing soon after can be postponed for 12–24 hours after birth. Some people may like to apply oil before giving bath to the baby. The bath is given by the trained birth attendant/health worker (female) or a nurse depending upon the situation. The bath is given with soap and warm water to remove the vernix, meconium and blood clots, etc. In winters, the repeat bath can be postponed by 2–3 days.

Physical Examination

The immediate physical examination of the baby should be done by health worker assisting mother in delivery soon after the birth to identify any birth injury, malformations and general health condition of the baby. It includes:

- Observation of skin for cyanosis, pallor, jaundice and skin lesions.
- Observation of respiratory and heart rate, muscle tone, crying and other movements.
- Observation of any deformity, like harelip, cleft palate, imperforated anus, deformity of joints, etc.
- Observation of signs of cerebral irritation, such as twitching, convulsion, rigidity of neck and bulging of anterior fontanel.
- Observation of weight, height, circumference of head and thorax and temperature. Observation of any of the abnormalities made should be reported for immediate action.

High-risk factors which require urgent medical help are:

- Noisy and difficult breathing
- Cyanosis
- Birth injuries
- Imperforated anus
- Hypothermic or hyperthermal babies
- Persisting vomiting or diarrhea
- Twitching, convulsions, neck rigidity and difficulty in sucking.

Further detailed examination of the baby must be done by the pediatrician within 24 hours of birth. This examination would form the basis for continual healthcare to baby.

Breastfeeding

The breastfeeding should be started as soon as possible, preferably within an hour of birth. This helps in mother-child bonding and in establishing feeding. The colostrum, which is secreted out for a few days, is rich in protein, other nutrients and anti-infective factors. The breastfeed during this period provides good nourishment, and immunity against infections. The baby should be fed on demand. Bottle feeding should not be done as it is neither required nor safe for the baby. Strict instructions should be given to the mother and family.

Immediate Care of the Mother

After the baby is born and the placenta is delivered, it is very important that the mother is made comfortable and watched for any complications.

- The fundus is palpated, clots are expressed, and fundal height is measured
- The perineum is inspected for any laceration or tear, perineal care is given, napkin fixed
- Mother is made comfortable by removing the soiled linen, thorough cleaning and by keeping her warm, etc.
- Hot drink is given thereafter
- The vital signs are recorded.

The following instructions are given to the mother and family regarding mother; to take rest, to watch for bleeding, to maintain perineal hygiene, to take normal diet, to report in case there is any problem regarding baby; to let the baby sleep and handle as little as possible; watch for bleeding from the cord; to breastfeed the child, not to give anything else, even water, not to apply anything on the cord, and to report, in case there is any problem.

Postnatal Visits and Care

It is very important to give regular and frequent visits to postnatal mother when the delivery is conducted at home. Ideally, she should be visited twice a day for the first 3 days, thereafter once a day in the morning till the cord is off; after that, every alternate day till the 10th day, thereafter once in a week till 42 weeks. The last visit is done by the mother along with the baby in the postnatal clinic.

But this schedule of postnatal visit is not feasible. The health worker is expected to follow the undermentioned schedule:

- **1st visit:** Within 24 hours (on the second day if delivery was conducted by her)
- **2nd visit:** 5th or 6th day
- **3rd visit:** 10th day
- **4th visit:** 2nd–4th week
- **5th visit:** 6th–8th week (this visit is done in the clinic).

During these visits, both mother and baby are given care to meet their basic health needs.

When delivery is conducted in maternity home, a health center or hospital, ideally the discharge should be given after 5th day of delivery. Usually, the discharge is given within 24–72 hours. In any case, the mother and the baby require care and supervision of the health personnel. They should be given follow-up care on the similar schedule as mentioned above by the community health agency.

Care of the Mother

During each visit, the following actions are generally performed:

- General observation of the mother and the surroundings to assess the overall apparent health status of the mother, cleanliness, orderliness, etc.
- Observation of temperature, pulse rate, respiratory rate
- Examination of breasts, involution of uterus, lochia, perineum for any kind of abnormality
- Inquiring about micturition and bowel movements and any other problem, such as excessive bleeding, pain in the legs, etc.
- Observation of any abnormality in the abdomen, like painful and hard abdomen.

All these observations are done to detect any abnormality or any early indication of puerperal sepsis (infection of the genital tract) and be able to take appropriate action on time.

It should be seen that the mother:

- Takes adequate nutritious diet with plenty of proteins, including milk, legumes, green vegetables and fresh fruits. The total calories should be 2,500 to meet the energy requirements of lactation.
- Takes sufficient rest and sleep than usual to regain her normal health.
- Does the desired exercises to regain muscle tone of abdomen and pelvis, gets out of bed within 24 hours and gradually resumes her household responsibilities.
- Gets support of her husband and family in taking care of herself and her baby so that she feels physically, mentally and emotionally secure.
- Breastfeeds her baby as breast milk is the most safe, convenient and nutritious food for the baby.

The mother should be advised to:

- Use clean cloth or pad after cleaning the private parts with clean water and drying. The cloth or pad should be regularly changed to avoid infection.
- Take sufficient rest, sleep, and do the desired postnatal exercises.
- Take full diet with plenty of proteins, including milk, green vegetables and fresh fruits.
- Breastfeed the child on demand, and avoid giving bottle feed.
- Maintain personal hygiene and cleanliness of her surroundings.
- Follow small family norms. She should be motivated for spacing or limiting the size of family according to her family planning needs.
- Report any untoward signs and symptoms about herself, e.g., fever, unhealthy lochia, abdominal tenderness, painful legs, etc., and about her baby, e.g., fever, difficulty in breathing, yellowness, rejecting breastfeeds, convulsion, stiffness, loose watery stools and vomiting.
- Come for health checkup for herself and for her baby after 6 weeks.

Complications of the Postpartum Period

In India, most of the deliveries take place at home under unhygienic environment and mostly by untrained dais lacking the required obstetrics skill. Often various health hazards result in, such as perineal tears, cervical damage, prolapse and displacement of uterus, fetal distress, postpartum hemorrhage, etc. Thus, it is very important to have properly trained, skillful and qualified health workers, adequate facilities and well-linked referral units where skillful and efficient emergency care can be given to save the mother and baby.

Puerperal Sepsis

Puerperal sepsis is the infection of genital tract mainly due to infection during labor and after delivery, which may occur within 3 weeks after delivery. This can occur when preventive measures, like maintenance of personal hygiene, sanitary conditions, aseptic procedures, etc. for infection control are not followed before, during and after delivery. The clinical signs and symptoms which need to be monitored are—rise in temperature and pulse rate, pain and tenderness in lower abdomen and foul-smelling lochia. This may lead to inflammation of ovaries, fallopian tubes, endometrium, cervix and vagina. Many a times, leucorrhea may persist for years. Sometimes secondary sterility may follow after acute or chronic salinities. Chronic infection of cervix may predispose to cancer of the cervix. It requires proper preparation for confinement by the mother, conduct of deliveries by trained and skillful dais, midwives, etc. and the availability of equipment and supplies, etc.

Secondary Hemorrhage

This refers to bleeding per vagina, which occurs any time from 6 hours after delivery till the end of the puerperium. It may be due to retained placenta or its membranes.

Thrombophlebitis

This refers to infection of veins of legs. Often it is associated with varicose veins. There is tenderness and swelling on the leg and it looks pale.

Other Complications

These are mastitis and urinary tract infection.

Care of the Newborn During Each Postnatal Visit

During each postnatal visit, the following actions are generally performed to take care of the newborn baby.

- General observations of the following actions are generally performed to take care of the newborn baby
- Observation of temperature, pulse and respiration
- Observation of the eyes for any kind of abnormality, such as watering of eyes, soreness or any discharge, etc.
- Observation of the skin for change in color, generalized erythema or any lesion, etc.
- Observation of muscle tone, tendon reflexes, cries, etc.
- Observation of any sign of abnormality of abdomen, such as distension, tenderness, etc.
- Observation of the cord stump and the skin around the base. It should be seen that the cord is kept clean and dry and, if necessary, care of the cord is done

- The weight is checked and recorded
- It should be seen that the baby is:
  - Adequately clothed, kept clean, and protected from draughts.
  - Breastfed as and when the child cries (e.g., on demand) unless contra indicated.
  - Not given bottle feeds, water or anything else.
  - Allowed to sleep and rest most of the time and handled only when necessary.
- Mother should be enquired about any problem/complaint regarding baby.

Proper care of the newborn baby during postnatal period is very important to prevent neonatal deaths. About 50–60% of all infant deaths occur during the first month of life. Of these, >50% deaths occur during the first week of birth. The risk of deaths is the highest within 24–48 hours of the birth of the baby. The risk of neonatal deaths is found to be more in poor socioeconomic conditions and in the areas where maternal and child care facilities are inadequate and ineffective. It is, therefore, very important that the services of the trained personnel and support services are available for effective management of maternal and child health services to prevent maternal mortality, morbidity and perinatal and neonatal mortality and morbidity.

TERM, SMALL FOR GESTATIONAL AGE AND PRETERM, LARGE-FOR-DATE

Introduction

The newborn requires thorough skilled observation to ensure a satisfactory adjustment to extrauterine life. By through assessment, we can identify any abnormalities. We can identify term, preterm and post-term babies.

Definitions

- **Term:** The babies with gestational age between (37–41) weeks are called term babies (259–293) days.
- **Preterm (immature, born early, premature):** Preterm is defined as a baby with a gestation of <37 completed weeks (up to 36 weeks <259 days) are called preterm babies.
- **Post-term:** Babies with gestational age of 42 weeks or more are classified as post-term babies (294 days or more).
- **Small for dates (SFD):** These babies are small-for-gestational age light-for-dates, intrauterine growth retardation. Babies with a birth weight of <10th percentile for their gestational age are designated as SFD babies.
- **Appropriate for dates (babies appropriate for gestational age):** Babies with a birth weight between 10th and 90th percentile for the period of gestation.
- **Large for date (babies large for gestational age and heavy-for-date):** Babies with birthweight of >90th percentile for their gestational age. The babies >97 percentile for their gestation are considered high-risk and monitored for hypoglycemia. The term, preterm or post-term babies can be identified by assessment of gestational age.

Assessment of Gestation after Birth

The clinical assessment of gestation at birth by physical and neurological examinations of the baby is more reliable as compared to the method recommended for assessment of the baby in utero. As the gestation proceeds, the baby grows and matures physically and neurologically. The anthropometric measurements, such as weight, length, head and chest circumference are unreliable parameters of maturity because they may be adversely offered by IUGR. Head circumference and length are relatively spreading baby with intrauterine malnutrition as compared to weight and chest circumference.

Grouping the Baby into Preterm and Term (Physical)

Sole Creases

- **Preterm baby:** Single deep creases over anterior one-third of baby; no other deep crisis. The sole may be full of superficial crises.
- **Term babies:** So many deep sole crises.
- **Genitals:** In male babies, both the testes are at or above the external ring and scrotums are small with scanty rugosities. In girls, labia majora are widely separated with labia minora fully exposed and clitoris hypertrophied in term.
- **Breast nodules:** Breast nodules are <5 mm and nipples are small or absent. In small-for-dates babies, breast tissue may be definite or absent even when they are gestationally fully mature.
- **Ear cartilage:** Cartilage may be absent or deficient at places on folding the external ear. The recoil may be poor.
- **Hair:** Brownish, black, fussy or woolly in appearance with no difficulty identifying the individual hair fibers.

Depending on the degree of immaturity, the preterm babies may have shiny and oily plethoric skin, plenty of lanugos and edema. Neurologically, they are fewer less alert. Hypotonic and various neonatal reflexes and may be absent or incomplete. The neurological assessment is based on four fundamental observations.

Neurological Assessment

Muscle Tone

It progressively increases in utero as maturity proceeds. The tone in the newborn baby must be assessed by the following three parameters:

1. Posture or attitude
2. Passive tone (popliteal angle and scarf sign)
3. Active tone (traction response and recoil).

Joint Mobility

The degree of flexion at ankle and wrist (square window) is limited in preterm babies because of greater stiffness of joints in early gestation. As the term approaches, the joints become more flexible and relaxed to allow for easy molding during delivery.

Automatic Reflexes

A number of automatic reflexes appear at various specific ages of gestational maturity. More reflexes appear as early as 20–30 weeks but lack complete adduction phase till 38 weeks of gestation. Pupillary response to light is present after 30 weeks and infant may turn his head towards diffuse light during 32–36 weeks. Blink responses to glabellar tap may appear as early as 29 weeks; grasp response—30 weeks; rooting and coordinated sucking—34 weeks; strong grasp—36 weeks.

Fundus Examination

The disappearance of the anterior vascular capsule of the lens has been used to assess the gestational age. The anterior capsule of the lens has been used to assess the gestation by completely vascularized for the infant having <28 weeks. After 34 weeks of maturity, anterior capsular vessels are almost completely atrophied. Ophthalmic examination is, however, technically cumbersome in the newborn.

Physical assessment and neurological assessment are given clearly in **Tables 7.4 to 7.7 and Figure 7.1**.

Small-for-date Babies

These are classified as follows:

Malnourished Small-for-date (IUGR)

The fetus gets malnourished during later part of gestation due to placental dysfunction and appears long, thin and marasmic head circumference and brain weight are unaffected or minimal reduction, whereas other internal organs are grassy and shrunken. Head circumference is generally >3 cm bigger than chest circumference. Double skinfold thickness reduces.

Ponderal index (PI) = Weighing (long-thin cm) 3 × 1,000
Usually, it is <2 compare AGA infant

Here growth retardation is due to reduction of growth of size of cells. Number of cells are unaffected. Good nutrition can replace the actual growth.

Table 7.4: Scoring system for assessing prematurity.

Criteria	*0*	*1*	*2*	*3*
Skin texture (by inspection and pinching)	Very thin and glutinous	Smooth, medium, thickness with superficial peeling	Thick with peeling and cracking over hand and foot	
Lanugo examination of the back	Nil or scanty	Abdominal lanugo	Thinning lanugo at places	Scanty lanugo with areas of baldness
Plantar creases (assess after stretching the skin)	Nil	Faint red mark over anterior half of the sole	Deep indentation over anterior 1/3–1/2 of sale	Deep indentation throughout the sole
Breast nodule	Nil	Breast tissue <5 mm on both sides	Breast tissue 5–10 mm	>10 mm
Ear firmness	Pinna soft and easily folded, no recoil	Soft but some recoil is present	Some cartilage felt along the edge and recoil is instant	Pinna firm with definite cartilage throughout and instant recoil
Male genitalia	Neither testis is in the scrotum	At least one testis is in the inguinal canal and can be pulled down to the scrotum	At least one testis is present in the scrotum	
Female genitalia	Labia majora widely separated	Labia majora partly covers the labia minora	Labia majora completely covers the labia minora	
Neurological assessment: Posture (observe with infant when quiet and when in supine position)	Arms and legs extended	Beginning of flexion of hips and arms extended	Stronger flexion of legs and some flexion of arms	Legs flexed and ablated while arms incompletely flexed
Arm recoil in a supine infant. The flexed forearm is extended by pulling its hands and then released	No recoil or only random movements	Arms return to incomplete flexion or slug response	Arms briskly return to full flexion	
Popliteal angle with infant in supine position; the thigh is held with knee-chest position by support in left hand and extended with right hand	180°	180–150	150–120	<120
Head and legs: With supine position, the baby is grasped and slowly pulled towards the shifting position. The position of head is observed in relation to trunk	Completely head-leg position	Partial head control	Able to maintain head in line with the body	
Glabellar tap: Tap sharply at the glabella (mid-point between eyes) and look for clear view of the eyes	Absent	Weak response	Brisk response	

Table 7.5: Relationship between combined score and gestational age.

Combined total score	*Gestation (weeks)*
9	28
10	29
11	30
12	31
13	32
15	33
16	34
17	36
18	35
19	36
20	37
21	–
22	38
23	–
24	–
25	39
26	40

Hypoplastic Small-for-date (Symmetric IUGR)

Intrauterine infections and certain genetic chromosomal disorders exert their advanced influence from early embryonic life and result in reduced growth potential of the fetus. The baby is proportionately small in all parameters, including the size. Ponderal index is >2 here.

Mixed Small-for-date Babies

They are the outcomes of advance intrauterine environmental influences operating from early or mid-pregnancy. These infants, though small for the period of their gestation, neither look obviously malnourished nor grossly hypoplastic. They show varying degrees of reduction in cell population and size. The constitutionally small babies of small mothers also fall under this category.

Common Determinants of IUGR

Maternal Correlates

- **Socioeconomic status**
  - *Racial and ethnic differences:* There is some evidence to suggest that there is genetic or constitutional predisposition for giving birth to LBW babies. In USA, the Caucasian child at birth weights >the child of the Negroid
- Previous history of spontaneous abortion, stillbirth or neonatal deaths is an important factor for the delivery of LBW baby
- **Antenatal care:** According to quality of antenatal care, the baby is born
- **Nutritional factors:**
  - Mother's height <145 cm
  - Prepregnancy weight <40 kg
  - Relative weight gain <7 kg
  - Energy and protein intake
  - Role of micronutrients.
- Placental dysfunctions and disorders
- Chronic systemic diseases
- Maternal infectious
- Maternal substance abuse
- Environmental pollutants.

Fetal Conditions

- Sex
- Chromosomal disorders
- Intrauterine infections.

Table 7.6: Ballard scoring system for assessment of gestation by assessing physical maturity.

Physical maturity of the ballard maturational assessment of gestational age

	–1	*0*	*1*	*2*	*3*	*4*	*5*
Skin	Sticky, friable, transparent	Gelatinous, red, translucent	Smooth pink, visible veins	Superficial peeling and/or rash, few veins	Cracking, pale areas, rare veins	Parchment, deep cracking, no vessels	Leathery, cracked, wrinkled
Lanugo	None	Sparse	Abundant	Thinning	Bald areas	Mostly bald	Sparse
Plantar surface	Heel-toe 40–50 mm: –1 <40 mm: –2	>50 mm no crease	Faint red marks	Anterior transverse crease only	Creases over anterior 2/3 of sole	Creases over entire sole	
Breast	Imperceptible	Barely perceptible	Flat areola no bud	Stippled areola 1–2 mm bud	Raised areola 3–4 mm bud	Full areola 5–10 mm bud	
Eye and ear	Lids fused Loosely: –1 Tightly: –2	Lids open pinna flat stays folded	Sl. curved pinna soft; slow recoil	Well-curved pinna soft but ready recoil	Formed and firm instant recoil	Thick cartilage ear stiff	
Genitals (male)	Scrotum flat, smooth	Scrotum empty, faint rugae	Testes in upper canal, rare rugae	Testes descending, few rugae	Testes down, good rugae	Testes pendulous, deep rugae	
Genitals (female)	Clitoris prominent and labia flat	Prominent clitoris and small labia minora	Prominent clitoris and enlarging minora	Majora and minora equally prominent	Majora large, minora small	Majora cover clitoris and minora	

Table 7.7: Maturity rating table.

Total score (Neuromuscular + Physical)	*Weeks*
–10	20
–5	22
0	24
5	26
10	28
15	30
20	32
25	34
30	36
35	38
40	40
45	42
50	44

Large-for-dates Babies

These babies need to be observed closely as they have a higher neonatal mortality as compared to the normally grown babies of identical gestation. The criteria for diagnosis include a birth weight of >90th percentile for the period of gestation.

Causes

- Genetic or constitutional
- Maternal diabetes mellitus and prediabetes
- Transposition of great vessels
- Hydrops fetalis
- Cretinism—weight is higher due to hyperthyroidism.

Skeletal Maturation

It causes administration of progesterone during pregnancy, and congenital adrenal hyperplasia.

Types

- **Wiedemann-Beckwith syndrome:** These babies have characteristic grooves into earlobes, macroglossia, exomphalos, visceromegaly and somatic overgrowth. They are prone to develop hypoglycemia due to hyperplasia of islet cells. Hypospadias, cleft palate, coloboma of the iris and capillary hemangioma may be associated. There is higher incidence of mental sequelae during childhood. In some patients, duplication of chromosome 11 has been demonstrated on karyotyping studies with banding technique.
- **Marshall-Smith syndrome:** The craniofacial characteristics include broad forehead with hypertelorism, micrognathia, long philtrum and mild microstomia.

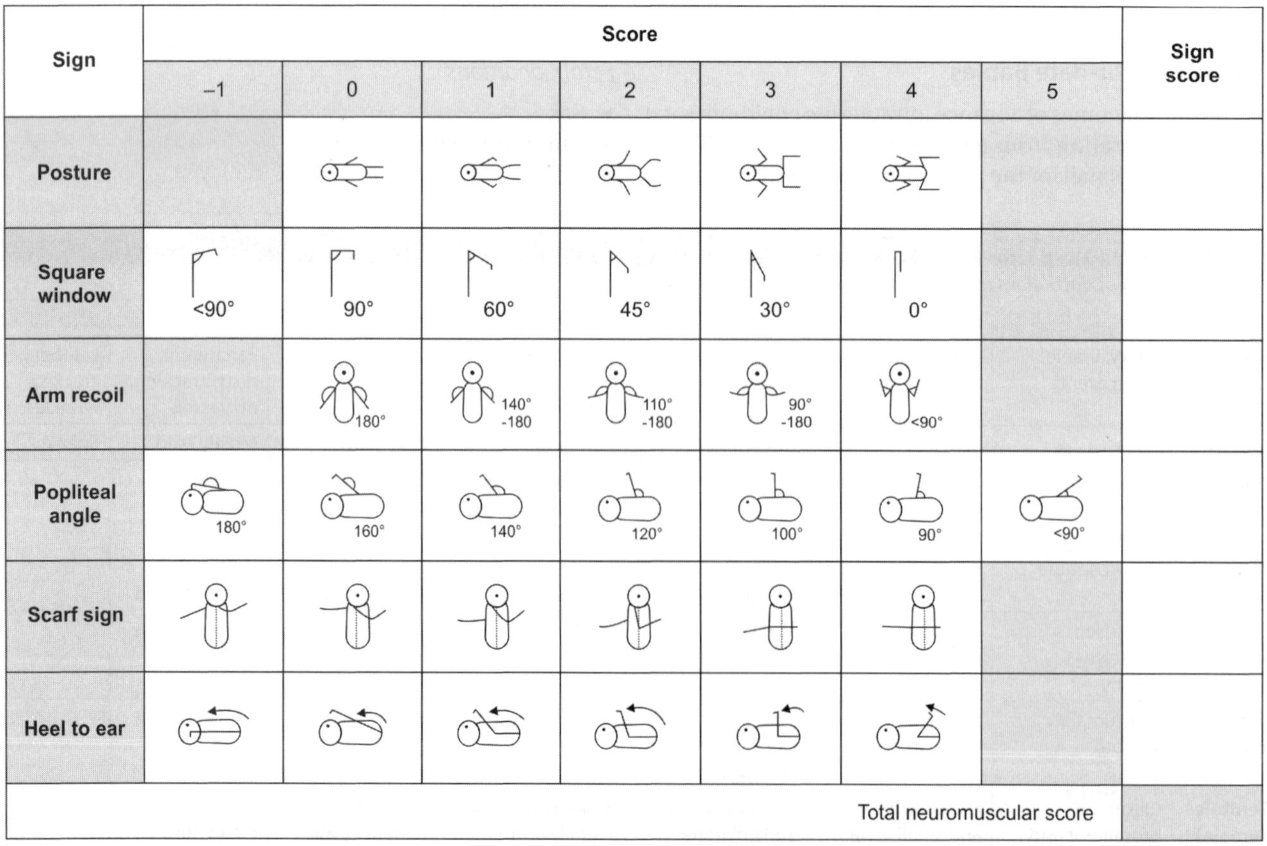

Sign	Score							Sign score
	–1	0	1	2	3	4	5	
Posture								
Square window	<90°	90°	60°	45°	30°	0°		
Arm recoil		180°	140°-180	110°-180	90°-180	<90°		
Popliteal angle	180°	160°	140°	120°	100°	90°	<90°	
Scarf sign								
Heel to ear								
							Total neuromuscular score	

Fig. 7.1: Neuromuscular maturity.

Cerebral Gigantism

It is a rare genetic disorder characterized by excessive physical growth during the first years of life and toumpanes. Excessive growth often starts in infancy and continues into the early teen years. The disorder may be accompanied by autism, mild intellectual disability, delayed motor, cognitive, and social development, hypotonia (low muscle tone), and speech impairments. Children with Sotos syndrome tend to be large at birth and are often taller, heavier, and have relatively large skulls (macrocephaly) than is normal for their age. Signs of the disorder, which vary among individuals, include a disproportionately large skull with a slightly protrusive forehead, large hands and feet, large mandible, hypertelorism and downslanting eyes. Clumsiness, an awkward gait, and unusual aggressiveness or irritability may also occur.

Management

The infants should be accorded special care depending upon their gestational maturity etiology of somatic overgrowth. They must be fed early with sugar-fortified food to maintain blood glucose level.

Post-term Babies (Gestational Age >42 Weeks)

Human placenta can generally sustain the growth of fetus up to 12 weeks; beyond this, it becomes dysfunctional to support the growth. Postmaturity is an important cause of placental dysfunction. The fetus is at an increased risk to suffer from hypoxia and birth asphyxia. In uterine passage of meconium passes grave hazards of respiratory distress due to massive meconium aspiration. Vernix caseosa and quantity of liquor begin to decrease around 36 weeks and almost disappear by 41 weeks of gestation. Lack of vernix in post-term infants forms desquamation and formation of deep sole creases. Skin, umbilical cord and nails may be stained yellow due to passage of meconium in utero. Skull bones are hard. The infant is alert at birth and shows advanced neurological development.

The common clinical problem in post-term babies includes congenital malformations, perinatal hypoxia, meconium aspiration, persistent pulmonary hypertension, hypoglycemia, hypocalcemia and polycythemia.

Management

Placental functions must be monitored to assess fetal well-being after 11 weeks. Fetal distress should be watched for. Oropharyngeal suctioning should be done only after head is delivered. Early feeding screen for blood glucose and application of oil and cold cream in dry area.

Common Health Problems in Neonates

Common health problems which can occur to neonates are as follows:

Hyperbilirubinemia

This condition refers to the excessive presence of bilirubin in the blood. It is indicated as pallor of the skin and eyes.

It is either due to physiological jaundice, RH or ABO incompatibility. Physiological jaundice usually disappears within 10 days with phototherapy. Jaundice due to RH incompatibility occurs within 24 hours and requires blood transfusion.

Hypothermia

The newborn baby may go into hypothermia within 1 hour of birth, with the temperature (axillary) falling below 36.5°C (97.7°F). This happens if proper precautions are not taken to prevent chilling of the baby. The women in the family and birth attendant should be made aware about drying the baby after birth, providing skin-to-skin contact with the mother and initiating breastfeeding within an hour of birth. Hypothermia is harmful to the newborn, increasing the risk of morbidity and mortality.

Neonatal Hypoglycemia

Blood glucose <30 mg/100 mL may occur within 48 hours of birth. This can be prevented by early feeding of the newborn baby.

Ophthalmia Neonatorum

Ophthalmia neonatorum is due to perinatal infection related to mothers caused by a variety of organisms.

These organisms include: *Neisseria gonorrhoeae*, *Chlamydia trachomatis*, *Candida*, *Streptococcus*, *Staphylococcus*, etc. Of these, *Neisseria gonorrhoeae* and *Chlamydia trachomatis* are the serious and important causes.

Ophthalmia neonatorum occurs in the absence of prophylactic care of the eyes at the time of birth of the child. The infection rate with prophylaxis ranges from 30–50%. Complications like corneal damage and blindness develop if early diagnosis and treatment are not done. For prevention of ophthalmia neonatorum, the following actions should be adopted:

- Recognition of gonococcal and chlamydial infections in pregnant women and their treatment.
- Use of eye prophylaxis in the newborn at birth. Eyes should be cleaned with boiled cool eye swabs carefully immediately after birth. Then apply either 1% tetracycline eye ointment or 1% freshly prepared silver nitrate solution.
- Training of all health workers and traditional birth attendants (TBA) regarding early recognition, treatment and referral of neonates with ophthalmia neonatorum.

Neonatal Tetanus (NNT)

NNT is a common killer disease. It is usually due to sepsis caused by unclean delivery and cord care. It is still quite common in the developing world. According to WHO estimates, there is considerable decline in the incidence of NNT and mortality due to NNT in the world. The greatest decline in NNT is observed in South-East Asian countries. According to the surveillance report in India, there has been a decline in the reported cases from 31,844 in 1987 to 4,811 in 1999 (decline by 84.9%). The decline is mainly due to significant increase in immunization coverage of antenatal mothers in the world and in India.

Ophthalmia neonatorum is a notifiable condition defined as any purulent discharge from the eyes of an infant within 21 days of birth or any inflammation that occurs in the eyes of an infant within 21 days of birth that is accompanied by discharges. The condition is associated with the mother during sexually transmitted diseases, such as gonorrhea, chlamydia in pregnancy or other sexually transmitted diseases. The causative organisms from vaginal canal are *Staphylococcus aureus, Streptococcus pneumoniae, Haemophilus influenzae, Escherichia coli, Klebsiella pseudomonas, Chlamydia trachomatis* and *Neisseria gonorrhoea.*

This condition can be prevented by antenatal screening, and detection of STD mother is very essential. Care of the eye as soon as possible may prevent such type of diseases. Wipe or clean with sterile cotton swabs in single stroke from the inner canthus to the outer canthus. Local cleaning and irrigation of the eye with normal saline and application of prophylaxis can protect the eye of an infant. In 1818, Crede used 2 percentile silver nitrate solution placed in the eye at birth. One percent tetracycline ointment was used, but sometimes it is resistant to gonococci than 0.5% erythromycin was used as prophylaxis. After that, it was observed that 2.5% povidone-iodine ophthalmic solution has proven to be very effective in prophylaxis of ophthalmic neonatorum.

Considering the preventable nature of NNT, WHO in 1989 has resolved to eliminate NNT by aiming to reduce the incidence to <one case per 1,000 live births by 1995. This goal was reaffirmed in 1999 and the target was extended to 2005. The same goal was accepted by the Indian Government. The following actions were implemented:

- 100% coverage of pregnant women with two doses of tetanus toxoid (TT).
- 100% clean deliveries.
- Surveillance of neonatal deaths and investigation of tetanus cases and deaths in the community.
- Use of information, education and communication strategies to promote five cleans, i.e., clean surface, clean hands, clean surroundings, clean blades/scissors, clean tie and clean cord.

Because of these measures, there was further decline in the number of reported cases of neonatal tetanus in 2009 (889).

Birth Asphyxia

Birth asphyxia is characterized by absent or depressed breathing at birth. In the developing countries, 3% of all newborn babies (3.6 million) develop moderate or severe asphyxia. Of these, about 84,000 die and approximately the same number of them develop severe epilepsy and mental retardation. Difficulty in initial breathing is due to a variety of reasons, such as prolonged or obstructed labor, prematurity, infection, etc. Often these can be anticipated.

The following actions should be taken to reduce neonatal deaths due to birth asphyxia:

- To keep ready the necessary equipment for the management of birth asphyxia.
- Clearing of the air passage immediately after the child is born.
- Ventilating with mask or bag and mask.
- Cardiac massage when bradycardia persists.
- Mouth-to-mouth breathing when necessary.
- Training of health workers, including TBAs in the assessment and management of birth asphyxia.

Infected Newborn

The child may be born with an infection present in the mother. The child may attain this infection either through transplacental circulations and/or during the course of pregnancy and delivery. The various infections which the child can have include tetanus, syphilis, gonorrhea, hepatitis B and C virus, and HIV.

Neonatal tetanus can be prevented by two doses of TT immunization of all pregnant women and by observing five cleans for all deliveries.

Congenital syphilis and gonorrhea can be prevented by early recognition of these diseases among the couples and their treatment and by observing clean and safe delivery practices during and after. But, usually these diseases are not reported and treated properly. It is also not possible to recognize the congenital syphilis because clinical signs do not occur soon after birth. But the treatment can be started in doubtful babies and especially in those cases where monitoring is not possible.

The newborn can be infected with hepatitis if the mother is a chronic carrier of hepatitis B virus. Transmission occurs through blood and genital secretions. Therefore, the newborn contracts infection during the immediate perinatal period. If the child gets the infection, he/she becomes a carrier and develops chronic hepatitis, cirrhosis or primary cancer of the liver during adulthood.

Perinatal transmission of hepatitis B can be prevented by seroprophylaxis (2 mL of specific anti-HBs gamma globulin) combined with anti-hepatitis B vaccination within 12 hours of birth. The vaccination must be repeated at 1 and 2 months and then at 1 year of age. Though it is found to be effective, but practically, it has not been found feasible, firstly, because it is difficult to identify and detect mothers who are carriers of this infection and, secondly, because of the high cost involved.

The newborn may also be infected with HIV if the mother is HIV-positive. About 30% of the babies born to HIV-positive mothers get infected with HIV. Like in hepatitis B, transmission occurs through blood and genital secretions. The risk of transmission depends upon the severity of infection in the mother. The possibility of transmission of infection through breast milk is also there. Therefore, whether to breastfeed the baby or not, it is to be considered for the survival of the child, especially for socioeconomically poor and underdeveloped people. BCG vaccination is contraindicated in these children and should not be given unless confirmed otherwise. Unlike hepatitis B, no preventative treatment so far is available for the newborn.

Oral Thrush

Oral thrush is characterized by white patches in the mouth. It is caused by candida albicans which is usually present in the vagina of some women. It is very important to maintain personal hygiene to prevent this infection.

Sepsis

The newborn baby is very susceptible to infection. Within a few hours of birth, staphylococcus may generate colonies on the baby's skin and in the nasal passages and may cause infection of the umbilical cord, skinfold, such as axilla and groin, nostrils, etc. The baby should be protected from being exposed to infection. Any person having any infection, such as upper respiratory infection, diarrhea, and skin infection should not be allowed to come in contact with the baby. Personal hygiene and general cleanliness need to be maintained.

CHILD HEALTH

Child health refers to a state of complete physical, mental and social well-being and not merely the absence of disease or infirmity in matters relating to growth and development of fetus during antenatal period and from birth of the baby till 5 years of age. It implies health care of the fetus during antenatal period, which refers to antenatal pediatrics, health care of neonates from birth to 28 days, care of infants up to 1 year, care of toddler from 1 year up to 2 years, care of preschool child from 2–5 years of age. The health of the children is also very important not only because they are the asset and future of their families and the nation but also because health status, health behavior and life style thus form during child hood determine the quality of life during the following years of life. The health of the children differs from place to place. It is assessed in terms of child morbidity and mortality. The factors which affect the health of children include poverty, ignorance, illiteracy, age, sex, environment, size of the family, malnutrition, lack of access to maternal and child health services, etc.

According to WHO, globally 30% of children under five are estimated to be stunted and 18% have low weight-for-height, and 43 million children are overweight. Nearly 9 million children die every year from preventable diseases and infections, the largest killer being the diarrheal disease. There are over 2 billion cases of diarrheal disease every year and is the leading cause of malnutrition amongst the children under five. According to NFHS-3, 60% of children have been brought to a health care facility with diarrhea, 69% have acute respiratory infection and 71% have presented with high fever.

Different Aspects of Child Health

Breastfeeding

Breast milk contains all types of nutrients which are essential for normal growth and development of child up to 6 months of age and should continue up to at least 2 years of age. It also provides high immunity power which can protect the child from many diseases. So, it is important for the mother to give breastfeeding to the baby soon after the child's birth and continue it exclusively for six months, which will prevent malnutrition and other diseases in the later life. Although exclusive breastfeeding prevents malnutrition on a large scale, many mothers are not practicing exclusive breastfeeding and colostrum feeding till now.

Weaning

For the first 6 months, the breast milk is sufficient for the baby's normal growth and development, but after 6 months, the baby requires additional food to meet the body's requirements as the breast milk alone cannot meet the requirements of the child. Therefore, supplementary feeding is essential along with breastfeeding.

Principles of introducing supplementary feeding to the child are:

- Start with semisolid to solid food. Small quantity to more according to the tolerance limit
- Start feeding soft boiled egg at 6–7 months and first give only yolk (yellow part). When the child starts tolerating, then the whole egg can be given at the completion of one year.
- The vegetables should be well cooked. Add a pinch of salt while feeding the child.
- Fruits should be well ripped, mashed or grinded.
- The consistency should be from thin to thick. Increase all solids' quantity until the child takes good five meals in a day, which are cooked for the family. Each meal should be finished at one go.

Now emphasis is also given on baby-led weaning (BLW). BLW means letting the baby eat solid food (rather than purees) from the start of weaning. Instead of being spoon-fed, they should be encouraged to explore food with their own hands, discovering taste and texture and eating as much or as little as they want. It is also a social experience, as babies join in with family mealtimes and eat the same food as everyone else. 'The core principle of baby-led weaning is to introduce babies to solid food at their own pace.' The idea is that you let the baby discover solid food by himself/herself, by giving him/her suitable family foods that he/she can suck, chew and initially play with. This is very different to the more traditional way of feeding, called 'puree or spoon-fed.' But the baby might not get all the nutrients he/she needs and it can be hard to know how much the baby is actually eating because much of his/her food ends up on the floor. That is why, the combination of both types of food can be advisable.

Immunization

Immunization is a process of protecting an individual from a disease through introduction of live or killed and attenuated organisms in the individual. Immunization against vaccine-preventable diseases is essential to reduce the child mortality, morbidity and handicapped condition. It is the means of protecting the largest number of people from various diseases. It gives resistance to an infectious disease by producing or augmenting the immunity. All the children should complete every immunization by following the National Immunization Schedule.

Growth Monitoring

The growth sprout is the highest during the first 5 years of life. Weight and height increase with age. In a normal child, the birthweight can double by the age of 5–6 months and triple by the age of 1 year. During the second year of life, the weight gain is about 2–2.5 kg from the period of infancy. During 3–5 years of age, the weight gain for the baby is 1.5–2 kg. Similarly, the length of the newborn is approximately 50 cm (20") at birth, which increases to 75 cm (29") at the age of one year. During the second year of life, the increase in height is about 10 cm (4–5") and the height increases to 6–7 cm (3") during 3–5 years. Regular weight-checking and comparison to the normal standard help to identify the degree of malnutrition and its related factors. The weight-checking can be done in the nearer hospitals, PHCs, subcenters or Anganwadis. Normally, every month, the weight of the child should be checked during the first year, and later, weight can be recorded at 3 months interval. The doctor should be consulted when the child's weight is reducing without any reason, weight is static for continuously 3 months or if there is any continuous illness.

Acute Respiratory Infections

Except during the neonatal period, ARIs are the most common causes of both illness and mortality in children under five, who average three to six episodes of ARIs annually regardless of where they live or what their economic situation is. However, the proportion of mild to severe disease varies between high- and low-income countries, and because of differences in specific etiologies and risk factors, the severity of LRIs in children under five is worse in the developing countries, resulting in a higher case-fatality rate. Upper respiratory tract infections are the most common infectious diseases. They include rhinitis (common cold), sinusitis, ear infections, acute pharyngitis or tonsillopharyngitis, epiglottitis, and laryngitis—of which ear infections and pharyngitis cause the more severe complications (deafness and acute rheumatic fever, respectively). Because most URIs are self-limiting, their complications are more important than the infections. Acute viral infections predispose children to bacterial infections of the sinuses and middle ear), and aspiration of infected secretions and cells can result in LRIs. ARIs control measures can be divided into four basic categories—immunization against specific pathogens, early diagnosis and treatment of disease, improvements in nutrition, and safer environments. The first two fall within the purview of the health system, whereas the last two fall under public health and require multisectoral involvement.

Diarrhea

Diarrhea is a very common problem in children. It is frequent, loose, or watery bowel movements (BMs) that differ from a child's normal pattern. Sometimes, diarrhea contains blood or mucus. Identifying mild diarrhea may be difficult because, in healthy children, the number and consistency of BMs vary with age and diet. For example, breastfed infants, who are not yet receiving solid food, often have frequent, loose stools that are considered normal. A sudden increase in number and looseness may indicate diarrhea in these infants. However, having watery stools for >24 hours is never normal. Children with diarrhea may lose their appetite, vomit, lose weight, or have fever. If diarrhea is severe or lasts a long time, dehydration is likely. Infants and young children can become dehydrated more quickly, sometimes in <1 day. Severe dehydration can cause seizures, brain damage, and death. Worldwide, diarrhea causes 2–3 million deaths a year, mostly in underdeveloped countries. In the United States, diarrhea accounts for about 9% of hospitalizations for children under 5 years old.

Worm Infestation

Worm infestation in children is very commonly seen in India. The common worm infestations are threadworm, roundworm and hookworm. It can lead to stomach pain after eating food, lack of appetite and poor digestion. The child looks weak and sick and becomes anemic. Whatever precaution is taken, there is chance of worm infestations among the under-five children as they play in soil and floor. Hence, to prevent worm infestations, which is the main factor of recurrent diarrhea and also resulting in malnutrition among the under-fives, deworming of children needs to be done every 6 months. Prevention and control of worm infestations includes thorough handwashing with soap and water before eating and after defecation, good personal hygiene, proper nail care, wearing of slippers, avoiding contact with pet animals, etc.

Malnutrition

Any nutritional disorders caused by inappropriate dietary intake is referred to as malnutrition, which is categorized under two groups—overnutrition, which means nutrition over and above the required limit, and undernutrition, which means insufficient dietary intake. Various reports reveal that malnutrition affects every fourth child worldwide. Around 800 million of people in the world are malnourished, out of which >half are under-fives. The prevention of malnutrition mainly depends upon the measures taken to improve nutritional status of mother and children. Malnutrition can affect growth and development, perceptual ability, social and behavioral development, mental development, IQ and also information processing and analytical capabilities. It can be prevented at the primary level by health promotion and highly nutritious diet for the pregnant and nursing mothers, promotion of exclusive breastfeeding up to 6 months, introduction of solids, food supplementation nutrition education, family planning, environmental sanitation and immunization. Other measures include early diagnosis and correction of malnutrition by regular weight monitoring, detection of deviation from normal, early detection and treatment of communicable diseases, deworming the children, health education to the parent and other family members.

NATIONAL POLICY FOR CHILDREN

The Government of India has adopted a Children's Policy in August 1974. According to this policy, the state has to provide adequate services to children, both before and after birth and through the period of growth, to ensure their full physical, mental and social development. The state shall progressively increase the scope of such services so that, within a reasonable time, all the children in the country enjoy optimum conditions for their balanced growth. As per the declaration, the development of children is considered an integral part of national development. The policy considers children as the 'nation's supremely important assets.' It spells measures to be adopted and priorities to be assigned to children's program. According to this, the focus areas of care are child health, child nutrition and welfare, welfare of the handicapped and destitute children. In line with the policy, a national-level children's board was established and the board is headed by the Prime Minister as its chairman. The board provides a forum to the issues relating to child welfare, purposeful development of children as useful members of the society. Based on the initiatives of the policy, the programs like ICDS, supplementary feeding programs nutrition and education, National's Children's Fund, instituting of National Awards for Child Welfare, welfare of the handicapped, CSSM program were initiated and edified.

Under-five Clinic

Under-five clinic is a center, where preventive, promotive, curative, referral and educational services are provided in a packaged manner to the under-five children under one roof. The services are provided by the trained nurses by which it becomes economical and available to a larger number of people.

Goal

The overall goal of the under-five clinics is to provide comprehensive health care to the young children as a separate specialized facility.

The under-five clinic is represented by a traditional logo of a triangle with four internal triangles representing different aspects and functions and an outer enveloping triangle as shown in the **Figure 7.2**. The functions of an under-five clinic was represents by its logo:

Functions of an under-five clinic: Based on the logo, the functions are classified as follows:

- **Care in illness:** Children are treated for acute and chronic illnesses and ailments of growth and development at these clinics. Nurses can play an important role in taking care of the sick children. Care in illness is the felt need of the mother and child for which any child is brought to the clinic. The usual illnesses encountered in children under five are fever, diarrhea, ARI, infections of the skin and helminthiasis. The facility should provide for essential laboratory investigations and X-ray facilities. The clinic should be backed by an effective referral mechanism.

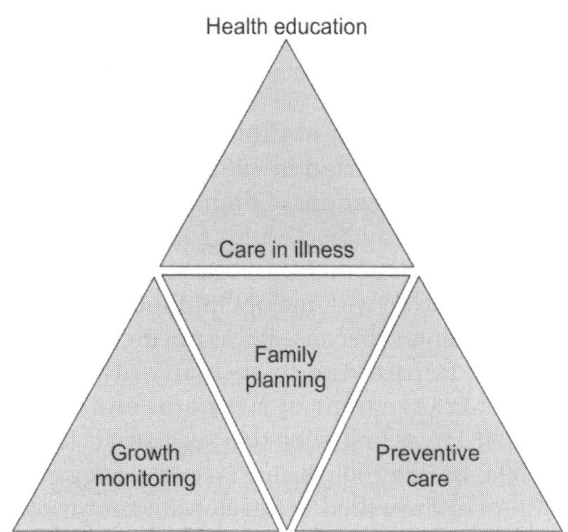

Fig. 7.2: Under-five clinic.

- **Growth monitoring:** This is one of the most important functions of the clinic. The child is weighed periodically, every month during the first year, every 2 monthly from 1–3 years of age, and every 3 monthly in 4th and 5th years. Besides weighing, measuring height, mid-arm circumference can also be carried out depending upon the availability of the trained manpower and equipment. The growth is plotted on the growth chart and any faltering in the growth is detected and suitable action initiated. The milestones are also recorded without any delay
- **Family planning:** Family planning is central to any program directed towards the women and children. The mothers are more receptive to family planning during early puerperium and lactation. The mother is counseled on the various options available, their merits and demerits, so that she can make a choice.
- **Health education:** The opportunity should be made use of to educate the mother on issues of child care, breastfeeding, nutrition, growth-monitoring, immunization and hygiene of safe water and food preparation.
- **Preventive care:** Preventive care includes all aspects which prevent the diseases. This involves primarily the immunization services during the first 5 years of life against different diseases, vitamin A supplementation and administration of iron supplementation and anthelmintic treatment to prevent anemia. The preventive care also provides for regular health check-up and use of ORS during diarrhea to prevent dehydration from developing.

INTEGRATED MANAGEMENT OF CHILDHOOD ILLNESS

Integrated Management of Childhood Illness (IMCI) is a strategy that was started in 1992 by the WHO and the United Nations International Children's Emergency Fund (UNICEF). The main objective for formulating this IMCI strategy was to reduce child mortality and morbidity which are associated with major childhood illnesses. This strategy was changed because it was not included newborn and become failure due to so many other grounds. Integrated Management of Neonatal and Childhood Illness (IMNCI) was first piloted in six districts from end of 2002 to 2004. Before 2000 during last 3 decades every year >10 million children died in developing countries before they reach their fifth birthday. Majority of such deaths are due to acute respiratory infections (mostly pneumonia), diarrhea, measles, malaria, or malnutrition—and often to a combination of these illnesses. According to National Family Health Survey, in India, common illnesses in children under 3 years of age include fever, acute respiratory infections, diarrhea and malnutrition and often in combination. Infant and childhood mortality are sensitive indicators of inequity and poverty. It is no surprise to find that the children who are most commonly and severely ill, who are malnourished and who are most likely to die of their illness belong to the most vulnerable and underprivileged populations of low-income countries.

Why an Integrated Evidence-based Syndromic-Approach to Case Management?

- In children under five years of age, pneumonia, diarrhea, malaria and neonatal infections are the most important causes of death. Malnutrition increases the risk of death and is associated with over two thirds of these deaths. Low birth weight and poor feeding are the major reasons for malnutrition in infants and children.
- IMNCI is an integrated approach that includes the assessment, classification and management of the major problems a sick infant or a child aged <5 years may have. It also includes assessment of nutritional and immunization status of all sick infants and children.
- In India, home visits for all newborns to teach the mother ways to prevent illnesses through exclusive breastfeeding and essential newborn care have been added to IMNCI. At these visits, mothers are also taught to recognize illnesses early and seek timely care. This entire package is referred to as community IMNCI.
- Every day, millions of parents seek health care for their sick children, taking them to health centers, pharmacists, doctors, hospitals and traditional healers. Surveys reveal that many sick children are not properly assessed and treated by these health care providers, and their parents are poorly advised. At first-level health facilities in low-income countries, diagnostic supports such as radiology and laboratory services are minimal or non-existent, and drugs and equipment are also scarce. These factors make providing quality care to sick children a serious challenge.
- Many well-known prevention and treatment strategies have already proven effective for saving young lives. Childhood vaccinations, oral rehydration therapy, effective use antibiotics, prompt treatment of malaria have save a millions of young lives from the serious disease like diarrhea, ARI, malaria and other killer diseases. Even modest improvements in breastfeeding practices have reduced childhood deaths.
- While each of these interventions has been successful, accumulating evidence suggests that an integrated approach is needed to manage sick children to achieve better outcomes. Child health programs need to move beyond single diseases to addressing the overall health and well-being of the child. Because many children present with overlapping signs and symptoms of diseases, a single diagnosis can be difficult, and may not be feasible or appropriate. This is especially true for first-level health facilities where examinations facilities and proper treatment facilities are not available.
- During the mid-1990s, the WHO, in collaboration with UNICEF and many other agencies, institutions and individuals, responded to this challenge by developing a strategy known as the IMCI.
- Although the major reason for developing the IMCI strategy stemmed from the needs of curative care, the strategy also addresses aspects of nutrition, immunization, and other important elements of disease prevention and health promotion.
- The objectives of the strategy are to reduce death and the frequency and severity of illness and disability, and to contribute to improved growth and development. This strategy has been expanded in India to include all neonates and renamed as 'IMNCI'. The guidelines represent an evidence-based, syndromic approach to case management that includes rational, effective and affordable use of drugs and diagnostic tools.

Components of the Integrated Approach

The IMNCI strategy includes both preventive and curative interventions which aim to improve the practices in providing healthcare services, the health system and at home. At the core of the strategy is integrated case management of the most common neonatal and childhood problems which are the most common causes of death.

The strategy includes three main components:

1. Improvements in the case-management skills of health care workers through the provision of locally-adapted IMNCI guidelines and activities to promote their use
2. Improvements in the overall health system required for effective management of neonatal and childhood illness
3. Improvements in family and community health care practices.

The Principles of Integrated Care

Depending on a child's age, various clinical signs and symptoms differ in their degrees of reliability and diagnostic value and importance. Therefore, the IMNCI guidelines recommend case management procedures based on two age categories:

Young infants age up to 2 months and children age 2 months to 5 years.

The IMNCI guidelines are based on the following principles:

- All sick young infants up to 2 months of age must be assessed for "possible bacterial infection/jaundice". Then they must be routinely assessed for the major symptom "diarrhea".
- All sick children age 2 months up to 5 years must be examined for "general danger signs" which indicate the need for immediate referral or admission to a hospital. They must then be routinely assessed for major symptoms: cough or difficult breathing, diarrhea, fever and ear problems.
- All sick young infants and children 2 months up to 5 years must also be routinely assessed for nutritional and immunization status, feeding problems, and other potential problems.
- Only a limited number of carefully selected clinical signs are used, based on evidence of their sensitivity and specificity to detect disease. These signs were selected considering the conditions and realities of first-level health facilities.

A combination of individual signs leads to an infant's or a child's classification(s) rather than a diagnosis. Classification(s) indicate the severity of condition(s). They call for specific actions based on whether the infant or child (a) should be urgently referred to a higher level of care, (b) requires specific treatments (such as antibiotics or antimalarial treatment), or (c) may be safely managed at home. The classifications can be identified by color-coded management chart.

THE IMNCI CASE MANAGEMENT PROCESS

Introduction to Color-coded Management Charts

Management charts include assess and classify chart, treat the young infant or child, counsel the mother chart. The assess and classify chart has four columns. "Assess" column lists what signs and symptoms to check and how to do it. "Signs" column summarizes the signs and symptoms present. "Classification" helps in classifying each illness the young infant or child has. "Identify Treatment" section lists appropriate treatment decisions for each classification **Flowchart 7.1**.

- The Assess and Classify chart is organized in three different colors red, yellow and green.
- The IMNCI guidelines address most, but not all, of the major reasons a sick infant or child is brought to a clinic. An infant or child returning with chronic problems or less.
- Does not include care at birth common illnesses may require special care. The guidelines do not describe the management of trauma or other acute emergencies due to accidents or injuries. They also do not cover care at birth.

Flowchart 7.1: IMNCI case management process.

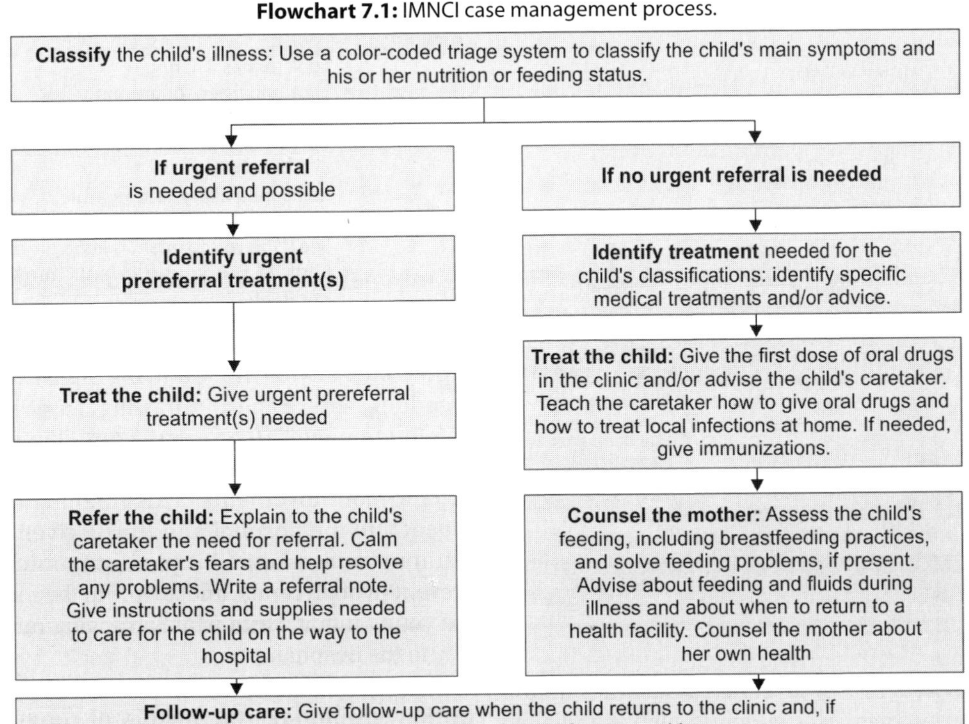

- IMNCI management procedures use a limited number of essential drugs and encourage active participation of caretakers in the treatment of infants and children.
- An essential component of the IMNCI guidelines is the counselling of caretakers about home care, including counselling about feeding, fluids and when to return to a health facility.

CASE MANAGEMENT OF SICK YOUNG INFANTS (0–2 MONTHS)

Young infants have special characteristics that must be considered when classifying their illnesses. They can become sick and die very quickly from serious bacterial infections. They frequently have the symptoms like slow movements, fever or low body temperature. Mild chest indrawing is normal in young infants because their chest wall is soft. For these reasons, you will assess, classify and treat the young infant somewhat differently than an older infant or young child **Flowchart 7.2**.

The assessment procedure for this age group includes a number of important steps that must be taken by the healthcare provider, including:

- History taking and communicating with the caretaker about the young infant's problem;

Flowchart 7.2: IMNCI case management process for the sick young infant up to 2 months of age.

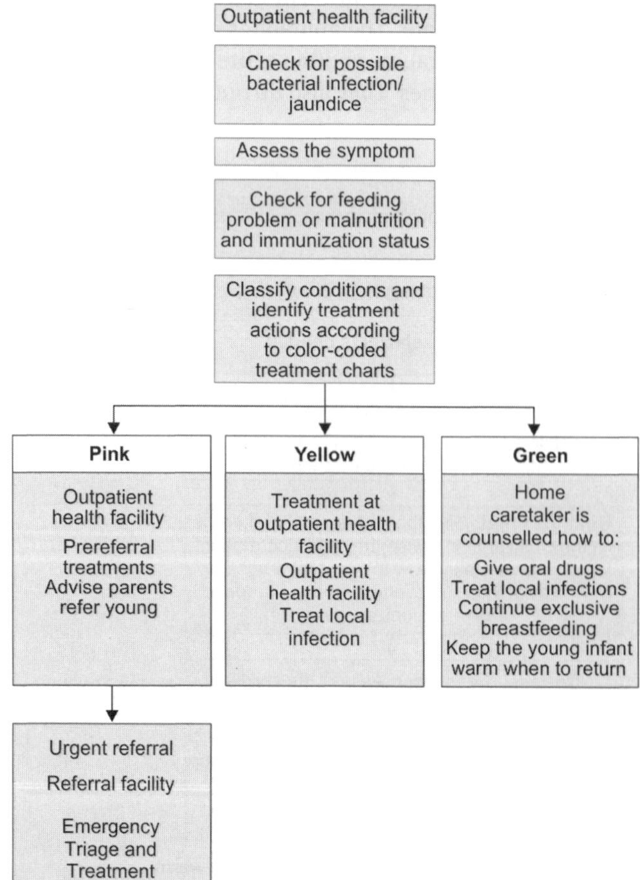

- Checking for possible bacterial infection/jaundice;
- Checking for diarrhea;
- Checking for feeding problem or malnutrition;
- Checking immunization status; and
- Assessing other problems.

History Taking and Communicating

It is critical to communicate effectively with mother of the infant or caretaker. Good communication skill is essential to ensure that common problems or signs of disease. Proper communication helps to reassure the mother or caretaker that the infant will receive appropriate care.

During History Taking

- Greet the mother and give a friendly smile.
- Ask the mother what the young infant's problems are.
- Listen carefully to what the mother tells you.
- Use words the mother understands.
- Give the mother time to answer the questions.
- Ask additional questions when the mother is not sure about her answer.
- Determine if this is an initial or follow-up visit for this problem.

Before starting assessment, select the case management chart for the young infant age up to 2 months chart.

Checking For Possible Bacterial Infection/Jaundice

There are two possible classifications for possible bacterial infection.

Ask	*Look, listen and feel*
Has the infant had convulsion	• Count the breaths in one minute. Repeat the count if elevated • Look for severe chest indrawing • Look for nasal flaring • Look and listen for grunting • Look at the umbilicus. Is it red or draining pus? • Look for skin pustules. Are there 10 or more skin pustules or a big boil? • Measure axillary temperature (if not possible feel for fever or low body temperature) • See if the young infant is lethargic or unconscious • Look at the young infant's movements. Are they <normal?

A sick young infant with *possible serious bacterial infection* is one with any of the following signs: convulsions, fast breathing, severe chest indrawing, nasal flaring, grunting, bulging fontanel, 10 or more many skin pustules or a big boil, fever, hypothermia, lethargy or unconsciousness, or <normal movements. This infant should be referred urgently to the hospital after being given the first dose of intramuscular ampicillin plus gentamicin, treatment to prevent hypoglycemia, and advice to the mother on keeping the young infant warm while arranging referral, and on the way to the hospital.

During assessing possible bacterial infection the health worker should take the history of convulsions of infant from the mother. The young infant must be quiet and calm during assessment. If the young infant is frightened, crying or angry, you will not be able to obtain an accurate count of the infant's breaths. If the infant breath 60 in a minute or >that it will be considered as fast breathing which will be confirmed after second count. During assessing chest indrawing when the young infant breathes IN, look at the lower chest wall (lower ribs). The young infant has chest indrawing if the lower chest wall goes IN when the infant breathes IN. In normal breathing, the whole chest wall (upper and lower) and the abdomen move OUT when the young infant breathes IN. When chest indrawing is present, the lower chest wall goes IN when the young infant breathes IN. Mild chest indrawing is normal in a young infant because the chest wall is soft. Severe chest indrawing is a sign of pneumonia and is serious in a young infant. Almost all neonates may have 'physiological jaundice' during the first week of life. Physiological jaundice usually appears between 48–72 hours of age, maximum intensity is seen on 4–5th day in term and 7th day in preterm neonates. Physiological jaundice does not extend to palms and soles, and does not need any treatment. Occurrence of jaundice in the first 24 hours of life and yellow discoloration of palms and soles at any time is always pathological and requires urgent referral. A sick young infant with local bacterial infection is the one with umbilicus red or draining pus or pus discharge from ear or <10 skin pustules. This infant may be treated at home with oral antibiotics but should be seen in follow-up after 2 days.

Classification and Identification of Treatment for Possible Bacterial Infection

• Convulsions or • Fast breathing (60 breaths per minute or more) • Severe chest indrawing or • Nasal flaring or • Grunting or • 10 or more pustules or a big boil or • Axillary temperature 37.5°C or above (or feels hot to touch) or temperature <35.5°C (or feels cold to touch) or • Lethargic or unconscious or • Less than normal movements	Possible serious bacterial infection	• **Give first dose of cotrimoxazole if able to take orally** • (½ pediatric tablet for an infant up to 1 month and 1 tablet for an infant 1–2 months) • Advise mother to continue breastfeeding • Warm the young infant by skin-to-skin contact if feels cold to touch • **Refer URGENTLY** to hospital
• Umbilicus red or draining pus or • Skin pustules <10	Local bacterial infection	• Give oral cotrimoxazole for 5 days • ½ pediatric tablet twice daily for an infant up to 1 month and 1 tablet for an infant 1–2 months • Teach mother to apply 0.5% gentian violet paint twice daily • **Follow-up in 2 days**

Diarrhea

A young infant is considered to have diarrhea if the stools have changed from usual pattern and are many and watery (more water than fecal matter). The normally frequent or loose stools of a breastfed baby are not diarrhea.

A young infant with diarrhea can be placed in one of the following 3 categories: (1) acute watery diarrhea; (2) dysentery (bloody diarrhea); and (3) persistent diarrhea (diarrhea that lasts >14 days). All young infants with diarrhea should be assessed for: (a) signs of dehydration; (b) duration of diarrhea; and (c) blood in the stool.

Clinical Assessment

All infants with diarrhea should be assessed to determine the duration of diarrhea, if blood is present in the stool and if dehydration is present. A number of clinical signs are used to determine the level of dehydration:

- **Infant's general condition:** Depending on the degree of dehydration, an infant with diarrhea may be lethargic or unconscious or look restless/irritable. Only infants who cannot be consoled and calmed should be considered restless or irritable.
- **Sunken eyes:** The eyes of a dehydrated infant may look *sunken*. In a severely malnourished infant who is visibly wasted, the eyes may always look sunken, even if the infant is not dehydrated. Even though the sign "sunken eyes" is less reliable in a visibly wasted infant, it can still be used to classify the infant's dehydration.
- **Elasticity of skin:** Check elasticity of skin using the skin pinch test. When released, the skin pinch goes back either *very slowly* (>2 seconds), or *slowly* (skin stays up even for a brief instant), or *immediately*. In an infant with severe malnutrition, the skin may go back slowly even if the infant is not dehydrated. In an overweight infant, or an infant with oedema, the skin may go back immediately even if the infant is dehydrated.

Based on a combination of the above clinical signs, children presenting with diarrhea are classified into three categories severe dehydration if he/she has any combination of two of the following signs: is lethargic or unconscious, is not able to drink or is drinking poorly, has sunken eyes, or a skin pinch goes back very slowly. Patients have severe dehydration if they have a fluid deficit >10% of their body weight.

After assessing and classifying the diarrhea infants with signs of severe or some dehydration should be referred to hospital. Infants with severe dysentery should be referred to hospital and a child who is not dehydrated should be treated at home.

Classification of Young Infant for Diarrhea

Blood in the stool	**Severe dysentery**	• **Give first dose of oral cotrimoxazole if able to take orally** • Refer URGENTLY to hospital • Advise mother to continue breastfeeding • Advise to keep the young infant warm

Contd...

Contd...

Two of the following signs: • Lethargic or unconscious • Sunken eyes • Skin pinch goes back very slowly	**Severe dehydration**	• Give first dose of oral cotrimoxazole • Refer URGENTLY to hospital with mother giving frequent sips of ORS on the way • Advise mother to continue breastfeeding • Advice to keep young infant warm
Two of the following signs: • Restless or irritable • Sunken eyes • Skin pinch goes back slowly	**Some dehydration**	
Not enough signs to classify as dehydration	**No dehydration**	• Give fluids to treat diarrhea at home (Plan A) • Advice home care • Follow-up in 2 days if not improving

Young infants with severe dehydration fluid deficit equal or >10% of their body weight require immediate IV infusion, nasogastric or oral fluid replacement according to WHO treatment guidelines described in Plan C. Infants with some dehydration have a fluid deficit equaling 5–10% of their body weight and require active oral treatment with ORS solution according to WHO treatment guidelines described in Plan B. Patients with diarrhea but no signs of dehydration usually have a fluid deficit <5% of their body weight. Although these children lack distinct signs of dehydration, they should be given more fluid than usual to prevent dehydration.

Plan B: Treat Some Dehydration with ORS

Give in clinic recommended amount of ORS over 4-hour period.

Age	**Up to 4 months**	**4 months up to 12 months**	**12 months up to 2 years**	**2 years up to 5 years**
Weight	<6 kg	6 – <10 kg	10 – <12 kg	12–19 kg
In mL	200–400	400–700	700–900	900–1400
No. of cups				

Feeding Problems and Malnutrition

Assessment of feeding in young infants has two parts. In the first part you ask the mother questions to determine if she is having difficulty feeding the infant, what the young infant is fed and how often. You also determine weight for age.

In the second part, if an infant has difficulty feeding, or is breastfed <8 times in 24 hours, or being given other foods or drinks, or low weight for age, then breastfeeding should be assessed. Assessment of breastfeeding in young infants includes checking if the infant is able to attach, if the infant is suckling effectively (slow, deep sucks, with some pausing), and if there are ulcers or white patches in the mouth (thrush).

The breastfeeding difficulties may include infrequent feeding of the young infant, not enough milk, sore nipples or the infant is not feeding well. If a mother says that the infant is not able to feed, watch her try to feed the infant to see what she means by this. An infant who is not able to feed may have a serious infection or other life-threatening problem and should be referred urgently to hospital. Based on the table given bellow the child should be assessed.

Ask:	**Look and feel:**
• Is there any difficulty feeding? • Is the infant breastfed? If yes, how many times in 24 hours? • Does the infant usually receive any other foods or drinks? • If yes, how often? • What do you use to feed the infant? • Does the mother have pain while breastfeeding?	• Assess breastfeeding if there is no indication for urgent referral: ▪ Ask the mother to put her infant to the breast. Observe the breastfeed for 4 minutes ▪ Is the infant able to attach well? • To check attachment, look for: ▪ Chin touching breast ▪ Mouth wide open ▪ Lower lip turned outward ▪ More areola visible above than below the mouth ▪ All of these signs should be present if the attachment is good ▪ No attachment at all ▪ Not well attached ▪ Good attachment • Is the infant suckling effectively (that is, slow deep sucks, sometimes pausing)? ▪ Not suckling at all ▪ Not suckling effectively ▪ Suckling effectively ▪ Clear a blocked nose if it interferes with breastfeeding. ▪ Look for ulcers or white patches in the mouth (thrush). If yes, look and feel for: – Sore nipples – Engorged breasts or breast abscess

Classification of Feeding Problem

Based on an assessment of feeding and weight, a sick young infant may be classified into three categories "not able to feed or possible serious bacterial infection or severe malnutrition" which is given bellow.

• Not able to feed or • No attachment at all or • Not suckling at all	Not able to feed—possible serious bacterial infection	• Warm the young infant by skin-to-skin contact if feels cold to touch • **Refer URGENTLY** to hospital
• Not well attached to breast or not suckling effectively or • <8 breastfeeds in 24 hours or • Receives other foods or drinks or • Thrush (ulcers or white patches in mouth)	Feeding problem	• If not well attached or not suckling effectively, teach correct positioning and attachment • If breastfeeding <8 times in 24 hours, advise to increase frequency of feeding • If receiving other foods or drinks, counsel mother about breastfeeding more, reducing other foods or drinks, and using a cup and spoon

Contd...

Contd...

• Breast or nipple problems		• If not breastfeeding at all, advise mother about giving locally appropriate animal milk and teach the mother to feed with a cup and spoon • If thrush, teach the mother to apply 0.25% gentian violet paint twice daily • If breast or nipple problem, teach the mother to treat breast or nipple problems • **Advise mother to give home care** (Breastfeed infant exclusively, keep infant warm, apply nothing to cord, ask mother to wash hands and explain danger signs in the infant) • **Follow-up in 2 days**
No other signs of inadequate feeding	No feeding problem	• Advise mother home care • Praise the mother for feeding the infant well

MANAGEMENT OF CHILDREN AGE 2 MONTHS UP TO 5 YEARS

Assessment of Sick Children

The assessment procedure for this age group includes a number of important steps that must be taken by the healthcare provider, including: (1) history taking and communicating with the caretaker about the child's problem; (2) checking for general danger signs; (3) checking main symptoms; (4) checking for malnutrition; (5) checking for anemia; (6) assessing the child's feeding; (7) checking immunization status; and (8) assessing other problems.

Good communication techniques and an integrated assessment are required to ensure that common problems or signs of disease or malnutrition are not overlooked which has already been discussed during assessment of young infants **Flowchart 7.3**.

Flowchart 7.3: IMNCI case management process for the sick child from age 2 months up to 5 years.

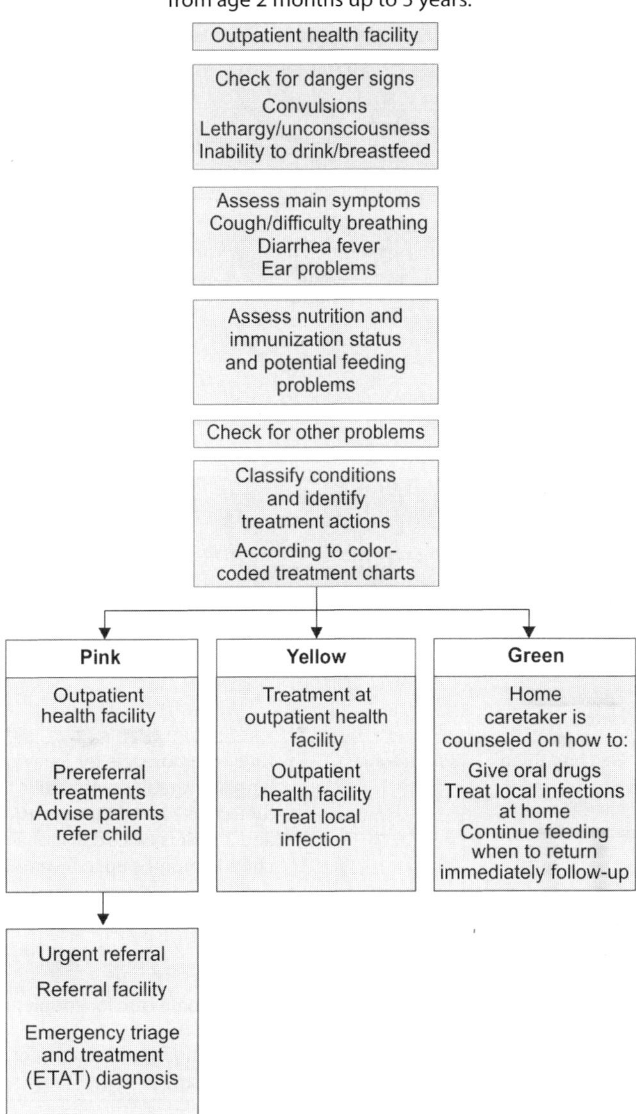

Check for General Danger Signs

Some children may present with serious, non-specific signs called "general danger signs" that do not point to a particular diagnosis. For example, a child who is lethargic or unconscious may have meningitis, severe pneumonia, cerebral malaria or another severe disease. Great care should be taken to ensure that these general danger signs are not overlooked because they suggest that a child is severely ill and needs urgent attention **(Fig. 7.3)**.

Cough or Difficult Breathing

A child with cough or difficult breathing may have any severe respiratory infection or pneumonia. Pneumonia is an infection of the lungs. Both bacteria and viruses can cause pneumonia. In developing countries, pneumonia is often due to bacteria. The most common are *Streptococcus pneumoniae* and *Hemophilus influenzae*. Children with bacterial pneumonia may die from hypoxia (too little oxygen) or sepsis (generalized infection). Three key clinical signs are used to assess a sick child with cough or difficult breathing that are respiratory rate, which distinguishes children who have pneumonia from those who do not; lower chest wall indrawing, which indicates severe pneumonia; and stridor, which indicates those with severe pneumonia who require hospital admission.

If the child's age is	*The child has fast breathing if you count*
2 months up to 12 months 12 months up to 5 years	50 breaths per minute or more 40 breaths per minute or more

Assessment	*Classification*	*Identify treatment and treat the child*
Any general danger sign or chest indrawing	Severe pneumonia or very severe disease	• Give first dose of cotrimoxazole • **Refer URGENTLY** to hospital

Contd...

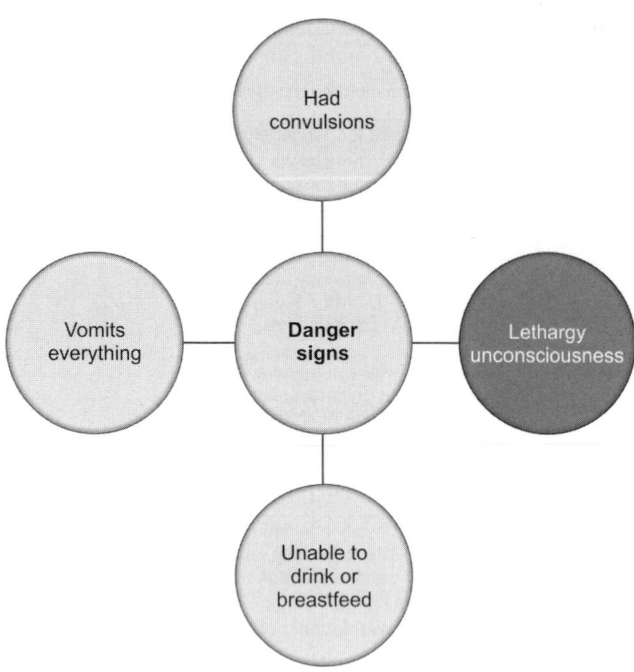

Fig. 7.3: General danger signs of sick children.

Contd...

Fast breathing	Pneumonia	• Give cotrimoxazole for 5 days. 2 pediatric tablet twice daily for a child 2 up to 12 months and 3 tablets twice daily for a child 12 months up to 5 years • **Follow up in 2 days** • Advise home care for cough or cold • Follow-up in 2 days
No signs of pneumonia or very severe disease	Cough or cold	• Advise home care for cough or cold • If coughing for <30 days, refer for assessment

Assess and Classify Diarrhea

Diarrhea should be routinely checked in every young infant and sick child brought to the clinic. Frequent passing of normal stools in not diarrhea. The number of stools normally passed in a day varies with the diet and age of the child. In many regions diarrhea is defined as three or more loose or watery stools in a 24-hour period. Though the disease pattern is same in case of both young infant and sick child extra point i.e., "Child's reaction when offered to drink" and the general danger signs will be assessed in case of sick child. The classification will be differ based on assessment.

Assessment	*Classification*	*Identify treatment and treat the child*
Diarrhea for 14 days or more	Severe persistent diarrhea	Refer to hospital
Blood in the stool	Dysentery	• Give cotrimoxazole for 5 days • 2 pediatric tablet twice daily for a child 2 up to 12 months and 3 tablets twice daily for a child 12 months up to 5 years • Follow-up in 2 days
Two of the following signs: • Lethargic or unconscious • Sunken eyes • Not able to drink or drinking poorly • Skin pinch goes back very slowly	Severe dehydration	**Refer URGENTLY** to hospital **with** mother giving frequent sips of ORS on the way
Two of the following signs: • Restless, irritable • Sunken eyes • Drinks eagerly, thirsty • Skin pinch goes back slowly	Some dehydration	• Give fluid and food for some dehydration (Plan B) • Follow-up in 2 days if not improving
Not enough signs to classify as some or severe dehydration	**No dehydration**	• Give fluid and food to treat diarrhea at home (Plan A) • Follow-up in 2 days if not improving

Fever

All sick children should be checked for fever. Fever is a very common condition and is often the main reason for bringing children to the health center. It may be caused by minor infections, but may also be the most obvious sign of a life-threatening illness, particularly malaria (especially lethal malaria *P. falciparum*), or other severe infections, including meningitis, typhoid fever, or measles.

Clinical Assessment

Body temperature should be checked in all sick children brought to an outpatient clinic. Children are considered to have fever if their body temperature is above 37.5°C axillary (38°C rectal). In the absence of a thermometer, children are considered to have fever if they feel hot. Fever also may be recognized based on a history of fever **(Fig. 7.4)**.

A child presenting with fever should be assessed for:

- **Risk of malaria:** The National Anti-Malaria Program has defined areas of high and low malaria risk in the country.
- **Duration of fever:** Most fevers due to viral illnesses go away within a few days. A fever that has been present every day for >seven days can mean that the child has a more severe disease such as typhoid fever. If the fever has been present for >seven days, it is important to check whether the fever has been present every day.
- **Bulging fontanelle and stiff neck:** Bulging fontanelle or a stiff neck may be a sign of meningitis, cerebral malaria or another very severe febrile disease. If the child is conscious and alert, check stiffness by tickling the feet, asking the child to bend his/her neck to look down or by

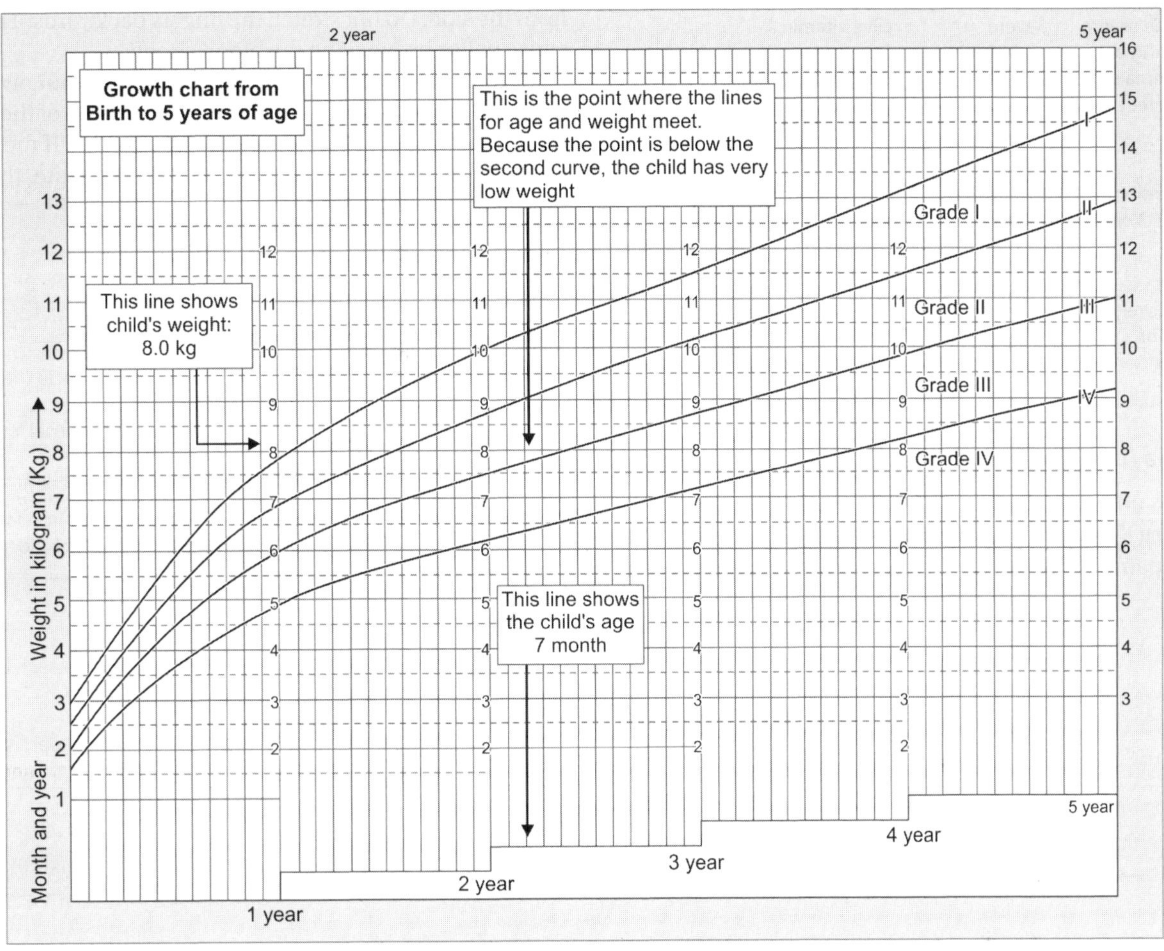

Fig. 7.4: Growth chart from birth to 5 years of age.

very gently bending the child's head forward. It should move freely.

- **Runny nose:** When malaria risk is low, a child with fever and a runny nose does not need an antimalarial. This child's fever is probably due to a common cold.
- **Measles:** Considering the high risk of complications and death due to measles, children with fever should be assessed for signs of current or previous measles (within the last 3 months).

Classification for Fever

• Any general danger sign or • Stiff neck	Very severe febrile disease	• Give first dose of cotrimoxazole • Give first dose of antimalarial as per NAMP guidelines after making a smear • Give one dose of paracetamol in clinic for high fever • Refer URGENTLY to hospital
Fever (by history or feels hot)	Malaria	• Give antimalarials as per NAMP guidelines after making a smear • Give one dose of paracetamol in clinic for high fever • Advise extra fluids, continue feeding and advise about danger signs • Follow-up in 2 days if fever persists • If fever is present every day for >7 days, refer for assessment

Malnutrition

A sick child can be malnourished, but you or the child's family may not notice the problem. A child with malnutrition has a higher risk of many types of disease and death. Even children with mild and moderate malnutrition have an increased risk of death. When assessing a child for malnutrition we have to assess signs suggesting malnutrition that are look for visible severe wasting, look for oedema of both feet and determine grade of malnutrition by plotting weight for age. Children with severe malnutrition exhibiting visible severe wasting or edema of both feet are at high risk of death from various severe diseases and need urgent referral to a hospital where their treatment can be carefully monitored. Children with very low weight for age also have a higher risk of severe disease and should be assessed for feeding problems. Children who are not very low weight for age and who show no signs of severe malnutrition are classified as having not very low weight. Because children <2 years old have a higher risk of feeding problems and malnutrition than older children do, their feeding should be assessed. When assessing the weight per age the weight should be monitored and plotted in growth chart. You will identify children whose weight for age is below the second curve of a weight for age chart.

• Visible severe wasting or • Oedema of both feet	Severe malnutrition	• Give vitamin A • Prevent low blood sugar by breastmilk, other milk/water with sugar (4 tsf sugar per cup) • Keep the child warm. • Refer URGENTLY to hospital
Malnutrition grade 2, 3 or 4	Very low weight	• Assess and counsel for feeding • Follow up in 14 days (if feeding problem, follow up in 5 days)
Normal weight for age or malnutrition grade 1	Not very low weight	• If child is <2 years old, assess and counsel for feeding • If feeding problem, follow-up in 5 days

Anemia (Look for Palmar Pallor)

Pallor is unusual paleness of the skin. It is a sign of anemia.

To see if the child has palmar pallor, look at the skin of the child's palm. Hold the child's palm open by grasping it gently from the side. Do not stretch the fingers backwards. This may cause pallor by blocking the blood supply.

Compare the color of the child's palm with your own palm and with the palms of other children. If the skin of the child's palm is pale, the child has some palmar pallor. If the skin of the palm is very pale or so pale that it looks white, the child has severe palmar pallor.

Classify Anemia

Here is the classification table for anemia:

Severe palmar pallor	Severe anemia	Refer to hospital
Some palmar pallor	Anemia	• Give iron folic acid therapy for 14 days • Assess and counsel for feeding • Follow-up in 14 days
No palmar pallor	No anemia	Give prophylactic iron folic acid if child 6 months or older

CHAPTER 8

Community Health Planning and Organization

INTRODUCTION

Plan is a deliberate attempt to spell out how the resources of a country should be put to use. It has some general and specific goals which are to be achieved within a specific period of time. The general goals of a plan are growth, modernization, full employment, self-reliance and equity. But all Plans may not give equal importance to all of them. Each plan can have some specific goals like improvement of agriculture. For example, our first five-year plan was geared up to improving the state of agriculture and the second to improving the industry. Health is an important contributory factor in the utilization of manpower and in the upliftment of the economic condition of the country. Every government plans for the improvement and maintenance of all the subsectors of health. Establishing health planning in India is a key to improving the health of the Indian population. The Ministry of Health and Family Welfare has been facilitating health needs in India by establishing various schemes and organizations.

The Constitution of India had considered health as every human being's right and an asset for the overall socioeconomic development. The Government of India and the Planning Commission give considerable importance to health in five-year plans.

HISTORICAL OVERVIEW OF PLANNING

As the healthcare delivery system has grown in the past 66 years, emphasis in health planning and evaluation has increased factors that have fostered increased interest in planning and evaluation, advance healthcare technology and consumer education, increased health care expectation has got pressure, professional conflicts focus on preventive care, urbanization, increased health risks, personnel shortage and increased healthcare casts.

- In 1920, the American Public Health Association Committees in administrative practice emphasized planning and evaluation.
- In 1944, American Hospital Organization established a committee for reorganized planning for health services.
- The year 1960 was marked by the great society programs of President Johnson. The social, economic and health programs grow out of great society to meet the people's needs.
- In 1965, the regional program legislation was passed to upgrade the quality of tertiary health care.
- In 1966, 89th Congress passed the comprehensive health planning and public health service adamants.
- In 1974, National Health Planning and Resource Development Act was passed.
- In 1980, a new federation became the catch phrase of the 1980s and emphasis was placed on cost shifting, cost reduction and more competition within the healthcare system. President Ronald Reagan proposed doing away the federal government's rule in health planning in 1981.

PLANNING OF A PROGRAM

A program management consists of assessing, planning, implementing and evaluating the process involved in the life of a program. As the healthcare delivery system has grown in the past 60 years, emphasis is on health planning and evaluation.

Definition of a Program

A program is an organized response designed to meet the assessed needs of individuals, familiar groups' communities by reducing or eliminating one or more health problems.

—Stanhope, 2003

A program is a sequence of activities designed to implement policies and accomplish objectives. A program gives a step-by-step approach to guide the action necessary to reach the predetermined goals.

Benefits of Program Planning

- Program planning is referred to as strategic planning. Systematic planning meets the clients' needs and provides benefits for the client, and the employing agency.
- Planning focus and attention on what the organization and health care provide or are attempting to do for the clients.
- To understand the relationship between the different activities of the program and the knock-on effects of changes to one part of the plan on other parts.

- Minimizing the risk to the program by using the plan as a tool to control and monitor delivery
- Ensuring that individual program and activity plans work within the constraints of the program
- Ensuring a demonstrably coherent approach to the delivery of service
- Managing expectations in terms of overall programming timescales
- Planning assists in identifying the resources and activities that are essential in meeting the objectives of the client services
- Planning the reduction of ambiguity
- Planning the aligning of responsibilities to the specific provider to meet the program objectives
- Planning also reduces uncertainty
- Planning helps the provider and the agency to anticipate events
- Finally, planning allows for quality decision-making and better control over the actual program result.

Health Program Planning

Health planning is a part of national development planning. Health planning is necessary for the economic utilization of material, manpower and financial resources. The purpose of health planning is to improve a health service which is affected by the governmental control over licensure funding by the social structure, by the cultural and belief system in which the program must function. Program planning is essential to meet the federal, state and local government mandates for funding, funding guidelines and internal agency requirements.

Health Needs and Demands

The purpose of health planning is to meet the health needs and demands of the people. Health needs have been defined as 'deficiencies in the health that call for preventive, curative control or eradication measures'. The health needs can be assessed during the whole community surveillance, or surveillance of any particular diseases, etc. The need for medical care, safe water supply, adequate nutrition, immunization, family planning—all are community health needs. It may be mentioned that the health needs as seen by the people are not exactly the same as seen by the experts. By analyzing the health needs and problems of the community, the program can be planned.

Resources

The term 'resource' is widely used in health planning. Resource means an economic or ductive factor required to accomplish an activity, or as a means to undertake an enterprise and achieve the desired outcome. Three most basic resources are manpower, money and materials. Other resources include skills, knowledge, techniques, and the time needed or available for the performance to support of action directed towards specific.

Objectives, Targets and Goals

Objectives, targets and goals should be clear before planning of a program. A number of ways are used to describe the end result of planning—objectives, target and goal.

- **Objectives:** It is the planned end-point of all the activities. It is either achieved or not achieved.
- **Target:** It is the measurement of how successfully to reach the program objective. The targets often report to discrete activities, such as the number of blood films collected or vasectomies done.
- **Goal:** Goal is defined as the ultimate desired state towards which objectives and resources are directed. It is an indicator of whether your aim is achieving its objective or not. A goal is described as a term what is to be attained, the intent to which it is to be attained, and the population.

PLANNING PROCESS

According to WHO, the health planning process has been defined as the underlying process of defining community health problems, identifying unmet needs and surveying the resource to meet these needs, establishing priority goals that are relative and feasible and projecting administrative actions to accomplish the purposes of the proposed program. This definition reveals the various steps. The steps always follow cyclic process, so it is also termed as planning cycle. Before starting planning any program or policy, preparation is necessary which is termed as preplanning which also follow some steps.

Preplanning

Preplanning is the preparation for planning. Before developing any plan to conduct any program, some important necessary preconditions which needs to follow-up. They are as follows:

Government Interest

Any plan for the health and welfare of the country must be based on the strong political will as manifested by the clear directives or policies given by the political authority.

Legislation

The social and health policies formulated may have to be translated into location. An example may be cited of the enactment of the Medical Termination of Pregnancy Act (1971) by the Indian Parliament to protect the health of the mothers.

Organization for Planning

There should be an organizational structure for the implementation of the various parts of the plan. Organization may be in the form of organization structure means the infrastructure and man power required for conducting the program.

Administrative Capacity

One of the essential preconditions of planning is the administrative capacity for proper coordination of activities and implementation of the plan at all levels.

Planning

Planning is the broad foundation on which much of the management is based.

Planning may be defined as the process of analyzing a system or defining a problem, assessing the extent to which the problem exists as a need formulating goals and objectives to alleviate or ameliorate those identified needs, examining and choosing from among the alternation strategies, initiating the necessary action for its implementation and monitoring the system to ensure proper implementation of the plan and evaluating the results of intervention in the light of the stated objectives.

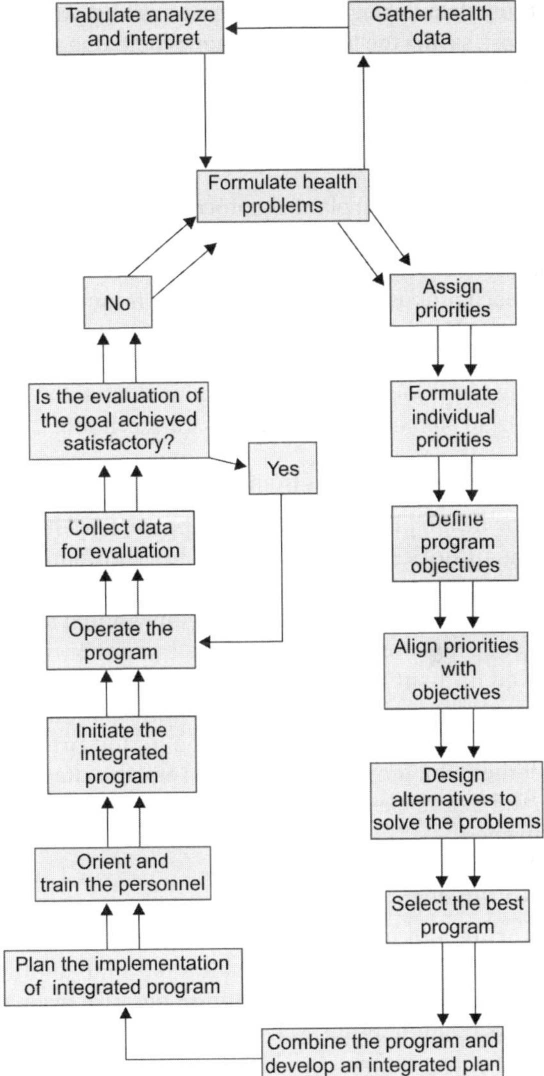

Fig. 8.1: Planning cycle.

STEPS OF PROGRAM PLANNING

The first step in health planning is the analysis of the health situation. It involves the collection, assessment and interpretation of information in such a way as to provide a clear picture of health situation. The following items of data are the minimum essential requirements for health planning.

Analysis of the Health Situation

The first step in health planning is the analysis of the health situation. It involves the collection, assessment and interpretation of information in such a way as to provide a clear picture of the health situation **(Fig. 8.1)**. The minimum requirements are as follows:

- The population, its age and structure
- Statistics of morbidity and mortality
- The epidemiology and geographical distribution
- Medical care facilities
- The technical manpower of various training facilities available
- Attitude and belief of people on health-related factors.

The analysis and interpretation for the above data brings out the health problems and the health demands.

Establishment of Objectives and Goals

After analysis of the health situation, the next step in the planning process is to determine what to accomplish during the planning period means establishment of objectives. Objectives must be established at all levels. At the upper level, the objectives are general and in the successive lower levels, they become more specified. Objectives may be short-term or long-term in setting. These objectives and resources are important factions. Objectives are not only a guide to action but also yardsticks to measure the work after being done.

Assessment of Resources

For planning any program assessment of resource is very essential. So the resources to achieve objectives need to be determined. The term 'resource' implies manpower, money and materials and time needed. The human resources should be skillful, knowledgeable and training received for the implementation of a health program. Budgetary assessment and planning must be done like who is funding agency and how much time required to achieve objectives. Proper distribution of time is also important because nowadays time is an important resource which need to be considered. During planning the optimum uses of resources must be planned. These resources are assessed and verified between balance struck what is required and what is available.

Fixing Priorities

Once the problems, resources and objectives have been determined and resources also planned the next step is the establishment of priorities. Establishment of priorities can be done in order of importance of magnitude, cost-effectiveness and consequences of the problems. So in fixing priorities, the attention is paid to the financial constraints, mortality and morbidity data through which diseases can be prevented at a low cost, saving the lives of younger people when there has been considerable social investment and also political and community interest and pressure.

Write-up the Formulated Plan

The next major step in planning process as the preparation of the detailed plan or plans. The plan must be complete in all respect for the execution of a project.

For each proposed health program, the resources (inputs) required are related to the result of (output) expected. Each stage of the plan is defined casted and time needed to implement is specified. The plan must contain working guidance to all those responsibilities for execution.

Programming and Implementation

Once the health plan is selected and approved by the policy-making authorities, programming and implementation are begun. Plan execution depends upon the existence of an effective organization. The organizational structure must incorporate the well-defined procedures to be followed and sufficient delegation of authority to, and fixation of responsibility of, different workers for achieving the predefined objectives during the period prescribed. Sometimes pilot project may launched and the effectiveness observed before execution of the final project to check the effectiveness.

Monitoring and Evaluation

Monitoring and evaluation tell us as to how much we achieved our objectives. The evaluation plan should be developed before the implementation because evaluation is also an ongoing process, which can start when we just implement the program.

DEVELOPING AN EVALUATION PLAN

There are four main steps to developing an evaluation plan:
1. Clarifying program objectives and goals
2. Developing evaluation questions
3. Developing evaluation methods
4. Setting-up a timeline for evaluation activities

Clarifying Program Objectives and Goals

Setting goals or objectives is the 1st step of planning process but before evaluation we should clarifying it that what are the main things should be accomplished and how it should be accomplished. Clarifying these will help us in identifying which major program components should be evaluated. One way to do this is to make a table of program components and elements.

Developing Evaluation Questions

For our purposes, there are four main categories of evaluation questions. Let's look at some examples of possible questions and suggested methods to answer those questions.

- **Planning and implementation issues:** How well was the program or initiative planned out, and how well was that plan put into practice?
  - *Possible questions:* Who participates? Is there diversity among participants? Why do participants enter and leave your programs? Are there a variety of services and alternative activities generated? Do those most in need of help receive services? Are community members satisfied that the program meets local needs?
  - *Possible methods to answer those questions:* Monitoring system that tracks actions and accomplishments related to bringing about the mission of the initiative, member survey of satisfaction with goals, member survey of satisfaction with outcomes.
- **Assessing attainment of objectives:** How well has the program or initiative met its stated objectives?
  - *Possible questions:* How many people participated? How many hours are participants involved?
  - *Possible methods to answer those questions:* Monitoring system (see above), member survey of satisfaction with outcomes, goal attainment scaling.
- **Impact on participants:** How much and what kind of a difference has the program or initiative made for its targets of change?
  - *Possible questions:* How has behavior changed as a result of participation in the program? Are participants satisfied with the experience? Were there any negative results from participation in the program?
  - *Possible methods to answer those questions:* Member survey of satisfaction with goals, member survey of satisfaction with outcomes, behavioral surveys, interviews with key participants.
- **Impact on the community:** How much and what kind of a difference has the program or initiative made on the community as a whole?
  - *Possible questions:* What resulted from the program? Were there any negative results from the program? Do the benefits of the program outweigh the costs?
  - *Possible methods to answer those questions:* Behavioral surveys, interviews with key informants, community-level indicators.

Developing Evaluation Methods

Once evaluation questions is ready the evaluator wants to answer the evaluation questions, so the next step is to decide which methods will best address those questions. Some common evaluation methods are generally monitoring and feedback system, member surveys about the initiative, goal attainment report, behavioral surveys and interviews with key participants. In this step of evaluation plan which method will be the best will be analyzed and determined.

Setting-up a Timeline for Evaluation Activities

In this stage timeline for each activity will be determined. When evaluation need to begin, when the key evaluation questions will set-up and type of evaluation measures to be used to answer them (i.e., what kind of data will be needed to answer the question?). Type of data collection (i.e., what evaluation methods you will use to collect this data) and when do feedback and reports need to be provided. In the evaluation phase soon after implementation evaluation will be started with the evaluation plan. Monitoring and evaluation for the effectiveness of the program depicts the shortcoming which will help in modify the planning for actual implementation stage. This implementation and evaluation may be carried out for a small scale helps in modification of planning. Monitoring is the day-to-day follow-up of activities during their implementation to ensure that they are proceeding as planned and are on schedule. It is a continuous process of observing, recording and reporting on the activities of the organization or project.

Monitoring, thus, consists of keeping a track of the course of activities and identifying the deviations and taking corrective action if excessive deviation occurs and evaluation is the terminal assessment at the end. The purpose of evaluation is to assess the achievement of the stated objectives of a program. It is adequacy, it is efficiency and it is acceptance by all portions involved. While monitoring is confirmed today or by the ongoing operations, evaluation is mostly concerned with the final outcome and with the factors associated with it.

GENERAL STEPS OF EVALUATION PROCESS

Planning and evaluation may be carried out for a program or for an organization or for any policies at the large scale. Some common steps must be followed for evaluation of any activities which are described **(Fig. 8.2)**.

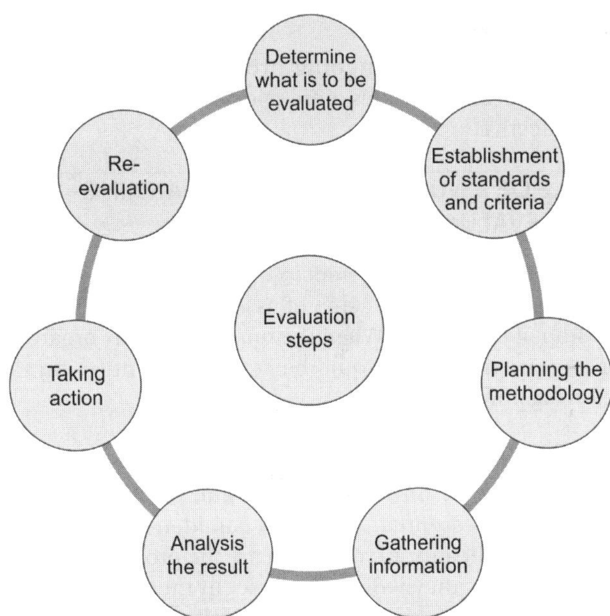

Fig. 8.2: Evaluation process.

Determine What is to be Evaluated

Generally speaking, there are three types of evaluation:

1. **Evaluation of structure:** This is the evaluation of whether facilities, equipment, manpower and organization meet the standards accepted by experts as good.
2. **Evaluation of process:** The process of medical care includes the problem of recognition, diagnostic procedures, treatment and clinical management, care and prevention. The environment in which the various activities of the program are carried out is evaluated by comparing with a predetermined standard. An objective and systematic way of evaluation by the physician's performance is known as 'medical audit.'
3. **Evaluation of outcome:** This is concerned with the end-result whether the person gets benefits from health services or not.

Establishment of Standards and Criteria

Standards and criteria must be established to determine how the desired objectives have been attained. Standards and criteria must be developed in accordance with the focus of the evaluation of the structural criteria, e.g., physical facilities and equipment.

Process criteria, e.g., every prenatal mother must have 6 check-ups. Outcome criteria, e.g., alteration in the patient's health status, etc.

Planning the Methodology

A format in keeping with the purpose of evaluation must be prepared for gathering the desired information. Standards and criteria must be included at the planning stage.

Gathering Information

Evaluation requires the collection of data or information. The type of information required may include political, cultural, economic, environmental and administrative factors influencing the health situation as well as the mortality and morbidity statistics. It may also concern health and related socioeconomic policies, plans and programs as well as the extent, scope, and use of the health systems, services and institutions.

Analysis of Results

The analysis and interpretation of data and feedback to all individuals concerned should take place within the shortest time possible once the information has been gathered. In addition, opportunities should provide for discussing the evaluation results.

Taking Action

For evaluation to be truly productive, emphasis should be placed on actions designed to support, strengthen or otherwise modify the service involved. This may also call for shifting priorities, revising objectives or development of new programs or services to meet the previously identified needs.

Re-evaluation

Re-evaluation is an ongoing process aimed mainly at rendering health activities more relevant, more efficient and more effective.

ROLE OF A NURSE IN PROGRAM PLANNING AND EVALUATION

The role of a nurse is different in different steps of program planning—from the first step of assessing the needs to the last step of evaluation. When the nurse is actually organizer for any program she should be keeping attention on the following points:

Assessing the Client's Needs

Before going for any health program, planning health assessment is essential. The nurse can identify the client's needs during health survey—what are the problems a client faced and how they will solve these. In the assessment of client's needs, she should find out the following facts:

- Who is the client?
- What needs are to be met?
- How is the clients' population to be served?
- Where are they located?
- Are any other programs addressing the same need?
- Why is the need not being met?

Establishing the Program

After assessing the need, the next step is establishing the program. In establishing the program, the nurse will decide about the following:

- What factors should be included?
- Who will be included and who will not be included and why?
- What are the causes which are excluded from the program?
- Is the program feasible, i.e., whether the program can be done or not?

Establishing the Objectives

Here the main responsibility of the nurse is selection of the objective. According to the problems and needs of the client, the objectives will be selected. The nurse should be aware about what objectives to be achieved and what are the expected outcomes of those.

Selecting the Resources

In selecting the resources, the nurse should check the resources, manpower, money and material that should be arranged.

Fixing Priorities

The nurse should prioritize the problems according to their severity, magnitude or financial constraints. She should divide the problems according to their mortality and morbidity data. Diseases can be prevented at low cost and saving the life of younger people can be prioritized first.

Selecting the Solution

In selecting the solution, the nurse should check whether the desire outcome will be achieved or not by selecting a particular program. She should select the solution and decide about the solutions that involve more risk and the solutions that involve low risk or are free of risk.

Implementation

Here in this stage she will actually implement the program. She will also monitor weather the program is running smoothly or not. She can monitor continuously the effectiveness of the program and the problems arises during the program for which she can found out solutions which will help her in later when the program will be planned in large scale.

Evaluation

- The nurse should evaluate how much the goal is achieved.
- Day-to-day follow-up activity or continuous monitoring should be done.
- The monitoring should be clubbed with feedback where the goal is not achieved.

In an evaluation, the nurse should evaluate the whole structure, process and outcomes of the program. She should select the evaluation tool. The standard and criteria must be fixed before the evaluation. She should gather all the required information about the program. Then she has to check how much the goal is achieved, whether it is fulfilled or partially fulfilled, in which area the goal is not achieved and what feedback is necessary. Then she should work on to strengthen that area for achieving the maximum outcomes.

Evaluation is also an ongoing process which runs parallel with planning. If any goal is not achieved, we will modify the whole planning process. **Table 8.1** shows history of planning India.

Table 8.1: History of planning India.

Time	*Health plan*
1934	Visvesvaraya planned in the book of 'The planned economy of India'. He was an Engineer, Ex-Diwan of Mysore and Bharat Ratna recipient
1938	Nehru's Congress plan. But not implemented due to world war II
1944	Bombay plan by noted industrialists such as JRD Tata, GD Birla, Kasturbhai Lalbhai et al.
1944	Sriman Narayan Agrawal's Gandhian plan
1945	MN Roy's 'people's plan'—with socialist leanings
1950	Jayprakash Narayan's Sarvodaya Plan based on Vinoba Bhave's philosophy
1950, March 15	Cabinet resolution to form Planning Commission
1952, August	National Development Council (NDC) made by Cabinet resolution
2014, August	Modi shuts down Planning Commission
2015, January	Government notified the formation of NITI Aayog—National Institution for Transforming India

HEALTH PLANNING IN INDIA

The economy of India was based in part on planning through its five-year plans, which were developed, executed and monitored by the planning commissions. The Planning Commission was set up in March 1950 by a resolution of the Government of India. The commission's original mandate was to raise the standard of living of ordinary Indians by efficiently exploiting the country's material and human resources, boosting production, and creating employment opportunities for all. With the Prime Minister as the ex-official Chairman, the Commission has a nominated Deputy Chairman, who has the rank of a Cabinet minister. The eleventh plan completed its term in March 2012 and when the twelve plan is underway, Prime Minister Narendra Modi has replace the Planning Commission with 'National Institution for Transforming India Aayog' or NITI Aayog. NITI Aayog has allowed the development of domain expertise which allows us the chance to increase the specificity of functions given to institutions. Specific to the planning process, there is a need to separate as well as energize the distinct 'process' of governance from the 'strategy' of governance. The new institution will be a catalyst to the developmental process; nurturing an overall enabling environment, through a holistic approach to development going beyond the limited sphere of the Public Sector and Government of India. This will be built on the foundations of an empowered role of States as equal partners in national development; operationalizing the principle of Cooperative Federalism.

THE NATIONAL HEALTH PLANS

First Five Year Plan (1951–56)

The First Indian Prime Minister, Jawaharlal Nehru presented the First Five-year Plan to the Parliament of India on 8th December 1951. The first plan sought to get the country's economy out of the cycle of poverty. The plan addressed, mainly the agrarian sector, including investments in dams and irrigation. Agriculture sector was hit hardest by the partition and needed urgent attention. During the first five year plan target growth was estimated 2.1% but the actual growth rate achieved is 3.6%.

Aim

- To fight against diseases, malnutrition, and unhealthy environment
- To build up health services for rural population and for mothers and children in order
- To improve general health status of the people.

Priorities

- Safe water supply and sanitation
- Control of malaria
- Health care of rural population
- Health services for mothers and children
- Education, training and health education
- Self-sufficiency in drugs and equipments
- Family planning and population control.

The Health Outlay

The total plan budget of 206.8 billion INR was allocated to seven broad areas:

- Irrigation and energy (27.2%)
- Agriculture and community development (17.4%)
- Transport and communication (24%)
- Industry (8.45%)
- Social services (16.64%)
- Land rehabilitation (4.1%)
- Others (2.5%)

The target growth rate was 2.1% annual gross domestic product (GDP) growth; the achieved growth rate was 3.6%. During the first five year plan the net domestic product went up by 15%.

A sum of ₹140 crores was allocated for health programs during the first five year plan which was 5.9% of the total outlay (₹2356 crores) for the entire development plan.

Major Development

- To meet the identified priority areas.
- The objectives are presented below according to year-wise sequence.

The Year 1951

It was started with outlay of ₹2,356 crores. BCG Vaccination Programme was initiated in the country to prevent and control tuberculosis.

The Year 1952

- A Pilot project of Community Development Programme was launched in 55 project areas on 2nd October, the birthday of Mahatma Gandhi to get rid of three ills from the society namely poverty, ill health and ignorance through bovver, all development of the rural areas.
- The central council of health was set up.
- Primary Health Centres were set up to render health services in rural areas.
- Virus Research Centre was set up in Pune.
- 'Auxiliary Nurse Midwife' (ANM) training was started to train ANM to function in a network of subcenter and Primary health centers in the rural areas and provide comprehensive Maternal Child Health (MCH) and Family Welfare services under the district supervision of lady health visitors/public health nurse at the block level.

The Year 1953

- The community development program was extended to National level on 2nd October and was called as community development and National Extension Service Programme.
- National Malaria Control Programme was launched.
- National Smallpox Eradication Programme was launched.

- National Family Planning Programme was launched.
- A committee was set up to draft a model Public Health Act for the country.

The Year 1954

- The contributory central Government Health scheme was started at Delhi.
- The central social welfare Board was set up.
- The National Leprosy Control Programme was launched.
- The National Water Supply and Sanitation Programme was launched.
- The prevention of Food Adulteration Act was enacted.
- VDRL Antigen Production center was set up at Kolkata.
- Shetty committee was constituted by the Government of India in 19th May 1954 to survey the existing facilities for nursing services and emoluments available to nurses, to assess minimum requirements of nurses in the country and to overcome the shortage of nurses and improve service conditions.

The Year 1955

- The National Filaria Control Programme was launched.
- A Filaria Training center was set up at Ernakulum, Kerala.
- The Central Leprosy Teaching and Research Institute was started at Chingelput, Madras (Chennai now).
- National TB sample survey was started.
- The minimum marriage age of 18 years for boys and 15 for girls was prescribed by Hindu Marriage Act.

With all these developments, health and medical facilities improved. Health services were rendered to rural population from the primary health centers (PHC).

Second Five Year Plan (1956–61)

The second five year plan focused on industry, especially heavy industry. Domestic production of industrial products was encouraged, particularly in the development of the public sector.

Aim

- To expand existing health services to bring them within the reach of all people.
- To promote progressive improvement of Nation's health.

Priorities

The priorities of the second five year plan were:

- Establishment of Institutional facilities for rural as well as for urban population.
- Development of technical manpower.
- Control of communicable diseases.
- Water supply and sanitation.
- Family planning and other supporting programs.

The Health Outlay

An outlay of ₹225 crores was allocated for the second five year plan for health programs which was 5.0% of the entire outlay for the total development plan. This proportionate outlay was less than the first five year plan by 9%.

The Major Developments

The major developments of the second five year plan in accordance to priorities areas were as under.

The Year 1956

- Draft Model Public Health Act was prepared by the committee and published.
- Director, Family planning was appointed at the center.
- The Demographic Training and Research Centre was established in Mumbai.
- The central Health Education Bureau was set up at the center.
- The immoral Traffic Act was enacted.
- The Tuberculosis Chemotherapy Centre was set of at Madras (Chennai).
- The RCA project was launched by the central Government with the support of Ford Foundation.
- The pilot project of Trachoma Control Programme was launched.

The Year 1957

The demographic research centers were established in Delhi, Kolkata and Madras (Chennai).

The Year 1958

- The National Malaria Control Programme was converted into National Eradication Programme.
- The National Tuberculosis survey was completed.
- The Leprosy Advisory committee of the Government of India was launched.
- A three tire structures were recommended as self-governing bodies at villages, districts and tehsils.

The Year 1959

- The Mudaliar Committee was set up by the Government of India to undertake the review of developments that have taken place since the submission of Bhore Committee's report and to make recommendations from further developments and expansion of health services.
- Panchayati Raj was introduced in Rajasthan.
- The Nutrition Research Laboratory at Coonoor was shifted to Hyderabad.
- The National Institute of Tuberculosis was established at Bengaluru.
- A central expert committee was constituted under the ICMR to study the problem of smallpox and cholera in India. The committee recommended programs for their eradication.

The Year 1960

Pilot projects of smallpox eradication were started.

- Pilot study of smallpox eradication
- A national nutrition advisory committee was formed

- Vital statistics were transformed from DGHS to registrar general of India.

Third Five Year Plan (1961–66)

Aim

To remove the shortages and deficiencies which were observed at the end of the 2nd five year plan in the field of health. These were pertaining to institutional facilities especially in rural areas, shortages of trained personnel and supplies, lack of safe drinking water in rural areas and inadequate drainage system.

Outlay: Total: ₹7500 crores, For health programmes: ₹342 crores (4.3%).

Achievements

- Mudaliar committee report submitted and published (1961).
- Setting up central institute of family welfare.
- Smallpox eradication, goiter control, beginning of national school health programmes.
- Establishment of national institute of communicable diseases, Delhi.
- Mukherji committee report regarding strategies for family planning (1965) and Jungalwala committee report (1967) on health services were also published during this plan.
- Trachoma Control Programme and Chadah committee report on malaria eradication was also presented during this period.

Plan Holiday: 1966–69: 1966 and 1968 (Famine Years)

The 4th FYP which was to commence from 1966 was postponed till 1969. India faced two wars one with China in 1962 and then with Pakistan in 1965. Economic difficulties disrupted the planning process in the mid 1960s. The uncertain economic situation in the country came as a huge set back to the economy as defense expenditure increased sharply and there was negative impact on industrial and agriculture growth. This intervening period was covered by annual plans with an outlay of 6756 crores, of which 316 crores (4.7%) were allotted for health programmes. Three annual plans guided development between FY 1966 and FY 1968 while plan policies and strategies were re-evaluated.

Fourth Five Year Plan (1969–73)

Aim

To strengthen PHC network in the rural areas for undertaking preventive, curative, family planning services and to take over the maintenance phase of communicable diseases.

Outlay: Total: 16774 crores, For health programmes: 1156 crores (7.2%).

Achievements

- Chittaranjan mobile hospitals (1970)
- Postpartum Family Planning Programme (1970)
- Medical termination of pregnancy facility (1971)
- Multipurpose health workers scheme (1973)
- National programme of minimum needs (1973).

Fifth Five Year Plan (1974–79)

Aim

To provide minimum level of well integrated health, MCH and FP, nutrition and immunization to all the people with special reference to vulnerable groups especially children, pregnant women, and nursing mothers, through a network of infrastructure in all the blocks and well-structured referral system.

Outlay: Total-37250 crores, For health programs-3277 crores (8.8%).

Achievement

- Rural health scheme (1977)
- Integrated child development scheme (1975)
- Community health workers scheme (1977)
- National Malaria Eradication Programme was replaced by modified plan of operation (1977)
- 20 point programme (1975)
- India was declared free from smallpox (1975)
- National Programme for Prevention of blindness (1976)
- Shrivastava committee report on providing three tier health services in rural areas was submitted (1976)
- ICDS was launched, National health and family planning institute were set up (1977) and India accepted Alma-Ata declaration (health for all)
- Reorientation of medical education scheme (1977)
- Expanded programme of immunization (1978)
- Parliament approved child marriage restraint act (1978).

Sixth Five Year Plan (1980–85)

Aim

To work out alternative strategy and plan of action for primary health care as part of national health system, which is accessible to all section of society.

Outlay: Total-97500 crores, For health programs-1822 crores (1.87%).

Achievements During 6th FYP

- Alma Ata Declaration on PHC-1979
- HFA/2000 AD-1981
- National health policy-1983
- The national drinking water and sanitation decade-1981
- Leprosy Control Programme switched over to Leprosy Eradication Programme-1983 Guinea worm Eradication Programme—1983
- Government of India pledged to provide safe drinking water.
- Air pollution prevention Act and National health policy were also announced (1983).
- Bhopal gas tragedy (1984) was registered as a catastrophe from the perspective of public health.

Seventh Five Year Plan (1985–90)

Aim

To plan and provide primary health care and medical services to all with special consideration of vulnerable groups and to attain health for all by 2000 AD.

Outlay: Total 180,000 crores, For health programmes- 3392 crores (1.9%).

- Universal Immunization Programme (1985) and Safe Motherhood Programme were launched.
- National Aids Control Programme (1989) was started.
- Control of Acute Respiratory Infection Programme (1990).

Annual Plans (1990–1992)

The Eighth Plan could not take off in 1990 due to the fast changing political situation at the center and the years 1990–91 and 1991–92 were treated as Annual Plans. The Eighth Plan was finally formulated for the period 1992–1997.

Eighth Five Year Plan (1992–97)

Aim

To continue organization and strengthening of health infrastructure and medical services accessible to all especially to vulnerable groups and those living in tribal, hilly, remote rural areas etc.

Outlay: Total-79,800 crores, For health programs-7576 crores (9.5%).

'Health of all': Government paid special attention to provide health services to the most needy, poorest and impoverished segment of society.

- Indian system of medicine were encouraged.
- Act on infant feeding and Infant foods (1992).
- Child Survival and Safe Motherhood (CSSM) Programmes started (1992).
- Reproductive and Child Health Programme (1994).
- Announcement of revised National Drug Policy (1995).
- Revised national TB Control Programme (1997).
- IGNOU started a three year Postbasic BSc Nursing Programme (1995).

Ninth Five Year Plan (1997–2002)

Aim

'Growth with Social Justice and Equity' same as 8th FYP. Nursing education and nursing services have been given a high priority in order to bridge the large gap between requirement and availability of nurses and ensure quality of nursing training. Efforts are made to meet the increasing demand for nurses with specialized training in specialty and subspecialty areas intensive medical and surgical care in hospitals and for public health nurses in healthcare system. Ninth five year plan targets have included fulfilling the health requirement of women, adolescents and children, improving the quality of services and increasing the coverage.

Outlay: Total-859,200 crores, For health programs-10818 crores (1.25%).

Achievements During 9th FYP

- Intensive Pulse Polio immunization Programme (1999)
- National Population Policy (2000)
- National health policy (2000)
- Guinea worm disease was eradicated.
- Planned Parenthood, control of STDs/STIs and AIDS/HIV.
- Finding the shortcoming and faults in conducting national health programme and removing them.
- Recognizing the basic structure of family welfare.
- Paying special attention to IEC training, the trainers at the National and District levels.
- Giving specific importance to RCH.
- Increasing health awareness in community and making efforts for setting up of education commission in health services for medical, dentistry, pharmacy and nursing personnel.
- Arranging funds for the female health workers at subcenters.

Tenth Five Year Plan (2002–2007)

Aim

- To improve the efficiency of existing health care infrastructure at primary, secondary and tertiary care setting
- To attain universal primary education
- Gender equality

Outlay: Total-9,21,291 crores, For health programs-9,253 crores (1%).

New Initiatives in the Tenth Plan

- The Reproductive and Child Health Programme, Phase II (2005–10)
- Janani Suraksha Yojana Support for six tertiary-level institutions on the lines of AIIMS, Delhi in the six backward states of Bihar, Madhya Pradesh, Odisha, Rajasthan, Chhattisgarh and Uttaranchal
- Integrated Disease Surveillance Project National Mental Health Programme
- A Capacity Building Project Expanding outreach of AYUSH
- Two new national programs: National Programme on Diabetes and Cardiovascular Diseases and National Programme on Hearing and Speech Impairment.

Recommendations

- Implementation of a National Rural Health Mission
- Implementation of a National Mission on Sanitation and Public Health Provide access to maternity health Insurance and community risk pooling. Systematization of insurance at secondary health care levels through reform of the CGHS.
- Institutionalization of public private partnerships in health care.
- Set up of a Public Health Development Authority.
- Set up of a National Authority for Drugs and Therapeutics.

Task Force

- Attain 8% GDP growth per year.
- Reduction of poverty ratio by 5% points by 2007.
- Providing gainful and high-quality employment at least to the addition to the labor force.
- All children in India in school by 2003; all children to complete 5 years of schooling by 2007.
- Reduction in gender gaps in literacy and wage rates by at least 50% by 2007.
- Reduction in the decadal rate of population growth between 2001 and 2011 to 16.2%.
- Increase in Literacy Rates to 75% within the Tenth Plan period (2002 to 2007).
- Making proper linkage between the primary, secondary and tertiary care.
- Developing appropriate referral system by utilizing IT and communication.
- Increasing the involvement of voluntary and private organizations in improving healthcare system.
- Increasing the efficiency of existing healthcare system in all sectors: government, private or voluntary.
- Improvement in quality of undergraduate/postgraduate education.

Eleventh Five Year Plan (2007–2012)

Aim

- Achieve an overall growth rate of 7.6%.
- Reduce poverty levels from 38 to 25%
- Achieve the literacy rate of 84% by the end of the Plan and reduce gender gap in literacy to 14%.
- Achieve reduction in dropout rate from 46.8% in 2003–04 to 20% by 2011–12 and eliminate gender disparity in elementary education.
- Bring down population growth rate to 1.62% by 2012.
- Reduce infant mortality ratio to 28 and maternal mortality ratio to 1 per 1000 live births.
- Reduce Total Fertility Rate to 2.1.
- Provide clean drinking water for all by 2009 and ensure that there are no slip-backs.
- Reduce malnutrition among children of age group 0–3 to half its present level.
- Reduce anemia among women and girls by 50% by the end of the plan.
- Raise the sex ratio for age group 0–6 to 935 by 2011–12 and to 950 by 2016–17.
- Ensure that at least 33% of the direct and indirect beneficiaries of all government schemes are women and girl children.
- Ensure that all children enjoy a safe childhood, without any compulsion to work.

Steering Committees

Planning Commission has constituted a High Level Expert Group (HLEG) on universal health coverage, seven Working Groups and Two Steering Committees to define the appropriate strategy for the Health sector for the XII Plan.

The Steering Committee on Health has identified following structural problem with the health sector:

- **Identifying structural problems:** The healthcare system in the country suffers from inadequate funding. There are several structural problems identified in health sectors too, like, the lack of integration between different programs in the social sector, minimum or no use of traditional systems of Medicines, feeble regulatory-systems for drugs as well as for medical practice and in proper public health management. A sound health system also requires the active participation of communities in preventive and promotive health care, on which the progress has been uneven.
- **National health outcome goals for the twelfth plan:** The Steering Committee on Health in its report has recommended health system for the 12th Plan should prioritize the making of the system responsive to the needs of citizens and the attainment of financial protection for the health care of households. More specifically, the national health outcome goals, which are meant to reflect the broader commitments during the 12th Plan.

Task Force

Planning for Human Resources in the Health Sector.

Working Groups

- Health Informatics including Tele-Medicine
- Public Health Services (including Water and Sanitation)
- Health on Women and Children
- Health Systems Research, Biomedical Research and Development and Regulation of Drugs and Therapeutics
- Population stabilization
- Integrating nutrition with health
- Clinical Establishments, Professional Services Regulation and Accreditation of Health Care Infrastructure
- Access to Health Systems including AYUSH
- Communicable and Non-Communicable Diseases
- Health Care Financing including Health Insurance
- Public Private Partnership to improve healthcare delivery.

The Planning Commission was charged with the responsibility of making assessment of all resources of the country, augmenting deficient resources, formulating plans for the most effective and balanced utilization of resources and determining priorities.

12th Five Year Plan

Introduction

The eleventh plan completed in March 2012 and the twelfth plan start from April 2012. With a renewed commitment to public health. That are:

- The directive principles of state policy in the constitution of India mandate 'improvement of public health' as one of the primary duties of the state.
- The central and state government have been taking proactive steps to promote health of the people by creating

a network of public healthcare facilities, which provide free medical services, and also proactively control the spread of diseases.

- The prime minister in his independence day speech (2011) stressed upon the need to provide access to improved health services to all.
- Government has decided to increase its total health expenditure to 2.5% of GDP by the end of twelfth plan.
- A high-level meeting chaired by prime minister also decided that the planning commission be requested to allocate adequate resources for the health sector to achieve the target, for which it could seek cooperation of the state.

Objectives of Health System

- Lower mortality, raise of expectancy.
- Lower morbidity, raise quality of healthy life lived.
- Financial protection.
- Choice to consumer.
- Welfare state: Principle of state society.
- Health is a state subject: Public health and sanitation; hospital and dispensaries.
- Items in concurrent event list are vital statistics, medical education, medical profession, food and drug, population control, spread of infectious disease across state.

12th Plan Strategy

- Strengthening the public sector health care.
- Substantially increase in healthcare expenditure.
- Efficient financial and managerial system.
- Coordinated delivery of services.
- Expansion of skilled human resource.
- Prescription drugs reform.
- Effective regulation through a public health cadre.
- Inclusive agenda.
- Pilots on universal health care.

Goals of 12th 5 Year Plan

- Reduce maternal mortality from 212 to 100
- Reduce IMR from 44 to 25
- Reduce underweight children below 3 years from 40 to 23%
- Increase child sex ratio from 914 to 950
- Reduce levels of anemia among women from 55 to 28%
- Reduce total fertility rate from 2.5 to 2.1
- Reduce poor households' out-of-pocket expenditure on health.

Policy Prescription

Reduction of Maternal Mortality Ratio (MMR)

- At historical rate of decline, India is projected to have an MMR of 149 by 2015 and 127 by 2017.
- An achievement of millennium development goal (MDG) of reducing MMR to 109 by 2015 would require a further acceleration rate of decline, the country can achieve the MMR of 75 by 2017.

Reduction of Infant Mortality Rate (IMR)

- At historical rate of decline, India is a project to have an IMR of 38 by 2015 and 34 by 2017.
- To achievement of the MDG of reducing IMR to 27 by 2015 would require an event further acceleration of this historical rate of decline. If this accelerated rate is sustained, the country can achieve an IMR of 19 by 2017.

Reduction of Total Fertility Rate (TFR)

India is on track for the achievement of a TFR target of 2.1 by 2017, which is necessary to achieve net replacement level of unity, and realize the long cherished goal of national population policy of 2000.

Prevention and Reduction of Underweight Children Under 3 Years

- Underweight children are at a risk of mortality rate and also morbidity rate. At the current rate of decline, the prevalence of underweight children is expected to be 29% by 2015, and 27% by 2017.
- The achievement of the MDG of reducing undernourished children under 3 years to 26% by 2015 would require an acceleration of this historical rate of decline.

Prevention and Reduction of Anemia among Aged 15–49 Years

- Anemia, the underlying determinate of MMR and LBW, is preventable and treatable by a very simple intervention.
- The prevalence of anemia has shown a rising trend (58.8% in 2007) which need to be prevent and reduced to 28%, which is half the current levels, by the end of 12th plan.

Raising Sex Ratio in the 0–6 Years Age Group

Like anemia child sex ratio is showing a deteriorating trend, and needs to be targeted for priority attention.

Prevention and Reduction of Burden of Diseases

- These add to the burden of diseases, reduce longevity, add to health expenditure and are very amenable to public health and preventive measure.
- Target of these conditions can be set by the MOHFW as robust systems are put in place to measure their burden.

Reduction of Households 'Out-of-Pocket' Expenditure from 71 to 50% of Total Healthcare Expenditure

Out-of-pocket expenditure on health care burden on families, particularly the poor ones. These need to be lowered to tolerable level in the 12th plan.

NATIONAL INSTITUTION FOR TRANSFORMING INDIA AAYOG

The National Institution for Transforming India Aayog or NITI Aayog is a Government of India policy think-tank established by Prime Minister Narendra Modi to replace

Table 8.2: Functional differentiation between planning commission and NITI Aayog.

Planning Commission	*NITI Aayog*
Design Five year plans	Design national agenda, and cooperative federalism
Decide two 'money' matters: 1. How much money to give to each state for centrally sponsored schemes (CSS) 2. How much money to give for each state's own state-five-year-plans	• Mostly work as a 'policy-formulation-hub'. The Press release is 'silent' on money/funding. So, most probably it'll be left to finance ministry • Some experts believe Interstate council will decide money allocation to states, then finance ministry will release the fund
3. States/UT were represented in National Development Council 4. PC framed FYP=>went to Cabinet=>NDC approved FYP=>Tabled in parliament	• States/UT represented in Governing council. But no specific mention about whether they can approve/reject/amend NITI Aayog's proposals?
5. One size fits all, top-down socialist planning by Armchair Nehruvian economists and IES cadre officers (Indian Economic Service)	• Press release talks about participatory planning but how exactly will they do that? No specific details laid out • IES officers are rarely invited in Modi's meetings • But given the entry of Free market economists and Technocrats, most probably it'll be an 'indicative planning + core planning', i.e., after inputs of state governments, a broad outline with selected targets, limited subsidies and monitoring through ICT

the Planning Commission. India has undergone a paradigm shift over the past six decades— politically, economically, socially, technologically as well as demographically. The role of Government in national development has seen a parallel evolution. Keeping with these changing times The Government has replaced Planning Commission with a new institution named NITI Aayog (National Institution for Transforming India. NITI will include leaders of India's 29 states and seven union territories). But its full-time staff—a Deputy Chairman, Chief Executive Officer and experts—will answer directly to the Prime Minister of India, who will be chairman. The Planning Commission was constituted on 15.3.1950 through a Government of India Resolution, and has served India well. India, however, has changed dramatically over the past 65 years. While this has been at multiple levels and across varied scales, the biggest transformatory forces are demographic and economical change, influence of private enterprise, globalization, development of States and Advancements in technology which urge to change in planning process. There are some functional differentiation between planning commission and NITI Aayog which are described in **Table 8.2**.

NITI Aayog and Healthcare Sector

India's progress in health outcomes has been slower in comparison to other countries with comparable incomes and at a similar stage of development. For instance, infant mortality rate (IMR) in India has declined by 50% from 1990 to 2012, while the decline in countries such as Bangladesh (67%), Nepal (66%) and Cambodia (60%) has been steeper for the same period.

NITI Aayog in its report on 'Health System in India, Bridging the Gap between Current Performance and Potential', has pointed out that the healthcare needs to access efficient systems are adequate funding resources. The country's polio elimination, lowering fertility rate, decrease in HIV prevalence, fall in malaria fatality are attributed to National Rural Health Mission (NRHM) through deployment of additional human resources, over 18,000 ambulances for free emergency response, and cash transfers to one crore women annually.

Currently, there is an absence of standard treatment guidelines. There is need to create a reliable routine clinical processes with accountability structures. There should be measurable improvements in quality of care focusing on patient safety, comfort, satisfaction, and clinical outcomes. Indian healthcare systems must place data systems that ensure monitoring, continual certification, verify processes of outcomes, and patient experiences, providing access to maternal healthcare services.

The government has consistently struggled to provide GDP for health care and was banking on increasing investments in public sector health care, it said, adding it was an astounding leap of faith fraught with potentially unfortunate consequences—that free services will be rationed as per budget/manpower availability.

Aims of NITI Aayog in Challenging Health Care

The NITI Aayog's health division has observed glaring issues in health care with limited budget allocation. Disparity in health care exists across states and there is an excessive focus on vertical disease control programs and inadequate attention to health system strengthening. Enormous challenges are facing the sector with limited funds. The government will need to look at maximizing returns from available financial resources and also increase investments in health, views the NITI Aayog health division. The NITI Aayog's views are in contrast to the redrafted National Health Policy. The policy had recommended investing 2.5% of gross domestic product (GDP) on health care by 2020 and investing most of it in public health care systems, using the private sector only to fill the gaps. It had laid down general taxation as the route to mobilize resources, including a health cess along the lines of an education cess.

The policy has objected to increasing investments and focusing on the public health sector as well as providing free drugs and diagnostics, as suggested in the updated draft National Health Policy of the National Democratic Alliance (NDA) government.

It has recommended that the private sector and insurance-based models be given a greater role in a public health system that would require people to pay for health services. The government's think tank, in its letter to the health ministry, has suggested that the recently launched insurance schemes of the government should be the basis for reworking the health policy.

While advocating against free health services to the people, the NITI Aayog has asked that a contributory sickness fund will be created. People would contribute to this fund and through it they will be able to purchase health services from private and public sectors, according to their choice.

The draft health policy, in contrast, had noted that public services provided a greater bang for the buck. 'The public sector is value for money as it accounts for less than 30% of total expenditure, but provides for about 20% of outpatient care and 40% of in-patient care. This same expenditure also pays for 60% of end-of-life care (RGI estimates on hospital mortality), and almost 100% of preventive and promotive care and a substantial part of medical and nursing education as well.'

Giving examples of developing countries which have a higher proportion of public health services the policy said, 'Health outcomes and financial protection are closely related to absolute and relative levels of public health expenditure. It would be desirable but ambitious if India could aspire to a public health expenditure of 4% of GDP, but most expert groups have estimated 2.5% as being more realistic. At such levels of expenditure, 'purchasing,' would have to be mainly from public providers for efficient use of resources with purchasing from private providers only for supplementation.' The NITI Aayog has raised several objections against increasing investments and dependence on public health infrastructure. The draft health policy had said India's investments in health sector, at large, and in public health sector, specifically, are much lower than in most other developing countries that had delivered better health statistics.

The government think tank said, The NITI Aayog policy document does not specifically indicate a framework for engaging private sector providers, barring expressing intent of regulating their quality through appropriate legislation or seeing the private sector as a resource for filling critical gaps in the public sector. The government's think tank, in its letter to the health ministry, has suggested that the recently launched insurance schemes of the government should be the basis for reworking the health policy. But it noted: 'Yes, we might say that the benefit package could be comparatively generous; but it is an issue which can be dealt with as the government gets more financial leewa.

The role of states in the planning commission era was limited. The states annually needed to interact with the planning commission to get their annual plan approved. They had some limited function in the National Development Council. Since NITI Aayog has all chief ministers of states and administrators of UT in its Governing Council, it is obvious that states are expected to have greater role and say in planning/implementation of policies. The top down approach is reversed in NITI Aayog. It will develop mechanisms to formulate credible plans to the village level and aggregate these progressively at higher levels of government. The provision of regional council is there in NITI Aayog to address local/regional development issues. One of the new functions of NITI Aayog is to address the need of the National Security in the economic strategy. How this is to be done is yet to be watched. While the planning commission formed Central Plans, NITI Ayog will not formulate them anymore. It has been vested with the responsibility of evaluating the implementation of programs. In this way, while NITI Aayog retains the advisory and monitoring functions of the Planning commission, the function of framing Plans and allocating funds for Plan assisted schemes has been taken away. The governing council, which has all chief ministers of states and administrators of the Union Territories sounds much like the National Development.

INVOLVEMENT OF STAKEHOLDER IN HEALTH PLANNING

Stakeholders are people or organizations invested in the program, interested in the success of the program through evaluation, and/or with a stake in what will be done with the results of the evaluation. Representing their needs and interests throughout the process is fundamental to good program evaluation. Stakeholders are individuals and organizations that have an interest in or are affected by your evaluation and/or its results. Stakeholders provide a reality check on the appropriateness and feasibility of your evaluation questions, offer insight on and suggest methods to access the target populations, provide ongoing feedback and recommendations, and help make evaluation results actionable.

Who are the Stakeholders?

Key stakeholders who can involve in health programs fall into three major groups:

1. **Those involved in program operations:** Management, program staff, partners, funding agencies, and coalition members.
2. **Those served or affected by the program:** Patients or clients, advocacy groups, community members, and elected officials.
3. **Those who are intended users of the evaluation findings:** Persons in a position to make decisions about the program, such as partners, funding agencies, coalition members, and the general public or taxpayers. If we will implement an STD screening program then the different types of stakeholder should be involved in planning the program are discussed in **Table 8.3**.

Table 8.3: Definition and examples of different types of stakeholders.

Types of stakeholders	*Definition*	*Examples*
Implementers	Those directly involved in the operations of the STD program	• STD director • STD program manager • Staff (field operation manager, frontline supervisor, Disease Intervention Specialist (DIS), service providers, health educations, laboratory technicians, clerical staff, among others volunteers and consultant)
Decision makers	Those in a position to do or decide something about the STD program	• STD director • STD program manager • Health department director
Participants	Those being served or affected by the STD program	• Clients/patients • Community members • Community-based organizations (CBOs) • Health service providers/STD clinic staff

Why Stakeholders are Important to an Evaluation?

Stakeholders can help an evaluation before it is conducted, while it is being conducted, and after the results are collected and ready for use. Because so many public health efforts are complex and because public health agencies may be several layers removed from frontline implementation, stakeholders take on particular importance in ensuring that the right evaluation questions are identified an d that evaluation results will be used to make a difference. Stakeholders are much more likely to support the evaluation and act on the results and recommendations if they are involved in the evaluation process. Conversely, without stakeholder support, your evaluation may be ignored, criticized, resisted, or even sabotaged.

Use the evaluation standards to help identify those stakeholders who matter most. Give priority to those stakeholders who:

- Can increase the credibility of your efforts or your evaluation
- Are responsible for day-to-day implementation of the activities that are part of the program
- Will advocate for or authorize changes to the program that the evaluation may recommend
- Will fund or authorize the continuation or expansion of the program.
- Involve stakeholders in key activities throughout the planning and implementation of the evaluation.
- Some of these activities can include:
  - Identifying and prioritizing program activities that need to be evaluated.
  - Overcoming resistance to evaluation and identifying the benefits.
  - Developing evaluation questions that are grounded in the perceptions, experiences, and interests of stakeholders.
  - Selecting appropriate and acceptable evaluation methods.
  - Reviewing evaluation findings and making program recommendations.
  - Disseminating and using evaluation findings for program improvement.

NATIONAL HEALTH POLICY

Introduction

Health policy is the expression of what health care system should be, so that it can meet the health care needs of the people. The Ministry of Health and Family Welfare, Government of India evolved a National Health Policy in 1983 to attain the objective of 'health for all by 2000 AD'. Health policy is not only linked with health but it also gives an emphasis on other social developmental areas, like education, employment, population, economics, etc.

Evolution

- During the British Period, for the services of elite people, interest was paid to improve medical services through hospitals and dispensaries. There is rapid growth of drug industry, commercialization. Public health was highly neglected, resulting in high mortality and morbidity.
- After independence, health services were based on the directions of the Bhore Committee and then the subsequent committees.
- The formal health policy was formulated in the year 1983.

National Health Policy (NHP), 1983

The policy provided political commitment and support to the administration in taking decisions and actions which were essential for attaining HFA through primary health care approach.

Primary Objectives

To attain the goal of HFA by 2000 AD, by establishing an efficient health care system, which is accessible to all citizens, especially vulnerable groups, like women, children and the underprivileged.

- It strongly stresses on:
  - Primary health care infrastructure
  - Coordination with health-related services
  - Active involvement of voluntary organization
  - Provision of essential drugs and vaccines
  - Qualitative improvement in health and family planning services
  - Provision of adequate training
  - Medical research on common health problems.
- It has the following key elements:
  - Creation of greater awareness of health problem by the community

Table 8.4: Targets and achievements of health indicators by 2000 AD.

Indicator	*Targets by 2000 AD*	*Achievement*
CBR	21	26.1
CDR	9	8.7
IMR	<60	70
PMR	30.35	44.2
Under-five mortality	10	23.7
MMR	<2	4
Life expectancy	64	64.6
Family size	2.8	3
NRR	1	1.5
Couple protection rate	60	43.5
Annual growth rate	1.22	2.1
TT for pregnant	100	79
DPT	85	92.5
Polio	85	93.4
BCG	85	99.1

- Supply of safe drinking water and basic sanitation using technologies that people can afford
- Reduction of existing imbalance in health care by concentrating rural health infrastructure
- Establishing dynamic HMIS which will help in health planning and implementation of health programs
- Providing legislative support to health protection and promotion
- Concerned action to combat widespread malnutrition
- Research in alternative methods of health care delivery and low-cost health technologies
- Greater coordination of different systems of medicine.

Table 8.4 shows targets and achievements of health indicators by 2000 AD.

Note: Evaluation of the progress for HFA is done on the basis of achievement of the targets which are defined globally by WHO and nationally by the respective government.

This is a substantial progress by 2000 AD. There has also been a decline in vaccine-preventable diseases due to an improvement in the immunization coverage. Smallpox, Guinea worm, and polio have been eradicated countrywide. Water-borne diseases are also much less than before.

Note: But TB, malaria, malnutrition, diseases related to lifestyle, like DM, HTN are still major public health problems.

Factors Interfering with Progress Towards HFA

- Insufficient political commitment
- Failure to achieve equity in access to all primary health care elements
- Low status of women
- Slow socioeconomic development
- Unbalanced distribution and weak support for human resources
- Widespread inadequacy of health promotion activities
- Weak health information system and no baseline data
- Pollution, poor food, safety, and lack of water supply and sanitation
- Rapid demographic and epidemiological changes
- Inappropriate use and allocation of resources, high-cost technologies
- Natural and manmade disasters.

National Health Policy, 2002

Introduction

Considering the kind and level of progress, the barriers and the change in health problems, and the circumstances, the Health and Family Welfare Department felt it necessary to formulate a new health policy.

Objectives

To achieve acceptable standard of good health amongst the general population of the country.

Approaches

- To increase the access to the decentralized public health system by establishing new infrastructure in deficit areas and upgrading the infrastructure in the existing institution
- Increasing importance would be given to ensuring equitable access to health services across the country
- Emphasis will be given to increasing the aggregate public health instrument through a substantially increased contribution by the central government to strengthen the capacity of public health administration at the state level
- **PPP:** The contribution of the private sector in providing health services would be much enhanced, particularly for that particular section of the society which can afford to pay for services
- Primacy will be given to preventive 7 first-line curative initiatives at the primary level
- Emphasis will be given on rational use of drugs within the allopathic system
- Increased access to the tried and tested system of traditional medicine will be ensured. **Table 8.5** shows goals to be achieved by 2000–2015.

National Health Policy, 2002—Policy Prescription

Financial Resources

- Taking into account the gap in health care facilities. It is planned under the policy to increase health sector expenditure to 6% GDP, with 2% of GDP being contributed as public health involvement by the year 2010.
- For public health investment, the central government's contribution would rise to 25% from the existing 15% by 2010.

Equity

In order to meet the various types of inequities and imbalances between regions, i.e., rural and urban, the most

Table 8.5: Goals to be achieved by 2000–2015.

Goals	*Target time (years)*
Eradication of polio and yaws	2005
Eliminate leprosy	2005
Eliminate kala-azar	2010
Eliminate lymphatic filariasis	2015
Achieve zero-level growth of HIV/AIDS	2007
Reduce mortality by 50% on account of TB, malaria and other vector- and water-borne diseases	2010
Reduce prevalence of blindness to 0.5%	2010
Reduce IMR to 30/1000 and MMR to 100/1 lakh	2010
Increase utilization of public health facilities from current level of <20 to >75	2010
Establish an integrated system of surveillance, national health accounts and statistics	2005
Increase health expenditure by government as a percentage of GDP from 0.9% to 2% increase share of central	2010
Increase central grants to constitute at least 25% of total health-spending	2010
Increase state sector health-spending from 5.5 to 7% of the budget	2005
Further increase to 8%	2010

cost-effective method is to strengthen the existing outlay and opening the additional public health service outlets.

Delivery of National Health Programs

In this policy, the central government designs health program with active participation of the state government. The central government provides functional, technical, monitoring and evaluation services.

- Optimal utilization of public health infrastructure at primary level.
- Vertical programs for control of major diseases, like TB, malaria, HIV/AIDS, RCH, immunization, etc. to be continued till moderate level prevalence is reached.
- The rural health staff should be available for the entire range of public health activities.

State Public Health Infrastructure

- It recognizes the need for frequent in-service training of public health MOs and paramedics
- Additional financial resources are placed for strengthening of primary health structure for attaining the improved public health outcomes on an equitable basis
- It also recognizes the practical need for levying reasonable user-charges for certain secondary and tertiary public health care services for those who can afford to pay.

Extending Public Health Services

This policy envisages that in the context of the availability and spread of allopathic graduates in their jurisdiction, the state government would consider the need for expanding a pool of medical practitioners as well as Indian system of medicine and homeopathy.

- Simple services/procedures can be provided by such practitioners outside their discipline in underserved areas.
- Regulation in standard in paramedical disciplines would be done by establishment of their statutory professional council to maintain standard of their training to register them and monitor their performances.
- Involvement of nurse practitioner.
- NHP-2002 recognizes the need for the states to simplify the recruitment procedure and rules for contact employment in order to provide trained medical manpower in the underserved areas.
- Rigorous enforcement of mandatory 2-year rural posting before awarding the graduate degree.

Role of the Local Self-Government Institutes

Implementing public health programs through local self-government. The state government to consider and decentralize implementation of health programs by 2005. Financial incentives will be provided by the central government.

Norms for Health Care Personnel: Minimal statutory norms for the deployment of doctors and nurses in medical institutions need to be introduced urgently under the provision of IMC Act respectively **(Table 8.6)**.

Education of Healthcare Professionals

Setting up medical grants commission for funding the new medical colleges and for upgradation of the existing government medical colleges to ensure standards. Revision and modification of the existing curriculum to include course content on geriatric disorder, and contemporary medical research.

To enable fresh graduates to contribute effectively for providing primary health services as a physician of the first contact.

Table 8.6: Suggested norms for healthcare personnel.

Category of personnel	*Norms suggested*	
Doctors	1 per	3500 population
Nurses	1 per	5000 population
Health worker (female and male)	1 per	5000 population in plain area and 3000 population in tribal and hilly areas
Trained dai	1 per village	
Health assistant (male and female)	1 per	30,000 population in plain area and 20,000 population in tribal and hilly areas
Health assistant (male and female)		Provides supportive supervision to 6 health workers (male/female)
Pharmacists	1 per	10,000 population
Laboratory technicians	1 per	10,000 population

Need for a Specialist in Public Health and Family Medicine

In order to alleviate the acute shortage of medical personnel with specialization in the disciplines of public health and family medicine, the policy envisages the progressive implementation of mandatory norms to raise the proportion of postgraduate seats in the discipline.

Nursing Professional

In the interest of patient care, it was emphasized to improve nurse vis-à-vis doctor/bed ratio.

- Increasing the number of nursing personnel
- Improvement of the skill level of the nurses
- Increasing the ratio of the degree-holding nurses, vis-à-vis diploma-holding nurses
- NHP, 2002 recognizes a need for the central government to stabilize the setting up and running of training facility for nurses on a decentralized basis and the establishment of super specialist nurses for the tertiary-level hospitals.

Use of Generic Drugs and Vaccines

- Need-based treatment regimen in both public and private sectors by providing some essential drugs of generic nature.
- Universal immunization program for preventable diseases by supply of vaccines in affordable prices.

Urban Health

Migration has resulted in urban growth, which is likely to go up to 33%. It anticipates the rising vehicle density, which leads to serious accidents. In this direction, NHP, 2002 has recommended an urban primary health care structure as under.

First Tier

- Primary center covers 1 lakh population
- It functions as an OPD facility
- It provides essential drugs
- It will carry out the national health programs.

Second Tier

- General hospital, a referral to primary center, provides the care
- The policy recommends a fully equipped hub and spoketrauma care network to reduce accident mortality.

Mental Health

It envisages:

- Establishment of decentralized mental health services for ameliorating the more common categories of disorders
- Upgradation of physical infrastructure (development of IPD) at government expenses so as to secure human rights of patients and with mental health problems.

IEC

- Establishing IEC policies which maximize the dissemination of information to those population groups which cannot be effectively approached through the mass media alone. The focus would be given on interpersonal communication of information and use of folk and other traditional media.
- Involvement of NGOs, setting specific targets, development of modules for dissemination of information.

School Health

Priority is given to school health programs aiming at:

- Preventive health education
- Regular health check-up
- Promotion of health-seeking behavior among children.

Health Research

- NHP, 2002 noted the aggregate annual expenditure on health ₹80,000 crores and that on research ₹1150 crores is quite low.
- The policy envisages an increase in government-funded health resources to a level of 1% total health spending by 2005 and up to 2% by 2010.
- New therapeutic drugs, especially for TB, malaria, HIV/AIDS and vaccines for tropical diseases are given priority.

Role of the Private Sector

- This policy welcomes participation of the private sector in all areas of health activities, i.e., primary, secondary and tertiary
- Cooperation of nongovernmental practitioners in National Disease Control Program
- Application of IT in the telemedicines in tertiary health care centers.

Role of the Civil Society

It recognizes a significant contribution made by the NGOs and other institutions of the civil society in making available the health services to the community.

National Disease Surveillance Network

Full operationalization of an integrated disease control network from the grassroot level to the central government level by 2005.

Health Statistics

Statistical methods to be put in place to enable the periodic updation of these baseline estimates:

- Complete baseline estimation of incidence of TB, malaria and blindness by 2005
- Establishing long-term baseline estimates for noncommunicable diseases
- Estimation of health cost on a continuation basis
- Need to establishing national health accounts confirming to the 'source-to-user' matrix structure.

Women's Health

This policy emphasize on women health because for reducing IMR, MMR, child mortality and morbidity status women health is important. The identification of specific programs targeted for women's health like RCH programme, Kisori Suraskha yojana, etc., should be emphasizes.

Medical Ethics

- In order to ensure that the common patient is not subjected to irrational or profit-driven medical regimens, a contemporary code of ethics be notified and rigorously implemented by the medical council of India
- Medical research in certain disciplines, such as gene manipulation and stem-cell research should have some discipline and guidelines that should be constantly reviewed and updated.

Enforcement of Quality Standard for Food and Drugs

Food and drug administration should be progressively strengthened in terms of both laboratory facilities and technical expertise.

Regulation of Standards in Paramedical Discipline

Regulation of standards in paramedical discipline would be done by establishment of their statutory professional council to maintain standards of their training to register them and monitor their performance.

Environmental and Occupational Health

Periodic screening of health conditions of the workers, particularly for high-risk health disorders associated with their occupation.

Providing Medical Facilities to Users from Overseas

- To capitalize on the comparative cost advantage enjoyed by domestic health facilities in the secondary and tertiary sectors.
- Providing such health services on a payment basis to service seekers from overseas.

National Health Policy, 2017

Introduction

Health policy is the expression of what health care system should be so that it can meet the health care needs of the people. The National Health Policy of 1983 and the National Health Policy of 2002 have served well in guiding the approach for the health sector in the Five-Year Plans. Now 14 years after the last health policy, the context has changed in four major ways. First, the health priorities are changing. Although maternal and child mortality have rapidly declined, there is growing burden on account of non-communicable diseases and some infectious diseases. The second important change is the emergence of a robust health care industry estimated to be growing at double digit. The third change is the growing incidences of catastrophic expenditure due to health care costs, which are presently estimated to be one of the major contributors to poverty. Fourth, a rising economic growth enables enhanced fiscal capacity. Therefore, a new health policy responsive to these contextual changes is required. And NHP 2017 is built on the progress made since the last NHP 2002.

The primary aim of the National Health Policy, 2017, is to inform, clarify, strengthen and prioritize the role of the Government in shaping health systems in all its dimensions—investments in health, organization of healthcare services, prevention of diseases and promotion of good health through cross sectoral actions, access to technologies, developing human resources, encouraging medical pluralism, building knowledge base, developing better financial protection strategies, strengthening regulation and health assurance.

Objectives

- Improve health status through concerted policy action in all sectors and expand preventive, promotive, curative, palliative and rehabilitative services provided through the public health sector with focus on quality.
- Assuring availability of free, comprehensive primary health care services, for all aspects of reproductive, maternal, child and adolescent health and for the most prevalent communicable, non-communicable and occupational diseases in the population.
- Ensuring improved access and affordability, of quality secondary and tertiary care services through a combination of public private participation. Enable private sector contribution in making health care systems more effective, efficient, rational, safe and affordable.
- Strengthening the trust of the common man in public health care system by making it predictable, efficient and patient centric, affordable and effective, with a comprehensive package of services and products that meet immediate health care needs of most people.

Goal

The prime goal of this policy is the attainment of the highest possible level of health and well-being for all at all ages, through a preventive and promotive health care orientation in all developmental policies, and universal access to good quality health care services without any financial hardship.

Key Principles of NHP 2017

- **Professionalism, integrity and ethics:** The health policy commits itself to the highest professional standards, integrity and ethics to be maintained in the entire system of health care delivery in the country, supported by a credible, transparent and responsible regulatory environment.
- **Equity and affordability:** Reducing inequity would mean affirmative action to reach the poorest by minimizing disparity on account of gender, poverty, caste, disability, other forms of social exclusion and geographical barriers. It would imply greater investments and financial protection for the poor who suffer the largest burden of disease and health care should be accessible and affordable to everyone.

- **Universality:** Systems and services should be designed to be universally available for the entire population—including special groups and exclusions on social, economic and on other grounds of health care should be prevented.
- **Patient-centered and quality of care:** Gender sensitive, effective, safe, and convenient healthcare services to be provided with dignity and confidentiality with all standards and guidelines at all levels of facilities and a system to ensure that the quality of healthcare is not compromised.
- **Accountability:** Financial and performance accountability, transparency in decision-making, and elimination of corruption in healthcare systems, both in public and private should be assured.
- **Inclusive partnerships:** A multisectorial approach with partnership and participation of all non-health ministries and communities including partnerships with academic institutions, not for profit agencies, and health care industry as well.
- **Pluralism:** Patients who so choose and when appropriate, would have access to AYUSH care providers based on documented and validated local, home and community-based practices.
- **Decentralization:** Decentralization of decision-making to a level as is consistent with practical considerations and institutional capacity. Community participation in health planning processes, to be promoted side by side.
- **Dynamism and adaptiveness:** Constantly improving dynamic organization of health care based on new knowledge and evidence with learning from the communities and from national and international knowledge partners is designed.

Specific Goals and Objectives

- **Life expectancy and healthy life:**
  - Increase life expectancy at birth from 67.5 to 70 by 2025.
  - Establish regular tracking of Disability Adjusted Life Years (DALY) Index as a measure of burden of disease and its trends by major categories by 2022.
  - Reduction of TFR to 2.1 at national and subnational level by 2025.
- **Mortality by age and/or cause:**
  - Reduce under-five mortality to 23 by 2025 and MMR from current levels to 100 by 2020.
  - Reduce infant mortality rate to 28 by 2019.
  - Reduce neonatal mortality to 16 and stillbirth rate to "single digit" by 2025.
- **Reduction of disease prevalence/incidence:**
  - Achieve global target of 2020 which is also termed as target of 90:90:90, for HIV/AIDS i.e., 90% of all people living with HIV know their HIV status—90% of all people diagnosed with HIV infection receive sustained antiretroviral therapy and 90% of all people receiving antiretroviral therapy will have viral suppression.
  - Achieve and maintain elimination status of Leprosy by 2018, Kala-Azar by 2017 and Lymphatic Filariasis in endemic pockets by 2017.
  - To achieve and maintain a cure rate of >85% in new sputum positive patients for TB and reduce incidence of new cases, to reach elimination status by 2025.
  - To reduce the prevalence of blindness to 0.25/1000 by 2025 and disease burden by one third from current levels.
  - To reduce premature mortality from cardiovascular diseases, cancer, diabetes or chronic respiratory diseases by 25% by 2025.
- **Coverage of health services:**
  - Increase utilization of public health facilities by 50% from current levels by 2025.
  - Antenatal care coverage to be sustained above 90% and skilled attendance at birth above 90% by 2025.
  - More than 90% of the newborn are fully immunized by one year of age by 2025.
  - Meet need of family planning above 90% at national and subnational level by 2025.
  - 80% of known hypertensive and diabetic individuals at household level maintain "controlled disease status" by 2025.
- **Cross sectoral goals related to health:**
  - Relative reduction in prevalence of current tobacco use by 15% by 2020 and 30% by 2025.
  - Reduction of 40% in prevalence of stunting of under-five children by 2025.
  - Access to safe water and sanitation to all by 2020 (Swachh Bharat Mission).
  - Reduction of occupational injury by half from current levels of 334 per lakh agricultural workers by 2020.
  - National/State level tracking of selected health behaviour.
- **Health finance:**
  - Increase health expenditure by Government as a percentage of GDP from the existing 1.1–2.5% by 2025.
  - Increase State sector health spending to >8% of their budget by 2020.
  - Decrease in proportion of households facing catastrophic health expenditure from the current levels to 25%, by 2025.
- **Health infrastructure and human resource:**
  - Ensure availability of paramedics and doctors as per Indian Public Health Standard (IPHS) norm in high priority districts by 2020.
  - Increase community health volunteers to population ratio as per IPHS norm, in high priority districts by 2025.
  - Establish primary and secondary care facility as per norms in high priority districts (population as well as time to reach norms) by 2025.
- **Health management information:**
  - Ensure district-level electronic database of information on health system components by 2020.
  - Strengthen the health surveillance system and establish registries for diseases of public health importance by 2020.

- Establish federated integrated health information architecture, Health Information Exchanges and National Health Information Network by 2025.

Policy Thrust

- **Ensuring adequate investment:** The policy proposes a potentially achievable target of raising public health expenditure to 2.5% of the GDP in a time bound manner. It envisages that the resource allocation to States will be linked with state development indicators, absorptive capacity and financial indicators.
- **Preventive and promotive health:** The policy articulates to institutionalize intersectoral coordination at national and subnational levels to optimize health outcomes. This is in line with the emergent international "Health in All" approach as complement to Health for All.
- **Organization of public health care delivery:** The policy proposes seven key policy shifts in organizing health care services
  - In primary care—from selective care to assured comprehensive care with linkages to referral hospitals
  - In secondary and tertiary care - from an input oriented to an output-based strategic purchasing
  - In public hospitals—from user fees and cost recovery to assured free drugs, diagnostic and emergency services to all
  - In infrastructure and human resource development—from normative approach to targeted approach to reach under-serviced areas
  - In urban health—from token interventions to on-scale assured interventions, to organize Primary Health Care delivery and referral support for urban poor. Collaboration with other sectors to address wider determinants of urban health is advocated.

National Health Programs

- **RMNCH + A:** This policy aspires to elicit developmental action of all sectors to support Maternal and Child survival and endorses the national consensus on accelerated achievement of neonatal mortality and stillbirth rates through improved home-based and facility-based management of sick newborns and it affirms commitment to pre-emptive care to achieve optimum levels of child and adolescent health. It gives special emphasis to the health challenges of adolescents and long-term potential of investing in their health care. The scope of Reproductive and Sexual Health should be expanded to address issues like inadequate calorie intake, nutrition status and psychological problems
- **Interventions to address malnutrition and micronutrient deficiencies:** Malnutrition, especially micronutrient deficiencies, restricts survival, growth and development of children. Micro-nutrient supplementation, food fortification, screening for anemia and public awareness.
- **Universal immunization:** Priority would be to further improve immunization coverage with quality and safety, improve vaccine security as per National Vaccine Policy 2011 and introduction of newer vaccines based on epidemiological considerations. The focus will be to build upon the success of Mission Indradhanush and strengthen it.
- **Control of communicable diseases and non-communicable diseases:** The policy recognizes the interrelationship between communicable disease control programmes and public health system strengthening. The prime focus is on control of TB, HIV and AIDS, vector-borne diseases and elimination of leprosy, etc., and the policy recognizes the need to halt and reverse the growing incidence of chronic diseases.
- **Mental health:** This policy will take into consideration the provisions of the National Mental Health Policy 2014 with simultaneous action on the following fronts:
  - Increase creation of specialists through public financing and develop special rules to give preference to those willing to work in public systems.
  - Create network of community members to provide psychosocial support to strengthen mental health services at primary level facilities and
  - Leverage digital technology in a context where access to qualified psychiatrists is difficult.
- **Population stabilization:** The National Health Policy recognizes that improved access, education and empowerment would be the basis of successful population stabilization.
- **Women's health and gender mainstreaming:** There will be enhanced provisions for reproductive morbidities and health needs of women beyond the reproductive age group (40+)
- **Gender-based violence (GBV):** Women's access to healthcare needs to be strengthened by making public hospitals more women friendly and ensuring that the staff have orientation to gender-sensitivity issues.
- **Emergency care and disaster preparedness:** Better response to disasters, both natural and manmade, requires a dispersed and effective capacity for emergency management. It also requires regular strengthening of their capacities in close collaboration with the local self-government and community-based organizations. The policy supports development of earthquake and cyclone resistant health infrastructure in vulnerable geographies.
- **Mainstreaming the potential of AYUSH:** For persons who so choose, this policy ensures access to AYUSH remedies through colocation in public facilities.
- **Tertiary care services:** The policy affirms that the tertiary care services are best organized along lines of regional, zonal and apex referral centers.
- **Human resources for health:** This policy recommends that medical and paramedical education be integrated with the service delivery system, so that the students learn in the real environment and not just in the confines of the medical school. The key principle around the policy on human resources for health is that, workforce performance of the system would be best when we have

the most appropriate person, in terms of both skills and motivation, for the right job in the right place, working within the right professional and incentive environment.

- **Medical education:** The policy recommends strengthening existing medical colleges and converting district hospitals to new medical colleges to increase number of doctors and specialists, in States with large human resource deficit. The policy recognizes the need to increase the number of postgraduate seats and policy proposes financial and non-financial incentives, creating medical colleges in rural areas; preference to students from under-serviced areas, realigning pedagogy and curriculum to suit rural health needs, mandatory rural postings, etc.
- **Nursing education:** The policy recognizes the need to improve regulation and quality management of nursing education. Other measures suggested are—establishing cadres like Nurse Practitioners and Public Health Nurses to increase their availability in most needed areas. Developing specialized nursing training courses and curriculum (critical care, cardiothoracic vascular care, neurological care, trauma care, palliative care and care of terminally ill), establishing nursing school in every large district or cluster of districts of about 20 to 30 lakh population and establishing Centers of Excellence for Nursing and Allied Health Sciences in each State.

Implementation Framework and Way Forward

A policy is only as good as its implementation. The National Health Policy envisages that an implementation framework be put in place to deliver on these policy commitments. Such an implementation framework would provide a roadmap with clear deliverables and milestones to achieve the goals of the policy.

- In National Health Programs—integration with health systems for program effectiveness and in turn contributing to strengthening of health systems for efficiency.
- In AYUSH services—from stand-alone to a three dimensional mainstreaming

NATIONAL HEALTH PROTECTION MISSION/ AYUSHMAN BHARAT SCHEME

It was observed that the healthcare in India is largely underpenetrated with government expenditure at around 1.25% of the GDP (Gross Domestic Product) and nearly 55–60 million Indians are pushed into poverty every year to meet medical needs. The hospitalization expenses for critical ailments had shot up by 300% over a decade. An estimated 6 million families sink into poverty each year due to hospitalization.

Ayushman Bharat is a fundamental restructuring of the manner at the primary, secondary and tertiary care levels of health services, in which beneficiaries can access it easily. Ayushman Bharat represents a transition from segmented, sectoral and fragmented program implementation models towards a comprehensive, holistic, need-based healthcare system. It encapsulates a progression towards promotive, preventive, curative, palliative and rehabilitative aspects through access of Health and Wellness Centers (HWCs) at the primary level and it provides provision of financial protection for access of curative care at the secondary and tertiary levels through engagement with both public and private sector **(Fig. 8.3)**.

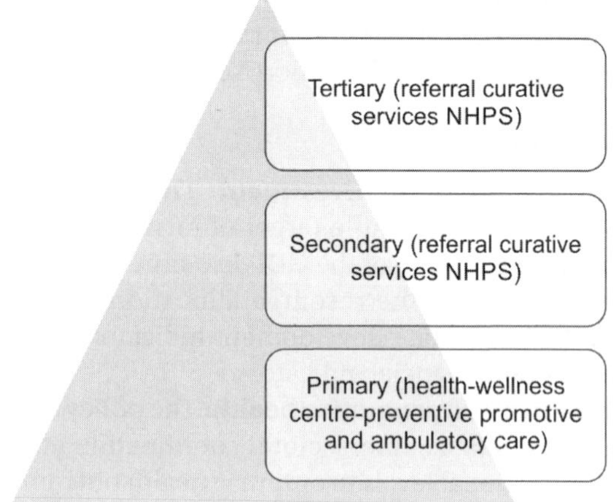

Fig. 8.3: Services Under National Health Protection Scheme at different level.

It is a flagship scheme of Government of India, which was launched as recommended by the National Health Policy 2017, to achieve the vision of Universal Health Coverage (UHC). This initiative has been designed to meet Sustainable Development Goals (SDGs) and its underlining commitment, which is to "leave no one behind."

Ayushman Bharat is an attempt to move from sectoral and segmented approach of health service delivery to a comprehensive need-based health care service. This scheme aims to undertake path breaking interventions to holistically address the healthcare system (covering prevention, promotion and ambulatory care) at the primary, secondary and tertiary level. The two inter-related components of Ayushman Bharat are:

- Health and Wellness Centres (HWCs)
- National Health Protection Scheme

Health and Wellness Centre

The first component, pertains to creation of 1,50,000 Health and Wellness Centres. The National Health Policy, 2017 has envisioned Health and Wellness Centres as the foundation of India's health system. Under this 1.5 lakh centers will bring health care system closer to the homes of people. These centers will provide Comprehensive Primary Health Care (CPHC), **(Fig. 8.4)** covering both maternal and child health services and non-communicable diseases, including free essential drugs and diagnostic services. The Budget has allocated ₹1200 crore for this flagship programme. Contribution of private sector through CSR and philanthropic institutions in adopting these centers is also envisaged. The first Health and Wellness Centre was launched by the Hon'ble Prime Minister at Jangla, Bijapur, Chhattisgarh on 14 April 2018.

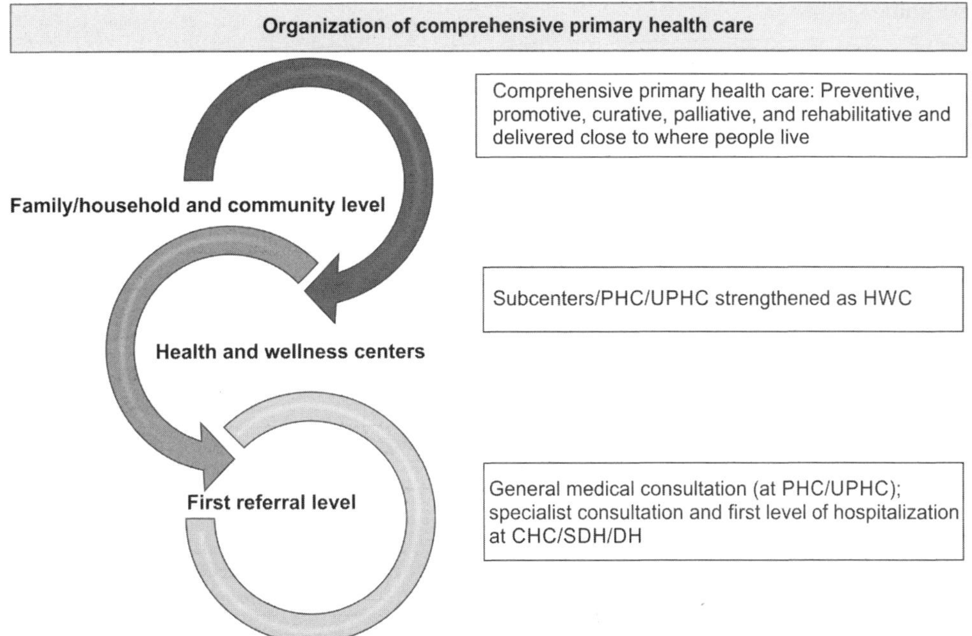

Fig. 8.4: Provision of comprehensive primary health care at different level.

In order to ensure delivery of Comprehensive Primary Health Care (CPHC) services, existing Subhealth Centres covering a population of 3000–5000 would be converted to Health and Wellness Centres (HWC), with the principle being "time to care" to be no more than 30 minutes. Primary Health Centres in rural and urban areas would also be converted to HWCs. Such care could also be provided/complemented throughout reach services, Mobile Medical Units, health camps, home visits and community-based interaction, but the principle should be a seamless continuum of care that ensures the principles of equity, quality, universality and no financial hardship. The HWC at the subhealth center level would be equipped and staffed by an appropriately trained Primary Health Care team, comprising of Multipurpose Workers (male and female) and ASHAs and led by a Mid-Level Health Provider (MLHP). Together they will deliver an expanded range of services. In some states, subhealth centers have earlier been upgraded to Additional PHCs. Such Additional PHCs will also be transformed to HWCs **(Fig. 8.5)**. A Primary Health Centre (PHC) that is linked to a cluster of HWCs would serve as the first point of referral for many disease conditions for the HWCs in its jurisdiction. In addition, it would also be strengthened as a HWC to deliver the expanded range of primary care services. The Medical Officer at the PHC would be responsible for ensuring that CPHC services are delivered through all HWCs in her/his area and through the PHC itself. The number and qualifications of staff at the PHC would continue as defined in the Indian Public Health Standards (IPHS). For PHCs to be strengthened to HWCs, support for training of PHC staff (Medical Officers, Staff Nurses, Pharmacist, and Lab Technicians), and provision of equipment for "Wellness Room", the necessary IT infrastructure and the resources required for upgrading laboratory and diagnostic support to complement the expanded ranges of services would be provided. States could choose to modify staffing at HWC and PHC, based on local needs. The HWC would deliver an expanded range of services. These services would be delivered at both SHCs and in the PHCs, which are transformed as HWCs. The level of complexity of care of services delivered at the PHC would be higher than at the subhealth center level and this would be indicated in the care pathways and standard treatment guidelines that will be issued periodically.

Expanded Range of Services

- Care in pregnancy and child-birth.
- Neonatal and infant health care services.
- Childhood and adolescent health care services.
- Family planning, Contraceptive services and other Reproductive Health Care services.
- Management of Communicable diseases including National Health Programmes.
- Management of Common Communicable Diseases and Outpatient care for acute simple illnesses and minor ailments.
- Screening, Prevention, Control and Management of Non-Communicable diseases.
- Care for Common Ophthalmic and ENT problems.
- Basic oral health care.
- Elderly and palliative health care services.
- Emergency Medical Services.
- Screening and basic management of mental health ailments.

In many states, the Primary Health Centre would serve as the first point of referral and administrative hub for subhealth centers. However, in certain states, the subhealth center is

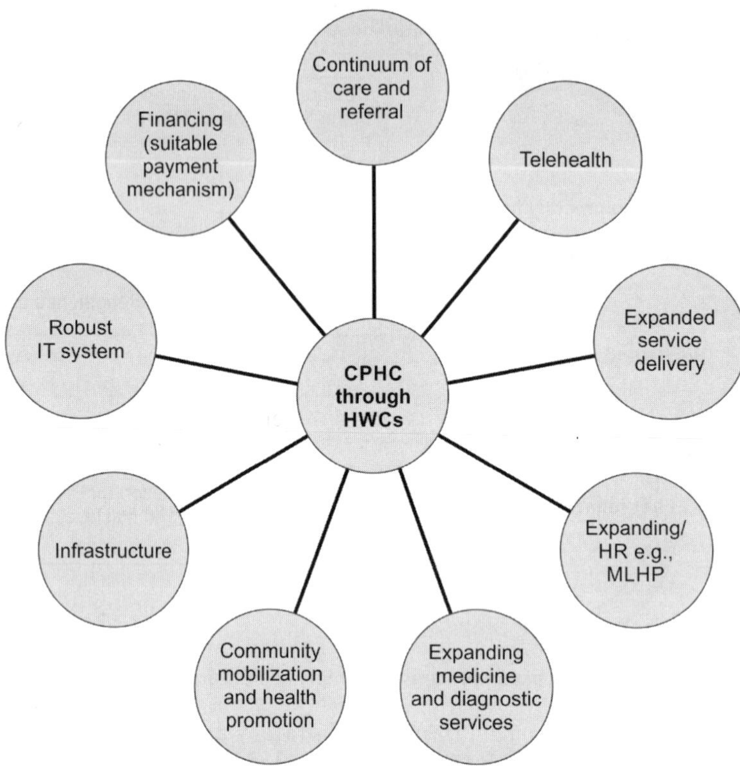

Fig. 8.5: Key elements of comprehensive primary health care through HWC.

linked directly to the Community Health Centre (CHC) at the block level (which in some blocks is a role performed by the Block PHC). Across all contexts however, it must be ensured that administrative, technical/mentoring and referral support be provided by a MBBS Medical Officer in a facility that is in geographic proximity to the cluster of HWCs and is equipped to manage referral support for HWC. This could therefore be either a PHC or a CHC.

Similarly, in the urban context, the Urban Primary Health Centres or Urban Health Posts, where they exist, would be strengthened as HWCs to deliver Comprehensive Primary Health Care. The norm of One MPW (F) per 10,000 population supported by four to five ASHAs, will enable outreach services, preventive and promotive care and home and community-based services. Therefore, in the urban context, the team of MPWs (F) and ASHAs would be considered equivalent to a frontline provider team with the first point of referral being the UPHC catering to about at 50,000 population. All the key principles of HWCs indicated above will be applicable to PHCs in urban areas.

In planning for HWCs, states need to pay close attention to improving geographic accessibility, ensure the full complement of staff at each level, enable regular capacity building and supportive supervision, ensure uninterrupted supply of medicines and diagnostics, and maintain a continuum of care seamlessly linking people to various levels of care so that the services offered at the primary health care level fully meet the promise of expanded range and commensurate outcomes.

Key Inputs of a Health Wellness Centre

The ***key inputs*** to be provided at a HWC are as follows:

1. **Primary healthcare team** to deliver the expanded range of services.
   a. *At the upgraded SHC:* The upgraded SHC should equip with one Midlevel provider, at least two (preferably three) multipurpose workers—two female and one male, and team of ASHAs at the norm of one per 1000.
   b. *At the strengthened PHC:* PHC must be strengthened as per IPHS standards. An additional nurse should be posted where cervical cancer screening is being undertaken/planned. In PHCs that are not envisaged to provide inpatient care, the existing nurses should receive modular training in certificate course for primary care. In urban areas, the team would consist of the MPW- F for coverage of 10,000 population and one ASHAs for coverage of 2500.
2. **Logistics:** Adequate availability and accessibility of essential medicines and diagnostics to sustain the expanded range of services, to resolve more and refer less at the local levels, and to enable dispensation of medicines for chronic illnesses as close to communities as possible.
3. **Infrastructure:** There should be sufficient room and space for outpatient care, for supply of medicines, adequate spaces for display of communication material of health messages including audio-visual aids, provision of diagnostic services, and appropriate community

spaces for wellness activities, including the practice of Yoga and physical exercises.

4. **Digitization:** The team members of HWC should be equipped with tablets/smart Phones to serve a range of functions. These functions include population enumeration and empanelment, enable quality follow-up, record delivery of services, family and population health profile, facilitate referral/continuity of care and create an updated individual, and generate reports required for monitoring at higher levels.
5. **Use of telemedicine/IT platforms:** Use of tele-consultation at all levels, would to improve referral advice, seek clarifications, and undertake virtual training including case management support by specialists should be ensured.
6. **Capacity building:** Mid-Level Health Providers will be trained in a set of primary healthcare and public health competencies through an accredited training program that combines theory and practicum with on the job training. Other service providers at health wellness center (HWC) will also be trained appropriately to deliver the expanded range of services.
7. **Health promotion:** Development of health promotion material and facilitation of health promotive behaviours among healthcare providers through engagement of community level collectives such as—Village Health Sanitation and Nutrition Committee (VHSNCs), Mahila Arogya Samiti (MAS) and Self-Help Groups (SHGs), and creating health ambassadors in schools. Enabling behaviour change communication to address lifestyle-related risk factors and undertaking collective action for reducing risk exposure, improved care seeking and effective utilization of primary health care services.
9. **Community mobilization:** Community mobilization can be encouraged for action on social and environmental determinants, which require intersectional convergence and build on the accountability initiatives under NHM so that there is no denial of health care and universality and equity are respected.
10. **Linkages with mobile medical units:** Linkages with Mobile Medical Units (MMU) could serve to improve access and coverage in remote and underserved areas where there is difficulty in establishing HWCs. In such cases, medicines and other support could be provided to frontline workers, with periodic MMU visits. MMUs could also be linked to nearby HWCs, where medical consultation could be arranged on scheduled days, for those unable to travel to referral sites.

Essential Outputs of Health Wellness Centre

- **The health wellness center (HWC) database:** Population enumeration and empanelment implies the creation and maintenance of database of all families and individuals in an area served by a HWC. This is planned such that every individual is empanelled to a HWC. This also involves active communication to make residents aware of this facility.
- **Health cards and family health folders:** These are made for all service users to ensure access to all health care entitlements and enable continuum of care. The health cards are given to the families and individuals. The family health folders are kept at the HWC or nearby PHC in paper and/or digital format. This ensures that every family knows their entitlement to healthcare through both HWC and the Pradhan Mantri Jan Arogya Yojana or equivalent health schemes of state and central government.
- **Increased access to services:** HWCs would provide access to an expanded range of services. The availability of services would evolve in different states gradually, depending on three factors—the availability of suitably skilled human resources at the HWC, the capacity at district/subdistrict level to support the HWC in the delivery of that service, and the ability of the state to ensure uninterrupted supply of medicines and diagnostics at the level of HWC. States will also have the flexibility to expand the range of service to address local health problems as defined by disease prevalence.

Outcomes of Program

- **Improved population coverage:** Active empanelment and HWC database will improve the population coverage. The HWC database would enable HWC staff to monitor and identify the left out population and improve coverage of national health programs.
- **Reduced out of pocket expenditure and catastrophic health expenditure:** Improved access to expanded services closer to the community, assured availability of medicines and diagnostic services and linkages for care coordination with Medical Officers/Specialists across levels of care will reduce financial hardships faced by community.
- **Risk factor mitigation:** Health promotion efforts by primary health care team would support in addressing the risk factors for diseases.
- **Decongestion of secondary and tertiary health facilities:** A strong network of HWCs at the subdistrict level would facilitate resolving more cases at primary level and reduce overcrowding at secondary and tertiary facilities for follow-up cases as well as serve a gate keeping function to higher level facilities.

Impact

- **Improved population health outcomes:** Improved availability, access and utilization will in turn contribute to equitable health outcomes measured through periodic population based surveys for key indicators listed in Section 10.1- Monitoring.
- **Increased responsiveness:** Provision of care by primary care team will be based on principles of family led care including dignity and respect for individuals and communities with particular focus on marginalized, information sharing, encouraging participation, including

intersectoral collaboration that will lead to increased trust building, comfort in access to care and enable addressing social and environmental determinants. While not all inputs can be provided immediately, the state needs to have a road map for HWC strengthening, in which some inputs can be added in an incremental manner. However, addition of the services for chronic conditions with requisite HR who is trained, and with the medicines and diagnostics would be a critical first step. The centers which do not fulfil all criteria but have only initiated expanded service delivery, would be referred to as "HWCs - progressive," and have a clear time-line to become "fully functional HWC", i.e., with the entire complement of the primary health care team, and delivery of the expanded range of services, identified for Comprehensive Primary Health Care.

Organization of Service Delivery

Family/Household and Community level	*Health and Wellness Centres*	*First Referral Level*
The ASHA and MPW will undertake house visits supported and supplemented by the MPWs for community mobilization for improved care seeking, risk assessments, screening, follow-up for primary and secondary prevention, counselling and increasing supportive environment in families and community. ASHAs can also support in follow-up for compliance to treatment and instructions from clinicians, through regular home visits, and assist in conducing meetings of patient support groups. Community platforms such as Village Health and Nutrition Days (VHNDs), Village Health Sanitation Nutrition Committees (VHSNCs), Mahila Arogya Samities (MAS), would be leveraged.	The HWC must be kept open with services available for at least six hours in the day. Outreach services and home visits of the team members should be so scheduled that someone is available at the HWC for the general OPD and follow-up for those with chronic illness. Follow-up of chronic illness could also be organized in the form of patient group meetings on fixed days at the HWC, for example a meeting for Hypertension/ Diabetes patients on Wednesday afternoons and elderly care on Thursdays, etc.	Referral care and sites will vary with each illness, its care pathways and availability of specialists. For consultations on acute illness, it is the MO in the PHC or the specialist in CHC/DH, either physically or through teleconsultation as appropriate. Over time, states will progress to establishing an FRU at the CHC level, and every DH having the full complement of specialist access required to provide referral support to the expanded range of services

National Health Protection Scheme

The "National Health Protection Scheme," presented as one of the largest government-sponsored health insurance schemes in the world, and was announced by the finance minister during the budget speech in parliament. The union cabinet under the prime minister approval and the launch of this scheme meant to benefit more than 10 crore poor and vulnerable families which targets 50 crore of individuals, with a family cover of ₹5 lakhs per family per year. The National Health Policy 2017 aimed at providing universal health care and quality services to all at an affordable cost, which was in line with the Sustainable Development Goal 3 of universal health care. The National Health Protection Scheme (NHPS) is an ambitious project of the government of India, aimed at providing quality health care to the poor and vulnerable families, and achieving its commitment on universal health care. The Pradhan Mantri Jan Arogya Abhiyaan (Ayushman Bharat) has been announced by the hon'ble Prime Minister on 15 August 2018 in his independence day speech and rolled out on 25 September 2018 and. An official website 'abnhpm.gov.in' has been launched by the government of India for the mission. This program will incorporate the on-going centrally sponsored schemes–Rashtriya Swasthya Bima Yojana (RSBY) and the senior citizen health insurance scheme.

Features and Benefits of the Scheme

- A cover of up to ₹5 lakh is available for the beneficiary family every year.
- The scheme can be utilised to get primary, secondary, and tertiary healthcare services.
- The benefits of the scheme can be availed at any government hospital or empanelled private hospital.
- The eligibility of beneficiaries targeted towards the poor, deprived rural families and identified occupational category of urban workers' families based on the Socio-Economic Caste Census (SECC) 2011 data.
- Package model will be followed to make payments. The package will be defined by the government-in-charge in terms of payment of total costs, specific services, and procedures.
- An Ayushman Bharat National Health Protection Mission will be established for effective coordination between the Central and the state governments.
- The scheme covers about 40% of the country's population who are poor and vulnerable.
- All expenses incurred by the beneficiary from his pocket during the hospitalization will also be covered.
- The cost incurred during the pre and post-hospitalization period will be covered.
- The insurance provides cashless hospitalization facility.
- Daycare treatment expenses are covered by the scheme.
- The insurance scheme covers all pre-existing health conditions.

Follow-up of medical examinations up to 15 days are also covered to ensure that the patients have recovered completely.

Beneficiaries

Beneficiary households under the AB-NHPS will be based on the deprivation and occupation status of the family, drawn from the Socioeconomic and Caste Census database.

Eligibility Criteria for Rural Families

There are six deprivation criteria to identify the rural families that are eligible for the benefits of the scheme. They are:

1. Families that do not have an earning adult member aged between 16 and 59 years.
2. Households headed by female members having no adult male members aged between 16 and 59 years.
3. Households with a single room having makeshift walls and roof.
4. Households belonging to the Scheduled Castes and Scheduled Tribes categories.
5. Households that have disabled members with no able members offering support.
6. Landless households with manual labor as their basic source of income.

In addition, the following households are automatically eligible:

- Destitute families who rely on alms.
- Families of manual scavengers.
- Households without proper shelter.
- Families of bonded labor.
- Primitive and particularly vulnerable tribal groups.

Eligibility Criteria for Urban Families

An urban family must belong to one of the listed occupational categories to be eligible for the scheme:

- Street vendors, cobblers, and hawkers.
- Domestic workers.
- Rag pickers and beggars.
- Construction site workers, plumbers, masons, painters, welders, and security guards.
- Coolies.
- Sweepers, sanitation workers, and gardeners.
- Transport workers such as conductors, drivers, cart pullers, and others.
- Artisans, home-based workers, handicraft workers, and tailors.
- Washermen and watchmen.
- Electricians, mechanics, repair workers, and assemblers.
- Peons, helpers, shop workers, delivery assistants, attendants, and waiters.

Eligibility Criteria for Hospitals

Similar to setting eligibility criteria for beneficiaries, the government has framed eligibility criteria for a hospital to be empanelled. The criteria are:

- The hospital must be registered with state health agencies.
- Qualified medical and nursing staff must be available 24/7.
- The hospital must have a minimum of 10 in-patient beds.
- The medical facility must have an accessible washroom.
- An interoperable IT system should be in place to manage data.
- A complete record of Ayushman Bharat patients must be maintained and shared with the government as per the requirement.
- Ambulance and other emergency services must be available.
- A dedicated medical officer should be appointed to take care of AB-NHPS operations.
- There should be a blood bank and testing laboratory in the vicinity.
- The medical facility must have all the equipment and technical necessities.
- The hospital must have facilities such as regulated water, electricity, and biomedical waste disposal.

COMPREHENSIVE PRIMARY HEALTH CARE

In 1978, at an international conference convened by the World Health Organization (WHO) and UNICEF (United Nations Children's Fund) in Kazakhstan, the 134 members of the World Health Assembly of World Health Organization ratified the Declaration of AlmaAta (World Health Organization, 1978). The declaration committed member states to supporting Primary Health Care (PHC) as a policy to achieve the WHO definition of health as a "state of complete physical, mental and social well-being and not merely the absence of disease or infirmity" (WHO, 2006A).

The declaration's lack of concrete guidelines resulted in an attempt by the recognized authorities in the health field to give some shape and form to the concept of Primary Health Care to lead to a definition for global health policy. The Alma-Ata declaration defined eight elements of PHC (World Health Organization, 1978, pp. 24–25). These were:

1. Education concerning prevailing health problems and the methods of identifying, preventing and controlling them.
2. Promotion of food supply and proper nutrition, an adequate supply of safe water and basic sanitation.
3. Maternal and child health care including family planning.
4. Immunization against major infectious diseases.
5. Prevention and control of locally endemic diseases.
6. Treatment of common diseases and injuries.
7. Promotion of mental health.
8. Provision of essential drugs.

However, no guidance on how to pursue these elements was provided. In an article in the prestigious New England Journal of Medicine, Julia Walsh and Kenneth Warren, who was then the director of health sciences at the Rockefeller Foundation, stated that though the vision and values of PHC were unquestionable, translating policy into practice needed refining. They put forward the concept of "selective primary health care" (SPHC) focusing on implementing policy for the diseases that had the highest prevalence and morbidity, highest risk of mortality, and greatest possibility of control in terms of the cost and effectiveness of the intervention. The advantages of selective PHC include: a rational, cost-effective way to prioritize disease problems; narrow scope, making it affordable for developing countries; and readily detectable results in the short term. Rejecting an interpretation of health as holistic and reflective of social justice and social determinants, SPHC put forward a view of health as dependent on vertical delivery of health services. It challenged the alternative "comprehensive Primary Health Care" (CPHC) approaches to health improvements, which included community participation, intersectoral collaboration, and appropriate technology. While WHO struggled with how to pursue a holistic approach to health, the co-sponsor of the Alma-Ata conference, UNICEF, chose to focus on specific interventions, referenced by the acronym GOBI-FFF (Growth Monitoring, Oral Rehydration, Breast-feeding, Immunizations, Family Planning, Female Literacy, and Food Technology; United Nations Children's Fund, 2016). The Child Survival Revolution, the umbrella for GOBI, was considered a Selective Primary Health Care (SPHC) approach. It focused on maternal and child health and ignored the health of the wider population, including males and seniors. The debate over SPHC versus CPHC became a consistent theme in translating PHC into practice.

The National Health Policy, 2017 recommended strengthening the delivery of Primary Health Care, through establishment of "Health and Wellness Centres" in place of subcenters and PHCs as the platform to deliver Comprehensive Primary Health Care and policies called for a commitment of two thirds of the health budget to primary health care. Keeping view on this in February 2018, the Government of India declared that 1,50,000 Health and Wellness Centres (HWCs) would be created by transforming existing Subhealth Centres and Primary Health Centres to deliver Comprehensive Primary Health Care and declared this as one of the components (between two) of Ayushman Bharat. This was the first step in the conversion of policy articulations to a budgetary commitment. Based on the Report of the Primary Health Care Task Force, Ministry of Health and Family Welfare, Government of India while reiterating that as primary health care is the only affordable and effective path for India to Universal Health Coverage, it is also required to provide valuable insights to structure and processes required health systems which will enable to provide Comprehensive Primary Health Care (CPHC). It was also decided to construct Health wellness center for delivering Comprehensive Primary Health Care (CPHC). The delivery of CPHC through HWCs rests substantially on the institutional mechanisms, governance structures, and systems created under the National Health Mission (NHM). NHM, as part of health system reform in the country, in its nearly 12 years of implementation, has supported states to create several platforms for delivery of community-based health systems, expanding Human Resources for Health and infrastructure towards strengthening primary and secondary care. Though largely limited to a few conditions, NHM created mechanisms for expanded coverage and reach, and developed systems for improved delivery of medicines, diagnostics and improved reporting. About five years ago, these components were also introduced in urban areas. Thus, although the delivery of universal Comprehensive Primary Health Care, through HWCs builds on existing systems, it will need change management and systems design at various levels, to realise its full potential. The other component of Ayushman Bharat, namely the Pradhan Mantri Jan Arogya Yojana (PMJAY) aims to provide financial protection for secondary and tertiary care to about 40% of India's households. Its success and affordability rests substantially on the effectiveness of provision of Comprehensive Primary Health Care through HWCs. Together, the two components of Ayushman Bharat will enable the realization of the aspiration for Universal Health Coverage.

Development of Guidelines

Guidelines have been developed after consultation with policy makers and practitioners at national and state level and with technical experts. It also draws on implementation experiences of government, NGO and private sector in the delivery of Primary Health Care. These guidelines are developed to serve as a framework for operationalizing the multiple components required for the delivery of Comprehensive Primary Health Care services through the Health and Wellness Centres. These guidelines are anticipated to support program managers at state and district levels in rolling out Comprehensive Primary Health Care. They provide an overview of the systems requirements and strategies for change management to deliver CPHC. The use of these guidelines would enable the states to put in place the necessary design elements and subsystems required for Health and Wellness Centres to be created and deliver the health services expected of them. However, states have the flexibility to make necessary modifications based on their specific needs and capacities. The implementation of Comprehensive Primary Health Care would require substantial change management in processes for planning, service delivery, monitoring and financing and will require the active participation of several stakeholders including civil society, NGOs, academic and research agencies development partners, the private sector and, most importantly, the community. Operationalizing HWCs will be incremental in nature with contextual variations in models and processes evolving in different states. These guidelines do not cover grounds included in several other guidelines already issued but highlight areas in which transformation and change management is needed, besides clarifying key concepts related to Comprehensive Primary Health Care and Health and Wellness Centres. These guidelines are envisaged to be reviewed periodically and revised based on implementation lessons from the field so that they continue to provide meaningful and updated guidance to program implementers and inform policy adaptation and modification.

POPULATION DYNAMIC AND CONTROL

Introduction

The population in the earth is increasing very fast because of declining death rate and high birth rate. The first increasing population is creating problem in imbalance in the ecosystem affecting socioeconomic aspects and quality life. As population is the integral component of community health care, so it is very important to understand the size and structure of community.

Demography

Demography comes from Ancient Greek word *dēmos,* meaning 'the people', and-*graphy* means 'writing, description or measurement. Demography is the statistical study of populations, especially human beings. As a very general science, it can analyze any kind of dynamic living population, i.e., one that changes over time or space. Demography encompasses the study of the size, structure, and distribution of these populations, and spatial or temporal changes in them in response to birth, migration, ageing, and death. Based on the demographic research of the earth, earth's population up to the year 2050 and 2100 can be estimated by demographers. Demographics are quantifiable characteristics of a given population. In simple it is the study of changes (such as the number of births, deaths, marriages, and illnesses) that occur over a period of time in human populations. It is also the branch of science which deals with human population. There are three elements of Demography, such as:

Change in the Size of Population (Increase/Decrease)

Population change is analyzed by measuring the change between one population size to another. Global population continues to rise, which makes population change an essential component to demographics. This is calculated by taking one population size minus the population size in an earlier census. The best way of measuring population change is using the intercensal percentage change.

Structure/Composition of Population (Age/Sex Distribution)

Population composition is the description of population defined by characteristics such as age, race, sex or marital status. These descriptions can be necessary for understanding the social dynamics from historical and comparative research. This data is often compared using a population pyramid. Population composition is also a very important part of historical research.

Geographical Distribution of Population (State/Territory)

The geographical distribution of population can be described as National International local rural, urban and tribal. According to geographical distribution the disease can varies. By comparing different geographical areas we can identifying the geographical or other factors affecting health conditions.

Demographic Process

Demography is influenced by five processes, Such as:

Fertility

Fertility is the natural capability to produce offspring. As a measure, fertility rate is the number of offspring born per mating pair, individual or population. Human fertility depends on factors of nutrition, sexual vior, consanguinity, culture, instinct, endocrinology, timing, economics, way of life, and emotions. Fertility declines with age in both sexes. In women the decline is more rapid, with complete infertility normally occurring around the age of 50.

Mortality

Mortality means death. Mortality rate, or death rate, is a measure of the number of deaths (in general, or due to a specific cause) in a particular population, scaled to the size of that population, per unit of time. Mortality rate is typically expressed in units of deaths per 1,000 individuals per year.

Marriage

Mobility patterns vary by life course stage in part because changes in family size require residential adjustment. More fundamentally, family-building events are well recognized as a major cause of migration, and in particular migration is closely related to marriage. Marriage is a demographic process as it influence the population size not by only migration but by increasing the family size.

Social Mobility

Social mobility is defined as movement of individuals, families, households, or other categories of people within or between layers or tiers in an open system of social stratification. Open stratification systems are those in which at least some value is given to achieved status characteristics in a society. The movement can be in a downward or upward direction. Social mobility change the composition and geographical distribution of the population and influence demographic process.

Migration

Migration is one of the demographic processes that contribute to changes in the size of a population. Population size and growth may also be influenced by migration. A population may experience simultaneously both people migrating out and people migrating in. When net migration is positive the number of people moving into the population is greater than the number of people leaving the population. Migration leads to an increase in the population and contributes to population growth, in the same way as natural increase.

Demographic Cycle

There are 5 stages by which all the nation passes, such as:

First Stage (High Stationary)

This stage is characterized by high birth rate and high death rate which cancel each other and the population remain constant, e.g., India has this stage till 1920.

Second Stage (Early Expanding)

The death rate begin to decline and the birth rate remains unchanged, the death rate starts declining birth rates may even increase due to improved health conditions and decreased period of breastfeeding, many countries in South Asia and Africa are in this stage.

Third Stage (Late Expanding)

The death rate declines further and the birth rate start to fall. The population continues to grow because birth exceeds death, e.g., India, China, Singapore.

Fourth Stage (Low Stationary)

This stage is characterized by low birth rate and low death rate which results zero population growth, e.g., Austria, 1980–85.

Fifth Stage (Declining)

The birth rate falls below death rate. The population size starts declining. Some of east European countries like Germany and Hungary are in this phase.

THEORIES OF POPULATION

The theorizing about population (population size and change) have remained an important subject since time immemorial due to population explosion. Many of the ancient philosophers like Confucius (China), Kautilya (India), Ibn Khaldun (Arab), Plato (Greece) and modem thinkers like Adam Smith, David Richard and others, either directly or indirectly, have said somewhat significant on population issues.

Population explosion is a very big issues. The world population in 1798 was at nine million. That time different theorist realized that if a population rises above the 'carrying capacity' of an environment—it will struggle to survive. There is much debate about what the carrying capacity of Planet Earth is. The 'carrying capacity' is the potential of an area to support life long-term. The area must be able to provide food and water, space for living and shelter, essential resources for life and able to absorb waste and pollution. The different theorist had given different predictions about population which is termed as population theories.

Malthus' Theory

Thomas Robert Malthus (1766–1834) was the key figure to analyze the population statistics. His formulation on population was a landmark in the history of population theories. He generalized the relationship between population factors and social change.

The core principles of Malthus are:
- Food is necessary for human existence
- Human population tends to grow faster than the power in the earth to produce subsistence
- The effects of these two unequal powers must be kept equal.

Malthus argued that because of the strong attraction of the two sexes, the population could increase by multiples, doubling every twenty-five years. He contended that the population would eventually grow so large that food production would be insufficient.

Human capacity for reproduction exceeded the rate at which subsistence from the land can be increased. Malthus further wrote 'Population when unchecked increases in a geometrical ratio. Subsistence increases only in an arithmetical ratio.'

Malthus contended that the world's population was growing more rapidly than the available food supply. He argued that the food supply increases in an arithmetic progression.

1, 2, 3, 4, 5, 6.......................................and so on.

Whereas the population expands by a geometric progression.

1, 2, 4, 8, 16, 32..and so on.

According to him, the population could increase by multiples, doubling every twenty-five years. He said the gap between the food supply and population will continue to grow over time. Even though food supply will increase, it would be insufficient to meet the needs of expanding population. Moreover, the famine and other natural calamities cause widespread sufferings and increase the death rate, which is nature's check against population.

In brief, Malthus theory states that:
- Population is necessarily limited by the means of subsistence.
- Population invariably increases where means of subsistence increased, unless prevented by some very powerful and obvious checks.
- These checks, and the checks which repress the superior power of population and keep its effects on a level with the means of subsistence, are all resolvable into moral restraint, vice and misery.

Malthus based his above arguments on man's two basic characteristics essential to the maintenance of life:
- The need for food, and
- The passion between sexes.

It was the second which led people to marry at a relatively early age and would result in such a large number of births that the population would double itself in few years if unchecked by misery and vice.

Malthus referred to two classes of checks which kept population down:

- **Positive means:** He spoke of positive check means increase of death rate due to different causes like famine (hunger), war, pestilence and vicious customs about women and disease condition. Malthus suggested that once this ceiling (catastrophe) had been reached by population explosion, further growth in population would be prevented and positive check will occur. He said that there is a rule 'what goes up, must come down'. When population exceeds carrying capacity, population increase crashes.

- **Negative means:** He suggested as an alternative that birth rate may be decreased through preventive measures such as late marriage (postponing marriage until later age), moral restraint, and chastity (abstinence). He contended that without such restraints the world would face widespread hunger, poverty and misery.

The 'positive' and 'preventive' checks which occur in human population to prevent excessive growth relate to practices affecting mortality and fertility respectively. Malthus saw the tension between population and resources as a major cause of the misery of much of the humanity. He was not, however, in favor of contraceptive methods, since their use did not generate the same drive to work hard as would a postponement of marriage.

Malthus argued that the positive and preventive checks are inversely related to each other. In other words, where positive checks are very effective, the preventive checks are relatively less effective and vice versa.

Criticism

Malthus' views have been widely challenged on many grounds. The main criticisms about his theory are as under:

- The validity of his two sets of ratios has been questioned by his critics. It is argued that population has rarely grown in geometrical proportion and means of production have rarely multiplied in arithmetic progression.
- Malthus overemphasized the 'positive' checks and did not visualize the role of 'preventive' checks like contraceptives and family planning. Neo-Malthusists argued for the adoption of birth control within marriage. Human inventions in the fields of birth control, health and nutrition and agriculture have helped to a great extent to strike a balance between human reproduction and food supply.
- Malthus was also severely criticized for ignoring the role of changing technology and the consequent transformation in socioeconomic set-up of a society. He did not fully appreciate the extent to which improved agricultural technology and crop fertilization could sustain large population.
- Both the positive checks of hunger and disease referred to by Malthus do not operate today, except the terrible disaster sometimes caused by Tsunami, Katrina, Rita and floods or rains in desert areas like Banner and Jaisalmer in August 2006.
- But catastrophe of this nature in any part of the world is immediately rushed to the affected place from surplus areas all over the world. A marked decline in the death rate even in the developing countries is a significant factor in the context of the population spurt. Moreover, natural calamities referred to above have occurred in underpopulated areas also and thus there was no causal relationship between positive checks and overpopulation.
- Malthus also failed to realize even the biological limitations that a population cannot grow beyond a certain limits.

Neo-Malthusians Theory

Neo-Malthusians Robert Kaplan and Thomas Fraser expanded Malthus' ideas to more than just food, but to also include energy resources. They agree that there are absolute limits on food supply, energy and other resources. Furthermore, they suggest that the problem is intensified by the disproportionate consumption of such resources by so-called developed (industrialized) actions. This formulation has been challenged by other researchers. The Club of Rome was a gathering of scientists who said in 1972 that unless the population of the earth was restricted by population control policies, then humanity faced a disastrous future with food shortages a certainty within 100 years. These theorists are known as Neo-Malthusians (new Malthusians').

Ester Boserup (1965)/Julian Simon (1981): The belief in human ingenuity to come up with solutions at times of crisis. These two theorists claim that rising populations are not a problem. In fact, Boserup suggested that it was at times when there were food shortages following periods of population growth, that people were forced to come up with better ways of producing food in order to survive. Summed up best by the phrase: Necessity is the mother of invention. Julian Simons supported this approach and suggested that governments should NOT try to influence populations. As resources become scarce, humans use their brain power to develop new technologies, substitute materials, or more efficient ways of using resources—so they do not run out. As a result, mankind is better off after periods of resource shortage as we develop better ways or innovation but Boserup admits overpopulation can lead to unsuitable farming practices which may degrade the land. Population pressure as one of the reasons for desertification in the Sahel region (so fragile environments at risk) and the potential consequences of Green Revolution.

Marx's Response to Malthus' Theory

Karl Marx went one step further and argued that starvation was caused by the unequal distribution of the wealth and its accumulation by capitalists. It has nothing to do with the population. Population is dependent on economic and social organization. The problems of overpopulation and limits to resources, as enunciated by Malthus, are inherent and inevitable features associated with the capitalist system of production.

Marx's contention that food production could not increase rapidly was also debated when new technology began to give farmers much greater fields. French sociologist E Dupreel (1977) argued that an increasing population would spur rapid innovation and development to solve problems, whereas a stable population would be complacent and less likely to progress.

During the depression of the 1930s, the debate changed somewhat because the birth rate fell sharply in industrial (western) nations. Some predicted that human species would die out. Schemes were proposed to encourage families to have more children by giving them allowances for each child born. The birth rate rose sharply after World War II, especially in the underdeveloped nations like India, Africa and Bangladesh. Birth control programs were instituted to control the population so as to eliminate starvation.

Despite the criticisms, the Malthusian thesis gained widespread currency during his lifetime. His ideas had profound effects on public policies, on the classical and neo-classical economists, on demographers and evolutionary biologists led by Charles Darwin.

Theory of Demographic Transition

Demographic transition is a term, first used by Warren S Thompson (1929), and later on by Frank W Notestein (1945), referring to a historical process of change which accounts the trends in births, deaths and population growth that occurred in today's industrialized societies, especially European societies. This process of demographic change began for the most part in the later 18th century.

Demographic transition should not be regarded as a 'law of population growth,' but as a generalized description of the evolutionary process. In simple terms, it is a theory which attempts to specify general laws by which human populations change in size and structure during industrialization. It is frequently accepted as a useful tool in describing the demographic history of a country.

The theory postulates a particular pattern of demographic change from a high fertility and high mortality to a low fertility and low mortality when a society progresses from a largely rural agrarian and illiterate society to a dominant urban, industrial, literate and modern society.

It is typically viewed as a three-stage process:

- That the decline in immortality comes before the decline in fertility
- That the fertility eventually declines to match mortality
- That socioeconomic transformation of a society takes place simultaneously with its demographic transformation.

The demographic transition theory is characterized by conspicuous transition stages.

The transition from high birth and death rates to low rates can be divided into three stages (some scholars like Haggett, 1975 have divided into four or five stages):

- **Pretransition stage:** High and fluctuating birth and death rates with little population growth.
- **Stage I:** High birth rates and declining death rates with rapid population growth.
- **Stage II:** Low birth and death rates with slow population growth.
- **Stage III:** Birth and death rates both decline appreciably leading to zero population growth.

The theory holds that pre-industrial societies were characterized by stable populations which had both a high death rate and birth rate. It postulates a little and slows population growth. The theory states that the high mortality rates characteristic of undeveloped areas will decline before fertility rates which are also high.

In the first stage of transition, death rates (especially the infant deaths) begin to fall as a result of advances in public health and sanitation as well as improvements in nutrition and food supply. Since the birth rate continues to remain high relative to the declining death rate, there is a rapid 'transitional' growth as we find in India today.

In the second stage, changes in social attitudes, the introduction of cheap forms of contraception and increases in life expectancy create social pressures for smaller families and for a reduction of fertility.

The diffusion of knowledge and cheap medical technology has brought many non-industrial societies into this stage of the demographic transition however, these societies have been unable to enter the third stage. The result has been very high rates of population growth in countries that are not experiencing corresponding economic growth.

In the last (third) stage of demographic transition birth and death rates decline appreciably which eventually becomes approximately equal, and in time it will result in zero population growth. Before this stage begins, there can be one more stage in which low birth and death rates lead to slow population growth.

The populations of advanced, urban industrial societies, which have entered the last stage, are now stable with low birth and death rates. In some cases (e.g. Eastern and Central Europe) birth rates have fallen so slow that the rate of natural increase was actually zero or negative. In this stage, the technical know-how is abundant, the deliberate controls on family planning are common and the literacy and education levels are also very high.

The growth pattern of human populations is thus held to be S-shaped, involving a transition from one type of demographic stability with high death rates to another type of plateau with low death and birth rates. Among the later demographers, Coale and Hoover further elaborated upon the role of development and modernization in the process of transition in demographic behavior, maintained that a society characterized by peasant economy is marked with very high birth and death rates.

Death rates are high because of lack of adequate nutritive food, primitive sanitary conditions and absence of any preventive and curative measures of control over diseases. A high birth rate, on the other hand, is a functional response to high death rates, particularly among infants and children.

In the present-day world, as would be true of any point in time, different countries of the world are at different stages of the demographic transition. In the opinion of Glenn Trewartha (1969), this is largely due to the dual nature of man.

According to him, biologically, man is same everywhere and is engaged in the process of reproduction but culturally man differs from one part of the world to another. It is the cultural diversity of man that gives rise to varying fertility patterns in different areas resulting in different stages of demographic transition discussed above.

Criticism

Although the theory of demographic transition has been appreciated widely by the demographers, it has been criticized on many grounds also. There are even critics who have gone to the extent of saying that it cannot be called a theory.

The main points of criticism are:

- Firstly, this theory is merely based upon the empirical observations or the experiences of Europe, America and Australia.
- Secondly, it is neither predictive nor its stages is segmental and inevitable.
- Thirdly, the role of man's technical innovations cannot be under-rated, particularly in the field of medicine, which can arrest the rate of mortality.
- Fourthly, neither does it provide a fundamental explanation of the process of fertility decline, nor does it identify the crucial variables involved in it.
- Fifthly, it does not provide a time frame for a country to move from one stage to another.
- Finally, it does not hold good for the developing countries of the world, which have recently experienced unprecedented growth in population due to drastic decline in death rates.

In spite of these criticisms and shortcomings, the demographic transition theory does provide an effective portrayal of the world's demographic history at macro level of generalizations. As an empirical generalization developed on the basis of observing the demographic trend in the West, the transition process for any country can easily be understood.

FACTOR INFLUENCING POPULATION INCREASE

The two major factors influencing population increases are decrease death rate and increase birth rate. There are a lot of causes which are related to decrease death rate and increase birth rate which are described below.

Decrease Death Rate

The death rate in India has been declining since 1921. In 1901, the average death rate was 43 per thousand and it declined to 8.5 per thousand in 2000–01. The major cause for declining death rate are:

Control of Epidemics

Epidemics such as plague, smallpox, TB and malaria which at one time used to cause a toll of heavy deaths, now have been effectively controlled. So death rate has reduced to a large extent.

Urbanization of Population

In 1911, hardly 10.3% of population lived in urban areas. The percentage of population living in towns and cities went up to 26 in 1991 and 27.8 in 2001. Better health, hygiene and sanitation facilities in the town are expected to have lowered the death rate.

More Medical Facilities

Medical facilities have increased in different parts of the country. Communicable diseases like diphtheria, tuberculosis and malaria have been properly controlled. During Five Year plans more than ₹2000 crore was spent on medical facilities.

Spread of Education

Literacy among woman is progressing rapidly. Educated women bring up their children with utmost care. They will provide regular and complete immunization and become conscious in caring their children. This rapidly brings down the infant mortality rate. Working women enjoy better economic status and as such they are healthier.

Late Marriage

Minimum eligible age for marriage has been fixed at 21 years for men and 18 for women by law. It has done away with the evil of early marriage. It has helped in reducing the death rate of women and children.

Control Over Famine

Besides the famine of 1943, no other serious famine has occurred in this century. Although famine like conditions emerged in 1987 in states of Gujarat, Rajasthan, Haryana, Bihar and Madhya Pradesh yet these were effectively combated to cause any serious loss of life.

Balanced Diet

People are now getting more and more nutritive and balanced diet than before. Government is also paying more attention to it. This has helped in reducing death rate.

Decline in Social Evils

Due to spread of education several social evils like purdah system, drugging of the female children are on the decline. This has reduced the death rate.

Change of Habits

People's habits have undergone a quite change. They now pay more need to health and cleanliness. This has kept the death rate low. In brief decline in death rate has been more than birth rate.

Better Sanitation and Community Health Schemes

These have increased average lifespan. (According to World Bank Report, average lifespan of man was 60.4 years during 1988–95 period, while it was 55 years during 1980–85 period and 50 years during 1970–71.) According to 2011 census, life expectancy of an Indian is 69.89 years.

Improvement in Agriculture

It included mechanization of agriculture; use of disease free, hybrid and high yielding varieties of seeds; and use of fertilizers and pesticides, etc. These have tremendously increased food production and availability. This has guaranteed adequate food for all.

Better Living Standards

Better living standards can change the lifestyle and helps to have a healthy lifestyle. Better living standards can helps in improving economic status and educational label of the people which has a direct significant relationship with health.

High Birth Rate

Universal and Early Marriages

In India universal marriage is a social custom. Early marriages are one of the major cause for the high birth rate. According to the law it is not permissible for girls to get married before the age of eighteen years and boys before twenty-one years. But in many rural and backward areas people are married early and even child marriages are prevalent. As the child-bearing capacity is more at an early age, birth rate tends to be higher. This generally leads to a larger number of children being born. Increase in social awareness is the only way to solve this problem.

Poverty and Illiteracy

Poverty and illiteracy are two other factors. Children are seen as additional working hands in poorer families. It is felt that they can contribute to the family's income and also support their parents in their old age. In reality, in a larger family it is harder to provide proper food, nutrition, and education for all the children. Thus, more children are condemned to being illiterate. Illiteracy, especially amongst women again leads to a larger number of children.

Preference of a Male Child

In Indian society, more importance is given to the male child as certain religious duties have to be performed only by sons. So they go for more and more child expecting a son to come. This leads to a high birth rate.

Climatic Factor

India is a hot country. In the hot climate girls get puberty at an early age which lengthens the fertility period. In the cold countries, girls get puberty late which reduces their effective period to produce children. In India, this climatic factor along with other socioeconomic factors has in a high birth rate.

High Infant Mortality

Infant mortality rate is very high in India due to hunger, malnutrition and poor living conditions. So the fear of early death of their infants encourages the parents to have more children.

Inadequate Supply of Family Welfare Services

There is inadequate supply of family welfare services, e.g., contraceptives. Poverty and ignorance discourage people from using contraceptives to practise small family norms. It adds to high birth rate.

Inadequate Recreational Facilities

Due to poverty, people have very little entertainment facilities. Sex is the only entertainment with most of the people. So birth rate increases.

Effect of Religion

In India, religion plays a major role in large size families. In Hindu family a son is must to provide continuity to family legacy. Similarly in Muslim families family planning is not allowed and it is against their religion which helps in increasing birth rate.

Agricultural Occupation

India is an agricultural country. Even children get some sort of work in agriculture. Thus they do not prove to be burden on the family. So rural population in India has the tendency to have large families.

Joint Family System

India is mainly an agricultural country. The social structure is dominated by the joint family system. An additional child born causes no immediate hardships to the parents. This factor is also responsible for high birth rate.

Dependency of Women

Generally, India is a male dominated country and females are generally dependent upon men. The urge to have a sex of male without using family planning methods can lead to high birth rate.

Illiteracy and Ignorance

According to census collection 2011 the literacy rate in India is 74.4%. Illiterate or poorly literate people have a lot of misconception regarding the adverse effects of different methods of family planning and these type of people resisst to change which otherwise leads to increase birth rate.

SOURCES OF DEMOGRAPHY

Population Census

It is the main source of demographic data worldwide. Census is the process of collecting, compiling, evaluating and disseminating demographic data at a specified time covering all persons in a country or in a well delimited part(s) of a country. Most countries, nations and states carry out their population censuses after every ten years as per United Nations recommendation provide information on size, composition, spatial distribution and information on fertility and mortality in countries that may not have fully developed their vital registration system. Censuses are carried out on either de facto or dejure basis. On de facto basis a person is enumerated where he/she is found whilst on dejure basis a person is enumerated at their usual place of residence.

National Sample Survey

The most flexible of all data collection methods which can investigate almost every demographic variable is National sample survey. Household surveys in particular are key source of data on special phenomenon and they provide a mechanism for supplying data that may not be met by censuses and VRS due to the fact that censuses cannot be frequently carried out. This is a dual record system, enumeration of births and deaths by an enumerator and independent survey every 6 months by investigator supervision. This surveys provide a basis for updating some census information at national or other large domains may examine such topics as fertility, mortality and morbidity. The overall cost of a survey is generally lower compared to a census. In general sample surveys produce statistical information of better quality because, as stated earlier, it is more feasible to engage better and well-trained enumerators.

Registration of Vital Statistics

Vital registration systems (VRSs) are part of administrative records and are another major source of demographic data. VRSs provide vital demographic information on a number of issues amongst which there is migrations, deaths, births, marriages, divorces, adoptions. VRSs in developing countries are still lagging behind. The majority of African countries do not have adequate civil registration and vital statistics systems, hence unable to produce current and continuous fertility and mortality statistics, including causes of death statistics at national and subnational countries with developed VRSs however are able to produce periodic reports on vital demographic events like the number of live births by sex, date, place and time of birth, number of deaths by sex.

Statistical Survey

The term health survey is used for surveys relating to any aspects of health morbidity, mortality, nutritional status, etc. When the mean variable to be studied in disease suffered by the people, the survey is referred as morbidity survey. The statistical survey is specially related the data on vital statistics like birth rate, death rate and fertility rate, etc.

Demographic Studies

Study conducted on demography also provide data about the population's education, occupation, etc. The demographic studies provide information about the latest demographic changes occurring from time to time.

Records

Records used in almost every country and a common example of such are health statistics from hospitals. Their reliability in providing accurate demographic data depends upon the completeness of the administrative recording process and the competence of reporting. Administrative recorded are a very cost effective data source in developing countries but unfortunately in most of the very same developing countries, have not yet fully developed their administrative recording systems.

Analysis and Interpretation of Data

The demographic data collected by any means needs to analyze and interpret. After analysis the collected data are need to be arranged in tables, charts, diagrams, graphs, pictures and curves to stress important points.

Tabulation

The table is a set of data arranged in rows and columns. Almost any quantitative information can be organized into a table. Tables are useful for demonstrating patterns, exceptions, differences, and other relationship. The table must have Title, Numbering, Clear and Concise data and headings of columns or rows. Tables should not be too large and presented data must be writte chronologically, alphabetically or geographically.

Charts

The analyzed data can be presented by different types of charts namely bar charts, pie charts and line diagrames, etc. (The charts and diagrams detail explained in Chapter 3 under the heading of presentation of epidemiological data).

Interpretation of Data

The data collected is analyzed and then interpreted so that interpretations can be generalized to public. The data interpreted should be in rate, ratio, percentage, mean, median, mode and normal curve. The demographic data can be analyzed and interpreted in forms of mainly rate and ratios.

Demographic Rates and Ratio

Birth Rate

Birth rate is a good indicator of demography, which tells about whether the birth rate is increasing or decreasing as compared to other countries as well as death rate. It is calculated by:

$$\text{Birth rate} = \frac{\text{Number of live births during the year}}{\text{Estimated mid-year population}} \times 1000$$

Death Rate

Death rate provides information about the age at which death is occurred and also about the cause of death.

$$\text{Death rate} = \frac{\text{Total no. of deaths during the year}}{\text{Estimated mid-year population}} \times 1000$$

Total Fertility Rate

Total fertility rate is the average number of children a women would have if she is to pass through its reproductive years bearing children at the same rate as women in each age group.

General Fertility Rate

It is defined as the number of live births per 1000 estimated mid year female population in reproductive age in a given year.

$$GFR = \frac{\text{No. of live births in an area during the year}}{\text{Mid-year female population in reproductive in same area in same year}} \times 1000$$

Net Reproduction Rate

Net Reproduction Rate (NRR) is defined as the number of daughters a newborn girl will bear during her lifetime assuming fixed age-specific fertility and mortality rates.

Ratio

- **Child woman ratio:** It is the number of children 0–4 years of age per 1000 women of child-bearing age, usually defined as 15–49 years of age.
- **Pregnancy ratio:** No of pregnancies in a year:Married women in reproductive age.
- **Abortion ratio:** Number of all types of abortion:Number of live births.

WORLD POPULATION TREND

At the beginning of the Christian era, nearly 2,000 years ago, world population was estimated to be around 250 million. Subsequent estimates of the world population and rates of increase are given in **Table 8.7**. After 1800 AD the world population to reach one billion. The second billion came after 130 years (around 1930 AD). If we will check carefully we can observe the third billion in 30 years (around 1960), the fourth billion in 15 years (in 1974), the fifth billion in 12 years (in 1987), and the sixth billion in 12 years (1999). The 7th billion came in 2014 (after 15). It is expected to reach 8 billion by 2025. Trends on increase of population of SEAR countries is shown in **Table 8.8**.

Table 8.7: World population.

Year	Population (million)	Average annual growth rate (%)
1750	791	—
1800	978	0.4
1850	1,262	0.5
1900	1,650	0.6
1950	2,526	1.1
1960	3,037	1.79
1970	3,696	1.92
1975	4,066	1.89
1908	4,432	1.72
1987	5,000	1.63
1991	5,385	1.7
1998	5,884	1.6
2000	6,054	1.4
2003	6,313	1.1
2007	6,655	1.4
2008	6,734	1.2
2010	6,908	1.23
2014	7,238	1.2
2016	7,418	1.2
2018	7,621	1.2
2019	7,715	1.1
2020	7,794	1.1

Birth Rate

It refers to the number of live births per 1,000 on estimated midyear population in a defined area per year. World's birth rate falls to 18.2 during mid 2019 and India's birth rate falls to 20 in 2020 **(Table 8.9)**.

Fertility rate of different countries had declined a lot if we compare the fertility rate of different countries between 1970 census and 2010 census **(Fig. 8.6)**. In 2020 crude birth rate has been reduced to below 20. We can observe a great achievement but still when comparing to other countries India requires to reduce population growth. In all these countries fertility declined due to Govt. Attitude towards growth, spread of education, increased availability of contraception and marked change in marriage pattern.

Table 8.8: Trends on increase of population of SEAR countries (in million).

Country	1991	Mid-2020
India	843.9	1,400.0
Bangladesh	118	169.8
Bhutan	1.5	0.7
Indonesia	187.7	271.7
Maldives	0.221	0.5
Myanmar	42.5	54.7
Nepal	19.6	30.0
Sri Lanka	17.4	21.9
Thailand	56.4	66.5

Table 8.9: Total fertility rates in selected development and developing countries from 1994 and 2020.

Country	1994	2020
India	3.7	1.8
Bangladesh	3.9	2.1
Nepal	4.8	1.9
Sri Lanka	2.3	2.2
Myanmar	3.6	2.2
China	1.9	1.7
Pakistan	5.5	3.6
UK	1.8	1.8
USA	2.0	1.8
Japan	1.5	1.4
Switzerland	1.5	1.5

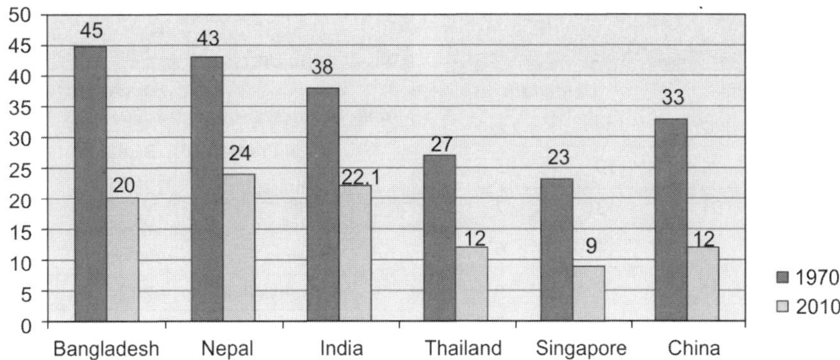

Fig. 8.6: Comparison of fertility rate in different countries (1970 census and 2010 census).

Death Rate

Death rate means number of death per 1,000 estimated mid-year population in a year in a defined area.

The death rate of world as well as countries have declined. Mainly the death rate is affected by IMR under five mortality rate which has been declined because of improved maternal and child health services, expanded program on immunization, diarrheal disease, respiratory diseases, etc. According to SRS 2020 survey the crude death was 6 per thousand population. **Figure 8.7** shows comparison of death rate in different countries. **Table 8.10** shows reduction in birth and death rates in selected countries, 1990-mid-2020.

Table 8.11 shows birth and death rates in selected development and developing countries in mid-2020.

Growth Rate

It is rate at which a population increase or decrease in a given year because of natural increase and net migration.

The world's population has declined from 1.92% in 1970 to 1.23% in 2010. Approximately 95% of growth is occurring in developing countries.

$$\textbf{Growth rate} = \frac{\textbf{(B - D)} \pm \textbf{(I - E)}}{\textbf{Total mid-year population}} \times \textbf{100}$$

DEMOGRAPHIC TRENDS IN INDIA (TABLES 8.12 AND 8.13)

Demographic characteristics provide an overview of its population size, composition, distribution, change, etc. Population statistics is measured by the indicators that measure size, sex ratio, density and dependency ratio. Similarly vital statistics is measured by the indicators like birth rate, death rate, natural growth rate, life expectancy at birth, mortality and fertility rate.

With a population of 1400.2 million in the year mid 2020, India is the 2nd most populous country in the world, where as 7th in land area, i.e., it supports 17.5% population but only 2.4% of land area. The population growth rate varies in different parts of the world. The striking difference is between the developing and developed countries of the world. According to the UN's World Population Dashboard, China still had slightly more people than India at the end of 2022 i.e., 1.45 billion, compared to India's 1.41 billion. But China's population has stabilized and is set to shrink, while India's is still growing.

India's population is steadily increasing since 1921. India's population is 238 million in 1921 and become double in 60 years, i.e., 439 million in 1961 and also double again after 30 years (846 million) in 1991. It crosses 1 billion mark on May 2000 and is projected to reach 1.53 billion in 2050. This will make India most populous country in this world by suppressing China.

Age-sex Composition

The age-sex composition of India's population is shown in **Table 8.14**. In the age group 0–14 years male population is

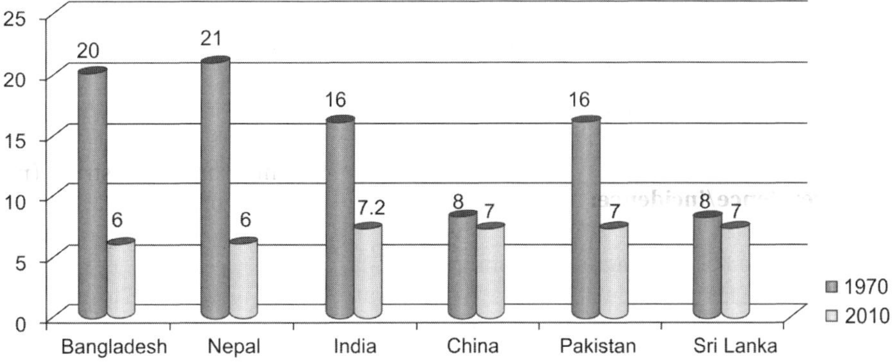

Fig. 8.7: Comparison of death rate in different countries.

Table 8.10: Reduction in birth and death rates in selected countries, 1990-mid-2020.

Country	Birth rate		Death rate	
	1990	2020	1990	2020
Bangladesh	35	21	10	5
Nepal	38	21	13	7
India	31	20	11	6
Sri Lanka	21	15	7	6
Thailand	19	10	8	8
Singapore	18	9	5	5
China	23	10	8	7
Pakistan	40	28	11	6

Table 8.11: Birth and death rates in selected development and developing countries in mid-2020.

Country	Birth rate	Death rate
India	20	6
Bangladesh	21	5
Pakistan	28	6
Sri Lanka	15	6
Thailand	10	8
Myanmar	18	8
Nepal	21	7
China	10	7
Japan	7	11
Singapore	9	5
UK	11	9
USA	12	9

Table 8.12: Census (1901–2011).

Year	Population	Annual growth rate (%)	Decadal growth rate (%)
2011	1,210,854,977	0.56	0.75
2001	1,028,737,436	-0.3	-0.31
1991	846,421,039	1.4	11.00
1981	683,329,097	1.33	14.22
1971	548,159,652	1.25	13.31
1961	439,234,771	1.96	21.64
1951	361,088,090	2.20	24.80
1941	318,660,580	2.22	24.66
1931	278,977,238	2.16	23.87
1921	251,321,213	1.7	21.52
1911	252,093,390	1.64	17.66

Table 8.13: Ranking of most populous states by projected population size 2020.

Rank	States	Population 2020 (000)	Percent to total Population of India 2020
1.	Uttar Pradesh	231,425	16.7
2.	Maharashtra	128,711	9.0
3.	Bihar	105,377	7.8
4.	Andhra Pradesh	90,949	6.5
5.	Madhya Pradesh	82,134	5.9
6.	Rajasthan	76,759	5.5
7.	Tamil Nadu	70,617	5.0
8.	Gujarat	65,532	4.7
9.	Karnataka	64,410	4.6
10.	Odisha	43,732	3.1

Table 8.14: Percent distribution of estimated population by Age and sex, India (2018).

Age group	Population percentage		
	Total	Males	Females
0–4	8.0	8.2	7.8
5–9	8.6	8.8	8.4
10–14	9.3	9.5	9.1
15–19	10.2	10.4	10.0
20–24	10.8	10.5	11.0
25–29	10.1	9.9	10.2
30–34	8.4	8.5	8.4
35–39	7.3	7.2	7.3
40–44	6.2	6.2	6.2
45–49	5.3	5.3	5.3
50–54	4.2	4.3	4.2
55–59	3.5	3.4	3.6
60–64	3.0	2.9	3.0
65–69	2.1	2.1	2.2
70–74	1.4	1.3	1.5
75–79	0.9	0.8	0.9
80–84	0.5	0.4	0.5
85+	0.3	0.2	0.3
Total	100.0	100.0	100.0

about 1.2% more than female, whereas in the age group more than 60 population, percentage of female population is 0.7% more than male population. The proportion of population in the age group 0-14 years is higher in rural areas (27.5%) than in urban areas (22.6%), for both male and female population. The proportion of population below 14 years of age is showing decline, whereas the proportion of elderly in the country is increasing.

Sex Ratio

Sex ratio is defined as the number of female per 1,000 males. Population growth and economic development of a nation depend on a great extent on sex composition. The sex composition of a country depends upon sex

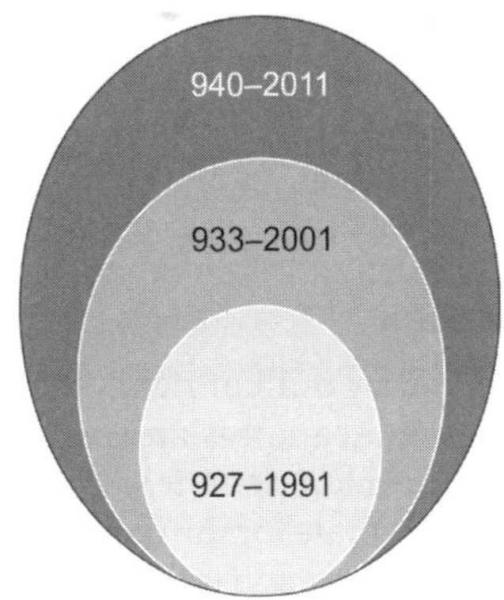

Fig. 8.8: Sex ratios in India in different census.

selective migration, mortality and sex ratio at birth. The causes of decline in sex ratio are generally strong male child preference, gender inequity, neglect of girl child, female infanticide, female feticide, easy availability of sex determination test, abortion services, child marriage, economic dependence and low status of the women in the family. A low sex ratio indicates strong male-child preference and consequent gender inequities, neglect of the girl child resulting in higher mortality at younger age, female infanticide, female feticide, higher maternal mortality and male bias in enumeration of population.

Sex ratio at birth: Sex ratio at birth can be affected by sex-selectivity and female feticide at birth. The sex ratio at birth for India for the year 2016–2018 has been estimated at 899. It varies from 900 in rural areas to 897 in urban areas. Among the different bigger states, the sex ratio at birth varies from 958 in Chhattisgarh to 843 in Haryana. In the rural areas, the highest and lowest sex ratio at birth are in the states of Chhattisgarh (976) and Haryana (840) respectively. The sex ratio in urban areas varies from 968 in Madhya Pradesh to 810 in Uttarakhand. **Figure 8.8** shows sex ratios in India in different census. **Table 8.14** shows percent distribution of estimated population by age and sex, India (2018). **Table 8.15** shows the variations of sex ratio at birth by residence in the bigger states of the country.

Table 8.15: Sex ratio at birth by residence in India (2016–2018).

	No. of females per 1000 males		
Bigger states	*Total*	*Rural*	*Urban*
Andhra Pradesh	920	930	898
Assam	925	927	905
Bihar	895	896	883
Chhattisgarh	958	976	881
Delhi	844	960	841
Gujarat	866	866	865
Haryana	843	840	847
Himachal Pradesh	930	932	891
Jammu and Kashmir	927	930	917
Jharkhand	923	932	888
Karnataka	924	949	881
Kerala	957	967	947
Madhya Pradesh	925	914	968
Maharashtra	880	878	881
Odisha	933	940	891
Punjab	890	878	908
Rajasthan	871	874	860
Tamil Nadu	908	913	903
Telangana	901	918	875
Uttar Pradesh	880	865	934
Uttarakhand	840	851	810
West Bengal	941	947	923
India	899	900	897

Dependency Ratio

Dependency ratio is generally determined by the ratio of person in dependent age group (under 15 years and over 64 years) to those in the economically productive age group (15–64 years). It is expressed as the number of person in the dependent age groups to 1000 person in the economically productive age group. It is generally two types:

1. Young age dependency ratio: 0–14 years
2. Old age dependency ratio: 65 years and more

The societal dependency ratio and reflects the need for a society to provide for their younger and older population groups. The dependency ratio can be subdivided into young age dependency ratio (0–14 years); and old age dependency ratio (65 years and more). These ratios are, however, relatively crude, since they do not take into consideration elderly or young persons who are employed or working age persons who are unemployed. It is given by the formula:

$$\text{Total dependency ratio} = \frac{\text{Population of 15 to 64 years}}{\text{Population of 15 to 64 years}} \times 100$$

For India, the dependency ratio for the year mid-2020 is calculated as:

Percentage (%)of population in 0–14 years age group = 26.2%

Percentage (%) of population above 65 years of age = 6.6%

Percentage (%) of population in 15–64 years age group = 67.3%

$$\text{Total dependency} = \frac{26.2 + 6.6}{67.3} = 48.736\%$$

The young age dependency ratio is 26.2%, and old age dependency ratio is 6.6% for the year mid 2020.

Urbanization

By definition, urban population is the number of persons residing in urban localities. The definition of urban locality varies from country to country. In Indian context, the urban areas are the "Towns (places with municipal corporation, municipal area committee, town committee, notified area committee or cantonment board); also, all places having 5,000 or more inhabitants, a density of not less than 1,000 persons per square mile or 390 per square kilometer, pronounced urban characteristics and at least three-fourths of the adult male population employed in pursuits other than agriculture".

As per population totals for the year 2019, the urban population stands at 471.828 million (34.5%). Mumbai is the highest populous city with 12.69 million followed by Delhi 10.927 million, Bengaluru comes third with 5.104 million, Kolkata 4.631 million is fourth and Chennai (4.328 million) is fifth. Fig. 3 indicates the level of urbanization in the country.

Causes of Urbanization

- Natural growth
- Migration from village for employment opportunity
- Attraction for better living conditions
- Availability of better social services like education, transportation, medical facilities, entertainments, etc. **Table 8.16** shows urban scenario in India.

Density of Population (Fig. 8.9)

It means No. of population living in 1 square kilometer. Though decadal growth rate is decreasing but density of population continuously increasing in India. There are a lot of factors which affecting the density of population has written below:

Factors Affecting Density of Population

- Climate of specific region
- Amount of rainfall
- Availability of water and electricity
- Natural composition of land
- Types of surface layer of land
- Stage of economic development
- Transportation facility
- Sociocultural environment
- Security of life and property

Table 8.16: The urban scenario in India.

Administrative Units	*Census 2011*	*2020*	*Increase*
No. of states/UTs	35	37	2
No. of districts	640	741	101
No. of subdistricts	5,924	6,553	629
No. of villages	640,867	664,369	23,502

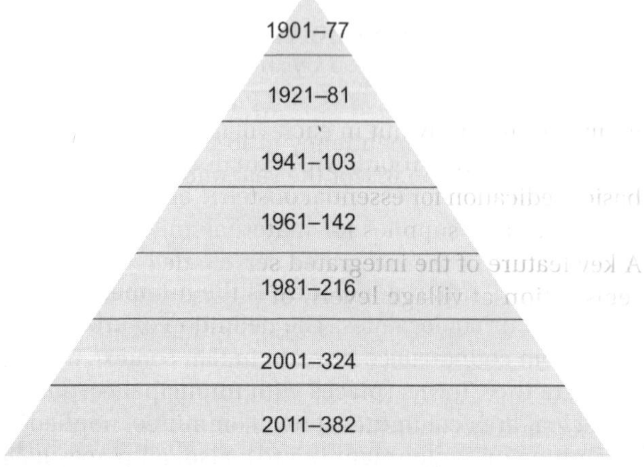

Fig. 8.9: Density of population in India.

Literacy and Education

In 1948, it was declared by human right that everyone has a right for education. Education is an crucial element for economic and social development. It was decided in 1991 census, to use the term literate for the population relating to 7 years of age and above. A person is deemed as literate if he or she can read and write with understanding any language. The same concept also continuing till 2011 census. Government has made the literacy compulsory up to the age of 14 years. According to 2011 census the male literacy rate is 82.14 where as the female literacy ratio is 65.46. Kerala occupy top rank of 93.91. On the other hand Bihar has the lowest literacy rate, i.e., 63.82, than Arunachal Pradesh 66.9%. Odisha has 73.45% out of which male literacy is 82.40 and female is 64.36%.

Life Expectancy

Life expectancy or expectation of life—at a given age is the average number of years which a person of that age may expect to live, according to the mortality pattern prevalent in that country. Demographers consider it as one of the best indicators of a country's level of development and of the overall health status of its population. Life expectancy at birth has continued to increase globally over the years. For 1950–1955, the combined life expectancy at birth for both sexes were 46.5 years. Five decades later by 2008, it was 69 years, an increase of 22.5 years. In 2020 life expectancy of India is 68 years. The life expectancies of different countries have been shown in **Table 8.17**.

NATIONAL POPULATION POLICY, 2000

To control the population explosion national population policy, 2000 has been developed.

In 1952, India was the first country in the world to launch a national program emphasizing family planning

Table 8.17: Expectation of life at birth in years, in selected countries 2020.

Developing countries	*2020*		*Developing countries*	*2020*	
	Male	*Female*		*Male*	*Female*
Nepal	67	70	UK	79	83
Bangladesh	71	74	USA	76	81
Myanmar	64	69	Sweden	81	85
India	68	70	Switzerland	82	85
Sri Lanka	74	80	Russian Federation	68	78
Thailand	73	80	Japan	81	87
Pakistan	67	71	Singapore	81	85

to the extent necessary for reducing birth rates 'to stabilize the population at a level consistent with the requirement of national economy'. After 1952, sharp declines in death rates were, however, not accompanied by a similar drop in birth rates. The National Health Policy, 1983 stated that replacement levels of total fertility rate (TFR) should be achieved by the year 2000. On 11th May, 2000, India is projected to have 1 billion (100 crore) people, i.e., 16% of the world's population on 2.4% of the globe's land area. In that time for stabilizing population become an essential requirement for promoting sustainable development with more equitable distribution. However, for making reproductive health care accessible and affordable for all, as of increasing the provision and outreach of primary and secondary education, extending basic amenities, including sanitation, safe drinking water and housing, besides empowering women and enhancing their employment opportunities the population policy has been emerged.

Objectives

Immediate Objectives

To address the unmet needs for contraception, health care infrastructure and health personnel and to provide integrated service delivery for basic reproductive and child health care.

Medium-term Objective

To bring the TFR to replacement level by 2010, through vigorous implication of intersectoral operational strategies.

Long-term Objective

To achieve a stable population by 2045, at a level consistent with the requirements of sustainable economic growth, social development and environmental protection.

Sociodemographic Goals

As per NPP, 2000, the goals to be achieved by 2010 are as follows:

- Address the unmet needs for basic reproductive and child health services, supplies and infrastructure
- Make school education up to the age 14 free and compulsory, and reduce drop out at primary and secondary level to below 20% for both boys and girls.
- Reduce infant mortality rate to below 30 per 1000 live births
- Reduce maternal mortality ratio to below 100 per 100,000 live births
- Achieve universal immunization of children against all vaccine preventable diseases.
- Promote delayed marriage for girls, not earlier than the age of 18, preferably after 20 years of age.
- Achieve 80% of institutional deliveries and 100% deliveries by trained persons.
- Achieve universal access to information/counseling, and services for fertility regulation and contraception with a wide basket of choices.
- Achieve 100% registration of birth, death and pregnancy.
- Contain the spread of AIDS and promote greater integration between the management of RTI, STI and the NACO.
- Prevent and control communicable diseases.
- Integrate Indian System of Medicine in the provision of RCH services and in reaching out to households.
- Promote vigorously the small family norm to achieve replacement level of TFR.
- Bring about convergence in implementation of related social sector programs so that family welfare becomes a people centered program.

Strategic Themes

Decentralized Planning and Program Implementation

The 73rd and 74th Constitutional Amendments Act, 1992, made health, family welfare, and education a responsibility of village panchayats. The panchayati raj institutions are an important means of furthering decentralized planning and program implementation in the context of the NPP 2000. However, in order to realize their potential, they need strengthening by further delegation of administrative and financial powers, including powers of resource mobilization.

Convergence of Service Delivery at Village Levels

Efforts at population stabilization will be effective only if we direct an integrated package of essential services at village and household levels. Below district levels, current health infrastructure includes 2,500 community health centers, 25,000 primary health centers (each covering a population of 30,000), and 1.36 lakh subcenters (each covering a population of 5,000 in the plains and 3,000 in hilly regions). Inadequacies in the existing health infrastructure have led to an unmet need of 28% for contraception services, and obvious gaps in coverage and outreach. Health care centers are over-burdened and struggle to provide services with limited personnel and equipment. Absence of supportive supervision, lack of training in interpersonal communication, and lack of motivation to work in rural areas, together impede the healthcare provider in providing reproductive and child health services, and contribute to poor quality of services and an apparent insensitivity to client's needs. The service should reach at door step by universalize coverage and outreach of antenatal, natal and postnatal health care. An equipped maternity hut in each village should be set up to serve as a delivery room, with functioning midwifery kits, basic medication for essential obstetric aid, and indigenous medicines and supplies for maternal and new born care. A key feature of the integrated service delivery will be the registration at village levels, of births, deaths, marriage, and pregnancies. Each village should maintain a list of community midwives and trained birth attendants, village health guides, panchayat sewa sahayaks, primary school teachers and anganwadi workers who may be entrusted with various responsibilities in the implementation of integrated service delivery.

Empowering Women for Improved Health and Nutrition

The complex sociocultural determinants of women's health and nutrition have cumulative effects over a lifetime. Discriminatory childcare leads to malnutrition and impaired physical development of the girl child. Undernutrition and micronutrient deficiency in early adolescence goes beyond mere food entitlements to those nutrition-related capabilities that become crucial to a woman's well-being, and through her, to the well-being of children. The positive effects of good health and nutrition on the labor productivity of the poor is well documented. To the extent that women are over-represented among the poor, interventions for improving women's health and nutrition are critical for poverty reduction. Impaired health and nutrition is compounded by early childbearing, and consequent risk of serious pregnancy related complications. Women's risk of premature death and disability is highest during their reproductive years. Malnutrition, frequent pregnancies, unsafe abortions, RTI and STI, all combine to keep the maternal mortality ratio in India among the highest globally.

Child Health and Survival

Infant mortality is a sensitive indicator of human development. High mortality and morbidity among infants and children below 5 years occurs on account of inadequate care, asphyxia during birth, premature birth, low birth weight, acute respiratory infections, diarrhea, vaccine preventable diseases, malnutrition and deficiencies of nutrients, including vitamin A. Infant mortality rates have not significantly declined in recent years.

Our priority is to intensify neonatal care. A National Technical Committee should be set up, consisting principally of consultants in obstetrics, pediatrics (neonatologists), family health, medical research and statistics from among academia, public health professionals, clinical practitioners and government. Its terms of reference should include prescribing perinatal audit norms, developing quality improvement activities with monitoring schedules and suggestions for facilitating provision of continuing medical and nursing education to all perinatal healthcare providers.

Meeting the Unmet Needs for Family Welfare Services

In both rural and urban areas there continue to be unmet needs for contraceptives, supplies and equipment for integrated service delivery, mobility of health providers and patients, and comprehensive information. It is important to strengthen, energize and make accountable the cutting edge of health infrastructure at the village, subcenter and primary health center levels, to improve facilities for referral transportation, to encourage and strengthen local initiatives for ambulance services at village and block levels, to increase innovative social marketing schemes for affordable products and services and to improve advocacy in locally relevant and acceptable dialects.

Under-served Population Groups

Urban Slums

Nearly 100 million people live in urban slums, with little or no access to potable water, sanitation facilities, and health care services. This contributes to high infant and child mortality, which in turn perpetuate high TFR and maternal mortality. Basic and primary health care, including reproductive and child health care, needs to be provided. Coordination with municipal bodies for water, sanitation and waste disposal must be pursued, and targeted information, education and communication campaigns must spread awareness about the secondary and tertiary facilities available.

Tribal Communities, Hill Area Populations and Displaced and Migrant Populations

In general, populations in remote and low density areas do not have adequate access to affordable health care services. Tribal populations often have high levels of morbidity arising from poor nutrition, particularly in situations where they are involuntarily displaced or resettled. Frequently, they have low levels of literacy, coupled with high infant, child, and maternal mortality.

Adolescents

Adolescents represent about a fifth of India's population. The needs of adolescents, including protection from unwanted pregnancies and sexually transmitted diseases (STD), have not been specifically addressed in the past. Programs should encourage delayed marriage and child-bearing, and education of adolescents about the risks of unprotected sex. Reproductive health services for adolescent girls and boys are especially essential in rural India.

Diverse Healthcare Providers

Given the large unmet need for reproductive and child health services, and inadequacies in healthcare infrastructure it is imperative to increase the numbers and diversify the categories of healthcare providers. Ways of doing this include accrediting private medical practitioners and assigning them to defined beneficiary groups to provide these services; revival of the system of licensed medical practitioner who, after appropriate certification from the Indian Medical Association (IMA), could provide specified clinical services.

Collaboration with NGOs and Private Sector

A national effort to reach out to households cannot be sustained by government alone. We need to put in place a partnership of nongovernment voluntary organizations, the private corporate sector, government and the community. Triggered by rising incomes and institutional finance, private health care has grown significantly, with an impressive pool of expertise and management skills, and currently accounts for nearly 75% of health care expenditures. However, despite their obvious potential, mobilizing the private (profit and nonprofit) sector to serve public health goals raises governance issues of contracting, accreditation, regulation, referral, besides the appropriate division of labor between the public and private health providers, all of which need to be addressed carefully. Where government interventions or capacities are insufficient, and the participation of the private sector unviable, focused service delivery by NGOs may effectively complement government efforts.

Mainstreaming Indian Systems of Medicine

India's community supported ancient but living traditions of indigenous systems of medicine has sustained the population for centuries, with effective cures and remedies for numerous conditions, including those relating to women and children, with minimal side effects. Utilization of ISMH in basic reproductive and child health care will expand the pool of effective health care providers, optimize utilization of locally-based remedies and cures, and promote low cost health care. Guidelines need to be evolved to regulate and ensure standardization, efficacy and safety of ISMH drugs for wider entry into national markets.

Contraceptive Technology and Research on Reproductive and Child Health

Government must constantly advance, encourage, and support medical, social science, demographic and behavioral science research on maternal, child and reproductive health care issues. This will improve medical techniques relevant to the country's needs, and strengthen program and project design and implementation. Consultation and frequent dialogue by Government with the existing network of academic and research institutions in allopathy and ISMH, and with other relevant public and private research institutions engaged in social science, demography and behavioral research must continue.

Providing Care for the Older Population

Improved life expectancy is leading to an increase in the absolute number and proportion of persons aged 60 years and above, and is anticipated to nearly double during 1996–2016, from 62.3 million to 112.9 million. When viewed in the context of significant weakening of traditional support systems, the elderly are increasingly vulnerable, needing protection and care. Promoting old age health care and support will help to reduce burden of the society and develop a healthy successful aging.

Information, Education, and Communication

Information, education and communication (IEC) of family welfare messages must be clear, focused and disseminated everywhere, including the remote corners of the country, and in local dialects. This will ensure that the messages are effectively conveyed. These need to be strengthened and their outreach widened, with locally relevant, and locally comprehensible media and messages. On the model of the total literacy campaigns which have successfully mobilized local populations, there is need to undertake a massive national campaign on population related issues.

Legislation, Public Support and New Structures

Legislation

As a motivational measure, in order to enable state governments to fearlessly and effectively pursue the agenda for population stabilization contained in the National Population Policy (NPP), 2000, one legislation is considered necessary.

Public Support

Demonstration of strong support to the small family norm, as well as personal example, by political, community, business, professional and religious leaders, media and film stars, sports personalities, and opinion makers, will enhance its acceptance throughout society. The government will actively enlist their support in concrete ways.

New Structures for NPP 2000

The NPP 2000 is to be largely implemented and managed at panchayat and nagarpalika levels, in coordination with the concerned state/Union Territory administrations. Accordingly, the specific situation in each state/UT must be kept in mind. This will require comprehensive and multisectoral coordination of planning and implementation between health and family welfare on the one hand, along with schemes for education, nutrition, women and child development, safe drinking water, sanitation, rural roads, communications, transportation, housing, forestry development, environmental protection, and urban development. Accordingly, the following structures are recommended:

National Commission on Population

National Commission on Population was Formulated on 11th May 2000 and reconstituted on Feb 2005. It presided over by the Prime Minister, will have the Chief Ministers of all states and UTs, and the Central Minister in charge of the Department of Family Welfare and other concerned Central Ministries and Departments, for example Department of Woman and Child Development, Department of Education, Department of Social Justice and Empowerment in the Ministry of HRD, Ministry of Rural Development, Ministry of Environment and Forest, and others as necessary, and reputed demographers, public health professionals, and NGOs as members.

Aims

- To review, monitor and give directions for the implementation of the National Population Policy.
- To promote synergy between demographic, educational, environmental and developmental programs.
- To promote intersectoral coordination in planning and implementation.

- First Meeting-23rd July 2005: Survey of all District to identify the weakness in Health Care Delivery System.

State Population Commission

Each state and UT may consider having a State/UT Commission on Population, presided over by the Chief Minister, on the analogy of the National Commission, to likewise oversee and review implementation of the NPP 2000 in the states/UTs.

Coordination Cell in the Planning Commission

The Planning Commission will have a Coordination Cell for intersectoral coordination between Ministries for enhancing performance, particularly in States/UTs needing special attention on account of adverse demographic and human development indicators.

Technology Mission in the Department of Family Welfare

To enhance performance, particularly in states with currently below average sociodemographic indices that need focused attention, a Technology Mission in the Department of Family Welfare will be established to provide technology support in respect of design and monitoring of projects and programs for reproductive and child health, as well as for IEC campaigns.

Promotional and Motivational Measures

- Panchayat and Zilla Parisads will be rewarded and honored for exemplary performance in achieving the above laid goals
- Balikasamridhi Yojana run by the department of Women and child development.
- For maternal benefit—₹500 is rewarded to mother who have delivered after 19 years of age
- Health insurance plan for the couple with BPI who under gone sterilization not less than 2 children will get insurance of ₹5000
- Establishment of self-help group at village level
- Opening of creche at rural and urban slum
- Local entrepreneur at villege level will be provided soft loan for provision of Ambulance services
- Voccational scheme for girl child
- Strict enforcement of child marriage restraint act
- Strict enforcement of prenatal diagnostic test.

Although there have been some spectacular achievements in the health sector, the overall picture is rather grim. While we have sophisticated world-class tertiary care facilities, our primary health care is riddled with problems due to a resource crunch and poor management of manpower and equipment. Communicable diseases, lifestyle diseases, accidents and injuries and newer emerging infections seem to have overwhelmed the health care industry.

The problem IMR/MMR is high and not declining fast enough, especially in rural areas and among the poor. High and prohibitive out of pocket expenditure makes access of poor people to health services difficult. Population stabilization is ineffective especially in a number of EAG States/CMP districts. Public health system is on the decline—poor governance, manpower shortages, ineffective service delivery.

The next problem is Involvement of community/PRIs/local government/user groups in health programs is weak. Mapping of people's health needs is not undertaken leading to people's needs being different from what the system has to offer. Convergence at Zilla Parishad level is weak-implications for wider determinants of health.

Large nongovernmental sector meets health needs of poor—at a price, often unethically, over prescription, syringe—saline syndrome. Government programmes have very little to do with the nongovernmental sector even though it is 4–5 times larger and can improve indicators/outcomes.

The health care conundrum 'There is growing evidence that the current health systems of nations around the world will be unsustainable if unchanged over the next 15 years'. Globally, health care is threatened by a confluence of powerful trends—increasing demand, rising costs, uneven quality, misaligned incentives. If ignored, they will overwhelm health systems, creating massive financial burdens for individual countries and devastating health problems for the individuals who live in them.

METHODS OF FAMILY SPACING

For family welfare, family planning is necessary. Family planning is the voluntary planning regarding childbirth by person or couples. Child birth should be according to their desire or choice not by chance.

Definition

- Planning for responsible parenthood is family planning.
- A way of thinking and living that is adopted voluntarily, upon the basis of knowledge, attitude and responsible decision by individual and couples in order to promote the health and family welfare of the family group and thus contribute effectively to the social development of a country.

Objectives

- To avoid unwanted births
- To bring about wanted births
- To regulate the interval between pregnancies
- To control the times at which birth occurs in relation to the ages of the parent
- To determine the no. of children in the family.

Table 8.18 shows achievement of NPP 2000.

Table 8.18: Achievement of NPP 2000.

Year	*CBR*	*IMR*	*TFR*
1997	27.2	71	3.3
1998	26.4	72	3.3
2002	23.0	50	2.6
2010	21.0	30	2.1

Scope of Family Planning Services

- Proper spacing between birth
- Limits number of birth
- Diagnosis of RTI
- Premarital examination/counseling
- Pregnancy test
- Providing services to unmarried mother
- Preparing for first birth
- Education about nutrition and finances
- Sex education
- Genetic counseling
- Education about parenthood
- Marital guidance
- Adoption services.

ASPECTS/ADVANTAGES OF FAMILY PLANNING

Family planning and health have a two way relationship. In developing country like India family planning affects the health services greatly.

Health Aspects

Women's Health

Pregnancy may endanger the mother's life. The risk is more when the mother grow older and more than 3–4 children. A woman's ability to choose if and when to become pregnant has a direct impact on her health and well-being. Maternal mortality and morbidity can significantly reduced by use of family planning method. It can be done by:

- *Protection from unwanted pregnancy* (leads to an induced abortion, if it will be criminal abortion then it will have higher health risk)
- *Reducing the number of birth* (repeated pregnancy increases maternal mortality and morbidity, toxemia, uterine atony and rupture, Placenta Previa, eclampsia and anemia)
- *Spacing the birth* (maternal mortality is higher below the age of 20 or above the age of 30–35). And if mother is explained significance of age in pregnancy then the mother can be protected from unnecessary pregnancies and many more health problems.

Health of Children

Family planning can prevent closely spaced and ill-timed pregnancies and births, which contribute to some of the world's highest infant mortality rates. It is also very important for growth and development of children. Children get good nutrition and their growth and development will be better. Child mortality and infectious disease will be less.

Economic Aspect

Increase in family size lowers the per capita income. The lower per capita income leads to low domestic savings lesser resources for economic development which further leads to small rate of economic development of family and community. Growth of individual, community and economy of nation depends upon small family norm. Small family is essential for growth in employment, consumption rate, per capita income and the total national income.

Social Aspect

Family planning method and small family norm make the social structure of nation progressive. Good education, good slandered of living and proper nutrition become the basis of good society and strong citizen.

Political Aspect

It affects the density of population. Political behavior is also influenced by the change in different pressure groups.

Small Family Norms

The family size plays an important role in health and welfare of individual, family and community.

In 1970s, the slogan for small family was 'two or three is enough'. In the concept of small family, has three aspects, such as:

1. Boy or girl—only two children
2. Second child after 3 year
3. Universal immunization.

NB: As per this target India has to be contained 1.3 billion by the year 2050, but India has already been achieved 1.2 billion by the year 2011.

The size of family affects:

Basic Human Needs

If the family will be large then the basic needs like food, clothing, shelter, basic education and primary care will be shared by all the member. The per capita income will get smaller which will not fully met the needs of family member. If the family size is small then the per capita share will be more and which will met the basic need of the family.

Income, Saving and Resources

If the family size will be large, per capita income will be no saving, so there will no further development of resources.

Quality and Quantity of Food

For large family size there will be low food quality and quantity. So it will not be able to meet the nutritive quantity.

Fragmentation of Family Land

In large family because of fragmentation of paternal land there will be low productivity, which will leads to migration from rural to urban slums.

Education

As in large family resources are low, so it will be very hard to give better education to each member of the family.

Health

It has been seen that large family have higher mortality and morbidity among mother and children. It is due to:

- **Early marriage and early pregnancy:** Premature birth, LBW, Ca cervix.
- **Frequent and too many pregnancies:** Ill health of mother and LBW, divided attention between children, economic hard ship, difficulty in meeting basic needs and unhappiness.
- **Late age pregnancies:** Congenital anomaly, Mongoloid child.

Some Terminology about Fertility

- **Eligible couple:** It refers to a currently married couple where in the wife is in the reproductive age group which is assumed to lie between age of 15–45 years.
- **Target couple:** The couple who have living 2–3 children, and family planning is largely directed to such couples.
- **Couple protection rate:** It is defined as the% of eligible couples effectively protected against child birth by one or the other approved methods of planning.

CONTRACEPTION

Contraception means prevention against pregnancy by using a varieties of methods. Some of the preventive methods to help women avoid unwanted pregnancies.

Table 8.19 shows classification of contraception.

Characteristics of Ideal Contraceptive

- Effective/reliable (in preventing pregnancy)
- Safe (safe for health and free from harmful effects)
- Simple (could be used without consultation or supervision of doctor)
- Reversible (should not obstruct pregnancy when desired)
- Affordable (should have long life and inexpensive)
- Feasible and acceptable

NB: No contraceptive have all the criteria, so it should left to the choice of couple to take appropriate one which is socioculturally acceptable.

Table 8.19: Classification of contraception.

Category	*Method*
• Spacing	
▪ Natural	• Coitus interrupts • Safe period • Abstinence • Others
▪ Barrier	
– Physical	• Condom • Diaphragm • Vaginal Sponge
– Chemical	• Foam tablets • Cream, jelly or paste • Suppositories • Soluble film
▪ Intrauterine device	• Lippes loop • Cu-T
▪ Hormonal	• Oral pill ▪ Combined pill ▪ Progestogen only pill ▪ Once a month only • Depot formulation (SR) ▪ Injectable ▪ Implants ▪ Vaginal rings
▪ Postconceptional	• Menstrual regulation • Menstrual induction • Abortion
• Terminal Sterilization	• Female sterilization • Male sterilization

NATURAL METHOD

Natural method do not involve the use of any man made device. These are useful for spacing of pregnancy. Natural methods of birth control, or natural family planning, are a type of birth control that relies on observations about the woman's body and menstrual cycle or the self-control of man.

Coitus Interruptus (Withdrawal Method)

Coitus interruptus, also known as the rejected sexual intercourse, withdrawal or pull-out method, is a method of birth control in which a man, during sexual intercourse, withdraws his penis from a woman's vagina prior to orgasm or ejaculation, and then directs his ejaculate (semen) away from the vagina in an effort to prevent deposition of semen in vagina.

Merit

- No cost
- It can be used by people who have objections to, or do not have access to, other forms of contraception.
- Does not require any device
- Helps to avoid adverse effects of other forms of contraceptions.

Drawback

- Requires self-control
- The pre-ejaculated fluid which contain sufficient sperm which may cause pregnancy.
- The semen deposited outside the vagina may risk of enter into genital tract.
- Failure rate more than 25%
- Couple are often dissatisfied
- Ineffective in the prevention of sexually transmitted infections.

Safe Period/Calender Method

This method based on the process of ovulation and menstrual cycle. It believes that ovulation occurs between 12–16 days before onset of menstruation. From the first day of menses to 9th day it is considered as safe period and from 10th–19th day it is unsafe. Generally before and after one week of menstruation is considered as safe period.

NB: The day of conception is calculated as:

- Shortest cycle-18 (First fertile period)
- Longest cycle-10 (Last fertile period)

Merits

- Does not require any man made device
- Accepted by Roman Catholic Church.

Drawback

- Greater deal of self-control
- Unsuitable who have irregular periods
- Safe for those couple who are educated and can calculate safe and danger period.
- The failure rate is high, i.e., 21%.

Abstinence

This is the only method of birth control which is completely effective. But complete abstinence is not practicable because suppression of sex leads to psychosocial problems.

Other Method of Periodic Abstinence

There are three methods which are based on physiologic changes associated with ovulation, and identification of fertile period.

Basal Body Temperature

At the time of ovulation there are some rise of BBT (0.3–0.5°C) because of increased production of Progesteron. This can be recorded by to women every day after waking up and before doing any activity in BBT thermometer. Abstinence is required till 3rd day after temperature rising days.

Demerit

- Abstinence is required throughout preovulatory period
- Requires control and cooperation of spouse
- Useful among literate people.

Merit

Does not require any artificial device.

Cervical Mucus Method

Recognition of fertile period/ovulation is done by the basis of change in mucus of cervix. During ovulation the mucous becomes watery, clear, smooth and slippery. It is of large quantity and like white part of egg. After ovulation due to the effect of progesterone mucus become thick and scanty.

Abstinence is required before ovulation, during ovulation and 3 day after ovulation.

Symptothermic Method

It is the combination of BBT, calender and cervical mucus method.

By following all this method the women can calculate the fertile period and maintain abstinence.

BARRIER METHOD

Barrier methods are those which prevent meeting of sperm with ovum.

Types

- Physical
- Chemical
- Combinition

Physical Barrier

Condom (Nirodh)

Nirodh is derived from a Sanskrit word means prevention. The Condom or Nirodh can used as a family planning method vas, it act as a barrier to prevent deposing semen in the vaginal wall. It is to be fitted on an erect penis before intercourse. Before wearing of condom air should be expelled from teat end to make a room for collection of semen. After coitus carefully withdrawn is essential and then it should be discarded safely to prevent spillages. Always a new one should be used each time. If the condom will use correctly at each intercourse it will provide 95% effective.

NB: The effectiveness of condom can be used by spermicidal jelly-survey shows 2–3% failure rate.

Merit

- Easily available
- Safe and inexpensive
- Do not require any medical supervision
- No side effects
- Protects from STI and STD
- Provide 95% effectiveness if used correctly.

Demerits

- If not used correctly them may tear or slip
- May have allergy to rubber
- Some unable to enjoy sex.

Diaphragm/Dutch Cap

It is a dome or shallow cup-shaped vaginal barrier. It is available in different size ranging from 5–10 cm diameter. It has two rim, the inner one should be placed at external os. Contraceptive cream or jelly can be applied on the rim and in both sides of diaphragm which can act as both spermicide and lubricant. It should be remain in vagina at least for 5 hr of post coital period.

Merits

- Diaphragm with spermicide is very effective
- No risk.

Demerits

- Assistance of doctor/health personnel is required for determination of size and demonstration
- Requires periodic checking
- As it remain in vagina for a long period then chance for toxic shock syndrome may occur.

Vaginal Sponge

The contraceptive sponge combines barrier and spermicidal methods to prevent conception.

Three brands are marketed: Pharmatex, Protectaid and Today. Pharmatex is marketed in France and the province of Quebec; Protectaid in the rest of Canada and Europe; and Today in the United States. Sponges work in two ways. First, the sponge is inserted into the vagina, so it can cover the cervix and prevent any sperm from entering the uterus. Secondly, the sponge is produced with spermicide already inside of it, which is used to prevent the sperm from moving. The sponges are inserted vaginally prior to intercourse and must be placed over the cervix to be effective. Generally it is 5 by 2 cm. It should be inserted before coitus and gives protection for 24 hours.

Demerits

- Some people are allergic to the spermicide used in the sponge.
- Women who use contraceptive sponges have an increased risk of yeast infection and urinary tract infection.
- Improper use, such as leaving the sponge in too long, can result in toxic shock syndrome.
- Failure rate 24–40%.

Chemical Barrier

In 1960s, before advent of IUD and oral pill, spermicidal vaginal gel are used widely. The chemical barriers have to be administered into the vagina 10 minutes prior to intercourse. Most chemical contraceptives contain a variety of substances like spermicides (sperm-killing substances) and/or lactic and citric acid which in combination act as spermicides and thus as contraceptives. They melt because of the body heat and transform into a viscous mass inside the vagina which acts as a barrier for the sperm cells. The effect however lasts for only one ejaculation. After the insertion of the chemical contraceptives a slight burning sensation may occur because of a possible irritation of the mucosa. Chemical contraceptives should never be used in combination with condoms because they can seriously damage the condoms' material. They are:

- Foam—foam tablet/foam jelly
- Cream, jelly or paste
- Suppository
- Soluble films.

Merits

- Free in health center
- Increase vaginal lubrication
- Easy to administer.

Demerits

- Must be inserted deep down where sperms are get accumulated
- Must be applied each times befor sex
- May cause irritation and burning
- Chemical contraceptive can't provide a sufficient protection from an unwanted pregnancy.
- Vaginal infections may increase by using these.

INTRAUTERINE DEVICES

These are the devices which are used in the uterine cavity. They are devices which are inserted to the uterus they halt conception in different ways some, help in the prevention of fertilization to take place while others disrupt normal ovulation patterns. It may be medicated or nonmedicated made up of polyethylene and the medicated one may contain either metal ions or hormones.

First Generation IUDs (Lippes, Spiral and Coil)

These are nonmedicated polythene material of different size and shape.

Lippes Loop: The lippes loop was invented by Lippe in 1962 in USA. It is double S-shaped device made up of polythene, which is nontoxic nontissue reactive and extremely durable. It contains small amount of barium sulfate which is visible by X-ray. The loop has attached thread made of fine nylon. Lippes is available in different sizes which is projects into vagina can be felt by mother. It is a an old method of IUD which is not used nowadays. It is available in ABCD size, latter is the largest.

- **Merits:** Have greater antifertility effect and lower expulsion rate.
- **Demerits:** Higher removal rate because of pain and bleeding.

Second Generation IUDs

It was found out that metallic copper had a strong antifertility effect. Copper IUD is available in many varieties they are more effective and can be left for a long time used by women worldwide. It was tried in 1970s. These are smaller which is easy to fit.

Advantages of Cu Devices

- Low expulsion rate
- Lower incidence of side effect—pain and bleeding
- Easier to fit even in nulliparous women
- Better tolerated by nullipara
- Increased effective
- Effective as postcoital contraceptive, if inserted within 3–5 days of unprotected sex.

Third Generation IUDs

These IUDs contain hormone which is released slowly in uterus. The hormone affects the lining of uterus and cervical mucus.

- **Progestasert:** It is a T-shaped device contain 38 mg of progesterone which releases @ 65 μgm/day. It is required to be replaced after 1 year.
- **Levonorgestrel:** This is a T-shaped device with poly-dimethylesiloxane 52 mg membrane around the stem which act as a steroid reservoir. It releases @ 20 μgm/day. It is to be replaced after 5 years.

Mechanism of Action

Mechanism of action of infertility is not yet clear. They do not inhibit ovulation mainly act on uterine cavity.

- Biochemical and histological changes in endometrium.
- There is a nonspecific inflammatory reaction along with biochemical reaction which has gametotoxic and spermolytic effect. From the macrophages prostaglandin releases which has antifertility effect.
- **Increased tubal mortality:** As a result of this the fertilized ovum migrate's to the uterus when the endometrium is not ready to receive.
- **Impaired sperm ascent:** Due to local chemical action that affect sperm vitality and migration.
- Copper prevent implantation by interfering the enzymatic action.
- The hormonal IUD suppress endometrium, cervical mucus becomes scanty, anovulation and insufficient luteal phase activity.

NB: Here sr. progesterone level does not rise.

Ideal candidate for IUD:
- Who has borne at least one child
- Has no history of pelvic diseases
- Has normal menstrual periods
- Is willing to check the IUD thread
- Has access for follow-up and treatment for potential problem
- Is an monogamous relationship.

Contraindication for IUD

- **Absolute:**
  - Suspected pregnancy
  - Pelvic inflammatory disease
  - Vaginal bleeding
  - Ca cervix
  - Previous ectopic pregnancy
- **Relative:**
  - Anemia
  - Menorrhagia
  - Purulent cervical discharge
  - Distortion of uterine cavity due to malformation, fibroid
  - Unmotivated person.

Table 8.20 shows classification of copper-T.

Timing of Insertion

- **Interval:** When the insertion is made in the interconceptional period, i.e., beyond 6 wk after child birth or birth, preferably 2–3 day after period is over. But it can be inserted any time during the cycle even during menstrual phase.
- **Postabortal:** Following termination of pregnancy by suction evacuation or D and E or following spontaneous abortion
- **Postpartum:** Device can be inserted before the patient can discharged from the hospital. It is preferable after 6 weeks.
- **Postplacental delivery:** Inserted following delivery of placenta. In this case expulsion rate is high.

Advantages

- Simple procedure
- Requires very few minute for insertion
- Once inserted stays in place till it is required for removal
- Reversible
- Highest continuation rate
- No need for continual motivation.

Side Effects

- Bleeding
- Pain
- Pelvic infection
- Uterine perforation
- Pregnancy
- Ectopic pregnancy
- Expulsion
- Cancer and teratogenicity
- Mortality.

Follow-up Care

- Provide motivation and emotional support
- Confirm the presence of IUD
- Diagnose and treat side effect
- Follow-up should be done 3 m–6 m–1 year interval
- Instruction should be given for fealing the thread, inform if there is any missed period.

Table 8.20: Classification of copper-T.

Type	*Name*	*Duration*	*Amount of copper*	*Rate of release*
Earlier device	Copper-7	4 years		
	Copper-T 200	3 years	215 sq mm Fine Cu wire wounded round the vertical stem	5 µgm/24 hr
Newer device	Variant of T device • Cu-T 220c • Cu-T 380A	10 years	380 mm^2 of a Cu wire wound around the stem of 176 mg and Cu sleeve on the horizontal arms of 66.5 mg	
	Multiload devices • Ml-Cu-250 • Ml-Cu-375	3 years		60–100 µgm/day
		5 years	375 mm^2 of Cu on a vertical stem	

HORMONAL CONTRACEPTION

Hormonal contraception refers to birth control methods that act on the endocrine system. These methods are composed of steroid hormones, although in India one selective estrogen receptor modulator is marketed as a contraceptive. The original hormonal method—the combined oral contraceptive pill—was first marketed as a contraceptive in 1960. In the ensuing decades many other delivery methods have been developed, although the oral and injectable methods are by far the most popular. Altogether, 18% of the world's contraceptive users rely on hormonal methods. Hormonal contraceptives are most effective if it is used correctly. Hormonal contraceptives mainly two types. They are oral pill and depot formulation.

Classifications

- **Oral pill:**
  - Combined pill
  - Progesterone only pill
  - Post coital pill
  - Once-a-month pill
  - Male pill
- **Depot formulation (slow release):**
  - Injectable
  - Subcutaneous implants
  - Vaginal rings.

Oral Pills

Combined pill: The pill is composed of two hormones, i.e., synthetic estrogen and progestogen in small doses. The main action of the combined pill is, estrogen inhibition of ovulation of ovum by blocking the secretion of gonadotropin from pituitary gland. The progestogen render the cervical mucus thick and scanty and thereby inhibit sperm penetration and also inhibit tubal motility and delay the transport of the sperm and of the ovum to the uterine cavity. This is to be taken orally from 5th day of menstruation to 21st day followed by 7 day break during which period will occur. If there is no bleeding then the women should be instructed to take next cycle pills.

The pills should be taken regularly and at fixed time. If anyone forgets to take a pill, then take immediately when she remembered and the next pill should be taken at usual times.

There are two types of pills which are available under the brand name Mala-N and Mala-D. Mala-N is available free from Government health center and Mala-D is retailer at price of ₹3.00 per pocket.

The constituents of the pills are:

- Mala-N
  - Norethisterone acetate........0.50 mg
  - Ethinyl estradiol..................0.04 mg
- Mala-D
  - D-norgestrol........................1.0 mg
  - Ethinyl estradiol.................0.03 mg
- Mala-N and Mala-D are available in pocket of 28 tablets. The first 21 white tablets are contraceptives pills and remaining seven pills are iron pills which are to maintain sequence and supplement iron.

Merits

- It is 100% effective if taken regularly.
- Easy to use
- Does not interfere with coitus.
- Reduce risk of anemia because menstrual bleeding is less by 50%.
- Reduce risk PID, ovarian and uterine cancer
- Protects from benign breast disorders, ovarin cysts and ectopic pregnancy.
- Because of regularly medical checkups any disease can be detected and treated early.
- It corrects pre-existing menstrual problems.

Demerits

- Failure rate increases if taken irregularly.
- Dizziness, nausea, vomiting, headaches, tenderness of breast, weight gain, these subsides follows continues use of 2–3 cycles
- Mild hypertension reverse back to normal 3–6 months stoppage of pills.
- Increased risk of cardiovascular diseases if the woman already at risk.
- Increase the risk of gallbladder diseases.
- Decreases in quantity of breast milk.

Progesterone only pill: Mini pill/Micro pill: It contains only progesterone, i.e., norethisterone and levonorgestrel. This is also known as mini pill and has to has to be taken daily from the 1st day of the cycle. Progestogen thickens cervical mucus thereby prevents sperm penetration, also makes endometrium unsuitable for implantation of fertilized ovum. This pill should be taken regularly at the same time of the day. These are to be taken throughout the menstrual cycle.

Advantages

- Have no adverse effect on lactation often called lactation pill.
- Easy to take as there is no on and off regime.
- Can be prescribed patients havings hypertenstion, diabetics.
- Reduces risk of PID.

Disadvantages

Less Effective

- **Postcoital contraception: 'morning after':** It is recommended 72 hr after unprotected sex specifically after rape, unprotected intercourse, contraceptive failure. Doses are generally:
  - Levonorgestrel, 75 mg within 72 hr of unprotected sex followed by 2nd tablet after 12 hr.

    Or

- 2 OCP containing 50 mcg of ethinyl estradiol within 72 hr of unprotected sex and the same dose after 12 hr.
  Or
- 4 OCP containing 30–35 mcg of ethinyl estradiol within 72 hr of unprotected sex and the same dose after 12 hr.
  Or
- Mifepristone 10 mg once within 72 hr.

- **Once a month Pill:** It contains quinestrol which is a long acting estrogen given in combination of short acting progesterone.
- **Demerit:** Pregnancy rate is too high. Irregular bleeding.
- **Male pill:** It contains gossypol which is a derivative of cotton seed oil.

MOA

- Preventing spermatogenesis
- Interfere with sperm storage and maturation
- Prevent sperm transport into the vas
- Affect constitutes of seminal fluid.

Mode of Action of Oral Pills

It prevent release of ovum from ovary by blocking the pituitary secretion of gonadotropin. Progesteron preparation makes the mucus thick and scanty, so inhibit sperm penetration. It also decrease sperm motility.

Effectiveness

If is taken according to prescription then it is 100% effective.

Merit

- High rate of safety against pregnancy
- Easy to use
- Easy availability and inexpensive
- Regularity in menstrual cycle and breast disease.

Demerit

- Missing the dose
- **Metabolic effect:** Weight gain, high BP, coagulation problem
- **Others like:** Breast tenderness, uneasiness, headache, liver disease, ectopic pregnancy, reduced lactation, delay pregnancy, irregular menstruation.

Depot Formation

- Implants are placed in the body filled with hormone that prevents pregnancy. It is a small, flexible plastic rods or capsules, the size of paper matchsticks that inserted under the skin in the arm as 15 minute outpatient procedure.
- Same mechanism as POPs
- 99.95% effectiveness rate.
- Irregular vaginal bleeding common but not harmful
  - *Norplant (I and II):* It has 3 or 6 cilastic capsule or rod implemented below skin/arm which gave 5 years effectiveness
  - *Injectable (progesteron only):*
    - DMPA: Intramuscular injection of depot Medroxyprogesteron acetate of 150 mg every 3 month. It is suitable above 35 years of age. It is given during first 5 day of menstrual cycle.
    - NET-EN: It is an IM injection of 200 mg norethisterone enanthate. It is given in an interval of 2 monthly.
    - DMPA-SC: A new lower dose formulation of DMPA, Depo subQ provera 104 injected under the skin. It given 3 month interval.

Merit: Safe, effective, acceptable, not affect the lactation, protects from heart disease and cancer.

Demerit: Irregular menstrual cycle, excessive bleeding, stress due to missed cycle.

- **NUVA RING:** Flexible contraceptive vaginal ring that contains the hormones estrogen and progesterone. The ring releases a continuous low dose of hormones that stops the ovaries from releasing an egg each month. Insert the ring in the vagina and leave it there for three weeks. Remove the ring for one-week ring-free period, on the same day of the week at about the same time. During the one-week break, you will usually have your menstrual period.
- **Ortho Evra (The Patch):** Transdermal contraceptive patch that contains estrogen and progesterone. It is thin, flexible, two inch square that is worn on the body. The increased hormone level caused by the patch stops the ovaries from releasing an egg each month and is 99% effective.
  - Apply patch one week on the same day each week for three weeks
  - Can wear it on bottom, abdomen or on the outside of upper arm
  - During week four do not wear the patch (your period will begin).

Postconceptional Method

These are the method which are used after the period is missed and pregnancy may or may not have occurred. This method helps in regulation or inducting menstruation and termination of pregnancy and aborting the fetus.

- **Menstrual regulation:** It is done 14 day of missed period when pregnancy is doubted but not confirmed. In this the uterine content is evacuated.
- **Menstrual induction:** It is done few day after induction by applying prostaglandin F2 under sedation which causes continuous uterine contraction for 7 min. It is followed by cyclic contraction for 3–4 hr followed by bleeding for a week
- **Abortion:** Termination of pregnancy before the fetus is viable. It may be legal or illegal but illegal is dangerous.

TERMINAL METHOD

Once the family is complete it is better to do Permanent sterilization. It is a surgical procedure where the reproductive function of a male or female is permanently destroyed. It is of following types:

Vasectomy

It is a permanent sterilization operation done in male where a segment of both vas difference are resected and ligated.

It is done as an OPD procedure under local anesthesia and takes hardly 15–20 minutes.

Types

- **No-scalpel vasectomy:** It is performed under LA.
  - Stretched skin over the vas, then punctured with a sharp pointed end of a forceps instead of using scalpel
  - Vas is dissected then ligated
- **Percutaneous vas occlusion:** It is an effective reversible method. Here polyurethane elastomers are injected into the vas. It solidifies and block the vas. This procedure is popular in China.
- **Open-ended vasectomy:** Here the abdominal end of the resected vas is coagulated and the testicular end is left open. This will prevent congestive epididymitis.

Limitation

Additional contraceptive is required for 2–3 month.

Merits

- Simple technique and can be done as an outdoor procedure
- Failure rate is only 15%
- Very few complications
- Cost effective.

Complications

- **Operative:** Pain, scrotal hematoma, wound infection.
- **Sperm granules:** It occures 10–14 days after operation. It may subside or recanalize the vas.
- **Spontaneous recanalization:** Rate is 0–6%. During the procedure doctor should explained about this and regular follow-up is required till 3 years.
- **Autoimmune response:** There may be an autoimmune response to sperm and antibody may be produced against that.
- **Psychological:** May be diminish sexual vigor, impotence, headache, fatigue.

Postoperative Advice

- He is not sterile immediately, it may take 30 ejaculation to be negative
- Use contraceptive till aspermia
- Avoid taking bath for first 24 hr
- Wear t-bandage
- Avoid cycling or heavy lifting for 15 days
- Remove stitch on the 5th day.

Tubectomy

It is the female sterilization, done by resecting small part of the fallopian tube and ligating the ends.

- **Laparoscopy:** It is done by abdominal approach through laparoscope. Once the tubes are visible, the falope ring or clips are applied to occlude the tube.
- **Minilap:** Under local anesthesia a small abdominal incision (2.5–3 cm) is made, tube resected then ligated.
- **Vaginal ligation:** Tubectomy is done through vaginal route by posterior colpotomy.

Guidelines for Sterilization

- The age of husband should not be less than 25 years and not more than 50 years
- Age of wife should not be less than 20 years or more than 45 years
- The motivated couple should have 2 children
- If the couple has 3 children then lower age limit can be relaxed.

NATIONAL HEALTH COMMITTEE

Introduction

The guidelines for national health planning were provided by a number of committees. Various committees of experts have been appointed by the government from time to time to render advice about different health problems. The reports of these committees have formed an important basis of health planning in India. The goal of National Health Planning in India is to attain Health for all. In 1940, the resolution adopted by the National Planning Committee based on the Sokhey Committee's recommendations, recommended integration of preventive and curative functions and the training of a large number of health workers. Bhore committee constituted in 1943 laid the framework on which the health care was eventually built in the independent India. The health care in India has since moved from bureaucratic government based top down approach to decentralized community based bottom-up system after the Panchayati Raj came into being.

Bhore Committee

During preindependence era, to improve the preventive, promotive and curative health services of country, a National Planning Commission was set up by the Indian National Congress in 1938. The rulers of that time, the British Empire realized the importance of Public Health and instituted the Health Survey and Development Committee which is known as Bhore committee.

Bhore committee was set up by the government of India in 1943 to investigate and recommend improvements to the Indian Public Health system. Under the chairmanship of Sir Joseph Bhore the committee made many landmark recommendations in its final report in 1946. It laid emphasis on integration of curative and preventive medicine at all levels and made comprehensive recommendations for remodeling of health services in India. The committee observed that, If the nation's health is to be built, the health program should be developed on a foundation of preventive health work and that such activities should proceed side by side with those concerned with the treatment of patients. The committee also stated that health and development are interdependent so improvement in sector other than health will also lead to improvement in health like water supply, sanitation improvement, nutrition, elimination of unemployment.

Guiding Principles

- No individual should be denied to secure adequate medical care because of inability to pay.
- Facilities for proper diagnosis and treatment should available and accessible.
- Health program must lay special emphasis on preventive work.
- As much medical relief and preventive health care should be provided to the vast rural population.
- Health services should be located close to the people to ensure maximum benefit to the community.
- Doctor should be a social physician protecting the people.
- Medical services should be free to all, without distinction.

Observations Made by the Committee

- Health status of the country as indicated by various indicators was poor.
- Mortality rates were very high.
- Life expectancy at birth was about 27 years.
- Incidence of communicable diseases was very high.
- Many of the health problems were preventable.

Recommendations

- Integration of preventive and curative services at all administrative levels.
- **Development of Primary Health Centers in 2 stages:** Short-term measures and long-term program
- Major changes in medical education which includes 3-month training in preventive and social medicine to prepare 'social physicians'.
- **As a short-term measure:** Primary health center should established to cover 40,000 population with 30 beds, 3 Subcenters and 2 medical officers, 4 public health nurses, 1 nurse, 4 midwives, 4 trained dais, 2 sanitary inspectors, 2 health assistants, 1 pharmacist, and 15 class IV employees.
- **As a long-term program (3 million Plan):** The primary health units with a 75 bedded hospital with 10,000–20,000 population; secondary health units with 650 bedded hospital; regional health units with 2,500 beds should established.

Mudaliar Committee (1962)

This committee known as the Health Survey and Planning Committee, Headed by Dr AL Mudaliar. This committee was appointed to assess the performance in health sector since the submission of Bhore Committee report and to provide guidelines for national health planning in context to 5 year plans. This committee found the conditions in PHCs to be unsatisfactory and the services provided by the PHCs are inadequate. This committee advised strengthening of the existing primary health centers before new centers were established. It also advised strengthening of subdivisional and district hospitals so that they could effectively function as referral centers.

The Health Survey and Planning Committee, popularly known as the Mudaliar Committee was set up towards the close of the Second Five Year Plan in 1959 and presented report on 1962 to survey the progress made in the field of health since submission of the Bhore Committee report and to make recommendations for future development and expansion of health services. The Mudaliar Committee found the quality of services provided by the primary health centers are inadequate.

Terms of Reference

- The assessment (or evaluation) in the field of medical relief and public health since the submission of the Health Survey and Development Committee's Report (the Bhore Committee).
- Review of the First and Second Five-Year Plan Health projects.
- Formulation of recommendations for the future plan of health development in the country.

Observations

- Basic health facilities had not reached at least half the nation.
- Gross mal distribution of hospitals and beds in favor of urban areas.
- Quality services provided by PHCs were grossly inadequate with poor functioning.
- Lack of referral system, and gross under staffing due to insufficient resources.

Recommendations

- Existing PHCs, to be strengthened before establishing new ones.
- Strengthening of subdivisional and district hospitals.
- PHC should not cater to more than 40,000 population.
- Curative, preventive and promotive services should be all provided at the PHCs.
- Consolidation of advances made in the 1st two 5 years plans.
- Regional organizations in each state.
- Strengthening of subdivisional and district hospitals to serve as central base of regional services.
- Constitution of All India Health services to replace the erstwhile Indian Medical service.
- Integration of medical and health services as recommended by the Bhore committee.

Chadha Committee (1963)

This committee was appointed under chairmanship of Dr MS Chadha, then Director General of Health Services, to advise about the necessary arrangements for the maintenance phase of National Malaria Eradication Programme. The committee suggested that the vigilance activity in the NMEP should be carried out by basic health workers (one per 10,000 population), who would function as multipurpose workers and would perform, in addition to malaria work, the duties of family planning and vital statistics data collection under supervision of family planning health assistants.

Terms of Reference

The committee should go into the details of the requirement related to the primary health centers, their planning, the necessary priority required according to the needs of the maintenance phase of the Malaria Eradication Programme. The committee should also consider the Staffing pattern required for the Malaria Eradication Programme but also for other health activities and the manner in which the technical and supervisory staff of the NMEP organization should be utilized after malaria eradication has been achieved.

Recommendations

- The Committee recommended that the vigilance operations in respect of the National Malaria Eradication Programme should be the responsibility of the primary health centers at the block level.
- The Committee also recommended that vigilance operations such as monthly home visits should be implemented through basic health workers. One basic health worker per 10,000 population was recommended.
- These workers were envisaged as 'multipurpose workers' to look after additional duties of collection of vital statistics and family planning, in addition to malaria vigilance.
- The Family Planning Health Assistants were to supervise 3 to 4 of these basic health workers.
- At the district level, the general health services were to take responsibility for the maintenance phase.

In a short time after implementation of MPHW scheme it was realized that malaria vigilance operations and family planning program could not be carried out satisfactorily. A committee known as Mukherjee committee was formed in 1965 and it recommended separate staff for Family planning activities so that malaria activities could receive undivided attention of its staff.

Mukherjee Committee 1965

The recommendations of the Chadha Committee, when implemented, were found to be impracticable because the basic health workers, with their multiple functions could do justice neither to malaria work nor to family planning work. The Mukherjee committee headed by then Secretary of Health Shri Mukherjee, was appointed to review the performance in the area of family planning. Multiple activities of the mass programs like family planning, smallpox, leprosy, trachoma, NMEP (maintenance phase), etc. were making it difficult for the states to undertake these effectively because of shortage of funds. A committee of state health secretaries, headed by the Union Health Secretary, Shri Mukherjee, was set up to look into this problem. The committee worked out the details of the Basic Health Service which should be provided at the Block level, and some consequential strengthening required at higher levels of administration.

Recommendations

- Posting of separate staff for the Family Planning program.
- The Family Planning assistants were responsible to undertake family planning duties only.
- The Basic health workers were to be utilized for purposes other than family planning.
- Delink the malaria activities from family planning so that the latter would receive undivided attention of its staff.

Jungalwalla Committee, 1967

This committee, known as the 'Committee on Integration of Health Services' was Set up in 1964 under the chairmanship of Dr N Jungalwalla, then Director of National Institute of Health Administration and Education (currently NIHFW) aimed to look into various problems related to integration of health services, abolition of private practice by doctors in government services, and the service conditions of Doctors. The committee defined 'integrated health services' as a service with a unified approach for all problems instead of a segmented approach for different problems. Medical care of the sick and public health program should be put under charge of a single administrator at all levels of hierarchy with due priority to each program.

Following steps were recommended for integration at all levels of health organization in the country:

- Unified Cadre
- Common Seniority
- Recognition of extra qualifications
- Equal pay for equal work
- Special pay for special work
- Abolition of private practice by government doctors
- Improvement in their service conditions.

The committee while gave sufficient indication for action to be taken but was neither careful to spell out steps and programs nor to indicate an uniform integrated set-up but left the matter to the states to work out the set-up. This committee also stated that 'integration should be a process of logical evolution rather than revolution'.

Kartar Singh Committee

The Kartar Singh Committee on Multipurpose workers developed by Govt. of India in 1973, laid down the norms about health workers in its report. The committee is headed by the Additional Secretary of Health. 'Committee is working on multipurpose workers under Health and Family Planning' constituted to form a framework for integration of health and medical services at peripheral and supervisory levels.

Recommendations

- Various categories of peripheral workers should be amalgamated into a single cadre of multipurpose workers (male and female)
- Appointment of MPW (F) in place of ANM.
- Appointment of MPW (M) the basic health workers, malaria surveillance workers, etc.
- PHCs to cover 50,000 pop.
- Each PHC to be divided into 16 subcenters.
- Each SC to cover 3000–3500 pop.
- 1 MPW (F), assisted by MPW (M) to be appointed at each SC.
- MPW to be initially started at places where Malaria control and Smallpox control program is going on.
- The Supervision of MPWS can be done by 1 Male Supervisor for 3–4 MPW (M) and 1 Female Supervisor for 3–4 MPW (F).
- LHV should be replaced by female supervisor.

Shrivastav Committee, 1975

Shrivastav Committee was set up in 1974 by 'Group on Medical Education and Support Manpower' to determine steps needed to reorient medical education in accordance with national needs and priorities and to develop a curriculum for health assistants who were to function as a link between medical officers and MPWs. To make any other suggestions to realize the above objectives.

Recommendations

- Immediate action for creation of bonds of paraprofessional and semiprofessional health workers from/within the community itself.
- Establishment of 2 cadres of health workers namely MPW and HA between the community level workers and MO I/C at PHC.
- Development of Referral Services Complex.

Establishment of a Medical and Health Education Commission for planning and implementing the reforms needed in health and medical education on the lines of University Grants Commission.

Committee felt that by the end of 6th 5 year plan:

- One multipurpose worker female (F) and one multipurpose worker male should be available to 5000 population.
- Heath assistant should be there at subcenter not at the PHC.
- One heath assistant (female) will supervise two multipurpose worker (female) only and one health assistant (male) will supervise two multipurpose worker (male) only.

Bajaj Committee, 1986

A expert committee for 'health manpower planning, production and management' was constituted under the chairmanship of Dr JS Bajaj, then member of planning commission, to tackle the problem of health manpower planning, production and management.

Recommendations

- Formulation of National Medical and Health Education Policy recommended for Formulation of National Health Manpower planning based on realistic survey.
- Formulation of National Health Manpower Policy.
- Establishment of an Educational Commission for Health Sciences (ECHS) on the lines of UGC.
- Establishment of Health Science Universities in various states and union territories.
- Establishment of health manpower cells at center and in the states.
- Carrying out a realistic health manpower survey.
- Vocationalization of education at 10 + 2 levels as regards, health related fields with appropriate incentives, so that good quality paramedical personnel may be available in adequate numbers.
- Uniform standard of medical and health science education by establishing universities of health sciences in all states.

Krishnan Committee, 1992

The committee under the chairmanship of Dr Krishnan reviewed the achievements and progress of previous health committee reports and also made comments on shortfalls. The committee address the problems of urban health and devised the health post scheme for urban slum areas. The committee had recommended one voluntary health worker (VHW) per 2,000 population with an honorarium of ₹100. Its report specifically outlines which services have to be provided by the health post. These services have been divided into outreach, preventive, family planning, curative, support (referral) services and reporting and record keeping. Outreach services include population education, motivation for family planning, and health education. In the present context, very few outreach services are being provided to urban slums.

INTERNATIONAL HEALTH AGENCIES

WORLD HEALTH ORGANIZATION (WHO)

WHO has its origin in April 1945 during conference at San Francisco to set up the United Nation. In 1946 it was approved by international conference of 51 nations in New York. WHO is a specialized, nonpolitical international health agency of United Nations. Its headquarter is in Geneva, Switzerland. The constitution of WHO came into force on 7th April 1948, which is celebrated every year as 'world health day'. The enjoyment of the highest attainable standard of health is one of fundamental rights of every human being without distinction of race, religion, political belief, economic or social condition' is the theme of WHO. The Activities of WHO in India are Malaria eradication, Control of communicable diseases, Health laboratory services, Manufacture of vaccines, Health statistics, Public health administration, RCH, Dental health, Medical rehabilitation, Quality control of drugs help in medical and nursing education.

Objectives

- Health is a state of complete physical, mental and social well-being and merely the absence of diseases of infirmity.
- The enjoyment of the highest attainable standard of health is one of the fundamental rights of every human being without distribution of race, religion, political belief, economic and social condition.
- The health of all peoples is fundamental to the attainment of peace and security and is dependent upon the fullest cooperation of individuals and states.
- The achievement of any state in the promotion and protection of health is of value to all.
- Unequal development in different countries in the promotion of health and control of disease, especially communicable disease.
- Healthy development of the child is basic importance.
- The extension to all people of the benefits of medical, psychological and related knowledge.
- Active cooperation on the part of the public are of the most importance in the improvement of the health of the health of the people.
- Governments have a responsibility for the health of their peoples which can be fulfilled only by the provision of adequate health and social measures.

Organization Structure

The WHO consists of three principle organ; the World Health Assembly, the Executive Board and Secretariat.

The World Health Assembly

The world health assembly is the 'Health Parliament' of Nations and the supreme governing body of the organization. It meets annually, usually in May, and generally at the headquarters in Geneva, but from time to time in other countries. The assembly is composed of delegates representing member states each of which has one vote. This is the highest administrative wing.

Functions of the Health Assembly

- To determine international health policy and programs.
- Top review the work of the past year.
- To approve the budget needed for the following year.
- To elect member states to designate a person to serve for three years on the Executive Board and to replace the retiring members.

Executive Board

The Executive Board had originally 18 members each designated by a member state. Subsequently the number was raised to 31. The members of the Board are to be 'technically qualified in the field of health.' One third of the membership is renewed every year, generally in January and shortly after the meeting of the world health assembly in May. The main work of the board is to give effect to the decisions and policies of the assembly. The board also has power to take action itself in an emergency such as epidemics, earthquakes and where immediate actions is needed. The main function of the board is to strengthen the decision and policies passed and approved by the world health assembly. It meets twice a year.

The Secretariat

The secretariat is headed by the director General is the chief technical and administrative officer of the organization. The primary function of the WHO secretariat is to provide member states with technical and managerial support for their national health development programmes. While in 1948, WHO staff counted 250 persons, in 1985 counted 4475 international public servants. The director has 5 deputies. Under the secretariat, there are 14 departments like survey, communicable diseases, health education, environment, budget, finance etc. The secretariat has different Regional organization in South-East Asia, Africa, America, Europe, Western Pacific and Eastern Mediterranean.

On 31 December, 1985 the WHO Secretariat comprised of the following divisions:

- Division of Epidemiological surveillance and Health Situation and trend assessment
- Division of Communicable diseases
- Division of Vector Biology and Control
- Division of Environmental Health
- Division of Public information and education for health
- Division of Mental Health
- Division of diagnostic, therapeutic and rehabilitative technology
- Division of Strengthening of Health Service
- Division of Family Health
- Division of Noncommunicable Diseases
- Division of Health Manpower Development
- Division of information systems support
- Division of Personnel and General Services
- Division of Budget and Finance.

Functions of the WHO

Prevention and Control of Specific Diseases

An important activity of WHO is epidemiological surveillance of communicable diseases.

Member states can also make use of the 'WHO Emergency Scheme for Epidemics' whenever necessary. The aim of international health regulations is to ensure maximum security against international spread of disease with the minimum interference with world traffic. The WHO has also paid attention in its program of work to noncommunicable disease problems such as cancer, cardiovascular diseases, genetic disorders, mental disorders, drug addiction and dental diseases. The activities of WHO have also branched out into the fields of vector biology and control, immunology, quality control of drugs and biological products, drug evaluation and monitoring and health laboratory technology.

Immunization against common diseases of childhood is now a priority program of the WHO.

Development of Comprehensive Health Services

WHO's most important function is to promote and support national health policy development and the development of comprehensive national health programs.

Health systems based on primary health care, the development of health manpower and utilization, building of long-term national capability.

WHO's main activities in 1980 were towards promoting national, regional and global strategies for the attainment of health for all.

Family Health

Family health is one of the major program activities of WHO since 1970, and is broadly subdivided into maternal and child health care, human reproduction, nutrition and health education. The chief concern is improvement of the quality of life of the family as a unit.

Environmental Health

Promotion of environmental health has always been an important activity of WHO. WHO advises governments on national programs for the provision of basic sanitary services. Recent activities are directed to protection of the quality of air, water and food; health conditions of work, radiation protection. A number of programs have been developed such as the 'WHO Environmental Health Criteria Programme' and 'WHO Environmental Health Monitoring Programme' towards improving environmental health.

Health Statistics

From 1947, WHO has been concerned with the dissemination of a wide variety of morbidity and mortality statistics relating to health problems. The data is published in the: (a) Weekly Epidemiological Record, (b) Health Statistics Quarterly and (c) World Health Statistics Annual. Readers interested in current data may obtain if from the chief statistics dissemination of statistical information, WHO, Geneva.

Biomedical Research

The WHO does not itself do research, but stimulates and coordinating research work. It has established a worldwide network of collaborating centers, besides awarding grants to research workers a research institutions for promoting research. Six topical diseases (malaria, schistosomiasis, trypanosomiasis, filarias, leishmaniasis and leprosy) are the target of the WHO special program for Research and training workers in the countries affected.

Health Literature and Information

WHO acts as a clearing house for information on health problems. It's publications comprise hundred, of titles on wide variety of health subjects. The WHO library is one of the satellite centers of the Medical Literature Analysis and Retrieval system of the US National Library of Medicine. The WHO has also a public information service both at headquarters and each of the six regional officers.

Cooperation with Other Organization

- WHO collaborates with the UN and with the other specialized agencies, and maintains various degrees of working relationships.
- Besides, WHO has also established relation with a number of international government organizations.

The Work of WHO in Nursing

- The functions of WHO include education of nurses and midwives, health visitors, auxiliary nurses—midwives and assisting in development of field services and training areas.
- Refresher courses for ward sisters, sister tutors, midwives and health visitors have been established and are held in various states.
- In order to standardizes the pattern of education and service, syllabus, programs of practical experience and procedure.
- An interesting development is the staff meetings among the hospitals or public health staff, and the interhospital tutors meetings, which help the program run more smoothly and ensure that they are established in family uniform manner.

INTERNATIONAL COUNCIL OF NURSES

The International Council of Nurses (ICN), founded in 1899 by Mrs Bedford Fenwick, is a federation of nonpolitical and self-governing national nurses associations. The headquarters are in Geneva, Switzerland. The main purpose of the ICN is to provide a means through which the national associations can share their interests in the promotion of health and care of the sick. It is an international association for all the nurses in the world. The ICN is a federation of more than 130 national nurses association.

Objectives

- To promote the development of Nurses Association.
- To assist National Nurses Association to improve the status of nurses within their countries.
- To assist National Nurses Association to improve the standard and competence of nursing.
- To serve as authorities voice for nurses and nursing internationally.

Membership

Membership is limited to one nursing organization per nation. In most cases, this is the national nurses' association such as the American Nurses Association, the Slovak Chamber of Nurses and Midwives or the Nursing Association of Nepal. ICN is a federation of more than 130 national nurses associations (NNAs), representing millions of nurses worldwide. ICN works directly with these member associations on issues of importance to the nursing profession. There is no individual membership to ICN. Nurses who are part of their national nurses association are automatically part of ICN. So all TNAI members can become member of ICN.

The Governing Body

The governing body of the ICN is the Council of National Representatives which is made up of the ICN Honorary Officers and the presidents of the national member associations. The council meets at least every other year and once every four years at the time of the ICN congress. The ICN Publishes the international Nursing Review on a quarterly basis. The Newsletter, which is published tens time a year. All nurses can become members of the ICN but not as individuals. The individual nurse becomes a member if her/his national nurses association is a member of the ICN. Nurses in India become members of the ICN when they become members of the TNAI. Affiliation fees of this membership are paid form a proportion of the membership fees paid to the TNAI. Membership in the ICN through the TNAI offers various benefits. A limited number of nursing student, may have their expenses paid in order to attend the congresses as observers. Among benefits to the graduate nurse are attendance of international congresses or conferences, the ICN exchange of privileges program, professional center. Nurses may receive publications about development in nursing and nursing education around the world. This helps the nurse become aware of being professionally related to international organizations such as the United Nations and the World Health Organization.

Activities

Three Goals and five core values guide and motivate all ICN activities.

The three goals are:

1. To bring nursing together worldwide.
2. To advance nurses and nursing worldwide.
3. To influence health policy.

The five core values are:

1. Visionary Leadership.
2. Inclusiveness.
3. Innovativeness.
4. Partnership.
5. Transparency.

Functions

- Promote the development of strong national nurses association.
- Assist at national level to improve standards of nursing.
- Review is a journal published quality by the ICN.
- Assist national Nurses Associations to improve the status of nurses.
- Take up nursing matters and serve as authoritative voice.
- Making the code of nurse.
- Formulating worldwide accepted definition of a nurse.
- Publishing A book of ethics 'The nurses Dilemma'.
- Developing Policy statement of health and social issue.
- Maintaining a register of professional qualification of people.
- Arranging exchange program for study and employment.
- Council meets one in two years and the ICN congress meets once in four years.
- Conducting seminars around the world to maintain relationship with other group to diseases and mental health problems.
- Publishing a number of professional periodicals from its headquarters Geneva.
- The bimonthly official journal and 'international Nursing review' are important journals lead in more than 100 countries.

The major activities can be divided into three major headings.

Development of Strong National Nursing Associations

Activities of the ICN are planned by the member associations, their elected representatives and the staff at headquarters appointed or approved by ICN's Board of Directors. Collectively the member association, and their representatives set goals for nursing education, practice, and research. The appointed staff to utilize resources to assist member associations, singly and collectively, in ways would enhance or strengthen their development. All aspects of ICN's programs and activities contribute directly or indirectly to the attainment of this objective—the development of strong national nursing associations.

Education and Practice

The ICN has always given high priority to assisting national nursing associations through programs, updating of standards for nursing education and practice. High technology in medical treatment and the increased understanding of primary health care needs in the world Focus ethical nursing questions and values relative to patient care, necessitating a careful review of standards of nursing practice. The ICN's definition of 'nurse' has been translated into many languages. ICN staff frequently participate in workshops and seminars of invitation form member associations. ICN supports the WHO goal of 'Health for All by year 2000 through primary Health care.

Social and Economic Welfare of Nurses

The International Labor Organization (ILO) and the World Health Organization, in promoting the status of nurses. In 1977 an international conference was promoting the status of nurses. In 1977 an international conference was convinced by the WHO/ILO with active involvement and Cooperation form the ICN.It is leading to the adoption of a series of conventions and recommendations pertaining to conditions of employment, life, and work of nursing personnel. ICN staff monitor the activities of the ILO in Geneva and endeavor to share pertinent information with its member associations through a regularly published newsletter, the socioeconomic news.

Blueprint for Future Action

- Developing the role and programs of the national nurses associations for influencing the development of health policy, standard setting for nursing education and practice, developing appropriate research activities and program development for socioeconomic welfare appropriate to that country.
- Influencing the development of policy affecting health and all heath workers through work with the WHO, ILO, UNICEF, and other international bodies.
- Maintaining the impetus of the socioeconomic welfare program for nursing.
- Implementing selected programs of international organizations as they related to national nurses associations and ICN's priorities.
- Developing efforts to convey realistic and positive image of today's nurses to the media.
- Maintaining links with other nursing groups.
- Reviewing the ICN code for Nurses to ensure continued relevance.
- Monitoring legislative issues of importance to nursing and nurses.
- Focusing ICN Publications and program efforts on these priority areas.

The International Council of Nurses provides a world stage for nursing and health priorities, characterized and defined by:

Credibility

The International Council of Nurses (ICN) is a long established and globally respected nongovernmental organization that leads in identifying and addressing the key issues on the nursing profession and how nurses impact the health and well-being of patients, families and populations.

Leadership

The organization delivers global leadership, ensuring that National Nursing Associations, through their collective action at the global level, add value to their own countries and to the worldwide nursing community. ICN provides its members the platform and the means to achieve common goals through collaborative action, working together for the benefit of society, the advancement of the profession and the development of its members. ICN and its members work with a wide range of nongovernmental organizations, governments, intergovernmental agencies, industry and key stakeholders so as to achieve maximum impact.

A Global Platform for Nursing Values

Working together ICN promotes the recognition of the value of care through the development of relevant research based policy and provides guidance and technical support to its members.

In addition, ICN membership provides benefits to its members in the following key areas:

Privileged Access to Critical and Current Information

Through environmental scanning, data collection and participation in high level fora, ICN continually identifies current and future trends that impact nursing, patient care and health systems. ICN uses many channels to share this critically important information with members, enabling members to react quickly to pressing issues and to plan strategically for the future.

In response to member needs and as a result of this scanning process, ICN regularly commissions leading edge monographs and other publications. In addition, it is the hub for a number of specialty area networks.

Influence and Advocacy

Through ICN, member nursing associations have a seat at many of the highest policy tables.

Intergovernmental activity: ICN is in official relations with a wide range of intergovernmental bodies and UN agencies, actively participating in and contributing to the policy development process of these bodies. For example, ICN routinely intervenes at the World Health Organization policy and agenda setting mechanisms—the Executive Board and World health Assembly. ICN successfully advocates for the inclusion of nurses in national delegations to these meetings and provide briefings and information material to its members who are part of their country delegations or the ICN delegation to the assembly.

Consultancy Services

ICN regularly, in response to member requests, comments on country legislation or policy directions and submits formal commentary and opinion on key topics to government ministries and other key national stakeholders. In addition ICN can provide expert consultancy to assist countries develop policy or legislation.

ICN International Forums and Topic Working Groups

Through ICN's various strategic and targeted forums and working groups, members have access to a range of events and activities that develop expertise in Professional Practice, Regulation and Socioeconomic welfare (ICN's 3 main pillars). Such activities strengthen the capacity to provide clear and informed leadership on matters of concern to their members, constituencies and the public.

Position Statements and Policy Papers

ICN provides regular position and policy guidance on key issues which members face in the areas of: Nursing Roles in Health Care Services; Social Issues; Health Care Systems; the Socioeconomic Welfare of Nurses; and the Nursing Profession.

Advocacy

ICN's extensive network of contacts in key leadership positions across sectors, and its capacity to mine and provide factual, accurate and reliable information on a broad range of issues, make the organization an active and effective advocate on key issues.

Recognition and Development

ICN's prestigious awards provide global recognition for the successful individuals nominated by members.

ICNs strategic direction is set by the Council of National Representatives. All member organizations have a voice and a role to play in the regular CNR meetings. In addition, member associations nominate and elect the ICN President and Board of Directors every four years. Participation in CNR and offering service to the Board of Directors provides an opportunity to contribute and further develop nursing knowledge and skills at the very highest level.

There is an opportunity for members to place their staff for short-term internships and sabbaticals so as to provide an opportunity to develop their skills and gain insights into the workings of our key partners.

As an ICN member association you can request endorsement for your associations' publications or policies.

Development Cooperation Projects

ICN's portfolio of innovative and effective international development projects provide members with a direct involvement—as implementers, beneficiaries or partners in on the ground projects impacting global health issues.

Financial Benefits

ICN members receive as part of the membership benefits:

- Free copies of all publications
- A preferential rate for bulk purchases
- Discounted rates on attendance at ICN Congress and Conferences
- Reduced charges for the award of ICN educational Credits (ICNECs) for national nursing association organized events.

ICN through its links with Industry, Inter-governmental agencies and the philanthropic sector is able to mobilize funding for certain projects that can then be prioritized towards member countries. For example, Leadership for Change, Wellness Centers, Clean Water Project, Mobile Library, Leadership in Negotiation, Positive Practice Environment Project and Girl Child Education fund.

UNICEF

The United Nations Children's Fund (UNICEF) is a United Nations Program that provides long-term humanitarian and developmental assistance to children and mothers in developing countries. It is one of the members of the United Nations Development Group and its Executive Committee. Its head quarter is at New York and It is a specialized agency of united nations. It was established in the year 1946, for rehabilitation of world war ravaged children.

In 1953, this was named as united nations children's fund after the end of emergency situations. but its short name retained as UNICEF. Its headquarter administered by an executive board of 30 nations. There are more than 200 country offices, 36-member Executive Board, by United Nations ECOSOC, for three-year terms. The Executive director has a five-year mandate. UNICEF is funded exclusively by voluntary contributions, and the National Committees collectively raise around one-third of UNICEF's annual income. This comes through contributions from corporations, civil society organizations around 6 million individual donors worldwide. They also rally many different partners - including the media, national and local government officials, NGOs, specialists such as doctors and lawyers, corporations, schools, young people and the general public—on issues related to children's rights.

Milestones of UNICEF

- **1946:** Focus on Food to Europe
- **1953:** UNICEF becomes permanent part Milestones (Cont.)
- **1959:** Declaration of the Rights of the Child Milestones (Cont.)
- **1961:** Education Milestones (Cont.)
- **1965:** Nobel Peace Prize Milestones (Cont.)
- **1989:** Convention on the Rights of the Child Milestones (Cont.)
- **2002:** Special Session on Children Milestones.

Objective

The main objective of UNICEF is the Improvement of health of mothers and infants.

There are threefold Mission of UNICEF:

- To ensure that basic nutrition, health, and education needs of children are met
- To give children the opportunity to expand their potential
- To create an international ethical standard of behavior toward children.

Functions

It plays the main role in all programs which benefits the children's health directly or indirectly the functions are:

- Child health (vaccine production)
- Child nutrition
- Family and child welfare
- Functions in India
- Development of rural health services
- Control of communicable diseases
- Immunization programs
- Applied nutrition program
- School health service
- Prevention of malnutrition
- Supply of audiovisual aids
- Helping in digging wells in rural areas

- Promoting child safety and safe mother hood programs.
- Reproductive and child health services
- Helps in medical education and training
- Arranging workshops
- Providing books and other education material to school of nursing
- Currently UNICEF is promoting a campaign known as GOBI to encourage 4 strategies for a child revolution
  - G-Growth charts to monitor child development
  - Oral rehydration to treat all mild and moderate dehydration
  - B-Breastfeeding
  - I-Immunization.

UNITED NATIONS FUND FOR POPULATION ACTIVITIES

The **United Nations Population Fund** (**UNFPA**), formerly the United Nations Fund for Population Activities, is a **United Nations** organization. UNFPA is the world's largest multilateral source of funding for population and reproductive health programs. The Fund works with governments and nongovernmental organizations in over 150 countries with the support of the international community, supporting programs that help women, men and young people UNFPA's work is guided by the Program of Action adopted by 179 governments at the International Conference on Population and Development in 1994. The conference agreed that meeting people's needs for education and health, including reproductive health, is a prerequisite of sustainable development.

Functions

The work of the UNFPA involves promotion of the right of every woman, man and child to enjoy a life of health and equal opportunity. One of their aims is to ensure that 'every pregnancy is wanted, every birth is safe, every young person is free of HIV and sexually transmitted diseases, and every girl and woman is treated with dignity and respect. Their work involves the improvement of reproductive health including creation of national strategies and protocols, and providing supplies and services to these minority groups, as well as internal migrants and refugees, the elderly and the handicapped. The organization has recently been known for its worldwide campaign against obstetric fistula and female genital mutilation. The UNFPA supports programs in more than 150 countries, territories and areas spread across four geographic regions: Arab States and Europe, Asia and the Pacific, Latin America and the Caribbean, and sub-Saharan Africa. Around three quarters of the staff work in the field. It is a member of the United Nations Development Group and part of its Executive Committee.

Achievements in India

- UNFPA gives financial support to India for extensive improvement in health and family welfare programmes.
- Area wise projects for intensive development of health and family welfare infrastructure and improvement in the availability of services in the rural areas have been under implementation in 11 district of Bihar and 4 district of Rajasthan.
- The UNFPA inputs are designed to develop national capability for the manufacture of contraceptives.
- To develop population education programs
- To conduct project in organized sector.
- To increasing the availability of health workers at the root level.
- Introduction of innovatives approaches to family planning and MCH care.

WORLD BANK

The **World Bank** is a United Nations international financial institutionis a specialized agency of UN. It was established with the purpose of helping less developing countries to raise their living standards.The powers of bank are vested in a board of governors. The bank gives loan for project which lead to economic growth. The projects are usually concerned with electric power, roads, railway, agriculture, water supply, education, family planning, etc that provides loans to developing countries for capital programs. The World Bank is a component of the **World Bank Group** and a member of the United Nations Development Group.

The World Bank's official goal is the reduction of poverty. According to its Articles of Agreement, all its decisions must be guided by a commitment to the promotion of foreign investment and international trade and to the facilitation of capital investment.

Many achievements have brought the Millennium Development Goals targets for 2015 within reach in some cases.

- **Eradicate extreme poverty and hunger:** Forty-five countries pledged US$ 25.1 billion in 'aid for the world's poorest countries', aid that goes to the World Bank International Development Association (IDA) which distributes the loans to eighty poorer countries. While wealthier nations sometimes fund their own aid projects, including those for diseases, and although IDA is the recipient of criticism, Robert B. Zoellick, the former president of the World Bank, said when the loans were announced on 15 December 2007, that IDA money 'is the core funding that the poorest developing countries rely on'.
- **Achieve universal primary education:** The percentage of children in school in developing countries increased from 80% in 1991 to 88% in 2005. Still, about 72 million children of primary school age, 57% of them girls, were not being educated as of 2005.
- **Promote gender equality:** The tide is turning slowly for women in the labor market, yet far more women than men—worldwide more than 60% - are contributing but unpaid family workers. The World Bank Group Gender Action Plan was created to advance women's economic empowerment and promote shared growth.

- **Reduce child mortality:** There is somewhat improvement in survival rates globally; accelerated improvements are needed most urgently in South Asia and Sub-Saharan Africa. Estimated 10 million-plus children under five died in 2005; most of their deaths were from preventable causes.
- **Improve maternal health:** Almost all of the half million women who die during pregnancy or childbirth every year live in Sub-Saharan Africa and Asia. There are numerous causes of maternal death that require a variety of health care interventions to be made widely accessible.
- **Combat HIV/AIDS, malaria, and other diseases:** Annual numbers of new HIV infections and AIDS deaths have fallen, but the number of people living with HIV continues to grow. In the eight worst-hit southern African countries, prevalence is above 15%. Treatment has increased globally, but still meets only 30% of needs (with wide variations across countries). AIDS remains the leading cause of death in Sub-Saharan Africa (1.6 million deaths in 2007). There are 300 to 500 million cases of malaria each year, leading to more than 1 million deaths. Nearly all the cases and more than 95% of the deaths occur in Sub-Saharan Africa.
- **Ensure environmental sustainability:** Deforestation remains a critical problem, particularly in regions of biological diversity, which continues to decline. Greenhouse gas emissions are increasing faster than energy technology advancement.
- **Develop a global partnership for development:** Emphasis is being placed on the Bank Group's collaboration with multilateral and local partners to quicken progress toward the MDGs' realization.WHO and world bank jointly carry out many projects like water supply, world food programme, population control, AIDS control, etc.

UNITED NATION DEVELOPMENT PROGRAMME (UNDP)

United Nation Development Programme (UNDP) is the United Nations global development network. It is funded entirely by voluntary contributions from member nations. Head quartered in New York City. UNDP was established in 1966 with the objectives of helping the poor countries in the development of human and natural resources. The project of UNDP provide necessary help in economic and social fields like agriculture, industry, science, health, hospital administration, nursing services, etc. Contribution for this project is made by the member countries of united nation in their annual meeting. UNDP advocates for change and connects countries to knowledge, experience and resources to help people build a better life. The organization has country offices in 177 countries, where it works with local governments to meet development challenges and develop local capacity. Additionally, the UNDP works internationally to help countries achieve the Millennium Development Goals (MDGs). Currently, the UNDP is one of the main UN agencies involved in the development of the Post-2015 Development Agenda. UNDP operates in 177 countries, working with nations on their own solutions to global and national development challenges. As they develop local capacity, they draw on the people of UNDP and its wide range of partners. This organization providing assistance to INDIA since 1974.

FOOD AND AGRICULTURE ORGANIZATIONS

The Food and Agriculture Organization (FAO) was established in 1945 in Quebec City, Quebec, Canada. In 1951, its headquarters were moved from Washington, DC, United States to Rome, Italy. The agency is directed by the Conference of Member Nations, which meets every two years to review the work carried out by the organization and to approve a Program of Work and Budget for the next two-year period. The Conference elects a council of 49 member states (serve three-year rotating terms) that acts as an interim governing body, and the Director-General, that heads the agency with head quarter at Rome. It is the united Nations 1st organization created to look after several areas of global cooperation.

The objectives of FAO are to help nation's living standards:

- To improve nutritional status of the people of all countries.
- To increase the output of agriculture, forestry, and fisheries.
- To improve status of rural population.

DANIDA

Danish International Development Agency (DANIDA), is the brand which the Ministry of Foreign Affairs of Denmark, uses when it provides humanitarian aid and development assistance to other countries, with focus on developing countries. Danish development assistance in the 1950s was nearly exclusively channeled through the United Nations. In 1962 Denmark established its first bilateral development assistance program for developing countries under the Ministry of Foreign Affairs. In 2010 about 40% of Denmark's bilateral assistance went to social sectors, including education and health. DANIDA also works in collaboration with the United Nations, the World Bank, regional development banks and the European Union. Danish international development agency has been helping in the development of the national blindness control program since 1978. This include development of manpower, establishment of managerial information system, supply of vehicles and appliances, health education material and information, etc. Danish government is giving grant for control of tuberculosis in tribal district of Odisha.

USAID

United States Agency for International Development (USAID) is a technical cooperation mission for international development was created in 1961. This is the United States

Federal Government Agency primarily responsible for administering civilian foreign aid. USAID has adopted as its mission statement to partner to end extreme poverty and to promote resilient, democratic societies while advancing the security and prosperity of the United States. USAID operates in Africa, Asia, Latin America and Europe. President John F Kennedy created USAID in 1961 by executive order to implement development assistance programs in the areas authorized by the Congress in the Foreign Assistance Act. The Congress updates this authorization through annual funds appropriation acts, and other legislation.

The USAID has been assisting in a number of projects designed to improve the health of India's people. These are:

- Malaria eradication
- Medical and nursing education
- Health education
- Water supply and sanitation
- Control of communicable diseases
- Nutrition and family planning
- Presently USAID helping in agricultural and family planning programs, with some reduction in aid in the general public health field.

INTERNATIONAL LABOR ORGANIZATION

The International Labor Organization (ILO) is a United Nations agency dealing with labor issues, particularly international labor standards and decent work for all 185 of the 193 UN member states are members of the ILO. In 1969, the organization received the Nobel Peace Prize for improving peace among classes, pursuing justice for workers, and providing technical assistance to other developing nations. The ILO registers complaints against entities that are violating international rules; however, it does not impose sanctions on governments.

It was established in 1919 to improve the labor and housing conditions of workers throughout the world. The Head quarter is in Geneva. The Governing Body decides the agenda of the International Labor Conference, adopts the draft program and budget of the organization for submission to the conference, elects the director-general, requests information from member states concerning labor matters, appoints commissions of inquiry and supervises the work of the International Labor Office.

Main Objectives

- To cooperate in maintaining peace in establishments by promoting social justice.
- To promote economic and social stability.
- To improve the housing and working conditions of labor through international efforts.
- To promote economic and social stability.
- To cooperate in maintaining peace by promoting social justice.
- There is a close collaboration between ILO and WHO in the field of heath and labor.

COLOMBO PLAN

The Colombo Plan was born out of a Commonwealth Conference of Foreign Ministers, held in Colombo, Sri Lanka, in January 1950. At this meeting, a plan was established to provide a framework within which international cooperation efforts could be promoted to raise the standards of people in the region. Originally conceived as lasting for a period of six years, the Colombo Plan was extended several times until 1980, when it was extended indefinitely. Initially it was called the Colombo Plan for Cooperative Economic Development in South and Southeast Asia. It has grown from a group of seven Commonwealth nations—Australia, Britain, Canada, Ceylon, India, New Zealand and Pakistan into an international organization of 27, including non-Commonwealth countries. When it adopted a new constitution in 1977, its name was changed to 'The Colombo Plan for Cooperative Economic and Social Development in Asia and the Pacific' to reflect the expanded composition of its enhanced membership and the scope of its activities.

At a meeting of the common wealth foreign ministers at Colombo in January 1950, a program was drawn up for cooperative economic development in South and South Eastasia. Colombo plan is providing help for industrial and agricultural development. The AIIMS New Delhi was made under Colombo plan with financial assistance from New Zealand.

The contribution of Canada in supplying cobalt therapy units to medical institutions in India was an important item of aid under the Colombo plan.

COOPERATIVE FOR AMERICAN RELIEF EVERYWHERE

Cooperative for American Relief Everywhere (CARE) is a secular, nongovernmental and a nonprofit organization. This was established in 1946 by American donors for sending food for war devastated, helpless and poor people of European countries. After end of war CARE spread its activities to help other countries. CARE carried out its programmes in India since 1950. Since 1971, CARE is assisting in the 'mid day meal scheme.' CARE extends cooperation in health, education, agriculture and professional training.

UNESCO

United National Educational, Scientific and Cultural Organization (UNESCO) is one of the specialized agency of united nations established on 16 November 1945. Its purpose is to contribute to peace and security by promoting international collaboration through education, science, and culture in order to further universal respect for justice, the rule of law, and human rights along with fundamental freedom proclaimed in the United Nations Charter. It is the heir of the League of Nations' International Committee on Intellectual Cooperation.

UNESCO has 195 member states and nine associate members. Projects sponsored by UNESCO include literacy, technical, and teacher-training programs; international science programmes; the promotion of independent media and freedom of the press, regional and cultural history projects; the promotion of cultural diversity; translations of world literature; international cooperation agreements to secure the world cultural and natural heritage (World Heritage Sites) and to preserve human rights, and attempts to bridge the worldwide digital divide. It is also a member of the United Nations Development Group. UNESCO pursue its objectives through 5 major programs such as Education, Natural science, Social and human science, Culture and Communication and Information and also implements its activities through the same five programs.

FORD FOUNDATION

The Ford Foundation is a New York headquartered, globally oriented private foundation with the mission of advancing human welfare. Created in 1936 by Edsel Ford and Henry Ford. The foundation makes grants through its headquarters and ten international field offices. For fiscal year 2011, it reported assets of US$ 10.0 billion and approved US$ 413 million in grants. The grants support projects that focus on reducing poverty and injustice; promoting democratic values; and advancing human knowledge, creativity and achievement. Ford Foundation is dedicated to the field of rural health services and family planning. In India the foundation provides help in short term training programs in community health, and pilot project of health services. It provided help in the water supply and drainage of sewage systems in Kolkata.

Current Issues, Initiatives and Goals

The foundation works on eight significant human welfare issues:

Democratic and Accountable Government

The foundation says: 'Effective public institutions are essential for societies to be safe, free and prosperous.' The process of governing must be more transparent, accountable and inclusive in order to achieve fairness and equity.

Economic Fairness

The foundation says: 'Expanding opportunities and providing fair and equitable ways for all people to earn a decent living and build economic resources is essential to creating prosperous societies.'

Educational Opportunity and Scholarship

The foundation says: 'In every society, people from marginalized and disadvantaged groups deserve an education that expands opportunity, guarantees quality, and achieves equitable results.'

Freedom of Expression

The foundation says: 'The free flow of information and ideas is essential to healthy, progressive societies. Our work offers space for creative expression and supports efforts to ensure that media systems and policies are open and equitable.'

Human Rights

The foundation says: 'Fulfilling the rights that belong to all people depends upon an active and engaged community and public officials and institutions committed to the inherent dignity and worth of every person.'

Metropolitan Opportunity

The foundation says: 'Equitable access to safe, affordable housing, efficient transportation, and good jobs is fundamental to building prosperous metropolitan areas.'

Sexuality and Reproductive Health and Rights

The foundation says: 'Sexuality and the right to reproductive health are fundamental to the human experience; all women and men should be able to exercise these rights free from coercion and violence.'

Sustainable Development

The foundation says: 'We believe that promoting greater access among the poor to natural resources is critical to achieving two interrelated goals: reducing global poverty and sustaining the quality of our environment.'

INDIAN RED CROSS

The Indian Red Cross Society is a voluntary humanitarian organization having a network of over 700 branches throughout India, The mission of the Indian Red Cross is to inspire, encourage and initiate at all times all forms of humanitarian activities so that human sufferings can be minimized and even prevented and this contribute to create climate for peace. The Red Cross is working by following Seven fundamental principles which include Humanity, Impartiality, Neutrality, Independence, Voluntary service, Unity: and Universality. The Indian Red Cross's programs are grouped into four main core areas these are Promoting humanitarian principles and values, Disaster response, Disaster preparedness and Health and Care in the Community. Red Cross promotes the Humanitarian values, which encourage respect for other human beings and a willingness to work together to find solutions to problems. Guiding and supporting the development of its Societies is one of the Red Cross's fundamental tasks and runs through these four core areas and others. Capacity building programs and activities include : management and volunteer training, improving branch structures, planning, fund-raising and gender equality creating the opportunity for Red Cross Societies to network. Other Major activities includes: hospital services, blood bank, HIV/AIDS programs, home for disabled servicemen, vocational training centers, tracing activities, maternity, child and family welfare, nursing, junior red cross activities, preparedness and prevention of communicable and infectious diseases, relief operations in fire, railway and other accidents and events.

THE KASTURBA SOCIETY MEMORIAL FUND

The Kasturba Gandhi National Memorial Trust (KGNMT) was established in 1945 as a result of a national endeavor, led by Mahatma Gandhi to address the issues of women in rural India.

With the backdrop of India's Freedom Struggle, KGNMT was founded by eminent people with collective effort of multiple anonymous masses at Kasturbagram (Indore). The KGNMT extending its various services and activities has spread its wings through 22 branches all over the country. Eminent people Mahatma Gandhi, Sri Vallabh Bhai Patel, Sri Thakkar Bapa, Dada sahib Mavlankar, Smt Prem Leela Thakarasi, Smt Laxmi N Menon, Sushri Maniben Patel and Dr Sushila Nayar have been the chairpersons of the Trust.

Mahatma Gandhi's universal and timeless vision of Sarvodaya finds its best practical expression in the Kasturba Trust as 'SARVODAYA' is reawakening of the spirit in harmony with nature and environment for all forms of life. Women and children are the backbone for our society. Constructive work among women and children is a primary and essential requirement for process of nation building as envisaged in 'SARVODAYA'.

'KGNMT' is marching ahead with Gandhiji's vision to strengthen women power and substantiating the empowerment creating adequate support to millions of women.

The 22 State Branches with more than 500 centers are spread throughout India. Some centers are reaching out to needy Women and Children in remote villages.

The KGNMT at Hydershakote, Hyderabad is one of the Branches set up by the KGNMT and is extending great help to destitute women and children.

HIND KUSHT NIVARAN SANGH

Hind Kusht Nivaran Sangh (Indian Leprosy Association) is an old and prestigeous body of people committed towards treatment, rehabilitation of leprosy patients and elimination of leprosy from India. Hind Kusht Nivaran Sangh was founded on 27th January 1925 with the name of Indian Council of British Empire Leprosy Relief Association (BELRA) with three objectives: (i) to carry out research on various aspects of leprosy; (ii) to provide short courses of training, treatment of leprosy; and (iii) to carry out propaganda. There were two headquarters, one located at Indian Red Cross Society Office, New Delhi (inaugurated by Sardar Bahadur Balwant Singh Puri) functioning as Administrative Office and the other headquarter working as Technical Office situated at the Department of Leprosy, School of Tropical Medicine and Hygiene, Calcutta under the leadership of Dr Ernest Muir. After the independence of India, The Indian Council of BELRA was renamed as Hind Kusht Nivaran Sangh (Indian Leprosy Association) and registered in 1950 under the Registration of Societies Act (XXI of 1860).

Present Activities of Hind Kusht Nivaran Sangh (Indian Leprosy Association)

- Production and distribution of health education and publicity material on leprosy.
- Publication of quarterly Indian Journal of Leprosy and a bimonthly news bulletin Kusht Vinashak for leprosy workers and the general public.
- Production and distribution of leprosy seals to create awareness about leprosy and help other organizations in raising funds for their work through the sale of these seals.
- Observance of Anti-Leprosy Day on the 30th January every year to create mass awareness about leprosy.
- Conducting training courses of nine months duration for physiotherapy technicians of at two leprosy training centers (Naini, Allahabad, Uttar Pradesh and Purulia, West Bengal).
- Organizing the All India Leprosy Workers Conference and Regional Leprosy Workers Conferences in collaboration with the state branches and other voluntary organizations.
- Providing assistance to voluntary organizations and leprosy patients.
- Maintaining a house called 'ShanthiIllam' at Vellore (Tamil Nadu) where leprosy patients who come for surgical treatment at the Christian Medical College and Hospital, Vellore are provided free boarding and lodging facilities.
- Running of two mobile leprosy treatment units in two districts of Delhi (North-East and West) with funds provided by the Government of India.
- Organizing exhibitions on leprosy in Delhi.

THE FAMILY PLANNING ASSOCIATION INDIA

The Family Planning Association India, is a registered charity in India. Established in 1949, the organization has 40 branches across the country that promote sexual health and family planning. It is the national affiliate of the International Planned Parenthood Federation Among other issues, the organization promotes reproductive choices, legal and safe abortion, education about sexually transmitted diseases and sexual and reproductive health.

THE INDIAN NURSING COUNCIL

The Indian Nursing Council (INC) is a national regulatory body. The Indian Nursing Council is an Autonomous Body under the Government of India, Ministry of Health and Family Welfare was constituted by the Central Government under section 3(1) of the Indian Nursing Council Act, 1947 of parliament in order to establish a uniform standard of training for nurses, Midwives and health visitors. The INC which was authorized by Indian Nursing Council Act 1947 was established in 1949 for the purpose of providing uniform standards in nursing education and reciprocity in nursing registration throughout the country. The act gives authority to prescribing curriculum for nursing education and recognizing qualifications of the institutions with teaching program for nursing. It is the only national legislation directly related to nursing practice, also provides a basis from which rules for nursing practice can be developed Among other responsibilities, this act gives authority to the Indian Nursing Council for prescribing curricula for nursing education and what the nurses are prepared to do. The INC uses the authority in nursing education but it delegates authority for control of nursing practice to state nurses registration council.

ALL INDIA WOMEN'S CONFERENCE

The All India Women's Conference (AIWC) is an organization based in Delhi. It was founded in 1927 by Margaret Cousins, as an organization dedicated to upliftment and betterment of women and children Mission AIWC was registered in 1930 under the Societies Registration Act, XXI of 1860.

Objectives

- To work for a society based on the principle of social justice, personal integrity and equal rights and opportunities for all.
- To secure recognition of the inherent right of every human being to work and to achieve the essentials of life, which should not be determined by accident of birth or sex but by planned social distribution.
- To support the claim of every citizen to the right to enjoy basic civil liberties.
- To stand against all separatist tendencies and to promote greater national integration and unity.
- To work actively for the general progress and welfare of women and children and to help women utilize to the fullest, one of the fundamental rights conferred on them by the Constitution of India.
- To work for permanent international amity and world peace.

Legislative Reforms Initiated By AIWC

- Sharda Act (1929)
- Hindu Women's Right to Property Act (1937)
- Factory Act (1947)
- Hindu Marriage and Divorce Act (1954)
- Special Marriage Act (1954)
- Hindu Minority and Guardianship Act (1956)
- Hindu Adoption and Maintenance Act (1956)
- The Suppression of Immoral Traffic in Women Act (1958)
- Maternity Benefits Act (1961)
- Dowry Prohibition Act (1961)
- Equal Remuneration Act (1958, 1976)

THE CENTRAL SOCIAL WELFARE BOARD

The Central Social Welfare Board was set up by a Resolution of Government of India dated 12th August, 1953 with the object of promoting social welfare activities and implementing welfare programs for women, children and the handicapped through voluntary organizations. Till 1969 the Board functioned as a limb of the Government and then it was registered as a charitable company under the Companies Act to give a legal status to the Board. The Board was given the dual responsibility of taking welfare services to the disadvantaged sections of society especially women and children, and also developing a nationwide infrastructure of voluntary agencies through which these services could be made available. In 1954 the State Social Welfare Advisory Boards were set up in the States and Union Territories to implement the programs of the Board and assist the Central Social Welfare Board in expansion and development of welfare services. The financial assistance to voluntary organizations under various schemes is given on the recommendations of the State Boards. Presently, there are 32 State Boards in different States and UTs. They are headed by nonofficial Chairpersons who are mostly renowned social workers. The Boards consist of nonofficial members, normally representing each major district of the State and are proportionately nominated by the Central Board and State Government. The State Boards advise the Central Board to take new initiatives for the promotion of voluntarism and strengthening of voluntary action at the State level. The State Boards are also a recommendatory body for the evaluation of the voluntary organizations for taking up programs of the Board. The expenditure on the State Board Establishment Budget is met on 50:50 basis (i.e., 50% by CSWB and 50% by the concerning State Government). Under this head, an amount of ₹460.00 lakhs has been released to State Boards during 2003–04 in installments as the Board has a 55-member General Body and a 15-member Executive Committee. The composition of the General Body are:

- All Chairpersons of State Social Welfare Advisory Boards (32)
- Representatives from the Parliament: two from Lok Sabha and one from Rajya Sabha.
- Five Professionals (one each from Law, Medicine, Social Work, Education and Social Development). Three eminent persons with extensive experience in social work.
- Representatives from Ministries/Departments/ Government of India, Department of Women and Child Development, Ministry of Finance, Department of Rural Development, Department of Education. Planning Commission, Ministry of Labor, Ministry of Social Justice and Empowerment Department of Family Welfare.
- Executive Director, Central Social Welfare Board.
- The members of educative committee are chairpersons of State Social Welfare Advisory Boards: 5 States by rotation.

TELEMEDICINE

Telemedicine is an upcoming field in health science arising out of the effective fusion of ICT with medical science having enormous potential in meeting the challenges of health care delivery to rural and remote areas. It is kind of system by the delivery of health care service done from a distance by all health care professionals using information communication technology for the exchange of different information. The term telemedicine has been derived from the Greek word 'tele' meaning at distance and medicine which is from the Latin word 'meden' meaning healing. Telemedicine is the used of modern telecommunications and information technology for the provision of clinic care to individuals at a distance and the transmission of information to provide that care, it includes the diagnosis, treatments, monitoring and education of patients using systems that allow ready access to expert advice and patients information no matter where the patient or relevant information is locate. Telemedicine relies on transfer of text, reports, voice, images and video, between geographically separated locations. Success relates to the efficiency and effectiveness of the transfer of information.

According to WHO

Telemedicine is the delivery of health care services where distance is a critical factors by all healthcare professional using information and communication technology for the exchange of valid information for diagnosis and treatment and prevention of disease and injuries, research and continuing education of healthcare providers all in the interest of advancing the health of individual and their community.

According to Willams

Telemedicine is defined as any health care provided to patient via technology across a distance. It also otherwise defined as the use of advance technologies to exchange health information and provide healthcare services across geographic area, time, social and cultural barriers.

The use of telecommunication is to provide medical information and services at may be as simple as to one health professional discussing a case over the telephone or as sophisticated as using satellite technology to broadcast or consultation between provides at two distant locations using video-conferencing equipment.

Americans Telemedicine Association Defines

'Telemedicine is the use of medical information exchanged from one site to another via electronic communications for the health and education of the patient or healthcare provider and for the purpose of improving patient care.' In plain speak telemedicine is a process by which a patient is able to communicate his problems, (along with, if necessary details of medical investigations) to a doctor many miles away and receive necessary and relevant medical advice.

Objectives

- To provide quality care to the people who are residing in remotest areas.
- To reduce the cost of health care services.

Areas of Telemedicine Applications

- Cardiology
- Home care
- Radiology
- Emergency care
- Surgery
- Dermatology
- Psychiatry
- Oncology
- Pathology
- Ophthalmology
- Hematology
- ENT
- Nephrology
- Prehospital care

Applications

It can be also used for:
- Tele health care
- Tele consultation
- Tele follow-up
- Tele education
- Disease surveillance and program
- Disaster management can be tackle
- Tele home health care to elderly people
- Continuous medical education
- Public awareness
- Tele mentored or procedures or surgeries.

Evolution of Telemedicine in India

- **1996:** Deployment of First Indigenously Developed Hospital Information System Software by CDAC Noida at SGPGIMS, Lucknow, UP
- **1999:** Indigenous Development of Telemedicine Technology and Pilot Deployments by DeitY, MCIT, Government of India at AIIMS, New Delhi, PGIMER, Chandigarh and SGPGIMS, Lucknow
- **2000:** SATCOM based Telemedicine Deployment by ISRO at Apollo Hospitals, Aragonda
- **2001:** First telemedicine network between three institutions AIIMS-New Delhi, PGI Chandigarh and SGPGI-Lucknow, First National Conference on Telemedicine was held and a Scientific Body for promotion of Telemedicine in the Country Telemedicine Society of India, was formed
- **2001–2003:** Major Medical Institutions (Government and Corporate) initiated Telemedicine activities and deployed hospital information system
- **2003–2004:** Deployment of SATCOM based TM nodes across the country by ISRO for Tele-education and Tele-consultation services
- **2005:** MoHFW constituted Indian Task Force for Telemedicine
- **2006:** Planning Commission approved budget for e-Health including Telemedicine in the 11th Five Year Plan School of Telemedicine and Biomedical Informatics (STBI) was set up at SGPGIMS, Lucknow by Government of UP PHFI was awarded Grant-in-aid to have MoHFW 'Healthy India' Website for Health Education from 2007–08 to 2012–13
- **2007:** STBI at SGPGIMS, Lucknow was made National Resource Centre for Telemedicine and Biomedical Informatics by DeitY Government of India MoHFW,

Government of India supported Tele-ophthalmology Project In many parts of the country MoHFW, Government of India supported Onco-NET Project
- **2009:** MoHFW, supported National Rural TM Network with ₹25–50 Lakh to start the pilot projects on Telemedicine
- **2010:** National Medical College Network Project Conceived. SGPGIMS was made National Resource Centre for Telemedicine by MoHFW, MCTS Launched by MoHFW, Government of India
- **2012:** EMR/EHR Standards by Expert Group of MoHFW establishment
- **2013:** Initiation of Process of establishment of NMCN with Open Tender Basis. MCIT Initiative of National Optical Fibre Network (2011) to provide high speed bandwidth connectivity up to every Gram Panchayat wherein 2,50,000 shall have connectivity. As a Pilot Project of Tele-consultation three sites (PHC/CHC) as one Telemedicine Centre each block have been connected with one medical college in the states for Telemedicine activities.

Growth of Telemedicine Applications

Services can be Provided by Telemedicine

Sometimes telemedicine is best understood in terms of the services provided and the mechanisms used to provide those services. Here are some examples:

- **Primary care and specialist referral services** may involve a primary care or allied health professional providing a consultation with a patient or a specialist assisting the primary care physician in rendering a diagnosis. This may involve the use of live interactive video or the use of store and forward transmission of diagnostic images, vital signs and/or video clips along with patient data for later review.
- **Remote patient monitoring,** including home telehealth, uses devices to remotely collect and send data to a home health agency or a remote diagnostic testing facility (RDTF) for interpretation. Such applications might include a specific vital sign, such as blood glucose or heart ECG or a variety of indicators for homebound patients. Such services can be used to supplement the use of visiting nurses.
- **Consumer medical and health information** includes the use of the Internet and wireless devices for consumers to obtain specialized health information and on-line discussion groups to provide peer-to-peer support.
- **Medical education** provides continuing medical education credits for health professionals and special medical education seminars for targeted groups in remote locations.
  - 2001: Teleradiology—still images
  - 2002: Teleradiology—still images
  - 2003: Telepathology, Teleophthalmology
  - 2004: Teleoncology, Telesurgery
  - 2005: Mobile telehealth—augmentation
  - 2006: Telemedicine for Primary healthcare.

What Delivery Mechanisms can be Used?

- **Networked programs** link tertiary care hospitals and clinics with outlying clinics and community health centers in rural or suburban areas. The links may use dedicated high-speed lines or the Internet for telecommunication links between sites. ATA estimates the number of existing telemedicine networks in the United States at roughly 200 providing connectivity to over 3,000 sites.
- **Point-to-point connections** using private high speed networks are used by hospitals and clinics that deliver services directly or outsource specialty services to independent medical service providers. Such outsourced services include radiology, stroke assessment, mental health and intensive care services.
- **Monitoring center links** are used for cardiac, pulmonary or fetal monitoring, home care and related services that provide care to patients in the home. Often normal land-line or wireless connections are used to communicate directly between the patient and the center although some systems use the Internet.
- **Web-based e-health patient service sites** provide direct consumer outreach and services over the Internet. Under telemedicine, these include those sites that provide direct patient care.

Types of Telemedicine

Real Time (Synchronous)

Real time telemedicine could be as simple as a telephone call or as complex as robotic surgery. It requires the presence of both parties at the same time and a communication link between them that allows a real time interaction to take place. Video-conferencing equipment is one of the most common forms of technologies used in synchronous telemedicine. There are also peripheral devices which can attached to the computer or the video conferencing equipment which can aid in an interactive examination. For instant, a tele-otoscope allows a remote physician to 'see' inside a patient's ear; a tele-stethoscope allows the consulting remote physician to hear the patient's heartbeat. Medical specialties conducive to this kind of consultation include psychiatry, family practice, internal medicine, rehabilitation, cardiology, pediatrics, obstetrics, genecology, neurology and pharmacy.

Store and Forward Telemedicine

Store and forward telemedicine involves acquiring medical data (like medical images, biosignals) and then transmitting this data to the doctor or medical specialist at convenient time for assessment offline. It does not require the presence of both parties at the same time. Dermatology (cf: teledermatology), radiology and pathology are the common specialties that are conductive to asynchronous telemedicine. A properly record Medical Record preferably in electronic form should be a component of this transfer. Telemedicine is most beneficial for population living in isolated communities and remote regions and is currently being applied in virtually all medical domains. Specialties that use telemedicine often use a 'tele' prefix; for example, telemedicine applied by radiologists is called Teleradiology. Similarly telemedicine as applied by cardiologists is termed as telecardiology, etc.

Categories of Services

Telemedicine can be provided three main categories of services. These are store-and-forward, remote monitoring and interactive services.

Store-and-forward

Telemedicine involves acquiring medical data (like medical images, biosignals, etc.) and then transmitting this data to a doctor or medical specialist at a convenient time for assessment offline. It does not require the presence of both parties at the same time. Dermatology (cf: teledermatology) radiology, and pathology are common specialties that are conducive to a synchronous telemedicine. A properly structured medical record preferably in electronic form should be a component of this transfer. A key difference between traditional in-person patient meetings and telemedicine encounters is the omission of an actual physical examination and history. The 'store-and-forward' process requires the clinician to rely on a history report and audio/video information in lieu of a physical examination.

Remote Monitoring

Remote monitoring also known as self-monitoring or testing, enables medical professionals to monitor a patient remotely using various technological devices. This method is primarily used for managing chronic diseases or specific conditions, such as heart disease, diabetes mellitus, or asthma. These services can provide comparable health outcomes to traditional in-person patient encounters, supply greater satisfaction to patients, and may be cost-effective.

Interactive telemedicine services provide real-time interactions between patient and provider, to include phone conversations, online communication and home visits. Many activities such as history review, physical examination, psychiatric evaluations and ophthalmology assessments can be conducted comparably to those done in traditional face-to-face visits. In addition, 'clinician-interactive' telemedicine services may be less costly than in-person clinical visit.

Advantages of Telemedicine

Advantages for Patients

Telemedicine has been growing rapidly because it offers four fundamental benefits:

- **Improved access:** For over 40 years, telemedicine has been used to bring health care services to patients in distant locations. People at remote areas get top class medical facility from reputed hospital. Not only does telemedicine improve access to patients but it also allows physicians and health facilities to expand their reach, beyond their own offices. Hospital can spread their reach in remote villages and serve people without much investment or without the infrastructure. Given the provider shortages throughout the world—in both rural and urban areas—telemedicine has a unique capacity to increase service to millions of new patients.
- **Cost efficiencies:** Reducing or containing the cost of health care is one of the most important reasons for funding and adopting telehealth technologies. Telemedicine has been shown to reduce the cost of healthcare by reducing travel cost and save time and increase efficiency through better management of chronic diseases, shared health professional staffing, reduced travel times, and fewer or shorter hospital stays.
- **Improved quality:** Studies have consistently shown that the quality of health care services delivered via telemedicine as good those given in traditional in-person consultations. In some specialties, particularly in mental health and ICU care, telemedicine delivers a superior product, with greater outcomes and patient satisfaction. Doctors can learn new technology by connecting foreign hospital.
- **Patient demand:** Consumers want telemedicine. The greatest impact of telemedicine is on the patient, their family and their community. Using telemedicine technologies reduces travel time and related stresses for the patient. Over the past 15 years, study after study has documented patient satisfaction and support for telemedical services. Such services offer patients the access to providers that might not be available otherwise, as well as medical services without the need to travel long distances.

Reduce Hospitalization and Save Time of Healthcare Provider

The patient can assess healthcare services at their residence. Generally the patient with minor illness and patient after care of postoperative condition need not came to hospital for minor consultation by which the time of healthcare provider can be saved.

Provide Patient Satisfaction

The patient used to like for treatment in their houses with presence of all relatives so this telemedicine helps in providing satisfaction to the patient by treating them in their own place.

Benefits for Doctors

- Excellent opportunity to share knowledge between physicians all over the world.
- Joint consultation with export physician and surgeons for better management of complicated cases.
- Local doctors can be updated at any time.
- Medical education in the form of teleconferencing.

Benefits for Government

- Reduces rush to medical facilities in cities.

- Improve monitoring facilities at rural centers.
- Increase reliance on Government Health care system.

Limitations of Telemedicine

- The overall cost of telecommunication system, especially data management apparatus and practical training of medical professionals is high.
- Virtual clinical treatment decreases human interaction among the health care professionals and patients that increases the risk of error in clinical services, if the service is delivered by inexperienced professional. Moreover, confidential medical information can be leaked through faulty electronic system.
- Telemedicine might take longer time for the difficulties in connecting virtual communication due to low internet speed or server problem. Moreover, this system cannot provide immediate treatment, such as, antibiotics.
- Low quality of health informatics records, like X-ray or other images, clinical progress reports, etc., run the risk of faulty clinical treatment.
- Telemedicine system requires tough legal regulation to prevent unauthorized and illegal service providers in this sector. Legal and ethical complications may arise.
- Shortage of computer trained healthcare professionals and lack of training facility with lack of IEC.
- Privacy and security concern is also there. Evidence based practice is not practiced.
- The uneducated and poorly educated people cannot be assess this.
- All type of care cannot be provided in this method.

TELENURSING

- Telenursing refers to the use of telecommunication and information technology for providing nursing services in health care whenever a large physical distance between patients and nurse or between a number of nurses. As a field it is a part of telehealth and has many points of contacts with other medical and nonmedical applications, such as telediagnosis, teleconsulation, telemonitoring, etc.
- Telenursing is achieving a large rate of growth in many countries due to several factors, such as:
  - The preoccupation in driving down the costs of health care.
  - An increase in the number of ageing and chronically ill population.
  - The increase in coverage of health care to distant rural, small or sparsely populated regions.
- Telenursing may help to solve increasing shortages of nurses, to reduce distance and save travel time and to keep patients out of hospitals. A greater degree of job satisfaction has been registered among telenursing.

Application

One of the most distinctive telenursing applications in home care. For example patients who are immobilized or live in remote area, citizens who have chronically ailments such as COPD, diabetes, CHD or disabilitating diseases (Parkinson's disease, Alzeimer's disease), etc., may stay at home and be visited and assisted regulatory by a nurse via, video conferencing, internet, video and phone, etc.

Still other applications of home care are the care of patients in immediate postsurgical situations, the care of wounds, handicapped individuals etc. In normal home health care one nurse is able to visit up to 5–7 patients/day but by using telenurisng one nurse can visit 12–16 patients in the same time.

A common application of telenursing is also used by call centers operated by managed care organizations which are staffed by registered nurses who act as case managers or perform patient triage. Infromation and conuseling as a means of regulating patient access and flow and decrease the use of emergency rooms. Telenursing can also involve other activities such as patient education, teleconsultations, examination of results of medical tests, and assistance to physicians in the implementation of medical treatment protocols.

Legal, Ethical and Regulatory Issues

Telenursing is freight with legal, ethical and regulatory issues as it happens with telehealth as a whole. In many countries interstate and inter country practice of telenursing is forbidden. The attending nurse must have a license both in her state/country or residence and in the state/country where the patient receiving telecare is located. Legal issues such as accountability and malpractice, etc. are also still largely an unsolved and difficult to address. In addition there are many considerations related to patient's confidentiality and safety of clinical data.

CHAPTER 9

Healthcare Delivery System in India

INTRODUCTION

Delivery of healthcare services concern is to develop a system which ensures need-based comprehensive health care services to people at large, especially those living in remote and backward areas, using the available resources as effectively as possible. India is a federal union comprising 28 states and 8 union territories, for a total of 36 entities. The states and union territories are further subdivided into districts and smaller administrative divisions. The states are largely independent in matters relating to the delivery of health care to the people. Each state has developed its own system of health care delivery, independent of the Central Government. The Central Government responsibility consists mainly of policy-making, planning, guiding, assisting, evaluating and coordinating the work of the State Health Ministries.

Health care delivery system is initially started from the central government of India. The scope of health services varies widely from country to country and is influenced by general and ever-changing national, state and local health problem, need attitude as well as the available resources. Health care should be accessible, acceptable, provide scope for community participation, should be comprehensive and affordable at low cost.

HEALTH SERVICES ORGANIZATION AT DIFFERENT LEVEL IN INDIA

The health services organization in the country extends from the national level to the subcenter level in the remote rural areas. Broadly, four levels of health organization may be distinguished. Sound administration is essential for the success of any public health program, whether at the national, intermediate or local level.

Central Level

The official organs of the health system at the national level consists of:

The Union Ministry of Health and Family Welfare

The Union Ministry of Health and Family Welfare is headed by the cabinet minister, and the ministers and deputy ministers of all the states are the members. The Union Ministry of Health and Family Welfare consists of three departments: Department of Health, Department of Family Welfare and Department of AYUSH. These are explained as follows:

- **Department of Health:** The Secretary to the Government of India is the head of the Department of Health and he is assisted by the Joint Secretary, Deputy Secretary, and a large number of administrative staff. This department deals with health care including awareness campaigns, immunization campaigns, preventive medicine, and public health. The bodies under the administrative control of this department are:
  - National AIDS Control Organisation (NACO)
  - 13 National Health Programs
  - Medical Council of India
  - Dental Council of India
  - Pharmacy Council of India
  - Indian Nursing Council
  - All India Institute of Speech and Hearing (AIISH), Mysuru
  - All India Institute of Physical Medicine and Rehabilitation (AIIPMR), Mumbai
  - Hospital Services Consultancy Corporation Limited (HSCC)
  - Food Safety and Standards Authority of India
  - Central Drugs Standard Control Organization
- **Department of Family Welfare (1966):** The Department of Family Welfare is headed by the Secretary to the Government of India and assisted by one Additional Secretary, one Commissioner of Family Welfare, and one Joint Secretary. The Department of Family Welfare (FW) is responsible for the aspects relating to family welfare, especially in reproductive health, maternal health, pediatrics, information education and communications, cooperation with NGOs and international aid groups; and rural health services. The Department of Family Welfare is responsible for:
  - 18 Population Research Centers (PRCs) at six universities and six other institutions across 17 states
  - National Institute of Health and Family Welfare (NIHFW), South Delhi
  - International Institute for Population Sciences (IIPS), Mumbai
  - Central Drug Research Institute (CDRI), Lucknow

- Indian Council of Medical Research (ICMR), New Delhi: Founded in 1911, it is one of the oldest medical research bodies in the world.

- **Department of AYUSH:** In concurrence to 11th five-year plan, this department is functioning with the Secretary to Government of India as the head and assisted by one Joint Secretary, one Director, four Advisors of Ayurveda, Yoga, Unani, Siddha and Homoeopathy. The Department of Ayurveda, Yoga and Naturopathy, Unani, Siddha and Homoeopathy (AYUSH) deals with ayurveda (Indian traditional medicine), yoga, naturopathy, Unani, siddha, and homoeopathy, and other alternative medicine systems. The Department of Indian Systems of Medicine and Homeopathy (ISMandH) was created in March 1995 and renamed as Department of Ayurveda, Yoga and Naturopathy, Unani, Siddha and Homoeopathy (AYUSH) in November 2003 with a view to providing focused attention to the development of Education and Research in Ayurveda, Yoga and Naturopathy, Unani, Siddha and Homeopathy systems.

  The department is charged with upholding education standards in the ISMandH colleges, strengthening research, promoting the cultivation of medicinal plants used, and working on Pharmacopoeia standards. The bodies under the control of the Department of AYUSH are research councils and educational institutions of Unani Medicine, Ayurveda, Siddha, Homeopathy, etc.

Functions of the Union Ministry of Health and Family Welfare

As set out in the Seventh Schedule of Article 246 of the Constitution of India, functions of the Union Ministry of Health and Family Welfare are classified under two the following two headings:

Functions under Union List

- International health relations and administration of port quarantine
- Administration of central institutes
- Regulation and development of medical, pharma, and nursing professionals, etc.
- Establishment and maintenance of drug standards
- Immigration and emigration
- Census collection and publication of other statistical data
- Regulation of labor in the working of mines and oil fields
- Co-ordination with state and with other ministries for the promotion of health
- Promotion of research through research centers and other bodies.

Functions under Concurrent List

- Prevention of communicable disease
- Prevention of adulteration of foodstuff
- Control of drugs and poisons
- Vital statistics
- Labor welfare
- Ports other than major
- Economic and social planning
- Population control and family planning.

The Director General of Health Services: Director General of Health Services (DGHS) is the principal adviser to the Union Government in both the medical and public health matters. He is assisted by Additional Director General of Health Services, a team of deputies and a large number of administrative staff. The Director General of Health Services, a repository of technical knowledge, is an attached office of this Ministry and the DGHS also renders technical advice on all medical and public health matters and in the implementation of various health schemes. In order to implement the policies and programs of the Ministry in an effective manner, there are three subordinate offices located at various places in the country which function directly under the Ministry. The Ministry is also administratively concerned with 29 autonomous/statutory bodies. There are also three Public Sector Undertakings under the administrative control of the Ministry. The directorate comprises three main units:

1. Medical care and hospitals
2. Public health
3. General administration:

The functions of the Director General of Health services are classified under two headings which are explained as follows:

1. General functions include:
   - Survey
   - Planning, coordination, programming, appraisal of all health matters in the country.
2. Specific functions:
   - International health relation and quarantine
   - Control of drug standards
   - Medical store depots
   - Postgraduate training
   - Medical education and medical research
   - Central Government health scheme
   - National health programs
   - Central heath education bureau
   - Health intelligence
   - National medical library.

The Central Council of Health and Family Welfare: The Central Council of Health and Family Welfare was set up by the Presidential order on 9th August, 1952. The Central Council of Health and Family Welfare was set up under Article 263 of the Constitution to provide support and advice to the Department of Health on policy formulation. The Ministry of Health and Family Welfare, Government of India, in collaboration with the WHO Country Office for India, has compiled and digitized the proceedings of all the Central Council meetings held from the year 1988 up to 2010. The Union Health Minister is the chairman of the Central Council of Health and Family Welfare, and the State Health Ministers are its members.

Functions of the Central Council of Health and Family Welfare:

- To consider and recommend the broad outlines of policies in regard to matters in all aspects including provision of preventive and curative services, environmental hygiene, nutrition, health education, and promotion of facilities for training and research.

- To make proposals for legislations in the field of activity relating to medical and public health matters as well as to lay down the pattern of development of the country as a whole.
- To establish any organization with the function for promoting and maintaining cooperation between the Central and State Health Administrations.
- To make recommendations to the Central Government regarding the distribution of the available grants for health purposes to the States and to periodically review the work done by using this fund.

State Level

There are at present 28 States and 8 Union Territories in India. Historically, the first milestone in State health administration was the year 1919, when the States (then known as provinces) obtained autonomy, under the Montague-Chelmsford reforms from the Central Government, in matters of public health. From 1921–22, all the States had created some form of public health organization. The Government of India Act, 1935 gave further autonomy to the States. The health subjects were divided three groups: federal, concurrent and state. The "state" which became the responsibility of the State included provision of medical care, preventive health services and pilgrimages within the State. The position has largely remained the even after the new Constitution of India came into force in 1950. The State is the ultimate authority responsible for health services operating within its jurisdiction. Each state its own health administration. In all the States, the management sector comprises the State Ministry of Health and a Directorate of Health.

- **State Ministry of Health:** State Ministry of Health consists of Minister of Health and Family Welfare, Deputy Minister of Health and Family Welfare, and Health Secretariat
- **Health Secretariat includes:**
  - Secretary-cum-Commissioner
  - Additional Secretary
  - Under-Secretary
  - Deputy Secretary
  - Administrative staff
- **State Health Directorate:** The State Health Directorate is functioned by Director of Family Welfare, Director of Health Services, and Director of Medical Education and Training. The State Health Directorate's functioning is assisted by a suitable number of deputy directors, regional director, all branches of public health, functional director and specialties in a particular field.

Functions

- Adequate medical and preventive services
- National health programs
- Control of CD
- **Health promotion activities:** MCH, immunization, school health services
- Control of food and drug adulteration
- Health services in jails
- Health education
- Vital statistics
- Information regarding incidence of notifiable diseases
- Medical, dental, nursing, etc., education and maintenance of standards, practice through statutory bodies
- Cooperation and coordination with the central health ministry
- Encourage AYUSH
- Effective distribution of vaccines
- Maintain storage of hospital drugs and appliances
- Study health problems and take steps to reduce morbidity
- Enact legislations dealing with public health and medical care
- Maintenance of regional laboratories for chemical and bacteriological examination.

DISTRICT LEVEL

The principal unit of administration in India is the district under a Collector. Most districts in India are divided into two or more subdivisions, each in-charge of an assistant collector. Each division is again divided into tehsils (talukas), in-charge of a tahsildar. A tahsil usually comprises between 200 to 600 villages. The rural areas of the district have been organized into blocks, known as community development blocks, the area of which may or may not coincide with tahsil. The block is a unit of rural planning and development, and comprises approximately 100 villages and about 80,000 to 1,20,000 population, in-charge of a Block Development Officer. Finally there are the village panchayats, which are institutions of rural local self-government.

Within each district there are six administrative divisions:

1. Subdivisions
2. Tehsils (taluks)
3. Community development blocks
4. Municipalities and corporations.
5. Villages
6. Panchayats.

For organizing health programme at district level the district officer with the overall control is designated as the chief medical and health officer (CM and HO) or otherwise known as chief district medical and public health officer. These officers are overall in-charge of the health and family welfare programmes in the district. They are responsible for implementing the programmes according to policies laid down and finalized at higher levels, i.e., State and Center. These DMOs/CMOs are assisted by Deputy CMOs/AHDO and programme officers. The number of such officers, their specialization, and status in the cadre of State Civil Medical Services differ from the State to State. Due to this, the span of control and hierarchy of reporting of these programme officers vary from state to state.

Responsibilities of the Chief District Health Officer/ Chief District Medical and Public Health Officer

- Planning and budgeting of health service and delivery infrastructure in the district
- Mobilizing resources for health service and delivery infrastructure in the district
- Monitoring and evaluating the health services in the district
- Procuring medical supplies and equipments
- Providing technical guidance and support supervision to health centers
- Managing and accounting for financial, medical supplies and other resources allocated to the district
- Coordinating the maintenance of health equipments and facilities
- Interpreting National Health Policy and integrating it to district health plans
- Tendering advice on health-related issues to district councils and other stakeholders
- Carrying and monitoring of health programs in the district
- Coordinating sensitization program about PHC in the communities
- Carrying out Human resource functions like identifying manpower needs, training, mentoring, coaching, promotions, leave, deployment and periodic assessment of health staff
- Managing Health research
- Enforcing the professional and service codes of conduct and ethics
- Preparing and submitting periodic reports.

URBAN LOCAL BODIES

Health organization in town area: After the 74th Amendment was enacted, there are only three categories of urban local bodies, which are explained as follows:

1. **Nagar Palika (Municipal Council):** In India, a Nagar Palika or Municipality or Nagar Nigam is an urban local body that administers a city with a population of 100,000 or more. However, there are exceptions to that, as previously the nagar palikas were constituted in the urban centers with population over 20,000. So, all the urban bodies which were previously classified as Nagar Palikas were reclassified as Nagar Palikas even if their population was under 100,000. Under the Panchayati Raj system, it interacts directly with the state government, though it is administratively a part of the district it is located in. Generally, smaller district cities and bigger towns have a Nagar Palika. Nagar Palikas are also a form of local self-government, entrusted with some duties and responsibilities, as enshrined and guided upon by the Constitutional (74th Amendment) Act, 1992.

   The members of the Nagar Palika are the elected representatives for a term of five years. The town is divided into wards according to its population, and the representatives are elected from each ward. The members elect a president among themselves to preside over and conduct meetings. A chief officer, along with officers, like an engineer, sanitary inspector, health officer and education officer, who come from the state public service, are appointed by the state government to control the administrative affairs of the Nagar Palika. The members of the Nagar Palika are the elected representatives for a term of five years. The town is divided into wards according to its population, and the representatives are elected from each ward. The members elect a president among themselves to preside over and conduct meetings. A chief officer, along with officers, like an engineer, accountant and auditor, sanitary inspector, health officer and education officer, who come from the state public service, are appointed by the state government to control the administrative affairs of the Nagar Palika.

   The Nagar Palika is responsible for the proper functioning and maintenance of:
   - Water supply
   - Hospitals
   - Roads
   - Street-lighting
   - Drainage
   - Fire brigade
   - Marketplaces
   - Records of births and deaths
   - Solid waste management.
2. **Nagar Panchayat (Notified Area Council, City Council):** A Nagar Panchayat or Notified Area Council or City Council is a form of an urban political unit in India comparable to a municipality. An urban center with more than 11,000 and less than 25,000 inhabitants is classified as a 'Nagar Panchayat'. Each Nagar Panchayat has a committee consisting of a chairman with ward members. Membership consists of a minimum of ten elected ward members and three nominated members. The NAC members of the Nagar Panchayat are elected from the several wards of the Nagar Panchayat on the basis of adult franchise for a term of five years. There are seats reserved for scheduled castes, scheduled tribes, backward classes and women. The councillors or ward members chosen by direct election from electoral wards in the Nagar Panchayat. The chairman is the head of the Notified Area Committee. The executive officer is the official in-charge of the Notified Area Council. The executive officers monitor the implementation of all the programs related to planning and development of the Notified Area Council with the coordination of NAC chairman and all ward members.

   The functions of a Nagar Panchayat are as follows:
   - Provide essential services and facilities to the urban area
   - Sanitation program in township
   - Street-lighting and providing roads in every wards and main roads of the town
   - Set up and run schools in the urban area. Execute programs for adult literacy and run city libraries
   - Water supplying to every ward of the urban area

- Drainage system to clear the solid and liquid wastes from the town
- Build culvert for underground drainage system
- Records of births and deaths.

3. **Nagar Nigam (Municipal Corporation):** Each Municipal Corporation has a committee consisting of a mayor with councillors. They are formed under the Corporations Act of 1835 of the Panchayati Raj system, which mainly deals in providing essential services in metropolitan cities. The number of councillors depends upon the area and population of the city with a minimum population of 3,00,000. Municipal Corporation members are elected from the several wards of the specific city on the basis of adult franchise for a term of five years. The largest corporations are in the six metropolitan cities of India, viz. Delhi, Mumbai, Kolkata, Chennai, Bengaluru and Hyderabad and among these, Mumbai is the most populous and largest metropolitan city of India. Mayor is the head of the Municipal Corporation. The Municipal Commissioner is the official in-charge of this organization. The Executive Officers monitor the implementation of all the programs related to planning and development of the corporation with the coordination of mayor and councillors.

   The functions of a Municipal Corporation are the proper functioning and maintenance of:
   - Water supply
   - Hospitals
   - Roads
   - Overbridges
   - Street-lighting
   - Drainage
   - Solid waste
   - Fire brigades
   - Marketplaces and
   - Records of births and deaths
   - It also helps in education and primary health care.

A town area committee is a semimunicipal authority constituted for the administration of small towns in India. They are assigned a limited number of civic functions like street lighting, drainage, roads, conservancy, etc. Town area committees were established by an Act passed by the state legislature. The Act mentions the composition, functions, and other matters related to the town area committee. The members may be partly elected and partly nominated by the state government, or wholly nominated, or wholly elected. In some states, District Collectors are given powers of surveillance and control over the Town area committees.

Panchayati Raj System

District Level—Zila Parishad

The instrument of local self-government at the District level is the Zila Parishad. The Chief Executive Officer (CEO), who is an IAS or a State Civil Service officer, heads the administrative machinery of the Zila Parishad. He may also be a District Magistrate in some states. The CEO supervises the divisions of the Parishad and executes its development schemes. The members of the Zila Parishad include all the heads of the Panchayat Samitis in the district, MPs, MLAs, representatives of the scheduled castes and scheduled tribes and cooperative societies. The Collector is a nonvoting member. The Zila Parishad is a supervisory and coordinating body. Its functions and powers vary from state to state. In Gujarat, the control of primary health centers is exercised by the Zila Parishads through the District Health Officer.

Block Level—Panchayat Samiti

Panchayat Samiti consists of 100 villages covering 80,000 to 1 lakh people. Which is a local government body at the tehsil (taluka) level in India. It works for the villages of the tehsil that together are called a Development Block. The Panchayat Samiti is the link between the Gram Panchayat (village council) and the Zila Parishad.

This Samiti consists of all Sarpanchs (heads) of the village panchayats in the Block, MLAs and MPs residing in the Block area, and the representatives of the scheduled castes and tribes. The Block Development Officer is the ex-officer (secretary of the Panchayat Samiti). The Panchayat Samiti supervises and gives technical assistance and guidance to the village Panchayats engaged in development work. The Samiti also acts as an agent of the State Government, which provides money for the developmental projects. Panchayat samiti should meet at least once in a month. The panchayat samiti is responsible for block development activities under the community development programme. The funds for the development activities are processes through panchayat samiti.

Village Level—Panchayat

- **Gram Sabha:** They meet at least twice in a year and elect the members of the Gram Panchayat. It constitutes a population of 5,000 to 15,000. There are 15 to 30 panchs as the members, who are headed by the sarpanch. Its term is up to 3 to 5 years. The Nyaya Panchayat in the village is a platform to resolve the disputes between villages/local group. Maintaining peace among the people is the basic purpose of the system of Panchayati Raj. It is an assembly of all the adults of the village.
- **Gram Panchayat:** It is the executive organ of the Gram Sabha. It is headed by a President-grade person known as Sarpanch or Mukhiya and there are 15 to 30 members in total. The members of the Panchayat are elected by the adults of the Gram Sabha and they hold the office for a period of 3 to 4 years. The functions of the Panchayat cover the entire field of civil administration, e.g., sanitation, street-lighting, control of disease, adult literacy, youth clubs, mahila samitis, improvement in health preventive and curative, measures during epidemics, maintenance of village schools, improvement of agriculture and cottage industries, etc. The panchayat Secretary helps the panchayat in its various activities.

- **Nyaya Panchayat:** It is the judicial organ of the Gram Sabha. There is one Nyaya Panchayat for a group of 5 village Panchayats. The Nyaya Panchayats try civil cases and minor criminal offences. They are empowered to impose fines up to ₹100.

HEALTHCARE DELIVERY IN INDIA

The concern of the delivery of healthcare services is to develop a system which ensures need-based comprehensive healthcare services to the people at large, especially those living in remote and backward areas, using the available resources as effectively as possible.

In 1997, the Government of India launched a rural health scheme based on the principle of 'placing people's health in people's hands'.

Purpose

The purpose of healthcare services is to improve the health status of the population.

Healthcare services, in general, are rendered by the Government through a network of health centers from the grass root level to the block level in the rural areas and also in urban areas. There are numbers of models developed for delivering health care. The easiest model has given in **Flowchart 9.1**.

HEALTH STATUS AND HEALTH PROBLEMS

An assessment of the health status and health problems is the first requisite for any planned effort to develop healthcare services. This is also known as 'Community Diagnosis'.

Following is the data required for health situation and defining the health problems: Morbidity and mortality statistics

- Demographic conditions of the population
- Environmental conditions which have a bearing on health
- Socioeconomic factors which have a direct effect on health
- Cultural background, attitudes, beliefs, and practices which affect health
- Medical and health services available
- Other services available.

HEALTH PROBLEMS IN INDIA

The health problems of India may be conveniently grouped under the following five heads:

1. Communicable disease problems
2. Noncommunicable disease problems
3. Nutritional problems
4. Environmental sanitation problems
5. Medical care problems
6. Population problems.

These are explained as follows:

Communicable Disease Problems

Infectious diseases caused by pathogens, such as bacteria, viruses, fungi and parasites are the major causes of morbidity and mortality all over the world. Epidemics due to these diseases disrupt the routine health services and cause public health emergencies. The lost productivity, the missed educational opportunities and the high health care costs caused by infectious diseases, thus, directly impact the growth of the society. Also, the indirect costs due to negative impact on domestic and international tourism and trade can be significant.

Children are particularly vulnerable to infectious diseases. Pneumonia, diarrhea and malaria are the leading causes of death among the children under five years of age.

Communicable diseases continue to be major problem in India. Diseases considered to be of great importance are—malaria, tuberculosis, diarrhea, and acute respiratory diseases.

Malaria

Malaria continues to be a major health problem in India. Although total malaria cases have declined compared to previous years, the proportion of *P. falcifarum* has increased. Malaria cases have increased in North East states, Madhya Pradesh, Chhattisgarh, Jharkhand, Odisha, Andhra Pradesh, Maharashtra, etc. During 2013 there were 0.8 million cases malaria (which included 0.44 million cases of Pf malaria) and 379 deaths.

- **Mode of transmission:** Vector transmission, direct transmission through blood transfusion, use of needle for injections in a drug-addict.
- **Incubation period:** It varies from 12 to 18 days, depending upon the species.
- **Clinical features:** There are three stages of malaria:
  1. *Cold stage:* Onset is with lassitude, severe headache, nausea, chilly sensation, temperature ranging from 39–41°C. Its period lasts from 15 minutes to 1 hour.

Flowchart 9.1: Healthcare delivery model.

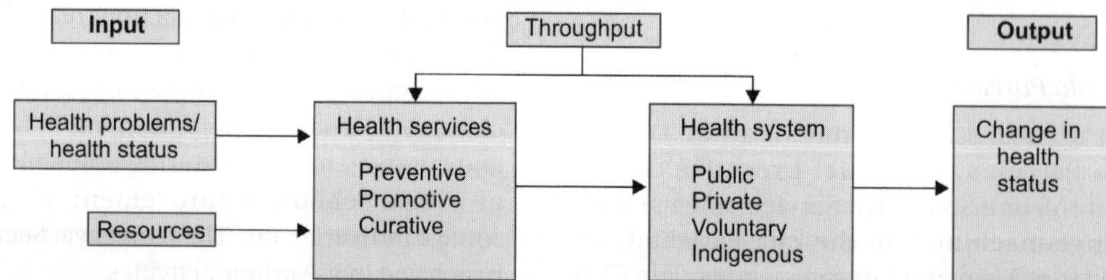

2. *Hot stage:* Skin is hot and dry to touch, intense headache, rapid respiration, period lasts from 2 to 6 hours.
3. *Sweating stage:* Fever comes down with profuse sweating, patient feels relaxed. Period lasts from 2 to 4 hours.

- **Management:** *P. vivax, P. ovale,* and *P. malariae* infections should be treated with chloroquine 600 mg, base followed by 300 mg in 6 hours. Later, 150 mg base 12 hourly for 2 more days. Check vitals 4 hourly. Maintain intake and output chart.

Tuberculosis

Tuberculosis remains a public health problem, with India accounting for one-fifth of the world incidence. Every year about 2.6 million persons develop tuberculosis, of which about 0.62 million are new smear positive highly infectious cases and about 0.24 million people die of TB every year. The emergence of HIV-TB coinfection and multidrug resistant TB has increased the severity and magnitude of the disease.

- **Causative agent:** *Mycobacterium tuberculosis*
- **Mode of transmission:** Droplet infection
- **Incubation period:** It may be weeks, months or years. Tuberculin-positive stage in 3 to 6 weeks' duration
- **Clinical manifestations:** Loss of weight, fatigue, cough with expectoration, hemoptysis, high fever, night sweats, dyspnea, chest pain, hoarseness of voice
- **Diagnostic measures:** Sputum test, X-rays, Mantoux test, family history and observing signs and symptoms
- **Treatment:** For 18–24 months, drugs used for standard treatment are: streptomycin injection isoniazid tablets (5 mg/kg), and thioacetazone tablets. Modern drugs as pyrazinamide (1500 mg), ethambutol (1200 mg), and rifampicin (450 mg) are available. Directly Observed Treatment, Short-course (DOTS) chemotherapy is prescribed. Nutritious diet is to be taken when the patient is on antituberculosis drugs. Safe disposal of sputum should be there. The patient should cover the mouth with clean cloth which is properly washed and dried in sunlight.

  The nursing measures are: The clothes, utensils, personal belongings of the patient should be kept isolated until the sputum becomes negative. Teach the patient about general hygiene, nutrition, and toxic effects of drugs.
- **Follow up:** Periodic check-up of the patient after treatment is important for at least 2 years.

Acute Respiratory Disease

It is one of the major causes of morbidity and mortality in children below 5 years of age. During 2013, 3.17 million episodes of ARI were reported with 3287 deaths.

- **Etiology:** Aspiration drug ingestion and overdose. Prolonged inhalation of high concentration of O_2, smoke, corrosive substances. Trauma, major surgery fat or air emboli.
- **Clinical manifestations:** Dyspnea hypoxemia
- **Assessment and diagnostic findings:** Severe hypoxemia intercoastal retraction crackles
- **Management:** O_2 administration antioxidant therapy. Corticosteroid therapy antisepsis agents nutritional therapy nebulization therapy chest physiotherapy suctioning mechanical ventilation. Reduce anxiety of patient provide rest.

Diarrhea

Diarrhea is one of the major causes of morbidity and mortality in children below 5 years of age. It continues in India due to poor environmental conditions. They are responsible for about 10.76 million cases of diarrhea each year. Outbreaks of diarrheal diseases (including cholera) continue to occur in India due to poor environmental conditions.

Causative agents:

- **Acute watery diarrhea:** Rota virus, *Salmonella, E. coli*
- **Acute bloody diarrhea:** Shigella, amoebiasis.

Mode of transmission: Fecal oral route.

Clinical Manifestations

- **Acute diarrhea:** An attack of sudden onset of diarrhea, lasting from 3 to 7 days or even up to 10 to 14 days. Passage of loose, liquid or watery stools, usually more than three times a day.
- **Inflammatory diarrhea:** Abdominal pain, fever, stools are frequent, blood-stained pus cells, mucus less in volume
- **Noninflammatory diarrhea:** Nausea, vomiting, abdominal pain, fever, voluminous and watery stools.

Confirmation of cause of diarrhea is done with the help of laboratory tests. As a community health nurse, notification to the local health authority is her responsibility. Assessment of dehydration and rehydration is done with the help of oral fluids, IV fluids, and ORS. Soft, easily digestible food is given. Breast milk is the best for infants and should be continued in diarrhea also. There should be a provision of safe water supply, sanitary latrines. Antibiotics as ciprofloxacin 500 mg 12 hourly for 3 days, metronidazole, etc., should be prescribed.

Leprosy

Leprosy is the year 2013–2014, total of 1.27 lakh new cases were detected, out of which child cases were 9.49% and deformity grade II and above was 4.14%. 51.48% of these cases are estimated to be multibacillary. All the state and union territories report cases of leprosy. However there are considerable variations not only between one state and another, but also between one district and another. With the prevalence rate of about 0.68 per 10,000 populations, India has achieved the goal of leprosy elimination at national level.

Causative agent: Mycobacterium leprae

Types: (a) Infectious type (lepromatous) and (b) Non-infectious type (tuberculoid)

Mode of transmission: Droplet and contact transmission.

Incubation period: 3–5 years

Clinical Manifestations

Common organs involved are nerve, eye, skin, bone and internal organs, hypopigmented patches and thickened nerves, nodules on skin, face, ears, and claw-hand deformity. In the late phase, loss of fingers, nasal depression, foot drop, claw toes, planter ulcers are seen.

Diagnostic Tests

- **Lepromin test:** 0.1 mL of lepromin ID on inner aspect of forearm is given. Reaction is read after 48 hours and on 21st day. If induration and redness are more than 10 mm at 48 hours, it is positive. On 21st day, nodule of more than 5 mm is positive. Skin tissue from ears, nasal smear, and skin patches for bacteriological examination.
  Management: Objectives for treatment are—to cure the patient, to prevent deformity and to interrupt the transmission of infections.
- **Multidrug therapy:** Rifampicin 600 mgm, Clofazimine 100–300 mgm. Dapsone: 100 mgm
- **Dapsone monotherapy:** Adult dose 100 mgm; in children aged 6–14, 50 mgm daily; below 6 years, 25 mgm daily.
  - *Examination of family members:* Early detect signs of leprosy as light-colored patches appear on skin. Tell the patient about the side effects of drugs, and that leprosy is not the result of sin or hereditary. If there is loss of sensation in hands, protect from burns, cuts, and wounds. Skin care, foot care, and eye care should be done. At an early stage, it may spread to others. If burns, cuts, and lesions are present, do not neglect as it can cause ulcers and eventually deformity.

AIDS

The problem of AIDS was increasing previously in magnitude. The problem now become stable. It is estimated that by the end of year 2012 there were about 2.08 million HIV positive cases in the country.

- **Causative agent:** Human immunodeficiency virus
- **Incubation period:** 6 months to 7 years
- **Mode of transmission:** Parenteral route, sexual transmission, and perinatal transmission

Clinical Manifestations

Loss of weight of more than 10% body-weight. Fever more than 1 month's duration, diarrhea, amenorrhea infections as herpes zoster, kaposi sarcoma, lymphoma, vasculitis, gingivitis, GI system symptoms include persistent diarrhea, colitis, dysphagia, perianal discomfort. Respiratory system symptoms are persistent cough, hemoptysis, pleural effusion. Neurological system include headache, dementia, visual impairment, meningitis, seizures hematological, renal, cardiac, endocrinal and reproductive manifestations. Hemiplegia, peripheral neuropathy, lymphoma.

Poliomyelitis

It is a highly infectious disease caused by polio virus.

- **Incidence:** Usually affects children below 5 years of age.
- **Incubation period:** 7 to 14 days.
- **Mode of transmission:** Feco-oral route, droplet infection.
- **Period of communicability:** Most infectious 7 to 10 days before and after onset of symptoms.
- **Clinical manifestations:** In the beginning stage, complaints of fever, headache, fatigue, restlessness, vomiting, diarrhea, cough and cold. Paralysis may occur in legs, face, larynx, esophagus, person may become permanently handicapped.
- **Diagnostic test:** By signs and symptoms, physical examination and study of virus.
- **Complications:** Paralysis or permanent deformity.
- **Management:** Symptomatic treatment and physiotherapy
- **Immunization:** It is essential to immunize every child against polio by 6 months of age. Two types of vaccines are inactivated polio vaccine, and oral polio vaccine. Kala azar, meningitis, viral hepatitis, encephalitis, enteric fever and helminthic infestations are other important communicable diseases in India as well as other countries. India consists of a small group of well-fed and a very large group of undernourished.

The specific problems in the country are: Protein energy malnutrition, nutritional anemia, low birthweight, xerophthalmia (nutritional blindness), iodine-deficiency disorders.

Filaria

The problem of filarial remains endemic in about 250 districts in 20 States and UTs. The population at risk is over 600 million. To achieve elimination of LF, the Govt. of India has launched nationwide Annual Mass Drug Administration (MDA) with annual single recommended dose of diethyl carbamazine citrate tablets in addition to scaling up home based foot care and hydrocele operations. In 2012, 250 endemic districts implemented MDA targeting a population of about 554 million with a coverage rate of 87%.

Other health problems include Kala-azar, meningitis, viral hepatitis, Japanese encephalitis, dengue fever, enteric fever and helminthetic infestations are among the other important communicable disease problems in India. The tragedy is that most of these diseases can be either easily prevented or treated with minimum input resources. In fact most of the developed countries of the world have overcome many of these problems by such measures as manipulation of environment, practice of preventive medicine and improvements of standards of living.

NONCOMMUNICABLE DISEASES PROBLEMS

Noncommunicable diseases (NCDs) are a group of diseases that affect individuals over a protracted period of time causing socioeconomic burden to the nation. The major noncommunicable diseases share four behavioral risk factors, that are unhealthy diet, lack of physical activity, and use of tobacco and alcohol. Factors contributing to the rise of NCDs also include ageing, rapid unplanned urbanization and globalization.

According to WHO 2021, Noncommunicable diseases (NCDs) kill 41 million people each year, equivalent to 71% of all deaths globally. Each year, more than 15 million people die from a NCD between the ages of 30 and 69 years; 85% of these "premature" deaths occur in low- and middle-income countries. 77% of all NCD deaths are in low- and middle-income countries.

Cardiovascular diseases account for most NCD deaths, or 17.9 million people annually, followed by cancers (9.3 million), respiratory diseases (4.1 million), and diabetes (1.5 million). These four groups of diseases account for over 80% of all premature NCD deaths. Tobacco use, physical inactivity, the harmful use of alcohol and unhealthy diets all increase the risk of dying from NCD.

Detection, screening and treatment of NCDs, as well as palliative care, are key components of the response to NCDs. Noncommunicable diseases (NCDs), also known as chronic diseases, tend to be of long duration and are the result of a combination of genetic, physiological, environmental and behavioral factors. The main types of NCD are cardiovascular diseases (such as heart attacks and stroke), cancers, chronic respiratory diseases (such as chronic obstructive pulmonary disease and asthma) and diabetes. NCDs disproportionately affect people in low- and middle-income countries where more than three quarters of global NCD deaths.

Nutritional Problems

Malnutrition

Malnutrition, specially under nutrition act as a major public health and nutrition challenge faced by many developing countries including India, stands as a consequence of several key social and economic factors such as lack of education, inadequate healthcare services and ill-informed cultural behaviors. More than 33% of deaths in 0–5 years are associated with malnutrition. High levels of malnutrition in children, particularly in those under the age of two, tend to prevail in those countries where levels of socioeconomic development are also low. It is estimated that improved feeding habits aimed to prevent or treat malnutrition could prevent 11 million child deaths globally per year. Thus, efforts to address this issue are of paramount importance and have political, economic and cultural implications across all levels of societies for many developing nations.

Nutritional Anemia

Iron deficiency anemia is the most common micronutrient deficiency in the world. It is a major health problem for adults as well as children, affecting almost 7 in 10 children age 6–59 months, affecting 55% of women and 24% of men. Anemia is considerably higher in rural areas, among children of women with no education, among scheduled castes and tribes, and among children in households in the lower wealth quintiles. The prevalence of children's anemia rises steadily with the mother's level of anemia, reaching 82% for children of mothers who are severely anemic. Children of mothers who are severely anemic are seven times as likely to be severely anemic as children of mothers who are not anemic.

- **Causes:** Iron deficiency, folic acid and vitamin B_{12} deficiency.
- **Signs and hazards:** Exhaustion, difficulty in breathing, suffocation, headache, blurring of vision, excessive sleep, paler skin, anorexia, edema, and cardiac problems. In some cases, the patient can also die.
- **Treatment:** It depends upon Hb level. Iron tablets 200 mg till it is controlled. Iron syrups for children. Blood transfusion in severe stage. For prevention, 180 mg ferrous sulfate, 0.5 mg folic acid tab is given for 2–3 months daily till Hb becomes normal.

Xerophthalmia

Vitamin A deficiency affects about 19 million pregnant women and 190 million preschool-age children, mostly from the World Health Organization (WHO) regions of Africa and South-East Asia. Infants and children have increased vitamin A requirements to support rapid growth and to help them combat infections. Xerophthalmia is a disorder of vitamin A deficiency which is also called 'nutritional blindness'. About 0.04% of total blindness in India is attributed to vitamin deficiency. Keratomalacia has been the major cause of nutritional blindness in children between 1 and 3 years of age.

- **Effects of vitamin A deficiency:** Night blindness, xerosis conjunctiva, xerosis cornea, Bitot's spots, keratomalacia, follicular hyperkeratosis.
- **Treatment and prevention:**
  - *Mild to moderate case:* 10 g of fat soluble vitamin A for period of 10 days.
  - *Severe case:* 50 g daily for a few weeks. Fortification of food with vitamin A. Protect children from PEM, diarrhea, measles and respiratory diseases.

Iodine Deficiency Disorder (IDDs)

Among all IDDs, Goiter is only the tip of the iceberg. Iodine deficiency results in physical and mental retardation. It affects people of all ages, both sexes and different socioeconomic status. It could result in abortion, stillbirth, mental retardation, deaf-mutism, dwarfism, squint, cretinism, goiter of all ages, neuromotor defect, etc. In our country, it is estimated that more than 200 million people are at risk of IDD, while the number of persons suffering from goiter and other iodine deficiency disorder is above 71 million.

- **Symptoms:** Swelling in the neck, usually painless but creates deformity. Breathing difficulty due to suppressed trachea.
- **Treatment:** Thyroidectomy prevented by regular use of iodized salt. Avoid goitrogenic food, like cabbage, cauliflower, and radish as these substances react with iodine present in food and make it unavailable.

Other nutritional problems: Other nutritional problems of importance are lathyrism, endemic fluorosis, and adulteration of food stuffs in certain parts of the country.

Environmental Sanitation Problems

The most difficult problem to tackle in this country is environmental sanitation problem, which is multifactorial and multifaceted. Main environmental problems in India are: Air and water pollution, depletion of natural resources, improper waste disposal and low level of sanitation, sound pollution, traffic pressure, degradation of land, industrialization and urbanization, radiation hazards, excessive use of fertilizers and chemicals in agriculture, destruction of forests. The cycle of increasing population, poverty, illiteracy, and unemployment further increases the environmental problems. The contamination of physical and biological components of the earth/atmosphere system to such an extent that the normal environmental processes are adversely affected is generally termed as 'environmental pollution'. Environmental hazards, like air, water, soil and noise pollution create different types of harmful effects not only to the Individual but also to the flora and fauna. For a healthy environment, the prevention and control of environmental hazards are highly essential.

Medical Care Problems

In India, national health policies are made but financial resources are considered inadequate to furnish the cost of running such services. In the rural areas, 74% population does not get benefit of modern curative and preventive health services. Approximately, 80% of health services are concentrated in the urban areas but with uneven distribution of doctors. Thus, the major medical care problem in India is inadequate distribution of the available health resources between the urban and rural areas, and lack of penetration of health services to social periphery.

Population Problem

The population problem is one of the biggest problems faced by our country. It has affected on all aspects of housing, health care, sanitation, and environment. The population is increasing very fast because of declining death rate and high birth rate. The first increasing population is creating problem in imbalance in the ecosystem affecting socio-economic aspects and quality life. While India's population growth has slowed remarkably over the last few years, it is still growing faster than China and is expected to surpass China in population by 2026, when both will have about 1.46 billion people. After 2030, India is expected to be the most populous country in the world. India is expected to reach its peak population of 1.65 billion people by 2060.

Healthcare Services

In the light of 'Health for All' by 2000, the goals to be achieved have been fixed in terms of mortality and morbidity reduction, increase in expectation of life, decrease in population growth rate, improvements in nutritional status, provision of basic sanitation, resources development and certain other parameters, such as food production, literacy rate, and reduction in the level of poverty. A comprehensive list of health services may be found in the report of WHO expert committee.

Health services should be:
- Comprehensive
- Accessible
- Acceptable
- Provide scope for community participation
- Affordable at low cost.

HEALTHCARE SYSTEM

Public Health Sector

Primary Health Care:
- Primary health centers
- Subcenters.

Hospitals/Health Centers

- Community health centers
- Rural hospitals
- District hospitals/health centers
- Specialist hospitals
- Teaching hospitals.

Central Government Health Scheme (CGHS)

Other Agencies

- Defense services
- Railways.

Private Health Sector

- Private hospitals, polyclinics, nursing homes and dispensaries
- General practitioners and clinics.

Indigenous Systems of Medicine (AYUSH)

- Ayurveda, Yoga and Siddha
- Unani and Tibbi
- Homeopathy
- Unregistered practitioners.

Voluntary Health Agencies

Voluntary health agencies which refers to any non-profit, nongovernmental agency, governed by lay or professional individuals, organized on a national, state, or local level whose main purpose is health related, and supported by voluntary public contributions, for example:
- Indian Red Cross Society
- Hind Kusht Nivaran Sangh
- Indian Council for Child Welfare
- The Kasturba Memorial Fund
- Family Planning Association of India
- All India Women's Conference.

National Health Programs

- National Programmes for Control of Communicable Diseases

- National Programmes for Control of Noncommunicable Diseases
- National Nutritional Programmes
- National Programmes Related to System Strengthening/ Welfare.

HEALTH SERVICES FOR THE RURAL AREAS

In India, generally there were 617 districts, 6345 blocks and 6,23,706 villages incorporating 581 District Hospitals (DHs), 4045 Community Health Centers (CHCs) and 22,370 Primary Health Centers (PHCs) in India in 2007. The health care in rural areas are included in service at the village level, at the subcenter level and at the primary health center level.

Village Level

At the village level, based on the VHG scheme the VHGs are chosen by the community. They serve as a link between the village, community and the Government health services system. These provide first contact between the individual and health system. These are voluntary health workers selected by the local community and trained locally for three months at the primary health centers and subcenters. After the completion of their training, they are given a manual, which gives them detailed instructions of what they should do and also a medical kit containing medicines worth ₹600 a year. The health guides (now mostly women) provide the first contact between the community and the official health system. It is proposed to train one health guide for every 1000 rural population. During the year 1981, the scheme was made 100% centrally sponsored under the Family Welfare Programme.

Guidelines for their Selection

- They should be permanent residents of the local community, preferably women
- They should have minimum formal education—at least 8th class
- They should be acceptable to all sections of the community
- They should be able to give at least 2–3 hours for community health work.

Responsibilities of VHGs

- Treatment of common minor ailments
- First aid during accidents and emergency
- Care to mothers and children
- Health education.

Local Dais/TBAs

These work under the supervision of FHW and provide services at the time of delivery in rural areas, health education on child care, immunization, nutrition and family planning.

Anganwadi Worker

Under the ICDS, one anganwadi worker is appointed per 1000 population.

Responsibilities

- Health check-up
- Supplementary nutrition
- Immunization
- Health education (nonformal)
- Referral services.

Accredited Social Health Activist (ASHA)

Under the NRHM, ASHA are being appointed to fulfill the gap in the rural health services in the states.

Criteria for Selection

- ASHA must be primarily a women resident of the village.
- ASHA should have effective communication Skills, leadership qualities.
- She should having minimum formal education up to 8th class.

Roles and Responsibilities of ASHA

- ASHA will create awareness on nutrition, basic sanitations, hygienic practice, and healthy living and utilization of family welfare services.
- She will counsel women on birth preparedness, importance of safe delivery, breastfeeding, immunization, contraception and prevention of RTIs/STIs.
- Accompany pregnant women and children requiring treatment/admission to the nearest PHCs/CHCs.
- Provide medical care for minor ailment and for DOTs under RNTCP.
- ASHA also acts as an adept holder for the provision of ORS, iron, folic acid, chloroquine, oral pills and condoms.
- Her role as a care provider, providing newborn care and management of common ailments, particularly childhood illness.
- Inform births and deaths in her village and also inform about any disease outbreaks to the subcenter/PHC.
- Work with the village and sanitation committee.

Roles and Integration with Anganwadi

- Organizing necessary events once/twice a month on health day
- AWWs will be depot-holder for drug kit and will be issuing it to the ASHA
- ASHA will support the AWWs in mobilizing pregnant women and lactating women and infant for nutrition supplement

Roles and Integration with ANM

She will take the help of ASHA in motivating the pregnant women for coming to the subcenter for initial check-up and taking full course of iron and folic acid tablets and TT injection.

Subcenters (SCs)

The subcenter is the most peripheral and first contact point between the primary health care system and the community. The Ministry of Health and Family Welfare is providing

100% central assistance. There are 1,45,272 subcenters functioning in the country as in March 2007. The entire Family Welfare Programme is being implemented through the Primary Health Care system. The Primary Health Care Infrastructure has been developed as a three-tier system with Subcenter, Primary Health Center (PHC) and Community Health Center (CHC) being the three pillars of Primary Health Care System. Progress of subcenters, which is the most peripheral contact point between the Primary Health Care System and the community, is a prerequisite for the overall progress of the entire system. The subcenter generally covers 5,000 population in general and 3,000 population in the hilly and tribal areas.

Staffing pattern:
- Health Worker (Female)/ANM 1
- Health Worker (Male) 1
- Voluntary Worker 1

Now under Ayushman Bharat scheme the subcenters has been modified to health wellness center and one CHO has been posted with a lots of responsibilities which has been discussed separately.

Functions

- Maternal and child health, family welfare, nutrition, immunization, diarrhea control and control of communicable diseases programmes.
- The subcenters are provided with basic drugs for minor ailments needed for taking care of the essential health needs of men, women and children.

Primary Health Centers (PHC)

These are the basic structural and functional units of the public health services in the developing countries. A typical Primary Health Center covers a population of 20,000 in hilly, tribal, or difficult areas and 30,000 population in plain areas with 6 indoor/observation beds. It acts as a referral unit for 6 subcenters and refer the cases to the 30-bedded hospitals and higher-order public hospitals located at the subdistrict and district level.

Each PHC has five or six subcenters staffed by the health workers for outreach services, such as immunization, basic curative care services, and maternal and child health services and preventive services. PHCs were established to provide accessible, affordable and available primary health care to people in accordance with the Alma Ata Declaration of 1978 by the member nations of the World Health Organization. PHC is the first contact point between village community and the medical officer. The activities of PHC involve curative, preventive, primitive and family welfare services. There are 22,370 PHCs functioning in the country as in March 2007. The staffing pattern of PHC has been given in **Table 9.1**.

Functions of PHCs

To provide an integrated curative and preventive health care to the rural population with an emphasis on preventive and promotive aspects of health care.

Table 9.1: The manpower of PHC.

Staff	*Type A*		*Type B*	
	Essential	*Desirable (Extra)*	*Essential*	*Desirable (Extra)*
Medical officer (MBBS)	1		1	1
Medical officer (AYUSH)		1		1
Accountant-cum-Data entry operator	1		1	
Pharmacist	1		1	
Pharmacist (AYUSH)		1		1
Nurse (Midwife)	3	1	4	1
Health worker (female)	1		1	
Health worker (male)	1		1	
Health assistant (female)/ lady health visitor	1		1	
Health educator		1		1
Laboratory technician	1		1	
Cold chain and vaccine logistic assistant		1		1
Multi-skilled group D worker	2		2	
Sanitary worker-cum-Watchman	1		1	1
Total	13	18	14	21

Provision of medical care:
- **OPD services:** Primary Health Centers provide total 6 hours of OPD services, out of which 4 hours in the morning and 2 hours in the afternoon for six days in a week. Time schedule will vary from state to state. Minimum OPD attendance is expected to be 40 patients per doctor per day. In addition to six hours of duty at the PHC, it is desirable that MO PHC shall spend at least two hours per day twice in a week for field duties and monitoring.
- **24-hour emergency services:** Appropriate management of injuries and accident, first aid, stitching of wounds, incision and drainage of abscess, stabilization of the condition of the patient before referral, dog-bite/snake-bite/scorpion-bite cases, and other emergency conditions. These services will be provided primarily by the nursing staff. However, in case of need, the medical officer may be available to attend to the emergencies on call basis.

Maternal Child Health Including Family Planning

- **Antenatal care:** One of the common functions of PHC under MCH care is antenatal care. Antenatal care includes early registration of all pregnancies ideally in the first trimester (before 12th week of pregnancy). However, even if a woman comes late in her pregnancy for registration, she should be registered and care given to her according to the gestational age. Record the tobacco use by all antenatal mothers. Minimum four antenatal check-ups

and provision of complete package of services. Suggested schedule for antenatal visits:
- *1st visit:* Within 12 weeks—preferably as soon as pregnancy is suspected—for registration of pregnancy and first antenatal check-up
- *2nd visit:* Between 14 and 26 weeks
- *3rd visit:* Between 28 and 34 weeks
- *4th visit:* Between 36 weeks and term.

Associated services like providing iron and folic acid tablets, injection Tetanus Toxoid, etc. (as per the Guidelines for Antenatal Care and Skilled Attendance at birth by ANMs and LHVs). Ensure at least one ANC, preferably on the 3rd visit, must be seen by a doctor. Minimum laboratory investigations, like hemoglobin, urine albumin and sugar, RPR test for syphilis and Blood Grouping and Rh typing, nutrition and health counseling, brief advice on tobacco cessation if the antenatal mother is a smoker or tobacco user and also inform about the dangers of second-hand smoke, identification and management of high risk and alarming signs during pregnancy and labor, timely referral of such identified cases to FRUs/other hospitals, which are beyond the capacity of medical officer, PHC to manage. Tracking of missed and left-out ANC, chemoprophylaxis for malaria in high malaria-endemic areas for pregnant women as per National Vector Borne Disease Control Programme (NVBDCP) guidelines.

- **Intranatal care (24-hour delivery services, both normal and assisted):**
  - Promotion of institutional deliveries
  - Management of normal deliveries
  - Assisted vaginal deliveries including forceps/vacuum delivery whenever required
  - Manual removal of placenta
  - Appropriate and prompt referral for cases needing specialist care
  - Management of pregnancy-induced hypertension, including referral
  - Prereferral management (obstetric first-aid) in obstetric emergencies that need expert assistance (training of staff for emergency management to be ensured)
  - Minimum 48 hours of stay after delivery
  - Managing labor using partograph.
- *Proficient in identification and basic first-aid treatment for PPH, eclampsia, sepsis and prompt referral (as per the 'Antenatal Care and Skilled Birth Attendance at Birth' Guidelines).*
- **Postnatal care:**
  - Ensure postnatal care for 0 and 3rd day at the health facility both for the mother and the newborn and sending direction to the ANM of the concerned area for ensuring 7th- and 42nd-day postnatal home visits. Three additional visits for a low birthweight baby (less than 2500 gm) on 14th day, 21st day and on 28th day respectively.
  - Initiation of early breastfeeding within one hour of birth.
  - Counseling on nutrition, hygiene, contraception, essential newborn care (as per the Guidelines of the Government of India on essential newborn care) and immunization.
  - Others: Provision of facilities under Janani Suraksha Yojana (JSY).
  - Tracking of missed and left-out PNC.
- **Newborn care:**
  - Facilities for Essential Newborn Care (ENBC) and Resuscitation (Newborn Care Corner in Labor Room/ OT, details of which are given in Annexure 3A).
  - Early initiation of breastfeeding within one hour of birth.
  - Management of neonatal hypothermia (provision of warmth/kangaroo mother care (KMC), infection protection, cord care and identification of sick newborn and prompt referral. Six Indian Public Health Standards (IPHSs) Guidelines for Primary Health Centers.
- **Care of the child:**
  - Routine and emergency care of the sick children including Integrated Management of Neonatal and Childhood Illnesses (IMNCI) strategy and inpatient care. Prompt referral of sick children requiring specialist care.
  - Counseling on exclusive breastfeeding for 6 months and appropriate and adequate complementary feeding from 6 months of age while continuing breastfeeding (as per the National Guidelines on Infant and Young Child Feeding, 2006 by Ministry of WCD, Government of India).
  - Assess the growth and development of the infants and under-5 children and make timely referral.
  - Full immunization of all infants and children against vaccine-preventable diseases as per the guidelines of the Government of India.
  - Vitamin A prophylaxis to the children as per the national guidelines.
  - Prevention and control of routine childhood diseases, and infections like diarrhea, pneumonia, and anemia, etc.
  - Management of severe acute malnutrition cases and referral of serious cases after the initiation of treatment as per the facility-based guidelines.

Family Welfare

- Education, motivation and counseling to adopt appropriate family planning methods.
- Provision of contraceptives, such as condoms, oral pills, emergency contraceptives, IUCD insertions.
- Referral and follow-up services to the eligible couples adopting permanent methods (tubectomy/vasectomy).
- Counseling and appropriate referral for couples having infertility.
- Permanent methods like tubal ligation and vasectomy/ NSV, where trained personnel and facility exist. Medical termination of pregnancies, essential counseling and appropriate referral for safe abortion services (MTP) for

those in need. Desirable MTP using manual vacuum aspiration (MVA) technique will be provided in PHCs, where trained personnel and facility exist. Medical Method of Abortion with linkage for timely referral to the facility approved for second trimester of MTP. Management of reproductive tract infections/sexually transmitted infections is essential, which can be done through the following methods:
- Health education for the prevention of RTIs/STIs
- Treatment of RTIs/STIs.

Nutrition Services (Coordinated with ICDS)

- Diagnosis of and nutrition advice to, the malnourished children, pregnant women and others.
- Diagnosis and management of anemia and vitamin A deficiency.
- Coordination with ICDS.

School Health

The teachers screen students on a continuous basis and ANMs/HWMs (a team of two workers) visit the schools (one school every week) for screening, treatment of minor ailments and referral. A doctor from CHC/PHC will also visit one school per week based on the screening reports submitted by the teams. Overall services to be provided under school health shall include:

- **Essential health service provision:** Screening, health care and referral: Screening of general health, assessment of Anemia/Nutritional status, visual acuity, hearing problems, dental check-up, common skin conditions, Heart defects, physical disabilities, learning disorders, behavior problems, etc. Basic medicines to take care of common ailments, prevalent among young school going children. Referral cards for priority services at district/subdistrict hospitals.
- **Immunization:** As per national schedule Fixed day activity Coupled with education about the issue.
    - *Micronutrient (Vitamin A and IFA) management:* Weekly supervised distribution of Iron-Folate tablets coupled with education about the issue Administration of Vitamin-A in needy cases. Deworming Biannually supervised schedule Prior IEC Siblings of students also to be covered.

Capacity-building

Monitoring and Evaluation

Mid-day meal in coordination with department of school education, Ministry of Human Resource Development.

Health-promoting Schools

- Counseling services
- Regular practice of yoga, physical education, and health education
- Peer leaders as health educators
- Adolescent health education—existing in a few places
- Linkages with the out-of-school children
- Health clubs, health cabinets
- First aid room/corners or clinics.
- Adolescent health care to be provided preferably through adolescent-friendly clinic for two hours once a week on a fixed day. Services should be comprehensive, i.e., a judicious mix of promotive, preventive, curative and referral services.

Core package—Essential Adolescent and Reproductive Health

Information, counseling and services related to sexual concerns, pregnancy, contraception, abortion, menstrual problems, etc. Services for tetanus immunization of adolescents, nutritional counseling, prevention and management of nutritional anemia, STI/RTI management, referral services for VCTC and PPTCT services and services for safe termination of pregnancy, if not available at PHC.

Optional/Additional Services (Desirable)

As per the local need, outreach services in schools (essential) and community camps (desirable), periodic health check-ups and health education activities, awareness generation and co-curricular activities.

Promotion of Safe Drinking Water and Basic Sanitation

- In a community, disinfection of water sources, like wells and tube wells and coordination with public health engineering department for safe water supply is very much essential to protect the people from different types of water-borne diseases.
- Promotion of sanitation including use of toilets and appropriate garbage disposal can prevent water pollution. Periodical testing of water quality using H_2S strip test (bacteriological) is also essential.
- Prevention and control of locally endemic diseases, like malaria, kala azar, Japanese encephalitis, etc.
- Collection and reporting of vital events.
- Health education and behavior change communication (BCC).

Training

- Imparting training to undergraduate medical students and intern doctors in basic health care.
- Orientation training of male and female health workers in various National Health Programmes including RCH, Adolescent health services and immunization
- Skill-based training to ASHAs.
- Initial and periodic training of paramedics in the treatment of minor ailments.
- Periodic training of doctors and paramedics through continuing medical education, conferences, skill-development trainings.
- All health staff of PHC must be trained in IMEP.
- **Others:**
    - There should be provision of induction training for doctors, nursing and paramedical staff.

- Whenever new/higher responsibility is assigned or new equipment/technology is introduced, there must be a provision of training.
- There must be a mechanism for ensuring quality assurance in training by training feedback and training-effectiveness evaluation.
- Appropriate placement for the trained person should be ensured.
- Trainings in minor repairs and maintenance of the available equipment should be provided to the user.

Basic Laboratory and Diagnostic Services

Essential laboratory services include the following:

- Routine urine, stool and blood tests (Hb%, platelets count, total RBCs, WBCs, bleeding and clotting time)
- Diagnosis of RTIs/STDs with wet-mounting, Grams-stain, etc.
- Sputum testing for mycobacterium (as per the guidelines of RNTCP)
- Blood smear examination (malarial)
- Blood for grouping and Rh typing
- RDK for Pf malaria in endemic districts
- Rapid tests for pregnancy
- RPR test for Syphilis/YAWS surveillance (endemic districts)
- Rapid test kit for fecal contamination of water
- Estimation of chlorine level of water using orthotoluidine reagent
- Blood sugar
- Blood cholesterol and ECG.

Validation of Reports

Periodic validation of laboratory reports should be done with external agencies like District PHC/Medical College for quality assurance, periodic calibration of laboratory and PHC equipment.

Monitoring and Supervision

- Monitoring and supervision of activities of subcenter through regular meetings/periodic visits, by LHV, health assistant male and medical officer, etc.
- Monitoring of all the National Health Programs by a medical officer with the support of LHV, health assistant male and health-monitoring activities of ASHAs by LHV and ANM (in her subcenter area)
- Health educator will monitor all IEC and BCC activities
- Health assistants (male) and LHV should visit subcenter once a week
- Checking for tracking of missed out and left out ANC/PNC, vaccinations, etc. during monitoring visits and quality parameters (including using partograph, AMTSL, ENBC, etc.) during delivery and postdelivery
- Timely payment of JSY beneficiaries
- Timely payment of TA/DA to ASHAs.

MO should visit all subcenters at least once in a month. This will be possible only if more than one medical officers is posted in the PHC.

Functional Linkages with Subcenters

There shall be a monthly review meeting at PHC chaired by MO (or in-charge), and attended by all the health workers (male and female). CHO posted on Ayushman Bharat scheme and health assistants (male and female), on the spot supervisory visits to subcenters, organizing village health and nutrition day at Anganwadi centers.

ASHAs and Anganwadi workers should attend monthly review meetings. Medical officer should orient ASHAs on selected topics of health care.

Mainstreaming of AYUSH

Provision of one AYUSH doctor and one AYUSH pharmacist has been made at PHC to provide choices to the people, wherever an AYUSH public facility is not available in the near vicinity. The AYUSH doctor at PHC shall attend patients for system- specific AYUSH-based preventive, promotive and curative health care and take up public health education activities including awareness generation about the uses of medicinal plants and local health practices. The signboard of the PHC should mention AYUSH facilities. AYUSH doctor should support in implementation of national health programmes after requisite training, if required. Locally available medicinal herbs/plants should be grown around the PHC.

From service delivery angle, PHCs may be of two types, depending upon the delivery caseload:

- **Type A PHC:** PHC with delivery load of less than 20 deliveries in a month
- **Type B PHC:** PHC with delivery load of 20 or more deliveries in a month.
- Select PHCs, especially in large blocks where the CHC is over one hour of journey away, may be upgraded to provide 24-hour emergency hospital care for a number of conditions by increasing the number of medical officers, preferably such PHCs should have the same IPHS norms as for a CHC.
- The manpower that should be available in the PHC is given in **Table 9.1**: For Type B PHCs, additional staff in the form of one MBBS medical officer (desirable, if the caseload of delivery cases is more than 30 per month), one staff nurse and one sanitary worker.

Community Health Centers

Healthcare delivery in India has been envisaged at three levels, namely primary, secondary and tertiary. The secondary level of health care essentially includes community health centers (CHCs) constituting the first referral units (FRUs) and the subdistrict and district hospitals. The CHCs were designed to provide referral health care for cases from the primary health center-level and for the cases in need of specialist care approaching the center directly. Four PHCs are included under each CHC, thus catering to approximately 80,000 populations in tribal/hilly/desert areas and 1,20,000 population for the plain areas. CHC is a 30-bedded hospital providing specialist care

Table 9.2: Manpower of Community Health Centers (CHCs).

Personnel	*No. required*	*No. desirable*	*Qualification*
Block Public Health Unit			
Block medical officer/medical superintendent	1		Senior-most specialist/GDMO, preferably with experience in public health/trained in professional development
Public health specialist	1		MD (PSM)/MD (CHA)/MD Community Medicine or Postgraduation degree with MBA/DPH/MPH
Public health nurse	1	1	
Specialty Services			
General surgeon	1		MS/DNB (General Surgery)
Physician	1		MD/DNB (General Medicine)
Obstetrician and gynecologist	1		DGO/MD/DNB
Pediatrician	1		DCH/MD (Pediatrics)/DNB
Anesthetist	1		MD (Anesthesia)/DNB/DA/LSAS-trained MO
General Duty Officers			
Dental surgeon	1		BDS
General duty medical officer	2		MBBS
Medical officer (AYUSH)			Graduate in AYUSH
Nurses and Paramedical			
Staff nurse	10		
Pharmacist	1	1	
Pharmacist (AYUSH)	1		
Laboratory technician	2		
Radiographer	1		
Dietician	1		
Ophthalmic assistant	1		
Dental assistant	1		
Cold chain and vaccine logistic assistant	1		
OT technician	1		
Multi-rehabilitation/Community-based rehabilitation worker	1	1	
Counselor	1		
Administrative Staff			
Registration clerk	2		
Statistical assistant/Data entry operator	2		
Administrative assistant	1		
Group D Staff			
Dresser (certified by Red Cross/St John ambulance)	1		
Ward boys/Nurses	5		
Driver	1	3	
Total	**46**	**52**	

(*Source:* Indian Public Health Standards (IPHS) Guidelines for Community Health Centers)

in medicine, obstetrics and gynecology, surgery, pediatrics, dental and AYUSH. The detail staffing pattern has been provided in **Table 9.2**. There are 4535 CHCs functioning in the country as on March 2010 as per the Rural Health Statistics Bulletin 2010. These centers are, however, fulfilling the tasks entrusted to them only to a limited extent. The launch of the National Rural Health Mission (NRHM) gives us the opportunity to have a fresh look at their functioning.

Functions of CHC

OPD Services and IPD Services

- **General:**
  - Medicine, surgery, obstetrics and gynecology, pediatrics, dental and AYUSH services
  - Eye-specialist services (at one for every five CHCs)
  - Emergency services
  - Laboratory services
  - National Health Programmes.

  Every CHC has to provide the following services:
- **Essential:**
  - *Care of routine and emergency cases in surgery:* This includes dressings, incision and drainage, and surgery for hernia, hydrocele, appendicitis, hemorrhoids, fistula, and stitching of injuries, handling of emergencies, like intestinal obstruction, hemorrhage, etc. Other managements including nasal packing, tracheostomy, foreign body removal, etc. Fracture reduction and putting splints/plaster cast.
  - *Care of routine and emergency cases in medicine:* Specific mention is being made of handling of all emergencies like, dengue hemorrhagic fever, cerebral malaria and others, like dog- and snake-bite cases, poisonings, congestive heart failure, left ventricular failure, pneumonias, meningoencephalitis, acute respiratory conditions, status epilepticus, burns, shock, acute dehydration, etc. In the case of National Health Programs, appropriate guidelines are already available, which should be followed:
    - Conducting daily OPD
    - Maternal Health.
  - Minimum 4 ANC check-ups including registration and associated services

As some antenatal cases may directly register with CHC, the suggested schedule of antenatal visits is reproduced below.

- **1st visit:** Within 12 weeks—preferably as soon as the pregnancy is suspected—for registration of pregnancy and first antenatal check-up.
- **2nd visit:** Between 14 and 26 weeks
- **3rd visit:** Between 28 and 34 weeks
- **4th visit:** Between 36 weeks and term.

24-hour delivery services including normal and assisted deliveries. Managing labor using partograph. All referred cases of complications in pregnancy, labor and postnatal period must be adequately treated. Ensure postnatal care for 0 and 3rd day at the health facility, both for the mother and the newborn and sending directions to the ANM of the concerned area for ensuring 7th- and 42nd-day postnatal home visits. Minimum 48 hours of stay after delivery, 3–7 days stay after delivery for managing complications. Proficiency in identification and management of all complications including PPH, eclampsia, sepsis, etc., during PNC. Essential and emergency obstetric care including surgical interventions, like cesarean sections and other medical interventions. Provisions of Janani Suraksha Yojana (JSY) and Janani Shishu Suraksha Karyakram (JSSK).

- **Newborn care and child health:** Essential newborn care and resuscitation by providing newborn corner in the labor room and operation theater (where cesarean takes place). Details of newborn corner given, early initiation of breastfeeding within one hour of birth and promotion of exclusive breastfeeding for six months.

Newborn Stabilization Unit

Counseling on infant and young child-feeding (IYCF) as per the IYCF guidelines. Routine and emergency care of sick children including facility-based IMNCI strategy. Full immunization of infants and children against vaccine-preventable diseases and Vitamin A prophylaxis as per the guidelines of Government of India, tracking of vaccination dropouts and left-outs, prevention and management of routine childhood diseases, infections and anemia, etc., management of malnutrition cases, and provisions of Janani Shishu Suraksha Karyakram (JSSK) as per the guidelines.

- **Family Planning:** Full range of family planning services, including IEC, counseling, provision of contraceptives, non-scalpel vasectomy (NSV), laparoscopic sterilization services and their follow-up, safe abortion services as per the MTP Act and MTP facility approved for the 2nd trimester of pregnancy.
- **National Health Programs (NHPs):** All NHPs should be delivered through the CHCs. Integration with the existing programs is vital to provide comprehensive services. The requirements for the important NHPs are being annexed as separate guidelines and following are the assured services under each NHP:

Under Integrated Disease Surveillance Project

CHC will function as a peripheral surveillance unit and collate, analyze and report information to the district surveillance unit.

Oral Health

Dental care and dental health education services as well as root canal treatment and filling/extraction of routine and emergency cases. Oral health education in collaboration with other activities, e.g., nutritional education, school health and adolescent health.

Other Services

School Health

Teachers screen students on a continuous basis and ANMs/HWMs (a team of two workers) visit the schools (one school every week) for screening, treatment of minor ailments and referral.

A doctor from CHC/PHC will also visit one school per week based on the screening reports submitted by the teams. Overall services to be provided under school health shall include the following health service provisions:

Screening, Health Care and Referral

Screening of general health, assessment of anemia/ nutritional status, visual acuity, hearing problems, dental check-up, common skin conditions, heart defects, physical disabilities, learning disorders, behavior problems, etc. Basic medicines to take care of common ailments prevalent among the school-going children. Referral cards for priority services at the district/subdistrict hospitals.

Immunization

As per the national schedule fixed-day activity, coupled with education about the issue.

Micronutrients (Vitamin A and IFA) Management

Weekly supervised distribution of Iron-folate tablets coupled with education about the issue and administration of vitamin A in needy cases.

Deworming

Biannually supervised schedule for deworming should be done. Prior to deworming through IEC, students should be well informed regarding it. Siblings of students should also be covered.

Health-promoting Schools

- Counseling services
- Regular practice of yoga, physical, education, health education
- Peer leaders as health educators
- Adolescent health education—existing in a few places
- Linkages with the out-of-school children
- Health clubs, health cabinets
- First aid rooms/corners or clinics.

Adolescent Health Care

To be provided preferably through adolescent friendly clinic for 2 hours once a week on a fixed day. Services should be comprehensive, i.e., a judicious mix of promotive, preventive, curative and referral services.

- **Adolescent and reproductive health:** Information, counseling and services related to sexual concerns, pregnancy, contraception, abortion, menstrual problems, etc.
- Services for tetanus immunization of adolescents
- Nutritional counseling, prevention and management of nutritional anemia
- STI/RTI management
- Referral services for VCTC and PPTCT services and services for safe termination of pregnancy, if not available at PHC.

Outreach Services in Schools (Essential) and Community Camps

Periodic health check-ups and health education activities, awareness generation and cocurricular activities.

Diagnostic Services

In addition to the lab facilities and X-ray, ECG should be made available in the CHC with appropriate training to a nursing staff/laboratory technician. All the necessary reagents, glassware and facilities for collecting and transport of samples should be made available.

In order to provide round-the-clock clinical services, there is a likelihood of the shortage of doctors in 8-hourly shift duties. This shortage can be compensated by resource pooling (Block Pooling Concept) of the available doctors posted at primary health centers covered under the CHC. Under the present scenario of the shortage of clinical manpower, *see* **Table 9.2,** it is suggested that the doctors of PHCs, in addition to attending to routine OPD duties at PHCs, may also do shift duties to provide emergency services. The following requirements are being projected based on the assumption that there will be average bed occupancy of 60%. The strength may be further increased if the occupancy increases with subsequent upgradation.

ROLE AND FUNCTION OF A HEALTH WORKER FEMALE

Maternal and Child Health

- Register and provide care to pregnant women throughout the period of pregnancy. Ensure that every pregnant woman makes at least 4 (four) visits for antenatal check-up including the associated services, such as IFA tablets, TT immunization, etc.
- Carry out all the investigations, like albumin, sugar, and hemoglobin levels.
- Refer all pregnant women to PHC/CHC for RPR test for syphilis and blood grouping.
- Refer the cases of abnormal pregnancy and cases with medical and gynecological problems to health assistant female or the primary health center.
- Conduct deliveries in subcenters, if facilities of a labor room are available and in her area when called for.
- Supervize deliveries conducted by dais and assist them whenever called for.
- Refer cases of difficult labor and newborns with abnormalities, help them to get institutional care and provide follow-up to the patients referred to or discharged from the hospital.
- ANM will identify the ultimate beneficiaries, complete necessary formalities and obtain necessary approvals of the competent authority before disbursement to the beneficiaries under Janani Suraksha Yojana (JSY) and, by 7th of each month, will submit accounts of the previous month in the prescribed format to be designed by the State. ANM will prepare a monthly work schedule in the meeting of all the accredited workers to be held on third Friday of every month, which is mandatory. The guideline under JSY is to be followed. In addition, ANM will hold weekly/fortnightly meetings with all the ASHAs of her area to guide and monitor them.

- Tracking of all pregnancies by name for scheduled ANC/PNC services.
- Make postnatal home visits on 0, 3rd, 7th and 42nd days for deliveries at home and subcenter and on 3rd, 7th, and 42nd days for institutional delivery. Postnatal visits are to be made for each delivery happened in her area and she should render advice regarding care of the mother, and care and feeding of the newborn.
- In case of low birthweight baby, a total of six postnatal visits are to be made on 0, 3rd, 7th, 14th, 21st and 28th days to screen for congenital abnormalities, assess the neonate for danger signs of sickness, etc. as per the IMNCI guidelines and appropriate referral.
- Initiation of early breastfeeding within one hour of birth, exclusive breastfeeding for six months and timely weaning at six months as per the Infant and Young Child Feeding Guidelines.
- Assess the growth and development of the infants and under-5 children, provide treatment for minor cases and make timely referral.
- Educate mothers individually and in groups in better family health including maternal and child health, family planning, nutrition, immunization, control of communicable diseases, and personal and environmental hygiene.
- Assist medical officer and health assistant (female) in conducting antenatal and postnatal clinics at the subcenter.

Family Planning

- Utilize the information from the eligible couple and child register for the family planning programme. She will be squarely responsible for maintaining eligible couple registers and updating those at all times.
- Spread the message of family planning to the couples and motivate them for family planning individually and in groups.
- Distribute conventional contraceptives and oral contraceptives to the couples, provide facilities and help the prospective acceptors in getting family planning services, if necessary, by accompanying them or arranging for the Dai/ASHA to accompany them to the hospital.
- Provide follow-up services to female family planning acceptors, identify side effects, give treatment on the spot for side effects and minor complaints and refer those cases that need attention by the physician to the PHC/hospital.
- IUCD insertion can be done by a trained ANM.
- Establish female depot holders, help the health assistant (female) in training them, and provide a continuous supply of conventional contraceptives to the depot holders.
- Build rapport with acceptors, village leaders, ASHA, Dais and others and utilize them for promoting family welfare programmes.
- Identify women leaders and train them with the help of the health assistant (female).
- Participate in Mahila Mandal meetings and utilize such gatherings for educating women in family welfare programmes.

Medical Termination of Pregnancy

- Identify the women requiring help for medical termination of pregnancy and refer them to the nearest approved institution.
- Educate the community of the consequences of unsafe abortion methods and septic abortion. Inform them about the availability of services for medical termination of pregnancy.

Nutrition

- Identify the cases of low birthweight, malnutrition among infants and young children (zero to five years), give the necessary treatment and advice and refer serious cases to the primary health center.
- Distribute iron and folic acid tablets as prescribed to the pregnant women, nursing mothers, adolescent girls and syrups to young children (up to five years) as per the national guidelines.
- Administer Vitamin A solution to children as per the guidelines.
- Educate the community about nutritious diet for mothers and children.
- Coordinate with Anganwadi workers.

Universal Immunization Programme (UIP)

- Immunize pregnant women with tetanus toxoid.
- Administer DPT vaccine, oral poliomyelitis vaccine, measles vaccine and BCG vaccine to all infants and children (hepatitis B in pilot areas) as per the immunization schedule.
- Ensure injection safety, safe disposal and record, report and manage minor and serious adverse event following immunization (AEFI). Submit monthly UIP reports, weekly surveillance reports (AFP, measles under IDSP). Serious AEFI and outbreak should be reported immediately.
- ANM is responsible for cold chain maintenance for vaccines during fixed and outreach sessions.
- Manage waste generated during immunization as per the Government of India/Central Pollution Control Board (CPCB) guidelines.
- Preparing work plan, estimating beneficiaries and logistics, preparing due list of expected beneficiaries in coordination with Anganwadi worker and ASHA/mobilizer on the session day and ensuring their vaccination through adequate mobilization.
- Maintain tracking bag/tickler box at each sub-center, file updated counterfoils and utilize them for follow-up.
- Tracking of dropouts and left-outs, records/reports (including MCH register and immunization card counterfoils), surveillance/reporting vaccine-associated paralytic poliomyelitis (VAPP) and AEFI incidents in the catchment area.

- Indent order of vaccines and logistics should be weekly based on the due beneficiary list. HW/alternate vaccinator should receive the required quantity of vaccine and logistics on the day of immunization and supply to the session site.
- Work plan indicating village, place, date and time of organizing proposed session, including the names of ASHA and AWW must be displayed at each subcenter.
- Posters/paintings on key messages, immunization schedule, positioning during vaccine administration, safe injection practices, VVM, AEFI awareness, use of hub-cutters.
- Village-wise dropout list for display at subcenter.
- Norm for due beneficiaries—three per session.

Communicable Diseases

- Notify the MO, PHC immediately about any abnormal increase in cases of diarrhea/dysentery, fever with rigors, fever with rash, flaccid paralysis of acute onset in a child <15 years (AFP), tetanus, fever with jaundice or fever with unconsciousness, minor and serious AEFIs which she comes across during her home visits, take the necessary measures to prevent their spread, and inform the health assistant (male)/LHV to enable him/her to take further action.
- Assist in carrying out control measures like anticholera inoculation, chlorination, distribution of ORS, DDT spraying, mass survey, etc.

Vital Events

Record and report to the health authorities the vital events including births and deaths, particularly of mothers and infants in her area.

Recordkeeping

- Maintenance of all the relevant records concerning mothers, children and eligible couples in her area.
- Register pregnant women, infants zero to one year of age, women aged 15–44 years under- and above-five children and adolescents.
- Maintain the records as regards the contraceptive distribution, IUD insertion, couples sterilized, clinics held at the subcenter and supplies received and issued.
- Prepare and submit the prescribed weekly/monthly reports to the Health Assistant (female).
- Maintaining passive surveillance register for the malaria cases.

Treatment of Minor Ailments

- Provide treatment for minor ailments, first-aid for accidents and emergencies and refer cases beyond her competence to the primary health center/community health center or the nearest hospital.
- Provide treatment as per AYUSH as needed at the local level.

Team Activities

- Attend and participate in the staff meetings at primary health center/community development block or both.
- Coordinate her activities with the health worker (male) and other health workers including the health volunteers/ASHA and dais.
- Coordinate with PRI and village health sanitation and nutrition committee.
- Draft annual Village Health Plan with the help of a health worker (male), panchayati raj institution (PRI) and village health and sanitation committees (VHSC) for submitting the same to the block.
- Meet the health assistant (female) each week and seek her advice and guidance whenever necessary. Maintain the cleanliness of the subcenter.
- Dispose medical waste as per the Infection Management and Environment Plan (IMEP) guidelines of the Government of |India.
- Organize, participate and guide in organizing the Village Health Nutrition (VHN) Days at the Anganwadi centers.
- Participate as a member of the team in camps and campaigns.

House-to-House Surveys

These surveys would be done once in April annually. Some of the diseases would require special surveys, but, at all times, not more than one survey per month would be expected. Surveys would be done with the support and participation of HW (male), ASHAs, Anganwadi workers, community volunteers, panchayat members and Village Health Sanitation and Nutrition Committee (VHSNC).

Role of HWF as a Facilitator of ASHA

Auxiliary nurse midwife (ANM) will guide ASHA in performing the following activities:

- She will hold weekly/fortnightly meeting with ASHA and discuss the activities undertaken during the week/fortnight. She will guide her in case ASHA had encountered any problem during the performance of her activities.
- ANM will act as a resource person for the training of ASHA.
- ANM will inform ASHA regarding date and time of the outreach session and will also guide her for bringing the beneficiary to the outreach session.
- ANM will participate and guide in organizing the Health Days at the Anganwadi centers.
- She will take the help of ASHA in updating eligible couple register of the village concerned.
- She will utilize ASHA in motivating the pregnant women for coming to subcenter for initial check-ups.
- ASHA will also help ANMs in bringing married couples to subcenters for adopting family planning methods.
- ANM will guide ASHA in motivating pregnant women for taking full course of IFA tablets and TT injections, etc.
- ANMs will orient ASHA on the dose schedule and side effects of oral pills.

- ANMs will educate ASHA on danger signs of pregnancy and labor so that she can timely identify and help beneficiary in getting further treatment.
- ANMs will inform ASHA on date, time and place for initial and periodic training schedule. She will also ensure that during the training, ASHA gets the compensation for performance and also TA/DA for attending the training.
- Train in salt testing using salt-testing kits.

The second ANM will follow similar job responsibilities as the above. It is to be ensured that one ANM out of the two is available at the subcenter. Another ANM will perform the field duties. The time schedule for their turn visits be prepared with the approval of the Panchayats involved.

ROLE AND FUNCTION OF A MALE HEALTH WORKER

The male health worker will make a visit to each family once a fortnight. He will record his visit on the main entrance to the house according to the instructions of the State/UT. His duties mainly pertain to different National Health Programmes, maintenance of records, school health, village sanitation, education and cancelling.

He will carry out all the activities related to various programmes in an integrated manner when visiting the village/households.

The roles of some major health programmes are described as follows:

National Vector Borne Disease Control Programme (NVBDCP)

- It may identify fever cases
- Make thick and thin smears of blood
- May give presumptive treatment
- Dispatch blood smears to the laboratory twice a week by post or personally
- Record results of examination of blood smears
- Should collect contact smears and mass survey smears when positive case is detected
- Arrange in focal spraying
- Assist or arrange for radical treatment of diagnosed Malaria cases
- Collect follow-up smears
- Educate community on the importance of blood smear examination of fever cases
- Insecticidal spraying and treatment of malaria cases.

National Leprosy Eradication Programme (NLEP)

- Impart health education on leprosy and its treatment to the community
- Refer suspected new cases of leprosy and those with complications to PHC
- Provide subsequent doses of MDT to patients to ensure regularity and completion of treatment and assist health supervisor in retrieval of absentee/defaulter
- Update the case cards at subcenters and treatment register at sector PHC
- Assist leprosy-disabled people in self-care practices, monitor them and refer them to PHC whenever required.

Revised National Tuberculosis Control Programme (RNTCP)

- Identify persons especially with fever for 15 days and above with prolonged cough or spitting blood and take sputum smears from these individuals. Refer these cases to the medical officer (MO), Public Health Center (PHC) for further investigations
- Check whether all the cases under treatment for tuberculosis are taking regular treatment, motivate defaulters to take regular treatment and bring them to the notice of the medical officer, PHC
- Educate the community on various health education aspects of tuberculosis program
- Assist the ASHA/similar village health volunteer to motivate the TB patients in taking regular treatment.

Universal Immunization Programme (UIP)

- Assistance to Human Welfare Foundation (HWF) for administering all UIP vaccines, like oral polio vaccine (OPV), Bacillus Calmette-Guérin (BCG), diphtheria, pertussis, and tetanus (DPT) vaccine, tetanus toxoid (TT) vaccine, measles, hepatitis B, Japanese Encephalitis (JE) vaccine, etc., to all the beneficiaries, including pregnant women and provision of Vitamin A prophylaxis as per the immunization schedule.
- Assistance to HWF for conducting VHN Day in coordination with other partners
- Assist the health assistant (male)/health assistant (female)/LHV in the school health program.
- Educate the people in the community about the importance of immunization against the various communicable diseases.
- To maintain record of fever cases diagnosed by blood slides/rapid diagnostic tests (RDTs) in M1 and prepare a subcenter report (M4) for all cases in the area, including those of ASHAs and FTDs and submit it to PHC
- To keep a record of supervisory visits in tour diary and submit to MO-PHC during monthly meetings for verification
- To keep records and reports as per the guidelines of NVBDCP
- Minutes of VHSNC decisions.

Village Health Sanitation and Nutrition Committee

MPW is expected to be a member of Village Health Sanitation and Nutrition Committee (VHSNC). He must take part in the meetings actively and lead the discussions. He must convey the importance of source-reduction activities.

Reproductive and Child Health Programme (RCHP)

- Spread the message of family planning to the couples and motivate them for family planning individually and in groups

- Distribute conventional contraceptives and oral contraceptives to the couples
- Help prospective acceptors of sterilization in obtaining the services, if necessary, by accompanying them or arranging for the ASHA/dai to accompany them to the PHC/hospital
- Provide follow-up services to male family planning acceptors, and refer those cases that need attention by the physician to PHC/hospital
- Build rapport with satisfied acceptors, village leaders, ASHA, dais and others and utilize them for promoting Family Welfare Programme
- Assist the health assistant (male) in training the leaders in the community and in educating and involving the community in Family Welfare Programme.

Communicable Diseases

- HIV/STI counseling, HIV/STI screening after receiving training
- Identify cases of diarrhea/dysentery, fever with rash, jaundice, encephalitis, diphtheria, whooping cough and tetanus, poliomyelitis, neonatal tetanus, acute eye infections and notify the health assistant (male) and MO PHC immediately about these cases
- Carry out control measures until the arrival of the health assistant (male) and assist him in carrying out these measures
- Educate the community about the importance of control and preventive measures against the communicable diseases and about the importance of taking regular and complete treatment.

Noncommunicable Diseases

- IEC activities for prevention and early detection of hearing impairment/deafness in health facility, community and schools, harmful effects of tobacco, mental illnesses, iodine deficiency disorders (IDD), diabetes, cardiovascular disease (CVD) and strokes
- House-to-house surveys to detect list and refer cases of hearing and visual impairment and maintain records
- Early detection of hearing impairment and cases of deafness and level-appropriate referrals
- Sensitization of ASHA/AWW/PRI about prevention and treatment of deafness
- Mobilizing community members for screening camps and assisting in conduction of screening camps if needed
- Motivation for quitting and referrals to Tobacco Cassation Center at District Hospital.
- Sensitization of ASHA/AWW/PRI about the noncommunicable diseases
- Identification and referral of common mental illnesses and epilepsy cases for treatment and follow them up in community
- Greater participation/role of community for primary prevention of noncommunicable diseases (NCDs) and promotion of healthy lifestyle
- Ensuring regular testing of salt at household level for the presence of iodine through Salt Testing Kits by ASHAs.

Environment Sanitation

- Chlorinate the public water sources, including wells at regular intervals
- **Educate the community on:**
  - The method of disposal of liquid wastes
  - The method of disposal of solid waste
  - Home sanitation
  - Advantage and use of sanitary type of latrines
  - Construction and use of smokeless chulhas
  - Coordination with village Health Sanitation and Nutrition Committee.
- **Primary medical care:** Provide treatment for minor ailments, first-aid for accidents and emergencies and refer cases beyond his competence to the nearest hospital or PHC/CHC.
- **Health education:** Educate the community and family about different aspects of health, nutrition, maternal and child health care, family planning and other services, which can be availed by the community people.
- **Nutrition:**
  - Identify cases of low birthweight and malnutrition among infants and young children (0–5 years) in his area, give the necessary treatment and advice or refer them to the anganwadi for supplementary feeding and refer serious cases to the PHC.
  - Educate the community about the nutritious diet for mothers and children utilizing locally available food.
- **Vital events:**
  - Enquire about births and deaths occurring in his area, record them in the births and deaths register, share the information with ANM and report them to the health assistant (male)/health assistant (female).
  - Educate the community on the importance of registration of births and deaths.
- **Recordkeeping and other miscellaneous functions:**
  - Survey all the facilities in his area and prepare/maintain maps and charts for the village
  - Prepare, maintain and utilize family and village records.
  - Assist the ANM to prepare and maintain the eligible couple as well as maternal and child health register.
  - Maintain a record of cases in his area who are under treatment for tuberculosis and leprosy.
  - Prepare and submit the prescribed monthly reports in time to the health assistant (male).
  - While maintaining passive surveillance register for malaria cases, he will record:
    - Number of fever cases
    - Number of blood slides prepared
    - Number of malaria-positive cases reported
    - Number of cases given radical treatment.
  - Prepare an annual Village Health Plan in association with ANM, PRI and VHSC members and submit the same to the block.

JOB RESPONSIBILITIES OF A HEALTH SUPERVISOR

Health Supervisor Male

There will be one health supervisor (male) for four health workers (male) to supervise the work of male health workers and provide adequate guidance to them making periodical visits as per the calendar of activities in his jurisdiction.

- He will check and supervise 10% of the work pertaining to detection of unregistered births, deaths, and take necessary action to improve the birth and death registrations in his jurisdiction. He will also review the work of each male worker in this regard.
- To arrange small group meetings and health education campaigns involving community and its leaders for spreading the message on health, nutrition and family planning practices to the eligible couples, especially males and carrying out health education measures in the area.
- To conduct the immunization as per schedule of all the male children of school-going age (i.e., 5 to 16) and female children of age 5 to 10 with the help of male health worker and maintain up-to-date registers thereafter.
- Check and supervise the immunization of preschool children conducted by the health worker (male).
- Check and supervise the work carried out by health workers under modified plan of operation of National Malaria Eradication Programme.
- Check and supervise the radical treatment given to all the malaria-positive cases in his jurisdiction.
- Organize and conduct in his area the insecticidal spraying operations for malaria, filarial, Japanese encephalitis, as per the instructions of the entomologists of the health unit district.
- Keep a close and vigilant watch to find out outbreaks of communicable diseases, such as acute diarrheal diseases, cholera, malaria, and fever with rash, Japanese encephalitis and food poisoning, etc. and report the occurrence of such diseases to the medical officer, PHC and DDHS and institute appropriate and adequate remedial and containment measures under the guidance and supervision of the medical officers of PHC.
- Attend the cases of minor ailments, fever with rash, etc., referred to by the health worker (male) and refer these cases further to the medical officer, PHC as per the guidelines issued from time to time.
- Supervise the work of the health worker pertaining to chlorination and disinfection of wells, improvement of environmental sanitation, construction of soakage pits, manure pits, sanitary latrines, and measures to avoid stagnation of water and breeding of mosquitoes, disinfection practices, etc.
- He will coordinate the activities with health supervisor (female) in all the campaigns and team activities and carry out surveillance activities in the area in the absence of male workers.
- Check the registers and records maintained by the health workers (male) periodically by actual physical verification and by field visits to assess the progress of work and correct the defects noticed in the field work and correct the defects noticed in the field work and maintenance of records.
- Assist the medical officer, PHC in the delivery of comprehensive health services, which includes family welfare and nutritional services to the community and school health services.
- Survey all the facilities in his area and collect general information about each village/locality and family in his area and maintain records and registers and send review reports and periodicals, and consolidated progress report prescribed to the medical officer, PHC.
- Maintain adequate supplies of materials, drugs, disinfectants and equipment, conventional contraceptives, etc., and supply to health worker (male) and check the stocks and stock registers.
- Attend staff meeting at the PHC for appraisal of progress of work.
- Educate the community on the importance and usefulness of registration of births and deaths and the method of registration.
- Provide treatment for minor ailments, provide first-aid for accidents and emergencies, and refer cases beyond his competence to the primary health center or the nearest hospital.
- Attend and participate in the staff meetings at a primary health center/community development block or both, coordinate his activities with the health workers (male) and female including the dais in regard to campaign activities. Meet with the health supervisor (female) and seek her advice and guidance whenever necessary.
- **Other duties:** He will maintain an inventory of all the equipment and instruments, furniture and other articles required for maternity and child welfare work in each subcenter and check the inventory at a specified period.

JOB RESPONSIBILITIES OF A MULTIPURPOSE HEALTH SUPERVISOR (FEMALE)

- There will be one health supervisor (female) for every four health workers. She will be responsible for the development of maternal and child health services in the area.
- She will conduct antenatal clinics, and well-baby clinics and toddlers' clinics at the PHC and at the maternity subcenters.
- She will arrange to give group talks to expectant mothers. During these talks, she will stress on personal hygiene and nutrition and environmental sanitation and mothercraft and child care practices.
- She will carry out home visits. During these visits, in addition to giving advice about maternity and child health, she will demonstrate simple procedure to relieve conditions, such as lousiness, scabies, sore eyes, etc., with the help and assistance of a health worker (female).
- She will visit once a week on fixed days each of the health subcenters. During these visits, she will conduct antenatal

and well-baby clinics. She will independently check some of the houses and find out omissions in antenatal care and postnatal care and under Maternal and Child Health Integrated Program.

- She will advise on family welfare practices.
- She will observe the work of multipurpose health worker (female) and dai during the clinic and home situation and help her improve her technical skills and human relationship.
- She will observe and supervise the work of multipurpose health worker (female) and dai. For this purpose, it will be necessary further to observe them and conduct one or two deliveries at homes.
- She will respond to the urgent calls from the health workers (female) or Dais.
- She will ensure that antenatal and postnatal and infant health cards are maintained for mothers and infant and toddler's cards for the children.
- She will scrutinize and approve the order for supplies and equipment by the multipurpose health worker (female).
- In abnormal cases, she will arrange for the transport to take expectant mothers to the hospitals.
- She will help in the training of indigenous dais.
- She will see that adequate equipment is provided and maintained for maternity and child care.
- She will check the health cards maintained by health worker (female).
- She will help the medical officer in the development of school health program and assist the medical officer in the medical examination of the girl students.
- She will conduct staff conferences with the multipurpose health workers (female) and child health.
- She will give an evaluation report of the work done in the field of maternal and child health.
- Each health supervisor should arrange to immunize 10% for the annual target of eligible children every month so as to achieve the annual target within the year. She will utilize the services of health workers (female).
- She should visit all the villages to impress the village community on the importance of DPT and polio and measles immunization among children.
- Apart from the immunization for children, the health supervisor must also give tetanus toxoid immunization for antenatal mothers and distribute vitamin A solution to children, and DTTA and TT to female school children from 10 to 16 years of age.
- She will coordinate with the male health worker and supervisor of the area concerned for campaign activities.
- She has to see that infant health cards and children cards are maintained. She will send her diary and returns relating to the immunization program and all activities to the medical officer, PHC.
- She will be responsible for the maintenance of records, and preparation and submission of reports and returns.
- She will sign in the wall chart on the day of her visit after enquiry and verification.
- She will discharge any other duties assigned by her supervisors delegated by the Director of Public Health and Preventive Medicine in regard to public health from time to time.

JOB RESPONSIBILITIES OF A STAFF NURSE AT PUBLIC HEALTH CENTER

Staff nurse will work in PHC only. The nature of job responsibilities is advised and based on the functional areas of the primary health center.

Outpatient Department

- Maintenance of cleanliness in and around PHC
- Organizing the registration counter and the medical officer consultation room
- Ensuring the distribution of OP tickets
- Arranging the medical officer's consultation with thermometer, tongue depressor, torch, kidney tray, lotion, BP apparatus, etc.
- Maintenance of substock
- She should supervise the work of cook-cum-waterman and sweeper in the arrangement and conduct of OPD.

Injection Room

- Responsible for sterilization of syringes/needles
- Responsible for administration of injections prescribed by medical officer
- Injections should be administered only by the staff nurse
- Medical officer may make alternate arrangements only in her absence
- Maintenance of stock of inventory of the injection room, including furniture, equipment and drugs
- Responsible for supervision of waterman and sweeper in maintenance of injection room.

Dressing Room

- Responsible for overall maintenance of dressing room
- Supervising the MNA/hospital workers in the work of cleanliness and maintenance of quality care in dressing room
- Maintenance of substock of inventory at the dressing room, including furniture, equipment and dressing materials.

Inpatient Ward

- Admission of patients/history taking/arrangements of laboratory
- Investigation/diet/temperature recording/administration of drugs
- Maintenance of cleanliness in the ward, including beds/lines
- Maintenance of substock of inventory at the inpatient wards, including furniture, equipment, drugs, linen, and diet.

Labor Ward

- Maintenance of cleanliness in the labor room
- Conduct of deliveries during her duty hours

- Maintenance of substock of inventory at labor room, including furniture/equipment/drugs
- Reporting births and deaths to health inspectors.

Minor Operation Theater

- Assisting medical officers in minor surgery
- Sterilization of dressing materials
- Maintenance of substock of inventory, including instruments, furniture, equipment, and linen
- Maintenance of substock of intrauterine devices (IUDs)—trained lady health visitors, health workers or medical officers will indent IUD from her for insertion in the operation theater at PHC.

Emergency Services

- Maintenance of emergency drug tray
- Duty of attending calls during night hours.

Administrative Issues

- The staff nurse is eligible to avail weekly off and casual leave as applicable to them.
- **Provision of residential quarters:** Project officer suggests that any vacant quarters of the primary health center may be allotted to staff nurse since most of them express their willingness to stay at the primary health center quarters.

Time Framing

- The sweeper and cook-cum-waterman should attend one hour before the operation starts, i.e., 6:30 AM to 7:30 AM. The sweeper should sweep and clean, swab the floor and keep the PHC ready for functioning.
- The cook-cum-waterman is responsible for filling up the water for sterilization equipment and he should be ready for issuing the operation tickets.
- The staff nurse should attend PHC work 6 hours before the operation starts.
- She should make rounds of the PHC and supervise the work done by the sweeper and cook-cum-waterman.
- Arranges operation injection room, etc., as per the specific functions mentioned above.
- She will attend the operation till 11 AM and thereafter inpatient care up to 1 PM.
- 1 PM to 3 PM: Rest hours (attend in emergency cases)
- 3 PM to 5 PM: Attend evening operation and inpatient care.

Night Duty

The cook-cum-waterman/sweeper/night watchman will be available at the PHC and call duty by the ANM (G), staff nurse, medical officer or whoever available during maternal and other emergencies. The primary health center should remain open for 24 hours.

Registers and Records to be Maintained by the Staff Nurse

- Indent registers for furniture, equipment, drugs, dressings, etc.
- Substock for expendable items, like injections, tablets, dressing materials and IUD
- Substock register for furniture equipment, drugs, linen, diet
- Inpatient/normal register
- Births and deaths register.

DISTRICT PUBLIC HEALTH NURSE

The District Public Health Nurse (DPHN) is responsible for planning, organizing and directing the public health program of jurisdiction where she is appointed.

- Participates in policy-making activities in regard to health care. She needs to learn and understand the organization and administration and state's public health programs are affected by quantity and quality of public health nursing service available in the rural areas.
- Evaluation of nursing services is done by district public nurse, who plans for continuously improving the quality of client care. The district public health nurse is attached to the district health office. She is directly responsible to the district health officer and delegates the responsibilities to all nursing personnel in the district community health field. She is supervised by a nursing officer at the directorate level.

District public health nurse works in close coordination with community health nursing, nursing tutors and hospital administration and other health workers.

Responsibilities as an Administrator

- Responsible for efficient implementation of policies and programs relating to nursing in public health
- Make recommendations to district health officer on requirements of nursing staff in public health field
- Staff development programs for educational promotional awareness
- Any indiscipline occurring in the community or nursing personnel
- Determine the need for supply and equipment for her section, and take part in budgetary planning
- Submit monthly report to District Health Officer at directorate level
- Field visits at least four times a day to each staff member in subcenters and primary health centers and to ensure the quality care, submit annual complete standard report for all primary health centers and subcenters, visits paid and recommendations for improvement of public health services.

Supervisory Responsibilities

- Conduct regular meetings and solving official as well as personal problems in the best possible way
- Encourage initiative and help in promoting professional growth of staff
- Interpretations of policies, plans and rules to the staff so as to regulate and develop the services

- Advice on organizing and planning of work, helping the individual staff members to evaluate the needs of their particular areas and to select priority for her work
- Help in improving the quality and quantity of health services by establishing good patterns of procedures and techniques
- Guidance to staff regarding use of records, report and the collection of statistical data and record-keeping system
- Ensure that public health nursing personnel have job descriptions, standing orders and understand their interpretations in the areas they went to.

Educational Responsibilities

- Organize the inservice education program for all the nursing staff
- Initiate and assist in planning and organizing the orientation program for the new staff
- Participate in community health field experience organized for nursing students of schools or colleges
  - Suggest in selection of areas for practical experience
  - Provide facilities and resources to students and staff
- Guide students during field experience.
- Help to supervise and guide the traditional birth attendants (TBAs)
- Keep her knowledge updated by reading, attending professional seminars and meetings, etc.

ROLES AND RESPONSIBILITIES OF A COMMUNITY HEALTH NURSE

Community health nurse represents most of the professional workers in the public health field, and nursing services are employed to implement or support the services offered to the community virtually.

Roles

- Community health nurse participates in planning, development and evaluation of the agency program as a whole, and advisement of technical knowledge of nursing has a big contribution to make in relation to determining the care and content of public health program.
- Application of nursing practice in public health field involves the use not only of technical and administrative skills with which the people are familiar but also the nursing skills which are interpersonal and organizational in character. The nurse not only provides homely, comforting services, treatment provided for the care of the sick or groups toward better health care, but she also uses epidemiologic as well as physiologic bases in her observation of the health status of the family or community.
- She uses administrative as well as clinical skills in organizing clinics, and recruiting and training volunteers.
- She considers the family as a service unit rather than an individual; hence, care is an important component of her functions.
- She plans her work and evaluates its effectiveness in terms of community as a whole.
- She provides nursing care to nonhospitalized sick, direct care or teaches the family member to give care to the sick.
- **Medical supportive activities:** Assisting with medical procedures, identifying, and reporting significant conditions or symptoms, providing inspectional services, e.g., examination of school students, during high incidence of communicable disease, routine observation of industrial workers exposed to specific occupational hazards and interpreting home or community factors. She prefers diagnostic testing procedures that can be done safely without medical supervision, e.g., collect specimens and blood slides.
- **Health counseling and teaching:** Family health counseling and teaching in all aspects of family care. Health counseling is the action taken to assist an individual to make and carry out his own plans to meet the health problems. Teaching may be a part of counseling and involves provision of information in such a way that family or individual learns how to apply this information in his own case and gains a serried health care.
- Control of environmental health hazard is an integral part of public health nursing observation and teaching helps to control the accidents, hazards at home, schools and industries prevent unnecessary exposure to injury or infection.

Responsibilities

General

- Responsible for organizing and conducting the health clinics, e.g., well baby clinic, antenatal clinic, family-welfare and general clinics, etc.
- Supervising, organizing and planning home visits for subordinate nurses and giving suggestions for improvement
- Organizing and encouraging the educational activities for improving quality care
- Will interpret the need of the nursing and health service to medical officer.

Administrative

- Responsibilities for the efficient implementation of the program.
- Outline the nursing requirements for nursing services and training programs.
- Responsible for ascertaining the need for supplies and equipment in her section and arrange for adequate maintenance.

Supervisory

- Promote harmony and efficiency within the team to improve the quality of work.
- Promote the professional growth of other staff and encourage initiative.

- Interpret the staff policies, plans and rules laid down for developing and regulating the service.
- Review the use of records, reports and collection of statistical data and advise wherever necessary.
- Describe each staff member's job description and interpret in the area of her own work.
- Home visit as per schedule to supervise the staff.
- Arrange orientation program of all new staff posted for training the unit area to acquaint them with the geography of the area, set-up, policies, and duties of different staff and channels of communication.

Plan and carry out continuous and effective inservice training program, and arranging monthly meetings for all nursing staff.

MIDLEVEL HEALTHCARE PROVIDER

India is alarming country for disease burden and to cover the huge gap in providing healthcare facilities, it requires the mid-level healthcare providers at different settings of the country. Indian community setting is in need to have access of affordable health care and government of India through National Health Mission (NHM) has declare the new pivotal role of community health officer (CHO) with its constructed roles and responsibilities for public health. A mid-level healthcare provider is defined as a health provider:

- Who is trained, authorized and regulated to work autonomously
- Who receives preservice training at higher education institution for at least a total of 2–3 years and
- Whose scope of practice includes (but is not restricted to) being able to diagnose, manage and treat illness, disease and impairments (including perform surgery, where appropriately trained), as well as engage in preventive and promotive care.

Trained and competent human resources are essential for an effective healthcare delivery system. There is a pressing need to strengthen health subcenters to provide Comprehensive Primary Care including for NCDs. Global evidence suggests that suitably trained (3–4 years duration) service providers can provide considerable primary care. As one of the measures to increase the availability of such appropriately qualified HR, especially in rural and remote areas.

On 13th November 2013, the Cabinet approved the introduction of a 3 and 1/2 year Bachelor of Science in Community Health (BSc CH) Course in India. However, the uptake for this course has been slow and if some Universities were to start the course, the first batch of professionals will be available for recruitment only by the end of the fourth year. On the other hand, qualified Ayurveda doctors and BSc/GNM qualified nurses are available in the system, who could be trained in public health and primary care through suitably designed 'Bridge Programmes in Community Health'. Such qualified human resource may function as Mid Level Health Care Providers and called 'Community Health Officers (CHOs)' and posted at health Subcenters; which could be develop as 'Health and Wellness Centers'.

Skill Required

- Public health skills
- General skills of biomedical waste management, medicine dispensation, medicine refills and injections, suturing of superficial wounds
- Laboratory skills
- Skills for management of common conditions—fever, aches and pains
- First aid stabilization care for common emergencies
- Maternal health skills
- Reproductive and adolescent health skills
- Newborn and child health skills
- Skills to use digital applications wherever applicable for reporting, inventory management, record maintenance and use population based
- Maintaining family health folders and individual health records
- Supportive supervision of field level functionaries.

Role and Responsibilities

Community health officer will bridge the gap between population and subcenter, primary health center and community health center. CHO's are permitted to serve the community independently to diagnose, manage and treat minor ailments and impairments and also engage in preventive. CHO is evolving concept in health care sector and their roles and responsibilities are purely population-oriented in public health. They are expected to provide specific service delivery, leadership, supervision, management and take pro-active role in all the activities at community level, organize various health program and activity in health promotion according the need.

Expanded Service Delivery

- Ensure that all households in the service areas are listed, empaneled and a database is maintained—in digital format/paper format as required by the state.
- Provide clinical care as specified in the care pathways and standard treatment guidelines for the range of services expected of the HWC.
- Clinical care provision would include coordinating for care/case management for chronic illnesses based on the diagnosis and treatment plan made by the Medical Officer/specialists who will initiate treatment for chronic diseases, dispense drugs as per standing orders by the medical officer.
- Coordination could be facilitated through processes such as telehealth.
- Focus attention in screening for chronic conditions on screening, enabling suspected cases confirmed and initiating treatment based on appropriate STGs or on basis of plans made by medical officer/specialists.

- As a team, ensure adherence, along with counselling and support as needed for primary and secondary prevention efforts. Such chronic conditions would include both non-communicable diseases and the chronic communicable diseases of tuberculosis, leprosy and HIV.
- Coordinate and lead local response to diseases outbreaks, emergencies and disaster situations and support the medical team or joint investigation teams for disease outbreaks.
- Support the team of MPWs and ASHAs on their tasks, including on the job mentoring, support and supervision and undertaking the monitoring, management, reporting and administrative functions of the HWC such as inventory management, upkeep and maintenance, and management of untied funds.
- Support and supervise the collection of population based data by frontline workers, collate and analyze data for planning and report the data to the next level in an accurate and timely fashion. Use HWC and population-data to understand key causes of mortality, morbidity in the community and work with the team to develop a local action plan with measurable targets, including a particular focus on vulnerable communities.
- Coordinate with community platforms such as the VHSNC/MAS/SHGs and work closely with PRI/ULB, to address social determinants of health and promote behavior change for improved health outcomes.
- Address issues of social and environmental determinants of health with extension workers of other departments related to gender-based violence, education, safe potable water, sanitation, safe collection of refuse, proper disposal of waste water, indoor air pollution, and on specific environmental hazards such as fluorosis, silicosis, arsenic contamination etc.
- Guide and be actively engaged in community health promotion including behavior change communication.

The Healthcare Services Provided by MLHP

Healthcare Services

- **Maternal health care:**
  - Prenatal care like antenatal check-up, screening for high risk, immunization and supplementation, child birth, postnatal care and if require referral to higher center.
  - *Neonate and infant health care:* Management of high-risk newborn, screening of congenital anomalies, IMNCI services, immunization.
- **Childhood and adolescent health care:** Adolescent health counselling, identification of drug abuse, detection of any deficiency, nutritional supplement and referral services.
- **Reproductive health care:** Family planning, prevention and management of STI, identification of gynecological problems and referral services.
- **Communicable diseases:** Diagnosis and treatment of vector or water borne diseases, provision of DOTs and DPMR (disability prevention and medical rehabilitation) services for leprosy along with referral services.
- **Illness and minor ailments:** Identification and management of fever, respiratory infection, diarrhea, cholera, skin rashes, pain, typhoid, etc.
- **Noncommunicable diseases:** Screening, prevention, control and management along with follow-up and maintenance of treatment modalities.
- **Eye and ENT:** Screening along with primary care of ophthalmic and ENT problem and referral services of any emergency.
- **Oral health:** Regular check-up and screening of oral health.
- **Geriatric and palliative care:** Health camp organization, routine check-up.
- **Emergency services:** Burn, injury, trauma along with first aid management
- **Mental health care:** Screening and counseling along with referral services, administrative and supervision services
- **Administrative services:** Guidance to other co-health workers and maintain inventory, report submission.
- **Supervision:** Supervision of national health program, ASHA, home visits, health promotion activities. Care pathway: Provide specific care according to standard treatment guidelines.
- **Case coordinator and manager:** Provide communication to higher authority regarding specific case, coordinate in care and management of care.
- **Disaster and outbreak of disease:** Local response to disease outbreak and early management of disaster.
- Education to community, speak about safe water, sanitation, disposal of waste, pollution control and identify environmental hazards and control.

The functions will be broadly classified following three major headings

1. Clinical functions: To provide ambulatory (out-patient) care and management.
2. Public health functions for health promotion, prevention and disease surveillance.
3. Managerial functions for efficient functioning of the Health and Wellness Centers.

HEALTHCARE INFRASTRUCTURE IN URBAN INDIA (FLOWCHART 9.2)

Previously healthcare delivery services in urban areas are restricted into tertiary level care which includes hospitals and medical colleges but after launching of NUHM health services has been reached in primary and secondary level.

As per report of Census 2011, it has been observed that the urban population consist of 37.7 cores which is 31.16% of the total population. In order to effectively address the health concerns of the urban poor population, the Ministry proposes to launch a National Urban Health Mission (NUHM). NUHM was approved by the Union Cabinet on 1st May, 2013 as a sub-mission under an overarching National Health Mission (NHM) for providing equitable and quality primary health care services to the urban

Flowchart 9.2: Healthcare delivery in urban area.

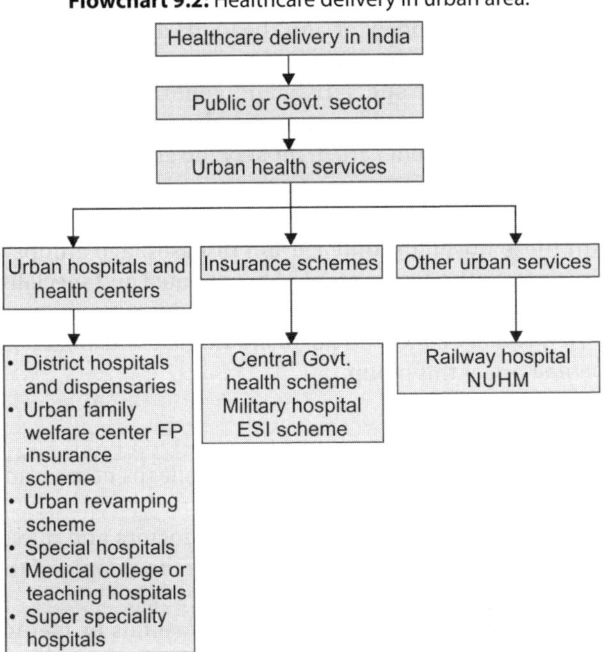

population with special focus on slum and vulnerable sections of the Society.

NUHM seeks to improve the health status by facilitating their access to quality primary healthcare. NUHM covers all the cities and towns with more than 50,000 population and district and state headquarters with more than 30,000 population.

Urban health program is being implemented through urban local bodies (ULBs), in seven metropolitan cities, viz., Mumbai, New Delhi, Chennai, Kolkata, Hyderabad, Bengaluru and Ahmedabad. For the remaining cities, the State Health department decides whether the urban health program is to be implemented through health department or any other urban local body.

The healthcare infrastructure in urban areas consists of the community health centers and primary health centers.

Population norms for urban health infrastructure:

- Community health centers—2,50,000 population (5 Lakh for metros)
- Primary health centers—50,000 population

Urban Primary Health Center

In order to provide comprehensive primary healthcare services, the National Urban Health Mission aims to establish urban primary healthcare centers, not as a standalone health facility, but as a hub of preventive, promotive and basic curative healthcare for its catchment population. Within its catchment area, the UPHC is responsible for providing the primary health care and public health needs of the population. The package of services envisaged at UPHC inclusive of preventive, promotive, curative, rehabilitative and palliative care. Further, in order to strengthen comprehensive primary health care across the country through "Ayushman Bharat-HWCs", states are upgrading their subcenters and primary health care centers as health and wellness centers (HWCs) across rural and urban areas. The UPHC is located preferably closer to slum or similar habitations. As on 31st March 2019, there are 3302 at the level of SC is functional in the urban areas of the country. Out of these SCs, a total of 98 SCs has been upgraded as HWCs.

Service provision: The UPHC's key responsibility is to provide comprehensive preventive, promotive, curative, rehabilitative, palliative care.

Services provided by UPHC include:

- OPD (consultation)
- Laboratory services
- Drugs and contraceptive dispensing
- Delivery of Reproductive and Child Health (RCH) services
- Preventive, promotive and curative aspects of communicable and noncommunicable diseases.
- Multispecialist services
- Minor surgical procedures
- Counseling and help desk
- Outreach activities
- Population-based screening

The hours of operation may be such so as to enable the urban working population to conveniently access the UPHC services. States may allot suitable timing, providing 8 hours of services, which are convenient to the community. It is recommended that the UPHC operates preferably from 12 noon to 8 PM or in dual shifts (i.e., 8 AM to 12 PM and 4 PM to 8 PM); Dual shift timing of UPHC could be flexible with the ability to be modified according to the catchment communities.

The package of services envisaged at UPHC inclusive of preventive, promotive, curative, rehabilitative and palliative care. Further, in order to strengthen comprehensive primary health care across the country through "Ayushman Bharat-HWCs", states are upgrading their primary health care centers++ as health and wellness centers (HWCs).

Urban Community Health Centers

Urban Community Health Center (UCHC) is set up as a referral facility for every 4-5 UPHCs. This is considered as secondary level health care. The UCHC caters to a population of 2,50,000 to 5 Lakhs. For the metro cities, UCHCs may be established for every 5 lakh population with 100 beds. In addition to primary healthcare facilities, it provides inpatient services, medical care, surgical facilities and institutional delivery facilities. It is a 30–50 bedded facility health center. The norms for urban CHC are same as rural CHCs. As on 31st March 2019, there are 350 UCHCs functional in urban areas of the India.

There are 350 UCHCs functional in the country as on 31st March 2019. About 96% of UCHCs are located in government buildings and 4% in rented buildings.

Urban Health and Wellness Centers

In order to ensure delivery of Comprehensive Primary Health Care (CPHC) services, for supervisory 4–5 UPHCs existing UPHCs would be converted to Health and Wellness Centers (HWC). Services could also be provided/complemented through outreach services, Mobile Medical Units, health camps, home visits and community-based interaction, but the principle should be a seamless continuum of care that ensures equity, quality, universality and no financial hardship.

At UCHCs there are 1,017 specialists, 713 GDMOs, 192 radiologists, 468 pharmacists, 447 lab technicians and 4,618 staff nurses available at UCHCs. There is a vacancy of 36.9% of specialists, 28.8% of GDMOs, 30.2% of radiographers, 13% of pharmacists, 17.3% of lab technicians and 17.6% of staff nurses at UCHCs. There is shortfall of 45.8% of total specialist, 24.6% of GDMOs, 48% of radiographers, 16% of pharmacists, 13.4% of lab technicians and 21.3% of staff nurses at UCHCs.

As on 31st March 2019, a total of 7919 SCs have been converted into HWC-SCs. Out of total 7919 HWC-SCs, 7,821 SCs has been converted into HWCs in rural areas and 98 SCs in urban areas. Also at the level of PHC, a total of 9,976 PHCs have been converted into HWC-PHCs. Out of total 9,976 HWCs, 8,242 PHCs has been converted into HWCs in rural areas and 1,734 in urban areas.

The Health Wellness Center at the Subcenter Level

The HWC at the SC level would be equipped and staffed by an appropriately trained Primary Health Care team, comprising of multipurpose workers (male and female) and ASHAs and led by a mid-level health provider (MLHP).

- The Medical Officer at the PHC would be responsible for ensuring that CPHC services are delivered through all HWCs in her/his area and through the PHC itself.
- For PHCs to be strengthened to HWCs, support for training of PHC staff (medical officers, staff nurses, pharmacist, and lab technicians), and provision of equipment for "Wellness Room", the necessary IT infrastructure and the resources required for upgrading laboratory and diagnostic support to complement the expanded ranges of services would be provided.
- States could choose to modify staffing at HWC and PHC, based on local needs.
- The first HWC was inaugurated by the hon'ble Prime Minister Shri Narendra Modi at Jangla in Bijapur, Chhattisgarh on 14th April 2018.

District Hospitals

Secondary healthcare refers to a second tier of health system, in which patients from primary health care are referred to specialists in higher hospitals for treatment. In India, the health centers for secondary health care include district hospitals and urban community health center at block level district hospital is a hospital complex engaged in the curative services for the population of the district. The medical superintendent or CMO heads the district hospitals. Each unit is under the charge of a senior specialist, who is assisted by junior specialists and general duty medical officers. The district hospital provides both ambulatory (OPD) and in-patient care in most of the general specialist.

Speciality Hospitals

- In these hospitals, only certain diseases, age groups or patients with specific problems are treated and specialists and specially trained nurses treat the patients.
- TB hospitals, children's hospitals, women's hospitals, etc., come under this group.

Teaching Hospitals

- Hospitals associated with medical colleges come under this category
- Along with teaching and training to doctors and nurses, these hospitals provide complete care to people of that area.
- At present there are 300 teaching hospitals or medical colleges in India (Till Dec 2009).

Super Speciality Hospitals or Institutes

- In these hospitals super specialists of different organs or diseases are trained and patients are also treated.
- All India Institute of Medical Science (AIIMS) is an example of such institute.
- Actually these institutes are center of excellence for health services.
- To enhance the super speciality urban health services and to decrease the patient load on AIIMS Delhi, Govt. of India has a plan to open such 6 (six) institutes in the various states.
- Selected places for proposed self-dependent AIIMS are; Jodhpur (Rajasthan), Bhopal (MP), Raipur (Chhattisgarh), Patna (Bihar), Bhubaneswar (Odisha) and Dehradun (Uttaranchal).
- Union Govt. has plan to take help of private sector in this context, to overcome the financial constraint. ₹999 crore has been allotted in the Tenth Plan outlay for the initial establishment of these AIIMS (2005).
- These institutes will be established under Pradhan Mantri Swasthya Suraksha Yojana (PMSSY).
- PMSSY has two components, in its first phase: (i) setting of 6 AIIMS like institutions and (ii) upgradation of 13 existing government medical college institutions. Out of 6 AIIMS like institutions, each institution will have a 960 bedded hospitals. The distribution of beds are as follows:
  - 500 beds for medical college hospitals
  - 300 beds for speciality/super speciality
  - 100 beds for ICU/accident trauma
  - 30 beds for physical medicine and rehabilitation
  - 30 beds for AYUSH
  - These institutions will provide health care in 42 speciality discipline.

- In the 2nd phase of PMSSY, it is proposed to set-up AIIMS like institution at: (i) Laigang Race-Bareilly (UP) and (ii) Talganj-Uttar-Dinajpur (WB).

HEALTH INSURANCE SCHEME

The MOHFW has advised to State/UT governments to prepare health insurance models as per their local needs. GOI will provide support to state governments for health insurance scheme/projects, under NRHM. There is no universal health insurance in India.

The different National Health Insurance Schemes in India are:

1. Rashtriya Swasthya Bima Yojana (RSBY)
2. Employees' State Insurance Scheme (ESIS)
3. Central Government Health Scheme (CGHS)
4. Family Planning Insurance Scheme
5. Aam Aadmi Bima Yojana (AABY)
6. Janashree Bima Yojana (JBY)
7. Universal Health Insurance Scheme (UHIS)

1. Rashtriya Swasthya Bima Yojana

Rashtriya Swasthya Bima Yojana (RSBY) has been launched by Ministry of Labour and Employment, Government of India to provide health insurance coverage for Below Poverty Line (BPL) families.

The overall objective of RSBY is to provide protection to BPL households from financial liabilities arising out of health shocks that involve hospitalization. Beneficiaries under RSBY are entitled to hospitalization coverage up to ₹30,000/- for most of the diseases that require hospitalization. Government has even fixed the package rates for the hospitals for a large number of interventions. Pre-existing conditions are covered from day one and there is no age limit. Coverage extends to five members of the family which includes the head of household, spouse and up to three dependents. Beneficiaries need to pay only ₹30/- as registration fee while Central and State Government pays the premium to the insurer selected by the State Government on the basis of a competitive bidding.

Unique Features of RSBY

The RSBY scheme is not the first attempt to provide health insurance to low income workers by the Government in India. The RSBY scheme, however, differs from these schemes in several important ways:

- **Empowering the beneficiary:** RSBY provides the participating BPL household with freedom of choice between public and private hospitals and makes him a potential client worth attracting on account of the significant revenues that hospitals stand to earn through the scheme.
- **Business model for all stakeholders:** The scheme has been designed as a business model for a social sector scheme with incentives built for each stakeholder. This business model design is conducive both in terms of expansion of the scheme as well as for its long run sustainability.
- **Insurers:** The insurer is paid premium for each household enrolled for RSBY. Therefore, the insurer has the motivation to enroll as many households as possible from the BPL list. This will result in better coverage of targeted beneficiaries.
- **Hospitals:** A hospital has the incentive to provide treatment to large number of beneficiaries as it is paid per beneficiary treated. Even public hospitals have the incentive to treat beneficiaries under RSBY as the money from the insurer will flow directly to the concerned public hospital which they can use for their own purposes. Insurers, in contrast, will monitor participating hospitals in order to prevent unnecessary procedures or fraud resulting in excessive claims.
- **Intermediaries:** The inclusion of intermediaries such as NGOs and MFIs which have a greater stake in assisting BPL households. The intermediaries will be paid for the services they render in reaching out to the beneficiaries.
- **Government:** By paying only a maximum sum up to ₹750/- per family per year, the Government is able to provide access to quality health care to the below poverty line population. It will also lead to a healthy competition between public and private providers which in turn will improve the functioning of the public healthcare provider.
- **Information Technology (IT) intensive:** For the first time IT applications are being used for social sector scheme on such a large scale. Every beneficiary family is issued a biometric enabled smart card containing their fingerprints and photographs. All the hospitals empaneled under RSBY are IT enabled and connected to the server at the district level. This will ensure a smooth data flow regarding service utilization periodically.
- **Safe and foolproof:** The use of biometric enabled smart card and a key management system makes this scheme safe and foolproof. The key management system of RSBY ensures that the card reaches the correct beneficiary and there remains accountability in terms of issuance of the smart card and its usage. The biometric enabled smart card ensures that only the real beneficiary can use the smart card.
- **Portability:** The key feature of RSBY is that a beneficiary who has been enrolled in a particular district will be able to use his/her smart card in any RSBY empaneled hospital across India. This makes the scheme truly unique and beneficial to the poor families that migrate from one place to the other. Cards can also be split for migrant workers to carry a share of the coverage with them separately.
- **Cashless and paperless transactions:** A beneficiary of RSBY gets cashless benefit in any of the empaneled hospitals. He/she only needs to carry his/her smart card and provide verification through his/her finger print. For participating providers it is a paperless scheme as they do not need to send all the papers related to treatment to the insurer. They send online claims to the insurer and get paid electronically.

2. Employees State Insurance Scheme

The Employees' State Insurance Scheme (ESIS) is an integrated measure of Social Insurance embodied in the Employees' State Insurance Act and it is designed to accomplish the task of protecting 'employees' as defined in the Employees' State Insurance Act, 1948 against the impact of incidences of sickness, maternity, disablement and death due to employment injury and to provide medical care to insured persons and their families. The ESI Scheme applies to factories and other establishments viz. Road Transport, Hotels, Restaurants, Cinemas, Newspaper, Shops, and Educational/Medical Institutions wherein 10 or more persons are employed. Employees of the aforesaid categories of factories and establishments, drawing wages up to ₹15,000/- a month, are entitled to social security cover under the ESI Act. ESI Corporation has also decided to enhance wage ceiling for coverage of employees under the ESI Act from ₹15,000–21,000/-.

- This programme provides health care to industrial labour and their families.
- This gives safely at the time of delivery, diseases, accidents, *etc.* Similarly if a labour dies in accident, family pension is given.
- For this scheme, money is contributed by the management as well as employees.
- Employees getting up to ₹50/-per day will not have to pay contribution also.

3. Central Government Health Scheme

The Central Government Health Scheme (CGHS) provides comprehensive health care to the CGHS beneficiaries in India. The medical facilities are provided through wellness centers (previously referred to as CGHS dispensaries)/ polyclinics under allopathic, ayurveda, yoga, unani, siddha and homeopathic systems of medicines.

Objective of the Scheme

- To give extensive medical facilities to central government employees and their family members.
- To save government from heavy expenses on medical refund.

Beneficiaries of Scheme

In the beginning, scheme was only limited to central government employees and their family members. With the extended programmes, new beneficiaries are:

- Central government employees and their family members.
- Members of parliament (present and former).
- Judges of Supreme Court and High Courts (present and retired).
- Freedom fighters.
- Pensioners of central government, semi-autonomous units or employees of semi-government organizations.
- Journalists
- Governors and Ex-vice Presidents.

Facilities under the Scheme

- Outdoor treatment facilities in all medical system.
- Emergency services in allopathy system.
- Free medicines.
- Facilities for laboratory tests and radiological investigations.
- Treatment facility for serious patients at their own homes.
- Specialist consultation facilities.
- Family welfare services.
- Treatment facilities in government or government recognized private hospitals where specialists are available.
- Facility for 90% advance payment, in case of need.

Coverage under the Scheme

Scheme was started in Delhi in the beginning. The scheme now covers besides Delhi, the cities of Mumbai, Allahabad, Meerut, Kanpur, Patna, Kolkata, Nagpur, Chennai, Hyderabad, Bangalore, Jaipur, Pune, Lucknow, Ahmadabad, Bhubaneswar and Jabalpur.

The scheme which started with 16 allopathic dispensaries in 1954 covering 2.3 lakh beneficiaries has now there are 9.34 lakhs card holders and 31.81 lakhs beneficiaries (2009). Under these schemes there are 247 allopathic hospitals, 82 dispensaries of AYUSH, 19 polyclinics, 65 laboratories, 21dental units and 4 Yoga centers (2009).

4. Family Planning Insurance Scheme

Government of India has launched family planning insurance scheme (FPIS) w.e.f. 29-11-2005 for acceptors of sterilization and indemnity insurance cover for doctors performing sterilization procedure both in Government and accredited private/NGO/Corporate health facilities.

MOHFW is also implementing a central sponsored family welfare linked health insurance scheme since 1981 to compensate the acceptors of the sterilization for the loss of wages for the day on which he or she attended the medical facility for undergoing sterilization.

5. Aam Aadmi Bima Yojana

Aam Admi Bima Yojana (AABY), a Social Security Scheme for rural landless household was launched on 2nd October, 2007. The head of the family or one earning member in the family of such a household is covered under the scheme. The premium of ₹200/- per person per annum is shared equally by the Central Government and the State Government. The member to be covered should be aged between 18 and 59 years. The insurances covered in Aam Admi Bima Yojana is given in **Table 9.3**.

Table 9.3: The insurances covered in Aam Admi Bima Yojana.

On natural death	₹30,000
On death due to accident/on permanent disability due to accident (loss of 2 eyes or 2 limbs)	₹75,000
On partial permanent disability due to accident (loss of one eye or one limb)	₹37,500

6. Janashree Bima Yojana

Janashree Bima Yojana (JBY) was launched on 10th August 2000. The Scheme replaced Social Security Group Insurance Scheme (SSGIS) and Rural Group Life Insurance Scheme (RGLIS). 45 occupational groups have been covered under this scheme **(Table 9.4)**:

Table 9.4: Forty five occupational groups on Janashree Bima Yojana.

Sl. No.	Occupation
1.	Beedi Workers
2.	Brick Kiln Workers
3.	Carpenters
4.	Cobblers
5.	Fisherman
6.	Hamals
7.	Handicraft Artisans
8.	Handloom Weavers
9.	Handloom and Khadi Weavers
10.	Lady Tailors
11.	Leather Tannery Workers
12.	Papad Workers Attached to SEWA
13.	Physically Handicapped Self-Employed
14.	Primary Milk Producers
15.	Rickshaw Pullers/Auto Drivers
16.	Safai Karmacharis
17.	Salt Growers
18.	Tendu Leaf Collectors
19.	Scheme for Urban Poor
20.	Forest Workers
21.	Sericulture
22.	Toddy Tappers
23.	Power Loom Workers
24.	Hilly Area Woman
25.	Food Stuffs Like Khandsari/Sugar
26.	Textile
27.	Manufacture of Food Products
28.	Manufacture of Paper Products
29.	Manufacture of Leather Products
30.	Printing
31.	Rubber and Coal Products
32.	Chemical Products like Candle Manufacture
33.	Mineral Products like Earthern Toys Manufacture
34.	Agriculturists
35.	Transport Drivers Association
36.	Transport Karmacharis
37.	Rural Poor
38.	Construction Workers
39.	Fire Crackers Workers
40.	Coconut Processors
41.	Aanganwadi Workers/Helpers
42.	Kotwal
43.	Plantation Workers
44.	Woman Associated with SHG
45.	Sheep Breeders

Contd...

Contd...

OTHER GOVERNMENT HEALTH SERVICES

In this, healthcare services for railway employees and military personnel may be included.

Defense Medical Services

- For defense services, there are separate hospital and health service system which provides medical care to military personnel and their family members.
- Defense health services come under armed force medical services (AFMS). They are responsible for providing all preventive, curative and promotional health services.
- Defense services have their own medical college, nursing college and nursing schools.

Railway Medical Services

- Indian railways are a biggest government organization with highest number of railway employees in the world.
- Railway provides wide range of health services to its employees through railway hospitals, clinics and health units.
- Similarly organizations like postal department, atomic energy department, etc., also provide limited health services to their employees. These services are usually linked to urban health services.

National Urban Health Mission

- Rapid urbanizations led to rapid increase in number of urban poor population, majority of which lives in slums.
- The need for improving the delivery of health care for the urban poor has been recognized by the National Health Policy (2000), the National Population Policy (2002) and the Eleventh Five Year Plan.
- However, policy prescriptions have not optimally translated into focused strategies for improving the health status of the urban poor.
- The proposed NUHM aims to improve the health status of the urban poor, particularly the slum dwellers and other disadvantaged sections by facilitating equitable access to quality health care with active involvement of the urban local bodies (ULBs) in cities with population one lakh and above and state capitals.
- The NUHM would be covering 21.07 core urban population with a special focus on 6.25 crore urban poor living in slums and spread over 430 cities.

PLANNING INSERVICE EDUCATION PROGRAM AND TEACHING

It is usually defined as a planned instructional or training program provided to the professional nurse by an employing agency in the employment setting and is designed to increase competence in a specific area.

Inservice education is a planned educational experience provided in the job setting and closely identified with services in order to help a person perform more effectively as a person and as a worker.

Identified Areas

- Human relation in health care
- Management techniques for nursing administrator
- Care in emergency of all specialties for staff nurses
- Educational technology for teachers of nursing.

Process of Planning of Inservice Education Program

When planning the inservice educational program, the following steps are involved:

- Identifying the learning needs of the personnel
- Setting goals and defining specific objectives
- Planning and organizing course and designing learning experience
- Assessing the available resources
- Establishing a workable budget
- Implementing plan of teaching
- Evaluating the program
- May restart the process.

Identifying the learning needs of the personnel: Determination of learning needs is one of the very important elements in the whole process of personnel development. A training activity/education program does not make any sense if it does not create enthusiasm in the nurse learner.

- **Definition of learning needs:** 'Need' refers to the difference between what a nurse is aware of, and what is desired or expected of her in a particular role.
  Need is a lack of knowledge, skills or attitude that prevents an employee from giving a satisfactory job performance.
- **Types of learning needs:** For clarity, let us divide the identification of learning needs under the three following headings:
  - Individual needs; for example, updating knowledge in any related field
  - Organizational needs enabling the staff to be efficient in work after going through the program
  - Community needs, providing knowledge in giving efficient care to the community, like prevention of AIDS or drug abuse, and encouraging breastfeeding.
- **Source of identifying the needs:** The needs can be identified from:
  - Learner
  - Supervisor and administrator
  - Client and patient who express what should be there and what is not there
  - Society and community while doing survey when the data reveals the need for immunization
  - Education to children regarding hygiene, etc.
  - Political commitment; for example, discussing awareness programs on AIDS
  - New technology and scientific knowledge, such as use of incubators, CPR, etc.
  - Continuing education coordinator as there is lot of sharing with various groups of participants from whom s/he can collect information regarding the 'felt need' of the nursing personnel.
- **Appropriate use to assess learning needs:**
  - Observation performance of nursing personnel will help to know the deficit in the performance of nursing procedure
  - Verbal communication also helps in assessing the learning needs of the learners
  - Written communication by questionnaire, slip technique in which the learner writes the topics for updating the knowledge, analysis of records and reports also helps in identifying the deficit area; incident reports and annual reports also help in identifying the learning needs. Job analysis can also be used in assessing the learning needs.
- **Sample proforma for assessment of learning needs:** Given below are three columns written as individual needs, organizational needs and societal needs. List the learning needs what you strongly feel you require to update your knowledge.
  Examples:
  Individual needs: Updating knowledge in nursing process
  Organizational needs: Developing/writing job description
  Societal needs: Education to a community about importance of personal hygiene
- **Common tools used to assess the learning needs:** Some of the common tools which can be used for assessment of learning needs are as follows:
  - Questionnaire
  - Rating scale
  - Checklist
  - Opinionnaire.

Questionnaire: We are trying to find out the learning needs of our ward sisters so that a continuous planning can be done to depute ward sisters for inservice education. This will enable the ward sisters to work effectively in the ward management.

Setting goals and defining specific objectives: Once the learning needs are identified, then the most important or felt need is decided for continuing the education. Let us take one of the needs for continuing education program, which is ward management. It is important to establish goals/purpose and define the specific objectives.

Purpose is the broad statement which gives direction in platinum and assists in the determination of appropriate objectives.

For example, the learning which is identified above the overall purpose is to enable the ward sisters to strengthen the concepts of ward management.

Objectives are established for overall program and for specific activities.

Let us discuss objectives for the above learning need. At the end of the ward management course, ward sisters will be able to:

- Develop the concept of ward management
- Strengthen knowledge in principles of administration
- Develop organizational plans and channels of communication
- Enlist the job responsibilities of ward sister
- Identify the methods of patient care
- Discuss the principles of supervision
- Develop plan for inservice education.

Planning and organizing course and designing learning experiences: Planning and organization are the relation of efforts and capacities of individuals and groups engaged upon a common task in such a way as to secure the desired objectives with the least friction and the most satisfaction for whom the task is done.

While planning the continuing education program, the following policies should be kept in mind:

- What content is to be included in continuing the education?
- The priorities given to the staff for attending it according to their placement
- Who will be accountable for the results of continuing the education?
- What methods of teaching will be used in continuing the education?
- What method of evaluation will be used?
- What qualification will be required of the resource persons?
- How will the resources and experts be identified and used?

Some of the policies discussed will help us in designing the program.

Let us go back to the following example:

Identification of learning need: 'Continuing education program on ward management for ward sisters'.

Objectives: Based on the objectives, let us identify the topics. Some of the topics are:

- Concept of ward management
- Principles of administration
- Principles of organization
- Job description
- Principles and methods of supervision
- Developing inservice education program.

While planning the program, we must always write the day, date, time, topic and resource person. The duration of the program will depend upon the budget. Any format can be used for planning the program. The programme schedule of an Inservice Education Program has been given in **Table 9.5**.

Theme: Continuing the education program on ward management

Table 9.5: Program schedule of an Inservice Education Program.

Monday 15.2.2016		Resource Person
9:00–10:00 AM	Registration	(Write the name of resource person)
10:00–11:00 AM	Inaugural session; Welcome address; Unfolding of theme objectives	Nursing person
	Inaugural speech	From funding agency
11:00–11:30 AM	Tea break	
11:30–1:00 AM	Concept of ward management	Principal, School of Nursing
2:00–4:30 PM	Principles of administration	Nursing superintendent

- **Participants:** 30 ward sisters
- **Date:** 10th July to 15th July, 2014
- **Time:** 9:00 AM to 4:30 PM
- **Venue:** College of Nursing, Berhampur
- **Coordinator:** Mrs 'X'
- **Purpose:** Write the example
- **Objectives:** As described, list all the objectives
- **Methods of teaching:** Lecture, discussion, role play, overhead transparencies, clinical visit, discussion with NS and ANS
- **Resource persons:** Names of those should be written here who are going to be the resource persons
- **Credit:** Certificate of attendance
- **Evaluation:** With the help of evaluation proforma.

This is just one day's example likewise the other days programme is finalized.

On the last day, half-day program is planned for the evaluation of workshop and the concluding session. The concluding session should include report of the workshop, concluding remarks and distribution of certificates.

Before confirming the program, there has to be a selection of the resources.

Selection of resources: Resources are categorized as financial resources, human resources, facilities, equipment and supplies.

- Financial resource is mainly the budget. For getting the finances, a proposal should be prepared. Three basic aspects of writing the proposal are:
    - *Getting ready:* Clarify the idea, discuss the idea, explore funding sources
    - Developing an overview, outline of the activity, plan in phases, build on resources
    - Producing the proposal, writing the proposal.

Guidelines for Writing the Proposal

- Name of the Director/organizer
- Name of the institution
- State the assessed problem/need
- Aim of the program

- Objectives of the program
- Duration of the workshop
- **Stipulate the participants:**
  - Type of group
  - Number of participants.
- **Funds required:**
  - Travelling allowances
  - Daily allowance
  - Honorarium allowances
  - Equipment and supplies
  - Technical and support staff.
- **Traveling allowances:**
  - Participants from far off distance
  - Participants from near distance
- Daily allowances/stipend
- **Honorarium:** Coordinator/Guest Lecturer/Resource Persons
- Finance for equipment and supplies/stationaries
- **Finance for technical staff/support staff:**
  - Human Resources should be assessed and utilized in the best possible manner and should be selected according to the size of the budget.
  - A speaker or resource person selected should have the following qualifications:
    - Familiarity with special needs of adult learner
    - Good knowledge of his/her assigned topic
    - Ability to conduct an effective session.

  Speaker can be selected from the faculty of the institution or from outside.
- Support staff, like clerk, technician, safaiwala, and serving persons should be available.
- **Equipment and supplies facilities:**
  - Calm and quiet place for workshop
  - Audiovisual equipment
  - Printed material, etc.

Implementing the program: Before implementing, check the following aspects:

- Organize a filing system (loose-leaf notebook) labeled accordingly.
- Determine the purpose of the workshop or conference.
- Determine who will undertake planning and direction.
- Determine time, place, and duration of workshop.
- Analyze the desired participants.
- Determine the possible dates for the workshop.
- Determine the possible locations for the workshop.
- Develop a time table.
- Develop a mailing list.
- Analyze methods of instruction.
- Determine the desired topical coverage.
- Determine the desired faculty.
- Determine the expenses to be met.
- Determine the funding arrangements.
- Develop a plan for controlling finances.
- Determine the place for workshop.
- Determine the accommodations required.

Now we need to develop the agenda:

- State the purpose of the workshop.
- State the desired learning outcome on the part of the participants.
- Determine the time available for the total workshop.
- Determine the topic coverage desired.
- Develop the realistic time allocations that can be adhered to.
- Allocate the time for registration.
- Allocate the time for opening remarks.
- Allocate the time for the introduction of speakers.
- Allocate the time for speakers.
- Allocate the time for discussion.
- Allocate the time for rest or coffee breaks.
- Allocate the time for the presiding officials.
- Allocate the time for the evaluation of the actions.
- Allocate the time for summation and adjournment.
- Develop the tentative agenda.

Prepare correspondence to the guest speakers:

- Letter or call of invitation, including consultant fee if appropriate.
- Outline coverage desired.
- Include courtesy copy of agenda.
- Query as to support requirements, e.g., 35 mm slide projector, 16 mm motion picture projector, remote controls, and lighting requirements.
- Determine whether any speaker may object to audience taping of his presentation.
- Include information as to sponsored and planned activities.
- When appropriate, carbon copy of correspondence may be sent to speaker's dean, administrator of employer.
- Develop teaching-learning strategies.

Evaluating the program: As the program is coming near to end on the last day, the evaluation of the following areas may be done by rating scale, questionnaire or opinionnaire:

- Evaluation of the program
- Evaluation of the facilities.

Guidelines for Evaluation of Continuing Education Program as Ward Management for the Ward Sisters

Instructions: Given below are statements. Tick mark (P) in any of the four columns given below according to your opinion.

Statements	*Strongly agree*	*Agree*	*Partially agree*	*Disagree*	*Strongly disagree*
The objectives of the programs were clearly stated					
The program was well-planned					
Concept of ward management was clear					
Principles of administration were covered adequately					

(All the topics may be covered like this.)

- AV aids selected were appropriate
- Group work was adequate
- Group discussions ware beneficial
- Nurses' responsibility in staff development and nursing audit.

Any other comments:

You may give remarks about food and accommodation.

REFERRAL SYSTEM

The system in which the patient is sent from the health center having fewer amenities to the health institution or treatment center, which has more resources, facilities and amenities, is called referral system. Thus, referral system is an essential component of healthcare system. From rural level to metropolises, and from health subcenters to specialist hospitals, all kinds of health facilities can be provided to the community through this system **(Flowchart 9.3)**.

Importance

- Providing diagnostic services to the patient and community.
- Providing specialist's services to the patient.
- Propagating the purposes of referral system among the health workers.
- Teaching the nursing personnel for reviewing of patients sent for referral.
- Preventing further complications and providing appropriate treatment.
- Sending or transporting the patient comfortably to the referral institute.

Selection of the Patient for Referral

Which patient should be sent for referral or what should be the basis of patient for referral system, this depends upon the resources available in the health center and the condition of the patient. Such patients can be divided into three categories:

Flowchart 9.3: Levels of referral system.

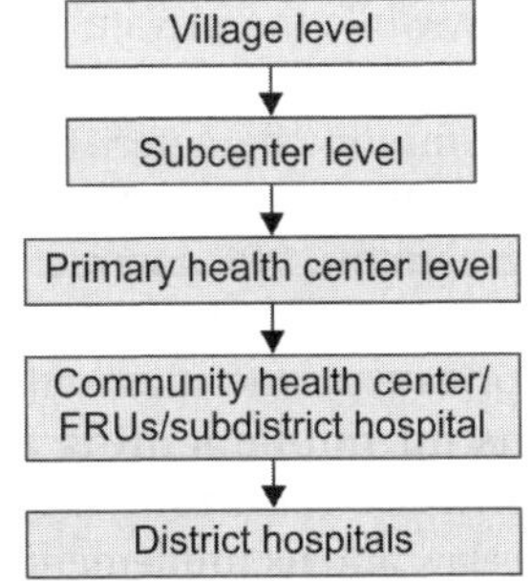

First Group or Fatal Patients

Such patients cannot survive despite the best treatment made available to them. So, to send them for treatment is the waste of time and money. Hence, it is better to give them appropriate treatment at the health center itself with the available resources. It is essential for the relatives of the patient to understand that owing to his fatal condition, it will not be beneficial to send the patient for referral.

Second Group or Serious Patients

The condition of such patients is considered serious but immediate treatment can save their lives. So, before sending them for referral, attempts should be made to reduce the seriousness of condition and only after that they should be sent for referral.

Third Group or General Patients

Though the diseases may be serious in such patients, still the condition of the patient is found to be normal. Delayed treatment may not threaten his life. Such patients can be immediately sent for referral. Similarly, after the surgery or in case diagnosis is not possible or for some special technique, the patient can be sent to a big or specialist hospital for consultation.

Thus, on the basis of a patient's condition, type of disease, objectives of treatment and the latest technique of treatment or the need of diagnosis, the case of the patient can be prepared for the referral system.

Although the levels of referral system are in the above-mentioned order, but a upgraded PHCs and CIICs are considered as First Referral Units (FRUs).

Interdisciplinary Referral System

When a patient cannot be treated, neither properly diagnosed nor satisfied with a particular pathy, then he can be referred to another type of therapy for the needful. This type of referral is called interdisciplinary referral system. It is very common in our country, where the patient shifts oftenly from allopathy to AYUSH (Ayurveda, Yoga and Naturopathy, Unani, Siddha and Homeopathy).

It is important to mention here that the Government of India is encouraging the availability of various treatment systems (therapies) under one roof. Some states are implementing this system in their selected hospitals, and this will more enhance the interdisciplinary referral system.

Responsibilities of Nurses in Referral System

- All nursing personnel working in subcenters, PHCs/CHCs or in district hospitals should have the knowledge of referral system. Patients should be carefully selected for the referral system.

- Nurses should be aware of their limitations and responsibilities in the referral system.
- In case of emergency, attempt should be made to save the life of the patient, and then only he should be sent for referral.
- Entries in the referral form or ticket should be clear and correct; related records should also be enclosed with it.
- While sending serious patients, life-saving equipment/ medicines should be arranged with him.
- If the facilities are available, then consultation for the patient can be procured through telephone, television network, medical transcription or internet (telemedicine), etc.
- As far as possible, the nurse should accompany the patient while sending him for referral.

PUBLIC PRIVATE PARTNERSHIP

Public private partnership (PPPs) have become more common not only in the after reckoning of the 2008 financial crisis, as governments are eager to leverage scarce public funds but have seen a rise in developing countries over the last two decades. More than 134 developing countries apply PPPs, contributing about 15–20% of total infrastructure investment. Widely utilized because of their purported advantages in off-budget funding, anticipated efficiency gains, and improved service quality, PPPs are a mechanism that governments regularly turn to in fulfilling their responsibilities regarding public infrastructure and service. PPPs, if implemented well, can help overcome inadequate infrastructure that constrains economic growth, particularly in developing countries. Infrastructure investments are known to accelerate much-needed growth in developing countries and reduce income disparities. But poor infrastructure is often a reflection of several constraints governments face.

Example: Insufficient public funds, poor planning, weak analysis underpinning project selection, or corruption infrastructure assets are also often poorly maintained.

PPPs can help overcome some of these challenges by mobilizing private sector sources, helping improve project selection and on-time and on-budget implementation and ensuring adequate maintenance. Although initially restricted to public infrastructure in the form of roads, railways, power generation, or water and waste treatment facilities, PPPs have increasingly moved into the provision of so-called "social infrastructure," such as schools, hospitals, and health services hold in developing countries PPPs may refer to informal and short-term engagements of non-governmental.

Concept of Public Private Partnership

"Public" would define Government or organizations functioning under State budgets. "Private" would be Profit/ Non-profit/Voluntary sector. "Partnership" would mean a collaborative effort and reciprocal relationship between Public-Private.

Public Private Partnerships (PPP) are collaborative efforts, between private and public sectors, with identified partnership structures, shared objectives, and specified performance indicators for delivery of health services between two parties.

It is an approaches to addressing public health problems through the combined efforts of public private and development organizations complimenting each other by contributing or sharing their core competency.

PPP means to bring together a set of actors for the common goal of improving the health of a population based on the mutually agreed roles and principles. **—WHO 1999**

It means that both parties have agreed to work together in implementing a program and that party has a clear role and say in how that implementation happens.

—Blagiscu and Young 2005

- It is a form of agreement that entails reciprocal obligations and mutual accountability, voluntary or contractual relationships, the sharing or investments and reputational risks and joint responsibility for design and execution.

  —World Economic Forum, 2005
- A useful way of engaging a wide range of stakeholders and NGO's in achieving the complex set off development objectives in health. **—ADBI, 2001**

Objectives of Public Private Partnerships

- Improving quality, accessibility, availability, acceptability and efficiency of health services
- Exchange of skills and expertise between the public and private sector and mobilization of additional resources
- Strengthening existing health system
- Widening the range of services and number of services providers.
- Universal coverage and equity for primary health care
- Set up common goals and objectives both private and public sectors and inciting joint decision-making process
- Understanding the strengths and weakness of both the public and private partners among themselves
- To generate a high-level of trust and confidence benefits to both the stakeholders.

Public Private Partnership Characteristics

Public Private Partnership (PPP) is a continually evolving process as partners look to refine the collaborative relationship. It is a contracted agreement between the government and a private sector partner. The government retains ownership of the facility, while the private partner does almost everything else, including building, fixing, maintaining or managing it. The common characteristics of Public Private Partnership (PPP) has been given in **Figure 9.1**.

- **Contractual agreement:** PPP contract means a mutually binding contract concluded between the contracting authority and private partner that set(s) forth the terms and conditions for implementing a PPP project, in accordance with the requirements and procedures provided by this law and its Implementing Regulations. A

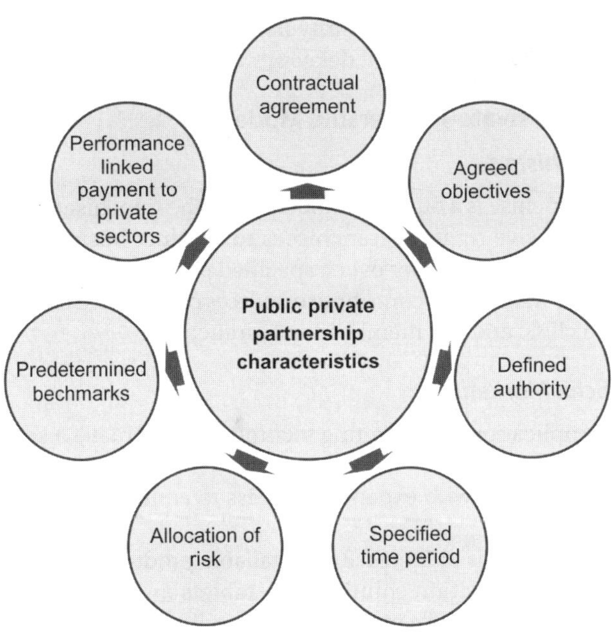

Fig. 9.1: Characteristics of public private partnership.

clear understanding between the partners about mutual benefits which will be written in contract. Regulatory framework that is followed and enforced to follow contract.

- **Agreed objectives:** In every contract there will be written objectives where both parties are responsible to achieve that by their mutual efforts. These objectives are mutually signed by both parties. With agreed objectives the assigned responsibilities will be written in same agreement. Mutual commitment to agreed objectives with accountability and responsibility set out for each partner. There will be clarity on incentives and penalties by achieving or not accomplishment of goals.
- **Defined authority:** A public-private partnership is a long-term arrangement between a government and private sector institutions. Typically, it involves private capital financing government projects and services up-front, and then drawing revenues from taxpayers and/or users over the course of the PPP contract. There should be clear defined authority and a clear understanding of the responsibilities and obligations between partners which will be also scribed in contract paper
- **Specified time period:** Always the agreement is applicable for a specific time period. It may extends days to years based on the types of agreement or services provided.
- **Allocation of risk:** There is well defined allocation of risk between the private sector and the public entity. The private partner faces availability risk if it cannot provide the service as promised. Demand risk occurs when there are fewer users than expected for the services.
- **Predetermined benchmarks:** Benchmarks means something that serves as a standard by which others may be measured or judged. In public-private partnership model there should be Predetermined Benchmarks by which the whole programme can be monitored and evaluated. There will be a strong management information system to evaluate whole performance.
- **Performance-linked payment to private sectors:** Public-private partnership model is a limited period of contractual arrangement where a private sector entity provides an asset or service which is traditionally provided by the government in return of some performance-based payment

Approaches of Establishing a Partnership

Conceptually, there are three approaches of establishing a partnership with the private sector, namely:

1. **Competitive bidding:** This refers to a well-designed bidding process to ascertain the capabilities of the service provider. The selection of the service provider is done amongst the bidders depending on the lowest bid in terms of operation and maintenance cost and highest equity premium and revenue share.
2. **Competitive negotiation:** This approach is a variant of the competitive bidding, difference being that the government negotiates the contract with the bidders. The negotiation can be direct or indirect type, which involves a master contractor who handles the dealings with all the subcontractors of the services. Hence, the government monitors the master contractor and not all subcontractors.
3. **Swiss challenge approach:** In this approach the government receives a proposal from the private sector stating all the details regarding its technical, financial and managerial capabilities and viability. If the proposal meets the priorities of the policy, then the government may invite counter proposals from other parties. In case a better proposal is received, the original proponent is given an opportunity to modify its proposal and the better of the two is selected.

Benefits of Public Private Partnerships (PPP)

- **Increase in efficiency:** When the existing services fails to reach all people or Government on its own cannot always fully address the most needy population and to set minimum standard for quality of services and legal regulation, pooling of resources can help in addressing the issues that cannot be addressed by a single entity. Upgrading the health infrastructure wherever the government's funding lacks will improve the quantity and quality of service.
- **Improved accessibility:** These partnerships work well when private sector technology and innovation combine with public sector incentives to complete work on time and within budget. The private entity working closely with public sector will expand the reach of the health services to hard to reach areas.
- **Improved affordability:** Only about 20% of Indian's have any form of health insurance. 16 PPP will reduce the burden of 80% out of pocket expenditure (OOPE) incurred on the people who are forced to seek services

from the unregulated private sector. For mutual benefits (cost, manpower and financial resources) and to improve Consumer's involvement in planning and monitoring of services, this is essential.

- **Risk sharing:** It will motivate the establishment of partnership with new and emerging private sector, unloading the burden and instead promoting the financial and operational risk sharing between the partners.
- **Improved coverage of national health programs:** Engagement with the private sector will not only promote the coverage of national health programs, but also assist in delivery of the services along with its monitoring and evaluation.
- **Implementation of standard treatment guidelines:** Partnership with the private healthcare professionals will aid in implementing similar standard treatment guidelines in both public and private health sectors thereby ensuring uniform quality of services.
- **Scale-up successful operational models:** Private sector expertise and successful experiences can be utilized in PPP projects implementation and vice- versa.
- **Global epidemic management:** In view of the current incidence of COVID-19, SARS and Dengue for Global epidemic management this is the ideal model. It is the result of increased global integration due to globalization.

Challenges in PPP

In the process of PPP, from planning to implementation, including monitoring and evaluation, there are a number of challenges need to be addressed.

- Of utmost importance is the assessment of needs based on which the PPP model is prepared. This will not only address the needs of the people, but also lead to enhanced participation of the community and reduce the opposition by the stakeholders.
- Achieving appropriate allocation of risks is another challenge. It calls for a robust analytic approach, involving both, individual project risks and aggregate PPP program risks, so as to assess the feasibility and terms based on which the risk may be allocated to the partners. This forms an essential part of strategic planning.
- A strong political commitment is a challenge that needs to be addressed and it calls for the development of PPP policy and institutional framework. This will enable managing communication and public acceptability of PPP.
- Clear messages for policy makers should be used to explain the rationale for PPPs. A PPP Unit can be useful in developing and supporting a communication strategy to underpin the PPP program based on sound technical and data input.
- The PPP Unit can also be available to provide answers to enquiries from parliamentary representatives and citizens. It is also required to manage the stakeholders, i.e., to look into the queries and concerns of those involved in the PPP program, so that the concerns can be addressed, better clarity be provided and acted upon appropriately without delay.

Public-Private-Partnership Models

Franchising

- Franchise is a business model where the franchiser grants exclusive rights to franchisees to conduct business in a prescribed manner over a specified period
- The franchisees contribute resources of their own to set up a clinic and pay membership to franchiser.

Social Marketing

- Application of marketing techniques to achieve a social objective
- Associated with expanding access to contraceptives and medicine
- The trend is to increase the available products, including oral rehydration solution, IFA tablets and other health products to make marketing more self-sustaining
- Social marketing and social franchise program in Bihar
- It combines social marketing with a clinic-based service delivery program and a franchisee program through which doctors in rural areas provide low-cost services
- Medicine centers sells condoms, pills and pregnancy test kit
- Supplies contraceptives to both rural and urban pharmacies and shops.

Contracting Out

- Contracting out refers to situation in which private providers receive a budget to provide services and manage a government health unit.
- Identify those government health clinics that need to be contracted out
- Vacancies for a long period, high absenteeism, and consistent low performance on all RCH indicators could be the critical criteria
- Telediagnosis and consultation in cardiac care and specialist care. Free diagnosis, medicines and treatment for BPL patients.

Contracting In

Hiring of one or more agencies or individuals to provide services.

Example: Hiring of medical specialists for certain days of the week in PHC or CHC.

Joint Ventures

- Joint venture companies are companies launched with equity participation of government and private sector.
- Joint venture companies, in most cases have not succeeded due to lack of understanding and trust between partners.

Example: The Rajiv Gandhi Super-specialty Hospital in Raichur Karnataka is a joint venture of Govt. of Karnataka and

Apollo Hospitals Group, with financial support from OPEC (Organization of Petroleum Exporting Countries).

Voucher Schemes

- Government of Andhra Pradesh has initiated Arogya Raksha Scheme in collaboration with New India Assurance Company and with private clinics.
- It is an insurance scheme fully funded by government.
- It provides hospitalization benefits and personal accident benefits to citizens below the poverty line
- The government paid an insurance premium of ₹75 per family to insurance company.

Running Mobile Health Units

- Mobile medical unit for a voucher is a document that can be exchanged for defined services as a token of payment
- Package can be bought, used when required and ensures privacy for the client.

Example: Chiranjeevi Yojna in Gujarat

Chiranjeevi Yojna Scheme

- Launched in Gujarat 2005
- **Aim:** Improve access of poor
- Families (BPL) to institutional delivery
- Form of partnership: Voucher scheme to involve private providers in delivering maternity care
- **Reasons for contracting:** High maternal mortality, low institutional delivery, involving large groups of private practitioners
- **Financing:** NRHM and state budget.

Build, Operate and Transfer (BOT)

- BOT models are highly successful in infrastructure development sector
- Financing of projects by government, subsidized land at prime locations
- These models are useful to establish large hospitals and ensure quality services at reasonable rates to poor people
- Vans go to identified central points on fixed days and provide primary health services to a cluster of villages.
- Vehicle, medical equipments, medicine will be provided by govt. and primary healthcare services will be provided by NGOs
- Bihar adopted the scheme under the name "Arogya Rath" and in Madhya Pradesh under the name "Deen Dayal Chalit Aspatal Yojana".

Community-based Health Insurance

- Government pays health insurance premium for families below poverty line. These families in turn are insured against expenses on health and hospitalization, up to a certain amount.
- Community members pay a minimum insurance premium per month and get insured against certain level of health expenditure
- Community-based schemes ensure that local needs and expectations of people are met.

Example: Rashtriya Swasthya Bima Yojna (RSBY).

ORGANIZATION AND ADMINISTRATION OF NURSING SERVICE

Sir William Osler said that the nurse is one of the greatest blessings of humanity. Nursing has a large, important and unique role in the healthcare delivery system of a country. Nursing care is extremely important for good patient outcome. The success of patient care depends upon the competence of the nursing staff. Nursing service is one service which must be maintained continuously throughout the 24-hour-period (round the clock), 365 days a year.

Nursing is defined as an art and science which involves the whole patient's body, mind and spirit, promotes spiritual, mental and physical health by teaching and by example; stresses health education and health preservation, as well as ministrations to the sick; involves the care of the patient's environment—social and spiritual as well as physical—and gives health care to the family and community as well as to the individual.

In a hospital, many variable factors influence the number of nurses which are needed in a ward in order to render a high quality of nursing care.

These factors are:

- The type of service, i.e., medical, surgical, obstetrics and gynecology, pediatrics, psychiatry, etc.
- The acuteness of the services and the rate of turnover in patients according to the degree or period of illness.
- The experience of the nurses who are to give the patient care.
- The number of non-nurses who are involved in the patient care, the quality of their work, their stability in services.
- The amount and quality of teaching which proceeds the assignment of personnel to the service as well as that given as inservice preparation.

Objectives of Nursing Service Administration

The first essential component of nursing service administration is the planning and it should be based on clearly defined objectives. The objectives of the nursing services department are as follows:

In Relation to Patient Care

The primary emphasis is on total patient care, that is:

- To give the highest possible quality of nursing care in terms of total patient's needs, which include physical, psychological, social and educational, and spiritual needs by collaborating with other health team members
- To assist the physician in providing medical care to the patients
- To provide preventive and rehabilitative services
- To provide round-the-clock nursing care to all the patients
- To render timely and appropriate nursing service to the emergency patients

- To provide cost-effective quality care as per the needs of the patients in a hospital
- Each patient should be treated with dignity and respect
- Each patient and family needs to be treated with compassion and concern
- Confidentiality and privacy of each patient should be maintained
- Constant monitoring and evaluation is of utmost importance to improve patient care continuously.

In Relation to Education

- Planning of education and training program for nurses is a must for professional growth and development needs through inservice education and research support
- To provide regular staff development in the inservice education and guidance services for all members of nursing staff
- To conduct regular orientation program for new entrants and for those who are on the job for a long time
- To conduct training for operating procedure of latest gadgets and on handling of sophisticated biomedical equipment.

In Relation to Administration and Organization

- To make regular supervision through rounds
- To ensure that the essential equipment are provided in functional status for nursing care services
- To provide regular flow of essential supplies for rendering quality nursing care
- To have a proper system of rotation of staff, provision for annual leave and days off for members of nursing staff without hampering patient care
- To ensure that nursing procedures, manuals and other manuals concerning nursing matters are available to the nurses for reference
- To establish a communication system for nursing personnel, other health workers, patients, health authorities, government authorities and public
- To ensure that each nurse identifies her job responsibilities and accountability
- Collective decision-making, progressive environment, utilization of current biotechnology
- Counseling for health personnel, patients and the public
- To provide financial personnel, patients and the public
- To provide financial resources and procure
- The formulation of policies, standards, goals, nursing services, education and practice
- To maintain proper documentation of the personnel employed in the nursing service.

In Relation to Research

- To establish a system for collection of essential information, research and studies concerning all aspects of nursing
- To encourage and support the nurses to conduct research projects/activities.

In Relation to Performance Appraisal

- Appraise the performance of nursing service personnel regularly against set standards and performance indicators objectively with a view to maintain quality nursing services.

  Nursing plays a pivotal role in the healthcare delivery system of the society. Odisha is the first state in the country to have a fully functional Directorate of Nursing with effect from 18th February, 2013. Directorate of Nursing is one of the Directorates within the Ministry of Health and Family Welfare. The Directorate of Nursing is the central body from which all the activities relating to nursing are managed. This includes all involving nursing and midwifery practices, providing primary health care and fulfilment of Millennium Development Goal on reduction of maternal and child mortality.

  Directorate of Nursing consists of the following functional wings:
- Nursing Council
- Nursing Board
- Nursing Management Support Unit (NMSU)
- Nursing Establishment and Administration.

The mandate: A fully functional and empowered Directorate of Nursing with:

- The best quality of education (including skills and competencies) being imparted in the nursing institutions
- Confident and competent Clinical Nursing services being rendered at the hospitals in the state
- A public health nursing cadre providing the best available services to public health in the field and ensuring the full benefits of all the government initiatives reach the beneficiaries as envisaged.

To strengthen the Directorate of Nursing, the following three broad areas are being strengthened:

1. Clinical nursing
2. Nursing education
3. Public health nursing

Placement of Nurses in a Healthcare Organization

The placement of nurses in a Healthcare Organization is given in **Flowcharts 9.4 and 9.5**.

At the Central and State Level

- At the central level, there is a post of nursing adviser in the medical division of DGHS
- Nursing Adviser is directly responsible to the Deputy Director General (medical)
- Nursing Adviser is assisted by nursing officer and support staff for all works
- She/he advises the DGHS, the Ministry of Health and Family Welfare as well as other ministries, other department like railways, labor, Delhi Administration/ Municipal Corporation of Delhi, etc.
- She/he also advises on all matters of nursing services, nursing education and research, etc.

Flowchart 9.4: Recommended organizational set-up of the Directorate General of Health Services (DGHS) and Institution under the Central Government (for Nursing Profession).

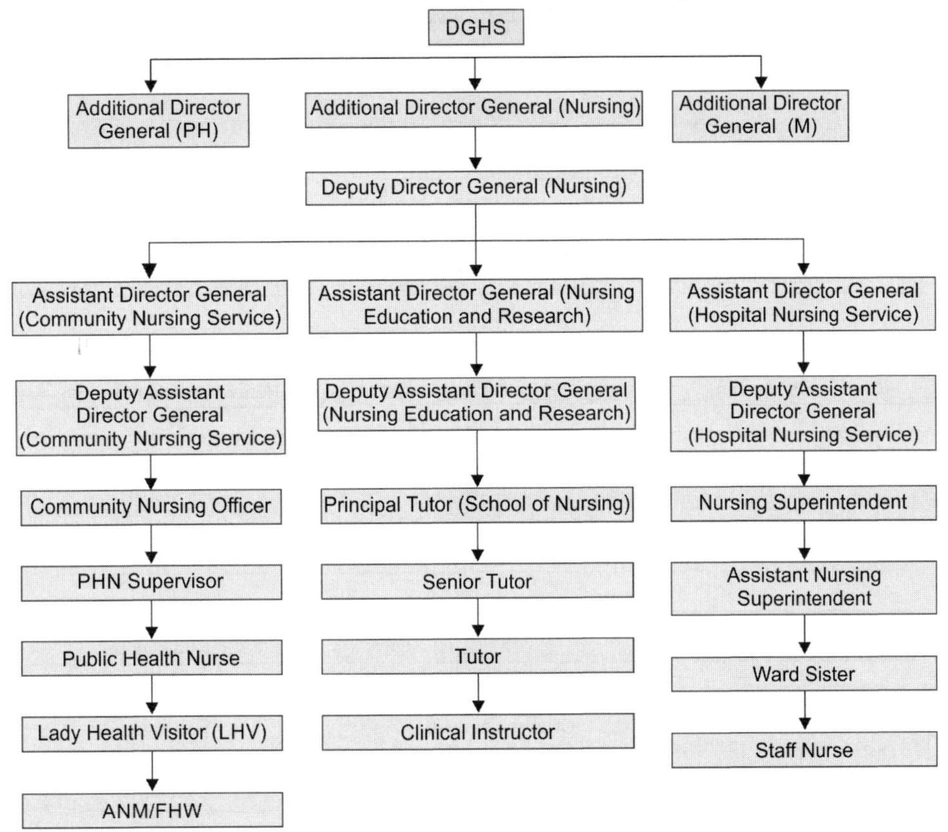

- Deputy Nursing Adviser at the rank of Assistant Director General (ADG-Nursing) in the Training division of the Department of Family Welfare.
- Presently, the Deputy Nursing Adviser deals with training of ANMs, dais, health supervisors, etc.
- In general, the high-power committee after careful examination of the organizational set-up at central, state, and district levels, found that the nursing positions in each of these settings are very low, designation-wise as well as salary-wise.
- They all have work responsibility but no limited authority and no uniformity for the nursing position.
- The committee recommended the organizational set-up at the central, state and district levels.

The recommended organizational set-up will need full administrative and financial support of the Government. It will look after the overall nursing components, development of nursing standards, norms, polices, recruitment, selection and placement rules for both hospital and community health nursing, etc., developments in specialty nursing, higher education in nursing and research, etc. These will promote professional autonomy and accountability.

At the District Level

In both the urban and rural areas of the district nurses, PHNs, LHVs, ANMs, etc., have played a vital role in providing healthcare services at various levels. They have been in the mainstream in providing primary healthcare services in the rural and urban areas from the very beginning.

Today, the ANM designated as a multipurpose health worker female is the key health worker rendering multipurpose healthcare services in the rural area. The professional nurses have a major role to play in providing support, guidance, supervision, etc. to ANMs [MPHW (F)].

The only professional public health nurse is at the district level in the district family welfare bureau, which is being created under the MPHWs' scheme and funded through the family welfare budget. Her major areas of responsibility are:

- Administration and management of nursing and midwifery services in the district
- Supervision and guidance of health supervisor/PHNS, etc.
- Inservice training program for nurses, PHNs, ANMs, and LHVs working in her district
- Attending to problems relating to health in her district, referred to her
- Participation in teaching program of the schools of nursing
- Helps in organizing community health nursing field experience for the nursing students
- Helps in collection and compiling reports from CHC/PHC in the district
- Conducts/assists in conducting field studies
- Plans and conducts evaluation program.

Flowchart 9.5: Recommended organizational set-up at the state and union territory level (for nursing profession).

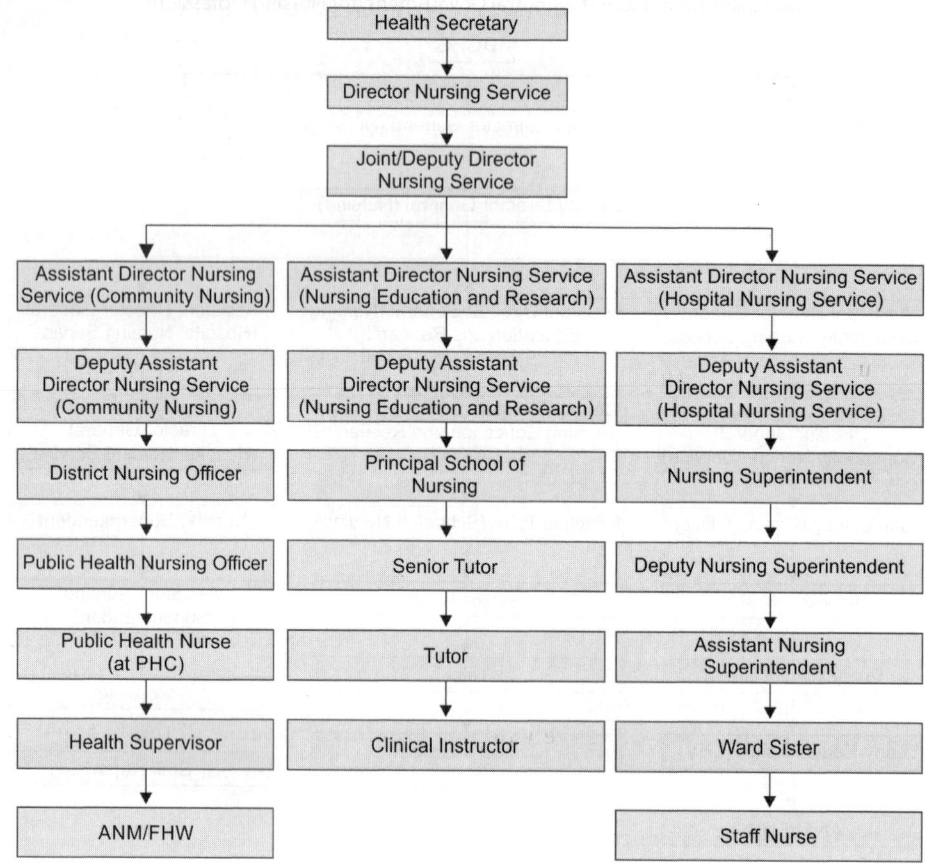

As reported by the high power committee on nursing, the district public health nurses face many problems, such as roles and functions not being clear, very low status being ascribed in the organizational set-up, transport not available for supervisory activities, lack of accommodation, nonpayment of travel allowance, etc. There is no coordination between the nurses at the district and state level in all the states, except in Maharashtra and West Bengal.

SYSTEM OF MEDICINE

It is a well-known fact that Traditional Systems of medicines always played important role in meeting the global healthcare needs. They are continuing to do so at present and shall play major role in future also. The system of medicines which are considered to be Indian in origin or the systems of medicine, which have come to India from outside and got assimilated in to Indian culture are known as Indian Systems of Medicine. There is a variety of system of medicine among which the allopathic medicine is quite effective in treating numerous physical ailments, but it is less effective in preventing illness, decreasing stress-induced illness, managing chronic disease and caring for the emotional and spiritual need of the individual. So, the number of clients seeking unconventional treatment has risen considerably. Though allopathic system of medicine is practiced in treating major disease and saving life still the contribution of other system is not negligible.

ALLOPATHIC MEDICINE

'Allopathic medicine' refers to the practice of conventional medicine that uses pharmacologically active agents or physical interventions to treat or suppress symptoms or pathophysiologic processes of diseases or conditions. It was coined by Samuel Hahnemann (1755–1843), a homeopath, in 1810. Although 'allopathic medicine' was rejected as a term by mainstream physicians, it was adopted by alternative medicine advocates to refer pejoratively to conventional medicine.

Allopathic medicine often refers to 'the broad category of medical practice that is sometimes called Western medicine, biomedicine, evidence-based medicine, or modern medicine'.

Allopathic medicine and allopathy (from the Greek prefix 'állos', 'other', 'different' + the suffix páthos, 'suffering') are terms coined in the early 19th century by Samuel Hahnemann, the founder of homeopathy, as a synonym for mainstream medicine. Allopathy was coined in 1842 by CFS Hahnemann to designate the usual practice of medicine.

Definition

Allopathic medicine is defined as 'the system of medical practice which treats disease by the use of remedies, which produce effects different from those produced by the disease under treatment.

Advantages of Allopathy

- Appropriate treatment
- During illness, it relives the systems
- Satisfaction of the treatment
- Get fast reliefs and miraculous care
- Advanced diagnostic methodology and treatment
- Large number of allopathic hospitals and easily accessible to people
- High-quality care can be provided.

Disadvantages of Allopathy

- Dangers of medication
- Overspecialization and technology.

There are three levels of healthcare service delivered by using allopathic medicine and treatment:

1. Primary-level Health Care
2. Secondary-level Health Care
3. Tertiary-level Health Care.

COMPLIMENTARY AND ALTERNATIVE SYSTEM OF MEDICINE

Definitions

Allopathic medicine has been dominant about 100 years. Allopathic medical care is particularly effective when aggressive treatment is needed in emergency. Allopathic has not been very effective in dealing with chronic illness. Increasingly, CAT is being used as an 'answer' to the problem of chronic illness.

A variety of terms have been used to describe health-related approaches that are considered outside the mainstream of the dominant system of health care. The terms currently used in Western cultures to describe such approaches include alternative, nontraditional, unconventional, holistic and natural. Currently, the most frequently used term to refer to such modalities and practices is complementary and alternative therapies.

Complementary and alternative medicine (CAM) includes various healing approaches and therapies that originate from around the world and that are not based on conventional Western medicine. These therapies are called alternative medicine when they are used alone and complementary medicine when they are used with conventional medicine.

Complementary Therapy

Complementary therapy is that therapy used in addition to conventional treatment recommend by the person's healthcare provider.

Alternative Therapy

It includes the same intervention as complementary therapies but frequently becomes the primary treatment that replaces allopathic medical care.

Objectives

- Relieve tension and other symptoms
- Relax, revitalize and nurture
- Improve circulation and revitalize
- Support psychoneuroimmunological response
- Release negativity and reaffirm positivity.

Principles

- Illness occurs if the body is out of balance
- Body can heal itself and maintain a healthy state if given the right condition.
- The whole person should be treated not just the disease or the symptoms.
- The gentlest therapies must be tried first before the harsher ones.
- There is no quick-fix since healing takes time.
- Natural products are preferable to synthetic ones.
- Complementary and alternative therapies are based on the body's innate ability to heal itself.
- Natural methods first. Complementary and alternative medicines do not rely on prescription drugs, surgery, and other conventional medical procedures. However, they do not discount the benefits that these procedures can provide when necessary.
- An individualized, comprehensive approach. Complementary and alternative medicine looks at the underlying cause of the problem and addresses the whole person (mind, body, emotions, spirit) without just masking the symptoms.
- The goal is to create optimum health. Complementary and alternative medicine focuses on preventing disease and helping someone feel the best they can as much as treating the disease.

Basic Terms/Concepts

Holism: It refers to the whole of the sick person including his mind, body, and the way of his living meaning that all these to be considered while treating the sick person and not just the symptoms of the disease.

Humanism: A system of thought that considers solving of the human problems with the help of religious beliefs. It emphasizes that the basis nature of humans is good.

Balance: A situation in which all the things exist in equal, correct or good amount.

Reasons to use alternative therapies:

- Reduce side effects of treatment
- Reduce side effects of disease
- Suggestions be family, friends and society
- Philosophical or cultural orientation
- Less expensive than conventional medicine
- Easier access to health food stores than physician
- Dissatisfaction with or loss of trust in conventional medicine
- Desire to treat the disease in a natural way
- Decrease the feelings of hopelessness and helplessness
- Improve the immune system
- Improve the quality of life.

Classification

Alternative Medical System

- Acupuncture
- Ayurveda
- Homeopathy
- Latin American practice
- Native American practice
  - Naturopathic medicine
- Traditional Chinese medicine.

Biologically Based Therapies

- Aroma therapy
- Macrobiotic diet
- Orthomolecular diet
- European phytomedicine
- Traditional Chinese herbal remedies
- Ayurvedic herbs.

Manipulative and Body-based Methods

- Acupressor
- Chiropractic medicine
- Feldenkrais method
- Tai chi
- Massage therapy
- Simple touch.

Mind-body Intervention

- Art therapy
- Biofeedback
- Meditation
- Imagery
- Music therapy
- Yoga
- Psychotherapy.

Energy Therapy

- Therapeutic touch
- Reiki
- Bioelectromagnetic therapy.

AYURVEDA

The word 'Ayurveda' means 'science of life' or 'practices of longevity'. Ayu (life) and veda (knowledge). It was taught by the creator, Brahma, to Daksha Prajapati and carried on by the wise men like Bharadwaja. Dhanvantari is an avatar of Vishnu, God of Ayurvedic medicine, an early Indian medical practitioner, surgeon, a discoverer and a researcher in the field of Ayurveda. Ayurveda is 'the complete knowledge for long life'; or ayurvedic medicine is a system of traditional medicine native to India and a form of alternative medicine. In Sanskrit, word 'āyus' means 'longevity', and 'veda' means 'related to knowledge' or 'science'. The earliest literature on Indian medical practice appeared during the Vedic period in India.

History

Early history of ayurveda asserts that around 1500 BC, ayurveda's fundamental and applied principles got organized and enunciated. In this historical construction, Ayurveda traces its origins to the Vedas, Atharvaveda in particular, and is connected to Hindu religion. Atharvaveda (one of the four most ancient books of Indian knowledge, wisdom and culture) contains 114 hymns or formulations for the treatment of diseases. Ayurveda originated in and developed from these hymns. In this sense, ayurveda is considered by some to have divine origin. It is originated especially in India and is one of the oldest medical systems in the world. Well established around 2500 to 600 BC, evolved into 2 schools—the School of Physicians and the School of Surgeons. Ayurveda is an Upaveda or annexure to the four main vedas (knowledge systems). Famous writings are Charaka Samhita by Sage Charaka regarding prevention and treatment of disease. Sushruta Samhita of Sage Sushruta deals with Ayurvedic surgical procedures. The Sushruta Samhita and the Charaka Samhita are encyclopedias of medicine compiled from various sources from the mid-first BCE to about 500 CE. They are among the foundational works of Ayurveda.

Concept and Basic Principles

Ayurveda says good health is the fundamental prerequisite to acquire materialistic, social and spiritual upliftment of a human being. No mental health without physical health is possible. Diseases result from imbalance in body. Ayurveda focuses on the prevention of disease, and surgical procedures, while restructuring a patient's lifestyle and provision of natural therapies to align it with the course of nature. It holds the importance of eating healthy foods. There are five basic elements—Pancha Mahabhootas, viz. earth (prithvi), water (jala), fire (agni), air (vayu), and space (akash), three humors (tridosha), viz. vata (resembles the classical elements—ether and air), pitta (fire), and kapha (water and earth) in our body. All the bodily processes are believed to be governed by a balance of the three doshas. Whichever dosha appears to dominate a person's behavior and physique is called his constitution type. There are also seven body tissues (saptadhatu), i.e., fluid components of the body (rasa), blood (rakta), muscle tissue (mamsa), adipose tissue (medas), bone tissue (asthi), bone marrow (majja), and reproductive elements (sukra), and three bio-wastes (trimalas), i.e., urine (mootra), feces (pureesha) and sweat (sweda). The essence of saptadhatu called ojas is responsible for immunity and strength. The essence of ayurveda is knowledge and awareness of the qualities of nature, called gurvadi gunah. The gurvadi gunah are listed in Vagbhata's Ashtanga Hridayam as: Guru (heavy), laghu (light), manda (slow), tikshna (quick, sharp), hima (cold), and ushna (hot).

Branches of Ayurveda

There are eight branches of the Ayurveda during the starting period and due to this, the Ayurveda is known as ashtanga. The eight specialties are Kayachikitsa (internal medicine), Balachikitsa (Pediatrics), Graha chikitsa-Bhoota Vidya (psychiatry), Urdhvanga chikitsa (treatment of eyes, ears, nose, throat and head), shalya chikitsa (surgery), Damstra chikitsa-Agada tantra (toxicology), Jara chikitsa-Rasayana (gerontology), Vrishya chikitsa- Vajikarana (aphrodisiacs). During the last 50 years, 16 specialties developed with an addition to eight specialties. The other eight specialties are Ayurveda Sidhantha (fundamentals of Ayurveda), Ras Shatra, Rachna Sharira (anatomy), Krya Sharira (physiology), Swasth vritta (SPM), Rog Nidan (pathology), Prasuti Tantra (obstetrics and gynecology), and Bhaishajya Kalpana (pharmaceuticals).

Diagnosis

- Examination of the patient, i.e., Rogi-pareeksha there are five influential criteria for diagnosis of disease that are identified. These are prodromal (precursory) symptoms, typical symptoms of the fully developed disease, observing the effect of therapeutic procedures, and the pathological process.
- Examination of the disease, i.e., Roga-pareeksha. This is achieved through tenfold examination of patients (dasavidha pareeksha) comprising of constitution (prakriti), disease susceptibility (vikriti), essence (sara), compactness (samhanana), anthropometry (pramana), compatibility (satmya), mind (sattwa), digestion capacity of food (aharasakti), physical strength (vyayamasakti), and age (vaya), with physical, urine, pulse, feces, tongue, eyes, skin, ear and examination of the functions.

Treatment

Therapeutic streams are as follows:
- Therapies with inexplicable mode of action (Daivavyapasraya chikitsa);
- Rationale treatment (Yukti vyapasraya chikitsa); and
- Preventive and remedial measures to psychic disorders (Satwavajaya chikitsa). Rely heavily on plant materials. Botanicals are mixed with metals, minerals or other naturally occurring substances. The diet regimen is as important as remedies. Prescribed doses of medicine are taken to cure them effectively. Ayurvedic medicines do not cause any side effects.

Treatment Procedures

Shodhana (Purification Treatment)—removal of the causative factors by Panchkarma (medically induced emesis, purgation, oil enema, decoction enema and nasal administration of medicines, external and internal oleation and induced sweating). Shamana (palliative treatment), suppression of vitiated humours (doshas). It is achieved by use of appetizers, digestives, exercise and exposure to sun, fresh air, etc.

Nidan parivarjan is to avoid the known disease-causing factors in diet and lifestyle of the patient, to refrain from precipitating or aggravating factors of the disease. Satvavajaya concerns mainly with the area of mental disturbances. It involves restraining mind from desires for unwholesome objects and cultivation of courage, memory, and concentration.

Rasayana therapy deals with promotion of strength and vitality. The integrity of body matrix, promotion of memory, intelligence, immunity against the disease, and the preservation of youth are some of the positive benefits credited to this treatment.

Diet Treatment

In Ayurveda, regulation of diet as therapy has a great importance. This is because it considers human body as the product of food. Lack of nutrients in food or improper transformation of food leads to a variety of disease conditions.

Pathya vyavastha (prescription of diet and activity) comprises indications and contraindications in respect of diet, activity, habits and emotional status. This is done with a view to enhance the effects of therapeutic measures.

Kshara sautra, a procedure using medicated thread, is a unique minimally invasive parasurgical measure being successfully practiced as a promising therapy for anorectal disorders.

Therapeutic Approach

Use of medicines, specific diet and prescribed activity routine are taken into consideration. One approach of treatment is that these three measures work by causing effect opposite to disease counteracting the symptoms called Vipreeta.

In the second approach, they exert effects similar to the disease process known as Vipreetarthkari.

For successful administration of a treatment, four things are essential. These are:
- **The physician:** He possesses technical skill, scientific knowledge, purity and human understanding, humility, wisdom and service to humanity.
- **The medicaments:** Food and drugs—adequate and with quality.
- **The nursing personnel:** Skillful, sympathetic, intelligent, and resourceful.
- **The patient:** Cooperative and obedient, and able to describe ailments.

YOGA

Yoga is a science as well an art of healthy living physically, mentally, morally and spiritually. While Ayurveda performs its panchakarma through the help of emetics, purgative Yoga performs them without the help of any drug, i.e., by developing full efficiency and control of eliminative systems of the body, which no other system of health care can do.

History

The tradition of Yoga was born in India several thousand years ago. Its founders were great saints and sages. Yoga has its origins in the Vedas, the oldest record of Indian culture. It was systematized by the great Indian sage Patanjali in the Yoga Sutra. The fundamental idea behind the practice of yoga is to unite the self/individual (Jiva) with the supreme/pure consciousness (Bramha). It is all about harmonizing the body with the mind and breath through the means of various breathing techniques, yoga postures and meditation/relaxation.

- **Physical posture:** It helps to strengthen and stretch the muscles. It improves mobility, flexibility and balance. This enhances circulation, digestion, respiration and elimination.
- **Breathing technique:** It mainly focuses on awareness of breath and promotes calm, and relieves stress and fatigue.
- **Relaxation technique:** It helps to ease tension.

Principles

Yoga means a holistic approach towards the cause and treatment of a disease. According to Yoga, most of the diseases, whether mental, psychosomatic or physical, originate in one's mind through wrong ways of thinking, living and eating, which is caused by attachment. The basic approach of Yoga is to correct the lifestyle by cultivating a rational, positive and spiritual attitude towards all life situations. Yoga emphasizes the development of brotherhood, harmony, and fraternity.

Yoga is classified under three major headings, such as:

- Patanjali yoga sutras
- Pranayama
- Meditation

But there are many different types of yogas:

- Vikrama yoga
- Hatha yoga
- Vinyasa yoga
- Kundalini yoga
- Ashtanga yoga
- Iyengar yoga
- Anusara yoga
- Restorative yoga
- Jivamukti yoga
- Prenatal yoga

Functions

- It helps to bring more oxygen to the blood and brain.
- It also helps to control prana or the vital life energy
- It purifies and disciplines both mind and body.

Benefits

- Positive results in treating depression.
- Deep breathing helps in control of premature ventricular contraction.
- Beneficial for treating breast cancer.
- Shows significant benefit in mood disturbances, GI disturbances, cognitive function.
- Regular yoga increases body's ability to use antioxidants.
- In case of diabetes, it increases nerve functioning and controls blood sugar.
- It increases hand grip strength among rheumatoid arthritis patients.
- Treating problems like asthma, back pain, and weight reduction.

Criticism

- Practice is impossible if there is limited mobility or flexibility.
- While attempting some of the postures of yoga before pre-exercise preparation, there is a possibility of getting injured.

UNANI

As an alternative form of medicine, Unani has found favor in Asia, especially India. It is close to Ayurveda. It is based on its natural and remarkable diagnostic methods and is affordable. The term 'Unani' is derived from 'Unan', which means 'Greece' in Arabic and Urdu.

History

In Greece, based on the teachings of Hippocrates (460 BC–377 BC), called the 'Father of Medicine' and his disciple Gallen and it developed into an elaborate medical system by the Arabs. In India, Unani system of medicine was introduced by Arabs. After independence, Unani received boost. Today, India is considered a world leader in Unani Medicine.

Concept and Basic Principles

Body is made up of four basic elements, i.e., earth, air, water, and fire, which have different temperaments, i.e., cold, hot, wet, and dry respectively. The body is made up of simple and complex organs. They obtain their nourishment from four humors, namely blood, phlegm, black bile and yellow bile. These humors also have their specific temperament. Disease occurs whenever the balance of humors is disturbed.

Six essentials are required for healthy state: (i) Air; (ii) Food and drink; (iii) Bodily movements and response; (iv) Psychic movement and repose; (v) Sleep and wakefulness; and (vi) Evacuation and retention. The human body has seven components having direct bearing on the health status. These are temperament (mizaj) of the patient; hereditary condition and effects; different complaints, signs and symptoms of the body; external observation; examination of the pulse (nubz); and urine and stool.

Diagnosis

Examination of the pulse for size, strength, speed, consistency, fullness, rate, temperature, constancy, regularity and rhythm, examination of the urine for odor, quantity, mature urine and urine at different age groups. Stool is examined for color, consistency, froth and time required for passage, etc.

Treatment

- Dietotherapy (Ilaj-bil-Ghiza) by administration of specific diets or by regulating the it. Regimental therapy mainly consists of drugless therapy, like exercise, massage, Turkish bath, douches.
- Pharmacotherapy (Ilaj-bid-Dawa) is done by use of herbal drugs derived from plants, animals and mineral origin.

Climatic therapy (Ilaj-bil-Hawa) based on the climatic changes and health.

SIDDHA

The Siddha system is therapeutic in nature. It is in use both in north India, called jhar phuk and siddha buti (medicine) Tantra, and in south India as Tamil traditional medicine. It is medicine that is perfect, to revitalize and rejuvenate dysfunctional disease-causing organs, capable of treating all types of diseases other than the emergency cases.

History

The origin of Siddha system is attributed to Lord Shiva Himself. In India, we have two distinct cultures—one is 'vedic' and the other one is 'tantric'. The sages of south India, who practiced tantrism were called Siddhars. Eighteen Siddhars were said to be there and sage Agasthiya is considered as a father figure of this medical system. This dates back to 3000 BC.

Branches of Siddha

Internal medicine is used through the oral route and is classified into 32 categories. External medicine includes certain forms of drugs and also certain applications, like nasal, eye and ear drops and also certain procedures, like leech application also classified into 32 categories.

Concept and Basic Principles

When the normal equilibrium of three humors (vatha, pitha, and kapha) is disturbed, a disease is caused. Under normal conditions, the ratio between these three humors (vatha, pitha and kapha) is 4: 2: 1 respectively. A particular disorder can be a Vatha, Pitta or Kapha type, or a blend of all three. The environment, climatic conditions, diet, physical activities, and stress are causes associated with diseases. It recognizes predominance of vatham, pitham and kapham in childhood, adulthood and old age respectively, whereas, in Ayurveda, it is totally reversed.

There are seven types of essential tissue. These tissue types are called dathus, which are the following—Rasa (lymph), Kurudhi (blood), Tasai (muscle), Kozhuppu (adipose tissue), Elumbu (bone), Majjai (marrow), Sukkilam and Artavam (sperm and menstrual fluids). Diet and lifestyle play a major role. This concept of the siddha medicine is termed as pathya and apathya, which is essentially a list of dos and don'ts. Summary of humors/elements stationed in a particular part of the human body and corresponding to a particular part of any plant is made.

Diagnosis

Astasthana-pariksa is done. This includes: Na (tongue), Varna (color), Svara (voice), Kan (ears), Sparisam (touch), Mala (stool), Neer (urine), and Nadi (pulse).

Treatment

All the factors leading to diseases are taken into account. Deal with the problems affecting the women's health, venereal diseases, chronic cases of liver, skin diseases, especially 'psoriasis', rheumatic problems, anemia, prostate enlargement, bleeding piles and peptic ulcer. Treatment is classified into three categories—(i) devamaruthuvum (divine method); (ii) manuda maruthuvum (rational method); and (iii) asura maruthuvum (surgical method). Practitioners have claimed that Siddha medicines are effective in reducing the highly debilitating problems that manifest themselves among patients of HIV/AIDS.

Types of Treatment Procedures

Therapeutic Approach

It involves the patient, the attendant, physician and medicine. When the physician is well qualified and the other agents possess the necessary qualities, even severe diseases can be cured easily. The treatment should be commenced as early as possible after assessing the course and cause of the disease.

Homeopathy

Homeopathy is a form of alternative medicine. It is based on the principle of 'like healing like' (Simile Similibus Curentur). Homeopathy believes that a sick person's symptoms are signs of the body's battle against illness and they try to stimulate, rather than suppress this reaction.

History

In the 16th century, the pioneer of chemical medicine, Paracelsus declared that 'small doses of what makes a man ill also cure him', anticipating homeopathy, but it was Hahnemann, who gave it a name and laid out its principles in the late 18th century. Homeopathy achieved its greatest popularity in the 19th century. Dr John Franklin Gray (1804–1882) was the first practitioner of Homeopathy in the United States, beginning in 1828 in New York City. As the time passed by, Homeopathy spread to various countries and came into India and became one of the important parts in the Indian Systems of Medicine.

Concept and Principles

- **Law of susceptibility:** It implies that a negative state of mind can attract hypothetical disease entities called 'miasms' to invade the body and produce symptoms of diseases. A miasm is an imputed 'peculiar morbid derangement of vital force'.
- **Law of similars, otherwise known as 'let like be cured by like':** It is believed that by inducing a disease through use of drugs, the artificial symptoms empowered the vital force to neutralize and expel the original disease and that this artificial disturbance would naturally subside when the dosing ceased.

Treatment

Homeopathic remedies are prepared by serial dilution with shaking by forceful striking, which homeopaths term as 'succussion', after each dilution under the assumption that this increases the effect of the treatment. Homeopathy uses many animal, plant, mineral, and synthetic substances in its remedies. Examples include Arsenicum album (arsenic oxide), Natrum muriaticum (sodium chloride or table salt), and Lachesis muta (the venom of the bushmaster snake).

Some modern homeopaths use remedies of 'imponderables' not originating from a material but from electromagnetic energy presumed to have been 'captured' by alcohol or lactose. Examples include: X-rays and sunlight. Some homeopaths also use techniques that are regarded by other practitioners as controversial. These include paper remedies, where the substance and dilution are written on a piece of paper and either pinned to the patient's clothing, put in their pocket, or placed under a glass of water that is then given to the patient.

Naturopathy

The origin of Indian Naturopathy could be traced right to the Vedic period, wherein Dietary discipline (Pathya and Ahara) and the principles of Health (Swastha Vurtha) described in Ayurveda have branched out and developed in the form of today`s Naturopathy. Naturopathy is a century-old healing discipline that fell from favor about 40 years ago, when drugs and technology became the norm.

History

Naturopathy has its origins in the Nature Cure movement of Europe. The ancient Greek 'Father of Medicine', Hippocrates was the first advocate of naturopathic medicine. Benedict Lust is known as the 'Father of US naturopathy' who also coined the term. He described the body in spiritual and vitalistic terms with 'absolute reliance upon the cosmic forces of a man's nature'. In 1901, Lust founded the American School of Naturopathy in New York.

Concept

The whole practice of Nature cure is based on the following three principles: (i) Accumulation of morbid matter; (ii) Abnormal composition of blood and lymph; and (iii) Lowered vitality. It also believes that human body possesses inherent self-constructing and self-healing powers. It does not believe in specific cause and specific treatment but takes into account the totality of factors. It believes in stimulating body's power to regain health with the help of earth, water, air, fire, and ether. Call to 'Return to Nature' and resort to living in harmony with the self, society and environment.

Diagnosis

Full life case history—covering all the facts of life, since birth. Facial diagnosis—the science of facial expressions by studying the various characteristic features upon the body. Iris diagnosis—study of iris indicating the condition of various visceral organs. Modern clinical diagnosis to some extent.

Treatment

- Water Therapy; Fire Therapy; Air Therapy
- Space Therapy; Mud Therapy; Food Therapy
- Massage Therapy; Acupressure; Magnetotherapy; Chromotherapy.

SOWA-RIGPA

'Sowa-Rigpa', commonly known as Tibetan or Amchi medicine, is the traditional medicine of the Himalayan region. Sowa-Rigpa means 'science of healing' and the practitioners of this medicine are known as Amchi (superior to all). In India, this system of medicine has been popularly practiced in Ladakh and Paddar-Pangay regions of Jammu and Kashmir, and also in Himachal Pradesh, Arunachal Pradesh, Sikkim, Darjeeling-Kalingpong (WB), and now in Tibetan settlements all over India and abroad.

History

It originated from India. It was amended and enriched with other medical traditions, like Chinese, Persian and Tibetan folk medicine to make it most effective and more suitable to the socioclimatic conditions of Tibet. From Tibet, the impact of Sowa-Rigpa along with Buddhism and other Tibetan art and sciences spread to the neighboring Himalayan regions, like Mongolia, Bhutan, Nepal, China and some parts of former Soviet Union, etc.

Concept

Sowa-Rigpa is a rich accumulation of science, art and philosophy with history of continuous practice and progress for more than 2,500 years. It is a science because it is based on systematical and logical framework of understanding the body, disease and its relationship with the environment. It is an art because the diagnostic techniques and composition of medicine, etc. are based on the creativity, immensity, delicacy and compassion of the medical practitioner. It is based on philosophy because it follows the key Buddhist principles of self-sacrifice, karma and ethics, etc.

Basic Principles

It is believed that whether we are physically healthy or not, all of us are sick until we attain Nirvana, and even though disease might not manifest. Ignorance gives rise to three basic illnesses: (i) Nespa-gsum (Tri-dosha/Three humours), i.e Dod-chags (desire/lust), root cause of lung problems (Air/Vata); (ii) Zes dang (anger), root cause of mkris-pa (Pitta, Bile); and (iii) Ti-mug (mental darkness), root cause of pad-kan (Kapha, Phlegm). The animate and inanimate phenomena of the universe are composed of same material basis of Jung-wa-lna (English—five elements; Sanskrit—Panch-mhabhuta), namely sa, chu, mai, rlung and nam-mkha (roughly translated as earth, water, fire, air and space; Sanskrit—Dharti, Jal, Agni, Vayu and Akash).

Diagnosis

Visual diagnosis—tongue examination and urinalysis; Diagnosis by touch—pulse (preparatory conduct, proper time for examination, place, pressure of physician's fingers, technique, constitutional pulse, astonishing pulse, general and specific pulse, death pulse etc.), temperature; Diagnosis by questioning—history of case, present condition, family background and changes in body.

Treatment

Diet, behavior, medicine and accessory/external therapies, minor ailments with regulation of diet and behavior. Medium state of condition can be treated with medicines, like decoction, powder, pills, purgatives, emetics, etc. Advanced stage diseases can be cured by the application of accessory/ external therapies, like massage, surgery, etc. Treatment of diseases is also possible under the three-humor basis. Buddhist rituals and mantras also play a very important role.

Golden Triangle Partnership

The Golden Triangle Partnership concept emerged in a National Workshop on Ayurveda Research organized at Chitrakoot from 24th to 26th May, 2003, where it was decided to set up an integrated technology mission for the development of Ayurveda and traditional medical knowledge based on synchronized working of modern medicine, traditional medicine and modern science with special budgetary support.

Modern Scenario

Increased side effects, lack of curative treatment for several chronic diseases, high cost of new drugs, microbial resistance and emerging diseases are some reasons for renewed public interest in Ayurvedic medicine. Global acceptance of Ayurveda is gearing up. Ayurveda physicians are in great demand in Germany, Russia, Singapore, Malaysia, the United States (US) and the West Asian countries. There has been increased interest among the healthcare professionals, researchers as well as the consumers about Ayurveda.

Ayurveda practices and disciplines should be closely examined by modern medicine. With the use of herbs, vegetable drugs, and natural practices, the Indian medicine has shown much value for western medicine to follow.

AROMA THERAPY

It is based on the theory that certain fragrances can change the way you feel and help them deal with stress or to help with fatigue.

The smell used in aroma therapy comes from plant oils, and they can be inhaled (breathed in) or used in baths or massages.

MACROBIOTIC DIET

A macrobiotic diet is a dietary regimen, which involves eating grain as a staple food, supplemented with other foods, such as local vegetables and avoiding the use of highly processed or refined food and most animal products. Macrobiotic diet planner also addresses the manner of eating and chewing thoroughly.

Historical Development

Christoph Wilhelm Hufeland, a German physician, in his book 'The Art of Prolonging Human Life' (1797) first used the word 'macrobiotics' in the context of food and health.

General guidelines for Japanese style macrobiotic diet include:

- **Whole cereal (Brown rice):** 40–60%
- **Vegetables:** 25–30%
- **Beans and legumes:** 5–10%
- **Miso soup:** 5%
- **Sea vegetables:** 5%
- **Traditional and natural processed food:** 5–10%.

Cooking Methods According to Various Seasons

- **In spring:** Lightly fermented, greens, steaming
- **In summer:** Lighter quality, greens, sweet corn, light grain, barley, summer pumpkin, steaming, etc.
- **In autumn:** Food with more concentrated quality, root vegetables, heavier grains, like millet and sweet rice
- **In winter:** Food with stronger and concentrated quality, round vegetables and roots, pickles, oilseeds, fried rice, and heavier grain.

Factors to be Considered

- Season, climate
- Age, sex, activity
- Health conditions

Complications

- Strict macrobiotic diet that includes no animal product may result in nutritional deficiency
- The deficiency may be worse for people with cancer, who may need more nutrition and calories
- Malnutrition among children.

ORTHOMOLECULAR DIET

This therapy is based on the promise that each individual has unique needs for various nutrients based in part on environmental pollution.

Focus

Achieving the nutritional balance by administering substances, like vitamins, minerals, essential amino acids and fats.

History

'Ortho' is a Greek word, meaning 'right'.

Dr FR Klenner was one of the first doctors to put this concept and put mega dose of vitamin C to a polio patient during 1948. In 1969, Linus Pauling championed in Vitamin C and other vitamin supplements for the prevention and care of the nervous diseases.

Treatment Modalities

- Physical examination and medical history: It includes extensive discussion on diet and lifestyle
- Blood test to see different levels of vitamin C and minerals in the body
- After evaluation, they prescribe vitamins in mega dose that is more than the RDA value
- They can titrate the amount and frequency of the therapy to fine-tune the treatment plan
- Treatment varies from person to person as they have unique biochemistry that is influenced by genetic variability and their absorption and effective process also vary.

Uses

- Vitamin C administration in case of polio
- Vitamin A in symptomatic HIV children
- Vitamin E in heart disease
- Copper therapy in behavioral disorders among children and schizophrenia
- Niacin in schizophrenia.

Limitations

Some nutrients, if taken in mega dose, may cause cancer.

Complications

- Coronary heart disease (CHD)
- Hypertension (HTN)
- Kidney stone
- Thrombophlebitis
- Peripheral neuropathy
- Jaundice and liver toxicity
- Spontaneous abortion
- Gout and ataxia.

EUROPEAN PHYTOMEDICINES

These comprise the use of plants as medicine based on traditional wisdom or understanding with scientific medicine.

Concepts

- The vital force and healing power of nature
- The treatment is not on the disease.

Practice

- It is a whole patient-centered approach in which the patient rather than the disease is the focus of the practitioner
- Background data of the client is collected by history taking (family, health, personal lifestyle)
- Therapy is directed on cause and not on symptoms.

Duration of Treatment

- Depends on individuals and their conditions
- Improvement in symptoms should be noted in an hour or a day for flu-like symptoms and 4–6 weeks in case of chronic illness.

Phytomedicine is Safe

It is very safe if prescribed by a fully qualified practitioner.

Uses

- Menstrual disorder
- Herat disease (Digoxin).

TRADITIONAL CHINESE HERBAL MEDICINE

The system of herbal medicine makes almost an exclusive use of herbal combination. This system is not designed to treat a specific illness, it is rather designed to treat an individual.

History

- In ancient herbology, focus was on the portion whose function was partly medicinal and partly magical, but it lacked theoretical basis
- During 2nd century BC and 2nd century AD, it gave emphasis on acupuncture only
- During 12th century AD, deeper principles of Chinese medicine fully applied to herbal treatment
- In China, Traditional Chinese Herbal Medicine (TCHM) is used alongside with conventional pharmaceutical treatment.

Principles

Health exists when the body is balanced and its energy is freely flowing. The term 'energy' refers to 'Qi', the life energy that is said to animate the body. The term 'balance' refers to the relative factor of 'yin and yang', i.e., the opposite force of the world. In an ideal state, both the yin and yang form a balanced state.

Usage

- Liver disease (hepatitis and cirrhosis)
- Sexual dysfunction in males
- Infertility among women
- Insomnia
- Cold and flu
- Diabetes mellitus, asthma, osteoarthritis
- Irregular menstruation
- Cancer
- Constipation.

Notes

- Acupuncture is often used along with herbs as a supplemental treatment
- Counsel to change the living situation, e.g., movement from basement to first floor/face the bed to south rather than north
- Exercise, e.g., Tai Chi and qigong are also recommended.

Safety Issue

- As multiple herbs are used, so risk for harm is more.
- May result in deposition of Hg, Pb as our body
- Coltsfoot (Tussilago farfara) used in Chinese cough syrup contains Pyrolizidine, which over time damages the liver.

ACUPRESSURE

- It has the same principles like acupuncture but without using needles.
- It is a traditional Chinese medical theory describing special acupoints or acupressure points that lie along the meridians or channels in your body.
- It is believed that through these invisible channels flows vital energy, or a life force called Qi.
- It is also believed that 12 major meridians connect to specific organ or network of organs, organizing a system of communication throughout your body. The meridians begin at finger tips, connect to your brain and then connect to an organ associated with certain meridians.
- If any one of the meridians is blocked or out of balance, illness can occur and acupressure can restore the balance.

Instruments Used for Acupressure

- Acuball
- Energy roller
- Power mat/pyramid mat
- Spine roller.

Uses

- Acupressure wrist band for motion sickness
- Postoperative nausea
- Low back pain
- Large intestine: LR4
- Liver: LR3
- Spleen: SP6.

CHIROPRACTIC MEDICINE

It is a branch of the healing art, which is concerned with human health and prevention of disease. Chiropractic medicine pays special attention to spinal biomechanics, musculoskeletal, neurological, vascular and nutritional relationship.

Evolution

It was developed by Daniel David Palmer in Lowa in 1895.

Principles

- It is a holistic therapy which recognizes the overall health of the patient and the bodies' innate ability to heal itself from physical, mental and emotional stress, and trauma.
- This branch of medicine is concerned with the relationship between spinal column, afferent and efferent nerve, and the entire nervous system.
- It is believed that the misalignment of the spinal cord affects other portions of the body and creates pain as well as musculoskeletal abnormality.
- According to Chiropractic medicine, pathologic disease may be influenced by:
  - Disturbances in the nervous system
  - Improper rest and lack of exercise
  - Genetic/hereditary factor
  - Inadequate or improper nutrition
  - Food tainted by fertilizers, pesticides, herbicides, preservatives, etc.
  - Air/water pollution
  - Stress and bodily trauma
  - Bacteria and viruses.

Palmer felt that the task of chiropractic was not to treat the condition but to remove the nerve interference caused by subluxation, so that the body's inherent capacity to heal itself would be restored.

Diagnosis

- History
- Physical examination
- Neuromuscular examination
- Biochemical/X-ray test
- Menstrual history
- Behavioral history.

Clinical Application

- **Osteology:** Neck and jaw pain, low back pain, osteoporosis, fracture, sprain
- **Joints:** Arthritis, sports injury
- **Vascular:** HTN, arrythmia, Raynaud's disease
- **Digestive:** Colic, hiccups
- **Respiratory:** Asthma, common cold, sinusitis
- **Urinary:** Bed-wetting
- **Reproductive:** Menorrhagia, impotence
- **Skin:** Postsurgical scar
- **Nervous system:** Depression, sleep disorder, convulsion, headache.

Limitation

Disease conditions, like cancer, muscle and bone cancer need referral to medical physician.

FELDENKRAIS METHOD

It is a unique and practical way to realize our potential fully.

- It is based on establishment of good self-image through awareness and correction of body movement that will enhance functioning.
- The technique integrates understanding physics of body movement pattern with an awareness of the way people learn, behave and interact.

Evolution

It is named after its originator, Moshe Feldenkrais (1904–1984), an engineer and physicist as well as a Judo teacher.

Benefits

- Relief from tension and muscle pain
- Eases breathing
- Greater relaxation and well-being
- Improved performance in music, drama, sports and dance
- Eases everyday activity
- Increased vitality.

TAI CHI

It is an ancient system of exercise that incorporates slow and graceful movement integrated with focused breathing and visualization to stimulate the flow of Qi, which further leads to increased self-awareness, vitality, oxygenation of blood, resistance to disease and improved sleep.

Principles

- It consists of sequence of standardized movements known as 'form'.
- The movement is precise and synchronized with breathing.
- It is done in slow velocity without use of special cloth/equipment.

Application

- Promotion of relaxation and better spinal flexibility
- Reduce pain
- Improve posture
- Increase balance and decrease fall.

MASSAGE THERAPY

In massage therapy, a trained therapist presses, rubs and otherwise manipulates the muscles and other soft tissues of the body. He often uses his hands and fingers. He may also use his elbow, forearm and feet.

History

- It evolved around 1000 years back in India, Egypt, and Greece
- In 1850s, two American physicians studied in Sweden and introduced massage therapy in USA.

Types

- **Sports massage:** Adapted to the need of the athletes
- **Swedish massage:** Uses long strokes, kneading, deep circular movements, vibration and tapping
- **Deep tissue massage:** Focuses on myofascial trigger points.

Effects of Massage

It has two types of responses:

1. **Mechanical response:** Results from pressure and movements as soft tissues are manipulated.
2. **Reflex response:** Stimulates the nerves.

Effects on Muscular System

- Relieves muscle tightness, stiffness, spasm
- Increases flexibility in muscle due to muscular relaxation
- Increases blood circulation, bringing more oxygen and nutrients to muscles. So, it reduces muscle fatigue and soreness.
- Promotes removal of toxins and waste products from the body.

Effects on CVs

- Improves circulation by promoting venous drainage.
- Dilates blood vessels and helping them to work more efficiently.
- Temporary decrease of blood pressure by dilating capillaries
- Decreases heart rate due to relaxation
- Reduces ischemia
- Enhances blood flow, deliver fresh oxygen and nutrients to tissue, remove CO_2 and toxins.

Effects on Lymphatic System

- Reduces edema by increasing lymphatic drainage.
- Strengthens immune system.

Effects on Nervous System

- Stimulates sensory receptors
- Parasympathetic nervous system stimulates, promotes relaxation and reduces stress.
- Reduces pain by releasing endorphins.

Effects on Skin

- Increases production of sweat and, thus, removes waste
- Improves skin color
- Increases elasticity of skin
- Improves sebum production—increases skin suppleness.

Effects on Respiratory System

- Deepens respiration—improves lung capacity
- Slows down rate of respiration due to reduced stimulation of sympathetic nerve.

Effects on GI System

- Increases peristalsis in large intestine—relieves constipation.
- Promotes activity of peripheral nervous system (PNS)—improves digestion.

Effects on Urinary System

Increases urinary output by improving circulation and lymphatic drainage.

Effects on Skeletal System

- Increases joint mobility by reducing thickening of connective tissue.
- Helps to free adhesion, break down scar tissue—restore ROM.

Uses

- Pain
- Sports injury
- Stress
- Anxiety
- Depression
- Relaxation.

Safety

- Avoid vigorous exercise in bleeding disorder, low platelet count.
- Avoid massage in areas of open wound, fracture, blood clot, skin infection, and osteoporosis.

Caution

- Consult with care provider
- Do not replace conventional therapy with massage
- Check the therapist's educational background, experience and other credentials.

MIND-BODY INTERVENTION

It includes variety of techniques designed to facilitate the mind's capacity to affect bodily function. It is based on the belief that thought, attitude, belief and emotions affect physical functioning. Interventions are generally designed to enhance control of physical functions through mental processes and manage the thinking process so that negative beliefs are replaced with positive attitude.

ART THERAPY (CREATIVE OR EXPRESSIVE ART THERAPY)

This therapy helps people manage their physical and emotional problems by using creative activities to express emotions. It provides a way for the people to be in terms with emotional conflicts, increase self-awareness and express unspoken and often unconscious concerns about their illness and their lives.

Note: It may be expressed by dance and other movements, drama, poetry, phototherapy and art methods.

History

The connection between art and mental health was first recognized in 1800. In 1922, a book was published—'Artistry of Mentally Ill'. In 1940, ideas from psychoanalysis and art were combined to release unconscious thoughts. In 1969, American Art Therapy Association was established.

Principles

- It helps the people express their hidden emotions, fears, anxiety and provides a sense of freedom.
- The art therapist works with patients individually or in groups. His job is to help patients express themselves through their creation and also to talk to the patients about their emotions related to the art.

Uses

- Bone marrow transplant patient
- People with eating disorder
- Emotionally impaired young people
- Disabled people
- Chronic illness
- Chemical addiction
- Sexually abused adolescents.

Complications

It is safe if it is conducted by a skilled therapist. But it may have harmful consequences if it is delayed the conventional treatment.

BIOFEEDBACK

It is a treatment technique in which people are trained to control their physiologic responses, like heart rate, body temperature, muscle tension and brain waves by using signals from their own body.

It is a technique in addition to relaxation intervention which assists an individual in learning how to control specific autonomic nervous system response.

History

The word 'Biofeedback' was coined in the late 1940s to describe laboratory procedure being used then to train experimental research subject to altered brain activity, blood pressure, heart rate and other bodily functions, which are involuntary.

Electromechanical instruments are used to measure or to provide information about neuromuscular and autonomic nervous system activity. Then the therapists help the individual to control his physiologic effect.

Biofeedback is often aimed at changing habitual reaction to stress that can cause pain or disease. Skin temperature and muscle tone provide information about relaxed state.

Instruments used are: EEG, ECG, EMG and galvanic skin response.

Desired physiologic state can be achieved by following relaxation techniques, imagery, etc.

Clinical Applications

- Migraine or tension headache
- Digestive system disorder
- Cardiac arrhythmias
- Raynaud's disease
- Epilepsy
- Paralysis.

Limitation

During relaxation therapy, repressed emotions may come up.

MEDITATION

- It is a certain way of concentrating that allows the mind and body to become very relaxed and focused.

- It is a self-directed practice for focusing, centering and relaxing the mind and body.
- It is any activity that limits stimulus input by directing attention to a single unchanging or repetitive stimulus that helps in relaxing the body and stilling the mind.
- It can be passive meditation (sitting meditation) or more active form of meditation (walking meditation).
- It is derived from the root word 'meditari' means consider or pay attention to something.

According to Bensor (1975), the components of meditation are:

- Quiet space
- Comfortable position
- Receptive attitude
- Focus of attention.

Clinical Applications

- Anxiety or tension state
- Hypertension
- Irritability
- Depression
- Stress disorder
- Chronic pain
- Drug abuse
- Chronic bereavement.

Merits

- It does not require any trained therapist or teaching.
- It helps in increasing oxygen uptake, reduction in blood pressure/heart rate, decreases muscle tone, improves memory, increases immune response and enhances peaceful state of mind.

Limitation

Regular practice is necessary.

IMAGERY (VISUALIZATION)

This technique uses the conscious mind to create mental images to stimulate physical changes in the body or to create a desired state. Desired state may include relaxation, enhanced sport performance, pain relief and immune modulation. It is a kind of relaxation training. It is divided into:

- **Self-directed:** Where individuals create their own mental image.
- **Guided:** In which a practitioner leads an individual to be through a particular scenario.
  - It begins with slow abdominal breathing.
  - It directs the client to visualize ocean wave coming to share with each inspiration and receding with each expiration.
  - Notice smell, sound and temperature that he/she is experiencing.

Clinical Applications

- Asthma
- Hypertension
- Functional urinary disorder
- Irritable bowel syndrome
- Chronic pain.

Limitation

Sometimes this may develop day-dreaming.

MUSIC THERAPY

It is a listening therapy, specially filtered classical music to improve ear, brain functions. A link is established between the sound we hear and our functioning in speech, learning, energy and stress. The classical music helps in:

- Improving ear functioning
- Recharging the cortex

Action

According to biochemical theory, music is a sensory stimulus that is processed through the sense of hearing. Sound vibrations are chemically changed into nervous impulses that activate either the sympathetic or parasympathetic nervous system.

Do's	*Don'ts*
Listening to it in a relaxed position, like lying down/sitting with headphone is effective	Listen to music while driving, eating, working, cooking, chatting
Listening to music for 20–30 minutes everyday for 6–8 weeks before going to bed is having a good healing effect	

Clinical Applications

- Decreases stress, anxiety and pain.
- Improves cognitive functioning.
- Alters mood states.
- Promotes relaxation and sleep.
- Enhances alertness.

Note: Preoperatively music can be used to decrease anxiety. During surgery or any procedure, music can be used to distract attention of the patients from their discomfiture. Study shows that the surgical patients exposed to music therapy require less analgesics and sedatives.

PSYCHOTHERAPY

It is derived from two words, i.e., 'psyche' meaning spirit, breath or soul, and 'therapia' meaning healing/medical treatment.

It is a therapeutic intervention contracted between a trained professional and a client, family, couple or group.

Aim

To increase the individuals sense of his/her own well-being.

Techniques

It is based on experiential relation-building dialogue, communication and behavior change that are designed to improve the mental health of a client.

Methods

It is done by written words, art work, drama, narrative story or music.

ENERGY THERAPIES

These involve the manipulation of energy fields. They focus on energy fields originating within the body (biofields) or those from other sources (electromagnetic fields). It includes:

- Reiki
- Therapeutic touch
- Healing touch.

Therapeutic Touch

It is a method of detecting and balancing human energy. It involves the conscious use of hands to direct or modulate human energy fields. Energy imbalance can be identified by the practitioner. The modulation of energy is achieved either by the therapeutic practitioner lightly touching the body or by maintaining the hands in a position a few centimeters away from the body and consciously directing the flow of energy.

Clinical Applications

- Wound healing
- Sleep promotion

Limitations

- Contraindicated in certain populations like who are sensitive to human touch or interaction.
- Old debilitating people.

Reiki

It is a Japanese technique for stress reduction and relaxation that also promotes healing. It is administered by 'laying on hand' and is based on the idea that an unseen 'life force energy' flows through us and is what causes it to be alive. If life force energy is low, then we are more likely to get sick or feel stressed, and if it is high, we are more capable of being happy and healthy.

The word 'Reiki' is derived from 'Rei' meaning god's wisdom/higher power and 'Ki' meaning life force energy. So, the word 'Reiki' means spiritually guided life force energy.

It treats body, emotion, mind and spirit, which causes relaxation, feeling of peace, securing and well-being.

Uses

To improve health and quality of life.

Purpose

- To help people realize that healing the spirit by consciously deciding to improve oneself is a necessary part of the Reiki healing experience.
- The client must accept responsibility for his healing and take an active part in it.

ROLE OF A NURSE

Nurses should have a good attitude towards CAM because they embrace a holistic approach to health, but they appear to lack a sufficient awareness about the risks and advantages of CAM and are apprehensive to discuss it with their patients. Nurses and other healthcare workers should be involved in starting or participating in a variety of research projects in this field. As a result, patients can get evidence based practice on a variety of topics. The nurse must have to know the use of CAM in symptomatic management of different diseases **(Table 9.6)**.

The role of a nurse in complementary therapy includes:

- **Assessment:** Assessment include history collection whether the patient has been used any form of this therapy knowingly or unknowingly. As the nurse documents the patient's pertinent medical history, CAM practices by asking open-ended questions, such as, "What do you use for reliving your migraine pain?" rather than "Do you use alternative medicine for your migraine pain?". The assessment includes assessing the patients' use of complementary therapy at their risk for complication or adverse interaction with conventional therapy. Assessment also includes assessing the conditions for which alternative therapy will be included. Now a days alternative medicine is utilized to treat a wide range of ailments, including diabetes, multiple sclerosis, dyslipidemia, and chronic pain but the nurse should have knowledge on this.
- **Make a triage:** The nurse has to determine for which cases complementary and alternative therapy can be used more. She can make a patient classifications based on risk of diseases and age of the person. CAM therapies are commonly used to treat pain, psychosocial problems, cardiovascular diseases, some chronic diseases like arthritis, symptomatic alleviation from cancer and other neurologic problems where allopathic treatment have

Table 9.6: Symptomatic management of different diseases.

Symptom	*Complementary medicine technique*
Pain	Acupuncture, chiropractic therapy, hypnosis, massage, music therapy, reiki
Nausea/vomiting	Acupuncture, aromatherapy, hypnosis, progressive muscle relaxation
Fatigue	Acupuncture, massage, meditation, reiki, Tai chi, yoga
High blood pressure	Aromatherapy
Hot flashes	Acupuncture
Headache	Chiropractic therapy
Muscle tension	Aromatherapy, massage
Anxiety/Stress/Fear	Aromatherapy, guided imagery, hypnosis, massage, meditation, music therapy, progressive muscle relaxation, prayer, Tai chi, yoga
Depression	Aromatherapy, guided imagery, progressive muscle relaxation

adverse effects. Similarly older persons appear to be more likely to use complementary and alternative medicine (CAM) than younger people for a variety of reasons. Here the nurses role is to decide for which cases to what extent this therapies can be used.

- **Provider for therapies:** As the nurse is providing comprehensive care in a holistic approach she can act as a resource person in providing CAM therapy. Nurses may choose to study CAM practices, become proficient in their use, and integrate their use into an existing nursing practice. However, nurses must keep in mind the legal implications of adding CAM therapies to their existing practice, to ensure they continue to practice within the legal boundaries of their license. Complementary and alternative therapy is commonly used to treat pain, psychosocial problems, cardiovascular diseases, lung diseases as well as to provide symptomatic alleviation for cancer discomfort, among other things. This is a treatment approach. Emphasizes on the individual's holistic care, with a special emphasis on client participation. The use of CAM in clients with neurological illnesses such dementia, multiple sclerosis, neuropathies, spinal cord injury, and epilepsy has been documented in the literature. Integrative medicine is a term that refers to the use of both traditional and alternative treatments. While CAM therapies aren't for everyone, treatments like acupuncture and healing touch therapies have been shown to aid with nausea, pain, and other cancer-related side effects. This all treatments can be provided by nurses but they should be well trained on these therapies before giving treatments.
- **Conducting research:** There is a need for efforts to promote research in the field of complementary and alternative therapy to address each practice individually, as well as a greater need for nurse researchers to collaborate with other members of the healthcare team to conduct quantitative and qualitative studies on various aspects of complementary and alternative therapies in order to build a body of evidence-based knowledge on the use of specific CAM therapies and their specific uses, effects, risks, and safety issues. Population surveys should be encouraged and supported by the mass media to raise knowledge and awareness about the practice of different complementary and alternative medicine modalities.
  - *Facilitator:* The nurse can act as a facilitator for complementary and alternative medicine where she thinks it is essential. For example, in relieving pain of a cancer patient or other chronic conditions. She can council the patient, family members regarding complementary and alternative medicine by considering the patient's health status and assess risks and benefits for providing treatment. She can advocate, and promote best possible care for the patient. It is required for her to take action in situations where patient safety and well-being are compromised. This includes notifying the prescriber of concerns, consulting with the healthcare team and recommending an appropriate healthcare provider to perform the procedure, etc.
- **Advocacy and policy making:** A nurse is also accountable to advocate for policies and procedures about complementary therapies that are driven for patient safety. When recommending a complementary therapy, it is necessary to ensure the patient has the necessary information to make an informed choice. Obtaining inform consent prior to performing the therapy is essential. A nurse must be aware of organizational policies regarding using complementary therapies. If there are no policies in place, she can work with her employer to develop policies around the use of complementary therapies. Professional nurses can offers a variety of choices in therapies to their patients as part of comprehensive care plan. The nurse can explain the role of the treatment in reducing the condition in comparison to other conventional treatment when explaining the therapies and the patients have their rights to choose the treatment for their own.

Nowadays the CAM therapies have increased significantly. Majority of people are using and seeking information about complementary and alternative therapies. This increasing interest comes not only from healthcare consumers but also from allopathic physicians, who have increasing concerns that current western medicine is not meeting the needs of their clients. The integrative medicine approach is consistent with the holistic approach that the nurses need to learn for practicing.

CHAPTER 10

National Health Program

INTRODUCTION

Before independence the communicable diseases are highly prevalent in India. The mortality rate due to different communicable diseases are also very high. After independence the National Government has undertaken several measures to improve health of the peoples. Several National Health Program has launched to control and eradicate the diseases and also get success. The programs also launched to improvement of sanitation, raising the nutritional status of the people. National Health Programs launched in India can be divided under some headings like as follows:

Programs for Communicable Diseases

- National Vector Borne Diseases Control Programme (NVBDCP)
- Revised National Tuberculosis Control Programme
- National Leprosy Eradication Programme
- National AIDS Control Programme
- Universal Immunization Programme
- National Guinea worm Eradication Programme
- Yaws Control Programme
- Integrated Disease Surveillance Programme.

Programs for Noncommunicable Diseases

- National Cancer Control Programme
- National Mental Health Programme
- National Diabetes Control Programme
- National Programme for Control and treatment of Occupational Diseases
- National Programme for Control of Blindness
- National Programme for Control of Diabetes, Cardiovascular Disease and Stroke
- National Programme for Prevention and Control of Deafness.

National Nutritional Programs

- Integrated Child Development Services Scheme
- Mid-day Meal Programme
- Special Nutrition Programme (SNP)
- National Nutritional Anemia Prophylaxis Programme
- National Iodine Deficiency Disorders Control Programme.

Programs Related to System Strengthening/Welfare

- National Rural Health Mission
- Reproductive and Child Health Programme
- National Water supply and Sanitation Programme
- 20-Points Programme.

NATIONAL VECTOR BORNE DISEASE CONTROL PROGRAMME

Introduction

The National Vector Borne Disease Control Programme (NVBDCP) is an umbrella program for prevention and control of Vector borne diseases. It is an integral part of NRHM. The Millennium Development Goal of halting and reversing the incidence of malaria and other vector borne diseases by the year 2015 toward reduction of poverty.

Earlier the Vector Borne Diseases were managed under separate National Health Programs, but now NVBDCP covers all 6 Vector borne diseases namely, Vector Borne Diseases Control Programme. It was launched in 2003–2004 by merging National Antimalaria Programme, National Filarial Control Programme and Kala-azar Control programmes. Japanese B Encephalitis and Dengue/DHF have also been included in this Program. Directorate of NAMP is the nodal agency for prevention and control of major Vector Borne Diseases. The basic approach for vector borne diseases control involves a strategy directed against the parasite and vector and to enlist the involvement of community in practicing various preventive measures. Prevention and control of Vector Borne Diseases under NVBDCP are Malaria, Lymphatic Filariasis, Kala-azar, Dengue, Chikungunya and Japanese encephalitis (JE).

Objectives

- Early diagnosis and prompt treatment.
- Reduction of death due to malaria
- To attain annual parasitic indices less than 01 per 1000 population.

- Integrated Vector Control (DDT Spray).
- Information, Education and Communication (IEC/BCC) for personal protection and Community Participation.
- Training and capacity building of Medical and Para-Medical Workers.
- Outbreak/Epidemic Preparedness and response.
- Supply and use of impregnated mosquito bed nets.
- Monitoring and evaluation including effective utilization and Computerized Management Information System.

The NVBDCP was launched with three main strategies, but in 2006–2007 it was being implemented under NRHM from 2007–2008.

Strategies for National Vector Control Programme

The basic approach for vector borne diseases control involves a strategy directed against the parasite and vector and to enlist the involvement of community in practicing various preventive measures such as:

- Disease management
  - Early detection and complete treatment
  - Strengthening of referral services
  - Epidemic preparedness.
- Integrated vector management (IVM)
  - Indoor residual spray (IRS)
  - Use of insecticide treated bed nets
  - Use of larvivorous fish
  - Antilarval measures in urban areas
  - Source reduction.
- Supportive intervention
  - Capacity building
  - Behavioral Change Communication (BCC)
  - Intersectoral collaboration
  - Operational research
  - Monitoring and evaluation
  - Vectors of malaria.

Major Activities

- **Epidemiological surveillance and disease management for reducing parasite load in the community:** Epidemiological surveillance and disease management can be done by early case detection through blood test by slide/RDT and further strengthening of existing surveillance system is important. Involvement of private pro-viders if possible in surveillance and disease management system prompt, effective and complete treatment should be provided as soon as possible. Strengthening of referral services for serious cases is essential. Be ready with epidemic preparedness and rapid response for sudden outbreak of cases. Monitoring of drug resistance is essential for further treatment.
- **IVM for reducing mosquito density:** Mosquito is the major vector which can transmit a lot of disease like Malaria, Lymphatic Filariasis, Dengue, Chikungunya and Japanese Encephalitis, etc. For reducing mosquito density the following activities are under taken.
  - Indoor Residual Spray (IRS) in selected high-risk areas
  - Use of larvivorous fish in perennial water bodies especially in urban areas including Nagar Panchayats
  - 100% coverage through LLIN of high-risk population
  - Antilarval measures in urban areas including use of biolarvicides
  - Use of chemical larvicides
  - Monitoring of entomological resistance
  - Effective entomological surveillance
  - Source reduction using minor engineering methods
  - Implementation of legislative measures.
- **Supportive interventions:** Supportive interventions includes a variety of aspects like Behavior Change Communication which is a process that motivates people to adopt and sustain healthy behaviors and lifestyles and it can been adopted as an effective strategy for community mobilization, health and environment education and various public outreach programs. Other interventions include Public Private Partnership and intersectional convergence, human resource development through capacity building, operational research including studies on drug resistance and insecticide susceptibility, Logistic Management Information System (LMIS) and monitoring and evaluation through periodic review/field visits and operationalization of web-based computerized National Antimalaria Management Information System (NAMMIS)/integration with HMIS of NHM, etc.
- **Strengthening of referral services:** For rapid transportation of severe malaria cases to the nearest health facility, transport available under NHM will be used and if not available, program will support transportation including mandays compensation for the volunteers for transporting the malarial cases (for Gomati, Dhalai, South and North District) Strengthening of referral centers by equipping them with requisite diagnostics and antimalarials for management of severe malaria cases.
- **Epidemic preparedness and rapid response included:**
  - Use of early warning system for detection epidemic
  - Strengthening of rapid response team in each health institutions.
  - For tackling outbreaks, adequate stocks of antimalarial drugs, diagnostics, insecticides, etc. will be provided by earmarking 25% buffer stock.
  - Fogging in the high-risk areas.
  - 10% of total NVBDCP fund to be kept for rapid response as reserve fund.
- **Source reduction through environmental modifications or biological measures:** Control of larval breeding would be done to limit the transmission of the VBDs. Clearing the margins of water bodies, deweeding to ensure proper water flow, and filling of small temporary water collections will be done to limit the breeding with the active involvement of VHSCs and spray squads under the umbrella of respective RKS. The spray squads may be compensated ensuring 150 mandays in a year.
- **Public private partnership (PPP) and intersectoral convergence:** Improving outreach services through

partnership with NGOs, FBOs, CBOs and local self-government (PRIs); flagging the issue of inter-sectoral convergence with state and district level departments like agriculture, urban development, education, information and cultural affairs, tribal and social welfare, railways, etc., to ensure support and incorporation of health impact assessment component in the projects under respective departments; and state level intersectoral meeting with the line departments.

- **Human resource development through capacity building:**
  - Training of the HR under IMCP-II as per need.
  - Continuation of performance based incentives to the programme personnel including ASHAs/ village level volunteers
  - Training of the Medical Officers, MPWs, MPS and other filed level staffs on control and prevention of Malaria/ Dengue/JE.
- **Logistic Management Information System (LMIS):**
  - Logistics will be supplied by the state NVBDCP as per the technical requirement.
  - State and District level supervision of use of logistics will be done by the appropriate level.
- **Monitoring and evaluation through periodic reviews/ field visits and web based MIS:**
  - The existing NAMMIS would be made fully functional by replacing all old computers and providing internet facility at district level.
  - Communication support, i.e., computer/laptop/ palmtop and communication systems like data-card, internet, mobile, telephone, etc., would be made available is need of the hour and to maintenance of records and timely reporting up to the block level (MTS level).
  - Integration of reporting of core indicators with the IDSP.
  - Establishing sentinel surveillance sites (SSS) at districts for Dengue/JE at all district hospital.
  - Periodic review at all levels and program evaluation at regular intervals.
  - Use of lot quality assurance sampling (LQAS) survey methodology at block level for monitoring the implementation of program and project activities.

MALARIA

History

At the time of independence, there were an estimated 75 million cases of malaria and 0.8 million deaths due to malaria were being reported annually. Government of India launched National Malaria Control Programme (NMCP) in 1953. Under this program indoor residual spray was being done with DDT twice a year. As a result, incidence of malaria cases came down from 75 million cases in 1953 to 2 million cases. In 1958 this control program was switched over to National Malaria Eradication Programme (NMEP), under which initially every house in the state was to be sprayed with DDT twice a year. Later on, spraying was withdrawn but surveillance activities were carried out vigorously. 1965, cases reduce to 0.1 million but again in early 1970, Resurgence of malaria started and in 1976, malaria cases reached 6.46 cases million. Due to this set back to the program a revised strategy was started called 'Modified Plan of Operation' (MPO) w.e.f. 1.4.1977. Under this all the rural population and towns having less than 40,000 populations were under active surveillance. Every dwelling unit is visited by health worker fortnightly to detect fever cases and to give presumptive treatment to them against malaria. Radical treatment was administered to declared positive cases. Again in 1997, World Bank assisted Enhanced Malaria Control Project was launched (EMCP). Provisional data for the year 2004 reveals the largest numbers of cases in the country were reported by Odisha, followed by Gujarat, Chhattisgarh, West Bengal, Jharkhand, Karnataka, Uttar Pradesh and Rajasthan and the largest numbers of deaths were reported by Odisha, followed by West Bengal, Mizoram, Jharkhand, Meghalaya, Karnataka, Tripura and Assam. 1.87 million cases of malaria (including 0.86 million *P. falciparum* cases) and 1006 deaths were reported from the country in 2003. The malaria control programme and other Vector Borne Diseases namely Kala-azar, Dengue, Lymphatic Filariasis, Japanese Encephalitis and Chikungunya were integrated into the National Vector Borne Disease Control Programme (NVBDCP) in 2002. New tools for malaria prevention and control were introduced under NVBDCP, i.e., monovalent RDTs for *P. falciparum* detection in 2005; ACT in 2006; Long-lasting insecticidal nets (LLIN)s in 2009; antigen detecting bivalent RDTs for detection of both *P. falciparum* and *P. vivax* in 2013; and newer insecticides and larvicides in 2014-15. New drug policy for Malaria has been implemented in 2010 and 2013. In 2017 National strategic for malaria elimination in India 2017-22 has been launched.

Milestone

- 1953—Launching of NMCP
- 1958—NMCP was change to NMEP
- 1965—Cases reduce to 0.1 million
- Early 1970—Resurgence of malaria
- 1976—Malaria cases 6.46 cases million
- 1977—MPO implemented
- 1997—World Bank assisted EMCP launched
- 1999—Renaming of NAMP
- 2002—Renaming of NAMP to NVBDCP
- 2005—Global fund assisted IMCP launched
- 2005—Introduction of RDT in program
- 2006—ACT introduced in areas showing chloroquine resistance in fm
- 2008—National Malaria Control Project launched
- 2009—Introduction of LLIN
- 2010—New drug policy for malaria
- 2012—Introduction of bivalent RDT
- 2013—New drug policy for 2013
- 2016—National framework for malaria elimination in India launch
- 2017—National strategic for malaria elimination in India 2017-22

Malaria is one of the major communicable diseases affecting mankind, caused by *Plasmodium* parasite, transmitted by the bite of infective female Anopheles mosquito. There are four *Plasmodium* species, *P. vivax* (Pv), *P. falciparum* (Pf), *P. malariae* (Pm) and *P. ovale* (Po).

Malaria is one of the serious public health problems in India. At the time of independence malaria was contributing 75 million cases with 0.8 million deaths every year prior to the launching of National Malaria Control Program in 1953. A countrywide comprehensive program to control malaria was recommended in 1946 by the Bhore Committee Report that was endorsed by the Planning Commission in 1951. The national program against malaria has a long history since that time.

In April 1953, Government of India launched a National Malaria Control Programme (NMCP) with the following objectives:

- To bring down malaria transmission to a level at which it would cease to be a major public health problem.
- An achievement was to be maintained by each state to hold down the malaria transmission at low level indefinitely.

Strategies Under NMCP

Principal operational activities under the control program comprised of residual insecticide spray of human dwelling and cattle sheds.

Malaria control teams were organized and directed by the state antimalaria organization to carry out surveys and to monitor the malaria incidence in the control areas.

Antimalarial drugs were made available for patients reporting to an institution.

Modified Plan of Operation (MPO)

In 1977 attempts at malaria eradication were given up and under the review policy, a Modified Plan of Operation (MPO) was adopted. Under this all the rural population and towns having less than 40,000 populations were under active surveillance. Every dwelling unit is visited by health worker fortnightly to detect fever cases and to give presumptive treatment to them against malaria. Radical treatment was administered to declared positive cases.

Objectives

- To prevent deaths due to malaria
- To reduce malaria morbidity
- To maintain agriculture and industrial
- Production through intensive antimalaria measures in such areas
- To consolidate the gains achieved so far.

Areas Having Annual Parasite Index (API) >2

Areas were reclassified based on the Annual Parasitic Incidence (API) as those having API >2 and those having < than 2 for operational purposes. Regular 2 rounds of insecticidal spray with DDT/Malathion/Synthetic Pyrethroids at the dose of 1, 2, 0. 5 mg/sq meter respectively. Entomological assessment for vector behavior and development of insecticidal resistance active and passive surveillance is carried out on regular basis every fortnight. Presumptive treatment to all fever cases and radical treatment to all slide positive cases is given. The principal activities are regular insecticidal spraying and entomological assessment. The supportive activities are active and passive surveillance, presumptive and radical treatment. Under the MPO guidelines these areas are given.

Areas Having Annual Parasite Index (API) <2

Regular spray is not carried out but 'focal' spray is carried out around falciparum cases detected during surveillance. Regular passive surveillance once in a fortnight treatment—All positive cases to receive radical treatment follow-up—All positive cases to be followed up for 1 year at monthly intervals after completion of radical treatment. Epidemiological investigation of all malaria positive cases. This may also include mass blood survey. In these areas, the principal activities are active and passive surveillance, and presumptive and radical treatment. The supportive activities are case follow-up, epidemiological investigation, and focal spraying where ever indicated. Surveillance in malaria essentially aimed at case finding and case confirmation. The efficacy of surveillance is determined by early identification of cases and prompt institution of radical treatment. The MPO strategy employs both active and passive surveillance mechanisms.

Active surveillance is carried out by multipurpose health workers who visit every house in their respective areas at fortnightly intervals. They enquire whether any one is suffering or has suffered from fever during the previous fortnight. In the event of a positive response a worker prepares a blood smear of suspected case making a thin and thick film on the same slide. The worker also gives a single dose presumptive chemotherapy to the case and makes the necessary entries in the stencil of the house card. He takes the blood smear to the primary health center (PHC) laboratory for microscopic examination, and in the event of positive report, he contacts the confirmed case and puts him on a course of radical chemotherapy.

The components of active surveillance are:

- Search for fever cases
- Collection of blood smears from fever cases
- Administration of appropriate presumptive treatment.

Malaria surveillance includes maintenance of ongoing watch over the status of malaria in a group or community. It provides a basis for measuring effectiveness of antimalaria program and helps control measures. Malaria surveillance presumes that every malaria case presents itself with symptoms of fever at some point of time during the course of infection. These all fever cases are examined for blood smears to know the malaria parasite load. Passive surveillance include screening the fever cases visiting the hospital for malaria by blood slides collection.

Urban Malaria Scheme

The proposal of urban malaria scheme (UMS) was sanctioned in 1971 when it was realized that urban malaria was a significant problem and if effective anti-larval measures were not undertaken in urban areas, the proliferation of malaria cases from urban to rural might occur in a bigger way. In this scheme, all the towns having more than 40,000 population and showing more than 2 API in last 3 years are to be covered. At present 131 towns and cities in 19 states and union territories are under the UMS. The breeding of mosquitoes is checked by carrying out Anti-larval operations regularly at weekly intervals in the following manner.

Source Reduction

Permanent and temporary breeding sources of mosquitoes are eliminated by filling of burrow pits, ditches, small irrigation canal and unused well.

Enhanced Malaria Control Project

Enhanced Malaria Control Project (EMCP) project was launched in April 1997 with the assistance of the World Bank. This is directly benefiting the six crore tribal population of the eight peninsular states covering 100 districts and 19 urban areas. However, the population living in other malaria endemic areas is also benefited, as the strengthening of the components of IEC, training and management information system have covered the entire country.

Annual parasitic incidence (API) is more than 2 for last 3 years.

Pf cases are more than 30% of the malaria cases; 25% population of the PHC is tribal; and the area has been reporting deaths due to malaria and also has the flexibility to direct resources to any needy areas in case of outbreak of malaria.

Objectives of EMCP

- Effective control of malaria to bring reduction in malaria morbidity
- Prevention of death due to malaria
- Consolidation of the gain achieved so far.

Strategies

- Early case detection and prompt treatment.
- Vector control by indoor residual insecticide spray in rural areas with API of 2 per 100 and above in the preceding three years with appropriate insecticide and by recurrent antimalaria in urban areas.
- Health education and community participation.

Components of EMCP

- Early case detection and prompt treatment
- Selective vector control legislative measures, personal protective measures
- Epidemic planning and rapid response and inter-sectoral coordination
- Institutional and management capacities strengthening
- Operation research
- Community participation.

Antimalaria Drug Policy

The National Antimalaria Drug Policy was drafted in 1982 to combat the increasing level of resistance to chloroquine detected in Pf. However, there was large scale malaria epidemics reported in recent times that has generated great concerns. An expert committee was formulated under the chairmanship of DGHS to revise the drug treatment policy and the committee submitted its recommendations. The Antimalaria Drug Policy was revised recently in 2013 and the recommended doses detail described in chapter communicable and noncommunicable diseases.

Insecticide Policy

DDT should be the insecticide of choice for residual spray. If resistance found to DDT then Malathion is the alternative choice. In case of resistance to both DDT and malathion then synthetic Pyrethroids is the choice.

Remote Sensing in Vector Borne Disease Control

Remote sensing (RS) technology is a tool for the surveillance of habitat, densities of vector species and even prediction of the incidence of disease that must be considered as new invention in the epidemiology of malaria and vector-borne diseases. Literal meaning of remote sensing is to sense any object from a distance. The human eyes and cameras also act as a remote sensing devices. However, scientist of NASA of USA used color infrared aerial photography to identify the habitats of a nuisance mosquito, *Aedes sollicitans* in 1971. The principle of RS rests on the fact that every object absorbs some part of radiation received from sunlight. Depending upon its physical and chemical properties, the object absorbs some part of radiation while the remaining part is reflected in specific wavelength of the electromagnetic spectrum (EMS). This reflected energy is channelized through a telescope to detectors/sensors present on board of the satellites. The sensors are sensitive to different bands of EMS. The sensors convert the light energy into electrical voltages produces two-dimensional discrete pictures. These are different for different objects and the satellite pass over a particular part of earth at the fixed time intervals repeatedly making it possible to monitor changes in the land use categories viz. water bodies, vegetation, forests, soil mapping, geology, crop estimation, detection of fire in forest, mines, oil sleek in sea, etc. Such data is generated in National Remote Sensing Agency, Hyderabad, in India. A feasibility study using satellite data in collaboration with the Indian Space Research Organization in and around Delhi was carried out and correlation of changes in the areas of land use features viz. water bodies and vegetations with mosquito density was found significant in some sites.

NATIONAL FRAMEWORK FOR MALARIA ELIMINATION IN INDIA

With observance of the success of the National Vector Borne Disease Control Programme (NVBDCP) in November 2014, the Asia Pacific Leaders Malaria Alliance (APLMA) representing 18 countries, including India, agreed to the goal of a region free of malaria by 2030. The APLMA Malaria Elimination Roadmap was endorsed in November 2015 in alignment with the WHO Global Technical Strategy for Malaria 2016–2030, and the Roll Back Malaria Partnership document Action and Investment to defeat Malaria 2016–2030. The NFME has clearly defined goals, objectives, strategies, targets and timelines and will serve as a roadmap for advocating and planning malaria elimination throughout the country in a phased manner.

Goals

In line with the WHO Global Technical Strategy for Malaria 2016–2030 (GTS) and the Asia Pacific Leaders Malaria Alliance Malaria Elimination Roadmap, the goals of the National Framework for Malaria Elimination in India 2016–2030 are:

- Eliminate malaria (zero indigenous cases) throughout the entire country by 2030; and
- Maintain malaria-free status in areas where malaria transmission has been interrupted and prevent re-introduction of malaria.

Objectives

- Eliminate malaria from all Category 1 and Category 2 states/UTs (26) with low and moderate-transmission of malaria by 2022
- Reduce the incidence of malaria to less than one case per 1000 population per year in all states/UTs and their districts and achieve malaria elimination in 31 states/UTs by 2024
- Interrupt indigenous transmission of malaria in all states/ UTs (Category 3) by 2027; and
- Prevent re-establishment of local transmission of malaria in areas where it has been eliminated and maintain malaria-free status nationally by 2030.

Strategic Approaches

Program Phasing

Malaria elimination in India will be carried out in a phased manner because various parts of the country differ in their malaria endemicity due to differences in their eco-epidemiological settings, socioeconomic conditions, health system development and malaria control accomplishments. Malaria incidence in high transmission areas (Category 3) must be lowered first before it is possible and rational to investigate each case. States/UTs will be subdivided into four categories with annual parasite incidence (API) as the primary criteria, and the annual blood examination rate (ABER) is secondary **(Table 10.1)**.

Table 10.1: Categories of states with annual parasite incidence (API).

S. No.	*Categories of states/UTs*	*Definition*
1.	**Category 0:** Prevention of re-establishment phase	States/UTs with zero indigenous cases of malaria
2.	**Category 1:** Elimination phase	States/UTs (15) including their districts reporting an API of less than 1 case per 1000 population at risk
3.	**Category 2:** Pre-elimination phase	States/UTs (11) with an API of less than 1 case per 1000 population at risk, but some of their districts are reporting an API of 1 case per 1000 population at risk or above
4.	**Category 3:** Intensified control phase	States/UTs (10) with an API of 1 case per 1000 population at risk or above

Milestones and Targets

By End of 2016

All states/UTs have included malaria elimination in their broader health policies and planning frameworks.

By 2020

- Transmission of malaria interrupted and zero indigenous cases and deaths due to malaria attained in all 15 states/ UTs under Category 1 (elimination phase) in 2014 (base year).
- All 11 states/UTs under Category 2 (pre-elimination phase) in 2014 enter into Category 1 (elimination phase).
- Five states/UTs under Category 3 (intensified control phase) in 2014 enter into Category 2 (pre-elimination phase).
- Five states/UTs under Category 3 (intensified control phase) in 2014 reduce malaria transmission but continue to remain in Category 3.
- An estimated reduction in malaria of 15–20% at the national level compared with 2014.
- Additionally, progressive states with strong health systems such as Gujarat, Maharashtra and Karnataka may implement accelerated malaria elimination programmes to achieve interruption of transmission and demonstrate early elimination followed by sustenance of zero indigenous cases.

By 2022

- Transmission of malaria interrupted and zero indigenous cases and deaths due to malaria attained in all 26 states/ UTs that were under Categories 1 and 2 in 2014.
- Five states/UTs which were under Category 3 (intensified control phase) in 2014 enter into elimination phase.
- Five states/UTs which were under Category 3 (intensified control phase) in 2014 enter into pre-elimination phase.
- An estimated reduction in malaria of 30–35% at the national level compared with 2014.

By 2024

- All states/UTs and their respective districts reduce API to less than 1 case per 1000 population at risk and sustain zero deaths due to malaria while maintaining fully functional malaria surveillance to track, investigate and respond to each case throughout the country.
- Transmission of malaria interrupted and zero indigenous cases and deaths due to malaria attained in all 31 states/UTs.
- Five states/UTs which were under Category 3 (intensified control phase) in 2014 enter into elimination phase.

By 2027

The indigenous transmission of malaria in India interrupted.

By 2030

- The re-establishment of local transmission prevented in areas where malaria has been eliminated.
- The malaria-free status maintained throughout the nation.

Focus on High Transmission Areas

The majority of malaria is being reported from states in the eastern, central and north-eastern part of the country, such as Odisha, Chhattisgarh, Jharkhand, Madhya Pradesh, Maharashtra, Tripura and Meghalaya. Most of these states are characterized by widespread hilly, tribal, forested and conflict-affected areas which are pockets of high malaria transmission. An aggressive scaling up of existing interventions, intensification of all malaria control activities and innovative strategies and partnerships will be carried out in these high endemic pockets to rapidly reduce malaria morbidity and mortality.

Special Strategy for *P. vivax* Elimination

According to the World Malaria Report 2015, more than 80% of the global *P. vivax* burden is contributed by 3 countries including India 1. This serious challenge to malaria elimination efforts within the country will require special measures to be undertaken, such as good quality microscopy to detect all *P. vivax* infections, operational research to estimate prevalence of G6PD deficiency in the population, appropriate vector control measures, and ensuring good compliance to 14-day radical treatment with primaquine in affected individuals.

District as the Unit of Planning and Implementation

Apart from the category to which they belong, each state/UT will be advised to further classify their districts so that even if a state/UT is not yet in the elimination phase, but has some districts with an API below 1 case per 1000 population at risk, those may be considered eligible for initiating elimination phase activities provided they meet the secondary criteria. In addition, states/UTs may also sub-classify districts into community health centers, community health centers into primary health centers, primary health centers into subcenters, and subcenters into villages for localized planning and implementation.

Key Interventions

In order to attain the stated goals, objectives, milestones and targets formulated under this national framework, key interventions and their specific packages have been identified. All activities, milestones and targets envisaged under the national framework are in line with global and regional goals set under the GTS, the APLMA Roadmap for Malaria Elimination Roadmap and the Action and Investment to defeat Malaria 2016–2030 document and in line with national goals and targets set under the Strategic Action Plan for Malaria Control in India 2012–2017.

Category 3 (Intensified Control Phase)

Key Interventions

- Massive scaling up of existing disease management and preventive approaches and tools, aimed at a significant reduction in the prevalence and incidence of malaria as well as associated deaths.
- Screening of all fever cases suspected for malaria.
- Classification of areas as per local malaria epidemiology and grading of areas as per risk of malaria transmission followed by implementation of tailored interventions.
- Strengthening of intersectoral collaboration.
- Special interventions for high-risk groups such as tribal populations and populations residing in conflict affected or hard-to-reach areas.
- One-stop centers or mobile clinics on fixed days in tribal or conflict affected areas to provide malaria diagnosis and treatment, and increasing community awareness with the involvement of other agencies and service providers as required.
- Timely referral and treatment of severe malaria cases to reduce malaria-related mortality.
- Strengthening all district and subdistrict hospitals in malaria endemic areas as per Indian Public Health Standards with facilities for management of severe malaria cases.
- Establishment of a robust supply chain management system.
- Maintenance of an optimum level of surveillance using appropriate diagnostic measures.
- Equipping all health institutions (primary health care level and above), especially in high-risk areas, with microscopy facilities and RDTs for emergency use and injectable artemisinin derivatives for treatment of severe malaria.

Category 2 (Pre-elimination Phase)

The states/UTs in pre-elimination phase are those close to entering the elimination phase. Therefore, malaria elimination interventions will be introduced with particular focus on setting up an elimination surveillance system and initiating elimination phase activities in those districts where the API has been reduced to less than 1 case per 1000 population at risk per year. The planning of elimination measures will be based on epidemiological investigation and classification of each malaria case and focus.

Category 1 (Elimination Phase)

In elimination areas, where transmission is focal and incidence/risk has become extremely low, all efforts will be directed at interrupting local transmission in all active foci of malaria.

- Mandatory notification of each case of malaria from the private sector, other organized government sectors or any other health facility.
- Adequate case-based surveillance and complete case management established and fully functional across the entire country to handle each case of malaria.
- Investigation and classification of all foci of malaria.
- A strict total coverage of all active foci by effective vector control measures.
- Early detection and treatment of all cases of malaria by means of active and/or passive case detection to prevent onward transmission.
- State and national level malaria elimination database established and operational.
- Implementation of interventions for effective screening, management and prevention of malaria among mobile and migrant populations.
- Establishment of an effective epidemic forecasting and response system.
- Ensuring rigorous quality assurance of all medicines and diagnostics.
- Setting up a national-level reference laboratory which will serve the following two functions.

All positive and a fixed percentage of negative slides will be referred to this laboratory for confirmation of diagnosis and cross-checking. After elimination has been achieved in each State/UT, 100% of cases will be notified to this laboratory for confirmation of diagnosis. The laboratory will be notified immediately on all positive cases of malaria by each state/UT through either SMS, e-mail or telephone with information on name, gender, address (village and district), date and type of testing and type of parasite for each positive case of malaria so that a national level database can be maintained.

Training of master trainers and accreditation/certification of microscopists as per Indian Public Health Standards shall also be undertaken at this laboratory.

Category 0 (Prevention of Re-establishment Phase)

The probability of malaria becoming re-established in a malaria free area varies with the level of receptivity and vulnerability of the area. If either of these factors is zero, the probability of malaria becoming re-established is zero even if the other factor has a high value. When importation of malaria due to the arrival of migrants from a malaria area coincides with increase in receptivity because of halted vector control measures or socioeconomic development of an area for example, re-establishment of malaria transmission is possible. In the absence of appropriate action, the area is likely to become malarious again and the duration is determined by the level of receptivity and vulnerability.

When any area, whether a state/UT or a district within a state/UT, has achieved malaria elimination, the specific objectives will be as follows:

- Detect any re-introduced case of malaria;
- Notify immediately all detected cases of malaria;
- Determine the underlying causes of resumed local transmission;
- Apply rapid curative and preventive measures;
- Prevent reintroduction and possible re-establishment of malaria transmission; and
- Maintain malaria-free status in these areas.

Cross-cutting Interventions

Some interventions will be common to all categories of states/UTs and are detailed below.

Policy and Planning

- Formation of a National Malaria Elimination Committee comprising of representatives from NVBDCP, WHO, research institutions, academia, private and civil society stakeholders for oversight of all malaria elimination activities in the country and form a technical working group as part of the National Malaria Elimination Committee for regular monitoring of progress.
- Revision of national guidelines for vector control, quality assurance, intersectoral collaboration, IEC/BCC and other relevant areas for prevention, intensified control and elimination of malaria.
- Revision of national or state level policy/legislation for all states and UTs planned for elimination to classify malaria as a notifiable disease.
- Formulation of a new surveillance and reporting strategy on the lines of China's '1-3-7' strategy18 for case notification, diagnosis, treatment and follow-up at the community level in a time bound manner. This will be different for each category of state/UT and based on the lines of 3Ts or Test, Treat and Track approach.
- Formulation of clear parameters for states/UTs to qualify for a certain category or transition from one category to another, as per stratification norms.

Monitoring and Evaluation

- Introduction of a new web-based reporting system to facilitate timely notification and analysis of malaria transmission and revision of monitoring and evaluation formats.
- Estimation of vector control coverage, including long-lasting insecticidal mosquito net (LLIN) or insecticide treated nets (ITN) use and indoor residual spraying (IRS) coverage, in each state/UT at district, subdistrict, block and village levels.

- Use of an annual scoring system for evaluating progress against elimination milestones and targets at national, state and district levels.
- Data validation by an external agency when any state/UT achieves malaria elimination or transitions from one category of malaria elimination into another and grading of all areas within a state/UT for endemicity or risk of malaria on the basis of fixed parameters.

Stratification

- Stratification of all states/UTs into four categories based on their API, APER and SPR and Substratification of all districts within each state/UT using the same criteria.
- Further stratification of CHCs, PHCs, SCs and villages within each district using the same criteria and implementation of strata-specific strategies.
- Feasibility assessment of each state/UT before planning elimination.

Surveillance

- **Entomological surveillance:** All entomological units in the country to be made functional and strengthened.
- Strengthening of routine surveillance for reducing malaria transmission in high transmission areas, and establishing case-based surveillance as a core intervention for elimination areas.

Quality Assurance

- Quality assurance of all medicines, diagnostics, treatment and vector control supplies as per internationally accepted standards.
- All malaria microscopy services in the country to be quality assured as per internationally accepted standards to ensure quality of services provided for malaria diagnosis.
- All testing facilities for malaria across states/UTs to be part of a national quality management network.
- Private sector laboratories providing malaria diagnosis in the country to be identified and laboratory technicians certified.

Intersectoral Collaboration

- Formulation of clearly defined roles and responsibilities for private providers, NGOs as well as other organized government sector organizations such as the Armed Forces, Central Reserve Police Force, Border Security Force.
- District-wide mapping of all private hospitals and NGOs in all states/UTs.
- Collaboration with private sector organizations and non-governmental organizations (NGOs) under the Corporate Social Responsibility (CSR) Act in every state/UT.
- Training and refresher trainings (continuing medical education) of private practitioners in malaria diagnosis, treatment and reporting as per national guidelines.
- Integration of data on malaria endemicity collected by private hospitals with the national Malaria Information System (MIS).
- Advocacy with private hospitals and practitioners on a regular basis to ensure adoption of national guidelines for diagnosis and treatment of malaria.
- Explore scope and establish collaboration with public works department for environmental management.

Cross-border Collaboration

- Screening of populations at international border crossings.
- Training of security personnel at international border crossings with provision of diagnostic and treatment facilities.
- Implementation of a mechanism for monthly data collection from international border areas and integration into national MIS.
- Joint planning and implementation of malaria prevention and control activities with neighboring countries.
- Sharing of information and policies for malaria prevention and control with neighboring countries.

Initiatives for Special Population Groups

- Implementation of the Tribal Malaria Action Plan (TMAP) for intensification of malaria prevention and control activities in tribal and ethnic population groups spread across different states/UTs. A total of 96 districts with an API of more than 1 case per 1000 people at risk and a tribal population of more than 25% are being included under this plan for intensified control measures. The following areas will receive special emphasis under TMAP.
- Strengthening of existing health systems and introduction of mobile-based surveillance where routine health services/facilities are not available.
- On the spot, species-specific treatment of all positive cases of malaria with a full course of antimalarials as per NVBDCP guidelines.
- Referral of severe cases to referral center/district hospital/any other health facility and follow-up of all positive cases.
- Prioritization of villages according to degree of risk, for example, a high proportion of Pf cases, type of vectors, forest-based economy or outdoor sleeping habits for appropriate vector control measures (IRS/LLIN or treatment of community-owned bed nets with insecticides).
- Training of mobile or migrant workers, military personnel, tribal or other population groups in malaria diagnosis and treatment.
- Instituting a mechanism for systematically collecting data from these population groups.
- Consideration of providing treatment to clinically indicative cases or standby treatment for small isolated population groups especially in hard-to-reach areas.

IEC/BCC

- Revision of IEC/BCC strategy with special emphasis on malaria elimination.
- This strategy will be tailored according to the endemicity of malaria in a region,

Innovation

Vector Control

- Promotion of LLINs using new approaches such as community awareness campaigns, regular surveys to assess utilization of LLINs by community health volunteers.
- Use of alternative methods of community-based vector control such as personal repellents, mosquito proofing of houses, use of vapour-phase insecticides, insecticidal wall linings, as per available evidence on their effectiveness on pilot basis in selected areas, according to indoor/outdoor transmission pattern of malaria. The decision regarding future use of these methods within the program will be based on the outcome of such pilot studies.
- Integration of malaria control into agricultural practices.
- Experimental hut facilities may also be established at one or two sentinel sites in each state/UT with relevant vector species for testing the efficacy of different vector control interventions.
  - To address malaria in outbreak and other special situations, standard operating procedures for outbreaks and other situations such as in the case of a natural disasters or emergencies, will be formulated and circulated to states/UTs.
  - Avenues for innovative financing to be explored for increasing and sustaining investments in malaria elimination efforts.
  - Innovative ways of service delivery such as integration with Ministry of Tribal Affairs for providing services to tribal populations, collaboration with NGOs, community-based organizations, other ministries and private sector organizations for reaching populations in hard-to-reach and conflict affected areas.

Capacity Building

- Preparation of annual training curricula and schedules for health officials at different implementation levels.
- Review of training status and schedules by program twice annually.
- Identification and training of a group of national level trainers in areas such as program implementation, management, supervision, quality assurance and supply chain management.

Research

- Facilitating research on devising methods to increase efficacy of IRS/LLIN such as through use of enhanced ingredients and new formulations.
- Surveys by states/UTs on behavior of mosquito vectors to better inform choices of vector control methods in different settings such as studies of vector feeding and resting behavior, malaria vector population dynamics.
- Surveys on community behavior such as resource use, means of livelihood, patterns of sleeping for better tailored IEC/BCC strategies and prevention, intensified control and elimination of malaria in different population groups.
- Longitudinal surveys on malaria vector population dynamics, community or district-based mosquito trapping schemes.
- Research on drug resistance monitoring, therapeutic efficacy studies.
- Cost-benefit analysis of interventions used for malaria elimination once every five years.

ELIMINATION OF LYMPHATIC FILARIASIS

Magnitude of the Problem

Filariasis has been a major public health problem in India next only to malaria. The discovery of microfilariae (mf) in the peripheral blood was made first by Lewis in 1872 in Calcutta (Kolkata). Indigenous cases have been reported from about 250 districts in 20 states/Union Territories. The North-Western States/UTs are known to be free from indigenously acquired filarial infection.

Cases of filariasis have been recorded from Andhra Pradesh, Assam, Bihar, Chhattisgarh, Goa, Jharkhand, Karnataka, Gujarat, Kerala, Madhya Pradesh, Maharashtra, Odisha, Tamil Nadu, Uttar Pradesh, West Bengal, Puducherry, Andaman and Nicobar Islands, Daman and Diu, Dadra and Nagar Haveli and Lakshadweep.

Signs and Symptoms of Filariasis

Lymphatic filariasis impairs the lymphatic system and can lead to the abnormal enlargement of body parts, causing pain, severe disability which causes social stigma. Symptoms may include itchy skin (pruritis), abdominal pain, chest pain, muscle pain (myalgias), and/or areas of swelling under the skin. Other symptoms may include an abnormally enlarged liver and spleen (hepatosplenomegaly), and inflammation in the affected organs.

National Filaria Control Programme: This programme was started in 1955. In 1998 the operational component was merged with Urban Malaria Scheme. In 2003–2004 it was merged with NVBDCP.

Filariasis has been a major public health problem in India next only to malaria.

Revised Strategy

In 1997, WHO and its Member States made a commitment to eliminate Lymphatic Filariasis (LF) as public health problem by 2020 through World Health Assembly Resolution WHA 50.29. The National Health Policy (2002) has set the goal of Elimination of Lymphatic Filariasis in India by 2015. Later extended to 2021. Subsequent to that Global Alliance to Eliminate Lymphatic Filariasis (GAELF) has been formed in 2000.

Twin pillar strategies of Mass Drug Administration (MDA) for interruption of transmission, i.e., no new case and Morbidity Management and Disability Prevention (MMDP) for catering the disease afflicted patients were adopted for elimination.

Mass Drug Administration (MDA)

- MDA started as mass campaign from 2004.
- Initially with single dose of DEC only.
- In the year of 2007 with DEC + Albendazole co-administration
- Form 2018 Triple Drug Therapy (IDA), i.e., DEC + Albendazole + Ivermectin is launched initially in five selected districts. Since elimination target is approaching first all the left out districts which are yet to achieve elimination will be brought under IDA.
- Accelerated Plan which include Triple Drug Therapy (IDA) was launched in the Global Alliance Elimination of Lymphatic Filariasis (GAELF) meeting held during 13th to 15th June 2018 by Hon'ble Union Health Minister and Hon'ble Minister of State. MDA has been observed in 151 districts, during 2019. The MoH and FW has approved the Triple Drug Therapy (IDA) implementation program in selective five districts named Arwal (Bihar), Simdega (Jharkhand), Varanasi (Uttar Pradesh), Nagpur (Maharashtra) and Yadgir (Karnataka) which has successfully implemented in these districts. Eleven more districts of Uttar Pradesh have implemented IDA during December, 2019. One district Tapi in Gujarat has implementing IDA in January 2020.

Morbidity Management and Disability Alleviation

Morbidity management is another pillar of strategy for ELF and states/UTs were advised on up-scaling home-based morbidity management of lymphedema cases and hydrocele operations. The process involved updating the line-listing of lymphedema and hydrocele cases in the districts. Demonstration and training on simple foot hygiene to affected persons and motivate them for self practice.

Since 2004, the states/UTs have reported 148,877 (2018) hydrocele operations. Different states have initiated management of lymphedema cases through demonstrating home-based foot hygiene method to patients at local levels.

KALA-AZAR

Kala-azar is a slow progressing indigenous disease caused by a protozoan parasite of genus *Leishmania*. In India *Leishmania donovani* is the only parasite causing this disease. The parasite primarily infects reticuloendothelial system and may be found in abundance in bone marrow, spleen and liver. Post kala-azar dermal Leishmaniasis (PKDL) is a condition when *Leishmania donovani* invades skin cells, resides and develops there and manifests as dermal lesions.

NATIONAL KALA-AZAR ELIMINATION PROGRAMME

Kala-azar has been a serious medical and public health problem in India since historical times. Bengal is the oldest known Kala-azar endemic area of the world. After the initial success, Kala-azar resurged in 70s. Concerned with the increasing problem of Kala-azar in the country, the Government of India (GOI) launched a centrally sponsored Kala-azar Control Programme in the endemic states in 1990–91. The program brought a significant decline in Kala-azar morbidity, but could not sustain the pace of decline for long.

Since 1992, after years of accelerated program implementation, the number of kala-azar cases in India has dropped by 97%. The National Health Policy-2002 set the goal of Kala-azar elimination in India by the year 2010 and due to not achieved the target once again National Health Policy-2017 set the goal to eliminate Kala-azar in India by the year 2017. But still according to National Center Vector Borne Disease Control in 2022 over all 435 people suffered in kala-azar and 35 death are reported.

Presently all programmatic activities are being implemented through the National Vector Borne Disease Control Programme (NVBDCP) which is an umbrella program for prevention and control of vector borne diseases and is subsumed under National Health Mission (NHM).

Goal

To improve the health status of vulnerable groups and at-risk population living in Kala-azar endemic areas by the elimination of Kala-azar so that it no longer remains a public health problem.

Target

To reduce the annual incidence of Kala-azar to less than one per 10,000 populations at block PHC level.

Objectives

To reduce the annual incidence of Kala-azar to less than one per 10 000 population at block PHC level by the end of 2015 by:

- Reducing Kala-azar in the vulnerable, poor and unreached populations in endemic areas;
- Reducing case-fatality rates from Kala-azar to negligible level;
- Reducing cases of PKDL to interrupt transmission of Kala-azar; and
- Preventing the emergence of Kala-azar and HIV/TB co-infections in endemic areas.

The Elimination Strategy

The national strategy for elimination of Kala-azar is a multipronged approach which is in line with WHO Regional Strategic Framework for elimination of Kala-azar from the South-East Asia Region (2011–2015) and includes:

- Early diagnosis and complete case management
- Integrated Vector Management and Vector Surveillance
- Supervision, monitoring, surveillance and evaluation
- Strengthening capacity of human resource in health
- Advocacy, communication and social mobilization for behavioral impact and inter-sectoral convergence.

Program Management

This is done for eliminating the human reservoir of infection through early case detection. Effective case management includes diagnosing a case early along with complete treatment and monitoring of adverse effects. This strategy will reduce case-fatality and will improve utilization of health services by people suspected to be suffering from the disease.

The starting point of early diagnosis is to follow uniform suspect case definition.

A 'suspect' case: History of fever of more than 2 weeks and enlarged spleen and liver not responding to antimalaria in a patient from an endemic area.

All patients with above symptoms should be screened with rapid diagnostic test and if found positive should be treated with an effective drug.

In cases with past history of Kala-azar or in those with high suspicion of Kala-azar but with negative RDT test result, confirmation of Kala-azar can be done by examination of bone marrow/spleen aspirate for LD bodies at appropriate level (district hospital) equipped with such skills and facilities.

Treatment: In 2010, the WHO Expert Committee on Leishmaniasis, and subsequently the Regional Technical Advisory Group (RTAG) of WHO South-East Asia Region (SEAR) recommended Liposomal Amphotericin B (LAMB) in a single dose of 10 mg/kg as the first choice treatment regimen for the Indian Subcontinent (ISC) within the current elimination strategy, given its high efficacy, safety, ease of use and assured compliance. The decision to use Liposomal Amphotericin B for Kala-azar was taken by the Technical Advisory Committee based on the available evidences and approved by Ministry of Health and Family Welfare, Govt. of India. In selected districts, Amphotericin B emulsion has been approved. The combination regimen (Injection Paromomycin-Miltefosine for 10 days) is also recommended. Miltefosine 28 days regime and Amphotericin B as multiple doses may also be used.

Within the Indian National Programme, assuming availability of drugs, appropriate training of health personnel, infrastructure and indication, the following drugs will thus be used in order of preference at all levels:

- Single dose 10 mg/kgbw Liposomal Amphotericin B (LAMB)
- Combination regimens (e.g., Miltefosine and Paromomycin)
- Miltefosine
- Amphotericin B deoxycholate in multiple doses.

Post Kala-azar Dermal Leishmaniasis (PKDL) patients are to be treated with (i) Liposomal amphotericin B: 5 mg/kg per day by infusion two times per week for 3 weeks for a total dose of 30 mg/kg, or (ii) Miltefosine: 100 mg orally per day for 12 weeks, or (iii) Amphotericin B deoxycholate: 1 mg/kg over 4 months 60–80 doses.

CONTROL OF DENGUE/DHF

Dengue is a viral disease which is transmitted by the infective bite of Aedes Aegypti. Man develops disease after 5–6 days of being bitten by an infective mosquito It occurs in two forms: Dengue fever and dengue hemorrhagic fever (DHF). Dengue fever is a severe, flu-like illness.

DHF is a more severe form of disease, which may cause death. Person suspected of having dengue fever or DHF must see a doctor at once.

Dengue/DHF

There was a major outbreak of Dengue/DHF in Delhi in 1996. Since then, many focal outbreaks have been reported from different areas of the country mainly from urban areas. This disease has been included in NVBDCP in 2003–2004. According to the data provided by National center for disease control DGHS (MoH and FW), till 31st May of 2022 there are total 10,172 dengue cases in India. Among them highest 2548 cases observed in Tamil Nadu.

Control Strategy

Public awareness and community involvement is the key issue in the strategy to control Dengue/DHF. All efforts should be made against the breeding of *Aedes egypti* mosquitoes by source reduction. Protection from mosquito bites. Early diagnosis and prompt treatment of cases. Vector control through insecticidal residual spray (IRS) with DDT up to 6 feet height from the ground twice annually. Early diagnosis and complete treatment and information education communication are essential for control of dengue and dengue hemorrhagic fever.

Chikungunya

Chikungunya (also called chikungunya virus disease or chikungunya fever), is a viral illness that is spread by the bite of infected mosquitoes. The disease resembles dengue fever, and is characterized by severe, sometimes persistent, joint pain (arthritis), as well as fever and rash. It is rarely life-threatening. Chikungunya occurs in Africa, India and Southeast Asia. It is primarily found in urban/periurban areas. There is no specific treatment for chikungunya. Prevention centers on avoiding mosquito bites in areas where chikungunya virus may be present, and by eliminating mosquito breeding site.

GOI Initiatives for Dengue and Chikungunya

Government of India has taken various steps for prevention and control of Dengue and Chikungunya in the country as detailed below:

- Developed a Long-term Action Plan for Prevention and Control of Dengue in the country and sent to the State(s) on January 2007 for implementation.
- National guidelines for clinical management of Dengue Fever, Dengue Hemorrhagic Fever, Dengue Shock

Syndrome has been sent to the State(s) April 2007 for circulation in all hospitals.
- Established Sentinel Surveillance Hospitals with laboratory support for augmentation of diagnostic facility for Dengue in endemic State(s) in 2007 which has been increased to 170 in 2009. All these are linked with 13 Apex Referral Laboratories with advanced diagnostic facilities for back up support.
- To maintain the uniformity and standard of diagnostics in these laboratories IgM, MAC, ELISA test kits are provided through National Institute of Virology (NIV), Pune. Cost is borne by GOI.
- Diagnosis of Dengue and Chikungunya is provided to the community at free of cost.
- Since 2007, every year in the 1st quarter Directorate of NVBDCP prepare the tentative allocation of test kits based on the previous epidemiological situation of Dengue and Chikungunya in the states and communicate to both NIV, Pune and States
- Kits are supplied by NIV, Pune on receipt of requirement from the respective states.
- Buffer stocks are also maintained to meet any exigency.
- State-wise allocation of Dengue and Chikungunya during 2010 was communicated to the states on 15th February 2010.
- Ensuring the diagnostic facility and availability of kits is the responsibility of the respective State Program Officers, NVBDCP.

JAPANESE ENCEPHALITIS

Japanese encephalitis (JE) is a viral disease which is transmitted by infective bites of female mosquitoes mainly belonging to *Culex tritaeniorhynchus, Culex vishnui* and *Culex pseudovishnui* group. However, some other mosquito species also play a role in transmission under specific conditions. JE virus is primarily zoonotic in its natural cycle and man is an accidental host. JE virus is neurotropic and arbovirus and primarily affects central nervous system. Japanese Encephalitis is becoming a health problem in a number of states especially in AP, TN, Kerala, Karnataka, WB, Assam, Bihar and Haryana. There was no national program for this disease and the affected states were managing the problem with the technical assistance from the center. This disease was included under the NVBDCP in 2003–2004.

Sign and Symptoms of JE

JE virus infection presents classical symptoms similar to any other virus causing encephalitis. JE virus infection may result in febrile illness of variable severity associated with neurological symptoms ranging from headache to meningitis or encephalitis. Symptoms can include headache, fever, meningeal signs, stupor, disorientation, coma, tremors, paralysis (generalized), hypertonia, loss of coordination, etc. Prodromal stage may be abrupt (1–6 hours), acute (6–24 hours) or more commonly subacute (2–5 days) In acute encephalitic stage, symptoms noted in prodromal phase convulsions, alteration of sensorium, behavioral changes, motor paralysis and involuntary movement supervene and focal neurological deficit is common. Usually lasts for a week but may prolong due to complications. Amongst patients who survive, some lead to full recovery through steady improvement and some suffer with stabilization of neurological deficit. Convalescent phase is prolonged and vary from a few weeks to several months. Clinically it is difficult to differentiate between JE and other viral encephalitis.

Control Strategy

Care of the patient to prevent sequelae development of a safe and standard vaccine.

Sentinel surveillance including clinical surveillance of suspected cases. Studies to identify high-risk cases epidemiological monitoring of the disease and effective implementation of preventive and control measures.

Strengthening early diagnosis and prompt case management at PHCs, CHCs and hospitals through training of medical and nursing staff.
- IEC for community awareness to promote early case reporting, personal protection, isolation of amplifier host, etc.;
- Vector control measures mainly fogging during outbreaks, space spraying in animal dwellings, and antilarval operation where feasible; and
- Development of a safe and standard indigenous vaccine. Vaccination for high-risk population particularly children below 15 years of age.

NATIONAL NUTRITION PROGRAMME

Under nutrition is by far most important single cause of illness and death globally accounting for 12% of all deaths and 16% of disability-adjusted life year lost. Low weight for age is associated more than half of all deaths in young children accounting for more than 6 million deaths per year. There are a variety of nutrition program against the micro and macronutrient deficiencies launched to control such nutritional problems. They are:
- Vitamin A Prophylaxis Programme
- Prophylaxis Against Nutritional Anemia
- Iodine Deficiency Disorder Control Programme
- Special Nutrition Programme
- Balwadi Nutrition Programme
- ICDS Programme
- Mid-Day Meal Programme
- Applied Nutrition Programme
- Tamil Nadu Integrated Nutrition Programme.

NATIONAL NUTRITION POLICY

The National Nutrition Policy (NNP), formulated by the Department of Women and Child Development, Government of India (GOI) was approved by the Cabinet in April 1993 and tabled in both houses of the parliament in August 1993.

Initially the policy is to monitor and evaluate the progress in implementing the World Declaration and plan of action for nutrition. However, it has been further developed to monitor country progress in developing, strengthening and implementing national nutrition plans, policies and programs, including multisectoral actions, development of dietary guidelines, undertaking of nutrition surveys, demographic and epidemiological data. The policy advocates a "comprehensive, integrated and inter-sectoral strategy for alleviating the multifaceted problem of malnutrition and achieving the optimal state of nutrition for the people". The National Plan of Action on Nutrition (NPAN) was released in 1995 to implement the National Nutrition Policy, which included strategies specifically to address the prevention and control of micronutrient deficiencies.

Aims of the National Nutrition Policy

The NNP is based on the conviction that reduction in malnutrition and improvement in nutritional status of the people will contribute significantly to development of human resources and the overall economic and social goals of the country.

The main aims of the NNP are:

- To draw attention to the urgent need to reduce malnutrition in the country, to highlight the need for inter-sectoral coordination to achieve nutritional goals,
- To orient relevant sectors to perceive nutrition as an outcome of their sectoral activities, and
- To identify short-term, intermediate and long-term strategies for achieving nutritional goals either through direct policy changes or indirect institutional or structural changes.

Nutrition Policy Instruments

Realizing the fact that nutrition is a multi-sectoral issue and needs to be tackled at various levels, the nutrition policy instruments focused on tackling the problem of nutrition both through nutrition interventions, for especially vulnerable groups, as well as, through various development policy instruments that will create conditions for improved nutrition. A direct intervention (short-term strategy) and an indirect policy instrument through long-term institutional and structural changes were advocated. Let us look at the nutrition policy instruments highlighting short and long-term measures.

Direct Short-term Intervention: The short-term measures focus on the following strategies:

1. **Nutrition intervention for especially vulnerable groups by:**
   - Expanding the nutrition intervention net through Integrated Child Development Services (ICDS) so as to cover all vulnerable children in the age group 0–6 years
   - Expanding the safety net for children—proper implementation of universal immunization, oral rehydration and ICDS services have been expanded to cover all vulnerable children in the age group 0–6 years
   - Improving growth monitoring between the age group 0–3 years in particular, with closer involvement of the mothers, in a key intervention
   - Reaching the adolescent girls through the ICDS so that they are made ready for a safe motherhood, their nutritional status is improved and they are given some skill upgradation training in home-based skills and covered by nonformal education, particularly nutrition and health education, and
   - *Nutrition of pregnant women to decrease incidence of low birthweight:* Under the policy the government has taken measures to improve the nutritional status of the pregnant mothers right from 1st trimester, supplementation of iron and folic acid, frequent health checkups etc.
   - Ensuring better coverage of expectant mothers, such coverage to include supplementary nutrition starting from first trimester of pregnancy to the first year after pregnancy.
2. **Food fortification:** Fortification of essential food items with appropriate nutrients is essential to avoid deficiency disorders like iodine deficiency, iron deficiency etc. Example, common salt with iodine or iron.
3. **Provision of low cost nutritious food:** Majority of the Indian population belongs to low socio-economic status and they cannot afford for the expensive food products. So there is a need to provide low cost and nutritious food products for the people to maintain and improve the health of the individual, family and the community by developing indigenous systems and with locally available foods. It also involves production and popularization of low cost nutritious foods from indigenous and locally available raw material, by involving women in this activity.
4. **Combating micronutrient deficiency in vulnerable group:** Control of micronutrient deficiencies among the vulnerable groups especially Vitamin A, Iron, Iodine, Folic acid among the pregnant, nursing mothers and children through various nutritional prophylaxis programs is essential. Example: Vitamin A Prophylaxis Programme, The Nutritional Anemia Prophylaxis Programme, etc. *Next, let us look at the indirect policy instruments.*

Indirect Policy Instruments

The long-term strategies for achieving the national goals through indirect institutional or structural changes includes:

- Ensuring food security, a per capita availability of 215 kg/person/year of food grains.
- Improvement in the dietary patterns by promoting the production and increasing the per capita availability of nutritionally rich foods.
- Policies for effective income transfers so as to improve the entitlement package of the rural and' urban poor by reorienting and restructuring the poverty alleviation programs (like Integrated Rural Development Programme) and employment generation schemes (like Jawahar Rozgar Yojana, etc.) to make a forceful dent on the purchasing power of the lowest economic

segments of the population and by ensuring an equitable food distribution, through the expansion of the public distribution system (PDS).

- Implementing land reforms.
- Health and Family Welfare.
- Basic nutrition and health knowledge, with special focus on wholesome infant feeding practices.
- Prevention of food adulteration, by strengthening/gearing up the enforcement machinery.
- Nutrition surveillance.
- Monitoring of nutrition programs.
- Communication through established media for effective implementation of the nutrition policy.
- Ensuring an effective, minimum wage administration.
- Community participation, by involving the community through their panchayats beneficiary committees or through actual participation, particularly of women, by promoting schemes relating to kitchen gardens, food preservation, etc., and generation of effective demand at the level of the community for all services relating to nutrition
- Education and literacy, and
- Improvement of the status of women.

The policy states that the measures enumerated above are to be administered through inter-sectoral coordination and activities. Next, we will look at how the National Nutrition Policy is being implemented.

National Policy Implementation

The nodal responsibility at the central level for policy implementation rests with the Ministry of Human Resource Development under the chairmanship of Secretary, Departments of Women and Child Development. Sectoral Ministries/Departments concerned like Agriculture, Food, Civil Supplies, Health and Family Welfare, Rural Development, Education and Environment, whose role is crucial for sustainable improvement in nutritional status of the population, be represented on the Inter Ministerial Coordination Committee. A National Nutrition Council is constituted in the Planning Commission with the Prime Minister as its President and concerned Union Ministers, a few State Ministers by rotation, and experts, representatives of nongovernmental organizations and grass root leaders (especially women) as its members. Further, the effective implementation of the NNP is dependent to a large extent on the State Governments Union Territory Administrations and the constitution of State Nutrition Councils. Its implementation focuses on following points:

Improving the purchasing power: One of the main causes of under nutrition is low purchasing power of the poor. So to increase their purchasing power, Government should generate jobs for them. Poverty alleviation program like Integrated Rural Development Programme and employment generation schemes like Jawahar Rozgar Yojana, Nehru Rozgar Yojana and DWCRA are to be reoriented and restructured. It is necessary to improve the purchasing power of the landless and the rural and urban poor by implementing employment generation programs.

Establishment of small and medium enterprises (SME): Small and medium enterprises are essential for dynamic economic growth and job creation. Improving access to finance for this sector will be key factor for growth.

Agriculture and rural development: Two-thirds of India's people depend on rural employment for their living. While the agriculture sector grew at only about 2.5% a year for a number of years, recent growth has touched 4.7% a year, facilitated by good monsoons, greater production of high-value crops, an increase in the minimum support prices for grains, and the rise in global prices for agricultural products. Rural livelihoods projects support the empowerment of the rural poor and the development of their livelihoods. Encouraging policies that promote competition in agricultural marketing will also ensure farmers receive better prices.

Informal sector jobs: While the services sector has been offering promising job opportunities for skilled workers, some 90% of India's labor force remains trapped in low-productivity jobs in the informal sector. India's labor regulations—among the most restrictive and complex in the world—have constrained the growth of the formal manufacturing sector, where these laws have their widest application. Better-designed labor regulations can attract more labor-intensive investment and create jobs for India's unemployed millions and those trapped in poor quality jobs.

Prevention of food adulteration: Government responsibility is to assure that food will not cause harm to the consumer when it is prepared and/or eaten according to its intended use. Under the provision of the PFA Act, the Government of India has promulgated PFA rules which specifies the following details like qualification, duties and functions of food analysts, food inspectors and central food laboratory. Procedure for drawing test samples and sending them to the analyst and laboratory. Specification for the identity and purity of food. Tolerance for contaminants, preservatives, emulsifiers and other additives.

Nutrition education: World Bank reports that Indonesia spent only 15% of its national budget on nutrition education and they reduced the prevalence of under-nutrition by 40%. Hence it is a very cost effective method in the Indian context also. The education strategies to make nutrition the central talking point are social marketing, communication for behavior change, advocacy. The services of nutrition specialists and local community leaders should be used to counsel about improving the dietary practices, sanitation and hygiene, encourage breastfeeding, birth spacing, deworming of children, gender sensitivity promoting use of fortified foods, mineral and vitamin supplements.

Recommendations of Policy

- Focus on 3–6 years age group children rather than since birth in ICDS because malnutritional ready sets in by then.

- Focus on mild to moderate malnutrition and not just on severe malnutrition.
- Establish regional, zonal centers with nutritionists/ scientists and use the expertise of biotechnologists and genetic engineers.
- Empower Panchayati raj institutions and form village level nutrition committees for microplanning and formulating short-term goals.
- A compulsory course on nutrition literacy at the UGC level.
- Form a nutrition council of India like MCI for quality management of training.
- Overnutrition, obesity and lifestyle related diseases are emerging as a threatening menace with rapid urbanization. The target population should be sensitized about this cause of concern.
- **Land reforms:** Implementing land reform measures so that the vulnerability of the landless and the landed poor can be reduced.
- **Health and family welfare:** Women's poor reproductive health in India is affected by a variety of sociocultural and biological factors. Thus, efforts to improve women's education, raise enrollment and attendance rates of girls in school and reduce the drop-out rate on the one hand and enhance women's income autonomy on the other are fundamental, in the long run, for improvements in women's and family health.
- **Nutritional surveillance:** Nutritional surveillance is necessary to understand the nutritional status of the people. The policy should be strengthened to conduct nutritional surveillance of children, adolescent girls, pregnant and lactating mothers. The nutritional surveillance should include the following: A. Anthropometry is relevant to program management for three reasons: (i) to identify target groups, (ii) in monitoring progress, and (iii) in assessing overall program effects. B. Indicators used must relate to the objectives of the program.
- **Research:** Research into various nutritional aspects should be developed to identify various deficiency disorders, planning and implementing the nutritional supplementation programs, develop extensive methods of food production, fortification of foods, production of nutritious food for low cost, etc. Minimum wage administration: To improve the purchasing power of the poor minimum wage legislation should be administered. Example at least 60 days leave for pregnant women by the employer in the last trimester.
- **Communication:** The department of National Food and Nutrition should take measures to communicate the public regarding the nutritional deficiency disorders, its prevention, and information regarding the nutritional programs through effective methods of information, education and communication. All the outreach health care centers should be provided with adequate facilities for this purpose.
- **Equal remuneration for women:** The Govt. of India should take measures to empower women by providing equal remuneration with that of men. So that she can fulfill the nutritional needs of the family.
- **Improvement of literacy, especially for women:** Women should be provided with basic education, since literate women will make the entire family as literates and she will fulfill the nutritional requirements of the family, so that nutritional status of the community can be maintained.
- **Improving the status of women:** Women should be empowered by providing basic education, equal preference for the women that of males, employment services, enhancing the health care services for the women, etc. Basic health and nutrition knowledge: To improve the purchasing power as well as the consumption of nutritional rich foods health education should be provided to the public especially women regarding the importance of nutrition for maintenance of health, various nutritional deficiency disorders, its prevention, *preservation and storage of nutrients while cooking etc.*
- **Monitoring of nutrition programs:** The Govt. of India through the Nutritional Monitoring Bureau supervises and evaluates the effective functioning of nutritional programs and recommends the necessary actions required to improve and maintain the health of all age groups.

VITAMIN A PROPHYLAXIS PROGRAMME

Vitamin A (VA) is an essential nutrient needed in small amounts for the normal functioning of the visual system, growth and development, maintenance of epithelial cellular integrity, immune function and reproduction. Severe deficiency of VA is known to produce corneal xerophthalmia, keratomalacia and blindness in children. Vitamin A deficiency (VAD) is mainly seen amongst the young children as they have high requirements due to increased physical growth and have low dietary intake. Further, episodes of illnesses, such as acute respiratory tract infection and measles, which deplete VA reserves from the body, are common in this age group.

A survey was carried out in five states such as Assam, Bihar, Odisha, West Bengal and Tripura which shows that the prevalence of bitot spot was 22%. Night blindness was 1.2–4.0% which indicating VAD is a public health problem in all 5 states. Vitamin A prophylaxis programme was initiated in 1970 with the specific aim of preventing nutritional blindness due to keratomalacia. The program was started as a 100% centrally sponsored program. It was launched as an urgent remedial measure to combat the unacceptably high magnitude of xerophthalmic blindness in the country reported in the 1950s and 1960s.

Under the national programme for prophylaxis against blindness in children, caused due to VAD every child has been provided prophylaxis against VAD in the oral five doses starting at 9 months with measures at a first dose (1 lakh IU) the 15 months a second dose (2 lakh IU) thin every six month (2 lakhs IU) till the age of 3 years which is termed as vitamin A.

In 2006, the age group of eligible children was revised as 6–59 months. This was done after reconsidering the recommendations of WHO, UNICEF and Ministry of Women and Child Development. The doses are administered by Anganwadi workers under the supervision of ANM. This program has been implemented.

Objectives

- To assess the magnitude of VAD in the project area.
- To assess and improve vitamin A status in school going children, adolescent boys and girls nonpregnant woman and geriatric population.
- To launch extensive information education and communication strategy through mass media to improve the dietary habits of the population.
- To coordinate with similar ongoing program being implemented in the country.

Control Measures

For eradicator control of VAD the health workers should trained properly. They should be able to diagnosis VAD. They should identify properly the sign and symptoms of night blindness, xerophthalmic (drying of conjunctive and cornea), Bitot's spot (occupation of foamy, cheesy material on the conjunctive. Corneal neurosis (ulceration), kerato-malaria (melting or wasting of cornea), corneal scar and Xerophthalmic fundus.

For prophylaxis according to this program vitamin A solution should be administered starting first dose. 1 lakh at 9 months than every 6 month 2 lakh IU vitamin A solution up to 5 years of age.

For treatment those are already suffered from VAD disorders should treated in case of children: two doses of 200000 (2 lakhs) IU vitamin A solution given 4 weeks apart and two doses should be given. However, WHO recommended another dose that should be given on the 2nd day after first dose. All doses the child will get at every level of health care delivery system. The child should be advised to consume vitamin A rich food such as papaya, carrot, butter, whole milk, egg yolk, green leaves, etc. Nutritional counseling should be given to the mother about vitamin A rich food.

Treatment to Mother

Around 40–50% antenatal mothers attending clinic and OPD showed vitamin A level less than 30 mg/dL which is inadequate.

Frank VAD is easy to identify however subclinical cases remain a problem for defection. Urinary ammonia nitrogen >0.5 indicative of inadequate status. Such women should treated with vitamin A that is not exceeding 10000 IU per day, till symptoms disappear or levels comes to normal. Excessive doses are potentially tonic and teratogenic.

Set Back of the Program

The Program suffered set back due to different causes that time. In Assam a 1 year boy died after consumption of vitamin A solution which belongs to few community.

This triggered panic among parents. Thousands of people rushed with their children to the nearest health center. Some of them complaining fever vomiting and diarrhea. All deaths and illness that occurred in children during following weeks were attributed to vitamin A. There is no evidence that vitamin A causes death, even if a child received twice the recommended amount. This program is now included in RCH Program. Vitamin A deficiency is compromising the immune system of approximately 60% of the developing world's under fives and leading to early deaths of an estimated one million young children each year. Presently, vitamin A supplementation (VAS) is implemented through the existing network of PHC and subcenters. The female multipurpose worker and other paramedics at the village level subhealth centers are responsible for administering vitamin A solution. The services of integrated child development services (ICDS) functionaries are also utilized for the implementation of the program. Monthly intensive drives are undertaken every 6 months to achieve universal coverage of those children who could not be covered during the routine visits of health functionaries.

Precautions for Vitamin A Administration

- Ensure dose limit not exceeded. Spoon provided with vitamin A solution to be used
  - 9–12 m 1 mL (100, 000 IU)
  - 13–59 m 2 mL (200, 000 IU)
- Do not administer vitamin A to a child who has received a dose in the last 1 month
- After opening the bottle of Vitamin A, write the date of opening on the label, use within 6–8 weeks
- Acute toxicity results from one or several closely spaced very large doses of vitamin A
- The signs are usually transient and disappear after a few days.
- Health workers should be aware of the transient side effects:
  - Loss of appetite
  - Bulging fontanelles
  - Drowsiness, increased intracranial pressure
  - Irritability, vomiting, excessive crying, restlessness.

Applied Nutrition Program

This program was started in 1963 by Government of India in collaboration with FAO, UNICEF, and WHO for improvement in nutritional status of pregnant and lactating women and children. The Applied Nutrition Programme (ANP) was introduced as a pilot scheme in Odisha in 1963 which later on extended to Tamil Nadu and Uttar Pradesh with the objectives of: (a) promoting production of protective food, such as vegetables and fruits and (b) ensure their consumption by pregnant and nursing mothers and children. During 1973, it was extended to all the state of the country. The nutritional education was the main focus and efforts were directed to teach rural communities through demonstration how to produce food for their consumption through their own efforts. The beneficiaries are children between 2 and 6 years and pregnant and lactating mothers. Nutrition worth of 25 paise per child per day and 50 paise per woman per day are provided for 52 days in a year. No definite nutrient content has been specified. The idea is to provide better seeds and encourage kitchen gardens, poultry farming, beehive keeping, etc., but this program does not produced any impact. The community kitchens and school gardens could not function properly due to lack of suitable land, irrigation facilities, and low financial investment.

Objectives

- To increase the production of protective foods, e.g., milk, fruits, vegetables, eggs, fish, etc.
- To encourage consumption of these foods by poor classes, children and mothers.
- To educate mothers, teachers, and nutrition workers regarding nutrition.
- To provide supplementary nutrition to vulnerable groups through local production of foods.

Activities of Applied Nutrition Programme

- Education and training in poultry, dairy, fishery, horticulture, home science, etc., were conducted by rural extension education centers.
- Development fields, coordination committees were constituted at the state, district, and block level.
- Production of protective foods.
- Give priority to local productions and demonstration of protective food.

NUTRITIONAL ANEMIA PROPHYLAXIS PROGRAMME

Started by Government of India under 4th five years plan. Iron and folic acid (IFA) tablets are distributed to young children and expectant mothers. Distribution of IFA tablets in free of cost is carried out in the community health centers (CHCs), MCH centers and hospitals. The beneficiaries are 'at risk' groups, i.e., pregnant women, lactating mothers, and children under 12 years. That time the children under 1 year are not consider for iron prophylaxis later children 6 months to 1 year also included in program.

Activities of Nutritional Anemia Prophylaxis Programme

The National Iron + Initiative is an attempt to look at the iron deficiency anemia comprehensively across all life stages including adolescents and women in reproductive age group who are not pregnant or lactating. There are some approaches to control Iron Deficiency Anemia under Nutritional Anemia prophylaxis programme. They are food-based approach, IFA supplementation, deworming and prevention of malaria. The Food-based approach included improve quantity and quality of diet and fortification of food the people need to improve food intake, iron fortified food and iron rich food. Dietary diversification is the long-term approach. Involves nutrition education and changes in dietary habits of the population. Improve absorption of iron by lowering inhibitor and increasing promoter concentrations. Encourage for green leafy vegetables and fruits and nonveg food like liver, egg, fish, meat. Grains—wheat, jowar, bajra, sprouted pulses, groundnut, sesame, jaggery, dried fruits alo adviced to take vitamin C rich foods help in absorption of iron. Citrus fruits (oranges, lemon), Indian gooseberry (Amla), apple, pear are rich in vitamin C which helps in iron absorption. Deworming in preschool children reduces anemia and improves weight gain and growth. WHO recommends that preventive deworming be bundled with preventive biannual Vitamin A supplementation programs to enhance the effectiveness of both interventions. The National Iron+ Initiative is an attempt to look at the Iron Deficiency Anemia comprehensively across all life stages including adolescents and women in reproductive age group who are not pregnant or lactating. Iron and folic acid supplementation can reduce anemia by 20–30%.

Prophylaxis with iron should be withheld in case of acute illness (fever, acute diarrhea, pneumonia, etc.), severe acute malnutrition (SAM) and in known case of hemoglobinopathy/history of repeated blood transfusion.

ANEMIA MUKT BHARAT PROGRAMME

The Ministry of Health and Family Welfare (MoH and FW) has launched Anemia Mukt Bharat Programme with special focus on the health and nutrition needs of children, adolescents, women of reproductive age group and pregnant mothers and lactating mothers. This will be achieved through six interventions, implementation of which will be facilitated by six robust institutional mechanisms. To facilitate seamless implementation of the interventions, a training tool kit has been developed which will be used to orient and train different stakeholders at various levels for effective implementation of Anemia Mukt Bharat (AMB) strategy. The reduction of anemia is one of the important objectives of the POSHAN Abhiyaan launched in March 2018. Complying with the targets of POSHAN Abhiyaan and National Nutrition Strategy set by NITI Aayog, the Anemia Mukt Bharat strategy has been designed to reduce prevalence of anemia by 3%age points per year among children, adolescents and women in the reproductive age group (15–49 years), between the year 2018 and 2022 **(Table 10.2)**.

Guiding principles:

- **Beneficiary-centered approach:** Commitment to improve health outcomes and reduce anemia prevalence among the target age groups
- **Inclusive partnerships:** Facilitate participation of all stakeholders to achieve the common goal
- **Accountability:** Commitment to inculcate accountability for service delivery among all service providers
- **Minimizing duplication:** Leverage existing institutional mechanism.

Table 10.2: Anemia Mukt Bharat—anemia reduction targets for 2022.

Age group	*Anemia prevalence (%)*	
	Baseline (NFHS 4)	*National target 2022 (at 3%age points per annum from baseline)*
Children (6–59 months)	58	40
Adolescent girls (15–19 years)	54	36
Adolescent boys (15–19 years)	29	11
Women of reproductive age	53	35
Pregnant women	50	32
Lactating women	58	40

SIX-SIX-SIX STRATEGY TO COMBAT ANEMIA FOR ANEMIA MUKT BHARAT

Six-Six-Six strategy to combat anemia for Anemia Mukt Bharat are 6-beneficiaries, 6-interventions and 6-Institutional mechanisms.

Six (6) beneficiaries: Six types of beneficiary includes under-five children (124 million Children 6–59 months), School going children 115 million, Adolescent boys and girls 30 million of Pregnant women (10–19 years), 17 million Women of reproductive age (20–24 years), 27 million of Lactating mothers. Children 6–59 months will be reached with biweekly IFA syrup by ASHA through home visits and mothers will be equipped with skills to provide biweekly IFA dose in households. School children 5–9 years will be provided weekly IFA (Pink) tablet in schools using spot feeding approach of IFA after the mid-day meal through teachers in Government aided schools and after lunch break in private schools. Out-of-school children between 5–9 years will be provided IFA tablets through ASHA during home visits. School-going adolescents 10–19 years will be provided weekly IFA (Blue) tablets by school teachers. Out-of-school adolescent girls 10–19 years will be provided IFA (Blue) tablets through quarterly Adolescent Health Day component of Rashtriya Kishore Swasthya Karyakram (RKSK) programme at Anganwadi centers. Women of reproductive age (WRA) who are not pregnant or non-lactating will be provided weekly IFA (Red) tablets. Pregnant women will be provided services under the strategy through antenatal care contacts (ANC clinics/VHND/PMSMA), receipt of IFA and Folic Acid tablets, screening and point-of-care treatment of anemia, and screening and prevention of malaria. Lactating women will be provided IFA tablets via the VHND platform when they bring their children for immunization.

Six (6) interventions: A key intervention is to give IFA to children, adolescents and women of reproductive age and pregnant women irrespective of anemia, under Anemia Mukt Bharat.

The **Table 10.3** delineates the dose and regime of Iron Folic Acid supplementation to be followed. **Tables 10.4 to 10.6** depicts the anemia management protocols of different age groups.

Table 10.3: Prophylactic dose and regime for iron folic acid supplementation.

Children 6–59 months of age	Biweekly 1 mL Iron and Folic Acid syrup. Each mL Iron and Folic Acid syrup containing 20 mg elemental Iron + 100 mcg of Folic Acid. Bottle (50 mL) to have an 'autodispenser' and information leaflet as per MoHFW guidelines in the mono-carton
Children 5–9 years of age	Weekly, 1 iron and folic acid tablet. Each tablet containing 45 mg elemental Iron + 400 mcg Folic Acid, sugar-coated, pink-color
School-going adolescent girls and boys, 10–19 years of age; out-of-school adolescent girls, 10–19 years of age	Weekly, 1 iron and folic acid tablet. Each tablet containing 60 mg elemental Iron + 500 mcg Folic Acid, sugar-coated, blue-color
Women of reproductive age (nonpregnant, non-lactating) 20–49 years (Under Mission Parivar Vikas)	Weekly, 1 iron and folic acid tablet. Each tablet containing 60 mg elemental Iron + 500 mcg Folic Acid, sugar-coated and red-color
Pregnant Women and Lactating Mothers (of 0–6 months child)	Daily, 1 iron and folic acid tablet starting from the fourth month of pregnancy (that is from the second trimester), continued throughout pregnancy (minimum 180 days during pregnancy) and to be continued for 180 days, post-partum. Each tablet containing 60 mg elemental Iron + 500 mcg Folic Acid, sugar-coated and red-color

Second intervention (deworming): Biannual mass deworming for children in the age groups between 1–19 years is carried out on designated dates - 10th February and 10th August every year under National Deworming Day (NDD) programme. The Anemia Mukt Bharat, also integrates deworming of women of reproductive age and for pregnant women as part of the NDD strategy.

The **Table 10.7** reiterates the deworming dose and regime to be followed.

Third intervention out of 6: Intensified year-round behavior change communication campaign (solid body, smart mind) including ensuring delayed cord clamping in newborns.

There is sufficient evidence that repeated engagement using consistent key messaging is required for any behavior to change, or to initiate new behavior so that it becomes a practice. The various behavior change communication activities of the strategy will address four key behaviors:

1. Compliance to iron folic acid supplements and deworming
2. Appropriate infant and young child feeding (IYCF) with emphasis on adequate and age-appropriate complementary foods for children 6 months and above
3. Increase intake of iron-rich, protein-rich and vitamin C-rich foods through dietary diversification/quantity/frequency and food fortification
4. Promoting practice of delayed cord clamping (by at least 3 minutes or until cord pulsations cease) in all health facility

Table 10.4: Anemia management protocol for children.

Who will screen and place of screening	ANM: VHND/subcenter/session site RSBK team: AWC/school Medical officer: Health facility
Periodicity	• RBSK/ANM: As per scheduled microplan • MO: Opportunistic
If Hemoglobin is 7–10.9 g/dL (mild and moderate anemia)	–
First level of treatment (at all levels of care)	3 mg of iron/kg/day for 2 months • For children 6–12 months (6–10.9 kg): 1 mL IFA syrup, once a day • For children 1–3 years (11–14.9 kg): 1.5 mL IFA syrup, once a day • For children 3–5 years (15–19.9 kg): 2 mL IFA syrup, once a day Line listing for all anemic children to be maintained by the ANM/ASHA/AWW
Follow-up	• Every month by ANM at VHND • Hb estimation after 2 months for completing 2 months of treatment to document Hb>= 11 g/dL • Monitoring by ASHA for compliance of IFA syrup every 14 days for a period of 2 months If hemoglobin levels have improved to normal level, discontinue the treatment, but continue with the prophylactic IFA dose
If no improvement after first level of treatment	In case the child has not responded to the treatment of anemia with daily dose of iron for 2 months, refer the child to the FRU/DH medical officer/pediatrician/physician for further investigation
If Hemoglobin is <7 g/dL (severe anemia)	–
Treatment	• Refer urgently to District Hospital/First Referral Unit • Management of severe anemia in children of 6–59 months is to be done by the medical officer at the First Referral Unit/District Hospital based on investigation
Target group B	Children 5–9 years
Who will screen and place of screening	RSBK teams will screen in-school and out-of-school children for anemia. All children with clinical signs and symptoms of anemia will be referred to SC/PHC for Hb estimation and further management
Periodicity	• Once a year • Opportunistic screening, e.g., routine Hb assessment of sick children presented to health facility
If Hemoglobin is 8–11.4 g/dL (mild and moderate anemia)	–
First level of treatment (at all levels of care)	3 mg of iron/kg/day for 2 months. Line listing of all anemic cases to be maintained in the school register for Iron Folic Acid supplementation and given to the ANM/LHV/Multiple Purpose Health Worker for designated area
Follow-up	• Class teacher/Nodal teacher at school to orient parents during Parent Teacher Meeting (PTM) for compliance of treatment • Parents to ensure follow-up of child after 30 days and 60 days at nearest SC/health facility • Follow-up by ANM/LHV/MPW of designated area, as feasible. • Hb estimation after completing 2 months of treatment to document Hb>= 11.5 g/dL • If hemoglobin levels have improved to normal level, discontinue the treatment, but continue with the prophylactic IFA dose
If no improvement after first level of treatment	In case the child has not responded to the treatment of anemia with daily dose of iron for 2 months, refer the child to the FRU/DH medical officer/paediatrician/physician for further investigation
If Hemoglobin is <8 g/dL (severe anemia)	–
Treatment	• Refer urgently to District Hospital/First Referral Unit • Management of severe anemia in children of 5–9 years is to be done by the medical officer at the First Referral Unit/District Hospital based on investigation

Table 10.5: Anemia management protocol for adolescents.

Target group	*All school-going adolescents 10–19 years in government/government-aided schools*
Who will screen and place of screening	In school premises by RSBK team
Periodicity	Annually
Mild and Moderate Anemia (Hb cut-off is 8–11.4 g/dL)	–

Contd...

Contd...

Target group	***All school-going adolescents 10–19 years in government/government-aided schools***
First level of treatment (at all levels of care)	Two IFA tablets (each with 60 mg elemental iron and 500 mcg folic acid), once daily, for 3 months, orally after meals.
Follow-up	• Line listing of all anemic cases to be maintained in the school register for Iron Folic Acid supplementation and given to the ANM/LHV/MPHW of designated area • Follow-up by ANM/LHV/MPHW of designated area, as feasible for the state • Parents to ensure follow-up of adolescent after 45 days to 90 days at the nearest subcenter/health facility • If hemoglobin levels have improved to normal level, discontinue the treatment, but continue with the prophylactic IFA dose
If no improvement after first level of treatment	If no improvement after three months of treatment (i.e., still in mild/moderate category), ANM/MO of nearest facility to refer adolescent to First Referral Unit (FRU)/District Hospital (DH)
If Hemoglobin is <8 g/dL (severe anemia)	–
First dose of treatment	Management of severe anemia in adolescents 10–19 years is to be done by the medical officer at FRU/DH based on investigation and subsequent diagnosis

Table 10.6: Anemia management protocol for pregnant women.

Periodicity	***At every ANC contact***
Target group	***Pregnant women registered for antenatal care***
If Hemoglobin is 10–10.9 g/dL (mild anemia)	
First level of treatment (at all levels of care)	• Two tablets of Iron and Folic Acid tablet (60 mg elemental Iron and 500 mcg Folic Acid) daily, orally given by the health provider during the ANC contact • Parental iron (IV Iron Sucrose or Ferric Carboxy Maltose (FCM) may be considered as the first line of management in pregnant women who are detected to be anemic late in pregnancy or in whom compliance is likely to below (high chance of lost to follow-up)
Follow-up	• Every 2 months for compliance of treatment by health provider during the contact • If hemoglobin levels have come up to normal level, discontinue the treatment and continue with the prophylactic IFA dose
If no improvement after first level of treatment	• If no improvement in hemoglobin (<1 g/dL increase) after one month of treatment, refer to First Referral Unit (FRU)/District Hospital (DH) by health provider • The case to be referred to FRU/DH for further investigations for cause of anemia and may be managed with IV Iron Sucrose/FCM
If Hemoglobin is 7–9.9 g/dL (moderate anemia)	
First level of treatment (at all levels of care)	• Two tablets of Iron and Folic Acid tablet (60 mg elemental Iron and 500 mcg Folic Acid) daily, orally given by the health provider during the ANC contact • Parental iron (IV Iron Sucrose or FCM) may be considered as the first line of management in pregnant women who are detected to be anemic late in pregnancy or in whom compliance is likely to be low (high chance of lost to follow-up)
Follow-up	• Every 2 months for compliance of treatment by health provider at regular ANC clinics/PMSMA/VHND platform. • The contact is to be utilized by the health provider to also conduct hemoglobin estimation of the anemic cases every month. If hemoglobin levels have come up to normal level, discontinue the treatment and continue with the prophylactic IFA dose.
If no improvement after first level of treatment	• If no improvement in hemoglobin (<1 g/dL increase) after two month of treatment, refer to First Referral Unit (FRU)/District Hospital (DH) by health provider • The case to be referred to FRU/DH for further investigations for cause of anemia and may be managed with IV Iron Sucrose/FCM
If Hemoglobin is 5.0–6.9 g/dL (severe anemia)	
First level of treatment	• Management of severe anemia in pregnant women will be done by the medical officer at PHC/CHC/FRU/DH • The treatment will be done using IV Iron Sucrose/Ferric Carboxy Maltose (FCM) by the medical officer • Immediate hospitalization recommended in the third trimester of pregnancy at a health facility where round-the-clock specialist care is available
Follow-up after first level of treatment	After the first level of treatment, monthly or as prescribed by the medical officer
Treatment protocol if no improvement	As prescribed by the medical officer
Note: For severely anemic pregnant women with hemoglobin less than 5 g/dL, immediate hospitalization irrespective of period of gestation where round-the-clock specialist care is available. This is to be done till normal level of hemoglobin is achieved	

Table 10.7: Dose and regime of different age group for deworming.

Dose and regime for deworming.	
Children 6–59 months of age	Biannual dose of 400 mg Albendazole (½ tablet to children 12–24 months and 1 tablet to children 24–59 months)
Children 5–9 years of age	Biannual dose of 400 mg Albendazole (1 tablet)
School-going Adolescent Girls and Boys, 10–19 years of age; Out-of-school Adolescent Girls, 10–19 years of age	Biannual dose of 400 mg Albendazole (1 tablet)
Women of Reproductive Age (nonpregnant, nonlactating) 20–49 years	Biannual dose of 400 mg Albendazole (1 tablet)
Pregnant Women and Lactating Mothers (0–6 months)	One dose of 400 mg Albendazole (1 tablet), after the first trimester, preferably during the second trimester

deliveries followed by early initiation of breastfeeding within 1 hour of birth.

Fourth intervention (Testing and treatment of anemia, with focus on pregnant women and school-going adolescents)

Screening and testing of anemia is important in all age groups so that appropriate treatment may be initiated as per the hemoglobin level of the individual. The current method of hemoglobin estimation in the field uses SAHLI's method, which needs to be replaced with newer advanced technologies for the available hemoglobin estimation.

6-Institutional Mechanisms

National Anemia Mukt Bharat unit: A National Unit will be established to support and monitor states for strategy implementation. The unit will monitor and anchor the strategy under the leadership of Joint Secretary (RMNCH+A) with technomanagerial support through a DC (CH) from Reproductive and Child Health (RCH) division. The State/UT should establish a state unit and designate a nodal officer. The State Unit will ensure accountability and effective implementation of the strategy. At the district level, under the supervision of the CMO/CDHO, the District Programme Officer under the National Health Mission will be in-charge of the day-to-day implementation of this strategy and the BMO/BHO will be the nodal officer at the block level.

Convergence with other ministries: Interministerial convergence under the strategy will be ensured via existing convergence platform under the POSHAN Abhiyaan. One of the targets under POSHAN Abhiyaan is 'anemia reduction by 3% per annum'. An Executive Committee under the Chairpersonship of Secretary, MoWCD, has been established via Government of India Letter No. NNM/50/2017-WBP8 dated 3 January 2018, wherein the Secretary, MoHFW, is a member. Therefore, all issues related to Anemia Mukt Bharat for which inter-ministerial convergence is needed should be discussed during this committee meeting. Similarly, State Executive Committee of POSHAN Abhiyaan should be Executive Committee of Anemia Mukt Bharat strategy.

Anemia Mukt Bharat dashboard and digital Portal–(one-stop shop for anemia): The Anemia Mukt Bharat portal (www.anemiamuktbharat.info) is a one-stop shop of materials developed under the Anemia Mukt Bharat strategy in one place, such as communication resource material, survey data, targets, state and district-wise denominators, and state and district-wise quarterly progress reports.

Intraministerial coordination: At the national level, the existing Rashtriya Kishor Swasthya Karyakram (RKSK) National Steering Committee will be expanded to include the National Anemia Mukt Bharat Steering Committee. The Steering Committee will have biannual convergent meetings in coordination with the respective divisions within MoHFW associated with the strategy chaired by the Secretary, Ministry of Health and Family Welfare, with invitation to other related Ministries such as Tribal Welfare (residential schools), Ministry of Woman and Child Development (POSHAN Abhiyaan), Ministry of Rural Development and Panchayati Raj (NRLM) and MHRD (Department of School Education and Literacy) and other experts as approved by the chair.

National Center of Excellence and Advanced Research on Anemia Control (NCEAR-A): All India Institute of Medical Sciences (Center for Community Medicine), New Delhi, will house the NCEAR-A. The Center will provide the following support to MoHFW:

- Provide technical inputs with focus on multisectoral approach for policy making, program guidelines and program implementation for anemia control programme in India.
- Address research needs including operational research for anemia control in India.
- Act as an apex reference laboratory for anemia screening and diagnosis at the national level.
- Facilitate periodic program review and capacity building of anemia control programme personnel and state-level institutes to strengthen program implementation including revising training components for service providers and program managers, teachers, ASHA and ANMs, and AWWs respectively with NCERT/DIET, SIHFW, NHSRC, and NIPCCD. At the state level, All India Institute of Medical Sciences (Center for Community Medicine/ Medical College/Nutrition College), can be designated as State Center for Excellence and Advanced Research for Anemia Control (SCEAR-A). SCEAR-A can help in trainings, monitoring and acting as the apex reference laboratory for anemia screening and diagnosis at the state level.

Strengthening Supply Chain and Logistics

The strategy plans to build upon the learning of implementing the National Iron Plus Initiative and Weekly Iron Folic Supplementation programmes and focuses on strengthening the procurement and supply chain mechanisms as these are key to effective implementation of these programs. Therefore, special emphasis is suggested for streamlining the supply chain mechanisms, to ensure uninterrupted supplies, states may consider: (a) introducing auto-indents at the district level, (b) provision for multi-year rate contracts (RC) and multivendor policy, (c) centralized procurement at the state level instead of district level procurement, and (d) Iron Folic Acid supplements and albendazole tablets included as part of the Essential Drug List (EDL).

MID-DAY MEAL PROGRAMME

Mid-day meal programme was launched in 1961 by ministry of education having main role is providing balanced diet to school children. In this program one-third of the children's daily food requirement can be fulfilled. CARE, UNICEF, and many international, national and voluntary agencies also give their contribution.

Aim of Mid-day School Meal

- To fulfill one-third nutrition requirement of school children in age group of 6–11 years of age.
- To create interest about school and education among children.
- To reduce absenteeism of children in school.
- Improving school attendance.

Principle of Mid-day School Meal

- One-third energy and half of protein requirement of the child should be met.
- The food should be free of cost.
- The food should be prepared in the school itself.
- Locally available food should be used in preparing the meal.
- Mid-day school meal program is a supplement and not substitute of home meal.

Mid-day Meal Scheme

Mid-day meal scheme was launched on 15 August 1995. It is a central sponsored scheme.

It was revised in 2004. It is also called as National Programme of Nutritional. Support to Primary Education. CARE, UNICEF, and many International, national and voluntary agencies also give their contribution in this program.

The main objective of the scheme is:

- To fulfill one-third nutrition requirement of school children in age group of 6–11 years of age.
- To create interest about school and education among children.
- To reduce absenteeism of children in school.
- Improving school attendance.

In this scheme center provides free supply of food grains through FCI to states.

The meal should supply of 100 g of grain per student per day which also contain at least 300 kcal and 12–15 g protein per day.

Suggestions for Preparing Mid-day Meal

- Food grains must be stored in a place away from moisture.
- Use whole wheat or broken wheat for preparing mid-day meal.
- Cereal pulse combination is necessary to have good quality protein.
- Leafy vegetables when added to any preparation should be thoroughly washed before cutting.
- Soaking of rice, dal, Bengal gram, etc., reduces cooking time.
- Cooking must be done with the lid to avoid loss of nutrients.
- Over cooking should be avoided.
- Only 'Iodized salt' should be used for cooking mid-day meals.

BALWADI NUTRITION PROGRAMME

The program was started in 1970 for the benefit of children in the age group of 3–6 years in the rural areas. Program was organized by central social welfare board.

Four National level organizations are given grants to implement the program. These are: Indian Tribal Caste Association, Indian council of child welfare, Kasturaba Gandhi National Memorial Trust and Harijan Sevak Sangh. The food supplement provides 300 calories of energy and 10 g of protein per child per day. Balwadis are being phased out because of the implementation of the Integrated Child Development Services (ICDS) programme.

ICDS PROGRAMME

The Integrated Child Development Services scheme integrates several aspects of early childhood development and provides supplementary nutrition, immunization, health check-ups, and referral services to children below 6 years of age as well as expecting and nursing mothers. Additionally, it offers nonformal preschool education to children in the 3–6 age group, and health and nutrition education to women in the 15–45 age group. ICDS was initiated in 1975 in 33 blocks and used below poverty line (BPL) as a criteria for delivery of services. Following a 2004 Supreme Court order, ICDS was expanded in 2005 to cover the entire country. Integrated Child Development Programme was started in 1975 by Ministry of social welfare. The beneficiaries are preschool children below 6 years, pregnant and lactating mothers. There is a strong nutrition component in this program in the form of supplementary nutrition, vitamin A prophylaxis and IFA.

Purpose for Initiation

- Routine MCH services not reaching target population
- Nutritional component not covered by health services
- Need for community participation.

Objectives of the ICDS Programme

- To improve the nutritional and health status of children of 0–6 years.

- To reduce the incidence of mortality, morbidity, malnutrition and school drop out.
- To enhance the capability of mother to look after the normal health and nutritional needs of the child through proper nutrition and health education.
- To lay the foundations for proper psychological, physical, and social development of the child.
- To achieve effective coordination of policy and implementation among various departments to promote child development.

Activities of Program

Under ICDS scheme there is a Anganwadi worker who is at the village level who deliver the services at Anganwadi center (AWC) especially. Each Anganwadi unit covers a population of about 1000. The work of Angan-wadi is supervised by Mukhyasevikas and the field supervision is done by the Child Development Project Officer (CDPO). The activities under ICDS Scheme mainly carried out by Anganwadi worker.

SUPPLEMENTARY NUTRITION PROGRAMME

This includes supplementary feeding and growth monitoring; and prophylaxis against VAD and control of nutritional anemia. All families in the community are surveyed, to identify children below the age of six and pregnant and nursing mothers. They avail of supplementary feeding support for 300 days in a year. By providing supplementary feeding, the Anganwadi attempts to bridge the caloric gap between the national recommended and average intake of children and women in low income and disadvantaged communities.

Types of Supplementary Nutrition

Children in the age group 0–6 months: For children in this age group, States/UTs may ensure continuation of current guidelines of early initiation (within 1 hour of birth) and exclusive breastfeeding for children for the first 6 months of life.

Children in the age group 6 months to 3 years: For children in this age group, the existing pattern of take home ration (THR) under the ICDS scheme will continue. However, in addition to the current mixed practice of giving either dry or raw ration (wheat and rice) which is often consumed by the entire family and not the child alone, THR should be given in the form that is palatable to the child instead of the entire family.

Children in the age group 3 to 6 years: For the children in this age group, State/UTs have been requested to make arrangements to serve Hot Cooked Meal in AWCs and mini-AWCs under the ICDS Scheme. Since the child of this age group is not capable of consuming a meal of 500 calories in one sitting, the States/UTs are advised to consider serving more than one meal to the children who come to AWCs. Since the process of cooking and serving hot cooked meal takes time, and in most of the cases, the food is served around noon, States/UTs may provide 500 calories over more than one meal. States/UTs may arrange to provide a morning snack in the form of milk/banana/egg/seasonal fruits/micronutrient fortified food, etc.

Immunization: Immunization of pregnant women and infants protects children from six vaccine preventable diseases-poliomyelitis, diphtheria, pertussis, tetanus, tuberculosis and measles. These are major preventable causes of child mortality, disability, morbidity and related malnutrition. Immunization of pregnant women against tetanus also reduces maternal and neonatal mortality.

Health check-up: This includes health care of children less than 6 years of age, antenatal care of expectant mothers and postnatal care of nursing mothers. The various health services provided for children by Anganwadi workers and PHC staff, include regular health check-ups, recording of weight, immunization, management of malnutrition, treatment of diarrhea, deworming and distribution of simple medicines, etc.

Referral services: During health check-ups and growth monitoring, sick or malnourished children, in need of prompt medical attention, are referred to the PHC or its subcenter. The anganwadi worker has also been oriented to detect disabilities in young children. She enlists all such cases in a special register and refers them to the medical officer of the PHC/Subcenter.

Nutrition and health education to women: Nutrition, Health and Education (NHED) is a key element of the work of the Anganwadi worker. This forms part of BCC strategy. This has the long-term goal of capacity-building of women especially in the age group of 15–45 years, so that they can look after their own health, nutrition and development needs as well as that of their children and families.

Nonformal education and preschool education of children: The nonformal and Preschool Education (PSE) component of the ICDS may well be considered the backbone of the ICDS programme, since all its services essentially converge at the Anganwadi. ICDS focuses on total development of the child. Its program for the 3 to 6 years old children in the Anganwadi is directed towards providing and ensuring a natural, joyful and stimulating environment, with emphasis on necessary inputs for optimal growth and development. The early learning component of the ICDS is a significant input for providing a sound foundation for cumulative lifelong learning and development. It also contributes to the universalization of primary education, by providing to the child the necessary preparation for primary schooling and offering substitute care to younger siblings, thus freeing the older ones, especially girls to attend school.

Therapeutic nutrition to the malnourished children: The malnourished children are given therapeutic nutrition. 300 kcal and 8–10 g of proteins are given to all the enrolled, at risk and moderately malnourished children. 600 kcal and 18–20 g of protein are given severely malnourished (Gr 111 and iv) 500 kcal and 18–20 g of protein to pregnant and lactating mothers.

Anganwadi center population norms: For Rural/Urban Projects between The area covers 400–800 population 1, 800–1600 population-2, 1600–2400 population-3 and thereafter multiples (in every 800 population 1). For Mini-150–400 population were established-in Tribal/Riverine/Desert, Hilly and other difficult areas/Projects 300–800 population covers 1 the Mini-AWCs covered 150–300 population.

Other Functions of AWW

- To elicit community support
- Make home visits
- Assist PHC staff
- Guide ASHA
- Assist in implementation of Kishori Shakti Yojana (KSY) helper
- Cook and serve food
- Clean the Anganwadi premises and check cleanliness of small children
- Bring small children to Anganwadi, hold weekly/ fortnightly meeting with ASHA
- Participate and guide in organizing the Health Days at AWC
- Utilize ASHA in motivating the pregnant women and married couples
- Guide ASHA in motivating pregnant women for full ANC Educate ASHA on danger signs of pregnancy and labor.

IODINE DEFICIENCY DISORDER CONTROL PROGRAMME

Iodine is an essential micronutrient. It is required at 100–150 μg daily for normal human growth and development. The disorders caused due to deficiency of nutritional iodine in the food/diet are called iodine deficiency disorders. Iodine Deficiency Disorders are a worldwide major public health problem. These affect a large segment of populations in all continents. As per information available, more than 1.5 billion people all over the world are at risk of IDD. The Government of India established the National Goitre Control Programme (NGCP) in 1962 at the end of the second Five-Year Plan. The objectives of NGCP were to identify the goiter-endemic regions of the country and supplement the intake of iodine to the entire population in these regions.

The objectives of NGCP were to conduct an initial baseline survey to identify the endemic and nonendemic districts based on goiter prevalence to produce and supply iodized salt to the identified endemic districts, to conduct an impact assessment of the program every 5 years to see the **effectiveness of the program.**

The NGCP primarily focused on the so called 'goiter belt' in the country which comprised the Himalayan and Tarai region in north and north-eastern parts of India. Subsequently, new evidence emerged that IDD was not limited to a few endemic foci in India and was reported from nearly every geographical region of the country. Based on the evidence from district IDD surveys carried out as per the guidelines of NGCP, situation analysis conducted by the Nutrition Foundation of India (NFI) and studies carried out by the Indian Council of Medical Research (ICMR) and the All India Institute of Medical Sciences (AIIMS), New Delhi team, it was decided to expand the activities of NGCP. In 1983 in the annual meeting of Central Council of Health, it was decided that all edible salt in India would be iodized by 1992. The process of iodization salt was started in a phased manner in the country from April, 1986. Iodized salt was brought under the revised Prevention of Food Adulteration (PFA) Act of 1988. There was a growing realization that iodine deficiency is not limited to goiter alone but could manifest in several other ways with far serious consequences. Available scientific evidence both from across the world and from India showed significant impact of iodine deficiency on early brain development, cognition and learning abilities of children. The World Summit for Children in 1990 endorsed the concept of 'IDD as a spectrum of diseases' and set up a target of global elimination IDD by year 2000. India was one of the participants and signatories of this declaration. The Government of India introduced an amendment in the National Plan of Action for Children to include universal access to iodized salt by 1995 as a specific goal. The nomenclature of the NGCP was changed to National IDD Control Programme (NIDDCP) in 1992 to emphasize the wider implications of iodine deficiency. In 1997-Sale and storage of noniodized salt banned in 2000. Central Government lifted ban on sale of noniodized salt in 2001. Complete ban on Sale and manufacture of noniodized salt for human consumption imposed in Odisha.

Objectives of NIDDCP

- To undertake surveys to assess magnitude of Iodine Deficiency Disorders.
- To supply Iodized salt in place of common salt.
- Resurvey after every 5 years to assess the extent of Iodine Deficiency Disorders and the impact of iodated salt
- To undertake monitoring of the quality of iodated salt.
- To conduct Health Education and Publicity.

Achievements of NIDDCP

The Government of India has issued notification banning the sale of noniodated salt for direct human consumption in the entire country w.e.f. 17th may, 2006 under the prevention of food adulteration act, 1954. There is no ban on the production of common salt per the same can be sold after iodization, iron fortification and can be used for preservation, animal, industrial and medicinal use with proper label declaration. Noniodated salt can be used for other industrial purposes. Annual production of iodated salt has been raised from 5 lakhs mt in 1985–1986 to 51 lakh mt in 2008–2009. 824 private manufactures have been licensed having annual production capacity of iodated salt more than 120 lakh MT. One IDD cell and one IDD monitoring lab have been sanctioned to all states/UTS. 31 states and union territories have established IDD cells. A national reference laboratory for monitoring of IDD has been set up at the biochemistry division of NICD. Four national laboratories at NIN, Hyderabad for south, AIIH and PH, Kolkata for east and

North-east, AIIMS, Delhi for west and NICD for north have been declared for training, monitoring, quality control of salt and urine testing at consumption level and thyroid function tests in the region.

Salt testing kits for creating awareness and monitoring at community level by ASHA is being distributed in all the districts. One IDD monitoring lab has been sanctioned to all states/UTs. Cash grants provided for surveys/resurveys health education and publicity.

NIDDCP has been included in 20 point program of prime minister. Standard of iodine content of salt fixed at production and consumption level at least 30 and 15 ppm respectively. Revised policy guidelines on national iodine deficiency disorders were printed out and distributed. Under PFA Act 1954, GOI issued notification banning the sale of noniodated salt-effect from 17th May 2006. As per policy decisions on NIDDCP, The Ministry of Health and Family Welfare IDD CELLS formulated at state and central level. 824 private salt production units licensed by Salt Commissioner 532 units commenced salt production

The Ministry of Railways is providing priority arrangements (CATEGORY 'B') for transport of iodated salt. Under PFA Act 1954, GOI issued notification banning the sale of noniodated salt-effect from 17th May 2006. NIDDCP included in the 20 points program of PM. Doordarshan, All India Radio, Directorate of Field Publicity, Song and Drama Division, Directorate of Advertising and Visual Publicity, State Health Directorate.

Pilot Project Against Micronutrient Deficiency

Correction of Malnutrition of Iodine, Iron, Zinc, Fluorine, 1995-Assam, Bihar, Odisha, West Bengal, Gujarat merged with NIDDCP. Objectives of pilot project to assess the magnitude of fluorosis/dental carries besides the Iron/Vitamin A deficiency in the project area. To assess and improve Iron/Vitamin A status in school going children, adolescent boys/girls, nonpregnant women, adult males and geriatric population. To launch extensive IEC strategy through mass media to improve the dietary habits to study Zinc level in various food products and soils. To coordinate with similar ongoing program being implemented in the country.

Universal iodization of salt has not been achieved even after a decade. Failure of legislation and restrictions of bans monitoring during transportation is usually not done regularly. Resistance for the consumption of iodized salt among elite and high section society. Retailers selling the noniodated salt. Low funding of the program.

Recommendations and Future Plans

Universal iodization of salt more strengthening of transportation of Iodized salt by roadways and railways. Boosting up of political and bureaucratic commitment difference in guidelines for assessment of IDD between Indian Government and International Organizations should be rectified. Increase the fund future plans to set up one IDD cell and IDD monitoring lab in each state and UT. To complete IDD survey of remaining districts of the states production and distribution of 52 lakh mt iodated salt extensive IEC campaign by associating doordarshan, All India Radio, Directorate of Field Publicity, Song and Drama Division, DAVP, private agencies, etc. Implementation, monitoring and evaluation of NIDDCP.

SPECIAL NUTRITION PROGRAMME

This program was started in 1970–1971 by the ministry of social welfare, Government of India. The beneficiaries include-children under 6 years of age, pregnant and lactating mothers and Tribal and backward rural areas.

Objective

The objective of the program is to improve the nutritional status of the preschool children, pregnant and lactating mothers of poor socioeconomic groups in Urban Slums, tribal areas.

The beneficiaries are given supplementary nutrition for 300 days in a year. Under this program, every child should receive 300 kcal and 10–12 g protein. The mother should get 20–25 g protein per day and 500 kcal per day. Severely malnourished children are provided 600 calories and 20 g protein per day. The main aim of the special nutrition program is to improve the nutritional status of the target groups. This program is gradually being merged into the ICDS programme.

UNIVERSAL PROGRAMME ON IMMUNIZATION

Introduction

After independence, Government of India has taken various steps to improve health level of citizens. Health is included in the concurrent list and hence, central government along with state governments take concurrent or coordinated measures to handle communicable, noncommunicable and other main diseases. These measures are called National Health Programs. These programs can decrease the mortality and morbidity rate. Immunization program is one of the most important National health programs to protecting an individual from a disease through introduction of live, or killed or attenuated organisms in the individual system.

Based on the experience with smallpox eradication programme in 1974, the WHO launched its "Expanded Programme on Immunization" (EPI) against six, most common, preventable childhood diseases, viz. diphtheria, pertussis (whooping cough), tetanus, polio, tuberculosis and measles. The word "Expanded" means expanding the number of diseases to be covered, expanding the number of children and target population to be covered, expanding coverage to all corners of the country and spreading services to reach the less privileged sectors of the society. Expanded programme on immunization (EPI) is a world health organization programme, with the goal to make vaccines available to all children throughout the world. While the WHO's programme is called EPI, the UNICEF in 1985 renamed it as "Universal Child Immunization" (UCI). There was absolutely no difference between these two. The goal was the same, i.e., to achieve universal immunization by 1990. EPI is regarded as the instrument of UCI. WHO certified India to be free of smallpox in March 1977. The government of India launched its EPI in 1978 with the objective of reducing the mortality and morbidity resulting from vaccine-preventable diseases of childhood, and to achieve self-sufficiency in the production of vaccines.

In 1985, the programme was modified as 'Universal Immunization Programme' (UIP) to be implemented in phased manner to cover all districts in the country by 1989–90 with the one of largest health program in the world. Universal Immunization Programme was started in India in 1985. It has two vital components: immunization of pregnant women against tetanus, and immunization of children in their first year of life against the six EPI target diseases.

It was renamed as Universal Immunization Programme in 1985 when its reach was expanded beyond urban areas. In 1992, it became part of Child Survival and Safe Motherhood Programme and in 1997 it was included in the ambit of National Reproductive and Child Health Programme. Since the launch of National Rural Health Mission in 2005, Universal Immunization Programme has always been an integral part of it.

Universal Immunization Programme (UIP) is one of the largest public health programs targeting close of 2.67 crore newborns and 2.9 crore pregnant women annually. It is one of the most cost-effective public health interventions and largely responsible for reduction of vaccine preventable under-5 mortality rate. Under UIP, immunization is providing free of cost against 12 vaccine preventable diseases: Nationally against 9 diseases-Diphtheria, Pertussis, Tetanus, Polio, Measles, Rubella, severe form of Childhood Tuberculosis, Hepatitis B and Meningitis and Pneumonia caused by Hemophilus Influenza type B. Sub-nationally against 3 diseases—rotavirus diarrhea, pneumococcal pneumonia and Japanese encephalitis.

Objectives

- To achieve 100% coverage with all UIP.
- Eradication of polio to maintain polio free state.
- To reduce seroprevalence of HBsAg to <1% among under fives.
- Elimination of neonatal tetanus and prevention of severe forms of TB.
- To maintain zero level of diphtheria.
- To reduce the incidence of whooping and bacteria meningitis due to *Haemophilus influenzae.*
- To improve quality of health services
- To achieve self sufficiency vaccine production
- To train health personnel.
- To supply cold chain equipment and establish good surveillance network.
- To ensure district-wise monitoring.
- To maintain immunization safety.
- To prepare for introduction of new vaccine.

Scope and Eligibility

- India has one of the largest Universal Immunization Programs (UIP) in the world in terms of the quantities of vaccines used, number of beneficiaries covered, geographical spread and human resources involved.
- Under UIP, all the vaccines are given free of cost to the beneficiaries as per the National Immunization Schedule.
- All beneficiaries' namely pregnant women and children can get themselves vaccinated at the nearest Government/Private health facility or at an immunization post (Anganwadi centers/other identified sites) near to their village/urban locality on fixed days.
- The UIP covers all sections of the society across the country with the same high quality vaccines.

Universal immunization was first taken up in 30 selected districts and catchment areas of 50 Medical Colleges in November 1985. The program has now been extended to all the districts and practice areas of all the 242 Medical Colleges, thus creating a base for wider coverage. The immunization services are being provided through the existing health care delivery system (i.e., MCH centers, primary health centers and subcenters, hospitals, dispensaries and ICD units).

Evolution of the Immunization Programme in India

Let us briefly discuss evolution of immunization programme:

- **1978:** Expanded Programme of immunization (EPI). It had limited reach and it was mostly in urban areas. Cold chain established.
- **1983:** TT for Pregnant woman
- **1985:** Universal Immunization Programme (UIP). For reduction of mortality and morbidity due to 6 VPD's. Indigenous vaccine production capacity enhanced. Measles added and typhoid removed focus on less than 1 year of age
- Phased implementation—all districts covered by 1989–90.
- Monitoring and evaluation system implemented.
- **1986:** Technology Mission on Immunization Monitoring under PMO's 20 point programme. Coverage in infants (0–12 months) monitored.
- **1990:** Vitamin A supplementation
- **1995:** Pulse polio immunization day
- **1997:** VVM introduced on vaccine
- **2002:** Hepatitis B started as pilot project in 33 districts of 10 states
- **2005:** National Rural Health Mission (NRHM)
- **2006:** JE Vaccine introduced
- **2007–8:** Hepatitis B extended to all districts of 10 states
- **2010:** Measles 2nd dose introduced
- **2011:** Hepatitis B vaccine universalized and Hemophilus influenza type B vaccine introduced. Open viral policy for immunization in UIP
- **2013:** Pentavalent expanded to nine states, 2nd dose of JE vaccine

- **2014:** India and south east Asia region declared polio free Mission Indradhanush started
- **2015:** Pentavalent expanded to all states, IPV introduced
- **2016:** Rota virus vaccine was introduced in 4 states in phase-1. Trivalent OPV was used throughout the world before April 2016. In April 2016, all countries using OPV switched to bivalent OPV
- **2017:** MR vaccine introduced. PCV phase launched
- **2020:** Covishield and Co-vaccine for preventing COVID-19 introduced.

Significant achievements have been made in India. At the beginning of the programme in 1985–86, vaccine coverage ranged between 29% for BCG and 41% for DPT. By the end of 2018, coverage levels had gone up significantly to about 90% for tetanus toxoid for pregnant women, about 92% for BCG, 89% for DPT 3 doses, 89% for OPV 3 doses, 89% of hepatitis B, 89% of HiB, 80% of MCV-2. Since then, there is a significant decline in the reported incidence of the vaccine preventable diseases as compared to their incidence in 1987 (**Table 10.8**).

Due to pandemic of COVID-19 the Global vaccination continues to decline in 2021 with 25 million children missing out on lifesaving vaccines, 2 million more than in 2020, and 6 million more than in 2019.

To strengthen routine immunization, Government of India has planned **the State Programme Implementation Plan (PIP)** part C. It consists of: Support for alternate vaccine delivery from PHC to Subcenter and outreach sessions.

- Deploying retired manpower to carry out immunization activities in urban slums and underserved areas, where services are deficient.
- Mobility support to district immunization officer as per state plan for monitoring and supportive supervision.
- Review meeting at the state level with the districts at 6 monthly intervals.
- Training of ANM, cold chain handlers, mid-level managers, refrigerator mechanics etc.
- Support for mobilization of children to immunization session sites by ASHA, women self-help groups, etc.
- Printing of immunization cards, monitoring sheet, cold chain chart vaccine inventory charts etc.

In addition, central government is supporting in supplies of auto-disposable syringes, downsizing the BCG vial from 20 doses to 10 doses to ensure that BCG vaccine is available in all immunization session sites, strengthening and maintenance of the cold chain system in the states, and supply of vaccine and vaccine van.

Table 10.8: Decline in reported vaccine preventable diseases from year 1987 to 2018.

Disease	*1987*	*2018*
Poliomyelitis	28,257	0
Diphtheria	12,952	11,720
Pertussis	163,786	18,006
NNT	11,849	181
Measles	247,519	20,815

Introduction of Hepatitis-B Vaccine

In 2010–2011, Government of India universalized hepatitis B vaccination to all States/UTs in the country. Monovalent hepatitis B vaccine is given as intramuscular injection to the infant at 6th, 10th and 14th week along with primary series of DPT and polio vaccines. In addition one dose of hepatitis B is given at birth for institutional deliveries within 24 hours of birth.

Introduction of Japanese Encephalitis Vaccine

The program was introduced in 2006 to cover 104 endemic districts in phased manner, using SA 14-14-2 vaccine, imported from China. Single dose of JE vaccine was given to all children between 1 to 15 years of age through campaigns. The JE vaccine is being integrated into routine immunization in the districts where campaign had already been conducted to immunize the new cohort of children by vaccinating with two doses at 9–12 months and 16–24 months.

Introduction of Measles Vaccine Second Opportunity

In order to accelerate the reduction of measles-related morbidity and mortality, second opportunity for measles vaccination is being implemented. The National Technical Advisory Group on immunization recommended introduction of 2nd dose of measles vaccine to children between 9 months and 10 years of age through supplementary immunization activity (SIA) for states where evaluated coverage of first dose of measles vaccination is less than 80%. In states, with coverage of measles vaccination more than 80%, the second dose of vaccine will be given through routine immunization at 16–24 months.

Introduction of IPV

IPV has been used successfully in the polio eradication programs in a few countries, notably in Scandinavia and the Netherlands, but until recently most countries have used the oral polio vaccine. IPV provides serum immunity to all three types of poliovirus, resulting in protection against paralytic poliomyelitis. In comparison to OPV, the protective efficacy of IPV is marginally better and the chances of any side effects are virtually nil. So on the basis of importance of this vaccine, IPV was introduced in November 2015 initially in 6 states, which was expanded across the country by April 2016.

Introduction of Pentavalent +Vaccine (DPT + Hep-B + Hib)

India introduced pentavalent vaccine containing DPT, hepatitis B and Hib vaccines in two states viz. Kerala and Tamil Nadu under routine immunization program from December 2011. DPT and hepatitis B vaccination require 6 injections to deliver primary doses. With the introduction of pentavalent vaccine, a new antigen, i.e., HiB has been added which protects against haemophilus influenza type

B (associated with pneumonia and meningitis) and the number of injections are reduced to 3. The vaccine has been expanded to 6 more states, i.e., Haryana, Jammu and Kashmir, Gujarat, Karnataka, Goa and Puducherry in 2012–13. Further expansion is planned to 11 states in October 2014 and rest of 16 states from April 2015.

Introduction of Rota-virus Vaccine

A vaccine to prevent rotavirus gastroenteritis was first licensed in the United States in 1998 but was withdrawn in 1999 because of its association with intussusception, a type of bowel blockage when the bowel folds into itself like a telescope. Again this vaccine was introduced in 2016 at Odisha, AP, Himachal Pradesh and Haryana and later it expand to the whole country. It will be given under UIP as 3 doses along with Penta.

Introduction of Measles Rubella Vaccine

Measles rubella campaign has been started in 2017 with the aims to sustain high population immunity against both measles and rubella besides maintaining high routine immunization coverage for both the antigens. The interval and need for follow-up campaigns will be determined based on routine immunization coverage and quality of MR campaigns, and must be guided by laboratory-supported MR surveillance data including epidemiology from across the states. The Measles-rubella (MR) vaccine used in immunization program is live attenuated vaccine and safe and effective. Measles vaccines are available either as single antigen vaccines or in combination with either rubella (MR) or mumps and rubella (MMR) vaccines and with mumps, rubella and varicella (MMRV) vaccine. When MR/MMR/MMRV vaccines are used, the protective immune response to each of the components remains unchanged.

MISSION INDRADHANUSH

The Government of India launched Mission Indradhanush on 25th December 2014, to cover children who are either unvaccinated or partially vaccinated against seven vaccine preventable diseases, i.e., diphtheria, whooping cough, tetanus, polio, tuberculosis, measles and hepatitis B. The goal is to vaccinate all under-fives by the year 2020. Under the programme, four special vaccination campaigns will be conducted between January and June 2015. Intensive planning and monitoring experience of pulse polio immunization program will be used.

Phases of Mission Indradhanush

- Mission Indradhanush Phase I was started from 7th April 2015 in 201 high-focus districts for four consecutive months. During this phase, more than 75 lakh children were vaccinated of which 20 lakh children were fully vaccinated and more than 20 lakh pregnant women received tetanus toxoid vaccine.
- The Phase II of Mission Indradhanush covered 352 districts in the country of which 279 are medium focus districts and remaining 73 are high-focus districts of Phase-I. During Phase II of Mission Indradhanush, four special drives of weeklong duration were conducted starting from October 2015.
- Phase III of Mission Indradhanush was launched from 7 April 2016 covering 216 districts. Four intensified immunization rounds were conducted for seven days in each between April and July 2016, in these districts. These 216 districts have been identified on the basis of estimates where full immunization coverage is less than 60% and have high dropout rates. Apart from the standard of children under 2, it also focused on 5-year-olds and on increasing DPT booster coverage, and giving tetanus toxoid injections to pregnant women.
- Phase IV of Mission Indradhanush was launched from 7 February 2017 covering the North-eastern states of Arunachal Pradesh, Assam, Manipur, Meghalaya, Mizoram, Nagaland, Sikkim and Tripura. It has been rolled out in rest of the country during April 2017. The four phases of Mission Indradhanush have reached to more than 2.53 crore children and 68 lakh pregnant women with life-saving vaccines.

Aims

Mission Indradhanush aims to immunize all children under the age of 2 years, as well as all pregnant women, against seven vaccine preventable diseases (like 7 colors of a rainbow/indradhanush). The diseases being targeted are diphtheria, whooping cough, tetanus, poliomyelitis, tuberculosis, measles, meningitis and hepatitis B. In addition to these, vaccines for Japanese encephalitis and *Haemophilus influenzae* type B are also being provided in selected states. In 2016, four new additions have been made namely Rubella, Japanese Encephalitis, Injectable Polio Vaccine Bivalent and Rotavirus. In 2017, Pneumonia was added to the Mission by incorporating Pneumococcal conjugate vaccine under Universal Immunization Programme.

Intensified Mission Indradhanush

To further intensify the immunization program, PM Narendra Modi launched the Intensified Mission Indradhanush (IMI) on 8 October 2017. Through this the Government aims to reach each and every child up to two years of age and all those pregnant women who have been left uncovered under the routine immunization program/UIP. The focus of special drive was to improve immunization coverage in select districts and cities to ensure full immunization to more than 90% by December 2018 instead of 2020.

Intensified Mission Indradhanush 2.0

It was a nationwide immunization drive to mark the 25 years of Pulse Polio programme (2019–20). It had targets of full immunization coverage in 272 districts spread over 27 States. It aimed to achieve at least 90% pan-India immunization coverage by 2022.

Intensified Mission Indradhanush (IMI) 3.0

The Government of India is committed to improve immunization coverage and achieve full immunization coverage of 90%. Launch of massive routine immunization campaigns, such as Mission Indradhanush (MI) and Intensified Mission Indradhanush (IMI), in part, reflects government's efforts under Universal Immunization Program to reduce child mortality and morbidity. To boost the routine immunization coverage in the country, Government of India introduced Intensified Mission Indradhanush-3.0 in 2021 to ensure reaching the unreached with all available vaccines and accelerate the coverage of children and pregnant women in the identified districts and blocks from February 2021-March 2021. Focus of the IMI 3.0 was the children and pregnant women who had missed their vaccine doses during the COVID-19 pandemic. Beneficiaries from migration areas and hard to reach areas were targeted as they might have missed their vaccine doses during COVID-19. As of April 2021, during the various phases of Mission Indradhanush, a total of 3.86 crore children and 96.8 lakh pregnant women have been vaccinated.

Intensified Mission Indradhanush 4.0

Intensified Mission Indradhanush 4.0 launched during February 2022. This programme have three rounds and will be conducted in 416 districts (including 75 districts identified for Azadi ka Amrit Mahotsav) across 33 States/UTs in the country. In the first round (Feb-April 2022), 11 states will conduct IMI 4.0. These are Assam, Uttarakhand, Gujarat, Jammu and Kashmir, Meghalaya, Mizoram, Nagaland, Rajasthan, Sikkim, Tripura and Chhattisgarh.

The others (22 states) will conduct the rounds from April to May 2022. These states/UTs include Himachal Pradesh, Maharashtra, Andhra Pradesh, Manipur, Arunachal Pradesh, Odisha, Bihar, Puducherry, Delhi, Punjab, Goa, Tamil Nadu, Haryana, Telangana, Jharkhand, Dadra and Nagar Haveli and Daman and Diu, Karnataka, Uttar Pradesh, Kerala, West Bengal, Madhya Pradesh, A and N Islands.

During immunization some guidelines the health workers should follow which are given in the forms of Dos and Don't during immunization **(Table 10.9)**.

PULSE POLIO IMMUNIZATION PROGRAMME

Pulse Polio Immunization Programme was launched in the country in the year 1995. Under this programme children

Table 10.9: Do's and Don'ts during immunization sessions.

Do's	*Don'ts*
Vaccination Schedule	
• It is safe and effective to give BCG, DPT, OPV and Measles vaccines at the same time to a 9-month-old child who has never been vaccinated. • Give BCG to infants less than 1 year of age (never give BCG to children above 1 year of age). • If a child is brought late for a dose, pick up where the schedule was left off. For example, if a child left with DPT-2 and comes at 13 months give DPT-3 and Measles.	Withhold the vaccine in case of illness such as cold, cough, diarrhea or fever
Cold Chain	
• Check VVM label of OPV vial before immunizing every child. • Keep the vaccines and diluents in a plastic bag or zipper bag in the center of vaccine carrier away from the ice packs. Make sure that the diluents are also at +2 to +8 centigrade before reconstitution. • Take one ice pack from vaccine carrier and keep reconstituted BCG and Measles vaccines only on the top of the ice pack.	• Leave vaccine carrier in sunlight; this spoils vaccines that are sensitive to heat and light. • Leave the lid open; this can allow heat and light into the carrier, which can spoil vaccines. • Drop or sit on the vaccine carrier; this can damage the carrier. • Carry vaccines in handbag as this can spoil vaccines that are sensitive to heat. • Keep the DPT, DT, TT and Hep.B vaccines on the ice pack during the session.
Vaccine Handling and Administration	
• Welcome beneficiaries. • Wash hands before conducting the session. • Verify beneficiary's record and age of the child. • Screen for contraindications. • Check label of the vial of T–Series vaccine before drawing the dose. • Use a sterile syringe and needle. • Use correct diluent for reconstitution of vaccine. • Give appropriate vaccine. • Use one child one syringe one needle norm. • Inject vaccine using the correct site and route for the vaccine, e.g., Intradermal in left arm for BCG: subcutaneous in Right arm for Measles; intramuscular in anterolateral aspect of thigh for DPT, DT and Hep. B. • Allow dose to self-disperse instead of massaging. • Explain potential adverse events following immunization and what to do. • Discuss with beneficiaries or parents about next visit.	• Use un-sterile syringe or needle for immunization. • Draw air into AD syringes. • Touch any part of the needle. • Recap the needle. • Leave the needle inside the vial. • Ever inject in the buttock, never do that. • Massage the vaccination site after vaccination. • Use reconstituted measles and BCG vaccine after 4 hours. • Use OPV vaccine with Stage 3 or 4 VVM or with expiry date.

Contd...

Contd...

Do's	*Don'ts*
Recording and Reporting	
• Fully document each immunization in the immunization card, daily reporting sheet and immunization register. Ask parents or guardians to bring the card on next visit. • Retain the counterfoil.	• Turn away beneficiaries for not bringing the card. • Leave any cell blank in immunization card.
Adverse Event Following Immunization (AEFI)	
• In case of serious AEFI refer the patient to appropriate health facility, inform your supervisor immediately document the type of vaccine(s), batch number, expiry date, and full address of the child. • Report all serious AEFI to the MOI/C.	Report minor reaction following vaccination (mild fever of less than three days, redness and pain).
Social Mobilization	
• Use vaccination card to remind parents when to return with their child. • Enlist community team like AWW, ASHA, NGOs and other community-based workers to remind parents of the importance of full immunization.	Leave any community meeting without communicating about immunization session days.

under five years of age are given additional oral polio drops in December and January every year on fixed days. These indicated days are called as National Immunization Days (NIDs).

The term 'pulse' has been used to describe this sudden, simultaneous, mass administration of OPV on a single day to all children 0–5 years of age, regardless to previous examination with cent percentage coverage.

Government of India conducted the first round of PPI consisting of two immunization days 6 weeks apart on 9th December 1995 and 20th January 1996. In India the peak transmission is from June to September. The dose of OPV during PPIs are extra doses which supplement, and do not replace the doses received during routine immunization services.

The first PPI conducted targeted all children under 3 years of age irrespective of their immunization status. Later on, as recommended by WHO, it was decided to increase the age group from under 3 to under 5 years.

An important improvement in PPI during 1998 has been the use of vaccine vial monitor. Color monitors labels are put on vaccine bottles. Each label has a circle of deep blue color. Inside it is a white square which changes color and gradually becomes blue, if vaccine bottle is exposed to higher temperature. When the color of white square becomes blue like that surrounding circle, the vaccine should be considered ineffective. This mechanism has been made mandatory in all vaccine procurements since 1998. This quality assurance will ensure that the children will have better protection against polio in 1999 and thereafter.

Strategies

- Conduct PPI days every year
- Sustain high-levels of routine immunization coverage
- Monitor OPV coverage at district level and below
- Improve surveillance
- Ensure rapid case investigation
- Arrange follow-up
- The term 'PULSE' has been used to describe this sudden, simultaneous, mass administration of OPV on a single day to all children 0–5 years of age, regardless of previous immunization.

Following recommendations from the **India Export Advisory Group on Polio Eradication (IEAG)**:

- Development and licensure of monovalent OPV1 (mOPV1) and mOPV3 for targeted use during SIAs based on surveillance data;
- Deployment of additional personnel to assist with intensified SIAs in the state of Bihar and UP and in Mumbai city;
- Social mobilization targeted at reaching population groups missed during previous SIAs;
- Use of mobile teams to vaccinate children at transit points (e.g., railway bus stations) and on moving trains;
- Increasing engagement and accountability of political leaders and of health staff at all levels.

With concept of PPI, there was reduction in the incidence of poliomyelitis but not satisfactory level. There were continuous outbreaks of poliomyelitis. In spite of PPI program during 1999 from oneday booth activity to three days programme called 'intensified Pulse Polio Immunization Programme' (IPPIP). It was intensified in order to detect and immunize the 'Missed and Eligible 'children, who were not immunized in the booth, on the first day of immunization program. To detect the missed and eligible children, all children who get OPV on the first day, are marked with gentian violet on the little finger. So it became an extra effort to reach the unreached.

On the second day 'House to House' visit is made by the health worker and mark by 'X' for those houses, which were locked, who were not cooperative or target child is not having gentian violet mark on the little finger and mark 'p' for those houses, where target children are immunized or target children are not available.

On the third day, visit is made only for those houses marked 'X' and immunize the missed and eligible children, mark the little finger with gentian violet, wipe off the 'X' mark and convert into 'P' mark.

Progress

Under PPI program, progress in India is in zigzag fashion. Following the widespread use of poliovirus vaccine in the mid-1950s, the incidence of poliomyelitis declined rapidly in many industrialized countries. In 1988, the WHO, together with Rotary International, UNICEF, and the US center for Diseases Control and Prevention passed the Global Polio Eradication Initiative with the goal of eradicating polio by the year 2000. The initiative was inspired by Rotary International's 1985 pledge to raise $120 million toward immunizing all of the world's children against the disease. The last case of wild poliovirus poliomyelitis in the Americas was reported in Peru, August 1991.

On 20 August, 1994, the Americas were certified as polio-free. This achievement was a milestone in efforts to eradicate the disease. In 1995, the Indian Government launched the Pulse Polio Campaign to eliminate polio. By 2001, 575 million children (almost one-tenth the world's population) had received some 2 billion doses of oral polio vaccine. The World Health Organization announced that Europe was polio-free on June 21, 2002, in the Copenhagen Glyptotek.

In 2002, an outbreak of polio occurred in India. By 2004, India had adopted strategies to increase ownership of polio vaccinations in marginalized populations, and the immunity gap in vulnerable groups rapidly closed.

Polio Eradication Progress in India

- South-East Asia Region of WHO has been certified polio-free. The Regional Certification Commission (RCC) on 27th March, 2014 issued a certificate which states that 'The Commission concludes, from the evidence provided by the National Certificate Committees of the 11 Member States, that the transmission of indigenous wild poliovirus has been interrupted in all countries of the region.
- India has achieved the goal of polio eradication as no polio case has been reported for more than 3 years after last case reported on 13th January, 2011.
- There are 24 lakh vaccinators and 1.5 lakh supervisors involved in the successful implementation of the PPI program.
- WHO on 24th February, 2012 removed India from the list of countries with active endemic wild polio virus transmission and on 27 March, 2014, WHO declared India a polio-free country with no case of disease being reported in the last 3 years.

Mopping-up

In addition, large scale multi-district mop-ups have been conducted. Mopping-up activities are usually the last stage in polio eradication. The strategies of 'mopping up' involves door-to-door immunization in high-risk districts, where wild polio virus is known or suspected to be still circulating. This strategy is being implemented in India. As a result only one case of polio was reported in 2011 in the month of January. As on 25th Feb. 2012, India was removed from the list of polio endemic countries, and on 27th March 2014, India was certified as polio-free country.

Steps Taken by the Government to Maintain Polio-free Status in India

- A unit called National Polio Surveillance Unit (NPSU) established in 1997 is located in New Delhi. NPSU is headed by a Program Manager who is an incumbent of WHO. So, the entire information system on surveillance is under the control of NPSU.
- All States and Union Territories in the country have developed a rapid response team (RRT) to respond to any polio outbreak in the country. An emergency preparedness and response plan (EPRP) has also been developed by all States indicating steps to be undertaken in case of detection of a polio case.
- Special booths are established in areas bordering neighboring countries like Wagah border and Attari train station in Punjab and Munabo train station in Barmer district of Rajasthan, to ensure that all children under 5 years of age coming from across the border are given polio drops.
- Government of India has issued guidelines for mandatory requirement of polio vaccination to all international travelers before their departure from India to polio-affected countries, namely Afghanistan, Nigeria, Pakistan, Ethiopia, Kenya, Somalia, Syria and Cameroon. The mandatory requirement is effective for travelers from 1st March, 2014.
- To reduce risk of importation from neighboring countries, international border vaccination is being provided to all eligible children round the clock. These are provided through special booths set up at the international borders that India shares with Pakistan, Bangladesh, Bhutan, Nepal and Myanmar. Environmental surveillance established in Mumbai, Delhi, Patna, Kolkata, Punjab and Gujarat.
- An extremely high-level of vigilance through surveillance across the country for any importation or circulation of poliovirus and VDPV is being maintained. A rolling emergency stock of OPV is being maintained to respond to any WPV or cVDPV.
- National Technical Advisory Group on Immunization (NTAGI) has recommended Injectable Polio Vaccine (IPV) introduction as an additional dose along with 3rd dose of DPT in the entire country in the last quarter of 2015 as a part of polio end-game strategy.

Acute Flaccid Paralysis Surveillance

Nationwide acute flaccid paralysis (AFP) surveillance is the gold standard for detecting cases of poliomyelitis. It is an essential strategy of PEI, which aims to look for wild poliovirus circulation in the community by investigating all possible polio cases.

The Role of AFP Surveillance

- **To identify high risk areas or groups:** AFP surveillance is surveillance for suspected or possible polio. Its purpose is to detect areas and groups where poliovirus transmission is occurring or likely to occur, and to allow supplementary immunization to be focused where it is needed.

- **To monitor progress:** AFP surveillance allows program managers to monitor progress and to determine whether strategies are implemented effectively or not.
- **To certify a country polio-free:** Certifying a country as polio-free requires that there are no reports of new cases of poliomyelitis caused by wild poliovirus for three successive years. It also requires evidence that a country can detect a case of paralytic polio should it occur. As an indicator of a country's ability to detect polio, at least 1 case of AFP per 1,00,000 children <15 years of age should be detected, even in the absence of polio.
- **Utilize data to choose supplementary strategies:** If AFP surveillance shows that wild poliovirus circulation is widespread in a country then NID should be implemented, while mopping-up immunization can be used if wild poliovirus circulation is limited to small foci.

The Role of the Laboratory in AFP Surveillance

- **To confirm polio by virus isolation:** Isolation and identification of poliovirus from feces is the best current method to confirm the diagnosis of poliomyelitis.
- **To trace the origin of a case:** Molecular techniques are available to characterize fully the poliovirus. Maintaining reference bank of the molecular structure of known viruses allows the geographic origin on new isolates to be traced. The laboratory will also determine whether isolated viruses are wild or vaccine-like.
- **To certify that polio has been eradicated:** In addition to AFP surveillance, this may include stool surveys of healthy children in high-risk areas and environmental surveillance.
- **To assess vaccine potency and efficacy:** The laboratory can perform potency tests on polio vaccine if circumstances indicate possible failure. A laboratory might participate in epidemiological serosurvey if knowledge of the antibody status of the population is important.

Types of AFP Surveillance

- **Routine surveillance for AFP, "zero reporting":** Immediate notification of AFP in children <15 years of age is required. AFP should also be included in the weekly and monthly reporting system. When no case of AFP is detected, reporting units should still send weekly and monthly reports indicating zero cases.
- **Active surveillance for AFP:** Active surveillance is a strategy to actively collect information by visiting health facilities. A designated person should make visits to sites likely to have cases of acute polio, such as hospitals and rehabilitation centers. An active surveillance is focusing mainly on hospitals because most children with sudden paralysis will be admitted to hospitals or end up in larger hospitals because of referrals.
- **Active AFP case finding:** Looking for AFP cases in the community.

The four steps of surveillance are:

1. Finding and reporting children with acute flaccid paralysis (AFP)
2. Transporting stool samples for analysis
3. Isolating and identifying poliovirus in the laboratory
4. Mapping the virus to determine the origin of the virus strain

YAWS ERADICATION PROGRAM

Introduction: Yaws is a disfiguring and debilitating nonvenereal disease caused by *Treponema pertenue* usually beginning in early childhood.

Yaws is an infection of the skin, bones and joints caused by the spirochete bacterium *Treponema pallidum.*

Geographic Distribution with Incidence and Prevalence

In Africa, e.g., Benin, Ghana, Ivory coast), there has been a great resurgence of yaws.

In America, reported yaws incidence is very low with small foci remaining in Brazil, Colombia, Ecuador, Guyana and Suriname.

Persistent low levels of yaws is reported in Sri Lanka and India.

About three quarters of people affected are children under 15 years of age, with the greatest incidence in children 6–10 years old. Therefore, children are the reservoir of infection.

In India, the disease has been reported from the tribal communities living in hilly forests and difficult to reach areas in 49 districts of 10 states, namely Andhra Pradesh, Assam, Chhattisgarh, Gujarat, Jharkhand, Madhya Pradesh, Maharashtra, Odisha, Tamil Nadu and Uttar Pradesh.

Mode of Transmission

Yaws is transmitted nonvenerally by:

- Direct contact
- Fomites
- Vector
- Transplacental, congenital transmission does not occur.

Clinical Features

Primary lesion 'mother yaw' appears as a large papule, about 6 cm in diameter, or as a vesicle on the knee or near the mouth. The lesion becomes macule and later a papilloma. Infected serious fluids exude from the lesion.

Secondary Stage

After 6–8 weeks, rashes resemble a raspberry and 'framboesia' develop. They fall off without pain. Periosteum and bone may be involved.

Tertiary or Later Stage

It occurs after about five years, destructive and often deforming lesions of the skin, bone and periosteum appear. The lesions of sole and palms are 'crab yaws'. The destructive lesions of soft palate, hard palate, and nose are called 'Gangosa'. Swelling by the side of the nose due to osteoperiostitis of the superior maxillary bone is called 'Goundu'.

The program was started in 1996–1997 in Koraput district of Odisha, then extended to endemic states as a centrally sponsored health scheme.

Objectives

Interrupting the transmission of yaws infection (no case in the country).

Eradication of yaws (i.e., no seroreactivity in children below 5 years of age) from the country.

Control of Yaws

Treatment

Treatment is based on the following observations:

- Treatment with a single injection of long-acting penicillin will cure infection
- The simultaneous treatment of all clinical cases
- Benzathine penicillin is the drug of choice in a dose (single intramuscular dose) 1.2 million units for adults and half of that dose 0.6 million units for children under 3 years of age.
- In penicillin-sensitive cases, erythromycin or tetracycline is used in recommended doses for a period of 15 days.

The WHO recommended three modes of treatments:

- **Total mass treatment:** In areas where yaws is hyper endemic (>10% prevalence of clinically active yaws) treatment is given to all irrespective of disease status of a person.
- **Juvenile mass treatment:** In mesoendemic communities (6%–10% prevalence), treatment is given to all cases and to all children under 15 years of age and other obvious contacts of infectious cases.
- **Selective mass treatment:** In hypoendemic (<5% prevalence), treatment is confined to cases in their households and other obvious contacts of infectious cases.
- Without treatment, about 10% of affected people develop disfiguring and disabling.

Complications: Deformities of the legs and nose-after 5 years. The disease and its complications cause school absenteeism and prevent adults from farming activities.

Prevention: There is no vaccine for yaws. Prevention is based on the interruption of transmission through early diagnosis and treatment of individual cases and mass or targeted treatment of affected populations or communities. Health education and improvement in personal hygiene are essential components of prevention. The number of reported cases has come down from 3500 during 1996 to zero during 2004. During 2009, till October, no new case has been reported. Yaws is not as vulnerable to eradication.

It can be easily prevented by health education, and improvement in personal hygiene is essential component of prevention.

NATIONAL AIDS CONTROL PROGRAMME

The first HIV case in the world was detected in 1981 at USA. The HIV/AIDS epidemic came to India in 1986 when the first case of HIV was detected in Chennai. Since then, the number of infected people has grown substantially and the HIV epidemic has travelled a long way, establishing itself with the greatest speed in the six high prevalence states of Andhra Pradesh, Maharashtra, Manipur, Nagaland, Karnataka and Tamil Nadu. The National AIDS Control Programme (NACP), launched in 1992, is being implemented as a comprehensive program for prevention and control of HIV/AIDS in India. Over time, the focus has shifted from raising awareness to behavior change, from a national response to a more decentralized response and to increasing involvement of NGOs and networks of People living with HIV (PLHIV).

The NACP Phase-I (1992–1999) started in 1992 was implemented across the country with the objective to prevent HIV transmission, decrease the morbidity and mortality associated with HIV infection, and minimize the socioeconomic impact of HIV infection in 1992, National AIDS Control Board and National AIDS Control Organization (NACO) were developed. The first phase focused on awareness generation setting up surveillance system for monitoring HIV epidemic measures to ensure access to safe blood and preventive services for high-risk group populations. NACP-I sought to provide certain services—education campaigns, protection of the blood supply, condom promotion, a system to monitor the prevalence of HIV, treatment for sexually transmitted diseases and limited treatment for AIDS-related conditions. Two components were added later—targeted interventions and 'intersectoral collaboration'.

In November 1999, the second National AIDS Control Project (NACP II) was launched to reduce the spread of HIV infection in India, and (ii) to increase India's capacity to respond to HIV/AIDS on a long-term basis.

- Below 5% of the adult population in high prevalence states
- Below 3% in states where the prevalence was moderate, and
- Below 1% and 2% in the remaining states where the epidemic was at a nascent stage.

NACP III was launched in July 2007 with the goal of Halting and Reversing the Epidemic over its five-year period.

NACP-IV (2012–2017) has been developed through an elaborate and extensive process. The process has adopted an inclusive, participatory and widely consultative approach with 15 working groups and 30 subgroups covering all thematic areas involving 624 representatives from central and state governments, representatives of high-risk group communities, people living with HIV/AIDS, civil society, subject experts, experts from NRHM and other government departments, development partners and other stakeholders. Regional and state-level consultations, and special studies/assessments were also undertaken to develop the strategic plan. Planning Commission Steering Committee has also been closely overseeing this entire process.

NACP-IV-Objectives

- Reduce new infections by 50% (2007 Baseline of NACP III)
- Provide comprehensive care and support to all persons living with HIV/AIDS and treatment services for all those who require it.

Key Strategies

- Intensifying and consolidating prevention services, with a focus on High-risk Groups (HRGs) and vulnerable population.
- Increasing access and promoting comprehensive care, support and treatment
- Expanding IEC services for (a) general population and (b) high-risk groups with a focus on behavior change and demand generation.
- Building capacities at national, state, district and facility levels
- Strengthening Strategic Information Management System

Key Priorities under NACP IV

- Preventing new infections by sustaining the reach of current interventions and effectively addressing emerging epidemics
- Prevention of Parent to Child transmission
- Focusing on IEC strategies for behavior change in HRG, awareness among general population and demand generation for HIV services
- Providing comprehensive care, support and treatment to eligible PLHIV
- Reducing stigma and discrimination through Greater involvement of PLHA (GIPA)
- De-centralizing rollout of services including technical support
- Ensuring effective use of strategic information at all levels of program
- Building capacities of NGO and civil society partners especially in states with emerging epidemics
- Integrating HIV services with health systems in a phased manner
- Mainstreaming of HIV/AIDS activities with all key central/state level Ministries/departments will be given a high priority and resources of the respective departments will be leveraged. Social protection and insurance mechanisms for PLHIV will be strengthened.

Package of Services Provided under NACP IV

Prevention Services

- Targeted Interventions for High-risk Groups and Bridge Population (Female Sex Workers (FSW), Men who have Sex with Men (MSM), Transgenders/Hijras, Injecting Drug Users (IDU), Truckers and Migrants)
- Needle-Syringe Exchange Programme (NSEP) and Opioid Substitution Therapy (OST) for IDUs
- Prevention Interventions for Migrant population at source, transit and destination
- Link Worker Scheme (LWS) for HRGs and vulnerable population in rural areas
- Prevention and Control of Sexually Transmitted Infections/Reproductive Tract Infections (STI/RTI)
- Blood Safety
- HIV Counseling and Testing Services
- Prevention of Parent to Child Transmission
- Condom promotion
- Information, Education and Communication (IEC) and Behavior Change Communication (BCC).
- Social Mobilization, Youth Interventions and Adolescent Education Programme
- Mainstreaming HIV/AIDS response
- Work Place Interventions

Care, Support and Treatment Services

- Laboratory services for CD4 Testing and other investigations
- Free First line and second line Anti-Retroviral Treatment (ART) through ART centers and Link ART Centers (LACs), Centers of Excellence (COE) and ART plus Centers.
- Pediatric ART for children
- Early Infant Diagnosis for HIV exposed infants and children below 18 months
- HIV-TB Coordination (Cross-referral, detection and treatment of co-infections)
- Treatment of Opportunistic Infections
- Drop-in Centers for PLHIV networks.

New Initiatives under NACP IV

- Differential strategies for districts based on data triangulation with due weightage to vulnerabilities
- Scale up of programs to target key vulnerabilities
  - Scale up of Opioid Substitution Therapy (OST) for IDUs
  - Scale up and strengthening of Migrant Interventions at Source, Transit and Destinations including roll out of Migrant Tracking System for effective outreach
  - Establishment and scale up of interventions for Transgenders (TGs) by bringing in community participation and focused strategies to address their vulnerabilities
  - Employer-Led Model for addressing vulnerabilities among migrant labor, i.e., Female Condom Programme
- Scale up of Multidrug Regimen for Prevention of Parent to Child Transmission (PPTCT) in keeping with international protocols
- Social protection for marginalized populations through mainstreaming and earmarking budgets for HIV among concerned government departments
- Establishment of Metro Blood Banks and Plasma Fractionation Center
- Launch of Third Line ART and scale up of first and second Line ART
- Demand promotion strategies specially using mid-media, e.g., National Folk Media Campaign and Red Ribbon Express and buses (in convergence with the National Health Mission)

NACP PHASE-IV EXTENSION (2017–2021)

The NACP Phase-IV (Extension) was first approved for the period of 2017–2020 and then further extended for one more year, i.e., 2020–21. Several gamechanger initiative were taken during NACP Phase-IV (Extension). The Phase started with the passing of the HIV and AIDS (Prevention and Control) Bill, 2017 and the launch of the 'Test and Treat' policy for HIV patients in April 2017. The Bill ensured equal rights for the people infected with HIV and AIDS in getting treatment and prevent discrimination of any kind. The Act came into force in September 2018. As the 'Test and Treat' policy was being scaled-up, the Program implemented "Mission Sampark" in 2017 to bring back People Living with HIV (PLHIV) who have left treatment after starting ART. 'Test and Treat' was complemented by the launch of universal viral load testing for on-ART PLHIV in February 2018. The year 2020–21 witnessed the onset of the COVID-19 pandemic. The national AIDS response was challenged in the initial months like any other aspect of life. However, the Program soon took many initiatives turning challenges into opportunities. IT systems were leveraged to enhance program review and capacity building. This resulted in improved inter and Intra-State coordination. Initiatives like multi-month dispensation and community-based ART refill ensured continuity in service provisions.

Context and Formulation of NACP Phase-V

The impact of the national AIDS response has been significant. The annual new HIV infections in India have declined by 48% against the global average of 31% (the baseline year of 2010). The annual AIDS-related mortalities have declined by 82% against the global average of 47% (the baseline year of 2010). The HIV prevalence in India continues to be low with an adult HIV prevalence of 0.22%. Despite the significant achievements and impact, there is no place for complacency given the country's commitment to ending the AIDS epidemic as a public health threat by 2030. HIV remains a national public health priority with new HIV infections happening at a rate higher than the desired level. The annual number of new infections among adults has declined by 48% since 2010, but still has a long way to go to achieve a 90% decline by 2030. The formulation of NACP Phase-V was necessitated by the need for continuous action and the vigil in context of the country commitment on ending of the AIDS epidemic as a public health threat by 2030. It was initiated in alignment with Fifteenth Finance Commission for 2021–26 of the Government of India. The formulation of NACP Phase-V coincided with formulation of UNAIDS Global AIDS Strategy 2021–2026, WHO Global Health Sector Strategies (GHSS) on HIV, viral hepatitis, and sexually transmitted infections for the period 2022–2030 and The Global Fund cycle of 2021–24. NACP Phase-V takes into account the global contexts, targets and strategies.

NACP PHASE-V (2021–26)

NACP Phase-V is a Central Sector Scheme, fully funded by the Government of India, with an outlay of ₹15471.94 crore. The NACP Phase-V aims to reduce annual new HIV infections and AIDS-related mortalities by 80% by 2025–26 from the baseline value of 2010. The NACP Phase-V also aims to attain dual elimination of vertical transmission, elimination of HIV/AIDS-related stigma while promoting universal access to quality STI/RTI services to at-risk and vulnerable populations.

The specific objectives of the NACP Phase-V are as below:

- HIV/AIDS prevention and control
  - 95% of people who are most at risk of acquiring HIV infection use comprehensive prevention
  - 95% of HIV positive know their status, 95% of those who know their status are on treatment and 95% of those who are on treatment have suppressed viral load
  - 95% of pregnant and breastfeeding women living with HIV have suppressed viral load towards attainment of elimination of vertical transmission of HIV
  - Less than 10% of people living with HIV and key populations experience stigma and discrimination
- STI/RTI prevention and control
  - Universal access to quality STI/RTI services to at-risk and vulnerable populations
  - Attainment of elimination of vertical transmission of syphilis.

Under NACP Phase-V, while the existing interventions will be sustained, optimized, and augmented; newer strategies will be adopted, piloted, and scaled-up under the program to respond to the geographic and community specific needs and priorities. The HIV and AIDS (Prevention and Control) Act, 2017 will continue to be the cornerstone of the national response to HIV and STI epidemic in NACP Phase-V. The Act will be the enabling framework to break down barriers driving delivery of a comprehensive package of services in an ecosystem free of stigma and discrimination.

Guiding Principles of NACP Phase-V (2021–26)

Eight guiding principles will be central to strategies and activities to attain the specific targets.

1. Keep beneficiary and community in center
2. Break the silos, build synergies
3. Augment strategic information-driven planning, implementation, monitoring, and mid-course corrections
4. Prioritize and optimize through high-impact program management and review
5. Leverage technology and innovation as critical enablers
6. Enhance and harness partnership
7. Integrate gender-sensitive response
8. Continue fostering technical arrangements and institutions
9. Collaboration with public and private sectors.

NACP Phase-V will build upon the systematized convergence with the existing schemes of Central Government including synergy with National health program, related line Ministries as well as State Governments through mainstreaming and partnership extending the reach of various HIV related services in a cost-neutral way. The collaboration framework of NACP Phase-V includes continued strategic engagement with private sector.

The Strategic Goals and Activities

Goal 1: Reduce Annual New HIV Infections by 80%

- NACP Phase-V will accelerate reduction in new annual HIV infections through a basket of strategies tailored to the high-risk, at-risk, and low-risk population groups.
- Continue and evolve the existing peer-led targeted interventions (TI) and Link Worker Schemes (LWS) strategies for integrated services
- Promote evidence-based comprehensive preventive packages tailored to location and population
- Strengthen the population size estimation and field epidemiological intelligence for coverage expansion and saturation
- Expand and intensify the coverage of NACP interventions including OST among Injecting Drug Users (IDU)
- Universalize the NACP interventions in prisons and other closed settings through a mix of service delivery models
- Pilot and scale models for community-based integrated service delivery models
- Redefine and expand coverage among the bridge population
- Develop and roll-out new generation communication strategy suitable to current context
- Cover 'at-risk' HIV negative through comprehensive prevention packages to keep them negatives
- Develop and scale-up sustainable models for 'at-risk' Virtual Population
- Maintain and augment the behavior change communications for general population
- Sustain focus on adolescent and youth population.

Goal 2: Reduce AIDS-related Mortalities by 80%

NACP Phase-V will build upon the strong momentum from previous phases and further accelerate the reductions on AIDS-related mortalities through strategies directed across care continuum.

- Maintain the existing models of HIV counseling and testing services (HCTS) and expand through strategic scale-up
- Develop and roll-out tailored communication campaigns focusing on risk perception and HCTS uptake
- Augment the existing HCTS models with efficient approaches for active case findings promoting early detections
- Appropriately adapt evidence-based newer technologies to supplement existing models
- Maintain existing care, support, and treatment (CST) services models and expand further through sustainable manner
- Continue provisions of high-quality ARVs through differentiated service delivery models improving through sustainable manner
- Focus on rapid ART initiation and advanced HIV disease management augmenting quality of care
- Suitably update the treatment guidelines periodically
- Address linkage loss at all levels
- Optimize the uses of public sector laboratories for viral load measurements
- Offer integrated service delivery packages to 'at-risk' people and PLHIV
- Prioritize sexual and reproductive health services for women at increased risk of HIV infection and women living with HIV
- Bring efficiencies and improve linkages through single window service delivery models
- Maintain and expand laboratory quality assurance system.

Goal 3: Eliminate Vertical Transmission of HIV and Syphilis

The NACP Phase-V takes into the account the global guidance towards elimination of vertical transmission of HIV and Syphilis.

- Augment comprehensive synergy with NHM for testing of pregnant women for HIV and syphilis
- Strengthen the primary prevention through coordinated actions
- Introduce and scale-up dual test kits (HIV and Syphilis) to fast-track progress on the dual elimination
- Strengthen linkage from screening facilities to confirmatory centers and subsequently to the treatment centers
- Strengthen retention and on-ART adherence among eligible WLHIV
- Prioritize family planning services for eligible PLHIV
- Strengthen the early diagnosis of infants and all children living with HIV (CLHIV)
- Engage with private sector augmenting their role in attainment of dual elimination
- Strengthen the strategic information in the context of HIV positive pregnant women/mother
- Prepare strategic roadmap to guide actions towards attainment of validation of elimination of vertical transmission.

Goal 4: Promote Universal Access to Quality STI/RTI Services to At-risk and Vulnerable Populations

NACP Phase-V will reinforce the STI/RTI component not only in terms of elimination of vertical transmission of HIV and syphilis but also to augment access to quality STI/RTI services through maximizing its system and opportunities for shared delivery models.

- Strengthen the strategic information on STIs
- Maintain the existing model of Designated STI/RTI Clinics (DSRCs) augmenting the role
- Develop and implement integrated communication strategies
- Dovetail dual testing at HCTS centers

- Promote active case findings facilitating early detections
- Improve collaboration with NHM on STI/RTI services provisions and reporting
- Strengthen and streamline private sector engagement on STI/RTI management
- Suitably update the STI/RTI management guidelines periodically
- Augment the laboratory capacities
- Strengthen the supply chain management.

Goal 5: Eliminate HIV/AIDS-related Stigma and Discrimination

- NACP Phase-V will build upon the gamechanger initiatives of NACP-Phase IV (Extension) to accelerate the progress on elimination of HIV/AIDS-related stigma and discrimination.
- Undertake bottom-up institutionalized community system strengthening
- Accelerate the notification of State rules and appointment of Ombudsman in the context of the HIV and AIDS (Prevention and Control) Act, 2017
- Undertake sensitization of related stakeholders on HIV/AIDS-related stigma and discrimination
- Design and implement communication strategy on elimination of HIV/AIDS-related stigma and discrimination
- Enhance strategic information on HIV/AIDS-related stigma and discrimination
- Engage with State governments promoting launch and scale-up of social protection schemes.

The HIV and AIDS (Prevention and Control) Act, 2017

The HIV and AIDS (Prevention and Control) Act, 2017 is a landmark legislation to provide for the prevention and control of the spread of HIV and AIDS and for the protection of human rights of persons affected by the HIV/AIDS. The Act aims to address stigma and discrimination so that people infected with and affected by HIV and AIDS are not discriminated in household settings, establishment settings and healthcare settings. The Act also reinstates constitutional, statutory, and human rights of people infected with and affected by HIV and AIDS. It also provides for a robust grievance redressal mechanism in form of Complaints Officer at establishments and Ombudsman at state level.

The HIV and AIDS (Prevention and Control) Act, 2017 will continue to be the cornerstone of the national response to HIV and STI epidemic in NACP Phase-V. The Act will be the enabling framework to break down barriers, driving delivery of a comprehensive package of services in an ecosystem free of stigma and discrimination.

FAMILY WELFARE PROGRAMS

Introduction

India is the second most populous country in the world with 2.5% of the world's land surface area has to accommodate about 16.7% of the world's population, on 2.4% of the world's surface area. The death rate stood at the level of 8 per 1000 and at the birth rate at 25 per 1000 in the mid 2003. The wide gap between the births and deaths if resulting in rapid rise of population. Realizing that high population growth is inevitable during the initial phases of demographic transition and the urgent need to accelerate the pace of the transition, India became the first country to formulate a National Family Planning Programme in 1952.

Aims of Family Planning

- Reduce MMR and IMR
- Curtail population growth
- Prevent pregnancies
- Improve health of mother and children.

Objectives

- Reduce birth rate
- Educate and motivate EC
- Increase literacy rate
- Raise marriageable age
- Access to good-quality services.

Historical Development

In 1923 first family planning clinic was established at Pune. In 1946 Bhore committee recommended for limitation of family size. During 1st 5 years plan National Family Planning Programme was launched. The Ist 5 years plan stated that 'the main appeal for family planning is based on considerations of health and welfare of the family. Family limitation or spacing of children is necessary and desirable in order to secure better health for the mother and better care and upbringing of children. During 2nd 5 years plan family planning and education integrated with community development. Measures directed to this end should, therefore, form part of the public health program during 3rd 5 years plan, clinic approach shifted to extensive education approach. Education to eligible couple regarding family planning method was given importance during the period between 1966 and 1969. A 'Cafeteria Approach' meaning choose whatever method of contraception you like was introduced by the Health and family welfare minister Prof. Chandrasekhar. A time bound target oriented approach was adopted to reduce the birth rate from 39 per thousand to 32 per thousand. Actually nothing remarkable could be achieved in this direction. By 1971, our population increased to 548 million. Emphasized on terminal method in the International Conference on Population and Development (ICPD) Increasing concern about the rapidly growing population led to the National Family Planning Programme being included as a priority sector program during the 5th plan. The massive sterilization drive of 1976 did result in eight million persons undergoing sterilization, but this did not have any perceptible impact on the birth rate, as the cases were not appropriately chosen. There was a steep fall in acceptance in the very next year. In 1978, the Expanded Programme of Immunization was initiated to improve coverage for the six vaccine preventable diseases. In 1979, the National Family Planning Programme was renamed as the National Family Welfare Programme and increasing integration of family planning services with those of maternal and child health and nutrition was attempted. The major thrust during the 1980s was to operationalize the WHO's Alma Ata declaration of health for all by 2000 AD (1978) by establishing a network of centers in urban and rural areas to provide essential primary health care. The network of postpartum centers was expanded to improve access to family welfare services. In 1983 the National Health Policy was formulated and provided comprehensive framework for planning, implementation and monitoring of health care services. The Universal Immunization Programme (UIP) started in 30 districts in 1986, was extended to cover 448 districts by the end of the 7th plan. The 1991 census showed that India was entering the opportunity window in demographic transition, when larger proportion of the population is in the age group of 20–40 years, when it will be possible to achieve a rapid decline in fertility and mortality. The report of the NDC Sub-Committee on population gave a new thrust and dynamism to the Family Welfare Programme. During the 8th plan, efforts were made under the child survival and Safe Motherhood initiative and the Social Safety Net programme to improve the access to maternal and child health services. In view of the massive interstate and intrastate differences in access to services and health indices, the Department of Family Welfare abolished the practice of setting centrally defined, method-specific targets for contraception. It was replaced by decentralized area-specific need assessment (community needs assessment approach), planning and implementing programs aimed at fulfilling these needs in 1997, the Department of Family Welfare initiated the reproductive and child health (RCH) programme aimed at providing integrated health and family welfare services to meet health care needs of women and children.

The NDC Sub-committee on Population recommended that there should be a paradigm shift in the Family Welfare Programme and the focus should be on:

- Decentralized area-specific planning based on need assessment.
- Emphasis on improved access and quality of services to women and children.
- Providing special assistance to poorly performing states/ districts to minimize the differences in performance.
- Creation of district-level databases on quality, coverage and impact indicators for monitoring the program.

The ICPD at Cairo in 1994 advocated a similar approach. A convergence between national (NDC Sub-Committee) and ICPD efforts improved funding of Family Welfare Programme during the 9th plan period.

REPRODUCTIVE AND CHILD HEALTH (RCH) PROGRAMME

It is the legitimate right of citizens to be able to experience sound reproductive and child health and therefore, the government of India is strive for obtaining reproductive and child health arrangements for the whole of the country's population. Reproductive and child health programme provide relevant services for assuring reproductive and child health to all citizens.

In the year 1994 International conference on population development (ICPD) was held at Cairo where 180 countries of the world participated and recommended the strategy of "Reproductive and child health." India launched the reproductive and child health programme in 15th October 1997 (phase-1). This programme was integration of CSSM + family planning + prevention and treatment of RTI and STD + adolescent health. The main aim of the program is to reduce infant, child and maternal mortality rates.

Reproductive health can be defined as " a state in which people have the ability to reproduce and regulate their fertility, women are able to go through pregnancy and child birth safely, the outcome of pregnancy is successful in terms of maternal and infant survival and well being, and couples are able to have sexual relations free of fear of pregnancy and of contracting diseases."

RCH PHASE-I THE MAIN OBJECTIVES OF THE PROGRAM IN ITS FIRST PHASE

- To improve the implementation and management of policy by using a participatory planning approach and strengthening institutions to maximum utilization of the project resources
- To improve quality, coverage and effectiveness of existing Family Welfare services
- To gradually expand the scope and coverage of the Family Welfare services to eventually come to a defined package of essential RCH services.
- Progressively expand the scope and content of existing FW services to include more elements of a defined package of essential
- Give importance to disadvantaged areas of districts or cities by increasing the quality and infrastructure of Family Welfare services.

Components of RCH Programme

The essential components recommended for nationwide implementation at all levels include:

- Community needs assessment approach (CNAA).
- Integrated package of services for mother and child.
- MTP services at PHC and safe abortion.
- Control and prevention of RTI/STI. Adolescent health.
- Services in urban slums
- Improving quality of services
- Unmet needs and subcenter action plans.
- Communication strategy in RCH.

- Gender sensitiveness.
- Greater involvement of Panchayati Raj institutions, non-governmental organization and community.

Components of Comprehensive RCH Care

- Effective maternal and child health care
- Increased access to contraceptive care
- Safe management of unwanted pregnancies
- Nutritional services to vulnerable groups
- Prevention and treatment of RTI/STD
- Reproductive health services for adolescents
- Prevention and treatment of gynecological problems.
- Screening and treatment of cancers, especially uterine, cervical and breast cancer.

Five Key Principles as the Basis of RCH Programme

1. Moving away from traditional approach of numerical, method-specific, contraceptive targets and incentives to a client-centered system of performance goals and measures.
2. Expanding the use of male and reversible contraceptive methods and broadening the choice of contraceptives.
3. Improving the breadth, availability and quality of services and involving communities for managing the public sector programs.
4. Strengthening the role of the private sector in the program.
5. Assuming adequate funding for the current program and for the expansion, which is implicit in adopting the reproductive health approach.

Highlights of the Program

This program is an integration of all programs related fertility regulation, maternal and child health and reproductive health. Types of services provided are client oriented, demand driven through decentralized participatory process and target free approach. Up-gradation of facilities, i.e., creation of first referral units given importance. Provision of specialist services for STD and RTI and also provision of out reach services for vulnerable groups are the main moto of this program.

Categories

For provision of better services the districts are categorized in three major categories. For weaker district more support was planned for providing. Based on crude birth rate and female literacy rate, the districts are categories in three major categories. Category A having 58 districts, category B having 184 districts and category C having 265 districts. All the districts covered in a phased manner over a period of 3 years.

Interventions in All Districts

- Child survival interventions, i.e., immunization, vitamin A (to prevent blindness), oral rehydration therapy and prevention of deaths due to pneumonia.
- Safe motherhood interventions, e.g., antenatal checkup, immunization for tetanus, safe delivery, Anemia Control Programme.
- Implementation of target free approach.
- High quality training at all levels.
- IEC activities.
- Specially designed RCH package for urban slums and tribal areas.
- District subprojects under Local Capacity Enhancement.
- RTI/STD Clinics at District Hospitals (where not available).
- Facility for safe abortions at PHCs by providing equipment, contractual doctors, etc.
- Enhancement community participation through Panchayats, women groups and NGOs.
- Adolescent health and reproductive hygiene.

Interventions in Selected States/Districts

- Screening and treatment of RTI/STD at subdivisional level.
- Emergency obstetric care at selected FRUs by providing drugs.
- Essential obstetric care by providing drugs and PHN/Staff Nurse at PHCs.
- Additional ANM at subcenters in the weak districts for ensuring MCH care.
- Improved delivery services and emergency care by providing equipment kits, IUD insertions and ANM kits at subcenters.
- Facility of referral transport for pregnant women during emergency to the nearest referral center through Panchayat in weak districts.

Service Package: For Mothers

Essential Obstetric Care

It is to provide the basic maternity services to all pregnant women through this, includes early registration mini-mum 3 antenatal check-up, safe delivery 3 postnatal check-up to monitor the postnatal recovery and to detect complications. Strengthening referral system, the component of RCH programme is more relevant for Assam, Bihar, Rajasthan, Odisha, Uttar Pradesh, Madhya Pradesh.

Emergency Obstetric Care

It is very essential to prevent maternal mortality and morbidity, traditional birth attendance should be maintained in conducting the delivery. To prevent maternal mortality and morbidity under CSSM programme 1748 the FRUs should be strengthened by supplying of kits and skilled manpower, Traditional Birth Attendants (TBA) are playing important role during delivery, Dai training also implemented in different states. The emergency obstetrics drug and equipment kits involves Kit-E-Laparotomy set, Kit-F-Mini-Laparotomy set, Kit-G-IUD insertion set, Kit-H-Vasectomy set, Kit-I-Normal delivery set, Kit-J-Vacuum extraction set, Kit-k-Embryotomy set, Kit-L-Uterine evacuation set, Kit-M-Equipment for anesthesia, Kit-N-Neonatal resuscitation set, Kit-O-Equipment and reagent for blood test and Kit-P-Donor blood transfusion set.

24 Hours Delivery Services at PHCs/CHCs

To promote institutional deliveries, provision has been made under the current RCH Programme, provision of additional honorarium to the staff to encourage round the clock delivery services at PHCs and CHCs. This was to ensure that at least one medical officer, nurse, and cleaner are available beyond normal working hours. Under this scheme, 226016 deliveries have been conducted as per reports received from the States. Deliveries by trained personnel in safe and hygienic surroundings are encouraged. Institutional deliveries are encouraged specially for women having complications. In case of complication referrals are made to First Referral Units for management of obstetric emergencies, three postnatal checkups are given to mothers after the delivery. Spacing of at least 3 years between children are encouraged.

RCH Camps

In order to provide RCH services to people living in remote areas where the existing services at PHC level are under utilized, a scheme for holding camps was initiated during 2000–2001. Initially 102 districts were selected in 17 States, i.e., Assam, Bihar, Chhattisgarh, Haryana, Jharkhand, Madhya Pradesh, Nagaland, Odisha, Rajasthan, Uttar Pradesh, Uttarakhand, Arunachal Pradesh, Manipur, Meghalaya, Mizoram, Sikkim and Tripura. During 2001–2002, 72 more districts were added to include all the states/UTs in the country under the scheme. Till now States have reported holding of 14565 camps.

For Children

Essential newborn care like keeping the baby warm, checking the baby's weight and giving the baby mother's first milk are encouraged. If the babies are premature or have low birth weight are provided special care. Babies with any complications refereed to the health center. Exclusive breastfeeding are encouraged for the first 6 months. Then introducing semisolid supplements in the 6th month, screen all children to identify those with severe grades of under-nutrition and treat them, administer massive dose of vitamin A supplements according to schedule, administer iron-folate supplements, if needed. Immunization are administered to every child meticulously to prevent death and disabilities. Early detection and management of ARI/diarrhea. Acute respiratory infection in children can be treated by cotrimoxazole tablets. Training of health care personnel in the early diagnosis of ARI and appropriate treatment. Diarrhea is one of the leading causes of death among children. Most of these deaths are due to dehydration, frequent passage of stools and can be prevented by the timely and adequate replacement of fluids. The Oral Rehydration Programme was started in 1986–1987 in order to prevent such deaths. Health education aimed at the rapid recognition and appropriate management of diarrhea has been a major component of the CSSM and RCH programme. The use of fluids available at home and oral rehydration solution (ORS) has resulted in a substantial decline in the mortality associated with diarrhea, from an estimated one million to 1.5 million children every year ORT.

For Eligible Couples

Promoting use of contraceptive methods among eligible couples is important to prevent unwanted pregnancies. Couples should be able to choose from various contraceptive methods including condoms, oral pills, IUDs, male and female sterilization. The couple was encouraged and motivated to choose appropriate contraceptive based on their health need.

It is estimated that in 1998, about 9% of maternal deaths were due to unsafe abortions. Available service data on MTPs indicate that following an initial rise in early 1980s, the number of reported MTP's hovered around 0.5–0.7 million in the 1990s. The estimated number of illegal induced abortions in the country is in the range of four to six million. There has not been any substantial decline in the estimated number of illegal abortions, reported morbidity due to illegal abortions or share of illegal abortions as the cause of maternal mortality. The management of unwanted pregnancy through early and safe, MTP services as envisaged under the MTP Act is an important component of the ongoing RCH programme. Safe services for medical termination of pregnancies should be encouraged for women desiring abortions.

Change in Manpower Structure

Additional ANMs: In order to improve delivery of services, all category C districts of 8 States of Uttar Pradesh, Bihar, Madhya Pradesh, Odisha, Haryana, Assam, Nagaland and Rajasthan were supported for providing additional ANMs in 30% of subcenters of these districts. The scheme has been extended to the remaining 6 North Eastern States during 1999–2000. In addition, Delhi is eligible for appointing 140 ANMs for extending services to slum areas. Till now States have reported appointing 6096 ANMs.

Public health/staff nurses: Under the program, Public Health/Staff Nurses were provided to 25% PHCs in C category districts and 50% PHCs in B category districts. Till now States have reported appointing 1784 Staff Nurses.

Laboratory technicians: To build the capacity of the First Referral Units for looking after the needs of emergency obstetric care and RTIs/STIs, the districts were being assisted to engage two laboratory technicians on contractual basis for doing routine blood, urine and RTI/STI tests. Till now States have reported appointing 464 LTs.

Private anesthetists: Under the RCH programme, FRUs are also being strengthened through supply of drugs in the form of emergency obstetric drug kits and skilled manpower on contractual and hiring basis. The subdistrict hospitals, CHCs and FRUs are entitled to hire services of Private Anesthetists for conducting emergency operations for which they are to be paid ₹1000 per case. The states have not been able to utilize the funds released to them, mostly due to the shortage of anesthetists.

Safe motherhood consultants: To alleviate the shortage of trained manpower in PHCs/CHCs and subdistrict hospitals, Government of India had assisted the States/UTs for engaging the doctors trained in MTP techniques (Safe Motherhood Consultants) to visit these institutions once a week or at least once a fortnight on a fixed day for performing MTPs and providing other service.

Other New Services

Treatment of RTI/STI

It is important to recognize that there are problems in the current programs for management of RTI. The Piot and Fransen model of RTI/STI management graphically sums up the problems in treatment of RTI. The model shows that about 40% of women have RTI/STI at any given time but only 1% complete full treatment of both partners even under optimal conditions. It is, therefore, hardly surprising that in spite of all the current efforts to improve treatment of RTI/STI patients, gynecologists and public health professionals feel that there has not been any substantial improvement in the situation over the last decade. However, it is important to persist with health education, providing ready access to diagnostic facilities and appropriate treatment.

Promotion Activities for Adolescents Health

Efforts to educate the girl, her parents and the community on the need to delay marriage. Programs for the early detection and effective management of nutritional (under-nutrition, anemia) and health (infections, menstrual disorders) problem in adolescent girls. Appropriate antenatal care to high-risk adolescent pregnant girls.

RCH PROGRAMME: PHASE II

RCH Programme Phase-II Launched on 1st April 2005.

Vision

- To bring about outcomes as envisioned in the Millennium Development Goals, the National Population Policy 2000 (NPP 2000), and the National Health Policy 2002
- Minimizing the regional variations in the areas of RCH
- Population stabilization through an integrated, focused, participatory program
- The RCH-II, a flagship program of the Government of India on Reproductive and Child
- Health, was launched in April 2005 under NRHM. This program has been reoriented and revitalized to give a pro-outcome and pro-poor focus. It aims at reducing the Maternal Mortality Ratio, the Infant Mortality Rate and Total Fertility Rate.

Components of RCH-II

- Maternal health
- Neonatal and child health
- Family planning
- Adolescent health
- Control of RTI and STDs.

Maternal Health Component

- Essential obstetric care
- Emergency obstetric care
- Safe abortion services
- Prevention and control of RTI/STDs.

Essential Obstetric Care and Emergency Obstetric Care

Institutional delivery: To promote institutional delivery in RCH Phase II, it is envisaged that 50% of the PHCs and all the CHCs would be made operational as 24-hour delivery centers, in a phased manner, by the year 2010. These centers would be responsible for providing Basic Emergency Obstetric Care and Essential Newborn Care and Basic Newborn Resuscitation services round the clock. The experiences of RCH phase-I indicate that giving incentive to health workers for providing round the clock services did not function well in most of the States. On the contrary there is the experience from Government of Andhra Pradesh and Tamil Nadu where round the clock delivery and newborn care services could be ensured by providing 3 to 4 staff nurses/ANM at the PHCs. Promotion of institutional deliveries 50% of the PHCs and CHCs made operational as 24-hours delivery centers.

NISHCHAY"- Pregnancy Detection Kit

Services for early detection of pregnancy: The Ministry of Health and Family Welfare (MOHFW), GOI, through National Rural Health Mission (NRHM) has introduced rapid home pregnancy test kits (Nishchay). Taking a holistic view of the concept, Nishchay is not a program for the promotion of the pregnancy test kit alone, but is an entry point to RCH and family planning services for women seeking quality and assured RCH and FP services. Nishchay pregnancy test kits are made available free of cost to all women in rural areas through the ASHAs, thus reaching out to women, who would otherwise have to travel great distances to confirm a pregnancy.

Skilled Birth Attendance

It is now recognized globally that the countries which have been successful in bringing down maternal mortality in their country are the ones where the provision of skilled attendance at every birth and its linkage with appropriate referral services for complicated cases have been ensured. The WHO has also emphasized that skilled attendance at every birth is essential to reduce the maternal mortality in any country.

The Policy Decisions

ANMs/LHVs/SNs have now been permitted to use drugs in specific emergency situations to reduce Maternal Mortality. They have also been permitted to carry out certain emergency interventions when the life of the mother is at stake. Emergency obstetric care operationalization of FRUs and skilled attendance at birth are the two activities which go hand inhand. In view of this, simultaneous steps have been taken to ensure tackling obstetric emergencies. It has been decided that all the First Referral Units (FRUs) be made operational for providing emergency and essential obstetric care during the second phase of RCH. Some of the steps taken are training of MBBS doctors in life-saving anesthetic skills for EmOC, establishing blood storage at FRUs and guidelines for operationalization of the FRUs. There is also a plan for training of MBBS doctors for management of obstetric cases, including cesarean section, etc. with the help of professional organizations such as FOGSI. The FRUs to provide 24 hours delivery services, emergency obstetric care, newborn care and emergency care of the sick child, full range of family planning services, safe abortion services, treatment of RTI and STI, blood storage facility, Essential laboratory services and referral (transport) services.

24×7 Hours Services by PHCs and CHCs

To provide the round the clock deliveries facility at health centers, 50% of PHC will be upgraded to provide essential and basic emergency obstetrics care. All upgraded CHC to act as FRU to provide comprehensive obstetric care. Basic Emergency obstetric care include Oxytocic's Anticonvulsants, Blood transfusion, Digital removal of products of conception including caesarean session must be available.

Strengthening Referral System

Time is an important factor for obstetric emergencies. During RCH I-funds were given to Panchayats for providing assistance to poor people no active involvement of Panchayats. In RCH II: Through involvement of Village health nutrition sanitation committee.(VHNSC). Referral transport systems, in general have been given emphasis across states; Madhya Pradesh and Gujarat has widespread availability and use of the Janani Express Yojana. Time is an important factor for obstetric emergencies. Women who undergo deliveries at home and develop complications often find it difficult to be transported to a referral unit. Under the current RCH Programme provision has been made to assist women from indigent families in 25% of the subcenter in selected States to provide a lump sum corpus fund to Panchayat through District Family Welfare Officers. Since, the scheme has been extended to all the States and UTs. Budgets have been released 16 States based on the proposals received from them.

New Initiatives

Training of PHC doctors in life-saving anesthetic skills for emergency obstetric care, a FRUs provision of adequate and timely Emergency Obstetric Care (EmOC) has been recognized globally as the most important intervention for saving lives of pregnant women who may develop complications during pregnancy or childbirth.

The operationalization of First Referral Unit at subdistrict/ CHC level for providing EmOC to pregnant women is a crucial strategy of RCH-II, which needs focused attention. It has not been possible to operationalize these FRUs till now due to various factors, the most pertinent, being shortage of specialist manpower, i.e., gynecologist and anesthetist, particularly at district and subdistrict level. The training shall be undertaken for only such number of MBBS doctors who are required for the operationalization of FRUs and CHCs and shall be limited to the requirement of tackling emergency obstetric situations only. In no way, it is the replacement of the specialist anesthetists. New initiatives have taken on following aspects:

Setting up of Blood Storage Centers (BSC) at FRUs

Timely treatment for complications associated with pregnancy is sometimes hampered due to nonavailability of Blood Transfusion services at FRUs. The Drugs and Cosmetics Act has been amended to facilitate establishment of Blood Storage Centers at such FRUs. Guidelines for these Blood Storage Centers (BSCs) have been prepared and disseminated to the states.

Improve Obstetric Management Skills

Government of India is also introducing training of MBBS doctors in Obstetric Management Skills. Federation of Obstetric and Gynecological Society of India has prepared the training plan for 16 weeks in all obstetric management skills including Cesarean section operation and is in the process of dissemination to the states.

Janani Suraksha Yojana

The National Maternity Benefit Scheme has been modified into a new scheme called Janani Suraksha Yojana. The new scheme has been launched with effect from 12.04.2005. The objectives of the scheme are reducing maternal mortality/ infant mortality through increased delivery at health institutions. While several interventions for improving maternal health have been under implementation through State/UTs, it is felt that effective care is possible by making available essential and emergency obstetric services, by way of focusing at increased institutional care, among women in below poverty line families.

Salient Features of the Janani Suraksha Yojana

- Janani Suraksha Yojana under the overall umbrella of the National Rural Health Mission integrates the benefit of cash assistance with institutional care during delivery, preceded with antenatal care and immediate postpartum care.
- The scheme will be a 100% centrally sponsored scheme.
- The benefit will be available to all women, both rural and urban areas, belonging to below poverty line (BPL) household and aged 19 years or above.
- The benefit will be available up to the first two live births. However low performing States (LPS) namely; Uttar Pradesh, Uttarakhand, Madhya Pradesh, Jharkhand, Bihar, Rajasthan, Chhattisgarh, Odisha, Assam and Jammu and Kashmir, the benefit will be extended up to the third child if the mother of her own accord chooses to undergo

sterilization in the health facility where she delivered, immediately after delivery.

- The Accredited Social Health Activist (ASHA) would work as a link health worker between the poor pregnant women and public sector health institution in the ten low performing states. ASHA would be responsible for making available institutional antenatal as well as postnatal care. She would also be responsible for escorting the pregnant women to the health center.
- All BPL pregnant women would be eligible to get cash benefits of ₹500/- per live birth on registration. However, the disbursement would be done at the time of delivery, irrespective of the place of delivery.
- Such eligible beneficiaries who deliver in health institutions would get an additional cash benefit of ₹200/- if they belong to rural areas and ₹100/- if they belong to urban areas of above mentioned ten low performing states.
- For the services provided by ASHA, in rural areas of all the ten low performing states, a package of assistance of ₹600/- has been provided. The package is toward meeting the cost of transportation for the pregnant women and the ASHA to reach the health center, transactional expenses for ASHA for her stay with the expectant mother in the health center during delivery and incentive money for ASHA. However, in urban areas the package of assistance for ASHA will be restricted to ₹200/- because of availability of better transport facilities, in comparison to the rural areas.
- In cases the pregnant women develops complications and requires cesarean sections, assistances up to ₹1500/- per case has been provided for hiring services of private experts where government specialist are not available in health institutions, to carry out the surgery in a Government medical facility.
- Acknowledging that infrastructural facilities in the public sector are not adequate, benefits under Janani Suraksha Yojana would also be available to eligible pregnant women delivering in the private hospitals/nursing homes/clinics duly accredited and recognized by the State/Union Territories Governments.
- The scheme would be implemented through the State and UT Governments.

Vandemataram Scheme

The scheme is continuing under public private partnership with the involvement of Federation of Obstetric and Gynecological Society of India and private clinics. The aim of the scheme is to reduce the maternal mortality and morbidity of the pregnant and expectant mothers by involving and utilizing the vast resources of specialists/trained workforce available in the private sector. The scheme intends to provide free antenatal and postnatal checkup, counseling on nutrition, breastfeeding, spacing of birth, etc., through public private partnership. This is a voluntary scheme wherein any OBG specialist, maternity home, nursing home, lady doctor/MBBS doctor can volunteer themselves for providing safe motherhood services. The enrolled doctors will display 'Vandemataram logo' at their clinic. Iron and folic acid tablets, oral pills, TT injection, etc. will be provided by the respective district medical officers to the 'Vandemataram doctors/clinics' for free distributions to beneficiaries. The cases needing special care and treatment can be referred to the government hospitals, who have been advised to take due care to the patients coming with Vandemataram cards. The details of the scheme, reporting format, etc. are available with District Medical Officers and Director of Family Welfare in the States.

Safe Abortion Services

- Increasing access to safe abortion services by popularizing manual vacuum aspiration (MVA) technique at PHC level for early pregnancy
- Control of RTI/STDs
- Planned and implemented in close collaboration with National AIDS control Organization (NACO)
- NACO is supporting to set up STD clinics up to the district level
- Each district are assisted by two laboratory technicians on contract basis for testing blood, urine for RTI/STD test to reduce maternal mortality and morbidity from unsafe abortion.
- Assistance from central government have been provided in the form of training of manpower, supply of MTP equipment, Provision for engaging doctors trained in MTP to visits PHCs on fixed dates to perform MTP.

Neonatal and Child Health Component

The Key Strategies under Neonatal and Child Health component are:

- Increase coverage of skilled care at birth for newborns in conjunction with maternal care—Pre-service IMNCI is underway in 62 medical colleges
- Implement a comprehensive IMNCI approach—a newborn and child health package of preventive, promotive and curative Currently being implemented in 193 out of 612 districts
- Navjaat Shishu Suraksha Karyakram
- Introduction of Hepatitis-B Vaccine in routine immunization.

Routine Immunization Monitoring System

Routine Immunization Monitoring System (RIMS) is a computerized implementation, to enter data, generate reports and perform queries. The system is presently developed in Microsoft ACCESS as a standalone CD version. It is user friendly and no special training is required to operate the system. Online system is under development in a different platform using other database and programming tools.

The data are collected at district level from PHCs/Reporting Units in the standard pre-designed UIP format and entered on five broad categories namely (A) Immunization and Vitamin A, (B) Vaccine Supply, (C) VPD Surveillance, (D) Status of Cold Chain Equipment and (E) AEFI (Adverse Event following immunization).

The system is capable of performing data analyses and generating useful reports for the use of UPI managers at all levels, i.e., district, state and national. RIMS will be very useful tool to monitor UIP program as reports from all the 600 districts will be collected in a short period and then analyzed automatically by the software.

IMNCI Approach

The IMNCI approach is the centerpiece of newborn and child health strategy in RCHI II. Integrated Management of Neonatal and Childhood Illness (IMNCI) Integrated Management of Childhood Illness (IMCI) strategy, which has already been implemented in more than 100 countries all over the globe, encompasses a range of interventions to prevent and manage five major childhood illnesses, i.e., Acute Respiratory Infections, Diarrhea, Measles, Malaria and Malnutrition. It focuses on preventive, promotive and curative aspects, i.e., it gives a holistic outlook to the program. Government of India recognizes the need to strengthen child health activities in the country. In order to do so and introduce IMCI in the country, a Core Group was constituted which included representatives from Indian Academy of Pediatrics (IAP), National Neonatology Forum of India (NNF), National Antimalaria Program (NAMP), Department of Women and Child Development (DWCD), Child-in-Need Institute (CINI), WHO, UNICEF, eminent Pediatricians and Neonatologists, and the representatives from Ministry of Health and Family Welfare Government of India. The Adaptation Group developed Indian version of IMCI guidelines and renamed it as Integrated Management of Neonatal and Childhood Illness (IMNCI).

"Navjaat Shishu Suraksha Karyakram"

- A new program on Basic Newborn Care and Resuscitation
- High Neonatal Mortality Rate despite substantial reduction in childhood and infant mortality
- Nearly two-thirds infant deaths each year occur within the first four weeks of life, and about two-thirds of those occur within the first week.
- Although childhood and infant mortality in India has reduced substantially during the last decade, the rate of neonatal mortality is still high. Nearly two-thirds infant deaths each year occur within the first four weeks of life, and about two-thirds of those occur within the first week. Thus, the first days and weeks of life are critical for the future health and survival of a child.

Aim

- To train health personnel in basic newborn care and resuscitation.
- Care at birth issues, i.e.,
  - Prevention of Hypothermia
  - Prevention of Infection
  - Early initiation of Breastfeeding and Basic Newborn Resuscitation.

Objective

To have a trained health personal in Basic newborn care and resuscitation at every delivery point.

To reduce perinatal asphyxia-related morbidity and mortality, Government of India launched a training program—Navjaat Shishu Suraksha Karyakram (NSSK) essential newborn care and resuscitation in 2009–10. The course was aimed to impart the basic skills required to manage common neonatal problems related to birth asphyxia, infections, hypothermia and breastfeeding. The program was rolled out across most states of India.

An evaluation of this training program revealed that knowledge to skill transfer of the trainees in the states ranged from good to average. It was recommended that the trainee selection criteria, prioritization, practical exposure and a quality training at the district level will ensure faster knowledge to skill transfer. Ensuring adequate number of trainers and dedicated training sites equipped with the required infrastructure and equipment/all training aids at the training site further add to the quality of training. Regular updates, refreshers, functional radiant warmers and self-inflating bags at the delivery points will enable the trainees in retaining the skills learnt in the training. Based on the above information the NSSK training package has been revised in the year 2020 using a training methodology, keeping adult learning principles in mind. A flip chart promoting participatory interactions with notes for the facilitator will be used during training. Better facilitator to participant ratio will also add to improving the quality of training. Emphasis for hands on practice of the skills is an effort to enable each participant to acquire the same skill set at the end of the training. The training duration remains as two days.

Revised NSSK package is a customized 2-days clinical update cum skill standardization training at identified training sites. (Preferably near SNCU/Newborn Care unit where the participants can be easily transferred for equipment demonstration) Facilitators: Trained pediatricians, medical officers and nurse tutors who have undergone master training can facilitate this training. For a batch of 24–28 participants, 4 facilitators shall be required. Eligibility of participants: All service providers working in the labor room, and involved with care of mother and the baby at time of birth are eligible for this training. Even SBA trained providers will be eligible for this training. Navjaat Shishu Suraksha Karyakram Batch Size: Each batch will be of 24–28 participants. The batch of the trainees is to be divided into group of 6–7 with one facilitator for the complete training. Sites of training: In each district, either the district hospital (DH) or/and a high case load subdistrict hospital should be the training site. One or more than one (depending on the size/need of the state), state level TOTs should be organized to develop a resource pool of trainers to continue trainings at the district level. The trainings should ideally be followed by mentoring visits. Training approach and role of trainers: The trainers will use participatory training methods based on adult learning principles to make the sessions interesting and at the same time ensure quality of training. To ensure clinical knowledge update, the trainers will present the information through interactive discussions and activities. To build competency, the trainers will demonstrate skills on anatomic models (humanistic approach) and facilitate learners to practice them using the relevant skills.

Village Health and Nutrition Days

The VHND is to be organized once every month preferably on Wednesdays, and if left out, on any other day of the same month at the anganwadi worker in the village. This will ensure uniformity in organizing the VHND. The anganwadi worker is identified as the hub for service provision in the RCH-II, NHM, and also as a platform for inter-sectoral convergence. VHND is also to be seen as a platform for interfacing between the community and the health system.

On the appointed day, ASHAs, AWWs, and others will mobilize the villagers, especially women and children, to assemble at the nearest AWC. The ANM and other health personnel should be present on time; otherwise the villagers will be reluctant to attend the following monthly VHND. On the VHND, the villagers can interact freely with the health personnel and obtain basic services and information. They can also learn about the preventive and promotive aspects of health care, which will encourage them to seek health care at proper facilities. Since the VHND will be held at a site very close to their habitation, the villagers will not have to spend money or time on travel. Health services will be provided at their doorstep. The VHSC comprising the ASHA, the AWW, the ANM, and the PRI representatives, if fully involved in organizing the event, can bring about dramatic changes in the way that people perceive health and health care practices.

Services to be provided:

- All pregnant women are to be registered.
- Registered pregnant women are to be given ANC.
- Dropout pregnant women eligible for ANC are to be tracked and services are to be provided to them.
- All eligible children below one year are to be given vaccines against six Vaccine-preventable diseases.
- All dropout children who do not receive vaccines as per the scheduled doses are to be vaccinated.
- Vitamin A solution is to be administered, to children.
- All children are to be weighed, with the weight being plotted on a card and managed appropriately in order to combat malnutrition.
- Anti-TB drugs are to be given to patients of TB.
- All eligible couples are to be given condoms and OCPs as per their choice and referrals are to be made for other contraceptive services.
- Supplementary nutrition is to be provided to underweight children.

Issues to be discussed with the community:

- Danger signs during pregnancy
- Importance of institutional delivery and where to go for delivery
- Importance of seeking postnatal care
- Counseling on ENBC
- Registration for the JSY
- Counseling for better nutrition
- Exclusive Breastfeeding
- Weaning and complementary feeding
- Care during diarrhea and home management
- Care during acute respiratory infections
- Prevention of malaria, TB, and other communicable diseases
- Prevention of HIV/AIDS
- Prevention of STIs
- Importance of safe drinking water.

Identification of cases that need special attention:

- Identify children with disabilities.
- Identify children with Grade III and Grade IV malnutrition for referral
- Identify severe cases of anemia.
- Identify pregnant women who need hospitalization.
- Identify cases of malaria, TB, leprosy, and Kala-azar.
- Identify problems of the old and the destitute.
- Pay special attention to the SC, ST, the minorities, and the weaker sections of society.

Data needs to be collected

- Compile data on the number of children with special needs, particularly girl children with disabilities.
- Report outbreaks of disease.
- Report/audit deaths of children and women.
- Compile data pertaining to the SCs, the STs, the minorities, and weaker sections of society that need services.

This day is mainly organized and conducted by ASHAs, Anganwadi workers and PRIs. They should understand their respective roles in providing their services effectively to the community during the monthly VHND. There are the checklists for ASHAs, AWWs, and ANMs to ensure that all the activities for which they are responsible are planned properly and carried out effectively, step by step. VHND if organized regularly and effectively can bring about the much needed behavioral changes in the community, and can also induce health-seeking behavior in the community leading to better health outcomes.

REPRODUCTIVE, MATERNAL, NEWBORN, CHILD AND ADOLESCENT HEALTH (RMNCH+A)

In order to bring greater impact through the RCH programme, it is important to recognize that reproductive, maternal and child health cannot be addressed in isolation as these are closely linked to the health status of the population in various stages of lifecycle. RMCH+A approach has been launches in 2013 and it essentially looks to address the major causes of mortality among women and children as well as the delays in accessing and utilizing health care and services. The RMNCH+A strategic approach has been developed to provide an understanding of 'continuum of care' to ensure equal focus on various life stages.

The health of an adolescent girl impacts pregnancy while the health of a pregnant woman impacts the health of the newborn and the child. As such, interventions may be required at various stages of lifecycle, which should be mutually linked. The reasons for adopting such a strategy can be understood when the available data is taken into account and the close inter-linkages between different stages of lifecycle are recognized.

Improving the maternal and child health and their survival are central to the achievement of national health goals under the National Health Mission (NHM). SDG Goal 3 also includes the focus on reducing maternal, newborn and child mortality. In the past years, innovative strategies evolved under the national program to deliver evidence-based interventions to various population groups. Following the Government of India's "Call to Action (CAT) Summit" in February, 2013, the Ministry of Health and Family Welfare launched Reproductive, Maternal, Newborn Child plus Adolescent Health (RMNCH+A) to influence the key interventions for reducing maternal and child morbidity and mortality. The RMNCH+A strategy is built upon the continuum of care concept and is holistic in design, encompassing all interventions aimed at reproductive, maternal, newborn, child, and adolescent health under a broad umbrella, and focusing on the strategic lifecycle approach. The RMNCH+A strategy promotes links between various interventions across thematic areas to enhance coverage throughout the lifecycle to improve child survival in India. The "plus" within the strategy focuses on:

- Inclusion of adolescence as a distinct life stage within the overall strategy.
- Linking maternal and child health to reproductive health and other components like family planning, adolescent health, HIV, gender, and preconception and prenatal diagnostic techniques.
- Linking home and community-based services to facility-based services.
- Ensuring linkages, referrals, and counter-referrals between and among various levels of health care system to create a continuous care pathway, and to bring an additive/synergistic effect in terms of overall outcomes and impact.

Goals/Aims of RMNCH+A Approach

Taking into account the progress made so far in maternal and child health, it is pertinent to establish the goals and targets for the implementation phase 2012–2017, after considering the main reasons for mortality and interventions proven to have an impact on them. The 12th Five Year Plan has defined the national health outcomes and the three goals that are relevant to RMNCH+A strategic approach as follows:

Health Outcome Goals established in the 12th Fiver Year Plan

- Reduction of Infant Mortality Rate (IMR) to 25 per 1,000 live births by 2017
- Reduction in Maternal Mortality Ratio (MMR) to 100 per 100,000 live births by 2017
- Reduction in Total Fertility Rate (TFR) to 2.1 by 2017.

Coverage targets for key RMNCH+A interventions for 2017

- Increase facilities equipped for perinatal care (designated as 'delivery points') by 100%
- Increase proportion of all births in government and accredited private institutions at annual rate of 5.6% from the baseline of 61% (SRS 2010)
- Increase proportion of pregnant women receiving antenatal care at annual rate of 6% from the baseline of 53% (CES 2009)
- Increase proportion of mothers and newborns receiving postnatal care at annual rate of 7.5% from the baseline of 45% (CES 2009)
- Increase proportion of deliveries conducted by skilled birth attendants at annual rate of 2% from the baseline of 76% (CES 2009).

In order to achieve these goals, that are ambitious, yet potentially feasible Lives Saved Tool (LiST), a computer-based application was used to estimate the coverage targets for key child health interventions. A subcommittee and an expert group were constituted to review the application of LiST in Indian context. The expert group ensured that the inputs to LiST are adapted to the Indian context and by undertaking an in-depth review of the impact of various newborn and child survival interventions.

To achieve systemic change by fostering high impact innovations to address key factors that contribute to maternal and child deaths such as:

- Early pregnancy
- Weak antenatal/postnatal care
- Unsafe deliveries
- Low nutrition levels
- Incomplete immunization
- Diarrhea and pneumonia.

Key Features of RMNCH+A Strategy

The RMNCH+A strategy approaches include:

- **Health systems strengthening (HSS):** Focusing on infrastructure, human resources, supply chain management, and referral transport measures. Health system strengthening and cross cutting interventions are described in **Table 10.10**.
- **Prioritization of high-impact interventions:** For various lifecycle stages
- **Increasing effectiveness of investments:** By prioritizing geographical areas based on evidence
- **Integrated monitoring and accountability:** Through good governance, use of available data sets, community involvement, and steps to address grievance
- **Broad-based collaboration and partnerships:** with ministries, departments, development partners, civil society and other stakeholders.

The overview of the key RMNCH+A interventions as a 'continuum of care' is provided in 5 × 5 Matrix for high impact RMNCH+A interventions **(Table 10.11)**.

Table 10.10: Health systems strengthening and cross-cutting interventions.

Health systems strengthening	*Cross-cutting interventions*
• Case load based deployment of HR at all levels • Ambulances, drugs, diagnostics, reproductive health commodities • Health Education, Demand promotion and Behavior Change Communication • Supportive supervision for monitoring and review including score cards based on HMIS • Public grievances redressal mechanism	• Bring down out of pocket expenses by JSSK, RBSK, etc. • ANMs and Nurses to provide specialized and quality care to pregnant women and children • Address social determinants of health through convergence • Focus on un-served and underserved villages, urban slums and blocks • Introduce difficult area and performance based incentives

Coverage Targets for Key RMNCH+A Interventions for 2017

- Increase facilities equipped for perinatal care (designated as 'delivery points') by 100%
- Increase proportion of all births in government and accredited private institutions at annual rate of 5.6% from the baseline of 61% (SRS 2010)
- Increase proportion of pregnant women receiving antenatal care at annual rate of 6% from the baseline of 53% (CES 2009)
- Increase proportion of mothers and newborns receiving postnatal care at annual rate of 7.5% from the baseline of 45% (CES 2009)
- Increase proportion of deliveries conducted by skilled birth attendants at annual rate of 2% from the baseline of 76% (CES 2009)
- Increase exclusive breastfeeding rates at annual rate of 9.6% from the baseline of 36% (CES 2009)
- Reduce prevalence of under-five children who are underweight at annual rate of 5.5% from the baseline of 45% (NFHS 3)
- Increase coverage of three doses of combined diphtheria-tetanus-pertussis (DTP3) (12–23 months) at annual rate of 3.5% from the baseline of 7% (CES 2009)
- Increase ORS use in under-five children with diarrhea at annual rate of 7.2% from the baseline of 43% (CES 2009)
- Reduce unmet need for family planning methods among eligible couples, married and unmarried, at annual rate of 8.8% from the baseline of 21% (DLHS 3)
- Increase met need for modern family planning methods among eligible couples at annual rate of 4.5% from the baseline of 47% (DLHS 3)
- Reduce anemia in adolescent girls and boys (15–19 years) at annual rate of 6% from the baseline of 56% and 30%, respectively (NFHS 3)
- Decrease the proportion of total fertility contributed by adolescents (15–19 years) at annual rate of 3.8% per year from the baseline of 16% (NFHS 3)
- Raise child sex ratio in the 0–6 years age group at annual rate of 0.6% per year from the baseline of 914 (Census 2011) the key RMNCH+A interventions as a 'continuum of care across lifecycle' is provided in the **Table 10.12**.

It must be recognized that the set of interventions described in this document are those that are shown to have high impact on reducing mortality and improving survival, and most of them have been part of the previous phase of NRHM. The effectiveness of these interventions is determined by the coverage achieved among the affected fraction of population as also the availability, accessibility, actual utilization of services and quality of service delivered. Therefore, it is important that 'Bottleneck Analysis' be carried out at various levels of planning, including the state and district level in order to prioritise attention to address specific

Table 10.11: 5 × 5 Matrix for high impact RMNCH+A interventions.

Reproductive health	*Maternal health*	*Newborn health*	*Child health*	*Adolescent health*
• Focus on spacing methods, particularly PPIUCD • Interval IUCD at all facilities including subcenters on fixed days • Doorstep delivery of contraceptive by ASHA • Maintaining sterilization services	• Use MCTS to ensure early registration of pregnancy and provide ANC • Detect high-risk pregnancies • Equip delivery points with trained HR • Add MCGH wings as per need	• Early initiation and exclusive breastfeeding • Home-based newborn care through ASHA • Essential newborn care and resuscitation services at all delivery points	• Complementary feeding, IFA supplementation and focus on nutrition • Diarrhea management at community level using ORS and Zinc • Management of pneumonia • Full immunization coverage	• Address teenage pregnancy and increase contraceptive prevalence • Introduce community-based services through peer education • Strengthen ARSH clinic
• Ensuring access to Pregnancy Testing kits and Strengthening safe abortion services	• Review maternal, infant and child deaths for corrective actions • Identify village with less institutional delivery load, distribute Misoprostol and incentive ANMs for domiciliary deliveries	• Equip special newborn care units with highly trained HR and other infrastructure • Community level use of Gentamicin by ANM	• Rashtriya Bal Swasthya Karyakram (RBSK): screening of children for 4Ds (birth defects, development delays, deficiencies and disease) and its management	• Weekly IFA Supplementation (WIFS) under national Iron Plus initiative • Promote menstrual hygiene

Table 10.12: Continuum of care across lifecycle and different levels of health system.

	Reproductive care	*Pregnancy and child birth care*	*Newborn and childcare*	
Clinical	• Comprehensive abortion care • RTI/STI case management, • Postpartum IUCD and sterilization; interval IUCD procedures • Adolescent friendly health services	• Skilled obstetric care and immediate newborn care and resuscitation • Emergency obstetric care • Preventing Parent to Child Transmission (PPTCT) of HIV • Postpartum sterilization	• Essential newborn care • Care of sick newborn (SNCU, NBSU) • Facility-based care of childhood illnesses (IMNCI) • Care of children with severe acute malnutrition (NRC) • Immunization	
	Reproductive health care	*Antenatal care*	*Postnatal care*	*Child health care*
Outreach/ Subcenter	• Family planning (including IUCD insertion, OCP and condoms) • Prevention and management of STIs • Peri-conception Folic acid supplementation	• Full antenatal care package • PPTCT	• Early detection and management of illnesses in mother and newborn • Immunization	• First level assessment and care for newborn and childhood illnesses • Immunizaton • Micronutrient supplementation
Family and Community	• Weekly IFA supplementation • Information and counseling on sexual reproductive health and family planning • Community-based promotion and delivery of contraceptives • Menstrual hygiene	• Counseling and preparation for newborn care, breastfeeding, birth preparedness • Demand generation • For pregnancy care and institutional delivery (JSY, JSSK)	• Home-based newborn care and prompt referral (HBNC scheme) • Antibiotic for suspected case of newborn sepsis • Infant and Young Child Feeding (IYCF), including exclusive breastfeeding and complementary feeding, • Child health screening and early intervention services (0–18 years) • Early childhood development • Danger sign recognition and care-seeking for illness • Use of ORS and Zinc in case of diarrhea	
	Intersectoral: Water, sanitation, hygiene, nutrition, education, empowerment			
	Adolescence/ Pre-pregnancy → Pregnancy → Birth → Newborn /postnatal → Childhood			

gaps in the delivery of a particular intervention or a set of interventions.

ADOLESCENT HEALTH SERVICES [RASHTRIYA KISHOR SWASTHYA KARYAKRAM (RKSK)]

The newly launched *Rashtriya Kishor Swasthya Karyakram (RKSK)* subsumes these components into a comprehensive program. Rashtriya Kishor Swasthya Karyakram (RKSK) was launched on 7th January 2014 to reach out to 253 million adolescents—male and female, rural and urban, married and unmarried, in and out-of-school adolescents as a part of RMNCH+A. Rashtriya Kishor Swasthya Karyakram is underpinned by evidence that adolescence is the most important stage of the lifecycle for health interventions.

The salient features of RKSK are:

- RKSK uses a health promotion approach and provides information, counseling and services to adolescent across level of care both in the community and at the facilities;
- The program expands the scope of adolescent health programming in India—from being limited to sexual and reproductive health, it now includes in its ambit nutrition, injuries and violence (including gender based violence), noncommunicable diseases, mental health and substance misuse and
- RKSK is a paradigm shift from the existing clinic-based services to promotion and prevention and reaching adolescents in their own environment, such as in schools and communities.

Key activities under the scheme include:

- Community-based Health education and outreach in the target population to promote menstrual health;
- Ensuring regular availability of Sanitary napkins to the adolescents;
- Sourcing and Procurement of Sanitary napkins;
- Storage and distribution of Sanitary napkins to the adolescent girls;
- Training of ASHA and nodal teachers in Menstrual Health and
- Safe disposal of sanitary napkins.

Adolescent health and nutrition status has an intergenerational effect. Therefore, adolescence is one of the important stages of the lifecycle in terms of health interventions. Adolescence is a period which maintain the major part of continuum of care. The nutritional deficiency, anemia during adolescence period can affect the health of the mother and baby in later life. Although adolescence is considered to be a healthy phase, more disease burden and almost 60% of premature deaths among adults can be associated with behavior or conditions that begin or occur during adolescence—for example, tobacco and alcohol use, poor eating habits, sexual abuse and risky sex. Considering the health of adolscents the selected program interventions for adolescents are:

- Adolescent nutrition; iron and folic acid supplementation
- Facility-based adolescent reproductive and sexual health services (Adolescent health clinics)
- Information and counseling on adolescent sexual reproductive health and other health issues
- Menstrual hygiene
- Preventive health checkups.

Adolescent Nutrition; Iron and Folic Acid Supplementation

As part of the new adolescent health strategy, in order to generate awareness, communication on consumption of balanced diet, nutritious food and inter-generational effects of malnutrition is deemed essential. It is proposed that nutrition education sessions be held at the community level using existing platforms like VHND, Kishori Diwas, school setting, Anaganwadi Centers (AWC) and Nehru Yuva Kendra Sangathan (NYKS). Nutritional counseling on a dedicated quarterly Adolescent Health Day (to coincide with Kishori Diwas in SABLA districts) is also proposed. To make deeper inroads, nutrition education is to be included in school curriculum, establishing working linkages with 'Sakshar Bharat' Abhiyan. Following the principle of 'continuum of care', the National Iron + Initiative provides a minimum service package for the management of anemia across life stages and at different levels of care. This initiative brings together existing programs for iron and folic acid (IFA) supplementation among pregnant and lactating women and children in the age group of 6–60 months, and proposes to include new age groups (adolescents ; women in reproductive age group).

Weekly Iron and Folic Acid Supplementation Scheme

The Weekly Iron and Folic Acid Supplementation (WIFS) scheme is a community-based intervention that addresses nutritional (iron deficiency) anemia amongst adolescents (boys and girls) in both rural and urban areas. It aims to cover adolescents enrolled in class VI–XII of government, government-aided and municipal schools as well as 'out of school' girls. The key features of the scheme are: (1) Supervised administration of weekly iron and folic acid supplements of 100 mg elemental iron and 500 mcg folic acid; (2) Screening of target groups for moderate and severe anemia and referral to an appropriate health facility; (3) Biannual deworming (Albendazole 400 mg) and (4) Information and counseling for improving dietary intake and preventive actions for intestinal worm infestation.

Adolescent Reproductive and Sexual Health Programme

Access to reproductive and sexual health information and services, including access to contraceptives and safe abortion services, delivered in an adolescent-friendly environment are critical to reducing incidences of STIs, unplanned and unwanted pregnancies and unsafe abortions.

In an effort to provide adolescent reproductive and sexual health information and services along the continuum of care, community-based intervention and demand generation initiatives will be linked to facility-based services across all levels of health system. Services at subcenter level will be provided by the ANM while an Adolescent Information and Counseling Center will be made functional by the Medical Officer and ANM at the Primary Health Center on a weekly basis. At the Community Health Center, District Hospital/Sub District Hospital/Taluk/Area Hospital and Medical College, Adolescent Health Clinics will provide services on a daily basis. A dedicated counsellor will be available on all days at higher-level facilities (Community Health Center onwards).

The National Adolescent Reproductive and Sexual Health strategy provides a framework for a range of sexual and reproductive health services to be provided to the adolescents. Services in adolescent health clinics will be available to all adolescents: married and unmarried, girls and boys, and will be further expanded and strengthened.

Special focus will be given to establishing linkages with Integrated Counseling and Testing Centers (ICTCs) and making appropriate referrals for HIV testing and RTI/STI management; providing comprehensive abortion care; and provision of information, counseling and services for contraception to both married and unmarried adolescents. The provision of contraceptives is to be made through this clinic, while ensuring continuous contraceptive supplies and services. These services will be linked to a strong community-based component for generating demand and mobilizing adolescents to the Adolescent Health Clinics.

Promotion of menstrual hygiene among adolescent girls in rural India: Menstruation is a normal body function. Despite this, generations of women have had to endure ill health, discomfort, lack of hygiene and even personal risk in trying to manage this normal function. The above-mentioned scheme promotes better health and hygiene among adolescent girls (aged 10 to 19 years) in rural areas by ensuring that they have adequate knowledge and information about the use of sanitary napkins. Through the scheme, high quality and safe products are made available to the girls and environmentally safe disposal mechanisms are made accessible. The sanitary napkins are provided under NRHM's brand 'Free days'. These napkins are being sold to adolescent girls by ASHAs. The scheme should also be seen as an opportunity to inform adolescent girls about sexual and reproductive health issues, nutrition, noncommunicable diseases and mental well being, and guide them to community-based counsellors and/or adolescent clinics in case of any queries or problems that need to be addressed.

Preventive health checkups and screening for diseases, deficiency and disability: The School Health Program addresses the need for preventive health checkups amongst school going children and adolescents. Bi-annual health screening is undertaken for students (6–18 years age group) enrolled in government and government-aided schools for disease, deficiency and disability, with referrals and linkages to secondary and tertiary health facilities, as required. The components of the School Health Program include screening, basic health services and referral; immunization; micronutrient supplementation (IFA, Vitamin A) and deworming. The new approach in the implementation of the School Health Program is to establish dedicated mobile health teams at block level. These teams will include two Medical Officers (MBBS/Dental/AYUSH qualified) and two paramedics (one ANM and any one of the following: Pharmacist/Ophthalmic Assistant/Dental assistant). These teams will be provided mobility support (dedicated hired vehicle) as per the approved norm of the state, equipment and medicines. School-going children and adolescents in need of secondary and tertiary care will be entitled to free treatment through Rastriya Swasthya Bima Yojna or State Health Insurance Scheme or NRHM. The School Health Program also requires a strong convergence with the Department of Education.

Social behavior change communication with focus on inter personal communication: The community level interventions involve selection of "Four Peer Educators (PEs) one per thousand population" to establish information and support network for adolescents in the community. The PEs will be trained in a comprehensive set of topics spanning the following issues: objectives of RKSK, roles and responsibilities of PEs, understanding adolescents as transition to adulthood, gender and sexual identity, health concerns of adolescents, peer pressure, emotional stress and other specific concerns of child marriages, gender based violence, child and ARSH rights etc.

Service to be provided at the Adolescent Health Day:

- **Information:** IEC and IPC on Nutrition, SRH, Mental Health, GBV, NCD and Substance misuse.
- **Commodities:** Sanitary Napkins, IFA, Albendazole, anti-spasmodic tablets and contraceptives.
- **Services:** Registration, general health check-up, (BMI, anemia and diabetes), referral to AFHCs (for counseling and clinical services.

NATIONAL HEALTH MISSION (NHM)

The National Health Mission (NHM) encompasses its two submissions, The National Rural Health Mission (NRHM) and The National Urban Health Mission (NUHM). The main programmatic components include Health System Strengthening, Reproductive-Maternal- Neonatal-Child and Adolescent Health (RMNCH+A), and Communicable and Noncommunicable Diseases. The NHM envisages achievement of universal access to equitable, affordable and quality health care services that are accountable and responsive to people's needs. The National Health Mission (NHM) was launched by the government of India in 2013 subsuming the National Rural Health Mission and National Urban Health Mission.

National Rural Health Mission (NRHM) was launched in April 12, 2005 to address the health needs of the underserved rural population especially women, children and vulnerable sections of the society and to provide accessible, affordable and quality healthcare. The National Urban Health Mission, (NUHM) was launched in May 2013 for serving urban vulnerable people and was subsumed with NRHM as a submission of the overarching National Health Mission (NHM). Many exclusive practices were encouraged like innovations in healthcare delivery practices, flexible financing to the states with strengthened monitoring and evaluation component for better health outcomes and health indicators of the states.

The 2nd vision of the NHM is "Attainment of Universal Access to Equitable, Affordable and Quality health care services, accountable and responsive to people's needs, with effective intersectoral convergent action to address the wider social determinants of health" and focuses on decentralized health planning, service delivery, creating knowledge hubs within district hospitals, strengthening secondary level care at district hospitals, expanding outreach services, improving community processes and behavior change communication, human resources development, public health management, and health management information systems. NHM particularly focuses on equity by prioritizing the health of tribal populations, those in Left Wing Extremism (LWE) and urban poor. A key outcome of NHM is to reduce Out of Pocket expenditures. Health outcomes, output and process indicators are monitored through large scale surveys conducted periodically with evaluations, use of HMIS data, and periodic reviews done. The main aim is to create a fully functional, decentralized and community owned system with greater intersectoral coordination so that wider social determinant factors affecting health of people like water, sanitation, nutrition, gender and education are also equally addressed.

NATIONAL RURAL HEALTH MISSION (NRHM)

Introduction

The National Rural Health Mission (NRHM) was launched on 12th April 2005, to provide accessible, affordable and quality health care to the rural population, especially the vulnerable groups. It aims to improve access of rural people especially poor women and children to equitable affordable accountable and effective primary health care. It aims at effective integration of health concerns with determinants of health like sanitation and hygiene, nutrition and safe drinking water through decentralized planning. It seeks decentralization of programs for district management of health. It aims to undertake architectural correction of health system to enable it to effectively handle increased allocation as promised under the National Common Minimum Programme and promote policies that strengthen public health management and services in the country. NRHM subsumes all existing programs like Reproductive Child Health, Immunization, National Disease Control Programme, and Integrated Disease Surveillance Project. It aims at integration of all vertical Family Health Programmes and strives for optimal utilization of funds and infrastructure and strengthening delivery of primary health care, through the existing health care system, though IMR/MMR is high and not declining fast enough, especially in rural areas and among the poor. High and prohibitive out of pocket expenditure make access of poor people to health services difficult. Major contributor to poverty and destitution of resources. Population stabilization is ineffective especially in a number of EAG States/CMP districts. Public health system was on the decline poor governance, manpower shortages, ineffective service delivery.

Definition

NRHM is a national effort at ensuring effective health care through a range of intervention at individual, house hold, community and most critically at the health system level.

Major Goal for NRHM

Major Goal for NRHM is to improve the availability and access to quality health care by people, especially for those residing in rural areas, the poor women and children.

For achieving this goal we have to:

- Reduce child mortality
- Improve maternal health
- Combat HIV/AIDS, malaria and other major diseases
- Ensure environmental sustainability.

Objective

The following are the major objectives of the National Rural Health Mission:

- Reduction in child and maternal mortality
- Universal access to public services for food and nutrition, sanitation and hygiene
- Universal access to public health care services with emphasis on services addressing
- Women's and children's health and universal immunization
- Prevention and control of communicable and non-communicable diseases, including locally endemic diseases
- Access to integrated comprehensive primary health care
- Population stabilization, gender and demographic balance
- Revitalize local health traditions and mainstream of AYUSH
- Promotion of healthy lifestyles.

Strategies of NRHM

Core Strategies

- Train and enhance capacity of Panchayati Raj Institutions (PRIs) to own, control and manage public health services at various level.
- Promote access to improved health care at household level through the female health activist (ASHA).
- Health plan for each village through Village Health Committee of the Panchayat.
- Strengthening subcenter through an untied fund to enable local planning and action and more Multi Purpose Workers (MPWs).
- Strengthening existing PHCs and CHCs, and provision of 30–50 bedded CHC per lakh population for improved curative care to a normative standard (Indian Public Health Standards defining personnel, equipment and management).
- Preparation and implementation of an intersectoral District Health Plan prepared by the District Health Mission, including drinking water, sanitation and hygiene and nutrition.
- Integrating vertical Health and Family Welfare programmes at national, state, block, and district levels
- Technical support to national, state and district health missions, for public health management.
- Strengthening capacities for data collection, assessment and review for evidence-based planning, monitoring and supervision. Formulation of transparent policies for deployment and career development of human resources for health.
- Developing capacities for preventive and promoting health care at all levels.
- Promoting nonprofit sector particularly in under-served areas.

Supplementary Strategies

- Regulation of private sector including the informal rural practitioners to ensure availability of quality service to citizens at reasonable cost.
- Promotion of public private partnerships for achieving public health goals
- Mainstreaming AYUSH (Ayurveda, Yoga, Unani, Siddha and Homeopathy)
- Reorienting medical education to support rural health issues including regulation of medical care and medical ethics.
- Effective and viable risk pooling and social health insurance to provide health security to the poor by ensuring accessible, affordable, accountable and good quality hospital care.

Plan of Action

The plan of action for NRHM developed based on eight components **(Fig. 10.1)**.

Components of NRHM

Component (A)

Accredited Social Health Activists

Accredited Social Health Activists is the first component under NRHM. Every village/large habitat (1000 population) will have a female ASHA. Chosen by and accountable to the Panchayat to act as the interface between the community and the public health system. ASHA would act as a bridge between the ANM and the village, must be primarily a women resident

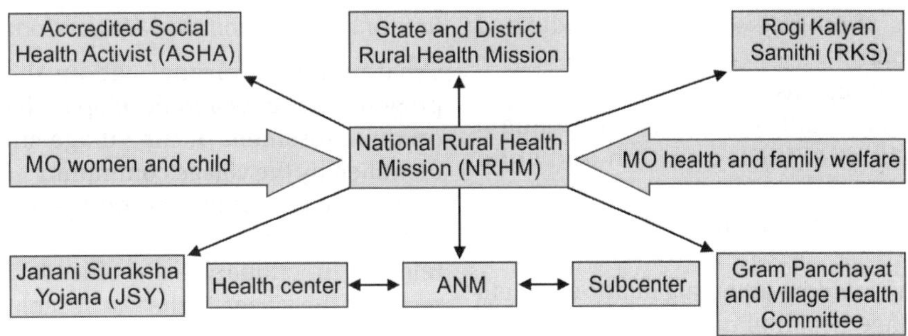

Fig. 10.1: Components of NRHM.

of the village—married/widow/divorced. She should be in the age group of 25–45 years, a literate woman with formal education up to 8th std. She will be an honorary volunteer, receiving performance-based incentives for promoting universal immunization, referral and escort services for RCH, construction of house hold toilets and other health delivery programs. She will be trained on a pedagogy of public health developed and monitored through a National Experts Group for best practices and implemented through active involvement of community health resource organizations. She will facilitate preparation and implementation of the Village Health Plan along with Anganwadi worker, ANM, functionaries of other departments, and self help group members, under the leadership of the Village Health Committee of the Panchayat. She will be promoted all over the country, with special emphasis on the 18 high focus states. The Government of India will bear the cost of training, incentives and medical kits. She will be given a drug kit containing both AYUSH and allopathic formulations for common ailments. The drug kit would be replenished from time to time.

Training for ASHA

Induction training of ASHA was planned for 23 days in a month, spread over 12 months. On the job training would continue throughout the year. Prototype training material to be developed at National level subject to State level modifications. Training will be given by the trainers including contact plus distance learning model. Training would require partnership with NGOs, ICDS, Training Centers and State Health Institutes.

Component (B)

Strengthening Subcenters

Each subcenter will have an untied fund for local action @ ₹10,000 per annum. This fund will be deposited in a joint bank account of the ANM and Sarpanch and operated by the ANM, in consultation with the Village Health Committee. Supply of essential drugs, both allopathic and AYUSH, to the subcenters. In case of additional outlays, MPW (Male)/ Additional ANMs wherever needed, sanction of new Subcenters as per 2001 population norm, and upgrading existing SC's, including buildings for SC's functioning in rented premises will be considered.

Component (C)

Strengthening PHCs

For quality preventive, promotive, curative, supervisory and outreach services, through adequate and regular supply of essential quality drugs and equipment to PHC's. Provision of 24-hour service in 50% PHCs by addressing shortage of doctors, especially in high focus states, through mainstreaming AYUSH manpower. Observance of standard treatment guidelines and protocols. In case of additional outlays, intensification of ongoing communicable disease control programs, new programs for control of noncommunicable diseases, supply of autodisabled syringes for immunization. Upgradation of 100% PHCs for 24-hours referral service, and provision of 2nd doctor at PHC level (1 male, 1 female) would be undertaken on the basis of felt need.

Component (D)

Strengthening CHCS for First Referral Care

Operationalizing 3222 existing CHCs (30–50 beds) as 24-Hour First Referral Units, including posting of anesthetists. Codification of new Indian Public Health Standards, setting norms for infrastructure, staff, equipment, management, etc. for CHCs. Promotion of Stakeholder Committees for hospital management. Develop, display and ensure compliance to Citizen's Charter at CHC/PHC level. In case of additional outlays, creation of new CHCs (30–50 beds) to meet the population norm as per census 2001.

Component (E)

District Health Plan

District Health Action Plan 2005–2012 is being prepared by each District. The key strategies suggested for DAP are as follows:

- Block will be the key level for development of decentralized plans so each block will be covered under the DAP and a block level plan will be prepared for each block in each district.
- Technical resource agency/groups will be identified for each block to assist in planning.
- A technical resource agency would be identified for the district to support the implementation of the DAP.

Four broad categories of programs have been indicated under NRHM.

1. RCH-II activities and programs
2. NRHM activities such as IPHS, Untied Funds, Janani Suraksha Yojana (JSY), AYUSH, nutrition and child development
3. National Disease Control Programme
4. Immunization.

District health plan would be an amalgamation of field responses through village health plans, state and national priorities for health, water supply, sanitation and nutrition.

- Health plans would form the core unit of action proposed in areas like water supply, sanitation, hygiene and nutrition. Implementing departments would integrate into 'District Health Mission' for monitoring.
- District becomes core unit of planning, budgeting and implementation.
- Centrally sponsored schemes could be rationalized/modified accordingly in consultation with states.
- Funds to district for effective integration of programs.
- All vertical Health and Family Welfare Programmes at district and state level merge into one common 'District Health Mission' at the district level and the 'State Health Mission' at the state level.
- Provision of Project Management Unit for all districts, through contract engagement of MBA, chartered accountant and data entry operator, for improved program management.

Component (F)

Under component F converging sanitation and hygiene activity has included. Total sanitation campaign (TSC) is presently implemented in 350 districts.

Components of TSC include IEC activities, rural sanitary marts, individual household toilets, Women sanitary complex, and School Sanitation Programme. Total Sanitation Campaign is also implemented through Panchayati Raj Institutions (PRIs). The District Health Mission would therefore guide activities of sanitation at district level, and promote joint IEC for public health, sanitation and hygiene, through Village Health and Sanitation Committee, and promote household toilets and School Sanitation Programme. ASHA would be given incentive for promoting household toilets by the mission.

Village Health Sanitation Committee (VHSC) and NRHM

The NRHM framework support decentralized planning and monitoring up to the grass root level.

Therefore it was decided to entrust village level committees, community-based organization for the planning, monitoring and implementation of NRHM activities into the 41000 revenue villages of the state. The VHSC will be the key agency for developing Village Health Plan and the entire planning of village Panchayat for NRHM.

This committee comprises of Panchayat representatives, ANM, MPW, Anganwadi workers, teachers, community health volunteers, ASHA.

Role of Villages Sanitation Health Committee Activities

Create public awareness about the essentials of health programs. Discuss and develop a Village Health Plan based on an assessment of the village situation and priorities identified by the village community.

Analyze key issues and problems related to village level health and nutrition activities, give feedback on these to relevant functionaries and officials. Present annual health report of the village in the Gram Sabha.

Participatory Rapid Assessment: to ascertain the major health problems and health-related issues in the village.

Estimation of the annual expenditure incurred for management of all the morbidities may also be done.

The mapping will also take into account the health resources and the unhealthy influences within village boundaries.

Component (G)

Strengthening Disease Control Programmes

National Disease Control Programmes for TB, Malaria, Kala-azar, Filaria, Blindness and Iodine deficiency and Integrated Disease Surveillance Programme shall be integrated under the mission, for improved program delivery. New initiatives would be launched for control of noncommunicable diseases. Disease surveillance system at village level would be strengthened. Supply of generic drugs (both AYUSH and Allopathic) for common ailments at village, SC, PHC/CHC level. Provision of a mobile medical unit at district level for improved outreach services.

Component (H)

Public-Private Partnership for Public Health Goals, Including Regulation of Private Sector

Since almost 75% of health services are being currently provided by the private sector, there is a need to refine regulation.

District Institutional Mechanism for mission must have representation of private sector.

Need to develop guidelines for Public-Private Partnership (PPP) in health sector. Identifying areas of partnership, which are need-based, thematic and geographic. Public sector to play the lead role in defining the framework and sustaining the partnership management plan for PPP initiatives at district/state and national levels. Task force to improve details/guidelines.

Component (I)

New Health Financing Mechanisms

A Task group to examine new health financing mechanisms, including Risk Pooling for Hospital Care as follows:

- Progressively the District Health Missions to move toward paying hospitals for services by way of reimbursement, on the principle of 'money follows the patient.'
- Standardization of services—outpatient, in-patient, laboratory, surgical interventions and costs will be done

periodically by a committee of experts in each state. A National Expert Group to monitor these standards and give suitable advice and guidance on protocols and cost comparisons.

- All existing CHCs to have wage component paid on monthly basis. Other recurrent costs may be reimbursed for services rendered from District Health Fund. Over the mission period, the CHC may move toward all costs, including wages reimbursed for services rendered.
- A district health accounting system is created to monitor the District Health Fund Management, and take corrective action. Adequate technical managerial and accounting support to be provided to DHM in managing risk-pooling and health security.
- Where credible Community-based Health Insurance Schemes (CBHI) exist/are launched, they will be encouraged as part of the mission. The Central Government will provide subsidies to cover a part of the premiums for the poor, and monitor the schemes. Which will be periodically evaluated for effective delivery.

Component (J)

Reorienting Health/Medical Education to Support Rural Health Issues

While district and tertiary hospitals are necessarily located in urban centers, they form an integral part of the referral care chain serving the needs of the rural people. Medical and paramedical education facilities need to be created in states, based on need assessment. Suggestion for Commission for Excellence in Health Care (Medical Grants Commission), National Institution for Public Health Management, etc.

Major initiatives under National Health Mission (NHM)

Some of the major initiatives under National Health Mission (NHM) are as follows:

Accredited Social Health Activists

Community Health volunteers called Accredited Social Health Activists (ASHAs) have been engaged under the mission for establishing a link between the community and the health system. ASHA is the first port of call for any health-related demands of deprived sections of the population, especially women and children, who find it difficult to access health services in rural areas.

Rogi Kalyan Samiti (Patient Welfare Committee)/ Hospital Management Society

The Rogi Kalyan Samiti (Patient Welfare Committee)/ Hospital Management Society is a management structure that acts as a group of trustees for the hospitals to manage the affairs of the hospital. Financial assistance is provided to these Committees through untied fund to undertake activities for patient welfare.

Mainstreaming of AYUSH

The NRHM seeks to revitalize local health traditions and mainstream AYUSH (including manpower and drugs), to strengthen the Public Health System at all levels. It is decided that AYUSH medications shall be included in the drug kit of ASHA. The additional supply of generic drugs for common ailments at SC/PHC/CHC levels under the Mission shall also include AYUSH formulations. At the CHC level two rooms shall be provided for AYUSH practitioner and pharmacist under the Indian Public Health Standards (IPHS) model. At the same time, single Doctor PHCs shall be upgraded to two Doctor PHCs by inducting AYUSH practitioner at that level.

Untied Grants to Subcenters have been used to fund grass-root improvements in health care. Some examples include:

- Improved efficacy of Auxiliary Nurse Midwives (ANMs) in the field that can now undertake better antenatal care and other health care services.
- Village Health Sanitation and Nutrition Committees (VHSNC) have used untied grants to increase their involvement in their local communities to address the needs of poor households and children.
- Involvement in their local communities to address the needs of poor households and children.

Health Care Contractors

NRHM has provided health care contractors to underserved areas, and has been involved in training to expand the skill set of doctors at strategically located facilities identified by the states. Similarly, due importance is given to capacity building of nursing staff and auxiliary workers such as ANMs. NHM also supports co-location of AYUSH services in Health facilities such as PHCs, CHCs and District Hospitals.

Janani Suraksha Yojana

Janani Suraksha Yojana (JSY) is a safe motherhood intervention scheme implemented by the Government of India. It was launched on 12 April 2005 by the Prime Minister of India. It aims to promote institutional delivery among poor pregnant women and to reduce neonatal mortality and maternal mortality. It is operated under the Ministry of Health and Family Welfare as part of the National Rural Health Mission. The Scheme integrates cash assistance with delivery and post-delivery care, particularly in states with low institutional delivery rates.

National Mobile Medical Units (NMMUs)

Many unserved areas have been covered through National Mobile Medical Units (NMMUs).

National Ambulance Services

Free ambulance services are provided in every nook and corner of the country connected with a toll free number and reaches within 30 minutes of the call.

Janani Shishu Suraksha Karyakram (JSSK)

As part of recent initiatives and further moving in the direction of universal healthcare, Janani Shishu Suraksha Karyakarm (JSSK) was introduced to provide free to and fro transport, free drugs, free diagnostic, free blood, free diet to pregnant women who come for delivery in public health institutions and sick infants up to one year.

Rashtriya Bal Swasthya Karyakram (RBSK)

A Child Health Screening and Early Intervention Services has been launched in February 2013 to screen diseases specific to childhood, developmental delays, disabilities, birth defects and deficiencies. The initiative will cover about 27 crore children between 0–18 years of age and also provide free treatment including surgery for health problems diagnosed under this initiative.

Mother and Child Health Wings (MCH Wings)

With a focus to reduce maternal and child mortality, dedicated Mother and Child Health Wings with 100/50/30 bed capacity have been sanctioned in high case load district hospitals and CHCs which would create additional beds for mothers and children.

Free Drugs and Free Diagnostic Service

A new initiative is launched under the National Health Mission to provide Free Drugs Service and Free Diagnostic Service with a motive to lower the out of pocket expenditure on health.

District Hospital and Knowledge Center (DHKC)

As a new initiative District Hospitals are being strengthened to provide Multispecialty health care including dialysis care, intensive cardiac care, cancer treatment, mental illness, emergency medical and trauma care etc. These hospitals would act as the knowledge support for clinical care in facilities below it through a tele-medicine center located in the district headquarters and also developed as centers for training of paramedics and nurses.

National Iron+ Initiative

The National Iron+ Initiative is an attempt to look at Iron Deficiency Anemia in which beneficiaries will receive iron and folic acid supplementation irrespective of their Iron/Hb status. This initiative will bring together existing programs (IFA supplementation for: pregnant and lactating women and; children in the age group of 6–60 months) and introduce new age groups.

Tribal TB Eradication Project

This project is launched by MoS Health Shri Faggan Singh Kulaste at Mandla on 20 January 2017 under NHM.

Roles and Responsibilities of ASHA

ASHA will be a health activist in the community who will create awareness on health and its social determinants and mobilize the community toward local health planning and increased utilization and accountability of the existing health services. She would be a promoter of good health practices.

She will also provide a minimum package of curative care as appropriate and feasible for that level and make timely referrals.

ASHA will take steps to create awareness and provide information to the community on determinants of health, such as nutrition, basic sanitation and hygienic practices, healthy living and working conditions, information on existing health services and the need for timely utilization of health and family welfare services.

She will counsel women on birth preparedness, importance of safe delivery, breastfeeding and complementary feeding, immunization, contraception and prevention of common infections including RTIs/STIs and care of the young child.

ASHA will mobilize the community and facilitate them in accessing health and health-related services available at the village/subcenter/PHCs, such as immunization, Antenatal Check-up (ANC), Postnatal Checkup (PNC), ICDS, sanitation and other services being provided by the government.

She will work with the Village Health and Sanitation Committee of the Gram Panchayat to develop a comprehensive village health plan. She will arrange escort/accompany pregnant women and children requiring treatment/admission to the nearest pre-identified health facility, i.e., Primary Health Center/Community Health Center/First Referral Unit (PHC/CHC/FRU).

ASHA will provide primary medical care for minor ailments, such as diarrhea, fevers, and first aid for minor injuries. She will be a provider of Directly Observed Treatment Shortcourse (DOTS) under Revised National Tuberculosis Control Programme.

She will also act as a depot holder for essential provisions being made available to every habitation like Oral Rehydration Therapy (ORS), Iron Folic Acid Tablet (IFA), chloroquine, Disposable Delivery Kits (DDK), oral pills and condoms, etc. A drug kit will be provided to each ASHA. Contents of the kit will be based on the recommendations of the expert/technical advisory group set up by the Government of India.

Her role as a provider can be enhanced subsequently. States can explore the possibility of graded training to her for providing newborn care and management of a range of common ailments particularly childhood illnesses. She will inform about the births and deaths in her village and any unusual health problems/disease outbreaks in the community to the Subcenters/PHCs.

She will promote construction of household toilets under Total Sanitation Campaign. Fulfillment of all the roles by ASHA is envisaged through continuous training and upgradation of her skills, spread over 2 years or more.

NRHM includes core and supplementary strategies with the components of ASHA, strengthening SC's, PHC's, CHC'S, district health plan, converging sanitation and hygiene, strengthening disease control programs, public-private partnership for public health goals including regulation of private sector, new health financing mechanisms, reorienting health medical education to support rural health issues.

NATIONAL URBAN HEALTH MISSION (NUHM)

The National Rural Health Mission (NRHM) is an initiative undertaken by the government of India to address the health needs of under-served rural areas and this program has been launched on 12 April 2005 by then Indian Prime Minister Manmohan Singh. The NRHM was initially tasked with addressing the health needs of 18 states that had been identified as having weak public health indicators. The Union Cabinet headed by Manmohan Singh vide its decision dated 1 May 2013, has approved the launch of *National Urban Health Mission (NUHM)* as a Submission of an overarching National Health Mission (NHM), with National Rural Health Mission (NRHM) being the other Submission of National Health Mission.

The National Urban Health Mission (NUHM) envisages to meet health care needs of the urban population with the focus on urban poor, by making available to them essential primary health care services and reducing their out of pocket expenses for treatment. This will be achieved by strengthening the existing health care service delivery system, targeting the people living in slums and converging with various schemes relating to wider determinants of health like drinking water, sanitation, school education, etc., implemented by the Ministries of Urban Development, Housing and Urban Poverty Alleviation, Human Resource Development and Women and Child Development.

Goals of National Urban Health Mission

- To improve the health status of the urban population specific need-based city and strengthen urban health care system to meet the diverse health care needs of the urban poor and other vulnerable sections by facilitating equitable access to quality health care.
- To implement institutional mechanism and management systems to meet the health-related challenges of a rapidly growing urban population.
- Partnership with community and local bodies for a more proactive involvement in planning, implementation, and monitoring of health activities.
- Availability of resources for providing essential primary health care to urban poor.
- Make Public health thrust on sanitation, clean drinking water, vector control, etc., by revising public health system.
- Partnerships with NGOs, for profit and not for profit health service providers and other stakeholders and encourage public private partnership.

The overall aim of NUHM is to improve the health status of the urban population but particularly of the poor and other disadvantaged sections, by facilitating equitable access to quality health care through a revamped public health system. Capacity of urban local bodies.

Urban Poor Population living in listed and unlisted slums. All other vulnerable population such as homeless, rag-pickers, street children, rickshaw pullers, construction and brick and lime kiln workers, sex workers, and other temporary migrants.

Strategies of NUHM

- **Improving the efficiency of public health system in the cities by strengthening, revamping and rationalizing existing government primary urban health structure and designated referral facilities**
  - The situational analysis has undoubtedly revealed that most of the existing primary health facilities, namely, the Urban Health Posts (UHPs)/Urban Family Welfare Centers (UFWC)/Dispensaries are not functioning optimally due to problems of human resources, infrastructure, diagnostics, referrals, case load, spatial distribution, and inconvenient working hours. The sub-mission NUHM therefore proposes to strengthen and revamp the existing facilities into an "Urban Primary Health Center" with outreach and referral facilities, to be functional for every 50,000 population on an average
  - The strategy has been made that to improve the efficiency of the existing system the NUHM would take steps to improve the efficiency of the existing system by making provision for a need-based contractual human resource, equipments and drugs. Provision of Rogi
  - Kalyan Samiti is also being made for promoting local action. For further strengthening the delivery of specialized OPD care, if need arises, they can utilize the services of specialist on weekly basis.
- **Promotion of access to improved health care at household level through community-based groups: Mahila Arogya Samitis:**
  - The 'Mahila Bachat Gat' scheme in Maharashtra and urban health initiatives in Indore and Agra have demonstrated the efficacy of women led thrift/self help groups in meeting urgent cash needs in times of health emergency and also empowering them to demand improved health services.
  - In view of the visible usefulness of such women led community/self help groups; it is proposed to promote such community-based groups for enhanced community participation and empowerment in conjunction with the community structures created under the Swarna Jayanti Shahari Rojgar Yojana (SJSRY), a scheme of the Ministry of Urban Development which seeks to provide employment to the urban poor
- **Strengthening public health through innovative preventive and promotive action**
  - Urban Poor face greater environmental health risks due to poor sanitation, lack of safe drinking water, poor drainage, high density of population etc. For solving the problem the Mission would also provide a framework for proactive partnership with NGOs/civil society groups for strengthening the preventive and promotive actions at the community level. The ASHA,

in coordination with the members of the MAS would promote proactive community action in partnership with the urban local bodies for improved water and environmental sanitation, nutrition and other aspects having a bearing on health.

- NUHM also provides for some untied funds at all levels for developing need-based innovative strategies for improved service delivery and public health action.

- **Increased access to health care through creation of revolving fund:** As substantiated by various studies the urban poor incur high out of-pocket expenditure often leading to poverty and impoverishment. To mitigate this risk, it is proposed to encourage Mahila Arogya Samitis to "save for a rainy day" for meeting urgent health needs.
- **IT enabled services (ITES) and e-governance for improving access improved surveillance and monitoring:** The availability of ITES in the urban areas makes it a useful tool for effective tracking, monitoring and timely intervention for the urban poor. The NUHM would provide software and hardware support for developing web based HMIS for quick transfer of data and required action. Mobile telephony will be used for data gathering and follow ups. The States would also be encouraged to develop strategies for affecting an urban disease surveillance system and a plan for rapid response in times of disasters and outbreaks.
- **Capacity building of stakeholders:** It was observed that many Counselors showing a clear proclivity for development of tertiary facilities. This skewed prioritization appears to have clearly affected the primary health delivery system in the urban local bodies, also adversely affecting skill sets of the workforce and limiting technical and managerial capacities to manage health. NUHM thus proposes to build managerial, technical and public health competencies among ULBs/Medical and Paramedical staff/Private Providers/Community level structures and functionaries of other related departments.
- **Prioritizing the most vulnerable amongst the poor:** It is seen that a fraction of the urban poor who normally do not reside in slum, but in temporary settlements or are homeless, comprise the most disadvantaged section. Under the NUHM special emphasis would be on improving the reach of health care services to these vulnerable groups among the urban poor, falling in the category of destitute, beggars, street children, construction workers, coolies, rickshaw pullers, sex workers, street vendors and other such migrant workers. Outreach services would target these segments consciously, irrespective of their formal status of resident ship etc.
- **Ensuring quality health care services:** NUHM would aim to ensure quality health services by (a) defining Indian Public Health Standards suitably modified for urban areas wherever required, (b) defining parameters for empanelment/regulation/accreditation of nongovernment providers, (c) developing capacity of public and private providers for providing quality health care, (d) encouraging the acceptance and enforcement of local public health acts, (e) ensuring citizen charters in facilities, (f) encouraging development of standard treatment protocols.

Targets to be Achieved

Process/throughput level indicators:

- Number cities/population where mission has been initiated
- Number of City specific urban health plans developed and operationalized
- Number of U-PHCs with outreach made operational
- Number of Cities/population with all slums and facilities mapped
- Number of Slum/Cluster level Health and Sanitation Day
- Number of MAS formed
- Number of U-PHCs with Program Managers
- Number of ASHAs trained and functioning.

Output level indicators:

- Increase in OPD attendance
- Increase in BPL referrals from U-PHCs/referral availed
- Increase in institutional deliveries as percentage of total deliveries
- Increase in complete immunization among children <12 months
- Increase in case detection for malaria through blood examination
- Increase in case detection of TB through identification of chest symptomatic
- Increase in referral for sputum microscopy examination for TB
- Increase in number of cases screened and treated for dental ailments
- Increase in ANC check-up of pregnant women
- Increased Tetanus toxoid (2nd dose) coverage among pregnant women
- Strengthened civil registration system to achieve 100% registration of births and deaths.

Impact level focus on urban poor:

- Reduce IMR by 40% (in urban areas) - National Urban IMR down to 20 per 1000 live births by 2017
- 40% reduction in U5MR and IMR
- Achieve universal immunization in all urban areas.
- Reduce MMR by 50%
- 50% reduction in MMR (among urban population of the state/country).

CONVERGENT ACTION IN URBAN AREAS

Institutional Framework

Resource Planning in NUHM

The National Urban Health Mission leverage on the institutional structures of the NRHM at the National, State and District level for operationalization of the NUHM. However, in order to provide dedicated focus to issues relating to Urban Health the institutional mechanism under the NRHM at various levels are strengthened for NUHM implementation.

- **State level:** There is a separate Urban Health Cell for NUHM at State level, reporting to State Mission Director.
- **District level:** At the District level the States may either decide to constitute a separate.

District Urban Health Missions/District Urban Health Societies or use the existing structure of the District Health Society/Mission under NRHM with additional stakeholder members.

At the district level, the management of NUHM activities may be coordinated by a District level. Urban Health Committee headed by the District Magistrate/Additional District Magistrate/Sub Division Magistrate based on whether the district is a district headquarters or a subdivision headquarter. This would help ensure better coordination with municipal departments like sanitation, water, waste management, especially in times of response to disease outbreaks/epidemics in the district.

Further for enhancing the Program Management, a District Program Management Unit may be established. The staff at the District PMU level may be as proposed below:

- Urban Health Data Manager/Coordinators.
- Urban Health Accounts Manager
- Consultant (Epidemiologist).

The National Urban Health Mission would promote participation of the urban local bodies in the planning and management of the urban health programs.

Service Delivery Infrastructure NUHM envisages setting up of service delivery infrastructure which is largely absent in cities/towns to specially address the healthcare needs of urban poor and provides:

- **Urban-Primary Health Center (U-PHC):** New U-PHCs are established as per gap analysis, as per norm of one U-PHC for approximately 50,000 urban populations. The new U-PHCs are preferably located within or near a slum for providing preventive, promotive and OPD (consultation), basic lab diagnosis, drug/contraceptive dispensing services, apart from counseling for all communicable and noncommunicable diseases.
- **Urban-Community Health Center (U-CHC) and Referral Hospitals:** 30–50 bedded U-CHCs are established for providing inpatient care. U-CHCs are set up in cities with a population of above 5 lakhs.
- **Outreach services:** NUHM also support engagement of ANMs for conducting outreach services for targeted groups particularly slum dwellers and the vulnerable population for providing preventive and promotive healthcare services at the household and community level.

Community Process

- **Mahila Arogya Samiti (MAS):** One Mahila Arogya Samiti will covers 250–1,000 beneficiaries and between 50–100 households and act as community-based peer education group in slums. So far 40132 MAS have been formed to facilitate community mobilization, monitoring and referral with focus on preventive and promotive care, facilitating access to identified facilities and management of grants received.
- **ASHA/Link worker:** One frontline community worker ASHA serves as an effective and demand- generating link between the health facility and the urban slum population. Each link worker/ASHA will have a well-defined service area of about 1000–2,500 beneficiaries/between 200–500 households based on spatial consideration. However, the states would have the flexibility to either engage ASHA or entrust her responsibilities to MAS. So far 31899 ASHAs have been identified.

Major Interventions Framed under NUHM

Planning

- Baseline survey, mapping of the urban slums, facility assessment and vulnerable assessment of the slums to be conducted in all identified cities/towns
- Establishment/upgradation/strengthening of the Urban Primary Health Centers (UPHCs) in every 50–60 thousand population.
- Establishment of one Urban Community Health Center (UCHC) comprising of 5–6 UPHCs or 2.5 urban populations in cities with above five lakh populations.
- Preparation of State Program Implementation Plan and City Implementation Plan
- Special focus to vulnerable population (authorized/listed slums, unauthorized slums, others like homeless, rag-pickers, street children, migrants, slum dwellers, rickshaw pullers, construction and brick workers deprived community and others)
- The migrant and poor living in the periurban areas (outside and adjacent) to the ULBs would be provided health services
- Establishment of "City Program Management Unit" with 1–3 human resource in 1 to 10 lakhs population cities/towns.
- Incorporate the noncommunicable disease as part of the Urban component of NHM.

Institutional Strengthening

- Reorganization of the State Health Mission with addition of Minister, Housing and Urban Development in Mission and concerned Secretary in the State society. The District Health Mission and City Health Mission would be formed accordingly.
- The MD, NRHM will also act as MD, NUHM.
- The State "Urban Health Cell" needs to be created within SPMU and DPMUs with adequate and appropriate HR.

Community Process

In the community process, Mahila Arogya Samiti (MAS) will be formed in the slums covering 50–100 households. Existing CBOs could be utilized for the same purpose. Provision of untied fund for MAS.

Engagement of Human Resources

- Engagement of ASHAs in 200–500 households in slum/1500 slum population.
- Engagement of ANMs in 10,000–12,000 urban population. They would have a clearly defined area of operation where they will be conducting outreach session as per the NUHM norms.

Coordination and Convergence

- Coordination of city level NUHM activities through the City Coordination Committee.
- The ULBs will involve in program implementation and State will take decisions regarding handover the capacity to cities/towns for management of the programs.
- Establishment of Inter and Inter sectoral convergence with various departments and schemes like RAY, JNNURM, BSUP, IHSDP, RAY, SJSRY, WCD, Education, Water supply and sanitation, etc.
- NUHM to provide a system for convergence of all Disease Control Programs, including communicable and non-communicable diseases (through integrated planning at the City level).

Budget

The Budget share between center and state would be 75% and 25% up to 2017. The funding pattern for North Eastern states and special category states of Jammu and Kashmir, Himachal Pradesh and Uttarakhand will be 90:10.

Others

- Engaging the private organizations/NGOs/public sector companies/commercial companies and utilization of their CSR funds for the urban poor.
- The Existing HIMS and MCTS will extend to urban areas and Integrated MIS (including health, nutrition, water, sanitation)
- MHU (Mobile Health Unit) or MMUs for migrants and urban poor.
- Mobile Sauchalaya (toilet)/Mobile shift toilet in unauthorized slums.
- All services in all facilities (urban and rural) should be free and withdrawal of user fees from the patient in Govt. hospitals.

NATIONAL RASHTRIYA BAL SWASTHYA KARYAKRAM (RBSK)

Ministry of Health and Family Welfare under the flagship National Rural Health Mission launched RBSK as structured health screening and management of childhood health conditions in February 2013. An operational guideline outlines the program. Health screening of school going children is a continued intervention under the School Health Program, and it is now being expanded to cover all children from birth to 18 years of age.

RBSK aims at early detection and management of the prevalent health conditions in children groups in 4 broad groups, '4Ds'-Defects at birth, diseases of childhood, deficiency and developmental delays including disabilities. A total of 30 conditions have been identified for screening and appropriate referral and management.

The services aim to cover all children of 0 to 6 years of age in rural areas and urban slums in addition to children enrolled in classes 1st to 12th in Government and Government aided schools. It is expected that these services will reach to about 270 million children in a phased manner.

The following mechanisms as per GOI operational guidelines will be used to reach children for health screenings:

- Community-based newborn screening at home through ASHAs for newborn till 6 weeks of age during home visit.
- Anganwadi center based screening by the dedicated mobile health teams for children 6 weeks to 6 years.
- Government and Government aided school based screening by dedicated mobile health teams for children 6 years to 18 years.
- Facility based newborn screening at public health facilities, by existing health manpower.

In addition to the community screening through mobile teams, an Early Intervention Center will be established at the District Hospital. The purpose of Early Intervention Center will be to provide referral support to children detected with health conditions during health screening in addition to establishing screening mechanism for detection of hearing, visual and other developmental delays and birth defects.

District Early Intervention Center (DEIC)

An Early Intervention Center will be established at the District Hospital. The purpose of Early Intervention Center is to provide referral support to children detected with health conditions during health screening. A team consisting of pediatrician, Medical officer, Staff Nurses, Paramedics will be engaged to provide services. There is also a provision for engaging a manager who would carry out mapping of tertiary care facilities in Government institutions for ensuring adequate referral support. Children and students presumptively diagnosed to have a disease/deficiency/disability/defect and who require confirmatory tests or further examination will be referred to the designated tertiary level public sector health facilities through the District Early Intervention Centers.

The Rationale for the RBSK Program

Out of every 100 babies born in this country annually, 6 to 7 have a birth defect. In Indian context, this would translate to 1. 7 million birth defects annually and would account for 9.6% of all newborn deaths. Various nutritional deficiencies affecting the preschool children range from 4% to 70%. Developmental delays are common in early childhood affecting at least 10% of the children. These delays, if not intervened timely, may lead to permanent disabilities with regard to cognition, hearing and vision.

There are also groups of diseases which are very common in children, e.g., dental caries, otitis media, rheumatic heart disease and reactive airways diseases which can be cured if detected early. It is understood that early intervention and management can prevent these conditions to progress into more severe and debilitating forms, thereby reducing hospitalization and resulting in improved school attendance.

The 'Child Health Screening and Early Intervention Services' will also translate into economic benefits in the long run. Timely intervention would not only halt the condition to deteriorate but would also reduce the out-of-pocket (OOP) expenditure of the poor and the marginalized population in the country. Additionally, the Child Health Screening and Early Intervention Services will also provide country-wide epidemiological data on the 4 Ds (i.e., Defects at birth, Diseases, Deficiencies and Developmental Delays including Disabilities). Such a data is expected to hold relevance for future planning of area specific services.

ANM and ASHAs

Field-level functionaries will be providers of information, services and commodities at the community level and make appropriate referrals to Adolescent Friendly Health Clinics (AFHCs) as and when required. They will serve as the first point of contact for the adolescents. These service providers will be instrumental in creating and enabling environment at the community level for adolescent health and development activities through existing platforms, such as AWCs, Sabla Kishori-Samooh, Teen Clubs and Village Health, Nutrition and Sanitation Committees (VHNSCs), and creating new platforms for service delivery such as organizing Adolescent Health Days (AHDs) every quarter. Community-based workers and volunteers will engage with parents and families of adolescents to increase awareness about the unique needs of this dynamic group.

Adolescent Health Day

Increase awareness among adolescents, parents, families and stakeholders about the determinants of adolescent health, such as nutrition, Sexual Reproductive Health (SRH), mental health, injuries and violence (including Gender-based violence), substance misuse and NCDs. Improve awareness of other adolescent health-related services, in particular Adolescent Friendly Health Clinics (AFHCs)/helplines. In addition, during Adolescent Health Day the counselor or the trained MO/ANM will hold group sessions with parents to provide information on topics related to adolescent health the Adolescent Health Day will be organized in every village once every quarter on a convenient day (preferably on a Sunday) following the VHND; in Sabla districts, this day should coincide with the existing Kishori Diwas. AWCs or community spaces may be used as venues for organizing the AHD. During an AHD, The following services will be provided:

- **Information:** IEC (Information Education and communication) and IPC (Interpersonal communication) on nutrition, Sexual Reproductive Health (SRH), mental health, Gender-based violence, NCD, substance misuse
- **Commodities:** Sanitary Napkins, IFA, Albendazole, anti-spasmodic tablets
- Contraceptives services
- Registration, general health checkup, (BMI, anemia, hypertension and diabetes), Referral to AFHCs (for counseling and clinical services).

NATIONAL LEPROSY ERADICATION PROGRAMME (NLEP)

Introduction

The National Leprosy Control Programme (NLCP) has been started since 1955. In 1983 Government of India redesignated into Leprosy Eradication Programme and introduced multidrug theraphy (MDT). The World Health Assembly in May 1991 adopted a resolution for global leprosy elimination as a public health problem by the year 2000. After the declaration of the global elimination, a target was reset for the remaining 15 countries to achieve elimination at the national level by the end of December, 2005. India was one of these countries. The National Health Policy of India 2002 also set the goal of leprosy elimination in India by the end of year 2005. In 12th plan Special action plan for 209 high endemic districts in 16 States/UTs Target to reduce the visible disabilities. In 2017 Sparsh Leprosy Awareness Campaign (SLAC) started for increasing the awareness, addressing high-level of stigma and discrimination—Convening special Grama sabha meeting.

Mission of National Leprosy Eradication Programme

To provide quality leprosy services free of cost to all sections of the population, with easy accessibility, through the integrated healthcare system, including care for disability after cure of the disease

Aims of NLEP

- Decentralization of NLEP to States and Districts.
- Leprosy Services integrated with General Health Care Services.
- Early diagnosis and prompt MDT treatment through routine and special efforts.
- Information, Education and Communication (IEC), also called "Behavioral Change and Communication (BCC) using local and Mass Media for reduction of Social Stigma and Discrimination.
- Renewed emphasis on Disability Prevention and Medical Rehabilitation (DPMR).
- Monitoring and periodic evaluation.
- Inter-sectoral collaboration.

Objectives

- To reduce the prevalence rate to less than 1/10,000 population at subnational and district level.

- To reduce Grade II disability% to < 1 among new cases at national level
- To reduce Grade II disability cases to < 1 case per million population at national level.
- Zero disabilities among new child cases
- Zero stigma and discrimination against persons affected by leprosy.

Program Strategy

- Integrated Leprosy services through General Health Care Services.
- Early diagnosis and prompt MDT treatment of new Leprosy cases through routine and special efforts.
- Carrying out household contact survey for early detection of cases.
- Involvement of Accredited Social Health Activists (ASHAs) in detection and completion of treatment of Leprosy cases on time.
- Strengthening of Disability Prevention and Medical Rehabilitation (DPMR) services.
- Information, Education and Communication (IEC), also called "Behavioral Change and Communication (BCC)" using local and Mass Media for reduction of Social Stigma and Discrimination, so that self reporting of the Leprosy disease to the Primary Health Centers (PHCs) is encouraged.
- Intensive monitoring and supervision at Primary Health Centers (PHCs)/Community Health Centers (CHCs).

Milestones of NLEP

- **1948:** Hind Kusht Nivaran Sangh
- **1955:** National Leprosy Control Programme
- **1970:** Definite cure in form of MDT was identified
- **1982:** WHO—study group recommended use of MDT
- **1983:** National Leprosy Eradication Programme, MDT started
- **1991:** World Health Assembly resolution to eradicate leprosy by 2000 AD
- **1993:** World Bank supports the MDT programme phase -NLEP1
- **1997:** Midterm appraisal of NLEP
- **1998–2004:** Modified Leprosy Elimination Campaign
- **2001–2004:** NLEP Project Phase II
- **2002:** Simplified Information system Introduced
- **2005:** Nationwide Evaluation of Project II
- **2005:** Dec Prevalence Rate of leprosy dropped to 0.95/10000 population, and India achieved elimination status Nationally
- **2005:** After Elimination, NLEP vertically run program services integrated with General Health Care System under newly launched National Rural Health Mission
- **2007:** Disability Prevention and Medical Rehabilitation Guidelines introduced for preventing disabilities at primary, secondary, and tertiary level
- **2007–2012:** XI Five Year Plan advocated inclusion of Persons Affected with leprosy in all decision making exercise
- **2012:** XII Five Year Plan adopted the Special Leprosy Action Plan for 209 High endemic districts in 16 States/UTs
- **2014:** Independent Evaluation of NLEP by World Health Organisation
- **2014:** Upgraded Simplified Information system implementation
- **2016:** Rights of Persons with Disabilities Act, 2016
- 2017–2019

  New Initiatives:
  - Active Case Detections Campaigns (14 days) in high endemic districts
  - Focused Leprosy Campaign (FLC) in low endemic districts
  - ASHA Based Surveillance for Leprosy Suspects (ABSULS)
  - Grade II Disability Epidemiological Investigation
  - Implementation of Post Exposure Prophylaxis (administration of Single Dose of Rifampicin)
  - Sparsh Leprosy Awareness Campaigns
  - Introduction of NIKUSTH - A real time leprosy reporting software across India
- **2019:**
  - External Evaluation of NLEP by World Health Organisation
  - Convergence of leprosy screening with Comprehensive Primary Health Care programme of Ayushman Bharat, to screen 30+ years population at HWCs
  - Convergence of leprosy screening with Rashtriya Bal Swasthya Karyakram (RBSK) to screen children (0–18 years) at Anganwadi Centers and Govt. schools
- **2020:**
  - Active Case Detection and Regular Surveillance (ACD and RS) guidelines rolledout.
  - Convergence of NLEP with Rashtriya Kishore Swasthya Karyakaram (RKSK) for counseling the children of teen age group (13–19 yrs) about leprosy at Adolescent Friendly Clinics

Activities under NLEP

- **Diagnosis and treatment of leprosy:** Free of cost Services for diagnosis and treatment (multidrug therapy) are provided by all public health care facilities like primary Health Centers, govt. dispensaries, CHC, DH and Medical colleges throughout the country. Difficult to diagnose, complicated cases, reaction cases and the cases requiring reconstructive surgery are referred to district hospital for further management. All drugs, diagnostics and surgical/nonsurgical interventions are provided free of cost to all patients of leprosy across the board.
- **Capacity building:** Training of general health staff like Medical Officer, health workers, health supervisors, laboratory technicians and ASHAs are conducted every year to develop adequate skills for diagnosis and management of leprosy cases.
- **IEC and counseling:** Intensive IEC activities are conducted to generate awareness which will help in reduction of stigma and discrimination associated with persons

affected with leprosy. These activities are carried through mass media, outdoor media, rural media and advocacy meetings. Major focus is also given on inter personnel communication.

- **Disability prevention and medical rehabilitation:** For prevention and management of disability, dressing material, supportive medicines and micro-cellular rubber (MCR) footwear are provided to leprosy patients. The patients are also empowered with trainings in self-care procedure for preventing aggravating disability to the insensitive hands/feet. Emphasis is also being placed on correction of permanent disability through reconstructive surgeries.
- **Supervision and monitoring:** Program is being monitored at different level through analysis of monthly progress reports, through field visits by the supervisory officers and program review meetings held at central, state and district level. For better epidemiological analysis of the disease situation, emphasis is put on assessment of New Case Detection and Treatment Completion Rate and proportion of grade II disability among new cases.
- **NGO services under SET scheme:** NGOs are getting grants from Govt. of India under Survey, Education and Treatment (SET) scheme. Various activities undertaken by the NGOs are IEC, Prevention of Impairments and Deformities, Case Detection and MDT Delivery. From Financial year 2006 onwards, Grant-in-aid is being disbursed to NGOs through State Health Societies.
- **Prioritization of the Districts to reduce the leprosy Burden:** The World Health Organization (WHO) facilitated an independent evaluation of NLEP from 1 to 14 November 2019. Districts were prioritized based on the leprosy burden. Annual new cases detected, ANCDR, G2D rate, prevalence rate during 2008–2018 were taken into consideration for categorization of the districts. Institutional framework and Program management for National Leprosy Eradication Programme (NLEP) at different level are described in **Table 10.13**.

Job Responsibilities of Health Personnel

- **Medical officer:**
  - Planning of NLEP activities
  - Case confirmation, treatment, lepra reaction Mx, referral of complications
  - On job training to PHC staff
  - Supervision and monitoring
  - Review of activities and feedback to DNT
- **ANMI MPHW/VHN:**
  - Suspect identification
  - Availability of MDT and providing MDT, compliance
  - Record Maintenance and Report Preparation
  - IEC activities
  - DPMR activities
  - Supervision of ASHA/AWW I Volunteer
  - Assist MO
- **ASHA/AWW**
  - Suspect identification and referral to PHC

Table 10.13: Institutional framework and program management (NLEP).

Level	Framework
Center level	• Ministry of Health and Family Welfare • DGHS • Central Leprosy Division - DDG (L) • Training Institutes - CLTRI, RLTRIs
State level	• State Health Society • State Leprosy Officer/State Leprosy Consultant
District level	• District Health Society • District Leprosy Officer/Deputy Director • District Nucleus Team (DNT)
Block level	• Block PHC/CHC - Rogi Kalyan samiti/PRI • Block Medical Officer/incharge MO CHC
PHC Level	• PHC-Rogi Kalyan samiti/Panchayati Raj Institution • Medical Officer
Subcenter level/ Health and Wellness Center	• Grama Panchayat • Male/Female Health Worker
Village level	• Village Health and Sanitation Committee • ASHA/AWW

  - Timely completion of treatment
  - Counseling and IEC
  - Contact Screening, support for active case detection campaigns.

Achievements as on 2021–22

A few major achievements under NLEP are as follows:

- Prevalence rate has decreased to 0.41per 10,000 population in 2020–21.
- Annual New Cases Detection Rate has declined to 4.58/100000 in 2020–21
- Child cases percentage among new cases detected has reduced to 5.76% in 2020–21.
- Percentage of Grade 2 Disability among new cases detected has decreased to 2.48% in 2020- 21.
- The G2D amongst new cases per million population is decreased to 1.14 per million population in 2020–21.

NB: Regarding management of leprosy the details has been given in chapter communicable and noncommunicable disease.

Sparsh Leprosy Awareness Campaign, 2017

Leprosy is a chronic infectious disease identified back thousands of years that has stigmatised the people affected since ancient times until now. This disability caused by this crippling disease does not only affect lives of a person affected with leprosy but also whole family of that person. Hence, in order to address the issue of high-level of stigma attached to leprosy and to increase awareness about various aspects of leprosy, a nationwide campaign called "Sparsh leprosy awareness campaign" was introduced under NLEP on 30th January 2017 on 'Anti-Leprosy day', 2017.

In order to provide the necessary stimulus to the activity a central level workshop was organized wherein prototypes of message of District Magistrate, appeal of Gram Sabha Pramukh and pledge of Gram Sabha Members were prepared on theme of early case detection and stop discrimination. In addition the guidelines of Sparsh Leprosy Awareness Campaign, 2017 and a 'Sparsh package' encompassing IEC materials, i.e., video spots, audio spots and posters etc., were prepared. All the prototypes, guidelines and 'Sparsh package' were shared with all States with instruction to distribute to all Gram Sabhas before 30th January, 2017.

Further, for better organization and management special committees at various administrative levels, i.e., State, District and Block level were formed.

The major activities undertaken in Gram Sabhas were:

- Message from District Magistrate on Leprosy disease (read by DM if available or by Gram Sabha Pramukh)
- Appeal from Gram Sabha Pramukh to all members for reduction of discrimination against persons affected with leprosy
- Undertaking of a pledge by all Gram Sabha members to not to discriminate with persons affected with leprosy,
- Felicitation of person affected with leprosy (if available) by Gram Sabha Pramukh and
- Question answer session using Frequently Asked Questions provided.

The event was facilitated by respective multi-purpose worker (MPWs), patwari, gramsevaik, school teacher, ASHA etc., at village level under supervision of Medical Officer of Primary Health Center (PHC). Using prototypes the activities were conducted in approximately 3.6 lakh villages as per the reports submitted by States.

In addition to the execution of Gram Sabha meetings as per the suggested activities mentioned above, States celebrated the SLAC, 2017 fortnight using innovative IEC activities to spread awareness regarding disease in the community.

NATIONAL PROGRAMME FOR CONTROL OF BLINDNESS

Prevention and control of blindness is one of the important health care programs in India. The National Health Policy document of the Government of India, 1983, stipulates that 'One of the basic human rights is the right to see. We have to ensure that no citizen goes blind needlessly, or being blind, does not remain so, if by reasonable deployment of skill and resources, his eye sight can be prevented from deterioration or if already lost, can be restored. National Programme for Control of Blindness (NPCB) was launched in the year 1976 as a 100% centrally sponsored vertical public health program. Two major surveys conducted to find out prevalence of blindness in the country. The first survey was done by the ICMR on a national sample in 1974 and arrived at the figure of 1. 38% prevalence rate for the economically blind. In the second survey conducted jointly by the NPCB and WHO in 1986–1989, the prevalence rate increased to 1.49%. The prevalence of blindness in other countries in the South East Asian region of WHO was around 0.8%. Rapid Survey on Avoidable Blindness conducted under NPCB during 2006–07 showed reduction in the prevalence of blindness from 1.1% (2001–02) to 1% (2006–07). Various activities/initiatives undertaken during the Five Year Plans under NPCB are targeted towards achieving the goal of reducing the prevalence of blindness to 0.3% by the year 2020. The Trachoma Control Programme started in 1963 was merged under NPCB in 1976. Nomenclature of the program was changed from National Programme for Control of Blindness to National Programme for Control of Blindness and Visual Impairment (NPCBVI) in 2017.

Evolution of the Program

National Programme for Control of Blindness was launched in the year 1976 as a 100% centrally sponsored vertical public health program. Major landmarks in the history of blindness control activities in India in chronological order are as follows:

- National Trachoma Control Programme was launched in 1963 to prevent and control trachoma
- A survey was undertaken by the ICMR in 1971–1974 to identify the main causes of blindness, which revealed that prevalence of blindness was 1.38% and cataract was the leading cause of blindness. Based on this survey, the GOI appointed a committee to formulate strategies to control blindness. A comprehensive NPCB was launched in 1976 with the goal of reducing prevalence of blindness to 0.3% by 2000 AD.
- DANIDA agreed to assist NPCB since 1978 (Phase I).
- National survey was undertaken by the GOI/WHO in 1986–1989. The survey revealed increase in prevalence from 1.38% to 1.49%. Cataract accounted for 80% of blindness. Decrease in blindness due to trachoma and malnutrition was noticeable.
- DANIDA assistance (Phase II) was launched in 1989. Midterm evaluation highlighted lack of management unit at the district level and lack of equipment as the main reasons for limited success.
- Pilot project in 5 districts implemented in 1991–1992 to assess effectiveness of District Blindness Control Societies.
- World Bank assisted Cataract Blindness Control Project was launched in 1994–1995 to control cataract blindness in seven states in the country. A Government of India project in Jammu and Kashmir and a DANIDA project in Karnataka were also launched in 1994–1995.
- Revised pattern of assistance under NPCB was launched to make it more effective in 1995 and again in 1997.
- DANIDA phase III project was launched in 1988.
- Midterm evaluation of World Bank project in 1997–98 indicated marginal (10–15%) fall in prevalence and lack of follow-up services, increase in proportion of IOL implants and superior outcomes after IOL surgery.
- Mega eye camps in underserved areas launched in the 50th year of India's Independence in 1997–1998.
- Expansion of the World Bank project components to the entire country was started in 1999. Presently, the goal set to be achieved under the NPCB is to reduce the prevalence of blindness from 1.49% to 0.3%. Nomenclature of the

program was changed from National Programme for Control of Blindness to National Programme for Control of Blindness and Visual Impairment (NPCBVI) in 2017.

Main objectives of the program in the 12th Five Year Plan period are:

1. To continue three ongoing signature activities, performance of 66 lacs cataract operations per year school eye screening and distribution of 9 lacs spectacles per year to school children suffering refractive errors; and collection of 50,000 donated per year for keratoplasty.
2. To reduce the backlog of avoidable blindness their identification and treatment of curable blind at primary secondary and tertiary levels, based on assessment of the overall burden of visual impairment in the country.
3. Develop and strengthen the strategy of NPCB for "Eye Health for All" and prevention of visual impairment. Through provision of comprehensive universal eye-care services and quality service delivery;
4. Strengthening and upgradation of Regional Institutes of Ophthalmology (RIOS) to become center of excellence in various subspecialties of ophthalmology and also other partners like Medical Colleges, District Hospitals, Subdistrict Hospitals. Vision Centers, NGO Eye Hospitals;
5. Strengthening the existing infrastructure facilities and developing additional human resources for providing high quality comprehensive eye care in all districts of the country:
6. To enhance community awareness on eye care and lay stress on preventive measures
7. Increase and expand research for prevention of blindness and visual impairment; and
8. To secure participation of voluntary organizations/private practitioners in delivering eye care.

Salient features/strategies adopted to achieve the objectives are:

1. Continued emphasis on free cataract surgery through the health care delivery system as well as by the involvement of NGO sector and private practitioners.
2. Emphasis on the comprehensive eye care programmes by covering diseases other than cataract, like diabetic retinopathy, glaucoma, corneal transplantation, vitreoretinal surgery, treatment of childhood blindness etc. These emerging diseases need immediate attention to eliminate avoidable blindness from the country.
3. Reduction in the backlog of blind persons by active screening of population above 50 years age, organizing screening eye camps and transporting operable cases to fixed eye care facilities.
4. Refractive error comprises a major part of avoidable blindness. Screening of children for identification and treatment of refractive errors and provision of free glasses to those affected and belonging to poor socio-economic strata.
5. Coverage of underserved area for eye care services through public-private partnership.
6. Capacity building of health personnel for improving their knowledge and skill in delivery of high quality eye services.
7. Information Education Communication (IEC) activities for creating awareness on eye-care within the community.
8. Regional Institutes of Ophthalmology and Medical Colleges of the states to be strengthened in a phased manner with latest equipments and training of manpower so that they can be upgraded as Centers of Excellence in the regions.
9. The district hospitals to be strengthened by upgrading infrastructure, equipment and providing adequate manpower like ophthalmologists and PMOAs on contractual basis and provide earmarked funds for basic medicines and drugs.
10. Continuing emphasis on primary healthcare (eye care) by establishing vision centers in all PHCs with a PMOA in position.
11. Multipurpose District Mobile Ophthalmic Units for better coverage.

Organizational Structure

At the national level, a National Programme Management cell has been established in the Directorate General of Health Services (DGHS), Department of Health in the Ministry of Health and Family Welfare. It has two wings viz: the technical wing in the DGHS which deals with the ophthalmic section and the administrative wing that deals with blindness control section. The Technical Wing is solely dealing with the NPCB. Senior officers of the administrative wing have blindness control as one of the functions. At the state level, each state has an ophthalmology cell in respective Directorate of Health Services devoted to the program implementation and monitoring. Gradually the process of setting up of a State Blindness Control Society in each state has been initiated. At the district level, District Blindness Control Society (DBCS) has been established in almost all the districts. It is the DBCS, which is responsible for planning and coordinating different agencies, and monitoring implementation of the program by pooling in all the resources available. Recurring funds are directly provided to the DBCS by the Government of India National Bodies for NPCB.

There are three bodies that have been constituted for monitoring, coordinating and development of the program.

1. National Blindness Control Board, chaired by the Union Secretary (Health) reviews the progress made under the program. Members include State Health Secretaries, Representatives of NGOs and DGHS.
2. National Programme Coordination Committee, chaired by Additional Secretary (Health) is the coordinating body represented by various government and nongovernment organizations involved in prevention and control of blindness in India. The committee also includes international funding agencies and representatives of professional organizations.
3. National Technical Advisory Committee, chaired by the Director General of Health Services with members consisting of leading ophthalmologists from government as well as from nongovernment sectors.

Major Activities

Disease Control

This part of the NPCB covers controlling of cataract, refractive errors in school going children and corneal blindness are the main target diseases for control. Activities undertaken for each of the target diseases are as follows:

Cataract

Identification of bilaterally blind persons, preparation of blind registers, screening for operable cataracts, performing surgery and follow-up services. The surgical services are available in the government, NGO, private fixed facilities (hospitals/institutions) as well as in eye camps. These services are free of cost for those who can not afford the costs.

Refractive Errors

Training of teachers in primary screening, secondary screening by ophthalmic assistant/teachers and provision of glasses for those who cannot afford.

Corneal Blindness

Prevention of VAD (supplementation integrated with immunization program), eye donation and corneal transplantation.

Other Diseases

Eye care facilities available in various sectors for management of glaucoma, infections, posterior segment disorders.

Achievements of NPCB

Recent surveys have confirmed higher success rates following cataract surgery with Intraocular lens implantation as compared to conventional surgery. Follow-up of operated cases was an important factor in those cases that had poor visual outcome following cataract surgery.

- There has been a significant increase in proportion of cataract surgeries with IOL implantation from <9% in 1994 to 93% in 2006–2007.
- During the year 2009–2010, 92.5% cataract surgeries were performed against the target set by Government of India, out of which 95% were with IOL implantation.
- 307 dedicated eye operation theaters and eye wards built in district level hospitals.
- Supply of ophthalmic equipment for diagnosis and treatment of common eye disorders.
- More than 2000 eye surgeons trained in IOL surgery and other super specialties.
- During the years 2009–2010, 109189 teachers were trained, 30862970 school children were screened, 1012918 children were detected with refractive errors, and 505398 children were provided free glass under school eye screening program.

Activities of National Programme for Control of Blindness and Visual Impairment (NPCBVI)

- Free Cataract Surgery at district hospitals and identified NGO eye hospitals/Pvt. Practitioners
- Eye Screening and Distribution of Free spectacles to School children and elderly
- Collection of Donated Eyes through network of eye banks and eye donation centers
- Diagnosis and Treatment of other eye diseases (glaucoma, childhood blindness, squint etc.) at District Hospitals and identified NGO eye hospitals
- Procurement and maintenance of Ophthalmic equipments at subdistrict/district Hospitals and Vision Centers (in public sector only from FY 2018–19).
- Training of Paramedical Ophthalmic Assistants posted at PHC/District Hospitals
- Strengthening of eye banks (in public sector only from FY 2018–19).
- IEC activities on promoting eye health, preventing eye diseases and increasing utilization of services.
- Provision of superspecialty and referral eye care services for diabetic retinopathy, Glaucoma, childhood blindness, retinopathy of prematurity and Keratoplasty (corneal transplantation) etc. at Regional Institutes of Ophthalmology and Medical Colleges.
- Construction of modular Eye OTs at RIOs for providing modern and tertiary level eye care services
- Training of eye surgeons in various specialties of Ophthalmology for skill development
- Provision for supply of MK Medium to Govt. Eye Banks through Dr RP Center, AIIMS, New Delhi for preservation of donated corneas and improve corneal utility rate.
- Conducting Surveys (blindness and visual Impairment Survey, Trachoma Survey, etc.) through identified institutions. The detail activities of program are given in table below:

Total No. of Cataract Surgery

Year	*Target*	*No. of cataract operations performed*	*% Achievement*
2016–17	66,00,000	64,81,435	98
2017–18	66,00,000	64,41,487	97
2018–19	66,00,000	66,85,476	101
2019–20	67,00,000	16,46,921	

Distribution of Free Spectacles Under School Eye Screening

	No. of free spectacles provided to school children suffering from refractive errors		*% Achievement*
Year	*Target*	*Achievement*	
2016–17	9,00,000	7,57,906	84
2017–18	9,00,000	7,98,411	88
2018–19	9,00,000	8,79,488	97
2019–20	10,00,000	82,590	

Collection of Donated Eyes for Corneal Transplantation

Year	No. of donated eyes collected		% Achievement
	Target	Achievement	
2016–17	50,000	65,135	130
2017–18	50,000	71,709	143
2018–19	55,000	68,007	123
2019–20	70,000	19,950	

Treatment/Management of Other Eye Diseases

Diabetic retinopathy, glaucoma, childhood blindness, keratoplasty, etc.

Year	Target	No. of cases treated	%
2016–17	72,000	4,04677	562
2017–18	72,000	5,48,448	761
2018–19	2,00,000	6,14,433	307
2019–20	6,00,000	1,88,507	31.42

Training of Eye Surgeons

Year	No. of eye surgeons trained in various specialties of ophthalmology
2016–17	121
2017–18	125
2018–19	129
2019–20	40

NATIONAL TUBERCULOSIS ELIMINATION PROGRAMME

Tuberculosis (TB) is an infectious disease caused by Mycobacterium tuberculosis. Tuberculosis commonly affects the lungs, but can also affect other parts of the body. It spreads from person to person through the air, when people who are infected with TB infection cough, sneeze or otherwise transmit respiratory fluids through the air.

About one-quarter of the world's population is estimated to be infected by TB bacteria but out of these only 5–15% of people will fall ill with active TB disease. The rest have TB infection with no illness and cannot transmit the disease. According to WHO, an estimated 9.9 million people fell ill with TB and 1.5 million people died globally in 2020, despite being a preventable and curable disease.

India notified more than 2.4 million TB cases in 2019, it continues to have the largest share of the global TB burden. India's National TB Elimination Programme (earlier known as Revised National TB Control Programme) is strengthened to meet the goal of ending the TB epidemic by 2025 from the country, five years ahead of the Sustainable Development Goals (SDG) for 2030. The National Strategic Plan for Tuberculosis Elimination 2017–2025 was developed to achieve the goal.

Tuberculosis (TB) control activities are implemented in the country for more than 50 years. The National TB Programme (NTP) was launched by the Government of India in 1962 in the form of District TB Center model involved with BCG vaccination and TB treatment. In 1978, BCG vaccination was shifted under the Expanded Programme on Immunization. A joint review of NTP was done by Government of India, World Health Organization (WHO) and the Swedish International Development Agency (SIDA) in 1992 and some shortcomings were found in the program such as managerial weaknesses, inadequate funding, over-reliance on X-ray, nonstandard treatment regimens, low rates of treatment completion, and lack of systematic information on treatment outcomes.

Around the same time in 1993, the WHO declared TB as a global emergency, devised the directly observed treatment—short course (DOTS), and recommended to follow it by all countries. After failure of NTCP, RNTCP was launched in 1997 based on WHO DOTS strategy recommended, and expanded across the country in a phased manner. The Government of India revitalized NTP as Revised National TB Control Programme (RNTCP) and DOTS was officially launched as the RNTCP strategy in 1997 and by the end of 2005 the entire country was covered under the program. The twin objectives of the program were:

- To achieve and maintain accuracy of at least 85% among new sputum positive (NSP) patients, and
- To achieve and maintain case detection of at least 70% of the estimated NSP cases in the community.

The Strategy of RNTCP are:

- Augmentation of organizational support at the central and state level for meaningful coordination
- Increase in budgetary outlay
- Use of sputum microscopy as a primary method of diagnosis among self-reporting patients
- Standardized treatment regimens
- Augmentation of the peripheral level supervision through the creation of a subdistrict supervisory unit
- Ensuring a regular uninterrupted supply of drugs up to the most peripheral level
- Emphasis on training, IEC, operational research and NGO involvement in the program.

The core element of RNTCP in Phase I (1997–2006) was to ensure high quality DOTS expansion in the country, addressing the five primary components of the DOTS strategy like Political and Administrative Commitment, Good Quality Diagnosis, Good Quality Drugs, Supervised Treatment to Ensure the Right Treatment, Given in the Right Way and Systematic Monitoring and Accountability.

During 2006–11, in its second phase RNTCP improved the quality and reach of services, and worked to reach global case detection and cure targets.

The RNTCP Phase II of the World Bank project has been approved by the CCEA for the period October 2006 to September 2011 for a total outlay of USD 256.9 million which includes credit from World Bank of USD 170 million and commodity assistance of anti-TB drugs from DFID through WHO for USD 62.5 million, and the balance by GOI. New financial norms in respect of certain expenditure heads have been approved by Cabinet Committee on Economic Affairs which have been implemented with effect from April 01, 2009.

The Global Fund has supported by grants. DOTS expansion in India under different rounds. DOTS expansion in the 3 States of Chhattisgarh, Jharkhand, and Uttarakhand (56 million populations) was supported by grants for USD 8.78 million under Round 1 of GFATM from April 2003–September 2006. In addition, the Round 2 of GFATM supported DOTS expansion in 56 districts of Bihar and Uttar Pradesh with a population of 110 million for USD 29.10 million (April 2004 to March 2009). Round 4 of GFATM is supporting strengthening of RNTCP implementation in the states of Andhra Pradesh and Odisha with effect from November 05 and January 2006 respectively for USD 26.63 million till March 2010. The RNTCP phase II is envisaged to consolidate the achievements of phase I, maintain its progressive trend and effect further improvement in its functioning and achieve TB related MDG goals while retaining DOTS as its core strategy.

All components of new Stop TB strategy are incorporated in the second phase of RNTCP. These are:

- *Pursue quality DOTS expansion and enhancement*, by improving the case finding are cure through an effective patient-centered approach to reach all patients, especially the poor.
- *Address TB-HIV, MDR-TB and other challenges*, by scaling up TB-HIV joint activities, DOTS Plus, and other relevant approaches.
- *Contribute to health system strengthening*, by collaborating with other health programs and general services.
- *Involve all health care providers*, public, nongovernmental and private, by scaling up approaches based on a public-private mix (PPM), to ensure adherence to the International Standards of TB care.
- *Engage people with TB, and affected communities* to demand, and contribute to effective care. This will involve scaling-up of community TB care; creating demand through context-specific advocacy, communication and social mobilization.
- *Enable and promote research* for the development of new drugs, diagnostic and vaccines. Operational research will also be needed to improve program performance.

These targets were achieved by 2007–08. Despite these achievements, undiagnosed and mistreated cases continued to drive the TB epidemic. TB was the leading cause of illness and death among persons living with HIV/AIDS and large number of multidrug resistant TB (MDR-TB) cases were reported every year. During this period for achievement of the long-term vision of a "TB free India", National Strategic Plan for Tuberculosis Control 2012–2017 was documented with the goal of 'universal access to quality TB diagnosis and treatment for all TB patients in the community'.

Significant interventions and initiatives were taken during NSP 2012–2017 in terms of mandatory notification of all TB cases, integration of the programme with the general health services (National Health Mission), expansion of diagnostics services, programmatic management of drug resistant TB (PMDT) service expansion, single window service for TB-HIV cases, national drug resistance surveillance and revision of partnership guidelines.

However, to eliminate TB in India by 2025, five years ahead of the global target, a framework to guide the activities of all stakeholders including the national and state governments, development partners, civil society organizations, international agencies, research institutions, private sector, and many others whose work is relevant to TB elimination in India is ***formulated by RNTCP*** as National Strategic Plan for Tuberculosis Elimination 2017–2025.

The program is accountable for the outcome of every patient treated. This is done using standard recording and reporting system, and the technique of 'cohort analysis'. The cure rate and other key indicators are monitored at every level of the health system, and if any area is not meeting expectations, supervision is intensified. The RNTCP shifts the responsibility for cure from the patient to the health system.

Sputum microscopy continues to be the primary tool for detection of infectious cases. Apart from sputum microscopy, RNTCP also uses standardized diagnostic algorithms to diagnose and treat all forms of TB wherein X-ray plays a supporting role. However in line with the stop TB strategy, the program is exploring all possible avenues with newer and innovative technologies for early detection of TB including use of LED fluorescent microscopes, liquid culture and line probe assay for diagnosis drug resistant TB, etc. Sufficient anti-TB drugs in patient wise boxes are made available at all the appropriate levels (Peripheral Health Institution).

NATIONAL STRATEGIC PLAN FOR TUBERCULOSIS ELIMINATION 2017–2025

RNTCP has released a 'National strategic plan for tuberculosis 2017–2025' (NSP) for the control and elimination of TB in India by 2025.

- **Vision:** TB-Free India with zero deaths, disease and poverty due to tuberculosis
- **Goal:** To achieve a rapid decline in burden of TB, morbidity and mortality while working towards elimination of TB in India by 2025.

The results framework impact, outcome indicators and targets for different years are described in **Table 10.14**.

Table 10.14: Results Framework (Impact and Outcome Indicators and Targets).

Impact indicators	*2015*	*2020*	*2023*	*2025*
To reduce estimated TB incidence rate (per 100,000)	217 (112–355)	142 (76–255)	77 (49–185)	44 (36–158)
To reduce estimated TB prevalence rate (per 100,000)	320 (280–380)	170 (159–217)	90 (81–125)	65 (56–93)
To reduce estimated mortality due to TB (per 100,000)	32 (29–35)	15 (13–16)	6 (5–7)	3 (3–4)
To achieve zero catastrophic cost for affected families due to TB	35%	0%	0%	0%

The results framework below highlights the core impact, outcome indicators and targets of the NSP that highlight the four thrust areas that include private sector engagement, plugging the leak from the TB care cascade, active TB case-finding among key populations (socially vulnerable and clinically high-risk) and specific protection for prevention from development of active TB in high-risk groups.

According to the NSP TB elimination have been integrated into the four strategic pillars of "Detect - Treat - Prevent - Build" (DTPB).

Detect

The first objective of NSP is to find all drug sensitive TB cases (DS-TB) and drug resistant TB cases (DRTB) with an emphasis on reaching TB patients seeking care from private providers and undiagnosed TB cases in high-risk populations (such as prisoners, migrant workers, people living with HIV/AIDS, contacts etc.). Early diagnosis and treatment of TB cases in the community is an important step in TB elimination, which will help in decreasing the risk of transmission of disease to others, poor health outcomes, and social and economic hardships of the patient and their family.

Notification of TB cases: Notification of all TB patients from all health care providers is made mandatory by Ministry of Health and Family Welfare, Government of India since 2012. All health care providers (clinical establishments run or managed by government (including local authorities), private, or NGO sectors, and/or individual practitioners) should notify every TB case to local health authorities (district health officer, chief medical officer of a district, and municipal health officer of a municipal corporation/ municipality) every month. With its amendment in 2015, all laboratories are also included to notify TB cases.

Till now, only medical practitioners, hospitals and laboratories were notifying TB patients to government health system, now according to 'Mandatory TB notification Gazette for private practitioners, chemists and public health staff' March 2018, all chemists will also inform about TB patients for whom they have dispensed the TB drugs. TB patients themselves are also encouraged to notify themselves. Every TB patient will be attempted to reach out by the local public health authority, namely, District Health Officer or Chief Medical Officer of a District and Municipal Health Officer of urban local bodies, so that the incentives and support to patients, families and communities can be properly extended.

Smear examination most widely used and acceptable testing tool resumptive TB cases referred to designated Microscopy Center (DMC) two samples within a day/in 2 consecutive days, one sample on the spot, under supervision, second sample at home (Morning sample) should be at least 2 mL and mucopurulent if transporting sample, should reach DMC and be examined as early as possible (within 2 days).

NIKSHAY: To facilitate TB notification, RNTCP has developed a case-based web-based TB surveillance system called "NIKSHAY" (https://nikshay.gov.in) for both government and private health care facilities. Future enhancements under NIKSHAY are for patients support, logistics management, direct data transfers, adherence support and to support interface agencies which are supporting program to expand the reach.

Public private partnership: For promotion of public-private mix (PPM) in TB prevention and care, private providers are provided incentives for TB case notification, and for ensuring treatment adherence and treatment completion. The incentives are provided through direct beneficiary transfer.

The incentives to the Private Sector TB Care Provider are as follows:

- ₹250/- on notification of a TB case diagnosed as per Standards for TB Care in India (STCI)
- ₹250/- on completion of every month of treatment
- ₹500/- on completion of entire course of TB treatment
- ₹2750/for notification and management of a drug-sensitive patient over 6–9 months as per STCI
- ₹6750/-for notification and correct management of a drug-resistant case over 24 months as per STCI.

Free drugs and diagnostic tests to TB patients in private sector: Free drugs and diagnostic tests are provided to TB patients seeking treatment from private health sector. There are two approaches for ensuring access to free drugs and diagnostic tests to TB patients in private sector, first is access to program—provided drugs and diagnostics through attractive linkages; and second is reimbursement of market-available drugs and diagnostics.

Significant cost reduction of select diagnostics is achieved by 'Initiative for Promoting Affordable and Quality TB Tests' (IPAQT). 131 private sector labs networked to provide four quality tests for TB at or below the 'ceiling prices.

For TB diagnosis more than 14,000 designated microscopy centers spread across the country. Cartridge Based Nucleic Acid Amplification Tests (CBNAAT)/Line Probe Assay (LPA) have been established at district levels for decentralized molecular testing for drug resistant TB. Reference laboratories have been established at state and national levels which provide culture and dug sensitivity test (DST) services as well as molecular diagnosis.

Treat

Next step under the program is initiation and sustaining all TB patients on appropriate anti-TB treatment wherever they seek care, with patient friendly system and social support. Provision of free TB drugs in the form of daily fixed dose combinations (FDCs) for all TB cases is advised with the support of directly observed treatment (DOT).

(DOT is a specific strategy, to improve adherence by any person observing the patient taking medications in real time. The treatment observer does not need to be a health-care worker, but could be a friend, a relative or a lay person who works as a treatment supervisor or supporter. If treatment is incomplete, patients may not be cured and drug resistance may develop).

Strategies

- **Initiation of appropriate treatment for all diagnosed TB patients.**
  - Provision of daily regimen for all TB patients
  - Introduction of shorter regimen for MDR TB
  - Incorporation of new treatment strategies with newer drugs
  - Effective strategy to ensure Standards for TB Care in India (STCI) for patients treated by private providers
- **Implementation of TB treatment services in health facilities and communities.**
  - Decentralization of treatment services through ICT support.
  - Promote appropriate treatment adherence mechanism including provision of mobility support to workers, patient enablers and insurance to TB patients, social support systems, nutrition support, ICT mechanisms, pharmacovigilance, etc.
  - Extend patient support services for patients in private sector which are the same as for patients in the public sector mentioned above.
  - Roll out of DST guided ITR in a phased manner for DRTB.
- **Regular and long-term follow-up and rehabilitation of all treated TB patients.**

Activities for treatment:

- **Treatment of patients in the private sector:** Once the patient is notified the responsibility of these will also be on the public sector to provide patient support that will ensure successful completion of treatment. This will include patient friendly adherence support, screening for co- morbidities and drug resistance. Mechanisms will be developed to ensure treatment regimens as per the STCI and quality assured drugs in the private sector. The mechanisms to ensure treatment regimens as per the STCI will include:
  - Effective use of Schedule 1 provisions
  - Use of reimbursement mechanisms
- **Treatment of DSTB:** The priorities of the current plan include change of regimen for DSTB using daily Fixed-dose combinations(FDC) as per patient's weight band with augmented continuation phase and intensified treatment support systems using ICT. This will be scaled up across India by the end of 2017 and also extended to the private sector in a phased manner over the next 5 years.
- **Treating drug resistant TB:** RNTCP will embark upon addressing all forms of drug resistant TB. The thrust areas in the treatment for DR-TB over the NSP period will include the following.
  - *Management of H Monopoly resistance:* H monopoly resistance is known to be around thrice as prevalent as RR-TB. It has been observed from programmatic data that nearly half of such patients treated with standard first line treatment failed and further half of them amplified to MDR-TB. Thus, a specific 9-12 month treatment regimen to manage H mono- poly resistance with available first line drugs substantiated with a fluoroquinolone and a second line injectable. This regimen will be scaled up across the country by end of 2017.
  - *Shorter MDR-TB regimen:* Since inception of PMDT services, RNTCP has witnessed a treatment success rate of just under 50% with the standard 24–27 months regimen. In 2016, WHO endorsed and recommended a shorter MDR-TB regimen for 9–11 months duration based on growing evidences of its effectiveness to improve treatment success particularly in RR-TB patients with additional resistance to fluoroquinolones and second line injectable. WHO also recommends prompt triaging of RR-TB patients with a simultaneously endorsed second line–line probe assay (SL-LPA) test to rapidly separate patients susceptible to fluoroquinolone and second-line injectables. Shorter MDR-TB regimen will be scaled up across the country by end of 2017 for all RR-TB patients.
  - *Newer drugs containing regimen:* In 2016, RNTCP introduced Bedaquiline with an optimized background regimen for management of RR-TB patients with additional resistance to fluoroquinolones and or second line injectables. Based on the early experiences of treating ~300 patients with Bedaquiline containing regimen, RNTCP will expand the access to Bedaquiline across India by the end of 2017. Simultaneously, RNTCP will also introduce another new drug Delamanid within 2017 after conditional approval from DCGI and undertake research with support of ICMR to evaluate the use of these newer drugs in combination therapy to reduce the duration of DR TB regimen to 4–6 months.
  - *DST Guided DR-TB Regimen:* RR-TB patients with additional resistance to fluoroquinolones and second-line injectable with or without resistance to any other first or second line drugs, but either not eligible or unfit or not consenting for newer drugs will be managed by appropriate regimen designed based on the DST results. This approach will also be scaled up along with Bedaquiline expansion across India by end of 2017.
  - *NTM treatment:* Nontuberculous Mycobacterium are environmental opportunistic microorganisms that can cause human disease with signs and symptoms similar to MTB. These organisms can affect the lungs or any other extrapulmonary sites. The diagnostic approach will require a mix of various diagnostic technologies like smear microscopy, rapid molecular tests, conventional culture and species identification while the treatment may vary with species. RNTCP will initiate addressing NTM and will be scaled up across India by end of 2018.
  - *Decentralization of DR-TB treatment:* As RNTCP intends to move to universal DST with CB-NAAT at every district, second line rapid molecular DST, Shorter MDR-TB treatment and DST guided treatment with or without newer drugs, the volumes of patients to be managed at centralized DR-TB centers will delay treatment initiation as well as loss to follow up. To mitigate this anticipated

loss and promote DR-TB treatment initiation within 24–48 hours, RNTCP will decentralize district DR-TB centers to initiate standard H mono-poly or Shorter MDR-TB regimen at every district level that will be established within close proximity of the CB-NAAT site while patients with additional resistance to second line drugs or drug intolerance or seriously ill patients needing regimen modification will be managed at the nodal DR-TB centers.

- *Palliative care and rehabilitation:* Patients with extensive drug resistance in whom an appropriate regimen could not be formed as per the WHO recommended regimen, even with addition of newer drugs and who need care beyond cure will be offered palliative care through the nodal DR-TB centers or at the community level under guidance of nodal DR-TB center. Necessary rehabilitative services including pain relief, surgery, prosthesis, psycho- social support, respiratory physiotherapy etc. Integration with existing network of Pallium India for knowledge and skill transfer to nodal DR-TB center will be explored. Any additional cost required for palliative care and rehabilitation will be covered under existing insurance scheme like NHPS.
- Prevention of relapse and development of DR in presumably pan sensitive first line treatment
- Extension of CP in cavitary and bilaterally/extensive disease
- Nutrition support
- Role of immunomodulators and vaccines both preventive and therapeutic
- PKPD studies
- Exploration of targeted drug delivery
- Exploration of nano- aerosol technology

- **Making care cascade monitoring a management priority:** Activities for ensuring care cascade monitoring for enhanced outcomes include the following:
  - Incorporation of local care cascade information into the district plans
    - Identification of active groups/local structures in villages/taluk/cities for supporting the care cascade.
    - Uptake of available RNTCP partnership options/ partnership guidelines
    - Collaboration with ongoing public health programs in the district for TB advocacy, ICF, care and management and subsequent rehabilitation of TB patients.
    - All stakeholders participating in the care cascade to be notified on Nikshay platform for direct benefit transfers, monitoring and notification of TB patients.
  - Sensitization of state and district officers on the need to budget supplementary activities required for care cascade support. These include administrative and health functionaries at all levels.
  - Regular monitoring to be undertaken through review meetings and onsite checklists at district and state level. Incorporation of "Care Cascade Check" indicators in the program management reports of the state and districts.
  - Trainings of program staff, partners, and volunteers on the reporting formats used for monitoring the care cascade. As the "e-gurukul" 9 system becomes operational, these trainings will be shifted on the electronic interface.
  - Patient feedback of service provided will be taken through the helpline "Call center" support. The information obtained will be shared with individual treatment supporter via "e-Nikshay" for remedial actions, if any.
- **Empower patients** with information, support structures and enablers/honorariums to initiate and sustain treatment
  - Each patient notified under the Nikshay platform starting from diagnosis, need to be enrolled for ICT enabled treatment adherence support and direct benefit transfers as per norms.
  - Patient support services will be linked with individual patient registry in e-Nikshay. Once the patient gets diagnosed by a public or private partner, the patient gets registered in e-Nikshay. Treatment information is further updated regarding the regimens, dosages, adherence mechanism and benefit schemes chosen. Accordingly timely alerts and feedback mechanism will get initiated through e-Nikshay.
  - The facility for ICT enabled benefit transfer through smart cards will be made available from the district TB office. In situations where the patient gets tested and treatment initiated somewhere else, support for patient enablers will get started based on the need for the same.
  - Through the e-Nikshay platform, automated reminders on treatment initiation, interruption and follow up will be sent to treatment provider and patients. In addition, SMS support services will also be made available for awareness, counseling and reminder alerts.
  - An offline app for patient education will be available for free download. Information regarding TB diagnostic and treatment services, enablers, grievance through call center support will be linked on the app through e-Nikshay.
  - Nutritional support/enabler honorarium linked to continuation on treatment through e-Nikshay.
  - Each District has been provided with a counsellor for providing necessary counseling. In addition, the Treatment supervisor and district accountant will monitor the availability of ICT enabled treatment adherence support and fund movement, respectively.
  - Several innovative models of involvement of patient support groups in rural areas has been found to be successful in providing a holistic approach to TB care. Such models will be replicated based on the availability of applicable norms
- **Expanding options for adherence monitoring:** Different choices for ICT based treatment adherence support mechanisms are as below:
  - *Mobile based "Pill-in-Hand" adherence monitoring tool:* In this mechanism, each time a patient takes a

dose of medication, a hidden number appears which is printed on the strip behind the drug. The patient need to send a missed call to a particular contact number with the digits appeared on drug package. This will be documented at a centralized ICT unit. And thus, an electronic treatment record of each patient will be maintained to monitor the treatment adherence.
   - S/he can also be providing the option of where in the patients treatment will be remotely followed up with help of Interactive Voice Response (**IVR**), **SMS** reminders. A call center has been established for care cascade and adherence monitoring
   - Specially designed **electronic pill boxes** or strips with GSM connection and pressure sensor can be used to monitor the pill consumption by tracking the weight of the remaining pills.
   - The treatment provider can use the **Patient Compliance toolkit;** a mobile app for patients to report treatment compliance using video, audio or text message.
   - **Automated pill loading system**, which will load the dosage as per the preprogrammed settings. Medication dispenser: a color-coded reminder system built in the dispenser that will hold drugs.
   - Treating doctors can be provided with **innovatively designed ICT enabled smart cards** to educate them on correct TB prescription methods. Doctors will then give these cards to TB patients, instructing them to SMS the server/customer care center (CCC) the unique code on the card which will register them on the network and also SMS the unique codes printed on their TB drugs as they take them. The CCC will then deliver phone interventions like reminders to take medicines, financial incentives, follow up calls, and TB health tips via SMS and phone balance recharge, mobile APP for scheduled dose reminders and alerts.
   - A Short Messaging service **(SMS) gateway** to be made available by which the patient can report day to day events like pill consumption, minor side effects or his need for help through simple and shortcut SMS templates. The gateway can allow incoming services in pre-recorded or Interactive Voice Response (IVR) mode to inform patients about their test results, as follow up reminders and as periodic counseling messages.
- **Direct Benefits Transfer (via Smart Cards):**
   - Since the very inception of the TB control programme in India, it has tried to adopt a holistic approach to treatment and patient care. Providing treatment enablers in the form of financial incentives and nutritional support can provide for increased adherence and treatment success rates. To meet these twin objectives of adherence and treatment support, the program has launched a "Direct Benefits Transfer (DBT)" scheme to financially aid TB patients.
   - There has been an increase in rural access to banking facilities over the years especially with the recent push through PM "Jan-Dhan Yojana". Subsequently DBT initiatives in social welfare schemes have also shown promise, making it prudent that the program too adopts a similar approach towards treatment enablers.
   - By using an ICT-based benefits transfer system, the program aims to prevent leakages and delays in transfer of benefits with effective targeting so that the benefits only flow to the intended beneficiary. The DBT is implemented via a smart card linked to AADHAR. This provides a tamper-proof storage of user and account identity. It allows for a comprehensive multisectoral multi-scheme benefit to the treatment care receiver. AADHAR linked smart cards will help streamline treatment when the patient comes in contact with the program at different locations. This smart card acts as single unique identifier for patients across private and public sector, insurance and across different central and state social welfare schemes that may become available to the treatment receivers over the course of his treatment. A smart card-based system can be implemented utilizing infrastructure set up for other public healthcare schemes like Rashtriya Swasthya Bima Yojana (RSBY).
   - A smart card provides improved patient identification, needed in the light of treatment incentives like financial support to be provided to the patients. At the same time from a programmatic point, it ensures increased administrative efficiency by providing medical records may be extended by 12–24 weeks in certain forms of TB like skeletal, disseminated TB based on clinical decision of the treating physician.
   - Patients eligible for retreatment should be referred for a rapid molecular test or drug susceptibility testing to determine at least rifampicin resistance, and preferably also isoniazid resistance status. On the basis of the drug susceptibility profile, a standard first-line treatment regimen (2HRZE/4HR) can be repeated if no resistance is documented; and if rifampicin resistance is present, shorter regimen for MDR-TB (multi drug resistant TB) regimen should be prescribed according to WHO's recent drug resistant TB treatment guidelines.

Prevent

With the objective to prevent emergence of TB in susceptible population various measures are indicated as:

- Scale up air-borne infection control measures at health care facilities
- Treatment for latent TB infection in contacts of bacteriologically-confirmed cases.

Address social determinants of TB through intersectoral approach.

- **Air borne infection control measures:** TB infection control is a combination of measures aimed at minimizing the risk of TB transmission within population and hospital and other settings. The foundation of such infection control is:
   - Early diagnosis, and proper management of TB patients.
   - Health education about cough etiquettes and proper disposal of sputum by patient. Cough etiquette means

covering nose and mouth when coughing or sneezing. This can be done with a tissue, or if the person does not have a tissue they can cough or sneeze into their upper sleeve or elbow, but they should not cough or sneeze into their hands. The tissue should then be safely disposed of.
  - Houses should be adequately ventilated.
  - Proper use of air borne infection control measures in health care facilities and other settings
- Contact tracing-Since transmission can occur from index case to the contact any time (before diagnosis or during treatment) all contacts of TB patients must be evaluated. These groups include:
  - All close contacts, especially household contacts
  - In case of pediatric TB patients, reverse contact tracing for search of any active TB case in the household of the child must be undertaken.
  - Particular attention will be paid to contacts with the highest susceptibility to TB infection
- **Isoniazid Preventive Therapy (IPT):** Preventive therapy is recommended to Children < 6 years of age, who are close contacts of a TB patient. Children will be evaluated for active TB by a medical officer/pediatrician and after excluding active TB he/she will be given INH preventive therapy
  - In addition to above, INH preventive therapy will be considered in following situation:
    - For all HIV infected children who either had a known exposure to an infectious TB case or are Tuberculin skin test (TST) positive (>=5 mm induration) but have no active TB disease.
    - All TST positive children who are receiving immunosuppressive therapy (e.g., Children with nephrotic syndrome, acute leukemia, etc.).
    - A child born to mother who was diagnosed to have TB in pregnancy will receive prophylaxis for 6 months, provided congenital TB has been ruled out. BCG vaccination can be given at birth even if INH preventive therapy is planned.
    - Close contacts of index cases with proven DR-TB (drug resistant-TB) will be monitored closely for signs and symptoms of active TB as isoniazid may not be prophylactic in these cases.
- **BCG vaccination:** It is provided at birth or as early as possible till one year of age. BCG vaccine has a protective effect against meningitis and disseminated TB in children.
- Addressing social determinants of TB like poverty, malnutrition, urbanization, indoor air pollution, etc. require inter departmental/ministerial coordinated activities and the program is proactively facilitating this coordination.

TB-HIV

Introduction

TB-HIV collaborative activities between Revised National Tuberculosis Control Programme (RNTCP) and Department of AIDS Control (DAC)/NACO started initially in the year 2001. Since then, TB-HIV activities have evolved in line with updated scientific evidences. National Framework for joint TB-HIV collaborative activities is developed under which National, State and District level coordinating mechanism were put in place. Components such as dedicated human resources, integration of surveillance, joint training, standard recording with reporting, joint monitoring with evaluation, operational research are strategically implemented. The key approach suggested as per the National Framework Nov 2013 is as below:

Strategic Interventions

- **Strategies for reducing the burden of TB among people living with HIV/AIDS**
  - *Intensified case finding activities in HIV care settings:* Program will emphasis on use of a simplified clinical algorithm for TB screening that relies on the absence or presence of four clinical symptoms (current cough, weight loss, fever and night sweats) to identify people eligible for further diagnostic work-up of TB. Also rapid molecular test CBNNAT will be offered to all presumptive TB cases among PLHIV for early diagnosis of TB in settings such as ART centers, Link ART Plus center (LAC+), Link ART center (LAC), Integrated Counseling with testing centers (ICTC) and Targeted Intervention Projects (By 2017)
  - *Airborne infection control in HIV/TB Care settings:* People living with HIV are at higher risk of developing TB and TB is cause of high mortality among PLHIVs. National Airborne Infection Control guidelines recommend implementation of AIC measures at all HIV/TB Care settings. These measures include:
    - Developing time bound action plan to implement AIC measures at all Centers.
    - Training of MOs and Nursing Staff in AIC guidelines
    - Risk assessment at all centers with recommendations of implementing AIC guidelines.
    - Health care workers surveillance for TB and appropriate AIC measures at all centers.
  - *TB prevention among PLHIV:* Isoniazid Preventive Therapy (IPT) Strategy for prevention of TB among PLHIV, to be implemented nationwide by 2017.
  - *Early initiation of ART:* All PLHIV with less than 500 CD4 count will be eligible for the ART. Considering this PLHIV already registered in Pre- ART care, additional one lakh fifty thousand patients will require to be started on ART. Additionally nearly 50,000 patients will be added annually per year.
- **Strategies for reducing the impact of HIV among TB patients**
  - **Provider initiated HIV testing and counseling (PITC) among presumptive TB cases** is now a policy. The implementation is being done in a phased manner, starting with high prevalent states and then in A and B category districts in rest of the country by 2017.

- *Early initiation of ART among HIV infected TB patients:* Systematic measures to extend financial support to the HIV-infected TB patient for travel to ART center for evaluation and treatment initiation. There will be a provision for travel support for HIV-infected TB patients to visit ART center. Efforts will be made to optimize outreach activity undertaken by different categories of NACP outreach workers.
- *Nutritional support for TB and HIV patients:* Linking all TB and HIV patients for nutritional support through PDS.
- **Implementation of daily anti TB regimen with 2 years of post-treatment follow-up**

- **Strategies for establishing mechanisms of Coordination**
  - *Improved surveillance:* Linking patient-wise database, implement a case-based, web-based electronic surveillance system to enable real time monitoring of inter-program linkages.
- **Strategies for high priority 20 selected districts**
  - *Early Diagnosis:* Increasing access to rapid diagnostics for PLHIV with clients accessing HIV testing services including strengthening Sputum Collection and transportation.
  - Innovative strategies for addressing local epidemics esp. in 20 high priority districts
  - Decentralized TB-HIV treatment delivery services through community led models
  - Strengthening social support and institutional support for co-infected patients
  - Private sector engagement in TB HIV Collaborative activities
  - Newer initiatives Community-based HIV testing, Test and Treat, implementation of Targeted Interventions strategies under NACP.

The implementation of TB HIV activities will require CBNAAT to be deployed at all ART/COEs Centers in the country for early diagnosis of TB (by 2015). Department of AIDS control to expand coverage of whole blood finger prick HIV screening test at all PHIs. General health system needs to provide storage facility for HIV testing kits, budget for implementation of AIC measures at HIV TB care settings (600 ART centers, LAC, ICTC), and budget for ART drugs. Availability of adequate stock of Isoniazid is to be ensured. E-Training module to be used for HIV care staff.

Build

Bold Policy Initiatives

National TB Policy and TB Bill

All efforts will be made to support a comprehensive TB bill placed in the parliament which will promote TB care as a rights issue and hasten the control of TB in the country. The various clauses of the bill will cover all aspects of TB prevention and care to protect, promote and fulfil the rights of persons with Tuberculosis during delivery of TB care and services and for matters connected therewith or incidental thereto and also to accelerate the response from every sector. Various stakeholders including academia, experts, and political establishments (inter-ministerial consultation) need to be consulted while formulating the bill.

The TB policy will be aligned to the National Health Policy. The necessary regulations under the TB policy, inter-alia, will include:

- Mandatory notification of all TB patients
- Assured access to quality diagnosis and treatment as a standard of care through all healthcare providers
- Regulation of use of diagnostic tests
- Regulation/Ban on sale of anti-TB drugs in open market
- Nonstigmatization for TB patients and families etc.
- Right to access to public health care
- Compensations
- Occupational screening, workplace interventions
- Enforcement (immigration/admission to educational institutions).

Market Based Regulation will also be part of the regulatory efforts and will include:

- Certification of C/DST Laboratories
- Establishing linkages with existing health insurance schemes of the government and at a later date with the Universal Health Coverage (UHC) of the Government.
- Regulate access to anti-TB drugs
- Incentives to the private providers
- Introduction of new anti-TB drugs.

The program also aspires for converting RNTCP into 100% central program in the long-term.

National TB Elimination Board

It is proposed to create an apex body to facilitate policy development, coordinate multi-sectoral involvement and overview the implementation of the strategy to move towards TB elimination. Proposed constituents include Prime Minister as patron, Union Minister Health and Family Welfare as Chairperson, Secretary Health as member secretary with other members including secretaries of related departments, representatives of affected communities, representatives of technical and donor partners, representatives from NGOs etc. Central TB Division will directly report to National TB Elimination Board (NTEB).

Similar structure at the State level (State TB Elimination Board) also needs to be created, with State specific changes as required. This structure will provide the highest level of political, administrative, social commitment to TB control at the local level where it is required the most. It shall also be the major medium for addressing issues of **health system strengthening.** This will enable local epidemiological features of the epidemic, local problems to be identified and local solutions to be implemented. The Board will **review performance** periodically. This will also enable the **multisectoral response** required for action on the social determinants of TB and its outcomes.

Restructure the TB Program Management Structure

The HR plan of RNTCP prefers posting of regular state staff for senior positions in RNTCP for e.g., MO STC, MO STDC, etc. In the event of unavailability of such at the state level, the program will hire staff on a contractual basis. Budgetary provisions have been made for such hirings.

The big ticket changes envisaged in the NSP include the following:

- **National level:** Creation of 4 divisions each in charge of key programmatic areas instead of the current CTD structure with a commensurate increase in staff strength including technical and operations staff.
- **State level:** Creation of 4 divisions to mimic the structure at the National level.
- **District level:** Unified cadre for supervision to provide one TB supervisor for every block.
- **Block level:** One community volunteer for communicable disease for every 1000 population to undertake community focused functions like active case finding, treatment support, etc. Program specific honorarium will be available to these functionaries.

Diagnosis of TB in RNTCP

Smear examination most widely used and acceptable testing tool resumptive TB cases referred to designated Microscopy Center (DMC) two samples within a day/in 2 consecutive days, one sample on the spot, under supervision, second sample at home (Morning sample) should be at least 2 mL and mucopurulent if transporting sample, should reach DMC and be examined as early as possible (within 2 days). The standardized treatment regimen based on the classification of patients are given in **Table 10.15**.

Types of Drug-resistant TB

Monoresistant

Resistant to any one TB treatment drug is **called as Monoresistant TB**.

Poly-resistant

Resistant to at least any two TB drugs (but not both isoniazid and rifampicin).

Multidrug-resistant

MDRTB refers to strains of the bacterium which are proven in a laboratory to be resistant to the two most active anti-TB drugs, isoniazid and rifampicin. Treatment of MDRTB is extremely expensive, toxic, arduous, and often unsuccessful.

Table 10.15: Classification of patients in categories for standardized treatment regimen in RNTCP.

Category	*Type of patient*	*Regimen*	*Duration in months*
Category I color of box: **RED**	New sputum positive, seriously ill sputum negative, seriously ill extrapulmonary	2 $(HRZE)_3$ 4 $(HR)_3$	6
Category II color of box: **BLUE**	Sputum positive relapse Sputum positive failure Sputum positive treatment after default	2 $HRZES)_3$ 1 $(HRZE)_3$ 5 $(HRE)_3$	8

DOTS has been proven to prevent the emergence of MDRTB, and also to reverse the incidence of MDRTB where it has emerged. MDRTB is a tragedy for individual patients and a symptom of poor TB management. The best way to confront this challenge is to improve TB treatment and implement DOTS (MDR TB) Multidrug-resistant is the resistant develop to at least isoniazid and rifampicin, the two best first-line TB treatment drugs.

Extensively Drug-resistant

Resistant to isoniazid and rifampicin, PLUS resistant to any fluoroquinolone and at least 1 of the 3 injectable second-line drugs (e.g., amikacin, kanamycin, or capreo-mycin).

NATIONAL MENTAL HEALTH PROGRAMME (NMHP)

Described in the Chapter 12: Community Mental Health Nursing.

INTEGRATED DISEASE SURVEILLANCE PROJECT (IDSP)

Background

Integrated Disease Surveillance Project (IDSP) is a decentralized, state-based surveillance program in the country. It is intended to detect early warning signals of impending outbreaks and help initiate an effective response in a timely manner. It is also expected to provide essential data to monitor progress of on-going disease control programs and help allocate health resources more efficiently. All outbreaks cannot be predicted or prevented. However, precautionary measures can be taken within the existing health infrastructure and service delivery to reduce risks of outbreaks and to minimize the scale of the outbreak, if it occurs. The effectiveness with which national programs are implemented and monitored, the alertness for identification of early warning signals and the capacity for initiating recommended specific interventions in a timely manner are important to achieve the bellow objectives.

Surveillance is the backbone of public health program and provides information so that effective action can be taken in controlling and preventing diseases of public health importance. In some cases action must be immediate - within hours - in order to prevent large scale epidemics and deaths (Cholera, meningitis, food contamination). In others, control and prevention activities are long-term response to information about disease such as tuberculosis, HIV and Noncommunicable Disease risk factors, for which action may be taken in weeks, months or even years.

All surveillance systems involve six key elements:

1. Detection and notification of health event
2. Investigation and confirmation (epidemiological, clinical, laboratory)
3. Collection of data
4. Analysis and interpretation of data
5. Feedback and dissemination of results

6. Response—a link to public health program specially actions for prevention and control.

Objectives

- To strengthen/maintain decentralized laboratory-based IT enabled disease surveillance system for epidemic-prone diseases
- To monitor disease trends and to detect and respond to outbreaks in early rising phase through trained Rapid Response Team (RRTs).

Program Components

- Integration and decentralization of surveillance activities through the establishment of surveillance units at Center, State and District level.
- Human Resource Development—Training of State Surveillance Officers, District Surveillance Officers, Rapid Response Team and other Medical and Paramedical staff on principles of disease surveillance.
- Use of Information Communication Technology for collection, collation, compilation, analysis and dissemination of data.
- Strengthening of public health laboratories.
- Intersectoral coordination for zoonotic diseases.

Data Management

Under IDSP data is collected on epidemic-prone diseases on weekly basis (Monday–Sunday). The information is collected on three specified reporting formats, namely "S" (suspected cases), "P" (presumptive cases) and "L" (laboratory confirmed cases) filled by Health Workers, Clinicians and Laboratory staff respectively. The weekly data gives information on the disease trends and seasonality of diseases.

Whenever there is a rising trend of illnesses in any area, it is investigated by the Rapid Response Teams (RRT) to diagnose and control the outbreak. Data analysis and actions are being undertaken by respective State/District Surveillance Units. In the month of February 2018, about 96% Districts have reported weekly disease surveillance data from districts.

Outbreak Surveillance and Response

CSU, IDSP receives disease outbreak reports from the States/ UTs on weekly basis. Even NIL weekly reporting is mandated and compilation of disease outbreaks/alerts is done on weekly basis. On an average 30–35 outbreaks are reported to CSU weekly. A total of 553 outbreaks were reported in 2008, 799 outbreaks in 2009, 990 outbreaks in 2010, 1675 outbreaks in 2011 and 1584 outbreaks in 2012, 1964 outbreaks in 2013, 1562 outbreaks in 2014, 1935 outbreaks in 2015, 2679 outbreaks reported in 2016 and 1714 outbreaks reported in 2017.

A total of 133 outbreaks reported from 1st January 2018 to 4th February 2018. Majority of outbreaks reported in 2018 were of Measles (28%), Chickenpox (23%), Food Poisoning (14%), Acute Diarrheal Disease (12%), Chikungunya (5%), Influenza-B (3%), Scrub typhus (3%), and Dengue (2%).

Media Scanning and Verification Cell

- Media scanning is an important component of surveillance to detect the early warning signals. Media scanning and verification cell daily receives an average of 2–3 media alerts of unusual health events which are detected and verified. A total of 4815 health alerts have been detected till 28th February 2018 since its establishment in July 2008. Majority of them were Acute Diarrheal Disease, Measles and Dengue. A total of 35 media alerts were scanned for any unusual from 1st February 2018 till 28th February 2018.
- The process of establishing Media Scanning and Verification Cells in all 29 States and 7 UTs is being undertaken right now.

Information and Communication Technology Network (ICT)

ICT plays an integral and most powerful role in implementing IDSP across the country. One of the important components of the program is data management, analysis and rapid communication in case of outbreaks.

Data Center

National Informatics Center (NIC) has installed Data Center Equipment at 776 out of 800 sites. The objective of Data Center is online data entry for speedy data transmission from Districts.

Training Center (NIC)

Training Center Equipments have been installed at 378 out of 400 sites. State to District communication is possible by NICs E-Learning Portal (http://e-learning.nic.in/lms), which has facility in managing live virtual classrooms for training (State/Area specific discussion on disease surveillance activities), e-learning, interactive electronic discussion (Chat rooms, Boards, Mailing Lists) and reviewing and monitoring program-related activities.

Training Center (ISRO)

- Indian Space Research Organization (ISRO) has installed training center at 367 out of 400 sites (EDUSAT/VSAT). Satellite connectivity is not available since Sept 2010. Recently, ISRO has allocated the bandwidth and has started migration of network from GSAT 3 to GSAT 12 to restart the satellite connectivity.
- SHOC (Strategic Health Operations center) established at CSU (IDSP), NCDC.

IDSP Portal

The IDSP portal is a one-stop portal (www.idsp.nic.in) which has facilities for data entry, view reports, outbreak reporting, data analysis, training modules and resources related to disease surveillance. About 96% of Districts are now reporting disease surveillance data in portal.

Training

The Training in IDSP is three-tiered:

- Master Trainers State and District Surveillance Officers and RRT members are trained at identified National level institutes.
- The Medical Officers and District Lab Technicians are trained by Master Trainers at State level.
- Health Workers and Lab Technician/Assistants at peripheral institutions are trained by District Surveillance officers/Medical Officers at District level.

Training of State/District Surveillance Teams has been completed in all 36 States/UTs.

The main focus of training for State level participants is on basics of disease surveillance, concepts of epidemiology and data management, whereas the District training focuses on correct procedures of data collection, compilation and reporting and outbreak response. A need-based special two-week Disease Surveillance and Field Epidemiology Training Programme (FETP) have been initiated for the District Surveillance officers. 770 District Surveillance Officers have already been trained in this special 2- week FETP.

State Health Societies were requested in June 2010 to recruit contractual manpower under IDSP. 455 Epidemiologists, 164 Microbiologists, 24 Entomologists, and 14 Veterinary Consultants have joined in States and Districts as per 28th February 2018. States has been requested to expedite the filling up the remaining contractual positions at the State/Districts levels. Induction training has been given to majority of them.

Strengthening of Laboratories

District laboratories are being strengthened for diagnosis of epidemic-prone diseases in a phased manner. Till date, 259 District Public Health Labs has been approved for strengthening, out of which 138 DPHLs are performing tests as per IDSP standards. These labs are being supported by trained manpower, funds for essential equipment and an annual grant of ₹4 lakhs per annum per lab for reagents and consumables.

A State-based referral laboratory network has been established by utilizing the existing functional labs in the identified medical colleges and other major centers in the states and linking them with adjoining districts for providing diagnostic services for epidemic-prone diseases during outbreaks. Presently this network is functional in 23 States/UTs involving 108 labs.

Prevention and Control of Avian/H1N1 Influenza

- 12 Laboratories are functional, for testing clinical samples of Influenza A H1N1 in different regions of the country.
- The Animal Component of Avian Influenza is being looked after by Ministry of Agriculture (Department of Animal Husbandry).

Table 10.16: Budget and Expenditure for IDSP is as under: (₹in crores/as on 28th February 2018).

Sl. No.	*Year*	*Budget Estimates (₹In crores)*	*Expenditure (₹In crores)*
1.	2010–11	35.00	48.98 (43.58 + 5.40*)
2.	2011–12	63.00	27.83
3.	2012–13	63.00	33.11
4.	2013–14	63.00	49.98**
5.	2014–15	63.00	55.65
6.	2015–16	64.35	64.44
7.	2016–17	68.35	63.05
8.	2017–18	68.35	57.13

Note:

- *₹5.40 crores released to North-East State Health Societies which has been diverted from Rural Family Welfare Services
- **The actual expenditure has been incurred for IDSP amounting to ₹36.52 Crores. In addition to that amount IDSP has released an amount of ₹13.44 Crores as Grant-in-Aid to State Health Societies on behalf of NVBDCP. So the total expenditure comes to ₹49.98 Crores.

Intersectoral Coordination with Animal Husbandry Department

25 states have included Veterinary Officers in the State and District Rapid Response Team to achieve inter-sectoral coordination to combat zoonotic diseases in India.

Finance

Budget and Expenditure for Integrated Disease Surveillance Project (IDSP) has been shown in **Table 10.16**.

TWENTY POINT PROGRAMME

Introduction

The twenty point programme (TPP) was launched by the Government of India in 1975. The TPP was initially launched by Prime Minister Indira Gandhi in 1975 and was subsequently restructured in 1982 and again on 1986. With the introduction of new policies and programs, it has been finally restructured in 2006 and it has been in operation at present. The programs and schemes under TPP-2006 are in harmony with the priorities contained in the National Common Minimum Programme, the Millennium Development Goals of the United Nations and SAARC Social Charter. The restructured program, called TPP-2006, was approved by the cabinet on 5th October, 2006 and operated.

The basic objective of the TPP is to eradicate poverty and to improve the quality of life of the poor and the under privileged population of the country. The program covers various socioeconomic aspects like poverty, employment, education, housing, health, agriculture and land reforms, irrigation, drinking water, protection and empowerment of weaker sections, consumer protection, environment, etc.

Goals

- Eradicating poverty

- Raising productivity
- Reducing income inequalities
- Removing social and economic disparities
- Although the TPP has been in existence for last 30 years, it is still relevant today as the desired objectives of eradication of poverty and improvement in the quality of life of the common man have yet to be completely attained
- Over the years, the need for restructuring the program has been felt in the light of achievements and experiences, as well as the introduction of several new policies and programs by the Government of India
- The restructured TPP-2006 has come into force with effect from 01.04.2007.

TPP-86: Scope and Coverage

The program covers various socioeconomic aspects like poverty, employment, education, housing, health, agriculture and land reforms, irrigation, drinking water, protection and empowerment of weaker sections, consumer protection, environment and responsible administration.

TPP-86: The Twenty Points

1. Attack on rural poverty
2. Strategy for rainfed agriculture
3. Better use of irrigation water
4. Bigger harvest
5. Enforcement of land reforms
6. Special programs for rural labor
7. Clean drinking water
8. Health for all
9. Two child norm
10. Expansion of education
11. Justice to SC and ST
12. Equality for women
13. New opportunities for youth
14. Housing for the people
15. Improvement of slums
16. New strategy for forestry
17. Protection of the environment
18. Concern for the consumer
19. Energy for the villages
20. A responsive administration.

TPP 86: Implementation

There is three tier monitoring mechanism for implementation of TPP 86.

- At the district level the program is monitored by District Planning Board, Panchayati Raj Institutions and other agencies.
- At the state level the program is monitored by different line departments and the state level monitoring committee.
- At the central level the program is monitored by the Central Administrative Ministries/Departments concerned with their respective schemes/programs. The Ministry of Statistics and Programme Implementation monitors the program in its entirety.

TPP-86: Reporting

Monthly progress report which covers physical achievements against the set targets for 20 crucial items. The information for monthly progress report is supplied by State/UTs. Capsule report based on the monthly progress report highlighting the main achievement. Half yearly progress Reports which covers all the 119 items of TPP. The information is supplied by Central Nodal Ministries/Departments.

Restructuring of Twenty Point Program

The need for further restructuring of TPP 86 is being felt constantly due to launching of several new schemes/ programs by the Central Government on the bases of new initiatives while some others are in the nature of replacement/modification of earlier schemes. Some of the existing programs are required to be deleted as they have lost their relevance in the present scenario or achieved the desired objectives. An exercise for restructuring of TPP is in progress in consultation with Central Nodal Ministeries and State/UT Administration.

TPP-2006

Approved by the cabinet on 5th October, 2006 and operated with effect from 1.4.2007. Twenty Point Programme consists of 119 items out of which 66 items are monitored against physical targets, 54 items are monitored on evaluatory basis.

TPP-06: The Twenty Points

1. Poverty eradication
2. Power to people
3. Support to farmers
4. Labor welfare
5. Food security
6. Housing for all
7. Clean drinking water
8. Health for all
9. Education for all
10. Welfare of SC, ST, Minorities and OBCs
11. Women welfare
12. Child welfare
13. Youth development
14. Improvement of slums
15. Environment protection and afforestation
16. Social security
17. Rural roads
18. Energization of rural area
19. Development of backward areas
20. IT enabled e-Governance.

TPP-2006: Implementation and Performance Appraisal

The programs and schemes under the TPP-2006 are in harmony with the priorities contained in the National Common Minimum Programme (NCMP). Schemes under this TPP are being implemented by concerned department of the state. Provision for the same is also made by the respective departments. Out of the funds allotted to these departments during the respective year. Physical targets under various items of the TPP are finalized by the concerned Nodal Ministries of Government of India, after consultation with the various departments of the State Government. Targets fixed for the state are further divided into district targets by the state. Performance of the districts is monitored at the state level by the Planning Department on the basis of the criterion adopted by the Ministry of Programme Implementation, Government of India and accordingly, ranking of the districts is decided by the state. On the basis of the ranking, incentives are given to districts based on their performance in a selected program and on the basis of sample survey of selected program.

MINIMUM NEEDS PROGRAMME

Introduction

The minimum needs programme (MNP) was introduced in the first year of the 5th 5 years plan. The objective of the program is to establish a network of basic services and facilities of social consumption in all the areas up to nationally-accepted norms, within a specified time-frame. The program is designed to assist in raising living standards and in reducing the regional disparities in development. The program is essentially an investment in human resources.

The basic needs of the people identified for this program based on which the program developed initially, there were eight components of MNP, viz. elementary education, rural health, rural water supply, rural electrification, rural roads, rural housing, environmental improvement of urban slums and nutrition. While adult education was added to the list of MNP components in the 6th plan, rural domestic energy, rural sanitation and public distribution system were added during the 7th plan.

Two basic principles are observed during the implementation of MNP:

1. The facilities under MNP are to be first provided in those areas which are at present undeserved so as to remove disparities among different areas
2. The facilities under MNP should be provided as a package to an area through intersectoral area projects to have a greater impact.

Objectives

The objectives are categorized under some special heading.

Elementary Education

- 100% enrollment in the age group 6–14 by 1990. It would be supplemented with nonformal education.
- 100% coverage of adults in the age group 15–35 by 1990 through nonformal education.

Rural Health

- One community health volunteer for a population of 1000 or a village by 1990.
- Establishment of one subcenter for a population of 5000 in plains and 3000 in tribal and hilly areas by 2000 AD.
- One PHC for 30,000 population in plains and 20,000 in tribal and hilly areas by 2000 AD.
- Establishment of one CHC for a population of one lakh or one CD Block by 2000 AD.

Rural Water Supply and Rural Roads

- 100% coverage of provision of safe drinking water in rural areas
- Linking up of all remaining villages with a population of 1500 and above and 50% of the total number of villages with population of 1000–1500 by 1990.

Rural Electrification

- At least 60% of the villages, in each State and Union Territory to be electrified by 1990.
- Housing assistance to rural landless laborers
- Provision of housing assistance to all landless labor households by 1990. Assistance to include house-site construction materials, drinking water well for a cluster of houses and approach road.

Environmental Improvement of Urban Slums

- Hundred percent coverage of the urban slum population by 1990. Facilities to include water supply, sewerage, paving of streets, storm water drains, community latrines. Areas inhabited by scheduled castes particularly scavengers would be given priority.
- Nutrition Programme under MNP includes: (i) Special Nutrition Programme (SNP) and (ii) the Mid-day Meals Programme (MDM). The objective of the Special Nutrition Programme are to provide the beneficiary 300 calories and 8–12 g of protein for the age-group 0–6 years, and 500 calories and 25 g of protein for pregnant women and nursing mothers. During the Sixth Plan, nutrition support was provided to 11 million beneficiaries in the on-going 1136 Integrated Child Development Scheme Projects and SNP centers outside ICDS areas.

Achievement

A review of these programs has been made in the relevant chapters in most cases, the physical and the financial targets have been achieved satisfactorily except in the area of rural sanitation.

- In the case of elementary education, over 90% of the children were enrolled and had access to a school. However, the literacy rate is about 50%. This is due to the high rate of dropouts at the primary level itself. The aim is eradication of illiteracy. Hence the achievement should be judged in terms of literacy rates and retention ratios and these have to be monitored.
- In the case of rural health, there is an extensive network of PHCs and subcenters but these have not been operationalized in terms of adequate staff or medicines. In any case, 'Health for All' means reduction in both

birth and death rates and control of diseases. Hence, the performance with respect to rural health should be judged in terms of a decline in the death rate, the infant mortality rate and the birth rate besides a reduction in morbidity due to illnesses and diseases.

- Similarly, under the rural water supply program the coverage of villages is not enough by itself. It is necessary to ensure that 40 liters of potable water per capita per day is available on a sustained basis and to ensure its quality upgradation by making it free from salinity and chemical and bacteriological contamination.
- In the case of rural domestic energy, lack of coordination between the fuel wood and improved chulha/stoves, subcomponents were found to be a major constraint. It is proposed to take up this program in the IREP blocks where effective coordination and monitoring will be ensured for families below the poverty line in the 8th 5 years plan.
- Electrification of villages may be achieved as per targets, but it is necessary to ensure that beyond the minimum quantum of power needed to meet domestic use and street lighting there is other economic uses of power, such as energization of pump sets, running small units of production, etc.
- In consideration of interstate variations, the literacy rate is as high as 90% in Kerala and as low as 38 to 39% in Bihar and Rajasthan, with the all India average at 52. With respect to female literacy rate, Kerala has an average rate of 87% with Rajasthan and Bihar of less than 25%. In the first instance, those states which are below the all India average need to be brought up to this average. Thereafter, the focus will have to shift toward bridging the gap between the top ranking states and the rest.
- While the All India average death rate is 11.9, in states like Himachal Pradesh, Bihar, Odisha and UP it is above 13.5. The infant mortality rate ranges between 26 in Kerala and 135 in UP. Birth rates are as low as 19.4 per thousand in Goa and as high as 39.2 per thousand in UP.
- In the case of rural roads, only about 10% of the villages with the population of 1500 and above still remain unconnected, though in Bihar, Mizoram and West Bengal their proportion is 34, 42 and 40% respectively. In the population category of 1000–1500, the target of covering 50% of the villages would have been exceeded with the exception of Mizoram covering 44%.
- Similarly, with respect to other components, there are certain interstate variations. Attention needs to be given to the states lagging behind in order that they achieve the national norms, and some mechanism needs to be devised for this. Some additional funds may also need to be provided to the states that have not achieved the national norms. However, the state Governments may have a tendency to withdraw their normal assistance from a sector if it is being funded by additional resources from the center. This needs to be guarded against.
- The planning and implementation of these programs should be integrated with other ongoing rural development programs at a decentralized level with the district as' the unit of planning. In addition, some provision should be made for basic village amenities as an integral part of the MNP with a certain amount of 'untied' funds allocated to the local level bodies for the implementation and maintenance of these amenities. These can include street lighting, a primary school building, community centers, hand pumps, fish ponds, social forestry, biogas, etc. The list can be an exhaustive one with the flexibility of spending funds left to the discretion of the village level organization.
- Provision of energy for subsistance and development in the rural areas have to be closely linked with the program for rural development. The following section discusses the importance of rural energy and the details of the Integrated Rural Energy Programme which was started as a plan scheme in the 7th plan, and is being intensified and expanded in the 8th plan.

CHAPTER 11

Communicable and Noncommunicable Diseases

INTRODUCTION

A disease is an abnormal condition affecting the body of an organism. It is often construed to be a medical condition associated with specific symptoms and signs. It may be caused by factors originally from an external source, such as infectious disease, or it may be caused by internal dysfunctions, such as autoimmune diseases. In humans, 'disease' is often used more broadly to refer to any condition that causes pain, dysfunction, distress, social problems, or death to the person afflicted, or similar problems for those in contact with the person. In this broader sense, it sometimes includes injuries, disabilities, disorders, syndromes, infections, isolated symptoms, deviant behaviors, and atypical variations of structure and function, while in other contexts and for other purposes these may be considered distinguishable categories. Diseases usually affect people not only physically, but also emotionally, as contracting and living with many diseases can alter one's perspective on life, and their personality.

CLASSIFICATION OF DISEASES

The disease can be classified in various ways. We can classify the diseases according to their cause (Infectious diseases, lifestyle diseases, Mental disorder, Organic disease); according to mode of transmission (Food borne illness, airborne disease); according to their period of infectivity (Acute disease and Chronic disease); according to their affecting parts (localized disease, disseminated disease and Systemic disease) and so on but the major classification of diseases is Noncommunicable disease and communicable disease.

Communicable Diseases and its Meaning

Communicable diseases are diseases that are the result of a causative organism spreading from one person to another or from animals to people. Some people may use the words contagious or infectious when talking about communicable diseases. These diseases affect people of all ages but more so children, due to their exposure to environmental conditions that support the spread. Communicable diseases are preventable if interventions are placed at the various levels of transmission of the disease.

In recent years our region also faces new and emerging diseases which are challenging public health as never before. Unfortunately, many of these diseases affect the poor and marginalized sections of society, and contribute not only to ill health and poverty at micro-level but also have serious socioeconomic implications at the macro-level. Health workers have an important role to play in the control of these diseases by applying effective and efficient management, prevention and control measures.

Classification of Communicable Diseases

- **Contact diseases:** The diseases which can transmitted through contact which include scabies, pediculosis, fungal skin infections, trachoma, acute bacterial conjunctivitis, etc.
- **Sexually transmitted diseases and HIV/AIDS:** Sexually transmitted diseases are communicable diseases caused by organisms, such as bacteria, viruses and protozoa, which are transmitted through sexual contact. Some of these organisms can also be transmitted from mother to fetus (vertical transmission), through blood transfusion and contaminated needles and syringes.
- **Vector-borne diseases:** The diseases which can transmit through vectors, such as relapsing fever, Bancroftian filariasis, onchocerciasis, yellow fever, trypanosomiasis, plague, schistosomiasis, dracunculosis, leishmaniasis and malaria are known as vector-borne diseases. A vector is an organism that transmits or carries a disease from one human to another or from one animal to another and in some cases from an animal to a human being.
- **Diseases caused by feco-oral contamination:** As the name suggests, feco-oral diseases are diseases that occur when the causative organisms which are excreted in the stools of infected persons (or less commonly animals) gain entry into the human host via the mouth, e.g., acute gastroenteritis, bacillary dysentery, *Campylobacter jejuni*, giardiasis, amebiasis, cholera, enteric fevers, food poisoning, poliomyelitis, viral hepatitis.
- **Helminthic diseases:** The diseases caused by different types of worms, such as cestodes (tapeworms), trematodes (flukes) and nematodes (roundworms) that can cause diseases like *Ascariasis, Enterobiasis, Trichuriasis,*

hookworm, Strongyloidiasis, Taeniasis, hydatidosis are known as helminthic diseases.
- **Airborne diseases:** Disease transmitted through air called airborne diseases, e.g., acute respiratory infections, meningitis (bacterial and fungal), tuberculosis and leprosy.
- **Zoonotic diseases:** Diseases that are caused by contact with animals or animal products, such as anthrax, brucellosis, rabies, hydatidosis, tetanus.

IMMUNITY AND IMMUNIZATION

Immunization is a process of protecting an individual from a disease through introduction of live or killed and attenuated organisms in the individual. Immunization against vaccine preventable disease is essential to reduce the child mortality, morbidity and handicapped condition. It means of protecting the largest number of people from various disease. It gives resistance to an infectious disease by producing or augmenting the immunity.

Immunity

Immunity is the security against a particular disease and non-susceptible to the invasive or pathogenic effects of foreign microorganisms or to the toxic effects of antigenic substances. The term immunity refers to the resistance exhibited by the host towards infection caused by microorganisms and their products (toxins). This is based on the property of self and non-self recognition. That means immunity is carried out by the process of recognition and disposal of non-self or materials that enter the body. Immune response is the reaction of the body against any foreign antigen. But protection against infection disease is only a part of it.

Host Defenses

Host against infection are at once local and systemic, nonspecific and specific, and humoral and cellular. It is difficult to identify any infectious agent that fails to stimulate multiple host defense mechanisms. The concept of overlapping host defenses is crucial to our understanding of susceptibility to infection. This overlapping underlies the reasonable measure of good health in the face of an apparently significant host immune defect.

There is a phase of passive immunity transmitted to the baby from the mother across the placenta. Maternal antibody transmitted to infant is gradually lost over a period of 6 months. Thus a large proportion of infants remain free from potent infection up to 3 months, or even longer. There is good evidence that this protective 'biological shield' is due to the presence of high levels of immunoglobulins lgM and especially lgG in the cord blood and plasma of infants born of immune mothers. It has been postulated that some other factors (breast milk, presence of fetal hemoglobulin), are also responsible for the transient protection of infants.

Specific Defenses

Specific defenses come into play, once microorganisms have breached local defense mechanisms. By virtue of these defenses, the host is able to recognize, destroy and eliminate antigenic material (e.g., bacteria, viruses, proteins, etc.) foreign to his own. A person is said to be immune when he possesses 'specific protective antibodies or cellular immunity as a result of previous infection or immunization, or is so conditioned by such previous experience as to respond adequately to prevent infection and/or clinical illness following exposure to a specific infectious agent'.

The specific defenses may be discussed for convenience under the following heads:
- **Active immunity:**
  - Humoral immunity
  - Cellular immunity
  - Combination of the above.
- **Passive immunity:**
  - Normal human Ig
  - Specific human Ig
  - Animal antitoxins or antisera.

Types of Immunity

Generally immunity is two types innate immunity and acquire immunity.

Innate Immunity

Innate immunity is the immunity which comes from genetic and constitutional make-up and it has no relationship with previous bacterial infection and immunization. The Immunity acts as first line of defense against infections, microorganisms, their products before they cause disease.

Acquired Immunity

The acquiring of immunity from outside source is known as acquired immunity. It is result of action of two major groups of cells.
1. Lymphocytes
2. Antigen presenting cells.

This immunity is initiated by the recognition of a foreign antigen and the response to this recognition. It is highly adaptive and has four important features.
1. Antigen specificity
2. Diversity
3. Immunological memory
4. Recognition self from non-self.

The acquired immunity is again classified into active immunity and passive immunity.

Active Immunity

Active immunity is produced by stimulating immunological defense mechanism through administration of antigen usually prior to natural exposure to infection. Active immunizing agents are also known as vaccine. It is the immunity which an individual develops as a result of infection or by specific immunization and is usually associated with presence of antibodies or cells having a specific action on the microorganism concerned with a particular infectious disease or on its toxin. In other words, active immunity depends upon the humoral and cellular responses of the host. The immunity produced is specific for a particular disease, i.e., the individual in most cases is immune to further infection with the same organism or antigenically related organism for varying periods depending upon the particular disease.

Active immunity may be acquired in three ways:

a. Following clinical infection, e.g., chickenpox, rubella and measles.
b. Following subclinical or inapparent infection, e.g., polio and diphtheria.
c. Following immunization with an antigen which may be a killed vaccine, a live attenuated vaccine or toxoid.

Passive Immunity

It is produced temporarily by supplying preformed exogenous animal or human antibody to suppress the disease, given soon after or prior to exposure of an infection. Acquiring of the antibodies passively from an immunized donor to a nonimmunized recipient is known as passive immunity. When antibodies produced in one body (human or animal) are transferred to another to induce protection against disease, it is known as passive immunity. In other words, the body does not produce its own antibodies but depends upon ready-made antibodies. Passive immunity may be induced.

1. By administration of an antibody-containing preparation (immune globulin or antiserum).
2. By transfer of maternal antibodies across the placenta. Human milk also contains protective antibodies, (IgA).
3. By transfer of lymphocytes, to induce passive cellular immunity—this procedure is still experimental.

Passive immunity differs from active immunity in the following respects:

a. Immunity is rapidly established.
b. Immunity produced is only temporary (days to months) till the antibody is eliminated from the body.
c. There is no education of the reticuloendothelial system.

Passive immunization is useful for individual who cannot form antibodies, or for the normal host who takes time to develop antibodies following active immunization.

Herd Immunity

When a critical portion of a community is immunized against a contagious disease, most members of the community are protected against that disease because there is little opportunity for an outbreak. Even those who are not eligible for certain vaccines, such as infants, pregnant women, or immunocompromised individuals—get some protection because the spread of contagious disease is contained. This is known as community immunity. It is the level of resistance developed in a community or group of people to a particular disease. In another way herd immunity implies group protection beyond that afforded by the protection of immunized individuals. That is, it concerns the freedom from infection of individuals within a herd by sole virtue of the influence of the herd structure on the transmission among individuals. Thus there is an unfortunate confusion over the definition of herd immunity.

Herd immunity provides an immunological barrier to the spread of disease in the human herd. For example, when an infectious disease is introduced into a group of population which population had a very low or no immunity, the attack and case fatality rates tend to be very high. The epidemic wave declined with a build-up of herd immunity following natural infection. Sometimes herd immunity can be obtained by mass immunization. There are three basic types of elements which contribute to herd immunity are:

1. Occurrence of clinical and subclinical infection in the herd
2. Immunization of the herd
3. Herd structure.

Herd structure is never constant. It is subject to constant variation because of new births, deaths and population mobility. An on-going immunization program will keep up the herd immunity at a very high level. The herd structure includes not only the hosts (population) belonging to the herd species but also the presence and distribution of alternative animal host and possible insect vectors as well as those environmental and social factors that favor or inhibit the spread of infection from host to host. The herd structure thus plays a decisive role in the immunity status of the herd.

Antigen

Any substance usually a protein, which can stimulate the production of antibodies and react specifically with those antibodies, may be a bacterium, pollen, grain, etc.

Antibody

A specific protein substance in the bloods that destroy or render inactive certain foreign substances, particularly bacteria and their product.

It may be developed naturally or in response to a specific antigen that has been introduced into the body.

Immunizing Agent

The immunizing agent may be classified as Vaccine, Immunoglobulin and Antisera.

Vaccines: Vaccines are immune-biological substances which produce specific protection against a given disease. It stimulates active production of protective antibody and other immune mechanism.

Vaccine are prepared from live attenuated organism, or inactivated or killed organisms extracted cellular fractions, toxoids or combination of these.

The ideal vaccine should induce permanent immunity, be free of toxic substances, and have minimal side effects, not produce disease to the recipient and be easy to administer.

Live Attenuated Vaccine

- **Bacterial:** BCG, typhoid (oral), plague.
- **Viral:** Oral polio, measles, mumps, rubella, yellow fever, chickenpox, influenza.
- **Rickettsial:** Epidemic typhus

Inactivated or Killed Vaccines

- **Bacterial:** Typhoid, cholera, pertusis, cs meningitis, plague
- **Viral:** Rabies, salk (polio), influenza, hepatitis-A and B, Japanese encephalitis.

Toxoid

Bacterial: Diphtheria and tetanus.

Vaccine Preventable Disease

The infectious diseases can be prevented by vaccines. Currently there are seven diseases against which vaccines are available:

- **Seven-killer vaccine preventable diseases are:** Poliomyelitis, tuberculosis, diphtheria, pertusis, tetanus, measles and hepatitis.
- **Other are:** Mumps, rubella, hemophilous influenza type B infection, typhoid, meningococcal meningitis, Japanese encephalitis, influenza, pneumococcal pneumonia, chickenpox, rota virus diarrhea, yellow fever, cholera, malaria, plague and rabies.

COLD CHAIN AND NATIONAL IMMUNIZATION SCHEDULE

Immunization schedule was planned according to the needs of the community which is relevant with existing community health problems. It must be effective, feasible and acceptable by the community. The immunization schedule has been changed from time to time and the most current immunization schedule is given in **Tables 11.1 and 11.2**. The WHO launched global Immunization program in 1974, known as Expanded Programme on Immunization (EPI) to protect all children of the world against six killer diseases but now it is seven killer diseases. In India, EPI was launched in January 1978. The EPI was now renamed as Universal Child Immunization, as per declaration sponsored by UNICEF. In 1985 November it is called Universal Immunization Programme (UIP).

Table 11.1: National Immunization Schedule.

Age	*Vaccines given*
Birth	Bacillus Calmette Guerin (BCG), Oral Polio Vaccine (OPV)-0 dose, Hepatitis B birth dose
6 Weeks	OPV-1, Pentavalent-1, Rotavirus Vaccine (RVV)-1, Fractional dose of Inactivated Polio Vaccine (fIPV)-1, Pneumococcal Conjugate Vaccine (PCV) -1
10 weeks	OPV-2, Pentavalent-2, RVV-2
14 weeks	OPV-3, Pentavalent-3, fIPV-2, RVV-3, PCV-2
9–12 months	Measles and Rubella (MR)-1, JE-1, PCV-Booster
16–24 months	MR-2, JE-2, Diphtheria, Pertussis and Tetanus (DPT)-Booster-1, OPV – Booster
5–6 years	DPT-Booster-2
10 years	Tetanus and adult Diphtheria (Td)
16 years	Td
Pregnant mother	Td-1, Td-2 or Td-Booster

The successful implementation of Universal Immunization Programme (UIP) will include the production of adequate quantities of vaccines, maintenance of continuous supply and maintenance of vaccine potency at the delivery end. As once the vaccines lose their potency, they can no longer protect individuals from disease. Vaccine potency cannot be regained once it is lost. Vaccines are preserved by maintaining a 'cold chain'.

Definition of Cold Chain

Cold chain is a system of storage, transport and distribution of vaccines in a potent state (at low temperature) from the manufacturer to the actual vaccination site.

The cold chain system is necessary because the vaccines are sensitive to heat. If the vaccines are exposed to heat, they will have shortened life. Loss their potency. So its need to maintain a temperature. More heat sensitive vaccine is polio. Least heat sensitive vaccines are: Measles, DPT, BCG, DT and Tetanus.

All vaccines retain this potency at temperature between 2 and 8°C among the vaccine polio is the most sensitive to heat requiring the storage at –20°C. So the vaccine must stay cold or maintain optimum temperature to the actual vaccination site.

Components of Cold Chain

The major components of cold chain are:

- **Apparatus:** These can be kept in 2 categories. First categories include those equipment, which keep the vaccines at 2 to 8°C and the other category has those equipment, which freeze the vaccines.
- **Supplies:** Vaccines and the solvent are the components of cold chain supplies. These are kept cool at low temperatures. Vaccines of polio, TB and measles can be kept in a frozen condition, but vaccines of DPT, DT, and TT lose their potency if kept in frozen condition.
- **Manual efforts:** It is necessary to train the people thoroughly about the equipment, supplies, transportation, communication those who are working with the manufacturer, health officer, health workers and those storing and transporting the vaccines.
- **Transportation:** To maintain the potency of vaccines, the rapid means of transport should be used a specific temperature is to be maintained; therefore heat resistant equipment should be used in the journey.
- **Communication:** A reliable and effective communication system is a must for the cold chain. All information and orders associated with cold chain should be immediately and clearly, sent and received.
- **Equipment of cold chain:** These equipment are designed to keep cold air inside and to prevent worm air from enter which protects vaccines from the heat when they are placed inside.

Table 11.2: immunization schedule for infants, children and pregnant women (vaccine-wise).

Vaccine	*When to give*	*Dose*	*Route*	*Site*
For pregnant women				
Tetanus and adult Diphtheria (Td)-1	Early in pregnancy	0.5 mL	Intramuscular	Upper arm
Td-2	4 weeks after Td-1	0.5 mL	Intramuscular	Upper arm
Td-Booster	If received 2 TT/Td doses in a pregnancy within the last 3 years*	0.5 mL	Intramuscular	Upper arm
For infants				
Bacillus Calmette Guerin (BCG)	At birth or as early as possible till one year of age	0.1 mL (0.05 mL until 1 month age)	Intradermal	Left upper arm
Hepatitis B - Birth dose	At birth or as early as possible within 24 hours	0.5 mL	Intramuscular	Anterolateral side of mid-thigh
Oral Polio Vaccine (OPV)-0	At birth or as early as possible within the first 15 days	2 drops	Oral	Oral
OPV 1, 2 and 3	At 6 weeks, 10 weeks and 14 weeks (OPV can be given till 5 years of age)	2 drops	Oral	Oral
Pentavalent 1, 2 and 3	At 6 weeks, 10 weeks and 14 weeks (can be given till one year of age)	0.5 mL	Intramuscular	Anterolateral side of mid-thigh
Pneumococcal conjugate vaccine(PCV)	Two primary doses at 6 and 14 weeks followed by Booster dose at 9–12 months	0.5 mL	Intramuscular	Anterolateral side of mid-thigh
Rotavirus (RVV)	At 6 weeks, 10 weeks and 14 weeks (can be given till one year of age)	5 drops (liquid vaccine) 2.5 mL (lyophilized vaccine)	Oral	Oral
Inactivated Polio Vaccine (IPV)	Two fractional dose at 6 and 14 weeks of age	0.1 mL	Intradermal two fractional dose	Intradermal: Right upper arm
Measles Rubella (MR) 1st dose	9 completed months-12 months. (Measles can be given till 5 years of age)	0.5 mL	Subcutaneous	Right upper arm
Japanese Encephalitis (JE)-1	9 completed months-12 months	0.5 mL	Subcutaneous (Live attenuated vaccine) Intramuscular (Killed vaccine)	Left upper arm (Live attenuated vaccine) Anterolateral aspect of mid thigh (Killed vaccine)
Vitamin A (1st dose)	At 9 completed months with measles–rubella	1 mL (1 lakh IU)	Oral	Oral
For children				
Diphtheria, pertussis and tetanus (DPT) Booster-1	16–24 months	0.5 mL	Intramuscular	Anterolateral side of mid-thigh
MR 2nd dose	16–24 months	0.5 mL	Subcutaneous	Right upper arm
OPV Booster	16–24 months	2 drops	Oral	Oral
JE-2	16–24 months	0.5 mL	Subcutaneous (Live attenuated vaccine) Intramuscular (Killed vaccine)	Left upper arm (Live attenuated vaccine) Anterolateral aspect of mid thigh (Killed vaccine)
Vitamin A (2nd to 9th dose)	16–18 months. Then one dose every 6 months up to the age of 5 years	2 mL (2 lakh IU)	Oral	Oral
DPT Booster-2	5–6 years	0.5 mL	Intramuscular	Upper arm
Td	10 years and 16 years	0.5 mL	Intramuscular	Upper arm

*One dose if previously vaccinated within 3 years

Note:
- JE Vaccine is introduced in select endemic districts after the campaign.
- The 2nd to 9th doses of Vitamin A can be administered to children 1–5 years old during biannual rounds, in collaboration with ICDS.
- PCV in selected states/districts: Bihar, Himachal Pradesh, Madhya Pradesh, Rajasthan and Uttar Pradesh (selected districts), and in Haryana as state initiative

Type of Cold Chain Equipment

Refrigerator

Ice lined refrigerator (ILR): ILR are top opening refrigerator, it is two types:
1. Electrolux: With ice tubes.
2. Vestfrost: With ice packs.

Deep freezer: Deep freezer is also top opening equipment. It is to be used for storing polio and measles vaccines and freezing of icepack pair of deep freezer and a vest-frost ILR connected to a common voltage stabiliser.

Defrosting of refrigerator: The temperature in the refrigerator can rise if there is a thick layer of ice around the freezer. It is, therefore, necessary to defrost the refrigerator periodically. This should be done if the ice in the freezer is more than 6 mm thick. Most refrigerators now have automatic defrosting switch. When the bottom is pressed, the cooling in the freezer compartment stops and the ice starts melting.

Dial thermometer: Dial thermometers have been provided to record the temperature in the refrigerators. One dial thermometer should be kept in each refrigerator, including ILRs. One person should be made responsible for recording the temperature. The booklet of 12 temperature recording forms should be kept on the top of the refrigerator and must be checked daily to see that the temperature is maintained.

Walk in Cooler

This is refrigerator of the size of a room (10′× 10′) all types of vaccines can be kept safe. At district health centers, vaccines are stored in these walk in coolers only.

These coolers have the arrangement to keep the vaccine at the appropriate temperature for long hours even if the supply is interrupted.

Cold Box

Cold boxes are means to transport large quantities of vaccines by vehicle to out-reach sites. It can keep vaccines cold up to one week with no power supplies.

Before using cold box, the nurse should ensure that it should be clean with no cracks and the lid closes tightly and has locks. When the vaccines are packed in a cold box, there should be ice or ice packs at the sides and on the top of the vaccines.

Cold Packs

These are flat bottles of plastic, which are filled with water. These are used in the vaccines carriers after freezing their water. These are kept in deep freezers for a minimum of 6 hours to freeze the water inside these.

Vaccine Carrier

These are suitable for carrying small quantities of vaccine to health subcenters, villages, satellite towns and small towns. These are made of heat resistant material and light in weight, therefore they can be carried easily in hand or on shoulder. Four packs of ice are kept in these, along all four sides. If the ice packs are completely frozen and lid of vaccine carriers is tightly closed, then the vaccine can be kept at a low temperature for two days, despite the outside temperature being 32–42°C. Vaccine carrier should be properly clean from inside, without any cracks and its lid should be properly closed.

Potency test: The process of investigating the effectiveness of vaccines is known as potency test. The vaccines should not lose its effectiveness, to ensure this, it is essential to conduct potency test. Lack of appropriate potency makes the vaccination a waste because then it will not be able to generate immunity.

Vaccine Sensitivity

- **BCG:** Relatively heat stable but sensitive to light. Not damaged by freezing.
- **OPV:** Sensitive to heat and light. Not damaged by freezing.
- **Measles:** Sensitive to heat and light. Not damaged by freezing.
- **DPT:** Relatively heat stable. Freezes at 3°C should not be frozen.
- **Hepatitis B:** Relatively heat stable. Freezes at 5°C should not be frozen.
- **DT:** Relatively heat stable. Freezes at 3°C should not be frozen.
- **TT:** Relatively heat stable. Freezes at 3°C should not be frozen.

Importance of Cold Chain

- Obtaining the vaccines from the manufacturers
- Storing and transporting the vaccines
- Maintaining the supply of vaccines
- Having information about essential equipment, supply of electricity, etc.
- Keeping the vaccines at a temperature suggested by manufacturer
- Protecting the vaccines from sunlight and antiseptic substances
- Maintaining the potency of vaccines by following all the above-mentioned points.

Cold Chain Issues in Field

Inadequate maintenance of cold chain equipment:
- High cold chain sickness rate
- Long response time to breakdown of equipment
- Not enough cold chain engineers/refrigerator mechanics in states and districts
- Lack of adequate training
- Lack of adequate equipment
- Voltage fluctuation, equipment not attached to stabilizers, lack of proper wiring and earthing
- Improper cleaning and defrosting of equipment.

Poor monitoring of the cold chain:
- Inadequate knowledge regarding cold chain maintenance by ANM and MPHW male

- Poor supervision and monitoring
- Shortage of accessories like thermometer, stabilizer, equipment stand, freeze tag, etc.
- Inadequate recording and documentation
- Power cuts/generator running/defrosting not documented in logbook
- Temperature charting not done regularly.

Methods of controlling cold chain:

- Keep the vaccine in appropriate conditions, as suggested by the manufacturer.
- Follow all the precautions while transporting the vaccine.
- Record the temperature of storage place twice a day and preparing the temperature chart.
- Maintain the equipment of cold chain and the appropriate functioning of its components, conducting potency test from time to time.
- Keep communication system effective and latest.
- Train all the people associated with vaccination (health officers, health workers, etc.) about the maintenance and controlled of cold chain.

EPIDEMIOLOGY OF COMMUNICABLE DISEASES

Smallpox (Variola)

Introduction

The word *variola* (smallpox) comes from the Latin word *varius*, meaning 'stained, ' or from *varus*, meaning 'mark on the skin'. The disease is also known by the Latin names *Variola* or *Variolavera*, derived from *varius* ('spotted') or *varus* ('pimple'). The disease was originally known in English as the 'pox or 'red plague'. Any confirmed case should be considered an international emergency and should be reported to public health authorities immediately. Smallpox was an infectious disease unique to humans, caused by either of two virus variants, *Variola major* and *Variola minor*. Smallpox are localized in small blood vessels of the skin and in the mouth and throat. In the skin it resulted in a characteristic maculopapular rash and later, raised fluid-filled blisters. Variola is stable outside the host and retains its infectivity. The last case of smallpox occurred in 1977 and was declared eradicated from the world in 1980.

Types

There are two major forms of smallpox, variola major and variola minor. Variola major is the more common and severe form, causing an extensive rash and a higher fever. The Variola major has an overall mortality rate of 30–35%. There are four forms of variola major (ordinary, modified, flat, and hemorrhagic). Variola minor is much less common and causes a less severe disease. The next few slides will better describe the various forms of variola major. In the discrete form of variola major smallpox disease, the pustules remain separate and distinct from one another. This is the most frequent form of smallpox.

Clinical Manifestation

Small red spots in the mouth and on the tongue are the initial signs of smallpox. Around the time the sores in the mouth breakdown, a rash appears on the skin, starting on the face. It then spreads to the arms and legs and then to the hands and feet. Usually the rash spreads to all parts of the body within 24 hours. As the rash appears, the fever usually falls and the person may start to feel better. The initial signs include a fever that subsides a bit upon the onset of the rash, which occurs after an incubation period of 7–17 days. The rash progresses through macules, papules, vesicles, pustules, and finally scabs. Fever, malaise, headache, prostration, backache, possibly abdominal pain and/or vomiting occur. The scabs fall off at the end of the 3rd or 4th week and the patient is no longer considered contagious.

Transmission

Transmission occurs through inhalation of airborne variola virus, usually droplets expressed from the oral, nasal, or pharyngeal mucosa of an infected person. It is transmitted from one person to another primarily through prolonged face-to-face contact with an infected person, usually within a distance of 6 feet (1.8 m), but can also be spread through direct contact with infected bodily fluids or contaminated objects (fomites) such as bedding or clothing. Rarely, smallpox has been spread by virus carried in the air in enclosed settings, such as buildings, buses, and trains. The virus can cross the placenta, but the incidence of congenital smallpox is relatively low. Smallpox is not notably infectious in the prodromal period and viral shedding is usually delayed until the appearance of the rash, which is often accompanied by lesions in the mouth and pharynx. The virus can be transmitted throughout the course of the illness, but is most frequent during the first week of the rash, when most of the skin lesions are intact. Infectivity wanes in 7 to 10 days when scabs form over the lesions, but the infected person is contagious until the last smallpox scab falls off.

Diagnosis

The clinical definition of smallpox is an illness with acute onset of fever greater than 101°F (38.3°C) followed by a rash characterized by firm, deep seated vesicles or pustules in the same stage of development without other apparent cause. If a clinical case is observed, smallpox is confirmed using laboratory tests.

Microscopically, poxviruses produce characteristic cytoplasmic inclusions, the most important of which are known as Guarnieri bodies, and are the sites of viral replication. Guarnieri bodies are readily identified in skin biopsies stained with hematoxylin and eosin, and appear as pink blobs. They are found in virtually all poxvirus infections but the absence of Guarnieri bodies cannot be used to rule out smallpox. The diagnosis of an orthopoxvirus infection can also be made rapidly by electron microscopic examination of pustular fluid or scabs. However, all orthopoxviruses exhibit identical brick-shaped virions by electron microscopy.

Definitive laboratory identification of variola virus involves growing the virus on chorioallantoic membrane (part of a chicken embryo) and examining the resulting pock lesions under defined temperature conditions. Strains may be characterized by polymerase chain reaction (PCR) and restriction fragment length polymorphism (RFLP) analysis. Serologic tests and enzyme linked immunosorbent assays (ELISA), which measure variola virus-specific immunoglobulin and antigen have also been developed to assist in the diagnosis of infection.

Chickenpox was commonly confused with smallpox in the immediate post-eradication era. Chickenpox and smallpox can be distinguished by several methods. Unlike smallpox, chickenpox does not usually affect the palms and soles. Additionally, chickenpox pustules are of varying size due to variations in the timing of pustule eruption: smallpox pustules are all very nearly the same size since the viral effect progresses more uniformly. A variety of laboratory methods are available for detecting chickenpox in evaluation of suspected smallpox case.

Chickenpox (Varicella)

Chickenpox or varicella is an acute, highly infectious disease cause by varicella-zoster. It is characterized by vesicular rash that may be accompanied by fever and malaise. It usually starts with vesicular skin rash mainly on the body and head rather than at the periphery and becomes itchy, raw pockmarks, which mostly heal without scarring. On examination, the observer typically finds skin lesions at various stages of healing and also ulcers in the oral cavity and tonsil areas.

Incidence and Prevalence

Primary varicella occurs in all countries worldwide. Varicella has a prevalence that is stable from generation to generation. As of 2010 it caused about 6,800 deaths, down from 11,200 in 1990.

In temperate countries, chickenpox is primarily a disease of children, with most cases occurring during the winter and spring, most likely due to school contact. It is one of the classic diseases of childhood, with the highest prevalence in the 4–10 years old age group. Like rubella, it is uncommon in preschool children. In temperate countries, most people become infected before adulthood, and 10% of young adults remain susceptible.

Epidemiological Determinants

Agent factors: Varicella zoster virus (VZV) is a DNA virus and is a member of the herpesvirus group. Like other herpesviruses, VZV has the capacity to persist in the body after the primary (first) infection as a latent infection. VZV persists in sensory nerve ganglia. Primary infection with VZV results in chickenpox. Herpes zoster (shingles) is the result of recurrent infection. The virus is believed to have a short survival time in the environment.

Varicella and herpes zoster occur worldwide. Some data suggest that in tropical areas, varicella infection occurs more commonly among adults than children. The reason(s) for this difference in age distribution are not known with certainty, but may be related to lack of childhood varicella infection in rural populations.

Reservoir

Varicella is a human disease. No animal or insect source or vector is known to exist.

Source of infection: The virus occurs in oropharyngeal secretions and lesions of skin and mucosa.

Infectivity

One to two days before the appearance of rash, and 4 to 5 days thereafter. Varicella is highly communicable, with an infection rate of 90% in close contacts until crusts fall off. Days 1 and 2 is most infective.

Host Factors

- **Age:** Chickenpox or varicella Primarily among children under 4 to 10 years of age group. Like rubella, it is uncommon in preschool children.
- **Immunity:** One attack gives durable immunity. Varicella is highly communicable, with an infection rate of 90% in close contacts.
- **Pregnancy:** It risk for the fetus. Varicella infection in pregnant women could lead to viral transmission via the placenta and infection of the fetus. If infection occurs during the first 28 weeks of gestation, this can lead to fetal varicella syndrome (also known as *congenital varicella syndrome*). Effects on the fetus can range in severity from underdeveloped toes and fingers to severe anal and bladder malformation.
- **Environmental factors:** In temperate areas, varicella has a distinct seasonal fluctuation, with the highest incidence occurring in winter and early spring. In the United States, incidence is highest between March and May and lowest between September and November. Less seasonality is reported in tropical areas.
- **Transmission:** Infection with VZV occurs through the respiratory tract. The most common mode of transmission of VZV is believed to be person to person from infected respiratory tract secretions. Transmission may also occur by respiratory contact with airborne droplets or by direct contact or inhalation of aerosols from vesicular fluid of skin lesions of acute varicella or zoster.

Varicella is highly contagious. It is less contagious than measles, but more than mumps and rubella. Secondary attack rates among susceptible household contacts of persons with varicella are as high as 90% (that is, 9 out of 10 susceptible household contacts of persons with varicella will become infected).

Control and Prevention

Hygiene measures: The spread of chickenpox can be prevented by isolating affected individuals. Contagion is by exposure to respiratory droplets, or direct contact with lesions, within a period lasting from three days prior to the onset of the rash, to four days after the onset of the rash. The chickenpox virus is susceptible to disinfectants, notably chlorine bleach (i.e., sodium hypochlorite). Also, like all enveloped viruses, VZV is sensitive to desiccation, heat and detergents. Therefore these viruses are relatively easy to kill in the environment.

Vaccine

The varicella vaccine is a live (attenuated) virus administered to protect against the viral disease commonly known as chickenpox caused by the varicella zoster virus (VZV). Another vaccine that is known as Zostavax is simply a larger-than-normal dose of Varivax, and is used in older adults to reduce the risk of shingles. Varicella vaccine is 70 to 90% effective for preventing varicella and more than 95% effective for preventing severe varicella. Furthermore, follow-up evaluations took place in the United States of children immunized that revealed protection for at least 11 years. People who do not develop enough protection when they get the vaccine may develop a mild case of the disease when in close contact with a person with chickenpox. In these cases, people show very little sign of illness. This has been the case of children who get the vaccine in their early childhood and later have contact with children with chickenpox. Some of these children may develop a mild chickenpox also known as breakthrough disease his vaccine is a shot given subcutaneously (under the skin). It is recommended for all children under 13 and for everyone 13 or older who has never had chickenpox.

Administration of Vaccine

Two doses of vaccine are always recommended. In the first case a first dose is administered at 12 to 15 months and a second dose at age 4–6 years. For people older than 13 the two doses are administered 4 to 8 weeks apart.

Contraindication: Seriously ill people, pregnant women, people who have experienced a serious allergic reaction to the varicella vaccine in the past, people who are allergic to gelatin, people allergic to neomycin, people suffering from an immune system disease, such as HIV, people receiving high doses of steroids, people receiving treatment for cancer with X-rays, drugs or chemotherapy, as well as people who have received blood products or transfusions during the past 5 months.

Treatment

Primary varicella infection in the healthy child is a rather benign disease that requires symptomatic therapy only. Oral acyclovir should be considered for healthy persons at increased risk of severe varicella infections. The symptoms of chickenpox in the pediatric population can be treated topically and with oral agents. Pruritus can be treated with calamine lotion or pramoxine gel; powdered oatmeal baths; or oral antihistamines. The nucleoside analog acyclovir (20 mg/kg PO qid for 5 d), though shown to decrease the symptoms and duration of primary varicella infection when administered within 24 hours of onset of symptoms, is not commonly prescribed for otherwise healthy children.

Adults and immunocompromised persons with chickenpox have a more complicated course than that occurring in children, and therefore, the condition necessitates a more aggressive pharmacotherapeutic approach. Intravenous acyclovir therapy is recommended for patients who are immunosuppressed or immunocompromised.

Varicella-zoster immune globulin (VariZIG) is indicated for use in highly susceptible, VZV-exposed immunocompromised or immunosuppressed populations. A live attenuated varicella vaccine (Oka strain) was approved by the FDA in 1995 for prophylactic use in healthy children and adults.

Measles (Rubeola)

An acute highly infectious disease of childhood caused by a specific virus of the group of myxoviruses. It is clinically characterized by fever and catarrhal symptoms of the upper respiratory tract (coryza, cough), followed by a typical rash.

Epidemiological Determinants

- **Agent factors:** Measles is caused by a virus known as RNA paramyxovirus. It is spread when an infected person coughs, sneezes, or shares food or drinks. The measles virus can travel through the air. This means that you can get measles if you are near someone who has the virus even if that person does not cough or sneeze directly on you. Source of infection is only source is a case of measles.
- **Infective material:** Secretions of the nose, throat and respiratory tract of infected person.
- **Secondary attack rate:** There is only one antigenic type of measles viruses.

Host Factors

- **Age:** Between 6 months and 3 years of age in developing countries where environmental conditions are generally poor and per children usually over 5 years in developed countries.
- **Sex:** Incidence equal both male and female.
- **Susceptibility and resistance:** Natural infection provides lifelong immunity. A history of prior measles infection should be confirmed serologically before vaccination is deferred as reports of clinical measles infection are not always accurate. Vaccination at 12 months of age produces a protective antibody in approximately 95% of recipients. The second dose of vaccine, recommended at 4 years, increases protection to approximately 99% of recipients.

Period of Communicability

Cases are infectious from slightly before the beginning of the prodromal period, usually five days prior to rash onset. They continue to be infectious until four days after the onset of the rash Highly infectious during the time of eruption of rashes.

Nutrition: Tend to be very severe malnourished child.

Environmental Factors

Epidemics of measles are common in India during winter and early spring.

Transmission

Measles transmission is airborne by respiratory droplet nuclei spread or it can be transmitted by direct contact with infected nasal or throat secretions. The virus can persist in the environment for up to two hours. Transmission has been reported to people whose only apparent source of infection was a room presumably contaminated with measles virus when it had been occupied by a patient with measles up to two hours earlier.

Incubation Period

The incubation period is approximately ten days, but varies from 7 to 18 days from exposure to the onset of fever. It is usually 14 days until the rash appears.

Signs and Symptoms

Measles typically begins with a mild to moderate fever, often accompanied by a persistent cough, runny nose, inflamed eyes (conjunctivitis) and sore throat. This relatively mild illness may last two or three days signs and symptoms appear 10 to 14 days after exposure to the virus. Tiny white spots with bluish-white centers on a red background found inside the mouth on the inner lining of the cheek (Koplik's spots) and skin rash. The rash consists of small red spots, some of which are slightly raised. Spots and bumps in tight clusters give the skin a splotchy red appearance. The face breaks out first, particularly behind the ears and along the hairline.

Over the next few days, the rash spreads down the arms and trunk, then over the thighs, lower legs and feet. At the same time, fever rises sharply, often as high as 104 to 105.8°F (40 to 41°C). The measles rash gradually recedes, fading first from the face and last from the thighs and feet.

Management of Measles

There is no specific treatment for measles. Treatment is supportive with particular attention to the possible complications of measles, particularly pneumonia and encephalitis.

The case should be immediately isolated to minimize any possible ongoing transmission. If the case requires hospitalization they should be nursed in an isolation room if possible preferably with negative pressure ventilation, using respiratory and standard precautions.

Cases not requiring hospitalization should be advised to stay at home until they are no longer infectious, usually the fifth day after rash onset. Children are excluded from school or child care for at least four days after the onset of the rash.

Prevention of Measles

Prevention of measles can done by active and passive immunization. Active immunization is done by using live attenuated vaccines. They are grouped into 2 groups like measles vaccines of single antigen and measles vaccines of multiple antigens. Measles vaccines of single antigen are of 2 types.

1. Aerolised vaccine (Edmonston Zagreb (EZ): Chick embryo vaccine; EZ human diploid cell vaccine)
2. Heat stable vaccine (containing either Schwartz strain or Moraten strain).

Measles vaccines of multiple antigens: MMR vaccine (Measles, Mumps, Rubella vaccine). All are tissue culture live attenuated, freeze dried vaccines. They are safe and effective.

Measles Vaccine

Measles is best prevented by active immunization. Only live attenuated vaccines are recommended for use; they are both safe and effective, and may be used interchangeably within immunization programs. Person to person transmission of measles vaccine strain has never been documented.

The vaccine is presented as a freeze dried products. Before use, the lyophilized vaccine is reconstituted with sterile diluents. Each dose of 0.5 mL contains ≥1000 TCID 50 (Tissue culture infective dose) live attenuated, Edmonston Zagreb strain of measles virus, propagated on human diploid cells. Measles vaccine may also contain sorbitol and hydrolyzed gelatin as stabilizers, as well as a small amount of neomycin, but it does not contain thiomersal. In general it is recommended that freeze dried vaccine be stored in a refrigerated condition. The diluents must not be frozen but should be cooled before reconstitution. Reconstituted measles vaccine loses about 50% of its potency after 1 hour at 200°C; it loses almost all potency after 1 hour at 370°C. The vaccine is also sensitive to sunlight, hence it is kept in colored glass vials. After reconstitution, the vaccine must be stored in the dark at 2–80°C and used within 4 hours.

Some important points about measles vaccine should be remembered. Those are:

1. **Age:** The principal problem of measles immunization is timing. Immunization is not recommended for children before 9 months of age because the vaccine will be rendered ineffective by the maternal antibodies, which will protect the children up to 9 months. The WHO expanded program on immunization recommends first dose of immunization at 9 month of age and second dose of immunization between 18 to 24 months of age. This recommendation has been adopted in India. The age can be lowered to six month if there is measles outbreak in the community. For infants immunized between 6 months and 9 months of age, a second dose should be administered as soon as possible after the child reaches the age of 9 months provided that at least 4 weeks have elapsed since the last dose.
   In countries where the incidence of measles has declined, the age of immunization is being raised to 12 months in order to avoid the blocking effect of persistent transplacentally acquired antibody.
2. **Administration route:** The reconstituted vaccine is generally injected subcutaneously, but it is also effective when administered intramuscularly.

3. **Immune response:** Measles vaccine induces both humoral and cellular immune responses comparable to those following natural infection, although antibody titers are usually lower. Also, lower average concentrations of maternal antibodies are found in infants born to vaccinated mothers when compared with naturally infected mothers. Following vaccinations, transient measles specific immunoglobulin (Ig) M antibodies appear in the blood and IgA antibodies appear in mucosal secretions; IgG antibodies persist in the blood for years. Vaccination also induces measles virus-specific CD4+ and CD8+ T lymphocytes.
4. **Reactions:** When injected into the body, the attenuated virus multiplies and induces a mild 'measles' illness (rash and fever) 5 to 10 days after immunization, but in reduced frequency and severity. This may occur in 15 to 20% of vaccines. The fever may last for 1–2 days and the rash for 1– 3 days. There is no cause for alarm. The vaccines now given rarely cause severe reaction. There is no spread of the virus from the vaccines to contacts.
5. **Immunity:** The vaccine has convincingly demonstrated to provide immunity to even severely malnourished children. Immunity develops 11 to 12 days after vaccination and appears to be of long duration, probably for life. Infants vaccinated at the age of 9 months show seroconversion of about 90%.
6. **Contacts:** Susceptible contacts over the age of 9 –12 months may be protected against measles with measles vaccine, provided that this is given within 3 days of exposure. This is because, the incubation period of measles induced by the vaccine is about 7 days, compared with 10 days for the naturally acquired measles.
7. **Contraindications:** Mild current infections are not considered a contraindication to vaccination, but it should be avoided if the patient has a high fever or other signs of serious disease. Measles vaccine alone, or in combination with other vaccines, should also be avoided by pregnant women. Being in the early stages of HIV infection is not a contraindication to measles vaccination.
   People with a history of an anaphylactic reaction to neomycin, gelatin or other components of the vaccine should not be vaccinated. Furthermore, measles vaccine is contraindicated in persons who are severely immune compromised due to congenital disease, severe HIV infection, advanced leukemia or lymphoma, serious malignant disease, treatment with high dose steroids, alkylating agents or antimetabolites, or who receive immune-suppressive therapeutic radiation.
8. **Adverse effect of vaccine:** Toxic shock syndrome (TSS) occurs when measles vaccine is contaminated or the same vial is used for more than one session on the same day or next day. The vaccine should not be used after 4 hours of opening the vial. TSS is totally preventable and reflects poor quality of immunization services. The symptoms of TSS are typical. Severe watery diarrhea, vomiting and high fever are reported within few hours of measles vaccination. There are usually a cluster of cases as all infants vaccinated from contaminated vials will be affected. This may cause death within 48 hours. Case fatality rates are high.

Measles and HIV

Given the serious course of measles in patients with advanced HIV infection, measles vaccine should be routinely administered to potentially susceptible, asymptomatic HIV positive children and adults. Vaccinations may be considered for those with symptomatic HIV infection if they are not severely immune-suppressed according to conventional definitions. In areas where there is a high incidence of both measles and HIV infection, first dose of measles vaccine may be offered as early as 6 months. Two additional doses of measles vaccine should be administered to these children according to the national immunization schedule.

Passive Immunization

This is done by human normal immunoglobulin. It is gamma globulin. It is nonspecific immunoglobulin. It is given for those young children who have come in contact with a case of measles and are not immunized. It is either prevents or modifies the attack of measles.

The dose recommended by WHO is 0.25 mL per kg of body weight. It should be given within 3 to 4 days of exposure. Given intramuscularly immunity lasts for about 3 weeks. Afterwards the contact is immunized actively. Just like active immunization, passive immunization is also generally not required for infants below six months of age, because of presence of maternal antibodies.

Treatment

There is no specific treatment for measles. Treatment is supportive with particular attention to the possible complications of measles, particularly pneumonia and encephalitis.

The case should be immediately isolated to minimize any possible ongoing transmission. If the case requires hospitalization they should be nursed in an isolation room if possible preferably with negative pressure ventilation, using respiratory and standard precautions.

Cases not requiring hospitalization should be advised to stay at home until they are no longer infectious, usually the fifth day after rash onset. Children are excluded from school or child care for at least four days after the onset of the rash.

Rubella (German Measles)

The name 'rubella' was derived from Latin, meaning *little red*. Rubella is also known as German measles because the disease was first described by German physicians in the mid-eighteenth century. Rubella or German Measles is an acute childhood infection, usually mild of short duration and accompanied by low-grade fever, lymphadenopathy and a maculopapular rash. The disease can last one to three days.

Epidemiological Determinants

- **Agent factors:** Rubella is caused by an RNA virus of the togavirus family.
- **Source of infection:** Clinical or subclinical cases of rubella.
- **Infective material:** Secretions of the nose, throat and respiratory tract.
- **Period of communicability:** Less communicable than measles probably because of the absence of coughing in rubella.

Host Factors

- **Age:** Mainly a disease of childhood particularly in the age group of 3 to 10 years.
- **Immunity:** One attack results in life-long immunity.
- **Environmental factors:** Occurs in a seasonal pattern.
- **Transmission:** Person to person by droplet infection.
- **Incubation period:** 2–3 weeks average 18 days.

Clinical Features

Rubella infection in a woman in the first 8 to 10 weeks of pregnancy results in death of or damage to the fetus in up to 90% of cases. Multiple defects are common (for example, deafness, blindness, brain and heart damage, and mental handicap) and late complications are being increasingly recognized. The risk lowers to about 10 to 20% if the mother gets rubella at 16 weeks gestation and defects are rare after 20 weeks.

In other people, rubella is a mild disease. The symptoms that is similar to those of flu. However, the primary symptom of rubella virus infection is the appearance of a rash on the face which spreads to the trunk and limbs and usually fades after three days. The facial rash usually clears as it spreads to other parts of the body. Other symptoms include low grade fever, swollen glands (suboccipital and posterior cervical lymphadenopathy), joint pains, headache and conjunctivitis.

The swollen glands or lymph nodes can persist for up to a week and the fever rarely rises above 38°C (100.4°F). The rash of German measles is typically pink or light red. The rash causes itching and often lasts for about three days. The rash disappears after a few days with no staining or peeling of the skin. When the rash clears up, the skin might shed in very small flakes where the rash covered it. Forchheimer's sign occurs in 20% of cases, and is characterized by small, red papules on the area of the soft palate.

Symptoms, particularly joint pains, are more severe in adults.

Complications

Rubella is a mild infection. Once you've had the disease, you're usually permanently immune. Some women with rubella experience arthritis in the fingers, wrists and knees, which generally lasts for about one month. In rare cases, rubella can cause an ear infection (otitis media) or inflammation of the brain (encephalitis).

However, in pregnancy rubella, the consequences for unborn child may be severe. Up to 90% of infants born to mothers who had rubella during the first 11 weeks of pregnancy develop congenital rubella syndrome. This can cause one or more symptoms, including symptoms in the infant may include cloudy corneas or white appearance to pupil, deafness, developmental delay, excessive sleepiness, irritability, low birth weight, intellectual disability, seizures, small head size, skin rash.

Prevention

The best way to avoid catching rubella is to be immunized with the measles, mumps and rubella (MMR) vaccine. The MMR vaccine is part of the routine childhood immunization program. First dose is usually given to a child when they are 12–13 months old. A second booster dose is given before they start school, usually between three and five years old.

It is possible to have the MMR vaccination at any age. If anybody already immunized, having the MMR vaccine again will not cause any harm to him.

Planning a Pregnancy

Before pregnancy an immunity test to rubella should done. If the test shows no immunity MMR vaccine should be taken before becoming pregnant. One should avoid pregnancy for one month after vaccination because MMR vaccine is made from weakened live viruses.

If pregnant a rubella immunity blood test action is required. If not immune to rubella, try to avoid anyone who has the rubella virus. The MMR vaccination can received after giving birth to protect against rubella in the future. The MMR vaccine can be given to breastfeeding mothers without any risk to their baby.

Limiting the Spread of Infection

Someone who has the rubella virus is infectious for one week before symptoms appear and for around four days after the rash first develops. The spread of infection can reduce by restricting the movement and avoiding contact with pregnant women for at least six days from the start of the rash.

Passive Immunization

Postexposure prophylaxis with immunoglobulins does not prevent infection in nonimmune contacts and is therefore not recommended for protection of women exposed to rubella. However it may reduce the likelihood of clinical symptoms which may reduce the level of maternal viremia and the risk to the fetus. Women who contract rubella during the first trimester of pregnancy but are determined to proceed with the pregnancy may be offered HNIG or rubella immunoglobulin. Dudgeon advocates the administration of HNIG to women who are determined to proceed to term. He suggests a dose of 1500 mg IM as soon as possible after exposure and 3 to 4 days later.

Mumps

An acute infectious disease by a specific virus which has a predilection for glandular and nervous tissues. Clinically, the disease is recognized nonsupportive enlargement and tenderness of one or both the parotid glands. It was a common childhood disease worldwide. It is still a significant threat to health in developing countries and outbreaks still occur sporadically in developed countries.

Epidemiological Determinants

Agent factors: Causative agent myxovirus parotiditis is a RNA virus of the myxovirus family. Virus in the family Paramyxoviridae are classified in two subfamilies, Paramyxovirinae and Pneumovirinae. The latter subfamily contains two genera, Pneumovirus and Metapneumovirus.

1. **Source of infection:** Both clinical and subclinical cases.
2. **Period of communicability:** Usually 4–6 days before the onset of symptoms and a week or more thereafter.

Host Factors

- **Age and sex:** Mumps is the most frequent cause of parotitis in children in the age group of 5–15 years. It affect both sex equally.
- **Immunity:** One attack, clinical or subclinical is assumed to induce lifelong immunity.

Environmental Factors

Endemic disease, cases occur throughout the year, but the peak incidence is in winter and spring.

Transmission

The virus most commonly is spread directly from one person to another via respiratory droplets. Less frequently, the respiratory droplets may land on fomites (sheets, pillows, clothing) and then be transmitted via hand-to-mouth contact after touching such items.

Clinical Manifestations

The incubation period ranges from 14–24 days, with a peak at 17–18 days. Approximately 30–40% of infections are subclinical In children, prodromal manifestations are rare but may be manifest by: Fever, Muscular pain (especially in the neck), Headache, Malaise, earache, discomfort with eating or drinking acidic food, Parotid pain (is most pronounced during the first few days of swelling), Trismus (spasm of the masticatory muscles) can occur. Other salivary glands, such as the submandibular and sublingual glands may also be involved. In 10–15% of patients only the submandibular gland(s) may be swollen, presternal edema can be notable. Morbilliform rash has been reported in association with mumps. Infection subsides within 7 to 10 days Adolescents and adults have more severe disease than young children.

Diagnosis

- Routine laboratory tests which shows leukopenia and lymphocytosis.
- Enzyme immunoassay for mumps immunoglobulin IgG and IgM antibodies.
- Culture of saliva, cerebrospinal fluid, blood, urine, brain, and other infected tissues.

Vaccine

The Centers for Disease Control and Prevention (CDC) recommends a combination vaccine (MMR) to children at 12 to 15 months of age with a booster dose at 4 to 6 years of age. During periods of possible epidemics, the booster dose may be administered after a minimum of 28 days following the initial vaccination. The MMR vaccination is designed to prevent measles, mumps, and rubella (German measles). Adults born after 1956 should receive at least one MMR vaccination. Those born prior to 1956 are generally found to have acquired natural immunity and no vaccination is necessary.

Those who should not receive the MMR vaccine include patient with a compromised immune system (HIV/AIDS, cancer, those receiving more than two continuous weeks of steroids) or who are allergic to any component of the vaccine, including gelatin or neomycin. MMR vaccines are very unlikely to produce a severe reaction to those who are egg white allergic. Daily use of inhaled steroids (such as those used to control certain pulmonary diseases, such as asthma, COPD, etc.) is *not* a contraindication to the MMR vaccine. Patients with a mild illness (e.g., the common cold) may safely receive the MMR vaccine. Conception should be avoided until at least 28 days following vaccination.

Treatment

The mainstay of therapy (regardless of age range) is to provide comfort for this self-limited disease. Taking analgesics (acetaminophen, ibuprofen) and applying warm or cold packs to the swollen and inflamed salivary gland region may be helpful.

Complications of Mumps

There are four serious complications of mumps which may occur without experiencing the classic involvement of the parotid gland.

1. **Meningitis:** More than half of patients with mumps will have meningitis, which may occur during any period of the disease. Generally patients make a full recovery without permanent side effects.
2. **Encephalitis:** Until the 1960s, mumps was the primary cause of confirmed viral encephalitis in the United States. Since the successful introduction of a vaccination program, the incidence of mumps encephalitis has fallen to 0.5%. Fortunately, most patients recover completely without permanent side effects.
3. **Deafness:** Preceding the mumps vaccination program, permanent nerve damage resulting in deafness was not

unusual. While occasionally bilateral, more commonly only one ear was affected.

4. **Orchitis:** This complication was the most common side effect to postpubertal males who contracted mumps. Severe was one-sided in most cases. Some affected testes atrophied (decreased in size), and some demonstrated impaired fertility. The 'common knowledge' of sterility was actually rare. Previous concerns regarding mumps orchitis and later testicular cancer have not been proven. (Ovarian involvement occurred in some postpubertal girls.)

Less frequent complications may include arthritis, infection of the pancreas, infection of the myocardium, and neurological conditions, e.g., facial palsy, Guillain-Barré syndrome, etc.)

Influenza

Influenza, commonly known as '**flu**', is an infectious disease of birds and mammals caused by RNA viruses of the family Orthomyxoviridae. Influenza is an acute respiratory tract infection caused by the influenza virus, which is of 3 types–A, B and C. The disease is characterized by sudden onset of chills, malaise, fever, muscular pain and cough.

Epidemiological Determinants

- **Agent factors:** Influenza is caused by Orthomyxovirus, a virus belonging to the MYXOVIRUS group and family orthomyxoviridae.
- **Reservoir of infection:** It exists in animal and birds
- **Source of infection:** Usually a case or subclinical case.
- **Period of infectivity:** Virus is present in the nasopharynx from 1 to 2 days before and 1 to 2 days after onset of symptoms.

Host Factors

- **Age and sex:** Affects all the ages and both sexes.
- **Human mobility:** It is an important factor in the spread of infection.
- **Immunity:** Antibodies are important in immunity against influenza.
- **Environmental factors:** Seasonal and overcrowding enhance transmission.
- **Transmission:** Person to person (droplet).
- **Incubation period:** 18 to 72 hours.

Signs and symptoms: Approximately 33% of people with influenza are asymptomatic.

Symptoms of influenza can start quite suddenly one to two days after infection. Usually the first symptoms are chills or a chilly sensation, but fever is also common early in the infection, with body temperatures ranging from 38 to 39°C. The Symptoms of influenza may include: Fever and extreme coldness (chills shivering, shaking (rigor), cough, nasal congestion, runny nose, Sneezing, bodyaches, especially joints and throat, fatigue, headache, irritated, reddened watering eyes, etc.

Control and Prevention

Vaccination: The influenza vaccine is recommended by the World Health Organization and United States Centers for Disease Control and Prevention for high-risk groups, such as children, the elderly, health care workers, and people who have chronic illnesses, such as asthma, diabetes, heart disease, or are immuno-compromised among others. In healthy adults it is modestly effective in decreasing the amount of influenza-like symptoms in a population.

Vaccines can cause the immune system to react as if the body was actually being infected, and general infection symptoms (cold and flu) can appear, though these symptoms are usually not as severe or long-lasting as influenza. The most dangerous adverse effect is a severe allergic reaction to either the virus material itself or residues from the hen eggs used to grow the influenza; however, these reactions are extremely rare.

Control measures includes good ventilation of public buildings, the avoidance of crowded places during epidemics, encouraging suffers to cover their faces with a handkerchief when coughing and sneezing.

Diphtheria

Diphtheria (dif-THEER-e-uh) is a serious bacterial infection usually affecting the mucous membranes of nose and throat. Diphtheria is a highly infectious and communicable disease caused by *Corynebacterium diphtheria* characterized by involvement of the respiratory system, local production of membrane and general symptoms caused by absorption of toxin. But the hallmark sign is a sheet of thick, gray material covering the back of throat, which can block the airway. The bacilli multiply locally, usually in the throat, and elaborate a powerful endototoxin which is responsible for:

- The formation of a grayish or yellowish membrane commonly over the tonsils, pharynx or larynx with well defined edges and the membrane cannot be wiped away.
- Marked congestion, edema and local tissue destruction.
- Enlargement of regional lymph node
- Signs and symptoms of toxemia.

Epidemiological Determinants

- **Agent factors:** *Corynebacterium diphtheriae* which is an **aerobic gram-positive bacillus.**
- **Source of infection:** Case or carrier. Case range from sub-clinical to frank.
- **Clinical cases:** Carrier may be temporary or chronic, nasal on throat carriers.
- **Infective material:** Nasopharyngeal secretions, discharge from skin lesions, contaminated fomites and possibly infected dust.
- **Period of infectivity:** Variable, until virulent bacilli disappear from discharges and lesions (usually 2 wks or less and seldom more than 4 wks).

Host Factors

- **Age:** Mostly affects 1 to 5 years children

- **Sex:** Both sexes are affected.
- **Immunity:** Inborn of immune mothers are relatively immune during first few weeks or months of life.

Environmental factors: Occurs in all season but winter month favor its spread.

Transmission

- Droplet infection
- Contamination of nasopharyngeal secretion
- Raw milk (served as a vehicle).

Portal of Entry

- Respiratory route
- Nonrespiratory route by skin where cuts and wounds.

Clinical Manifestations

The sign and symptom depends upon site of infection, immunization status and escape of toxin to circulation. Diphtheria is classified clinically on the basis of the anatomic location of initial infection and the diphtheria membrane:

Nasal Diphtheria

Initially resemble mild common cold with rhinorrhea and paucity of systemic symptoms.

Tonsillar and pharyngeal diphtherias (insidious and more severe): It accompanying symptoms and signs like anorexia, malaise, low grade fever and pharyngitis. Within 1–2 days a membrane appears in various extent (depending on the immune status of the host). Cervical lymphadenitis is variable. **'Bull Neck'** (edema of soft tissue of neck) is also observed.

Laryngeal Diphtheria

Downwards extension of membrane from pharynx to larynx and toxicity less prominent.

Incubation period: 2 to 6 days occasionally larger.

Diagnosis

Confirmation of diphtheria can be done by Schick test. Schick test is a test which identify *Corynebacterium diphtheriae* toxin. 0.1 mL of Schick test toxin is injected into the skin of one forearm (test site) and the same quantity of the same, but heat-inactivated, material into the skin of the other forearm (control site); those with toxin-neutralizing antibodies either will have no reaction at either injection site (negative test) or may have a pseudoreaction due to antibodies for substances (antigens) in the test materials other than diphtheria toxin; people lacking toxin-neutralizing antibodies may have a positive reaction, which consists of an area of redness appearing 24–36 hours at the test site only and persisting for 4–5 days.

Management of Diphtheria

The specific management of diphtheria is done by prompt initiation of treatment with antidiphtheritic serum (ADS), an antitoxin to neutralize the circulatory exotoxin. It is administered IM/IV after skin test. The dose of ADS depends upon the type of diphtheria, extent of membrane and degree of toxemia. ADS may be given as repeat dose for better improvement. Desensitization is needed in case of sensitivity to ADS. Close observation of the patient is very important to detect the untoward reactions and complications.

Antibiotic therapy, preferably penicillin or erythromycin, should be administered for 2 weeks to eradicate the bacilli and to stop production of diphtheria toxin. Only after 3 negative culture of the patient should be considered as free of bacteria and cured. Carriers also need effective treatment to prevent spread of infection.

Supportive measures include isolation of infected child, bed rest for 2 to 3 weeks, easily digestible diet with high calorie, drug therapy with antipyretics and sedative. In case of seriously ill patient IV fluid, oxygen therapy, nasogastric tube feeding may be needed for maintenance of fluid electrolyte and nutritional requirements. Frequent removal of oropharyngeal or nasal secretion is essential. Tracheostomy may be required in respiratory obstruction. Mechanical ventilation may be needed in case of respiratory failure. Cardiac complication should be detected early by close monitoring and necessary management should be initiated promptly.

During recovery phase, if Schick test is positive, diphtheria toxoid should be given since not all patients develop adequate immunity after the disease.

Prevention and Control

The most reliable preventive method of diphtheria is active immunization by DPT and DT to all children by universal coverage. Isolation of cases, disinfection of contaminated articles and chemoprophylaxis (with oral erythromycin for 7 days or single dose of benzathine penicillin) of all household contacts and carriers are important preventive measures to control the disease. All close contacts need to have Schick test and throat swab culture before administering chemoprophylaxis. Passive immunization with ADS may be given to the carriers with negative Schick test and positive culture with unknown immunization status.

Diphtheria Immunization

Current prophylactics are:

- **Combined or mixed vaccines:**
  - DPT (diphtheria - pertussis - tetanus vaccine)
  - DTPw (diphtheria, tetanus, whole cell pertussis)
  - DTPa (diphtheria, tetanus, acellular pertussis)
  - DT (diphtheria - tetanus toxoid)
  - dt (diphtheria - tetanus, adult type)
- **Single vaccine:**
  - FT (formal - toxoid)
  - APT (alum - precipitated toxoid)
  - PTAP (purified toxoid aluminum phosphate)
  - PTAH (purified toxoid aluminum hydroxide)
  - TAF (toxoid - antitoxin flocculus)
- **Antisera:** Diphtheria antitoxin.

DPT Vaccination

Universal immunization is the best measure to prevent diphtheria. The diphtheria toxoid vaccine, which is generally combined with the tetanus and pertussis vaccine, is currently recommended for administration to infants, adolescents, and adults. DPT also known as DTaP and DTwP) refers to a class of combination vaccines against three infectious diseases in humans: diphtheria, pertussis (whooping cough), and tetanus. The vaccine components include diphtheria and tetanus toxoids and killed whole cells of the organism that causes pertussis (wP).

DTwP (diphtheria and tetanus toxoids and whole cell vaccines): diphtheria vaccine is a toxoid (DT), containing diphtheria toxin inactivated by formalin and adsorbed on aluminum hydroxide that acts as an adjuvant. The quantity of toxoid contained in a vaccine is expressed as its limit of flocculation (Lf) content. The most commonly used vaccine containing DT is DTwP, a combination vaccine containing 20–3 Lf of DT, 5–25 Lf of tetanus toxoid (TT) and >4 IU of whole cell killed pertussis.

DTaP (diphtheria, tetanus, and a cellular pertussis vaccines): DTaP is a combined vaccine against diphtheria, tetanus, and pertussis, in which the component with lower case 'a' is acellular. The available DTaP vaccine contain inactivated pertussis toxin (PT) and one or more additional pertussis antigen, like filamentous hemagglutinin (FHA), pertactin, fimbrial protein and a nonfimbrial protein. Trials have demonstrated that the efficacy of these vaccines is similar to DTwP, but the risk of systemic and local side effects is reduced significantly. Each dose of vaccine contains at least 4 IU (10 to 25 mg) of PT component and 6.7–25 Lf of DT. The DTaP vaccine is not recommended as part of the National Program in India due to its cost. However the IAP recommends that the vaccine be offered to children when parents optional for it in view of the advantage of fewer side effects, or are reluctant to the administration of further doses of DTwP after an adverse effect with a previous dose while endorsing the continued use of the DTwP in the national program.

DTaP is a vaccine that helps children younger than age 7, develop immunity to three deadly diseases caused by bacteria: diphtheria, tetanus, and whooping cough (pertussis). Tdap is a booster immunization given at age 11 that offers continued protection from those diseases for adolescents and adults.

It must be noted that the contraindication for DTaP are the same as for DTwP; and the vaccine should not be administered if a previous dose of DTwP or DTaP was associated with immediate anaphylaxis, or the development of encephalopathy within 7 days of vaccination. These children should complete immunization with DT instead of DTwP or DTaP.

Reduced Antigen Acellular Pertussis Vaccine (Tdap) and Reduced Antigen Diphtheria Toxoid Vaccine (Td): Immunity against pertussis induced by natural infection or through immunization in infancy wanes by adolescence, resulting in a second peak of the disease in adolescence. Pertussis control is unlikely to be achieved if adolescents and adults remain susceptible to the disease, because they act as a source of infection to susceptible individuals. Immunity against diphtheria also wanes with time and the only effective way to control the disease is through immunization throughout life to provide constant protective antitoxin levels.

The availability of offers the prospect of reducing pertussis incidence in the community. The available Tdap vaccines in India contain 5 Lf of TT, 2 Lf of DT and 3 acellular pertussis components namely pertussis toxoid 8 μg, filamentous hemagglutinin 8 μg, and pertactin 2.5 μg. Contraindications to Tdap are the same as those listed for DTaP or DTwP. Unimmunized individuals should receive one dose of Tdap if older than 7 years; this is followed by 2 doses of Td vaccine at 1 and 6 months. In some countries, a single dose of Tdap is administered to all children at 10–12 years, followed by Td boosters every 10 years. Tdap may also be used as replacement for Td/TT vaccine booster in children above 10 years and adults of any age if they have not received Tdap in the past and 5 years have elapsed since the receipt of previous TT/Td vaccine.

Educational Measures

Educational measures include to inform the public and especially parents of young children about the hazards of diphtheria and the importance of immunization.

Control of patient, contacts and immediate environment: Early detection of both cases and carrier is essential.

Early notification by reporting to the local health authority

Isolation: Strict respiratory isolation for pharyngeal diphtheria and contact isolation for cutaneous diphtheria.

Until 2, cultures from both throat and nose or skin lesions taken at least 24 hours apart, and not less than 24 hours after cessation. Of antimicrobial therapy, fail to show diphtheria. bacilli.

Or when culture is impractical, isolation may be ended after 14 days of appropriate antibiotic.

Concurrent disinfection: Of all articles in contact with patients is essential.

Management of case:

- DAT and antibiotics to be started immediately without waiting for lab results
- Rest and observation, to cover the period of potential cardiac damage and paralysis
- Avoid limbs deformity and ensure joint mobility
- Tracheostomy and artificial respiration.

Management of contacts:

1. For those who are previously immunized, administer booster dose.
2. For those not immunized they should be cultured and given DAT followed by immunization later on.

Whooping Cough (Pertussis)

An acute infectious disease, usually of young children caused by *B. pertussis*. It is clinically characterized by an insidious onset with mild fever and an irritating cough, gradually becoming paroxysmal with the character 'Whoop' (loud crowing inspiration). The spectrum of disease varies from severe illness to typical and mild illness without whoop. The Chinese called it a 'hundred day cough'.

Epidemiological Determinants

Agent factors: *Bordetella pertussis* is an aerobic, nonspore forming, Gram negative coccobacillus. It has no known reservoir other than humans and is thought to be unable to survive in the environment for prolonged periods of time (Merkel, 1998). The *Bordetella* genus of the *Alcaligenaceae* family is comprised of seven different species, four of which cause upper respiratory tract infections in different host organism. *B. pertussis* invades its human host through entry into the respiratory tract where it colonizes to cause whooping cough, also known as pertussis, which was at one time a very common and potentially life-threatening infection for children. Today, whooping cough still effects 20–40 million people worldwide each year and causes between 200,000 and 400,000 fatalities.

Source of infection: Case

Infective material: Nasopharyngeal and bronchial sex reactions.

Period of infectivity: From a week after the exposure to about 3 weeks after the onset of paroxysmal stage.

Attack rate: 90% in unimmunized household contacts.

Host Factors

Age: High incidence 1–5 years of age.
Sex: More among females than male children.
Immunity: Adequate immunization is followed by immunity.

Environmental Factors

It occurs throughout the year, a season trend with more cases occurring during winter and spring months, due to overcrowding.
Transmission: Through droplet infection.
Incubation period: 7 to 14 days, but not more than 3 weeks.

Clinical Manifestations of Pertussis

- Usually affect children before vaccine available
- Clinical illness in 3 stages
  a. *Catarrhal phase:* Cold-like (coryza, conjunctival irritation, occasionally a slight cough) for 7–10 days
  b. *Paroxysmal phase*
    - Long duration (2–6 weeks); No fever
    - A series of rapid, forced expirations, followed by gasping inhalation the typical whooping sound.
    - Post-tussive vomiting common
    - Very young infants may present with apnea or cyanosis in the absence of cough
  c. *Convalescent phase:* During this convalescent stage, these coughing attacks continue to gradually decrease and usually disappear within 2–3 weeks.

Control

Prevention: Whooping cough can be prevented with the pertussis vaccine, which is part of the DTaP (diphtheria, tetanus, acellular pertussis) immunization. DTaP immunizations are routinely given in five doses before a child's sixth birthday. To give additional protection in case immunity fades, the American Academy of Pediatrics (AAP) now recommends that kids ages 11–18 get a booster shot of the new combination vaccine (called Tdap), ideally when they are 11 or 12 years old, instead of the Td booster routinely given at this age.

The Tdap vaccine is similar to DTaP but with lower concentrations of diphtheria and tetanus toxoid. It also should be given to adults who did not receive it as preteens or teens. The vaccine is also recommended for all pregnant women during the second half of each pregnancy, regardless of whether or not they had the vaccine before, or when it was last given.

- Identification and management of cases and contacts: Cases can be managed by early diagnosis, solation, disinfection of discharges and erythromycin 30–50 mg/kg/body weight in 4 divided doses for 10 days.
- **Contacts:** Infant and young children should kept away from cases.
- Active immunization
  - DPT
  - Pertussis vaccine
- Passive immunization.

MENINGOCOCCAL MENINGITIS

Meningococcal meningitis or cerebrospinal fever is an acute communicable disease caused by *N. meningitidis*. It usually begins with intense headache, vomiting and stiff neck and progresses to coma within a few hours. Meningococcal meningitis is a rare but serious infection which causes inflammation of covering of brain and spinal cord. Each year, approximately 1,000 people in the US get meningococcal disease, which includes meningitis and septicemia (blood infection).

Meningococcal meningitis can be fatal or cause great harm without prompt treatment; as many as one out of five people who contract the infection have serious complications. According to the Centers for Disease Control, about 15% of those who survive are left with disabilities that include deafness, brain damage, and neurological problems.

Epidemiological Determinants

- **Agent factors:** *N. meningitidis*
- **Source of infection:** Cases or carriers.
- **Period of communicability:** Until meningococci are no longer present in discharges from nose and throat.

Host Factors

- **Age and sex:** It is a disease of children and young adult of both sexes.
- **Immunity:** All the ages are susceptible.

Environmental Factors

- Outbreaks in dry and cold months of year.
- Overcrowding

Transmission: Droplet infection
Incubation period: Usually 3 to 4 days but may vary from 2–10 days.

Clinical Manifestation

The common features are headache, neck rigidity, sudden high fever. Other symptoms are photophobia (intolerance to bright light) and phonophobia (intolerance to loud noises). Small children often do not exhibit the aforementioned symptoms, and may only be irritable and look unwell. The fontanelle (the soft spot on the top of a baby's head) can bulge in infants aged up to 6 months. Other features that distinguish meningitis from less severe illnesses in young children are leg pain, cold extremities, and an abnormal skin color.

Meningitis caused by the bacterium *Neisseria meningitidis* (known as '*meningococcal meningitis*') can be differentiated from meningitis with other causes by a rapidly spreading petechial rash, which may precede other symptoms. The rash consists of numerous small, irregular purple or red spots ('*petechiae*') on the trunk, lower extremities, mucous membranes, conjunctiva, and (occasionally) the palms of the hands or soles of the feet. The rash is typically nonblanching; the redness does not disappear when pressed with a finger or a glass tumbler.

Diagnosis:

- *Laboratory test:* CRP, complete blood count, blood culture
- CT scan and MRI.

Management

Meningitis is potentially life-threatening and has a high mortality rate if untreated, delay in treatment has been associated with a poorer outcome. Thus, treatment with wide-spectrum antibiotics should not be delayed while confirmatory tests are being conducted. If meningococcal disease is suspected in primary care, guidelines recommend that benzylpenicillin can be administered before transfer to hospital. Intravenous fluids should be administered if hypotension (low blood pressure) or shock are present. In children routine intravenous fluids for two days may improve outcomes in those who arrive at hospital after being sick for some time. If necessary patient can be admitted in ICU. Seizures are treated with anticonvulsants.

Prevention and Control

1. **Behavioral:** Bacterial and viral meningitis are contagious. Both can be transmitted through droplets of respiratory secretions during close contact, such as kissing, sneezing or coughing on someone, but cannot be spread by only breathing the air where a person with meningitis has been. Viral meningitis is typically caused by enteroviruses, and is most commonly spread through fecal contamination. The risk of infection can be decreased by changing the behavior that led to transmission.
2. **Vaccination:** Routine vaccination against *Streptococcus pneumoniae* with the pneumococcal conjugate vaccine (PCV), which is active against seven common serotypes of this pathogen, significantly reduces the incidence of pneumococcal meningitis.
3. **Antibiotics:** Rifampicin, ciprofloxacin or ceftriaxone) can reduce their risk of contracting the condition, but does not protect against future infections.
4. Environment measures—avoid overcrowding.

Acute respiratory infections: It may cause inflammation of the respiratory tract anywhere from nose to alvedi, with a wide range of combination of symptoms and signs. It classifies:

1. **Upper respiratory tract infections (URTI):** It includes common cold, pharyngitis and otitis media.
2. **Lower respiratory tract infection (LRTI):** It includes epiglottitis, laryngitis, laryngotracheitis, bronchitis, bronchiolitis and pneumonia.

CORYZA (COMMON COLD)

Common cold is a mild, self-limiting viral infection. It spreads by direct contact with infectious secretions and inhalation of droplets of infected respiratory secretions. This is the reason why it spreads fast from a person to another, especially those within close proximity with an infected person.

Clinical Features

Clinically, many people are aware of the signs of this illness or so they think they do. Below are some of the common signs that will help you to make a clinical diagnosis of coryza.

Sneezing, headache, malaise, nasal discharge and sore throat. Adults may not have fever but young children frequently do. Initially the nasal discharge is clear, watery and profuse but later becomes thick.

Complications of Coryza

These complications usually are as a result of secondary infection and include:

- **Secondary bacterial sinusitis:** This causes blocked noses and plenty of thick mucus discharge from the nose. Normally it is a main cause of nuisance, since one has to keep blowing nose. In children it may cause blocked nose hence difficulty in breathing hence need to watch over them closely.
- **Otitis media:** This is the infection of the middle part of the year, may cause itchiness and discomfort to the affected ear.

Treatment

Various approaches have been proposed for the treatment of coryza. There are however basic rules to managing the condition.

- Antibiotics are not needed for uncomplicated colds;
- Symptomatic treatment is used for common colds. That is to treat fever, headache, running nose or any other symptom with medications suitable for the symptoms.

Symptomatic Treatment

Nasal obstruction: This can be treated with:

- Decongestant nasal drops. This is useful especially for young children who experience nasal block.
- Antihistamines like piriton (sedating) or cetirizine (nonsedating). This reduces the amount of mucus in the nose.

Cough: Cough can be irritating and if unchecked could lead to further damage of the mucus membranes lining the upper air way, resulting to secondary infections. It can be treated with preparations containing codeine or dextromethorphan. This minimizes the irritation that leads to cough reflex.

Sore throat: A sore throat is a nasty experience and in some people it may be painful to swallow and at time may lead to voice alteration or reduction. Various localized remedies have been tried some successfully others may be psychological. To treat this symptom you can use:

- **Warm saline gargles:** You can request the patient to prepare it domestically by using warm water and a tinge of salt in a glass/cup. Then gurgle for a couple of minutes two to three times a day. Usually it should clear in a day or two.
- **Lozenges containing a topical anesthetic:** These help to ease the soreness resulting to relative comfort within a couple of hours.
- **Drinks:** A sore dry throat can be due to a blocked nose causing you to sleep with your mouth open—probably snoring.
    - Drink lots of fluids—water or orange juice are good.
    - Sip warm drinks like a honey, lemon juice and hot water mixture.

FLU (INFLUENZA)

Influenza is caused by one of several different influenza viruses. The viruses are spread in the same way as those that cause common colds.

Epidemiological Determinants

- **Agent factors:** Microbial agents includes bacterias and viruses.
- **Host factors:** Age—higher in children than adults, Adult women experience more illness than men.

Risk Factors

- Climate
- Overcrowding
- Poor nutrition
- Low birth weight
- Intense indoor smoke pollution
- Low socioeconomic status.

Mode of transmission: Airbrone. It can transmitted by sneezing, coughing and touching.

Sign and Symptoms

- Fever
- Headaches
- Aches in the rest of the body
- Shivering and
- Feeling hot and cold than with colds
- Bodyaches
- Nose is not all drippy and runny like with a cold.

Diagnosis: The disease can be diagnosed on the basis of sign and symptoms and serum examination.

Treatment: Influenza has no specific treatment. Clinical assessment and physical examination should be done to classify the illness from common cold/cough to very severe respiratory disease. The schedule of treatment has been depicted in **Table 11.3**.

Table 11.3: Daily dose schedule of medications.

Age/weight	Pediatric tablet Sulfamethoxazole 100 mg and Trimethoprim 20 mg	Pediatric syrup (5 mL) Sulfamethoxazole 200 mg Trimethoprim 40 mg
<2 month (wt. 3–5 kg)	One tablet twice a day	Half spoon (2.5 mL) twice a day
2–12 months (wt. 6–9 kg)	2 tablet twice a day	One spoon twice a day
1–5 years (wt. 10–19 kg)	3 tablet twice a day	One and half spoon twice a day

Control

- Improving living conditions
- Better nutrition
- Reduce of smoke pollution indoors
- Better MCH care
- Immunization
- Acute respiratory disease control program in India.

SEVERE ACUTE RESPIRATORY SYNDROME

Severe acute respiratory syndrome (SARS) is a respiratory infection but its acuteness, rapid transmission and fatality had worried all over the world in the beginning of 2003. It is a viral disease caused by coronavirus. The most common symptoms in patient progressing to dizziness, cough, sore throat, fever, malaria, chills, headache, myelgia, running nose and resulting in respiratory distress. SARS has been called as flumonia because it spreads like flu and kills like pneumonia.

Epidemiological Determinants

- **Agent factors:** New strain of coronavirus.
- **Host factors:** Children are rarely affected.

- **Environmental factors:** International flights have been associated with transmission of SARS from symptomatic probable cases to passenger or crew.
- **Incubation period:** It has been estimated 2 to 7 days, commonly 3 to 5 days.

Transmission

Close contact with patient and infected materials.

Clinical Manifestation

The major symptoms of SARS are high fever (>38.5°C), dry cough, shortness of breath or dyspnea. Other associated symptoms are headache, muscular stiffness, loss of appetite, malaise, rashes, diarrhea, confusion, etc.

Diagnosis: There is no specific diagnostic test during early stage of infection. Clinical manifestation and X-ray chest shows pneumonia.

Treatment

- Strict isolation and barrier nursing is recommended.
- Symptomatic treatment with supportive care is needed.
- Sometimes antiviral (ribavirin) and high dose of corticosteroid shows effective.
- Health worker and visitor should use personal protective equipments.

Complication: If not managed in time, it may cause death.

Control and Prevention

- Prompt identification of patient with SARDS, their movement and contact.
- Effective isolation of SARS patients in hospitals.
- Appropriate protection of medical staff treating these patients.
- Comprehensive identification and isolation of suspected SARS cases.
- Exit screening of international travelers.
- Timely and accurate reporting and sharing of information with other authorities and/or government.

CORONA VIRUS DISEASE (COVID-19)

Corona viruses are important human and animal pathogens. At the end of 2019, a novel coronavirus was identified as the cause of a cluster of pneumonia cases in Wuhan, a city in the Hubei Province of China. It rapidly spread, resulting in an epidemic throughout China, followed by a global pandemic. In February 2020, the World Health Organization designated the disease COVID-19, which stands for coronavirus disease 2019.

The incidence of COVID-19 has been increased every minute as it is a highly contaminated disease. The death rate also high during first and second wave which is slowly declined due to administration of vaccination. There are Globally, till 5th August 2022, there have been 579,092,623 confirmed cases of COVID-19, including 6,407,556 deaths, reported to WHO. Data shows as of 1 August 2022, a total of 12,308,330,588 vaccine doses have been administered. COVID-19 history said in 12th December 2019 the 1st case of COVID-19 reported in Wuhan city, Hubei province of China. In 31st Dec', 2019; Chinese authorities alerted WHO about cases of Pneumonia of unknown ethology. On 01st Jan' 2020; Wuhan Seafood Market closed by Chinese authorities. In 3rd Jan, 2020; India notified by WHO regarding the outbreak 07 Jan, nCoV identified as the causative organism.

Epidemiological Determinants

Agent factors: The virus that causes COVID-19 is designated severe acute respiratory syndrome coronavirus 2 (SARS-CoV-2). If we analyze the term COVID-19, CO' stands for corona, 'VI' for virus, 'D' for disease, and 19 refers to 2019, the year in which it was first discovered. Coronaviruses are enveloped positive-stranded RNA viruses. Full-genome sequencing and phylogenetic analysis indicated that the coronavirus that causes COVID-19 is a beta-coronavirus in the same subgenus as the severe acute respiratory syndrome (SARS) virus. Corona viruses are spherical and pleomorphic (ability to change their morphology) enveloped particles with single strand of RNA. The envelope is covered with projecting glycoproteins, and surrounds a core consisting of matrix protein. The envelope glycoproteins are responsible for attachment to the host cell. The diameter of the viral particle varies from 60 to 140 nm. The Coronavirus Study Group of the International Committee on Taxonomy of Viruses has proposed that this virus be designated severe acute respiratory syndrome coronavirus 2 (SARS-CoV-2).

Incubation period: On average, symptoms showed up in the newly infected person about 5–6 days after contact. Rarely, symptoms appeared as soon as 2 days after exposure. Most people with symptoms had them by day 12. And most of the other ill people were sick by day 14. In rare cases, symptoms can show up after 14 days. So generally incubation period for COVID-19 is 1–14 days.

Host factors: The disease become more virulent among those having multimorbidity condition like who have suffered in diabetes mellitus, coronary heart disease, cancers and other chronic diseases. In 1st wave more older population affected and died where as in 2nd wave more younger population affected. It may be due to the nature of variant.

Diagnosis: Specially collection of upper respiratory specimens like nasopharyngeal and oropharyngeal swab have been collected for diagnosis of COVID-19. Though virus can be present in other specimen like collection from lower respiratory tract but it is not used generally for diagnosis. Specimens for virus detection should reach the laboratory as soon as possible after collection. Correct handling of specimens during transportation is essential. Specimens that can be delivered promptly to the laboratory can be stored and shipped at 2–8°C. The name of the test are real time reverse transcription–polymerase chain reaction (RT-PCR) for COVID-19 virus and Serology test (rapid antibody testing).

Mode of Transmission

- **Direct close contact:**
  - Through airborne droplets from one person to other.
  - Possible aerosolized transmission.
- **Indirect contact:** Contact with the surfaces where virus is settled in active form.

Different Phases in COVID-19

So far during the pandemic, several factors have had an impact on whether new COVID-19 cases are increasing or declining in particular locations. These factors include the effectiveness of vaccines over time, human behavior, infection prevention policies, changes to the coronavirus itself, and the number of people who are vulnerable because they have not developed some immunity, whether from natural infection or through vaccination. Due to mutation of different variant the symptoms, affected risk groups are different. Based on increase and decrease of case loads and variations it has been classified as different phases **(Table 11.4)**.

For instance, a large spike of COVID-19 cases occurred over the winter months of 2020–21 when people travelled and gathered for the winter holidays. The arrival of FDA-authorized vaccines in December 2020 helped bring new infection levels back down in many areas through the spring of 2021. Another surge began in July 2021 as the contagious delta variant began to circulate and eventually become dominant. Waning immunity and relaxation of public policies and infection prevention measures also played a role. This is known as second phase or 2nd wave. Delta was first identified in India in 2020 and later it led to the second wave of the coronavirus in the country claiming millions of lives. In late 2021 and early 2022 3rd phase started with the variant of omicron. Omicron was first identified from a specimen collected on 9 November 2021. The difference between delta and omicron has been depicted in **Table 11.5**. This variant has a large number of mutations, some of which are concerning.

Table 11.4: Difference between first and second wave.

Specific characteristics	*First wave*	*Second wave*
Causative organism	SARS-CoV-2 virus	Several mutants of SARS-CoV-2 virus
Knowledge about the disease	Less	More
Symptomatology	More related to respiratory system	Newer symptoms like gastrointestinal, etc., adding
Presentation	More severe	Lesser intense
Shortness of breaths	Less cases with breathlessness	More cases with breathlessness
Age profile of the patients	More older population	More younger population
Comorbidities	Patients with comorbidities affected more	Less
Drug availability	Acute shortage and black marketing	Available in the hospitals and pharmacies
Healthcare workers	Lesser trained people • Fear of acquiring infection • Not vaccinated	• More trained increased • Lesser fear to acquire infection • Mostly vaccinated

Table 11.5: Difference between delta and omicron.

Characteristics	*Delta*	*Omicron*
Symptoms	Delta may result in more severe symptoms if critical likely to lose their sense of smell	Omicron are less likely to lose their sense of smell. Experts reveal that fatigue, joint pain, cold and headaches are four common signs of omicron
Lung involvement	Lung involvement more	Lung involvement less
Multiplication	Less multiplies in the throat	Largely multiplies in the throat
Identification in India	Delta was first identified in India in 2020 and later it led to the second wave of the coronavirus in the country claiming millions of lives	First identified in Late 2021
Hospitalization	More Hospitalization	Less Hospitalization Omicron may cause milder cases in vaccinated individuals, and severe cases in unvaccinated
Incubation period	Comparatively longer incubation period	Omicron has a shorter incubation time than other variants

Prevention and Management

COVID-19 is a highly contagious deadly disease and in 1st phase the vaccines were not available, so strict infection control protocols have been applied by both center and state Government. In every health care set-up strict infection control technique have been followed. The Doctors, Nurses and other paramedic have been trained regarding care of COVID-19 patients.

For controlling of COVID-19 Govt. has taken many steps like, following strict lockdown guidelines, setting up extensive care and medical facilities, following rules of social distancing and self-quarantining, sealing of hotspots, arranging test kits, Isolation of patients, quarantine of risk cases, large scale testing of slum dwellers and other such low lying areas, and setting up R and D to work on potential antidote etc. At health care level these following points have given importance

- Applying standard precautions for all patients like hand hygiene, respiratory hygiene (etiquette), PPE according to the risk, safe injection practices, sharps management and injury prevention, safe handling, cleaning and disinfection of patient care equipment, environmental cleaning, safe handling and cleaning of soiled linen and waste management.

- Ensuring triage, early recognition, and source control
- Implementing empiric additional precautions for suspected cases of COVID-19 infection
- Implementing administrative controls
- Using environmental and engineering controls.

At the Community level the community health nurse must be concern about:

- Early identification of illness.
- Prevention of community spread and containment of disease.
- Care of patients with symptoms associated with Coronavirus Disease (COVID-19)
- Protection of self and other HCWs
- Health education
- Prevention of stigma.

Type of Treatments

The FDA has authorized certain antiviral medications and monoclonal antibodies to treat mild to moderate COVID-19 in people who are more likely to get very sick.

Antiviral treatments target specific parts of the virus to stop it from multiplying in the body, helping to prevent severe illness and death.

Monoclonal antibodies help the immune system recognize and respond more effectively to the virus.

The National Institutes of Health (NIH) provides COVID-19 Treatment Guidelines for healthcare providers to help them work with their patients and determine the best treatment options for them. Several options are available for treating COVID-19 at home or in an outpatient setting. People at home receiving treatment from healthcare provider by staying at home through counseling by phone. The different forms of treatments for different groups have been depicted in **Table 11.6**.

COVID-19 Vaccination

There are several COVID-19 vaccines validated for use by WHO (given Emergency Use Listing). The first mass vaccination program started in early December 2020 and the number of vaccination doses administered is updated on a daily basis on the COVID-19 dashboard.

The WHO Emergency Use Listing process determines whether a product can be recommended for use based on all the available data on safety and efficacy and on its suitability in low- and middle-income countries. Vaccines are assessed to ensure they meet acceptable standards of quality, safety and efficacy using clinical trial data, manufacturing and quality control processes.

As of 12 January 2022, the following vaccines have obtained EUL:

- The Pfizer/BioNTech Comirnaty vaccine, 31 December 2020.
- The SII/COVISHIELD and AstraZeneca/AZD1222 vaccines, 16 February 2021.
- The Janssen/Ad26.COV 2.S vaccine developed by Johnson and Johnson, 12 March 2021.
- The Moderna COVID-19 vaccine (mRNA 1273), 30 April 2021.
- The Sinopharm COVID-19 vaccine, 7 May 2021.
- The Sinovac-CoronaVac vaccine, 1 June 2021.
- The Bharat Biotech BBV152 COVAXIN vaccine, 3 November 2021.
- The Covovax (NVX-CoV2373) vaccine, 17 December 2021.
- The Nuvaxovid (NVX-CoV2373) vaccine, 20 December 2021.

The COVID-19 vaccines with WHO Emergency Use Listing (EUL) provide different levels of protection to infection, mild disease, severe disease, hospitalization and death. Research is ongoing by thousands of scientists around the world to better understand how new virus mutations and variants affect the effectiveness of the different COVID-19 vaccines.

In general, the COVID-19 vaccines are very effective at preventing serious illness, hospitalization and death from all current virus variants. They are less effective at protecting you against infection and mild disease than they were for earlier virus variants; but if you do get ill after being vaccinated, your symptoms are more likely to be mild.

COVID-19 vaccines are an important tool to stop the pandemic, but they will not do so on their own. Public health and social measures such as surveillance, contact tracing, isolation and individual protective behaviors such as staying at least 1 meter away from other people, wearing a properly fitted mask over your nose and mouth, avoiding poorly ventilated places and settings, staying home if unwell, covering coughs and sneezes and cleaning your hands frequently remain essential to breaking the chain of transmission.

Table 11.6: Different treatments for COVID-19.

Treatment	*Who*	*When*	*How*
Nirmatrelvir with Ritonavi (Paxlovid) Antiviral	Adults; children ages 12 years and older	Start as soon as possible; must begin within 5 days of when symptoms start	Taken at home by mouth (orally)
Remdesivir (Veklury) Antiviral	Adults and children	Start as soon as possible; must begin within 7 days of when symptoms start	Intravenous (IV) infusions at a healthcare facility for 3 consecutive days
Bebtelovimab Monoclonal antibody	Adults; children ages 12 years and older	Start as soon as possible; must begin within 7 days of when symptoms start	Single IV injection
Molnupiravir (Lagevrio) Antiviral	Adults	Start as soon as possible; must begin within 5 days of when symptoms start	Taken at home by mouth (orally)

TUBERCULOSIS

Tuberculosis has remained an enemy of human society. Tuberculosis is a specific infectious disease caused by *M. tuberculosis*. The disease primarily affects lungs and causes pulmonary tuberculosis. Tuberculous infection occurs when a person carries the tubercle bacilli inside the body, but the bacteria are in small numbers and are dormant. These dormant bacteria are kept under control by the body's defenses and do not cause disease. Many people have tuberculous infection and are well. Tuberculosis is a state in which one or more organs of the body become diseased as shown by clinical symptoms and signs. This is because the tubercle bacilli in the body have started to multiply and become numerous enough to overcome the body's defenses.

Tuberculosis is an airborne transmitted disease can affect any part of the body pulmonary TB—most common form 80% of TB cases.

Extrapulmonary TB: Any body part other than lungs Among Tuberculosis cases 10–15% risk of developing active TB disease in HIV infected persons. Among the three greatest causes of death among women aged 15–44 years. Pediatric cases constitute about 10–15% of all TB cases.

Magnitude of TB	Global	Indian
Incidence of disease	8.6 million	2.2 million
Prevalence of disease	12 million	2.8 million
Mortality	1.3 million	270,000
HIV prevalence among incident cases	13%	5%
Source: WHO Global Tuberculosis Report 2013		

Pathology

TB is a bacterial infection caused by *Mycobacterium tuberculosis* (M.tuberculosis) also referred to as tubercle bacilli. The *M. tuberculosis* is a Gram-positive aerobic bacterium. It is a small rod-like bacillus with a complex cell wall, which can withstand weak disinfectants and survive in a dry state for weeks, but can only grow in a host organism. It most commonly affects the lungs, producing pulmonary TB. However, transported by the blood or lymphatic system, the TB bacilli can infect almost any part of the body, including lymph glands, joints, kidneys, and bone—extrapulmonary TB. It is critical to understand the disease, its etiology and its epidemiology to develop a strong TB control programme. Early symptoms of pulmonary TB are often vague and easily attributable to other conditions, with the result that many cases of active, infectious TB can remain undetected for some time. Thus, the disease spreads from one person to another. TB is spread when an infectious person coughs, sneezes, talks or sings, releasing droplets containing the bacilli into the air. However, TB can also be spread when TB bacilli are aerosolized by treatments, such as irrigating a wound that is infected with TB. In either case, a susceptible person inhales the airborne droplets, which then traverse the upper respiratory tract and bronchi to reach the alveoli of the lungs. Once in the alveoli, alveolar macrophages take up the TB bacilli, holding some in the lungs, and transporting others throughout the body. Usually within 2–10 weeks, the immune response limits further multiplication and spread of the bacilli.

Epidemiological Determinants

Agent factors: TB is a bacterial disease caused by *Mycobacterium tuberculosis* (and occasionally by *Mycobacterium bovis* and *Mycobacterium africanum*). These organisms are also known as tubercle bacilli (because they cause lesions called tubercles) or as acid-fast bacilli (AFB). When sputum containing tubercle bacilli is stained with certain dyes and examined under the microscope, the bacilli look red. This is because they are acid-fast (they have kept the dye even after being washed with acid and alcohol). Tubercle bacilli can remain dormant in tissues and persist for many years.

Source of Infection

The most important source of infection is the patient with TB of the lung, or pulmonary TB (PTB), and who is coughing. This person is usually sputum smear-positive. Coughing produces tiny infectious droplet nuclei (infectious particles of respiratory secretions usually less than 5 μm in diameter and containing tubercle bacilli). A single cough can produce 3000 droplet nuclei. Droplet nuclei can also be spread into the air by talking, sneezing, spitting and singing, and can remain suspended in the air for long periods. Bovine source of infection is infected milk. Unpasteurized infected milk can also spread bovine tuberculosis milkborne *M. bovis* may infect the tonsils presenting as scrofula (cervical lymphadenitis), or the intestinal tract, causing abdominal TB.

Risk of Infection

An individual's risk of infection depends on the extent of exposure to droplet nuclei and his or her susceptibility to infection. The risk of infection of a susceptible individual is high with close, prolonged, indoor exposure to a person with sputum smear-positive PTB. The risk of transmission of infection from a person with sputum smear-negative PTB is low, and even lower from someone with extrapulmonary TB (EPTB). Patients are infective for risk of transmission as long as they remain untreated but after starting treatment after two months they will be no more infective.

Host Factors

- **Age and sex:** It affects all ages and more prevalent in males than in females.
- **Nutrition:** Malnutrition predisposing to this condition.
- **Immunity:** Man has no inherited immunity against TB.

Social Factors

Tuberculosis is a social disease with medical aspects. There are a varieties of social factors which includes poor quality of life like poorly ventilated housing, smoking, stress, social deprivation and poor social capital. Overcrowding population explosion, under nutrition, lack of education, large families, early marriages and lack of awareness are the factors for disease transmission.

From infection to development of a positive TB skin test reaction (the incubation period) is approximately 2 to 12 weeks. The risk for developing active disease is the highest in the first two years after infection and development of a positive TB skin test reaction.

Diagnosis

Sputum smear microscopy: To confirm active disease, the patient's sputum must be examined. *M. tuberculosis* is identified microscopically by its staining characteristics: It retains certain stains after being treated with acid solution. Therefore, it is classified as an 'acid-fast bacillus' (AFB). The most common staining technique is the Ziehl-Neelsen stain. AFB are stained bright red, which stands out clearly against a blue background. In addition, AFB can be visualized by fluorescent microscopy, and by an auramine-rhodamine stain. In addition, all specimen should be isolated and identified by means of a sputum culture. Culturing the specimen means growing the mycobacteria on media, substances that contain nutrients, in the laboratory. When the mycobacteria have formed colonies they can be identified.

Chest X-ray: Helpful in suspects found to be smear negative to look for cavitations, areas of consolidation and infiltration, enlargements of the hilar.

Computer Tomography (CT) and Magnetic Resonance Imaging (MRI): Useful for guiding the diagnosis process in some difficult cases, but frequently not available.

Tuberculin skin test: In this test, a substance called tuberculin is injected into the skin of the arm. Tuberculin is protein derived from tubercle bacilli that have been killed by heating. In most infected people, the immune system will recognize the tuberculin because it is similar to the tubercle bacilli that caused infection. This will cause reaction to the tuberculin. Tuberculin is used for diagnosing; it is not a vaccine.

Monoresistant TB: TB in patients whose infecting isolates of *M. tuberculosis* are confirmed to be resistant *in vitro* to one first-line anti-TB drug.

I-resistant TB: TB in patients whose infecting isolates are resistant *in vitro* to more than one first-line drug, other than isoniazid and rifampicin.

Multidrug resistant TB: It is active TB involving *M. tuberculosis* organisms that are resistant to at least both isoniazid and rifampicin, the two most powerful anti-TB agents. An MDR-TB strain can be resistant to more than these two antibiotics and in most cases it is resistant to other first-line drugs. Although MDR-TB varies widely across regions, it occurs in all geographical settings able to produce data and is therefore a world-wide problem. WHO estimates a global prevalence of one million MDR-TB cases, and some 300,000–600,000 new cases emerging every year. China, India and the Russian Federation account for 68% of the annual incidence of MDR-TB cases 15 of the estimated 300,000–600,000 new cases of MDR-TB, about half of them are new TB patients (primary drug resistance) and the other half have been previously treated (acquired drug resistance).

Extensive-drug resistant TB: It is defined as resistance to at least rifampicin and isoniazid, in addition to any fluoroquinolone, and to at least one of the three following injectable drugs used in anti-TB treatment: Capreomycin, kanamycin and amikacin. Extensively Drug-Resistant TB (XDR-TB) is a rare type of MDR-TB. XDR-TB is defined as resistance to rifampicin and isoniazid (which is the definition of MDR-TB), in addition to any fluoroquinolone, and at least one of the three following injectable drugs used in anti-TB treatment: capreomycin, kanamycin and amikacin. Because XDR-TB is resistant to first- and second-line drugs, patients are left with treatment options that are less effective. However, it can be identified early, can be treated and cured in some cases under proper TB control conditions. Successful treatment outcomes depend on the extent of the drug resistance, the severity of the disease and the immune response of the patient. Patients with pulmonary TB are referred to as either smear positive or smear negative. This is an important distinction as smear positive patients tend to have more advanced disease with more damage to their lungs so they cough up more infectious material and are therefore more contagious. Without treatment, the outcome of their disease is poorer than that of smear.

Diagnosis of Extrapulmonary TB

The diagnosis of extrapulmonary TB can be difficult as it is less common than pulmonary disease and there may be numerous differential diagnoses. It is therefore essential to recognize the general symptoms of TB that are common to both pulmonary and extrapulmonary TB. Specific symptoms for extrapulmonary TB vary according to the site of disease but severe pain is common—this can be excruciating when it causes destruction in bones and joints. In some cases, particularly with regard to lymph node TB, it may be possible to collect pus by aspirating the infected site. Biopsies may also be useful, but it is important to remember to send specimens for both histopathological as well as microbiological examination. If at all possible diagnosis should be based on culture positive specimen, or historical or strong clinical evidence consistent with active TB, followed by a decision by a clinician to treat with a full course of anti-TB chemotherapy. A list of diagnostic tests is included in the table above. There is likely to be varied availability of these tests especially, imaging, according to local resources.

Contact Tracing

In some countries contact tracing is initiated at the initial assessment. The patient provides a list of those people closest to him/her. These people are then invited for screening: A symptoms check, a tuberculin skin test and/or a chest X-ray. If resources are scarce, the patient is encouraged to identify anyone he knows who is showing signs or symptoms of the disease and to encourage them to come to the health clinic for investigation. As a minimum, all children under the age of five living in the patient's household are examined. Whatever the circumstances, this is a distressing process, since the patient may not want others to know that he has TB. Contact tracing offers a good opportunity to educate others about TB and address stigma, thus increasing the patient's support system. Contract tracing must always be conducted sympathetically, with the greatest possible effort to maintain confidentiality.

Chemotherapy

The WHO recommended formulations of anti-TB drugs and fixed-dose combinations (FDCs) of drugs appear in the *WHO Model List of Essential Medicines* (available at www.who.int/medicines/publications/essentialmedicines/en). The formulations and combinations of anti-TB drugs available in each country. To facilitate procurement, distribution and administration of treatment to patients, the daily dosage may be standardized for three or four body weight bands—for instance 30–39 kg, 40–54 kg, 55–70 kg and over 70 kg, as is done with the Global Drug Facility patient kits.

Long course regimen: 18 months of treatment was required to avoid relapses.

Short course chemotherapy: Short course regimens of 6 months duration that are highly recommended doses of first-line antituberculosis drugs for adults **(Table 11.7)**.

The antitubercular drugs are classified into two groups

1. **Bactericidal:**
   - Rifampicin 10–12 mg/kg body weight
   - Streptomycin 0.75 to 1 g
   - Pyrazinamide 30 mg/kg body weight divided in 2 or 3 doses/day
   - INH 4–5 mg/kg of body weight.
2. **Bacteriostatic drugs:**
   - Ethambutol 15 mg/kg body weight given in 2 to 3 times
   - Thioacetazone 2 mg/kg body weight.

Table 11.7: Treatment regimen of tuberculosis.

Drug	*Recommended dose*			
	Daily		*Three times per week*	
	Dose and range (mg/kg body weight)	*Maximum (mg)*	*Dose and range (mg/kg body weight)*	*Daily maximum (mg)*
Isoniazid	5 (4–6)	300	10 (8–12)	900
Rifampicin	10 (8–12)	600	10 (8–12)	600
Pyrazinamide	25 (20–30)	–	35 (30–40)	–
Ethambutol	15 (15–20)	–	30 (25–35)	–
Streptomycin	15 (12–18)		15 (12–18)	1000

Category IV (Dots–Plus) Treatment for MDR-TB

Recognizing that the diagnosis and treatment of MDR-TB is complex, RNTCP has developed national guidelines based on the WHO recommend international DOTS-Pus guidelines. Drug resistance may be suspected based on history of prior treatment (e.g., smear positive case after repeated treatment courses. Category II failure, etc.) and/or close exposure to a possible source case confirmed to have drug-resistant TB. As per guidelines the diagnosis of MDR-TB is at intermediate reference laboratories accredited to perform culture and drug sensitivity testing (DST).

Treatment regime: The treatment used is -6 (9) Km Ofx Eto Cs ZE+ 18 Ofx Eto CsE (Km—Kanamycin; Ofx—Ofloxacin; Eto—Ethinamide; Cs—Cycloserine; Z—Pyrazinamide; E—Ethambutol).

If results of second line DST from accredited laboratory are available, an individualized regimen may be used in such patients after obtaining a detailed history of previous anti-TB treatment.

Duration of treatment: At least six months of intensive phases should be given, extended up to nine months in patients who have a positive culture result taken at fourth month of treatment. Minimum 18 months of continuation phase should be given following the intensive phase. Treatment categories and sputum examination schedule in DOTS chemotherapy in India and management of patients who were smear-negative at diagnosis and who interrupt treatment has been given in **Tables 11.8 and 11.9**.

POLIOMYELITIS

Poliomyelitis is an acute viral infection caused by an RNA virus that can affect nerves and can lead to partial or full paralysis. It is primarily an infection, the human alimentary tract but the virus may infect the CNS in a very small percentage of cases resulting in varying degrees of paralysis and possibly death.

Epidemiological Determinants

- **Agent factors:** Polio virus which has 3 serotypes 1, 2 and 3.
- **Reservoir of infection:** Man
- **Infective material:** Viruses found in the faces and oropharyngeal sex reactions of infected person.
- **Period of communicability:** Cases most infectious 7 to 10 days before and after onset of symptoms.

Host Factors

- **Age:** Most vulnerable age is between 6 months and 3 years.
- **Sex:** 3 males to one female ratio.
- **Risk factors:** Precipitate an attack of paralytic polio in individual already with polio viruses.
- **Immunity:** The maternal antibodies gradually disappear during the first 6 months of life.
- **Environmental factors:** Occurs during rainy season
- **Mode of transmission:** It is mainly transmitted by fecal—oral route and Droplet infection.
- **Incubation period:** Usually 7 to 14 days.

Table 11.8: Treatment categories and sputum examination schedule in DOTS chemotherapy in India.

Treatment regimen			*Sputum examinations for pulmonary TB*			
Category of treatment	Type of patient	Regimen*	Pretreatment sputum	Test at month	If result is	THEN:
New cases Category 1 Red Box	New sputum smear-positive New Sputum negative New extrapulmonary** Sputum smear-positive treatment after default others	$2(HRZE)_3$ + $4(HR)_3$	+	2	-	Start Continuation phase, test sputum again at 4 and 6 months[#]
					+	Continue intensive phase, for one more month[#] Complete the treatment in 7 months
Previously treated Category II Blue Box	Sputum smear-positive Relapse*** Sputum smear-positive Failure*** Sputum smear-positive treatment after default others	$2(HRZES)_3$ + $4(HRZE)_3$ + $5(HRE)_3$	+	3	-	Start Continuation phase, test sputum again at 5 months and 6 months, completion of treatment[#]
					-	Continue intensive phase for one more month, test sputum again at 4 months if sputum is positive send sputum for culture and drug sensitivity as it might be a case of MD –TB[#]

*The number before the letters refers to the number of months of treatment. The subscript after the letters refers to the number of doses per week. H: Isoniazid (600 mg), R: Rifampicin (450 mg), Z: Pyrazinamide (1500 mg), E: Ethambutol (1200 mg), S: Streptomycin (750 mg). Patients who weigh more than 60 kg. receive additional rifampicin 150 mg. Patients more than 50 years old receive streptomoycin 500 mg. Patients in categories I and II, who have a positive sputum smear at the end of the initial intensive phase, receive an additional month of intensive phase treatment.

**Examples of seriously ill extrapulmonary TB cases are meningitis, disseminated TB, tuberculous pericarditis, peritonitis, bilateral or extensive pleurisy, spinal TB with neurological complications and intestinal and genitor-urinary TB.

***In rare and exceptional cases, patients who are sputum smear-negative or who have extrapulmonary disease can have relapse or failure. This diagnosis in all such cases should always be made by an MO and should be supported by culture or histological evidence of current, active tuberculosis. In these cases, the patient should be categorized as 'Other' and given Category II treatment.

#Any patient treated with Category I who has a positive smear at 5 months of treatment should be considered a failure and started on Category II treatment, afresh. If category I sputum smear-ve case fails to improve or if patient develops pulmonary signs and positive smear at the end of intensive phase, it is considered treatment failure. Start category II treatment and confirm failure by culture and perform DST.

Table 11.9: Management of patients who were smear–negative at diagnosis and who interrupt treatment.

Treatment received before interruption	*Length of interruption*	*Do a sputum smear examination*	*Result of sputum smear examination*	*Outcome*	*Re-registration*	*Treatment*
Less than 1 month	Less than 2 months	No	—	—	—	Resume treatment and complete all doses
	2 months or more	Yes	Negative	—	—	Resume treatment
			Positive	Default	New	Begin CAT I afresh
More than 1 month	Less than 2 months	No	—	—	—	Resume treatment and complete all doses
	More than 2 months	Yes	Negative	—	—	Resume treatment and complete all doses
			Positive	Default	Treatment after default	Begin CAT II treatment afresh

Risks include:
- Lack of immunization against polio
- Travel to an area that has experienced a polio outbreak.

Clinical Manifestation

There are three basic patterns of polio infection: subclinical infections, nonparalytic, and paralytic. Most people have subclinical infection, and may not have symptoms.

Subclinical infection symptoms
- General discomfort or uneasiness (malaise)
- Headache
- Red throat
- Slight fever
- Sore throat
- Vomiting.

People with subclinical polio infection might not have symptoms, or mild symptoms may last 72 hours or less.

Clinical poliomyelitis affects the central nervous system (brain and spinal cord), and is divided into nonparalytic and paralytic forms. It may occur after recovery from a subclinical infection.

Diagnosis

Physical assessment
- Abnormal reflexes
- Back stiffness

- Difficulty lifting the head or legs when lying flat on the back
- Stiff neck
- Trouble bending the neck.

Tests include:
- Cultures of throat washings, stools, or spinal fluid
- Spinal tap and examination of the spinal fluid (CSF examination) using PCR
- Test for levels of antibodies to the poliovirus.

Treatment

The goal of treatment is to control symptoms while the infection runs its course as there are no specific treatment for this viral infection.

People with severe cases may need life saving measures, especially breathing help. Symptoms are treated based on their severity. Treatment may include:
- Antibiotics for urinary tract infections
- Moist heat (heating pads, warm towels) to reduce muscle pain and spasms
- Analgesics to reduce headache, muscle pain, and spasms (narcotics are not usually given because they increase the risk of breathing trouble)
- Physical therapy, braces or corrective shoes, or orthopedic surgery to help recover muscle strength and function.

Prognosis

The prognosis depends on the form of the disease (subclinical, or paralytic) and the body area affected. Most of the time, complete recovery is likely if the spinal cord and brain are not involved. Brain or spinal cord is involved that lead to paralysis or death (from respiratory disorder). Disability is more common than death. Infection that is located high in the spinal cord or in the brain increases the risk of breathing problems.

Possible Complications

- Aspiration pneumonia
- Cor pulmonale (a form of heart failure found on the right side of the circulation system)
- Lack of movement
- Lung problems
- Myocarditis
- Paralytic ileus (loss of intestinal function)
- Permanent muscle paralysis, disability, deformity
- Pulmonary edema
- Shock
- Urinary tract infections.

Postpolio syndrome is a complication that develops in some patients, usually 30 or more years after they are first infected. Muscles that were already weak may get weaker. Weakness may also develop in muscles that were not affected before.

Prevention

Vaccination (oral polio vaccine) inactivated (salk) polio vaccine.

Strategies for polio eradication in India:
- Conduct pulse polio immunization days every year for 3–4 years or until poliomyelitis is eradicated.
- Sustain high level of routine immunization coverage.
- Monitor OPV coverage at district level and below.
- Improve surveillance capable of detecting all cases of AFP due to polio and nonpolio etiology.
- Ensure rapid case investigation, including the collection of stool samples for virus isolation.
- Arrange follow-up of all cases of AFP at 60 days to check for residual paralysis.
- Conduct outbreak control for cases confirmed or suspected to be poliomyelitis to stop transmission.

Mopping up

Mopping up involves door-to-door immunization.

Pulse polio immunization was started in 1995, in India, eradication programme has not yet reached the point where it can completely shift to mop-up activities.

VIRAL HEPATITIS

Viral hepatitis may be defined as infection of the liver caused by any of half dozen viruses.

Hepatitis–A

It is an acute infectious disease cause by hepatitis A virus. The disease is heralded by nonspecific symptoms such as fever, chills, headache, fatigue, generalized weakness and aches and pain, followed by anorexia, nausea, vomiting, dark urine, and jaundice.

Epidemiological Determinants

Agent factors: The hepatitis A virus is an enterovirus of the picornaviridae family. Following ingestion, HAV enters the bloodstream through the epithelium of the oropharynx or intestine. The blood carries the virus to its target, the liver, where it multiplies within hepatocytes and Kupffer cells (liver macrophages). *Virions* are secreted into the bile and released in stool. HAV is excreted in large quantities approximately 11 days prior to appearance of symptoms or anti-HAV IgM antibodies in the blood.

Resistance

Virus is fairly resistant to heat and chemicals especially resistant to detergent, acid (pH 1), solvents (e.g., ether, (chloroform, drying, and temperatures up to 60°C).

Reservoir of infection: Human cases are only reservoir of infection.

Period of Infectivity

The risk of transmitting HAV is greatest from the latter half of the incubation period until a few days after the onset of jaundice (i.e., from 2 weeks before to 1 week after the onset of jaundice), corresponding to a peak in transaminase levels in cases without jaundice. Most cases are not infectious after the first week of jaundice. Long-term carriage or excretion of the virus does not occur.

Infective Material

Mainly man's feces, blood, serum and other fluids are infective during the brief stage of viremia. HAV is excreted in the feces for about 2 weeks before the onset of jaundice and for up to one week thereafter.

Host Factors

- **Age:** Infection with HAV is more frequent among children than in adults.
- **Sex:** Both sexes are equally susceptible.
- **Immunity:** Immunity after attack probably lasts for life.

Environmental Factors

- Cases may occur throughout the year.
- Poor sanitation, overcrowding favor the spread of infection, giving rise to waterborne and food borne epidemics.

Modes of Transmission

- **Fecal oral route:** Infection is transmitted by the fecal-oral route from person to person or via fomites. Infectious food handlers may contaminate noncooked foods such as salads.
- Infection can also occur through ingestion of contaminated food or water. Filter-feeding shellfish such as oysters raised in contaminated waters may harbor the virus.
- **Parenteral route:** Hepatitis A can be transmitted by the parenteral route but very rarely through blood and blood products.
- Sexual transmission hepatitis A can also be transmitted through sexual transmission.

Incubation Period

Incubation period for hepatitis A is 15 to 45 days.

Diagnosis

- Demonstration of HAV particles or specific viral antigens in the feces.
- Demonstration of a rise in anti-HAV titer
- Detection of IgM antibody to HAV in the patients serum.

Prevention and Containment

Control of reservoir: As the reservoir of infection is a human being so control of reservoir of HAV is difficult because firstly there is prolong fecal shedding of the virus through defecation and open field defecation is highly present in rural area of India secondly low socioeconomic profile of the people leads them poor lifestyle and unhygienic practices and thirdly absence of specific treatment for the infected person.

Control of transmission: Control of transmission of HAV infection is possible by emphasizing on hygienic practices, The hygienic practices can be followed as such like:

- Handwashing before eating and after toilet
- Food hygiene
- Avoidance of fly breeding
- Sanitary disposal of excreta
- Purification of water and adequate supplies of safe drinking water.

Control of Susceptible Population

Vaccines: The best way to prevent hepatitis A is through vaccination with the hepatitis A vaccine. Vaccination is recommended for all children age 12 months and older, for travelers to certain countries, and for people at high risk for infection with the virus.

The hepatitis A vaccine is given as two shots, six months apart. The hepatitis A vaccine also comes in a combination form, containing both hepatitis A and B vaccine, that can be given to persons 18 years of age and older. This form is given as three shots, over a period of six months or as three shots over one month and a booster shot at 12 months.

The Centers for Disease Control and Prevention recommends the following individuals receive a hepatitis A vaccine:

- All children at age 1, or older children who did not receive the vaccine at age 1
- Laboratory workers who may come in contact with hepatitis A
- Men who have sex with men
- People planning travel to areas of the world with high rates of hepatitis A
- People who use illegal drugs, injected and noninjected
- People who receive treatment with clotting-factor concentrates
- People with chronic liver disease.

Immune Globulin

Immune globulin is a substance made from human blood plasma that contains antibodies that protect against infection. Immune globulin for Hepatitis A is given as a shot and provides short-term protection (approximately 3 months) against Hepatitis A. Immune globulin can be given either before exposure to the Hepatitis A virus (such as before travel to a country where Hepatitis A is common) or to prevent infection after exposure to the Hepatitis A virus. Immune globulin must be given within 2 weeks after exposure for the best protection.

Hepatitis-B

It is an acute systemic infection with major pathology in the liver, caused by hepatitis B virus and transmitted usually by the parenteral route.

Sign and Symptoms

Generally hepatitis B often has no symptoms. Sometimes people are not aware that they have the infection. About 1 out of 2 adults who have it never have hepatitis B symptoms. Usually the symptoms of hepatitis appear between six weeks and six months after infection. The symptoms include extreme tiredness, tenderness and pain in the lower abdomen, loss of appetite nausea, vomiting, pain in the joints, headache, fever, skin rashes, etc., and in later stage of hepatitis B symptoms include more severe abdominal pain, dark urine, pale-colored bowel movements. Jaundice—yellowing of the skin and eyes, etc.

Epidemiological Determinants

Agent factors: Agent is the Hepatitis B virus that infects the liver. The surface antigen is the first to be detected. It appears in the serum during the incubation period before biochemical evidence of liver damage or the onset of jaundice.

Reservoir of Infection

Man is the only reservoir of infection. Contaminated blood, body secretions such as vaginal secretions and semen of infected person are infected material.

- **Resistance:** Virus is quite stable and capable of surviving for days on environmental surfaces.
- **Period of communicability:** Virus is present in the blood during the incubation period (for a month before jaundiced) and acute phase of the disease.

Host Factors

- **Age:** Highest prevalence in the 20–40 years age group.
- **Risk group:** Includes recipients of blood transfusions, health care and laboratory personnel, homosexuals, prostitutes, percutaneous drug abusers, infants of HBV carrier mothers and patient who are immunocompromised.

Modes of Transmission

- **Parenteral route:** Parenteral route is the major route of transmission which include syringes, needles, IV infusion sets, contaminated blood and blood products, Improper sterilization of syringe needles and tubings can aid this transmission.
- **Perinatal route:** The name of the route of transmission indicates the transmission from mother to child may be during pregnancy, delivery or during postnatal period through breastfeeding. This can be prevented by proper diagnosis and vaccination before pregnancy.
- **Sexual transmission:** Hepatitis-B can be transmitted by both homosex and heterosex. The vaginal fluid, seminal fluid can infect with Hepatitis-B.
- **Other route:** Transmission from child to child, often called horizontal transmission, by blood sucking arthropods (e.g., Mosquito, bed bugs).

Incubation period for *Hepatitis-B* can extends from 45 to 180 days.

Prevention and Containment

Vaccine

Hepatitis B vaccine: The hepatitis B vaccine contains hepatitis B surface antigen (HBsAg) adsorbed on to aluminum hydroxide adjuvant. There is also a combined vaccine available with provides protection against hepatitis A and hepatitis B. This vaccine is safe and effective, but should not be seen as an alternative to a strategy of prevention of transmission.

Recommendation

The hepatitis B vaccination is recommended for the high-risk groups like:

- Those who may be exposed to blood or blood products through their occupation, e.g., healthcare workers, ambulance crews, carers of high-risk or known patients, and morticians.
- Travelers who intend to stay for long periods in high-prevalence areas.
- Those considered to be at risk of hepatitis B through their planned activities, e.g., volunteers undertaking manual work, taking part in contact sports, involvement with casual sex.
- Those individuals who change sexual partners frequently.
- Travelers with pre-existing medical conditions, who may be at higher risk of requiring medical procedures abroad, e.g., pregnancy. (Pregnancy is not a contraindication to immunization.)
- Injecting drug users.
- Partners and children of injecting drug users.
- Noninjecting drug users who live with injecting drug users.
- Individuals in residential accommodation for those with learning difficulties.
- People travelling to or going to reside in areas of high or intermediate prevalence.
- Hemophiliacs requiring treatment and those who are receiving regular blood or blood products.
- Prisoners and prison officers.
- Family contacts of those with chronic hepatitis B infection.
- Those patients with chronic kidney disease or chronic liver disease.
- All pregnant women should be screened for hepatitis B virus (HBV).
- If positive, the baby should receive vaccination soon after birth.
- Babies born to highly infectious mothers should also receive hepatitis B immunoglobulin.

The vaccine protects against the hepatitis B virus by making the body's immune system develop antibodies. The hepatitis B vaccine is given in a series of three shots:

1. 1st dose/mL at elected date
2. 2nd dose/mL 1 month later
3. 3rd dose/mL 6 months after the 1st dose.

Hepatitis B immunoglobulin: Hepatitis B immune globulin (HBIG) is a human immune globulin that is used to prevent the development of hepatitis B. HBIG is prepared from the plasma of donors who have high antibody levels of the hepatitis B surface antigen. It is extracted from the

Cohn fraction II During the process, viruses are deactivated, and in the final steps, solvents used in the preparation are removed. The preparation is tested for absence of HIV, HCV and herpes virus. Prevention of hepatitis B infection following parenteral exposure (e.g., needle stick), direct mucous membrane contact, or oral ingestion (e.g., pipetting accident); prevention of hepatitis B in infants born to hepatitis B surface antigen (HBsAg)-positive mothers; prevention of hepatitis B after sexual exposure to an HBsAg positive person; prevention of hepatitis B following household exposure to persons.

Other preventive measures: Measures to be taken include:
- Practise safe sex
- Avoid sharing intravenous drug paraphernalia
- Immunize at-risk individuals
- Wear gloves when exposed to blood or body fluids
- Clear up blood or body fluids, using warm water and detergent
- Ensure surgical instruments are disposable or adequately sterilized
- Handle 'sharps' safely
- Wear goggles if there is risk of infected material splashing into the eye
- Do not permit health care workers (who are positive for hepatitis B e antigen (HBeAg) to work in areas where they could be a risk to other.

Hepatitis C

Hepatitis C is part of a group of hepatitis viruses which is commonly found in infected blood. It is rarely found in semen (cum) and vaginal fluids. The virus is usually passed on through using contaminated needles and syringes or other items with infected blood on them and also be passed on through unprotected sex, especially when blood is present.

Hepatitis C (known as hep C or HCV) is part of a group of hepatitis viruses that attack the liver. Chronic hepatitis C can be serious and without appropriate treatment and care, can cause liver disease and liver cancer. Treatment, where available, can cure hepatitis C in most cases. Hepatitis C is a liver disease caused by the hepatitis C virus (HCV). The virus can cause both acute and in severity from a mild illness lasting a few weeks to a serious, lifelong illness. It is a major cause of liver cancer.

Epidemiological Determinants

Agent factor: Caused by hepatitis C virus which is 50–60 nm virus with a ss RNA belonging to Flaviviridae family, its envelope carry glycoprotein spikes.

Host Factor

High risk group:
- People who inject drugs
- People in prisons and other closed settings
- People who use drugs through other routes of administration (noninjecting)
- Men who have sex with men (MsM)
- Recipients of infected blood products or invasive procedures in healthcare facilities with inadequate infection control practices
- Children born to mothers infected with HCV
- People with HIV infection
- Prisoners or previously incarcerated persons
- People who have had tattoos or piercings.

Incubation period: 40–120 days

Mode of transmission: The infection can be spread by:
- Sharing needles and syringes, particularly when injecting drugs
- Medical and dental equipment that has not been properly sterilized
- The transfusion of unscreened blood and blood products.
- Unsterilized tattoo and body piercing equipment
- Sharing contaminated razors, toothbrushes or towels (this is rare).

It can be transmitted sexually, especially during **anal sex or other types of sex that may involve blood, although this is less common. The risk of hepatitis C infection is increased when** the sexual partner have another form of STI – especially which causes sores. People with HIV are more likely to get hepatitis C. The virus can also be passed on from a pregnant woman to her unborn baby.

Clinical Features

Many people with hepatitis C do not have any symptoms, especially during the first 6 months. The hepatitis C infection can go through two stages: acute and chronic. In the early 'acute' stage, these symptoms can include:
- Flu-like symptoms, tiredness, high temperature and aches and pains
- Loss of appetite
- Abdominal pain
- Yellowing of the eyes and skin (known as jaundice).

For some people the infection will clear without treatment.

In most cases an acute infection will develop into long-term 'chronic' infection. Chronic infection may not become apparent for a number of years until the liver displays signs of damage.

Symptoms vary but some of the most common include:
- Problems with short-term memory, concentration and completing complex mental tasks (often called 'brain fog')
- Depression or anxiety
- Mood swings
- Constantly feeling tired
- Nausea, vomiting or abdominal pain
- Dark urine and pale feces
- Jaundice
- Itchy skin
- Feeling bloated
- Joint and muscle pain.

Prevention

Primary Prevention

- Safe and appropriate use of health care injections.
- Safe handling and disposal of sharps and waste.
- Provision of comprehensive harm-reduction services to people who inject drugs including sterile injecting equipment and effective and evidence-based treatment of dependence.
- Testing of donated blood for HBV and HCV (as well as HIV and syphilis)
- Training of health personnel.

Secondary Prevention

- Education and counselling on options for care and treatment.
- Immunization with the hepatitis A and B vaccines to prevent coinfection from these hepatitis viruses and to protect their liver.
- Early and appropriate medical management including antiviral therapy.
- Regular monitoring for early diagnosis of chronic liver disease.

Treatment

Treatment for hepatitis C depends on how long you have had the virus. People with acute (short-term) infection do not always need treatment because their immune system may clear hepatitis C on its own. If you test positive during the acute stage, your doctor may ask you to come back after a few months to re-test and to see if you need any treatment. If any one develop chronic (long-term) infection, he/she will need treatment to help clear the virus. Treatment with drugs called direct-acting antivirals (DAAs) can cure hepatitis in most cases. These are usually taken for 8–12 weeks. There is chance of re-infection of Hepatitis C because it does not give lifelong immunity. WHO's updated 2018 guidelines recommend therapy with pan-genotypic direct-acting antivirals (DAAs). DAAs can cure most persons with HCV infection, and treatment duration is short (usually 12 to 24 weeks), depending on the absence or presence of cirrhosis. WHO recommends treating all persons with chronic HCV infection over the age of 12 with pan-genotypic direct-acting antivirals (DAAs).

Hepatitis D

Hepatitis D, also known as "delta hepatitis," is a liver infection caused by the hepatitis D virus (HDV). Hepatitis D only occurs in people who are also infected with the hepatitis B virus. Hepatitis D is spread when blood or other body fluids from a person infected with the virus enters the body of someone who is not infected. Hepatitis D can be an acute, short-term infection or become a long-term, chronic infection. Hepatitis D can cause severe symptoms and serious illness that can lead to life-long liver damage and even death. People can become infected with both hepatitis B and hepatitis D viruses at the same time (known as "coinfection") or get hepatitis D after first being infected with the hepatitis B virus (known as "superinfection"). There is no vaccine to prevent hepatitis D. However, prevention of hepatitis B with hepatitis B vaccine also protects against future hepatitis D infection.

Epidemiological Determinants

Agent Factor

Hepatitis D or Hepatitis delta is a type of viral hepatitis caused by the hepatitis delta virus (HDV), a small spherical enveloped particle that shares similarities with both a viroid and virusoid. HDV is considered to be a satellite (a type of sub viral agent) because it can propagate only in the presence of the hepatitis B virus (HBV). Hepatitis D virus (HDV) is a virus that requires hepatitis B virus (HBV) for its replication. Hepatitis D virus (HDV) affects globally nearly 5% of people who have a chronic infection with hepatitis B virus (HBV). The virion is spherical, 36–38nm particle with an outer coat composed of HBsAG surrounding ss RNA Genome.

Risk Group

HDV infection occurs when people become infected with both hepatitis B and D simultaneously (co-infection) or get hepatitis D after first being infected with hepatitis B (super-infection).

Populations that are more likely to have HBV and HDV coinfection include indigenous populations, recipients of hemodialysis and people who inject drugs.

The combination of HDV and HBV infection is considered the most severe form of chronic viral hepatitis due to more rapid progression towards liver-related death and hepatocellular carcinoma.

Incubation period: 2–12 weeks

Mode of transmission: The routes of transmission of hepatitis D are similar to those for hepatitis B. Infection is largely restricted to persons at high risk of hepatitis B infection, particularly injecting drug users and persons receiving clotting factor concentrates.

Clinical Features

The signs of HDV can include—jaundice, stomach pain, fatigue, joint pain, light -colored stool. Two type of infection are recognized:

1. In confection—delta and HBV transmitted at same time.
2. In superinfection—delta infection occurs in a person harboring HBV.

Diagnosis

- Immunofluorescence
- ELISA

Prevention

- The vaccine for hepatitis B protects against hepatitis D virus because of the latter's dependence on the presence of hepatitis B virus for it to replicate.

- In absence of a specific vaccine against delta virus, the vaccine against HBV must be given soon after birth in risk groups.
- Health education in case of superinfection
- Screening of blood donor.

Treatment

- Hepatitis D is generally considered the dominant virus over hepatitis B except in rare instances.
- pegylated interferon alpha is effective in reducing the viral load and the effect of the disease during the time the drug is given, but the benefit generally stops if the drug is discontinued.
- In May 2020, the Committee for Medicinal Products for Human Use of the European Medicines Agency approved the antiviral Hepcludex (bulevirtide) to treat hepatitis D and B. Bulevirtide binds and inactivates the sodium/bile acid cotransporter, blocking both viruses from entering hepatocytes.

Hepatitis E

Hepatitis E is inflammation of the liver caused by the hepatitis E virus (HEV). The virus has at least 4 different types: genotypes 1, 2, 3 and 4. Genotypes 1 and 2 have been found only in humans. Genotypes 3 and 4 circulate in several animals including pigs, wild boars and deer without causing any disease, and occasionally infect humans. The virus is shed in the stools of infected persons and enters the human body through the intestine. It is transmitted mainly through contaminated drinking water. The infection is usually self-limiting and resolves within 2–6 weeks. Occasionally a serious disease known as fulminant hepatitis (acute liver failure) develops, which can be fata.

Epidemiological Determinants

Agent: Hepatitis E is inflammation of the liver caused by infection with the hepatitis E virus (HEV). Hepatitis E has mainly a fecal-oral transmission route that is similar to hepatitis A, although the viruses are unrelated. HEV is a positive-sense, single-stranded, nonenveloped, RNA icosahedral virus and 29–32 nm diameter. It has been classified genus Herpes virus under the family caliciviridae.

Animal reservoir: Pigs I

Incubation period: 2–9 weeks

Mode of transmission: The hepatitis E virus is transmitted mainly through the fecal-oral route due to fecal contamination of drinking water. The risk factors for hepatitis E are related to poor sanitation, allowing virus excreted in the feces of infected people to reach drinking water supplies. Ingestion of undercooked meat or meat products derived from infected animals (e.g., pork liver); her baby.

Clinical Features

An initial phase of mild fever, reduced appetite (anorexia), nausea and vomiting, lasting for a few days; some persons may also have abdominal pain, itching (without skin lesions), skin rash, or joint pain.

- Jaundice (yellow color of the skin and whiteness of the eyes), with dark urine and pale stools; and
- A slightly enlarged, tender liver (hepatomegaly).
- In rare cases, acute hepatitis E can be severe, and result in fulminant hepatitis (acute liver failure); these patients are at risk of death. Fulminant hepatitis occurs more frequently.
- Cases of chronic hepatitis E infection have been reported in immunosuppressed people, particularly organ transplant recipients on immunosuppressive drugs.

Diagnosis

ELISA kits are available for IgG and IgM antibody.

Prevention

- No vaccine can prevent the hepatitis E virus.
- Do not drink water or use ice that you do not know is clean.
- Do not eat undercooked pork, deer meat, or raw shellfish.
- Wash your hands with soap and water after you use the bathroom, change a diaper, and before you prepare or eat food.
- Maintaining quality standards for public water supplies; and
- Establishing proper disposal systems for human feces.

Treatment

- There is no specific treatment capable of altering the course of acute hepatitis E. As the disease is usually self-limiting, hospitalization is generally not required. Most important is the avoidance of unnecessary medications. Acetaminophen/Paracetamol.
- Hospitalization is required for people with fulminant hepatitis, and should also be considered for symptomatic pregnant women. Immunosuppressed people with chronic hepatitis E benefit from specific treatment using ribavirin, an antiviral drug.

In terms of the diagnosis of hepatitis E, only a laboratory blood test that confirms the presence of HEV RNA or IgM antibodies to HEV can be trusted.

Hepatitis G

Hepatitis G virus (HGV) is a rare cause of hepatic inflammation. Although chronic infection and viremia have been documented, histologic evidence is rare, and serum aminotransferase levels are usually normal. At this time, reporting of HGV to the Minnesota Department of Health would be treated as anecdotal.

Epidemiological Determinants

Agent Factor

GB virus C (GBV-C) formerly known as hepatitis G virus (HGV) and also known as HPgV is a virus is a virus in the *Flaviviridae* family and a member of peg virus genus, is known to infect humans, but is not known to cause human disease.

HGV RNA has been found in patients with acute, chronic and fulminant hepatitis, hemophiliacs, patients with multiple transfusion and hemodialysis, IV drugs, addicts, and blood donor.

Mode of transmission: High prevalence is observed among subjects with the risk of parenteral exposures, including those with exposure to blood and blood products, those on hemodialysis, and intravenous drug users. Sexual contact and vertical transmission may occur. About 10–25% of hepatitis C-infected patients and 14–36% of drug users who are seropositive for HIV-1 show the evidence of GBV-C infection.

Laboratory detection:

- GBV-C RNA detection.
- Anti-GBV-C Antibody.

It is often found in co-infection with other viruses, such as HCV, HBV and HIV.

Many people with hepatitis do not have symptoms and do not know they are infected. Symptoms may appear after many year of exposure.

Signs and Symptoms

- Most infected persons are asymptomatic.
- Incubation period is unknown.

Long-term Effects

- HGV can cause chronic infection and viremia; however, there is no conclusive evidence to indicate that HGV causes fulminant or chronic liver disease.
- Co-infection with hepatitis B virus (HBV) or HCV does not seem to worsen the course or severity of disease

Prevention

No specific measures have been identified. But prevention of blood borne infection technique can be followed. Regular hand wash, care of sharp instrument, prevention of needle stick injuries, proper BMW management technique must be followed. Prevention of sexual transmission of diseases may be followed.

Treatment

Because GBV-C infection is not associated with clinical liver disease, no treatments have targeted GBV-C specifically. In HIV–HCV–GBV-C coinfected persons, peginterferon and ribavirin treatment led to sustained GBV-C clearance in 31% of patients, with no observable subsequent effect on the course of HCV or HIV infection. In patients coinfected with GBV-C and HCV who were treated with interferon and ribavirin, GBV-C RNA disappeared from serum during therapy but reappeared in all patients following discontinuation of therapy. Importantly, no effect of GBV-C infection was observed on the response to treatment of HCV infection.

CHOLERA

Cholera is an acute epidemic infectious disease caused by the bacterium vibrio cholerae. A soluble toxin elaborated in the intestinal tract by the bacterium activates the adenylate cyclase of the mucosa, causing active secretion of an isotonic fluid resulting in profuse watery diarrhea, extreme loss of fluid and electrolytes, and dehydration and collapse, but no gross morphologic change in the intestinal mucosa. This sudden onset of profuse, effortless, watery diarrhea and vomiting gives rise to rapid dehydration, muscular cramps and suppression of urine.

History of Cholera

Cholera was prevalent in the US in the 1800s, before modern water and sewage treatment systems eliminated its spread by contaminated water. Only about 10 cases of cholera are reported each year in the US and half of these are acquired abroad. Rarely, contaminated seafood has caused cholera outbreaks in the US. However, cholera outbreaks are still a serious problem in other parts of the world. At least 150,000 cases are reported to the World Health Organization each year.

The disease is most common in places with poor sanitation, crowding, war, and famine. Common locations include parts of Africa, South Asia, and Latin America. If you are traveling to one of those areas, knowing the following cholera facts can help protect you and your family.

Causes of Cholera

Vibrio cholerae, the bacterium that causes cholera, is usually found in food or water contaminated by feces from a person with the infection. Common sources include:

- Municipal water supplies
- Ice made from municipal water
- Foods and drinks sold by street vendors
- Vegetables grown with water containing human wastes
- Raw or undercooked fish and seafood caught in waters polluted with sewage.

Epidemiological Determinants

Agent factors: The organism that causes cholera is labeled as *V. cholerae.*

Infection material: Stools and vomit of cases and carriers.

Period of communicability: 7–10 days

Carrier of cholera: It may be defined as an apparently healthy person who is excreting V. cholera. It has 4 types:

1. Preclinical or incubatory carrier
2. Convalescent carrier
3. Contact or healthy carrier
4. Chronic carrier.

Host Factors

- **Age and sex:** It affects all ages and both sexes
- **Gastric acidity:** It is destroyed in an acidity of pH5 or lower.
- **Population mobility:** Movements of population results in increased risk of exposure to infection.
- **Economic status:** Higher incidence in low socio economic groups mainly to poor hygiene.

- **Immunity:** Natural infection confers quite effective immunity.

Environmental Factors

Poor environmental sanitation.

Mode of Transmission

- Fecally contaminated water.
- Contaminated food and drinks
- Direct contact.

Incubation period: From a few hours up to 5 days.

Clinical Manifestation

Symptoms of cholera can begin as soon as a few hours or as long as five days after infection. Often, symptoms are mild. But sometimes they are very serious. About one in 20 people infected have severe watery diarrhea accompanied by vomiting, which can quickly lead to dehydration. Although many infected people may have minimal or no symptoms, they can still contribute to spread of the infection.

Signs and symptoms of dehydration include:

- Rapid heart rate
- Loss of skin elasticity (the ability to return to original position quickly if pinched)
- Dry mucous membranes, including the inside of the mouth, throat, nose, and eyelids
- Low blood pressure
- Thirst
- Muscle cramps.

Diagnosing Cholera

One should consider the cholera diagnosis in all cases of severe watery diarrhea and vomiting especially with rapid dehydration and recent travel or consumption of shellfish. Lab tests include stool gram stain (gram negative rods) culture, dark field microscopy or stool PCR. People must begin treatment even before diagnostic work-up. 'Cholera cots,' cots with openings to allow fecal output into a bucket, are used to measure volumes of stool loss and fluid replacement needs.

Vaccination for Cholera

Active immunization against cholera is indicated only for individuals traveling to or residing in countries where cholera is endemic or epidemic. The primary immunizing course consists of two doses administered one week to one month or more apart. The **Table 11.10** summarizes the recommended doses for both primary and booster immunizations by age, volume (mL), and route of administration. The intracutaneous (intradermal) route is satisfactory for persons 5 years of age and older, but higher levels of antibody may be achieved in children less than 5 years old by the subcutaneous or intramuscular routes.

Table 11.10: Vaccination for cholera.

		Route and age		
Dose number	Intradermal	Subcutaneous or Intramuscular		
	5 years and over	6 months-4 years	5–10 years	Over 10 years
1 and 2	0.2 mL	0.2 mL	0.3 mL	0.5 mL
Boosters	0.2 mL	0.2 mL	0.3 mL	0.5 mL

Treatment options for cholera

- Because death from cholera is a consequence of dehydration, the disease is treated using oral rehydration therapy (ORT), which consists of large volumes of water mixed with a blend of sugar and salts. Prepackaged mixtures are commercially available, but wide distribution in developing countries is limited by cost. Therefore, homemade ORT recipes using common household ingredients and materials have been developed. Severe cases of cholera require intravenous fluid replacement.
- **Antibiotics** can shorten illness, but ORT is still necessary even when antibiotics are used. Do not use antidiarrheal medicines, since they prevent flushing of the bacteria out of the body.

Control of Cholera

- Verification of the diagnosis by bacteriological diagnosis.
- Notification of cases immediately to the local authority.
- Early case findings
- Establishment of treatment centers
- Rehydration therapy
- Oral rehydration
- Intravenous rehydration by RL solution
- Adjuncts to therapy: Antibiotics should be given as soon as vomiting has stopped, which is usually after 3 to 4 hours of oral rehydration.
- Epidemiological investigations
- Sanitation measures includes
  a. Water control
  b. Excreta disposal
  c. Food sanitation
  d. Disinfection.
- Chemoprophylaxis, e.g., Tetracycline-500 mg towards adult, 125 mg towards 4–13 years, 50 mg towards 0–3 years.
- Health education: The Health education in the community include food hygiene, water hygiene, safe disposal of excreta, vaccination and proper management of diarrheal diseases.

ACUTE DIARRHEAL DISEASES

Though the mortality rate for children under five suffering from acute diarrhea has fallen from 4.5 million deaths annually in 1979 to 1.6 million deaths in 2002, acute diarrhea continues to exact a high toll on children in developing countries. Diarrhea is defined as the passage of loose liquid or watery stools. These stools are passed more than 3 times a day.

There are three clinical types of diarrhea:

1. Acute watery diarrhea—lasts several hours or days, and includes cholera

2. Acute bloody diarrhea—also called dysentery
3. Persistent diarrhea—lasts 14 days or longer.

Causes

Infection: Diarrhea is a symptom of infections caused by a host of bacterial, viral and parasitic organisms, most of which are spread by feces-contaminated water. Infection is more common when there is a shortage of adequate sanitation and hygiene and safe water for drinking, cooking and cleaning. Rotavirus and *Escherichia coli* are the two most common etiological agents of diarrhea in developing countries.

Malnutrition: Children who die from diarrhea often suffer from underlying malnutrition, which makes them more vulnerable to diarrhea. Each diarrheal episode, in turn, makes their malnutrition even worse. Diarrhea is a leading cause of malnutrition in children under five years old.

Source: Water contaminated with human feces, for example, from sewage, septic tanks and latrines, is of particular concern. Animal feces also contain microorganisms that can cause diarrhea.

Other causes: Diarrheal disease can also spread from person-to-person, aggravated by poor personal hygiene. Food is another major cause of diarrhea when it is prepared or stored in unhygienic conditions. Water can contaminate food during irrigation. Fish and seafood from polluted water may also contribute to the disease.

Epidemiological Determinants

Agent Factors

1. Viruses
   a. Rotaviruses
   b. Astroviruses
   c. Adenoviruses
   d. Coronaviruses.
2. Bacteria
   a. *Campylobacter jejuni*
   b. *E. coli*
   c. *Shigella*
   d. *Salmonella*
   e. *Vibrio cholerae*
   f. *Vibrio parahaemolyticus.*
3. Others
   a. *E. hystolytica*
   b. Trichuriasis
   c. Intestinal worms.

Reservoir of infection: Man is the principal reservoir.

Host factors: Most common in children especially between 6 months and 2 years.

Environmental factors: Bacterial diarrhea occur temperature climate season.

Viral diarrhea occur during the winter season.

Medical Care

In 2003 the Center for Disease Control (CDC) put forth recommendations for the management of acute pediatric diarrhea in both the outpatient and inpatient settings including indication for referral.

Indications for medical evaluation of children with acute diarrhea include the following:

- Younger than 3 months
- Weight of less than 8 kg
- History of premature birth, chronic medical conditions, or concurrent illness
- Fever of 38°C or higher in infants younger than 3 months or 39°C or higher in children aged 3–36 months
- Visible blood in the stool
- High-output diarrhea
- Persistent emesis
- Signs of dehydration as reported by caregiver, including sunken eyes, decreased tears, dry mucous membranes, and decreased urine output
- Mental status changes
- Inadequate responses to oral rehydration therapy (ORT) or caregiver unable to administer ORT.

The report also includes information on assessment of dehydration and what steps should be taken to adequately treat acute diarrhea.

Treatment of dehydration due to diarrhea includes the following:

- **Minimal or no dehydration:**
  - Rehydration therapy—Not applicable
  - Replacement of losses
    - Less than 10 kg body weight—60–120 mL oral rehydration solution for each diarrhea stool or vomiting episode
    - More than 10 kg body weight—120–140 mL oral rehydration solution for each diarrhea stool or vomiting episode.
- **Mild-to-moderate dehydration:**
  - Rehydration therapy—Oral rehydration solution (50–100 mL/kg over 3–4 h)
  - Replacement of losses
  - Less than 10 kg body weight 60–120 mL oral rehydration solution for each diarrhea stool or vomiting episode
  - More than 10 kg body weight 120–140 mL oral rehydration solution for each diarrhea stool or vomiting episode.
- **Severe dehydration:**
  - *Rehydration therapy:* Intravenous lactated Ringer solution or normal saline (20 mL/kg until perfusion and mental status improve), followed by 100 mL/kg oral rehydration solution over 4 hours or 5% dextrose (half normal saline) intravenously at twice maintenance fluid rates.
  - *Replacement of losses:*
    - Less than 10 kg body weight 60–120 mL oral rehydration solution for each diarrhea stool or vomiting episode
    - More than 10 kg body weight 120–140 mL oral rehydration solution for each diarrhea stool or vomiting episode

- If unable to drink, administer through nasogastric tube or intravenously administer 5% dextrose (one fourth normal saline) with 20 meq/L potassium chloride.

Control of Diarrheal Diseases

Diarrheal Disease Control (DDC) Programme was started in 1980. The interventions are:

i. **Short-term:** Appropriate clinical management
   a. ORS
   b. Appropriate feeding
   c. Chemotherapy
ii. **Long-term:** Better MCH care practices
   a. Maternal nutrition
   b. Child nutrition.

Prevention

Key measures to prevent diarrhea include:

- Access to safe drinking-water
- Use of improved sanitation
- Hand washing with soap
- Exclusive breastfeeding for the first six months of life
- Good personal and food hygiene
- Health education about how infections spread
- Rotavirus vaccination
- Fly control.

Recommendations

The revised recommendations emphasize family and community understanding of managing diarrhea. When they become routine practice, caretakers will act quickly at the first sign of diarrhea, rather than waiting before treating the child. The aim is that the recommendations become routine practice both in the home and healthcare facility.

Mothers and Other Caregivers Should

- Prevent dehydration through the early administration of increased amounts of appropriate fluids available in the home, and ORS solution, if on hand
- Continue feeding (or increase breastfeeding) during, and increase all feeding after the episode.
- Recognize the signs of dehydration and take the child to a health care provider for ORS or intravenous electrolyte solution, as well as familiarize themselves with other symptoms requiring medical treatment (e.g., bloody diarrhea).
- Provide children with 20 mg per day of zinc supplementation for 10–14 days (10 mg per day for infants under six months old).

Healthcare Workers Should

- Counsel mothers to begin administering suitable available home fluids immediately upon onset of diarrhea in a child
- Treat dehydration with ORS solution (or with an intravenous electrolyte solution in cases of severe dehydration).
- Emphasize continued feeding or increased breastfeeding during, and increased feeding after the diarrheal episode.
- Use antibiotics only when appropriate, i.e., in the presence of bloody diarrhea or shigellosis, and abstain from administering antidiarrheal drugs.
- Provide children with 20 mg per day of zinc supplementation for 10–14 days (10 mg per day for infants under six months old).
- Advise mothers of the need to increase fluids and continue feeding during future episodes.
- Healthcare workers treating children for diarrhea are encouraged to provide caretakers with two 1-liter packets of the new ORS, for homeuse until the diarrhea stops. Caretakers should also be provided with enough zinc supplements to continue home treatment for 10–14 days. Printed material (including text and illustrations) with advice on preventing and treating diarrhea at home should accompany the ORS and zinc supplements.

Countries Should

- Develop a 3–5 year plan to reduce mortality rates from diarrheal diseases.
- Assess progress in controlling diarrheal diseases by monitoring usage rates of ORT/ORS, home-based treatment and zinc supplementation.
- Using the media and face-to-face communication, promote and refine messages on diarrhea prevention, home management of diarrhea and appropriate care-seeking.
- Prioritize improving the availability of the new ORS solution and zinc supplements through private and public channels.
- Craft suitable strategies to educate health care workers at all levels about using the new ORS and zinc supplements in treating diarrhea.
- Promote the availability of a zinc formulation that is cost-effective and easily administered to both infants and children.
- Identify obstacles to the use of ORS, zinc supplements and home-based treatments in managing acute diarrhea.

UNICEF, WHO and Other Partners will Support These Actions by

- Advocating, facilitating and investing resources to ensure country adoption and implementation of these revised recommendations.
- Working with governments and the private sector, including nongovernmental organizations and businesses, to rapidly disseminate these recommendations.
- Supplying new ORS and zinc supplements to countries that cannot manufacture them to quality standards.
- Helping with communication efforts aimed at enhancing prevention and management of diarrhea, including promoting routine use of new ORS and zinc supplements.

TYPHOID FEVER

Typhoid fever is the result of systemic infection mainly by *S.typhi* found only in man. The disease is clinically characterized by a typical continuous fever for 3 to 4 weeks, relative bradycardia with involvement of lymphoid tissues and considerable includes both typhoid and paratyphoid fever.

Epidemiological Determinants

Agent factors: *S. typhi* is the major cause of the enteric fever. It infecting the body via the Peyer's patches of the small intestine. The bacteria migrates to mesenteric lymph nodes and arrive via the blood in the liver and spleen during the first exposure. After multiple replication in the above locations, the bacteria migrates back into the Peyer's patches of the small intestine for the secondary exposure and consequently the clinical symptoms are seen. Inflammation in the small intestine leads to ulcers and necrosis.

Reservoir of infection

i. **Case:** It is a infectious as long as bacilli appear in stools or urine.
ii. **Carriers:** Temporary or chronic.

Source of infection

- Feces and urine of cases or carriers.
- Contaminated water, food, fingers and flies.

Host Factors

- **Age:** Typhoid fever may occur at any age but it is considered to be a disease mainly of children and young adults. In endemic areas, the highest attack rate occurs in children aged 8–13 years. In general Higher incidence was found in 5–19 years of age group.
- **Gender and race:** Typhoid fever cases are more commonly seen in males than in females. On the contrary, females have a special predilection to become chronic carriers.
- **Occupation:** Certain categories of persons handling the infective material and live cultures of *S. typhi* are at increased risk of acquiring infection.
- **Socioeconomic factors:** It is a disease of poverty as it is often associated with inadequate sanitation facilities and unsafe water supplies.
- **Environmental factors:** Though the cases are observed through out the year, the peak incidence of typhoid fever is reported during July–September. This period coincides with the rainy season and a substantial increase in fly population.

Social factors: Pollution of drinking water supplies, open air defecation, and urination, low standards of food and personal hygiene, and health ignorance.

Nutritional status: Malnutrition may enhance the suscepti-bility to typhoid fever by altering the intestinal flora or other host defenses.

Incubation period: Usually 10–14 days but it may be as short as 3 days or as long as 21 days depending upon the dose of the inoculums.

Reservoir of infection: Man is the only known reservoir of infection—cases or carriers.

Period of communicability: A case is infectious as long as the bacilli appear in stool or urine.

Mode of Transmission

The disease is transmitted by feco-oral route or urine—oral routes—either directly through hands soiled with feces or urine of cases or carriers or indirectly by ingestion of contaminated water, milk, food, or through flies **(Fig. 11.1)**. Contaminated ice, ice-creams, and milk products are a rich source of infection. It may be spread through poor hygiene habits and public sanitation conditions. Public education campaigns encouraging people to wash their hands after defecating and before handling food are an important component in controlling spread of the disease.

Carriers may be temporary or chronic: Temporary (convalescent or incubatory) carriers usually excrete bacilli up to 6–8 weeks. By the end of one year, 3–4% of cases continue to excrete typhoid bacilli.

Persons who excrete the bacilli for more than a year after a clinical attack are called chronic carriers.

Clinical manifestation: The symptoms become worsen by lingering treatment and the clinical manifestation in different weeks are as follows:

- **First week**: The disease classically presents with step-ladder fashion rise in temperature (40–41°C) over 4 to 5

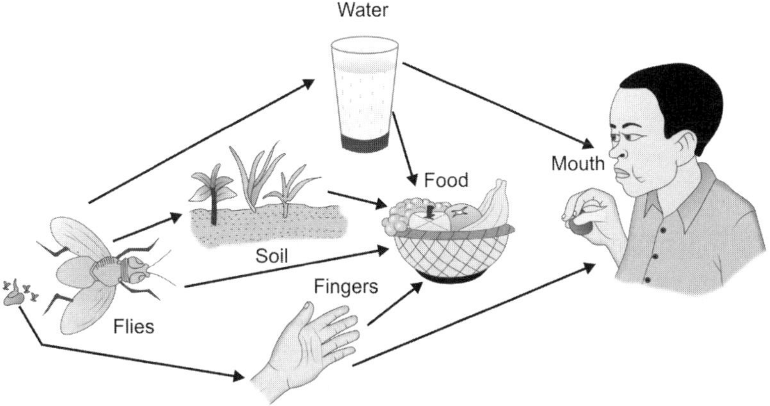

Fig. 11.1: Feco-oral route of transmission.

days, accompanied by headache, vague abdominal pain, and constipation.
- **Second week:** Between the 7th–10th day of illness, mild hepatosplenomegaly occurs in majority of patients. Relative bradycardia may occur and rose-spots may be seen.
- **Third week:** The patient will appear in the 'typhoid state' which is a state of prolonged apathy, toxemia, delirium, disorientation and/or coma. Diarrhea will then become apparent. If left untreated by this time, there is a high-risk (5–10%) of intestinal hemorrhage and perforation.

Diagnosis

A complete blood count (CBC) will show a high number of white blood cells.

A blood culture during the first week of the fever can show *S. typhi* bacteria.

Other tests that can help diagnose this condition include:
- ELISA urine test to look for the bacteria that cause Typhoid fever
- Fluorescent antibody study to look for substances that are specific to typhoid bacteria
- Platelet count (platelet count may be low)
- Stool culture.

Treatment

Fluids and electrolytes may be given by IV (into a vein). Or you may be asked to drink uncontaminated water with electrolyte packets.

Antibiotics are given to kill the bacteria. There are increasing rates of antibiotic resistance throughout the world, Chloramphenicol, Ampicillin, Amoxicillin, Trimethoprim and Sulfamethoxazole, Fluroquinolones are the drugs of choice for typhoid fever. In case of quinolone resistance—Azithromycin, 3rd generation cephalosporins (ceftriaxone) can be advisable.

Control of Typhoid Fever

Measures Directed to Reservoir

- **Cases:**
  - Early diagnosis
  - Notification of cases
  - Isolation
  - Treatment by chloramphenicol or cotrimoxazole amoxicillin and trimethoprim.
  - Disinfection of stools.
- **Carriers:**
  - Identification
  - Treatment by ampicillin with probe new (2 g/day for 6 weeks)
  - Surgery—cholecystectomy
  - Surveillance
  - Health education.

Measures at Routes of Transmission

a. Water sanitation
b. Food sanitation
c. Excreta disposal
d. Fly control.

Measures for Susceptibles

a. Immunoprophylaxis
b. Health education.

Measures for Health Promotion

- Keep the premises and kitchen utensils clean
- Dispose rubbish properly
- Keep hands clean and fingernails trimmed
- Wash hands properly with soap and water before eating or handling food, and after toilet or changing diapers
- Drinking water should be from the mains and preferably boiled
- Purchase fresh food from reliable sources. Do not patronize illegal hawkers
- Avoid high-risk food like shellfish, raw food or semi-cooked food
- Wear clean washable aprons and caps during food preparation
- Clean and wash food thoroughly
- Scrub and rinse shellfish in clean water. Immerse them in clean water for sometime to allow self-purification
- Remove the viscera if appropriate
- Store perishable food in refrigerator, well covered
- Handle and store raw and cooked food especially seafood separately (upper compartment of the refrigerator for cooked food and lower compartment for raw food) to avoid cross contamination
- Clean and defrost refrigerator regularly and keep the temperature at or below 4°C
- Cook food thoroughly
- Do not handle cooked food with bare hands; wear gloves if necessary
- Consume food as soon as it is done
- If necessary, refrigerate cooked leftover food and consume as soon as possible. Reheat thoroughly before consumption. Discard any adulterated food items
- Exclude typhoid carrier from handling food and from providing care to children
- Specific protection.

Three Types of Vaccines

1. Injectable Typhoid vaccine (Typhim -Vi, Typhivax)
2. The live oral vaccine (Typhoral)
3. TAB vaccine.

Injectable Typhim-VI

- This single-dose injectable typhoid vaccine, from the bacterial capsule of *S. typhi* strain of Ty21a.
- This vaccine is recommended for use in children over 2 years of age.
- Subcutaneous or intramuscular injection
- Efficacy: 64–72%.

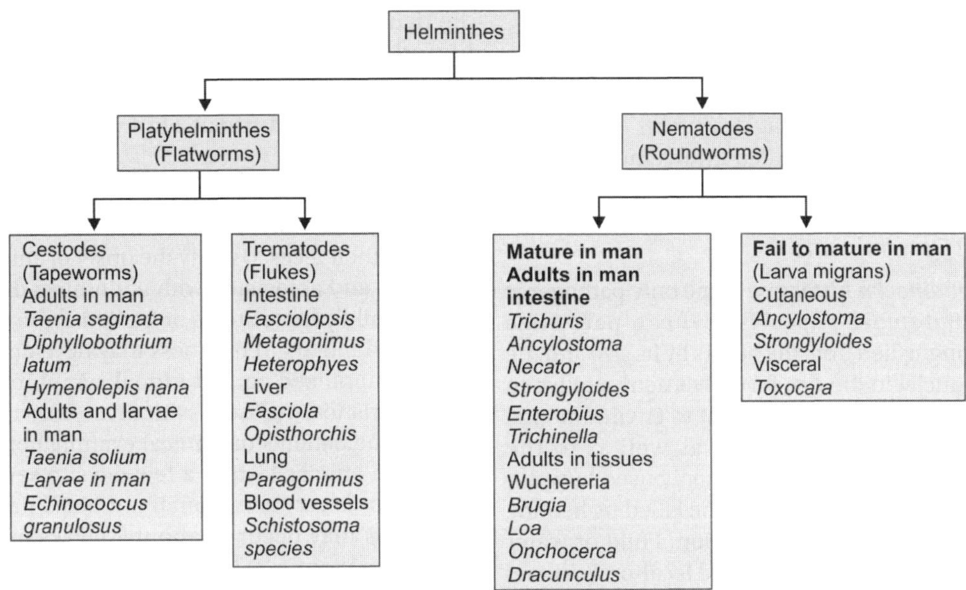

Fig. 11.2: A simplified classification of helminthic parasites of man.

Typhoral

- This is a live-attenuated-bacteria vaccine manufactured from the Ty21a strain of *S. typhi*.
- The efficacy rate of the oral typhoid vaccine ranges from 50–80%
- Not recommended for use in children younger than 6 years of age.
- The course consists of one capsule orally, taken an hour before food with a glass of water or milk (1st day, 3rd day and 5th day)
- No antibiotic should be taken during this period
- Immunity starts 2–3 weeks after administration and lasts for 3 years. A booster dose after 3 years.

Side Effects

Injectable Typhim -Vi: The most common adverse reactions are injection site pain, erythema, and induration, which almost always resolve within 48 hours of vaccination. Occasional fever, flu-like episodes, headache, tremor, abdominal pains, vomiting, diarrhea, and cervical pains have been reported.

Nausea, abdominal pain and cramps, vomiting, fever, headache, and rash or urticaria may occur in some instances but are rare.

HELMINTHIC DISEASES

According to the worms of medical importance the worms can be divided into three groups: Cestodes (tapeworms), trematodes (flukes) and nematodes (roundworms). However, according to their shape, worms are divided into two groups: flat or round. The flukes and the tapeworms are included in the group of the flatworms or *Platyhelminthes.* This is because they are usually flattened, bilaterally symmetrical, have no true body cavities, and are hermaphrodite. On the other hand, roundworms are zoologically distinct, more tubular and simple but the sexes are distinct. The classification is illustrated in **Figure 11.2**.

Adult tapeworms have no digestive systems. However, they absorb nutrients directly from the host's gut contents through their surfaces. An adult tapeworm has a small head (scolex) with two or four suckers and usually a circle of hooks by which it attaches to the host's intestinal wall. It also has a body (strobila) which is generally long and tape-like and consists of many units also referred to as proglottids. It is from the tape-like structure of its body that the tapeworm gets its name. The larval stages occur in various organs and tissues of vertebrate intermediate hosts.

The roundworms have a complete digestive system with a mouth and anus. Hookworms, *Ascaris*, *Trichuris* and *Strongyloides* are all soil-transmitted helminths. *Enterobius* is transmitted directly by the fecal-oral route. The final host of all the worms is man except for the dog tapeworm for which the human is an accidental intermediate host. The eggs of all the intestinal worms are excreted in stools.

Sanitary disposal of human feces is the preventive measure of choice because it will control most of these worm diseases with the exception of the hydatid disease, *Enterobius* and schistosomiasis.

AMEBIASIS

Amebiasis, or amebiasis, refers to infection caused by the amoeba *Entamoeba histolytica* gastrointestinal infection that may or may not be symptomatic and can remain latent in an infected person for several years, amebiasis is estimated to cause 70,000 deaths per year world wide. Symptoms can range from mild diarrhea to dysentery with blood and mucus in the stool. *E. histolytica* is usually a commensal organism. Severe amebiasis infections (known as invasive or *fulminant* amebiasis) occur in two major forms.

Entamoeba histolytica

The symptomatic group has been subdivided into:
- Intestinal disease varies from mild abdominal discomfort and diarrhea to acute fulminating dysentery.
- Extraintestinal amebiasis includes involvement of liver, brain, spleen, skin, etc.

Epidemiological Determinants

Agent factors: *Entamoeba histolytica* is the only pathogenic one of several *Entamoeba* species that can parasitize humans. It is distinguished from the others by its size and the fact that it has 4 nuclei in the cyst form. It is activated when cysts are ingested. The cysts are resistant to environmental conditions such as low temperature as well as to the normal concentration of chlorine commonly used in water purification. The parasite can, however, be killed by heating food or water to 55°C before consumption. Food or water contaminated with *E. histolytica* cysts and fecal-oral contact are the main means of infection.

Reservoir of infection: Untreated water and human feces used as fertilizer are important sources of infection. Food handlers passing amoebic cysts play a role in spreading the infection.

Period of communicability: As long as cysts are excrete, the period may be several years. If cases are unrecognized and untreated.

Host factors: It occurs at any age and sex.

Environmental factors: It is more closely related to poor sanitation and socioeconomic status than to climate.

Mode of transmission: Amebiasis is usually transmitted by the fecal-oral route, but it can also be transmitted indirectly through contact with dirty hands or objects. Infection is spread through ingestion of the cyst form of the parasite, a semi-dormant and hardy structure found in feces. Any nonencysted amebae, or trophozoites, die quickly after leaving the body but may also be present in stool: Since amebiasis is transmitted through contaminated food and water, it is often endemic in regions of the world with limited modern sanitation systems, including Mexico, Central America, Western South America, South Asia, and Western and Southern Africa.
- Fecal-oral route.

Pathology

The cyst is resistant to gastric acidity and digestive enzymes, and upon ingestion it excysts in the small intestine releasing 8 trophozoites. The emerging trophozoites take up residence in the ascending large bowel where they can live as a commensal (asymptomatic carrier) or begin penetrating the intestinal wall, causing small mucosal ulcerations which result in dysentery. The parasite penetrates through the submucosa and into the muscularis layer of the colon. If the muscularis layer becomes extensively involved scarring can result (ameboma). Invasion of the bloodstream by the trophozoites may lead to infection of the liver, especially the right lobe, lungs and brain. After a variable incubation period, a liver abscess may develop. Lung and brain metastasis are rare.

Incubation period: About 2 to 4 weeks or longer.

Clinical Features

Most infected individuals are asymptomatic and cysts are found in their feces. Usually the onset of amebic dysentery is insidious and associated with abdominal discomfort. There may be mildly loose stools or frank diarrhea with or without blood and mucus. Tenderness may develop over the cecum area. Generalized constitutional symptoms and signs are characteristically absent with fever only noted in about a third of the patients on clinical examination. The dysentery occurs in attacks lasting a few days to several weeks and recurrence is very common in untreated patients. Intestinal amebiasis may occur in about 2 weeks of infection or be delayed for months. When the ameba penetrate the intestinal wall, they multiply in the submucosa, causing bottle-shaped ulcers. From these ulcers, the ameba may be transported to the liver. An ameboma or amebic granuloma may result from repeated invasion in the colon. An ameboma may become very large, forming a hard swelling which is difficult to differentiate clinically from carcinoma.

Prevention and Control

Primary prevention:
- **Sanitation:** Safe disposal of human excreta couples with the elementary sanitary of washing hands after defecation and before eating is a crucial factor in the prevention and control of amebiasis.
- **Water supply:** Protection of water supplies against fecal contamination is equally clean bathrooms and toilets often; pay particular attention to toilet seats and taps. Replace solid soap in the toilet with liquid soap.
- **Food hygiene:** Environmental measures should also include the protection of food and drink against fecal contamination. Avoid sharing towels or face washers.
- Health education in the community regarding avoiding of open field defecation, maintaining food hygiene, hand hygiene and avoid eating street foods especially in public places where others are sharing sauces in one container, etc., ensuring that food handlers are not carriers. Avoid raw vegetables when in endemic areas, as they may have been fertilized using human feces.
- Good sanitary practice, as well as responsible sewage disposal or treatment, are necessary for the prevention of *E.histolytica* infection on an endemic level. *E.histolytica* cysts are usually resistant to chlorination, therefore sedimentation and filtration of water supplies are necessary to reduce the incidence of infection.

Treatment

E. histolytica infections occur in both the intestine and (in people with symptoms) in tissue of the intestine and/or liver. As a result, two different classes of drugs are needed to treat the infection, one for each location. Such antiamebic drugs are known as amebicides. An amebicide (or amoebicide) is an agent used in the treatment of amoebozoa infections. Among these agents are the following, linked to the infections they are used to treat metronidazole, or a related drug such as tinidazole, secnidazole or ornidazole is used to destroy amebae that have invaded tissue.

Several drugs are available for treating intestinal infections, the most effective of which has been shown to be paromomycin (also known as Humatin). *E. histolytica* infections occur in both the intestine and (in people with symptoms) in tissue of the intestine and/or liver. As a result, both tissue and luminal drugs are needed to treat the infection, one for each location. Metronidazole is usually given first, followed by paromomycin or diloxanide.

Ascariasis

An infection of the intestinal tract caused by the adult, *Ascariasis lumbricoides* and clinically manifested by vague symptoms of nausea, abdominal pain and cough.

Epidemiological Determinants

- **Agent factors:** Ascariasis is an infection caused by *Ascaris lumbricoides*, the largest intestinal roundworm, reaching up to 40 cm in length. It lives in the small intestine and the female produces up to 200,000 eggs which pass with feces daily. It is one of the commonest nematode infestations of the small intestine. It does not appear to depend so much on the climate, although it is more perennial in the damp and humid areas of the tropics. This explains why ascariasis is common in all areas of Africa. The reservoir of infection is human being.
- **Host factors:** Infection rates are high in children.
- **Environmental factors:** Ascaris is a 'soil-transmitted' helminth. Infection with the Ascaris parasite results when a person swallows food containing eggs of this parasite. The eggs have to be embryonated in soil before they are infective for a period of 8–50 days. The soil must be loose and not too dry. Oxygen must be available and the temperatures over 15°C.
- **Human habits:** Unwashed hands and children picking up things from the floor or ground and putting them into the mouth are common ways of acquiring Ascaris. In communities that use human feces as manure, the possibility of ingesting the eggs from foodstuffs grown using this manure is very high. Seeding of soil by ascaris eggs is also a human habit. Consumption of raw vegetables or half cooked vegetables or fruits from ground without washing properly can also transmit the diseases.
- **Period of communicability:** Until all fertile females are destroyed and stools are negative.
- **Mode of transmission:** Fecal oral route.
- **Incubation period:** About 2 months.

Clinical Features

The infection with ascaris is usually asymptomatic. There may be vague abdominal discomfort. Abdominal pain, diarrhea, vomiting and slight temperature. Complications may occur in very heavy infections or due to wandering worms.

In some instances young ascaris larvae migrate to the lungs via hepatic blood vessels causing tissue destruction and if their numbers are large, enlargement and tenderness of the liver results. Sometimes intestinal obstructions may occur at the ilio-cecal junction by a large ball of worms and appendix. A drug used previously for treatment of hookworm is tetrachloroethylene which caused wandering worms cause acute symptoms, like vomits worms, swelling of the glottis and larynx resulting in difficulties in breathing. The wandering worms can also cause blockage of bile ducts resulting in obstructive jaundice. If by chance the worms migrate into liver tissue that may result in formation of a liver abscess. They may enter bile or pancreatic duct and interfere with digestion. They also injure the intestine and cause peritonitis. Long term ascariasis may contribute to malnutrition states such as kwashiorkor and vitamin A deficiency. Sometime the larvae causes inflammation and hemorrhage in the lungs which results in pneumonia—may leads fatal.

Diagnosis

Diagnosis is by stool microscopy which should show the characteristic ascaris eggs. During the early lung phase, when eosinophilic pneumonia occurs, larvae can be found in sputum or gastric aspirates before diagnostic eggs appear in the stool. A plain abdominal radiograph may reveal masses of worms in gas filled loops of bowel in patients with intestinal obstruction.

Prevention and Control

Prevention includes environmental measures such as provision of adequate and safe water supplies, facilities for safe fecal disposal and prevention of fecal contamination of food. Discourage use of fresh human feces as farm manure. When human faces are used as fertilizers, they should first be composted as the temperature at the center of the heap usually exceeds 60°C. It is important to remember that temperatures in the outer layers of a well-made heap or in a poorly made heap may not reach 60°C and the feces should not be used as fertilizers. Composting the feces for 6 months will kill *ascaris* eggs. After this time the compost can safely be used as fertilizer. Generally vegetables should be thoroughly washed in a mild solution of potassium permanganate and properly cooked before use. During consumption of raw vegetables or fruits it should be washed properly and deepening in potassium permanganate solution or salt water for ten minute then used. Provision of safe drinking water, food hygiene habits and; health education regarding use of sanitary latrine, personal hygiene and proper behavioral pattern is essential for prevention of ascaris.

Treatment

Infections with *A.lumbricoides* are easily treated with a number of anthelmintic drugs. The drug of choice and their doses are:

- Pyrantel pamoate given as a single dose of 10 mg/kg
- Levamisole given as a single dose of 2.5 mg/kg
- Mebendazole given as a single dose of 500 mg
- Albendazole given as a single dose of 400 mg.

Ascariasis should always be treated to prevent potentially serious complications. Both mebendazole and albendazole are effective, but are contraindicated in pregnancy and in heavy infections in which they may provoke ectopic migration. Piperazine is safe in pregnancy. Mebendazole is the drug most commonly used in drug kits of the essential drug program because it is a broad-spectrum anthelmintic. All patients suspected of intestinal obstruction should be referred. Surgery may be necessary, if medical treatment does not respond. The symptoms of intestinal obstruction may resolve with anthelmintic treatment and intravenous fluids.

HOOKWORM INFESTATION

Hookworm infection in humans is caused by two types of hookworm: *Necator americanus* and *Ankylostoma duodenale*. The two species overlap in many tropical regions. In most areas, older children have the greatest incidence and intensity of hookworm infection. Hookworms need a hot humid climate for their development. A minimum temperature of 18°C is required and a soil temperature of 20–32°C is help to grow the virus more. Hookworm infection is therefore, most common in the hot, humid areas of Africa. Ancylostoma is found in Europe around the Mediterranean, on the West Coast of South America and in parts of China and India.

Necator is found over much of the Western Hemisphere, Africa and South east Asia. More than a billion people infected.

Clinical Manifestation

Infection with hookworm disease may vary from asymptomatic infection to a chronic debilitating disease caused by severe iron deficiency anemia, and in some cases loss of protein from the bowel leading to edema. Heavy worm burden, a prolonged duration of infection and poor iron intake all contribute to the development of hookworm disease. Many people (hookworm carriers) harbor the worms without any ill effects. The clinical manifestation can be categorized according to different stages of symptoms.

- **Invasion stage:** The skin, at the site of entry of filariform larva. Maculopapular lesions 'ground itch' or 'dew itch' itching, edema.
- **Migration stage:** Passage of the larvae in the lung leads to Hemorrhages and pneumonia, cough, fever, eosinophilia.
- **Intestinal stage:**
  - Sucking of blood by the worm **(iron-deficiency anemia)**

    Severe anemia leads to weakness as 0.15–0.26 mL of blood may be withdrawn by a ancylostoma in 24 hours and proximately 50% of the red blood cells are hemolyzed
  - Bleeding at the site of attachment and after movement to a new sites.
  - Intestinal ulcers: Flatulence, nausea, vomiting, diarrhea.

Diagnosis

- Diagnosis can be determined by looking for hookworm eggs in a recently collected stool sample.
- Blood tests for anemia and nutritional deficiencies, particularly iron, can help to confirm the diagnosis.

Epidemiological Determinants

Agent factors

- *Ancylostoma duodenale (old hookworms)*
- *Necator americanus (new hookworms)*

Adult worms live in the small intestine, mainly jejunum where attach themselves to the villi.

Reservoir of Infection

Human being is the main reservoir of infection and the Infective material is the fecal material containing ova of hook worm.

Period of Infectivity

As long as person harbory the parasite.

Host Factors

- **Age and sex:** All ages and both sexes are susceptible to infection.
- **Nutrition:** Malnutrition is a predisposing factor
- **Host:** Parasite balance.
- **Occupation:** The people working with field generally farmers having more chance to get the disease.

Environmental Factors

- **Soil:** Most suitable for the eggs and larvae
- **Temperature:** 24–23°C
- **Oxygen:** Required for growth and development
- **Moisture:** Necessary for survival
- **Rainfall:** 140 inches and above rainfall
- **Shade:** Shade protects pathogen
- **Human habits:** Open field defecation and not wearing foot wear during defecation.

Mode of Transmission and its Pathology

Hookwook enter the body, usually feet by penetrating the skin.

The eggs at the embryonic phases are passing out with feces. The eggs hatch into *rhabditi form* larvae which leave the feces and bury themselves in moist damp soil where they change into the infective sheathed *filariform* stage. The development from the noninfective *rhabditiform* larvae to the infective *filariform* stage occurs over a period of 1-week. The *filariform* larvae may attach themselves to grass or hide in the soil.

An infective *filariform* larva then penetrates the skin and reaches the lungs through the venous system and the right side of the heart. There they invade the alveoli and ascend the airways before being swallowed back and reaching the small intestine 3–5 days after penetrating the skin. The larvae develop into adults in the small intestine and stay attached onto the mucosa by hooks in their buccal cavity. The period from skin penetration to appearance of eggs in the feces is about 6 to 8 weeks, but it may be longer with *Ancylostoma duodenale*. Larvae of *Ancylostoma duodenale*, if swallowed, can survive and develop directly in the intestinal mucosa into adults. Adult hookworms may survive over 10 years but usually live 6 to 8 years for *A.duodenale* and 2 to 5 years for *Necator americanus*.

Incubation Period

The incubation period for *N. Americanus*—7 weeks and A duodenale 5 weeks to 9 months.

Effects of Disease

- **Individual:** It causes chronic blood loss and depletion of body's iron stores leading to iron deficiency anemia.
- **Community:** It exerts a significant and harmful effect on various aspects of the economy and quality of life of a community, especially in 3 major areas. These are:
  - Nutrition
  - Growth and development
  - Work and productivity
  - Medical care costs.

Treatment

Hookworms can be eradicated by the use of several safe and highly effective anthelmintic. The drug of choice is albendazole which is both ovicidal and larvicidal and the dose recommended 400 mg single dose in adults and children over 2 years old otherwise mebendazole is 500 mg single dose in adults and children can also be administered which is not recommended for children below 2 years old.

Correction of the anemia: For children worm infestation is the major cause of anemia which need to be corrected. Dietary supplementation, supplementation of IFA tablet according to body requirement.

Prevention and Control

Sanitary disposal of feces: Sanitary disposal of feces means construction of sanitary latrine in both rural and urban area, proper sewage treatment system, change of farming practice like not using the fecal waste as manure, etc., proper disposal of human and animal feces is more effective not only hook worm but also in preventing other fecal-oral transmission. It is best method in preventive in feco-oral transmission than food hygiene, provision of clean water, health education, or other preventive interventions. As a result, it is very important to achieve a high level of sanitation in displaced populations.

Health education regarding specially wearing shoes can help to prevent the hookworm larvae from penetrating the feet. Proper disposal of feces in areas away from habitations can prevent the occurrence of infective larvae in the environment. Avoidance of open field defecation and construction of latrine is also important.

DRACUNCULIASIS

Dracunculiasis or guinea worm disease is a vector-borne parasite disease, mainly of subcutaneous tissue (usually leg and foot) caused by the nematode parasite, dracunculus medinensis.

Epidemiological Determinants

Agent factors: The adult parasite inhabits the subcutaneous tissue mainly of the legs also of other parts of the body, including the head and neck.
Reservoir of infection: An infected person harboring the gravid female. The possibility of an animal reservoir exists but not proved.
Host factors: Host susceptibility universal.
Environmental factors: Water infested with cyclops.
Mode of transmission: Consumption of water.
Eradication: The eradication strategy comprises the following elements:
- Provision of safe drinking water
- Control of cyclops
- Health education of the public in matters relating to boiling drinking water through a double thickness cotton cloth for personal protection and prevention of water contamination by infected persons.
- Surveillance—active search for new cases.

Treatment of cases

The drugs available for this purposes are niridazole and metronidazole.

ARTHROPOD-BORNE INFECTIONS

DENGUE SYNDROME

Dengue viruses are arboviruses capable of infecting humans, and causing disease. The infections may be asymptomatic or may lead to:
- Classical dengue fever
- Dengue hemorrhage fever with shock.

Dengue fever is a common communicable disease characterized by occurrence of high fever, severe body aches and intense headache. It is a very common disease that occurs in epidemic form from time to time.

Delhi and parts of North India experienced a large number of cases of Dengue in 1996, 2003 and 2006. The disease is quite severe in young children as compared to adults. It is a disease which occurs throughout the world except in Europe and affects a large number of people. For example, it is estimated that every year, 2 crore cases of Dengue fever occur in the world. Death rate varies from 5 per 100 cases to 30 per 100 cases. Dengue fever is a self-limiting disease and represents the majority of cases of dengue infection. A prevalence of Aedes aegypti and Aedes albopictus together with the circulation of dengue virus or more than one type in any particular area tends to be associated with out breaks of DHF/DES.

Cause

It is caused by a virus (dengue virus) which has got four different types (Type 1, 2, 3, 4). Common name of the disease is 'break-bone fever' '(*Haddi Tod Bukhar*)' because of severe body and joint pains produced.

Spread

Just like in malaria, dengue fever is also spread by bites of mosquitoes. In this case, the mosquitoes are 'Aedes' mosquitoes which are very tough and bold mosquitoes and bite even during day time. This disease occurs more frequently in the rainy season and immediately afterwards (July to October) in India. The dengue virus is present in the blood of the patient suffering from dengue fever. Whenever an Aedes mosquito bites a patient of dengue fever, it sucks blood and along with it, the dengue virus injected into his body. The virus undergoes further development in the body of the mosquito for a few days. When the virus containing mosquito bites a normal human being, the virus is injected into the person's body and he/she becomes infected and can develop symptoms of dengue fever.

Incubation period: It means the time between bite of an infected mosquito and appearance of symptoms of dengue fever in the bitten person. Commonly, it is 5–6 days. However it can vary from 3–10 days.

Classical Dengue Fever

Classical dengue or 'break-bone fever' is an acute viral infection, caused by at least 4 serotypes of dengue virus.

The reservoir of infection is both man and mosquito. The transmission cycle is 'man-mosquito-man' (mosquito-man). Ades mosquito become infective by feeding on a patient from the day before onset to the 5th day of illness. After an extrinsic incubation period of 8 to 10 days, the mosquito becomes infective, it remains so for life.

All the ages and both sexes are susceptible to dengue fever. The onset is sudden with chills and high fever, intense headache, muscle and joint pains which prevent all movements. Within 24 hours retro-orbital pain, particularly on eye movements or eye pressure and photophobia develops. Other common symptoms include extreme weakness, anorexia, constipation, altered taste sensation, colicky pain and abdominal tenderness, dragging pain in inguinal region, sore throat and general depression. Fever is usually between 39°C and 40°C. The rash may be diffuse flushing, mottling or fleeting pin point eruptions on the face, neck and chest. The rash lasts for 2 hours to several days and may be followed by desquamation.

Dengue Hemorrhagic Fever (DHF)

DHF is a severe form of dengue fever caused by infection with more than one dengue virus. DHF is transmitted by A aegypti.

Following an incubation period of 4 to 6 days, the illness commonly begins abruptly with high fever accompanied by facial flushing and headache. It may (maculopapular) appear early or late in the course of illness.

Criteria for Clinical Diagnosis of DHF

- **Fever:** Acute onset, high continuous and lasting 2 to 7 days.
- **Hemorrhage manifestation:** Petechiae, purpura, ecchymosis, epistaxis, gum bleeding, hematemesis and/or melena. Based on the symptoms the Classification of dengue virus infection has been shown in **Figure 11.3**.

Grading

Grade I: Fever accompanied by nonspecific constitutional symptoms. The only hemorrhage manifestation is a position tourniquet test.

Grade II: Patient with spontaneous bleeding usually in the form of skin and or other hemorrhages in addition to the manifestations in grade I.

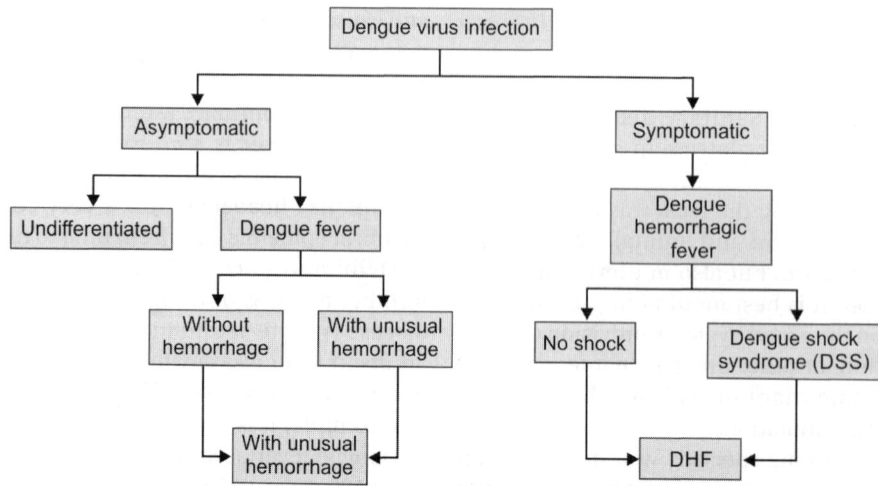

Fig. 11.3: Classification of dengue virus infection.

Grade III: Circulatory failure manifested by rapid and weak pulse, narrowing of pulse pressure or hypertension with the presence of cold clammy skin and restlessness.

Grade IV: Profound shock with undetectable blood pressure and pulse.

Laboratory Diagnosis

- Thrombocytopenia (1,00,000/mm^3 or less)
- Hemoconcentration—hematocrit increased by 20% more of baseline value.

Dengue Shock Syndrome

The clinical diagnosis is based on:
- All the above criteria, plus
- Shock manifested by rapid and weak pulse with narrowing of the pulse pressure or hypotension with the presence of cold, clammy skin and restlessness.

Treatment

If it is classical (simple) dengue fever, the patient can be managed at home. As it is a self-limiting disease, the treatment is purely supportive and symptomatic:
- Keep the fever low by giving paracetamol tablet or syrup as per health worker's advise.
- Avoid giving aspirin or disprin tablets to the patient
- If fever is more than 102°F, carry out hydrotherapy to bring down the temperature.
- Give plenty of fluids water, shikanji, etc., to the patient.
- Continue normal feeding. In fever, the body, infact, requires more food.
- Allow the patient to rest.
- If any of the symptoms indicative of DHF or DSS develop, rush the patient to the nearest hospital at the earliest where appropriate investigations will be carried out and necessary treatment instituted, e.g., transfusion of fluids or platelets (a kind of blood cells which become low in DHF and DSS).
- Replacement therapy can also initiated Children - 5% D in half strength and NS 5%—D 1/3 for infant can also be advisable.

Mosquito Control

Prevention of dengue fever is easy, cheap and better. What is required are some simple measures for:
- Preventing breeding of Aedes mosquitoes
- Protection from Aedes mosquitoes' bites.

Preventing Breeding of Aedes Mosquitoes

- Mosquitoes breed only in water sources such as stagnant water in drains and ditches, room air coolers, broken bottles, old discarded tyres, containers and similar sources.
- Do not allow water to remain stagnant in and around the house. Fill the ditches. Clean the blocked drains. Empty the room air coolers and flower vases completely at least once in seven days and let them dry. Dispose off old containers, tins and tyres, etc., properly.
- Keep the water tanks and water containers tightly covered so that the mosquitoes can not enter them and start breeding.
- Wherever it is not possible to completely drain the water off from room cooler, water tanks, etc. it is advised to put about two tablespoons (30 mL) of petrol or kerosene oil into them for each 100 liters of water.
- Put some types of small fish (Gambusia, Lebister) which eat mosquito larvae into these water collections. These fish can be obtained from the local administrative bodies (e.g., Malaria Officer's office in the area).

Protection from Aedes Mosquitoes' Bites

- Wherever possible, practicable and affordable, prevent entry of mosquitoes into the house by keeping wire mesh on windows and doors. Avoid areas of likely mosquito activity
- Ensure flyscreens in houses, caravans and tents are in good condition
- Use mosquito repellent sprays, creams, coils, mats or liquids to drive away/kill the mosquitoes. Use of *googal* smoke is a good indigenous method for getting rid of mosquitoes.
- Wear clothes which cover the body as much as possible. This is more relevant in case of children. Nickers and T-shirts are better avoided during the season of malaria and dengue fever, i.e., from July to October.
- Use insecticidal sprays in all areas within the house at least once a week. Do not forget to spray behind the photo-frames, curtains, calendars; corners of house, stores. Keep the surroundings of your house clean. Do not litter garbage.
- Do not allow wild herbs, etc. to grow around your house (at least in a radius of about 100 meters around your house). They act as hiding and resting places for mosquitoes.
- Do inform and take help from your local health center, panchayat or municipality in case you notice.
- Abnormal density of mosquitoes or too many cases of fever are occurring in your area.
- Use mosquito coils, or candle heated or gas operated devices using insecticide treated pads for patio and veranda or relatively sheltered or low wind outdoor situations.
- It is good to remember that Aedes mosquitoes bite even during daytime and hence you should take precautions against their bite during daytime also.
- If fencing of the doors and windows is not possible due to any reason, spray the entire house daily with pyrethrum solution.
- Dengue fever occurs most frequently in India in the months of July to October because this season provides very suitable conditions for breeding of mosquitoes. Hence all these preventive steps must be taken during the season.
- Lastly, it is advisable to always keep the patient of dengue fever under a mosquito net in the first 5–6 days of the illness so that mosquitoes do not have an access to him/

her. This will help in reduction in spread of dengue fever to other persons in the community.

MALARIA

Malaria is a protozoal disease caused by infection with parasites of genus plasmodium and transmitted to man by certain species of infected female anopheline mosquito. A typical attack comprises three distinct stages—cold storage, hot storage and sweating stage.

Epidemiological Determinants

Reservoir of infection: Human reservoir is one who harbors the sexual forms of the parasite.

Period of communicability: Four to five days after the infestation of pathogens.

Relapses: It relapse more than 3 years after the patients first attack.

Host factors

- **Age:** Malaria affects all ages.
- **Sex:** Males are more frequently exposed to the risk of acquiring malaria, than females because of the outdoor life they lead.
- **Pregnancy:** It increases the risk of malaria in women.

Socioeconomic development

Housing: Ill ventilated and ill lighted houses provide ideal indoor resting places for mosquitoes.

Population mobility

Occupation: Rural disease closely related to agriculture practices.

Human habits such as:

- Sleeping out of doors
- Nomadism
- Refusal to accept spraying of houses
- Replastering of wall.

Immunity: It is acquired only after repeated exposure to several years.

Environmental factors

- **Season:** July to November
- **Temperature:** 20 deg to 30 deg C
- **Humidity:** Relative humidity 60% considered necessary for mosquito
- **Rainfall:** Changes for breeding mosquito
- **Altitude:** 2000–2500 meters.

Man made malaria includes:

- Barrow pits
- Garden pools
- Irrigation channels
- Engineering projects.

Mode of transmission

a. Vector transmission
b. Direct transmission—accidently by IM or IV injection, e.g., blood transfusion
c. Congenital malaria.

Incubation period

Not less than 10 days.

Clinical features: Typical attack distinguish into 3 stages:

1. **Cold stage:** 39–41°C temperature, headache, vomiting, cold skin last for ¼–1 hours.
2. **Hot stage:** Burning off his clothes, hot and dry skin, intense headache, it last for 2 to 6 hours.
3. **Sweating stage**

General clinical features may include:

- Headache
- Chills
- Profuse sweating
- Muscle pains
- Joint pains
- Nausea, vomiting and diarrhea
- Irritability and refusal to feed
- Other findings are mild anemia and slash or splenic enlargement.

Diagnosis

Microscopy

Microscopy is the gold standard for the diagnosis of malaria parasites in the peripheral blood of the patient. Demonstration of malaria parasites can easily be done by obtaining thick and or thin blood slides from the patient.

Rapid Diagnostic Tests

Rapid diagnostic kits (RDTs) have been developed for malaria diagnosis. RDTs are used for the identification or exposure to malaria parasites by the detection of antibodies, parasite antigens, parasitic metabolic products or parasite enzymes. They usually use immune-chromatographic methods performed on lysed blood containing antigens/antibodies and other parasites metabolic products.

Under National Vector Borne Diseases Control programme the common National Guidelines for treatment of malaria as per the Drug Policy 2013.

Treatment

Treatment of *Vivax* malaria: Diagnosis of *vivax* malaria may be made by the use of RDT (Bivalent) or microscopic examination of the blood smear. On confirmation following treatment is to be given:

Drug schedule for treatment of *P. vivax* malaria:

1. **Chloroquine:** 25 mg/kg body weight divided over three days, i.e., 10 mg/kg on day 1, 10 mg/kg on day 2 and 5 mg/kg on day 3.
2. **Primaquine:** 0.25 mg/kg body weight daily for 14 days. Primaquine is contraindicated in infants, pregnant women and individuals with G6PD deficiency. 14 day regimen of Primaquine should be given under supervision. Dosage chart for treatment of *vivax* malaria has depicted in **Table 11.11**.

Table 11.11: Dosage chart for treatment of *vivax* malaria.

	Day 1		*Day 2*		*Day 3*		*Day 4 to 14*
Age	*CQ (150 mg base)*	*PQ (2.5 mg)*	*CQ (150 mg base)*	*PQ (2.5 mg)*	*CQ (150 mg base)*	*PQ (2.5 mg)*	*PQ (2.5 mg)*
<1 year	½	0	½	0	¼	0	0
1–4 year	1	1	1	1	½	1	1
5–8 year	2	2	2	2	1	2	2
9–14 year	3	4	3	4	1½	4	4
15 year and above	4	6	4	6		6	6
Pregnancy	4	0	4	0	2	0	0
(CQ: Chloroquine; PQ: Primaquine)							

Treatment of Falciparum Malaria

Diagnosis of *falciparum* malaria may be made by the use of RDT (Monovalent or Bivalent) or microscopic examination of the blood smear. It is imperative to start the treatment for falciparum malaria immediately on diagnosis. The treatment for falciparum malaria is as Follows ACT-AL coformulated tablet of Artemether (20 mg) Lumefantrine (120 mg) (Not recommended during the first trimester of pregnancy and for children weighing <5 kg).

In Other States

Artemisinin based Combination Therapy (ACT-SP): Artesunate (AS), available as 50 mg tablets are given for three days, and sulfadoxine-pyrimethamine (S-P) tablets, containing 500 mg sulfadoxine and 25 mg pyrimethamine are given for one day, as shown in the dosage chart below. All tablets for a day should be taken together, swallowed with water. In addition, Primaquine (PQ Large) tablets should be given on the second day.

Dose schedule for treatment of uncomplicated *P. falciparum* cases:

1. **Artemisinin-based Combination Therapy (ACT-SP)*:** Artesunate 4 mg/kg body weight daily for 3 days Plus Sulfadoxine (25 mg/kg body weight)—Pyrimethamine (1.25 mg/kg body weight) on first day.
   *ACT is not to be given in 1st trimester of pregnancy.
2. **Primaquine:** 0.75 mg/kg body weight on day 2.
   With the introduction of different colored Blister Packs for different age groups.
   Treatment by the field level staff has been made easy. The color code for different age groups for Packing of Tablet ACT + SP has been given in **Table 11.13:**

Treatment of uncomplicated *P. falciparum* cases in pregnancy:

1st trimester: Quinine salt 10 mg/kg 3 times daily for 7 days. Quinine may induce hypoglycemia; pregnant women should not start taking quinine on an empty stomach and should eat regularly, while on quinine treatment.

2nd and 3rd trimester: Area-specific ACT as per dosage schedule given above., i.e., ACT-AL in North Eastern States and ACT-SP in Other States. Recommended regimen chart for treatment of *P. falciparum* malaria has depicted in Tables **11.12 and 11.13.**

Primaquine (PQ) prevents transmission of falciparum malaria to others by its ability to kill gametocytes. PQ tablets

Table 11.12: Recommended regimen by weight and age group. The packing size for different age groups based on Kg bodyweight.

Coformulated tablet ACT-AL	*5–14 kg (>5 months to <3 years)*	*15–24 kg (≥ 3 to 8 years)*	*25–34 kg (≥ 9 to 14 years)*	*>34 kg (>14 years)*
Total Dose of ACT-AL	20 mg/120 mg twice daily for 3 days	40 mg/240 mg twice daily for 3 days	60 mg/360 mg twice daily for 3 days	80 mg/480 mg twice daily for 3 days
Pack size				
No. of tablets in the Packing	6	12	18	24
Dose	1 Tablet twice daily for 3 days	2 Tablet twice daily for 3 days	3 Tablet twice daily for 3 days	4 Tablet twice daily for 3 days
Color of the pack	Yellow	Green	Red	White
Primaquine 0.75 mg/kg body weight on day 2.				

Table 11.13: Dosage chart for treatment of falciparum malaria with ACT-SP.

	Day 1		*Day 2*		*Day 3*
Age	*AS*	*SP*	*AS*	*PQ*	*AS*
<1 year Pink Blister	1 (25 mg)	1 (250+12.5 mg)	1 (25 mg)	Nil	1 (25 mg)
1–4 year yellow Blister	1 (50 mg)	1 (500 + 25 mg each)	1 (50 mg)	1 (7.5 mg base)	1 (50 mg)
5–8 year green Blister	1 (100 mg)	1 (750 + 37.5 mg each)	1 (100 mg)	2 (7.5 mg base each)	1 (100 mg)
9–14 year red Blister	1 (150 mg)	2 (500 + 25 mg each)	1 (150 mg)	4 (7.5 mg base each)	1 (150 mg)
15 year and above white	1 (200 mg)	2 (750 + 37.5 mg each)	1 (200 mg)	6 (7.5 mg base each)	1 (200 mg)

ACT-AL: Artemisinin-based Combination Therapy-Artemether-Lumefantrine
ACT-SP: Artemisinin-based Combination Therapy (Artesunate + Sulfadoxine – Pyrimethamine)

should be taken after a meal; not on an empty stomach. Children less than the age of one year and pregnant women should not be given Primaquine. As pregnant women having falciparum malaria require different medicines, they should be directed to go to the nearest PHC or hospital immediately, without delay.

Treatment of mixed infections *(P.vivax + P.falciparum)* **cases:**

All mixed infections should be treated with full course of ACT and Primaquine 0.25 mg per kg body weight daily for 14 days.

In North-Eastern States: Treat with: Age-specific ACT-AL for 3 days + Primaquine 0.25 mg per kg body weight daily for 14 days.

In Other States: SP-ACT 3 days + Primaquine 0.25 mg per kg body wt. daily for 14 days.

Treatment of *P. ovale* and *P. malariae*: In India these species are very rarely found in few places. *P. ovale* should be treated as *P. vivax* and *P. malariae* should be treated as *P. falciparum*.

Treatment of mixed infections: All cases of mixed infection are to be treated as Pf as per the drug policy applicable in the area plus primaquine for 14 days. Dosage chart for treatment of mixed (vivax and falciparum) malaria with ACT-S is shown in **Table 11.14**.

Use of paracetamol: Paracetamol tablets are available as part of the ASHA kit also in the health facilities.

Paracetamol usually brings down fever from any cause within half an hour. However, paracetamol does not cure the disease that is causing the fever. So, its effect does not last long. The fever remains low for about 4–6 hours, and then the fever can rise again.

Paracetamol can be safely given at any age and even during pregnancy, in the dose shown in the dosage chart. In this dose, it can be given 3–4 times a day if needed.

If the fever is not very high, and the patient is able to tolerate the fever, there is no need to give paracetamol.

Initiation of treatment and advice to the patient/caretaker: Once a suspected case is diagnosed positive by RDT or microscopy, treatment is started. The first dose is always taken in the presence of the health volunteer/worker. The blister pack with remaining tablets is given to the patient/caretaker to take home with clear instructions.

Caution: If the patient is a child under 5 years or pregnant, ask the patient to wait for 15 minutes after taking the first dose. If it is vomited within this period, let the patient rest for 15 minutes, then give the first dose again, i.e., open a new blister-pack and discard what remains of the old. If the patient vomits the first dose again, it is considered a case of severe malaria, refer the patient immediate to the nearest Block PHC/CHC/Hospital.

Explain to the patient/caretaker: That if the treatment is not completed as prescribed, the disease may manifest again with more serious features and more difficult to treat.

To come back immediately, if there is no improvement after 24 hours, if the situation gets worse or the fever comes back.

That regular use of a mosquito net (preferably insecticide treated net) is the best way to prevent malaria.

Resistance to antimalarial drugs: Resistance can be defined as either the ability of a parasite strain to survive and/or multiply despite the administration and absorption of a drug given in doses equal to or higher than those usually recommended, but within the limits of tolerance of the patient.

In the last two decades, an increasing proportion of *Plasmodium falciparum* infections is proving to be resistant to chloroquine in India. Drug resistance is declared in a study area, when the proportion of treatment failures exceeds 10% of all falciparum infections. In these areas the decision has been taken to treat all Pf cases with the drug ACT instead of chloroquine.

Why does malaria parasite become resistant to antimalarials?

Drug resistance is a complex phenomenon, where by genetic mutation, a parasite acquires the ability to resist, partly or fully, the effects of one or more antimalarial drugs. When the resistant parasites are exposed to the drug, they multiply selectively. If parasites are resistant to the drug being used, the patient may not respond to treatment.

One of the commonest reasons for the development of drug resistance is that the parasites are exposed to insufficient amount of the drug due to:

- Low prescription dosage
- Lesser amount of drug dispensed
- Incomplete treatment taken by the patient
- Drug vomited out.

In such cases, most of the sensitive parasites are killed by even these small doses, but resistant parasites survive, multiply and spread to other people by mosquitoes. The

Table 11.14: Dosage chart for treatment of mixed (vivax and falciparum) malaria with ACT-S.

	Day 1			*Day 2*		*Day 3*		*Day 4 to 14*
Age	*AS tablet (50 mg)*	*SP tablet*	*PQ (2.5 mg)*	*AS tablet (50 mg)*	*PQ (2.5 mg)*	*AS tablet (50 mg)*	*PQ (2.5 mg)*	*PQ (2.5 mg)*
<1 year	½	½	0	½	0	½	0	0
1–4 years	1	1	1	1	1	1	1′	1
5–8 years	2	½	2	2	2	2	2	2
9–14 years	3	2	4	3	4	3	4	4
15 years and above	4	3	6	4	6	4	6	6

new patient then gets infection from the resistant malaria parasites and does not respond to the drug at all, or responds only partly. Meanwhile, the earlier patient may appear cured because most of the parasites were killed by the drug, and the symptoms abated.

Severe and Complicated Malaria

A case of uncomplicated malaria usually presents with fever, rigors, headache, body ache, fatigue, anorexia and nausea. Serious complications can arise in *P. falciparum* infection and rarely in *P vivax*. They may sometimes develop suddenly over a span of time as short as 12–24 hours and may lead to death, if not treated promptly and adequately. Severe malaria is clinically characterized by confusion, generalized convulsions or drowsiness with extreme weakness (prostration). The health worker can identify such cases and refer them to the nearest PHC as soon as possible.

Criteria for immediate referral to Primary Health Center:
- Persistence of fever after 24 hours of initial treatment.
- Continuous vomiting and inability to retain oral drugs
- Headache continues to increase
- Severe dehydration—dry, parched skin, sunken face
- Too weak to walk in the absence of any other obvious reason
- Change in sensorium, e.g., confusion, drowsiness, blurring of vision, photophobia, disorientation
- Convulsions or muscle twitching
- Bleeding and clotting disorders
- Suspicion of severe anemia
- Jaundice
- Hypothermia.

RABIES

Rabies is a serious often fatal zoonotic disease caused by a virus known as *Lyssavirus.* If the disease is not treated immediately it is invariably followed by death. Rabies is evenly distributed in the world although most of the deaths due to rabies are reported in developing countries. Rabies is transmitted by the virus laden saliva of a rabid animal (mainly dogs) introduced through a bite or scratch. The main reservoirs of the disease are wild animals such as mongooses, jackals and hyenas. These animals infect domestic animals including cattle, donkeys and horses, which in turn infect man. In North and South America, rabid bats have been known to infect humans. All warm-blooded animals are susceptible to rabies. Though it is 100% fatal, it is also 100% preventable:
- Rabies occurs in more than 150 countries and territories.
- It causes 50,000 to 60,000 deaths worldwide/year in rural areas of Africa and Asia.
- India contributes 20,000 deaths alone, i.e., about 2/lac population at risk/year.
- In Africa 24,000, i.e., about 4/lac population at risk.
- Majority of rabies victim are children under 15 years of age.
- More males (55.7%) than female (44.3%).
- Dogs remain the principal cause of animal bites and rabies cases are 90% and cat 7%.

Epidemiological determinants

Agent factors: Lyssavirus type 1 is a bullet shaped neurotropic RNA containing virus. Single-stranded neurotropic genus is Lyssavirus of the family rhabdoviridae.

Reservoir of Infection

Rabies exists in 3 epidemiological forms, urban rabies, wildlife (sylvatic) rabies and bat rabies.

Source of Infection

The source of infection to man is the saliva of rabid animals.

Host Factors

All warm blooded animals including man are susceptible to rabies. Rabies in man is a dead-end infection.

Mode of Transmission
- Animal bites—person-to-person
- Licks
- Aerosols.

Clinical Presentation

- The earliest symptoms usually consist of increasingly severe pain in the bite wound, depression, irritability, nausea, sore throat, headache and loss of appetite.
- Later, two clinical presentations emerge Furious rabies, whereby the infected person develops convulsions, intense fear of death and irrational excitement, which alternates with periods of alertness and calmness. The patient is also unable to tolerate noise, bright light and cold drought (aerophobia—fear of cold air). There is increased reflexes, muscle spasms, excessive sweating, dilatation of pupils, excessive salivation and lacrimation. The patient develops intense hydrophobia (fear of water) because of the intense pain experienced when swallowing water due to spasms of the pharyngeal muscles. This stage is also known as the 'furious' rabies stage and it lasts for 2–3 days and sometimes for 5–6 days. Death usually occurs due to cardiac or respiratory failure during a convulsion.
- The next stage is the *paralytic rabies* stage which is characterized by paralysis of muscles causing paraplegia, quadriplegia and coma. Patients who reach this stage do not survive for more than a week.

Incubation Period

Usually 3–8 weeks but can last several years. The incubation period of rabies ranges from 2 weeks to 1 year, with an average of 2–3 months. The length of the incubation period is influenced by the following factors:
- **The size of the bite:** The deeper the bite the shorter the incubation period
- **Distance of the wound from the brain:** The nearer the wound is to the brain the shorter the incubation period
- **Type of wound:** If the wound is big with extensive the tissues damage the shorter the incubation period.

Diagnosis

Usually rabies is diagnosed from history and physical examination which confirms the dog bite. This may be accompanied by unusual behavior. Presence of Negri bodies in the brain of a suspected rabid dog that has bitten a person presenting with above symptoms is a confirmation of the disease.

Management

There is no cure for rabies once the disease has started. It is however possible to prevent it from reaching this stage by the bite wound should immediately and thoroughly be washed with soap or detergent and flushed with water to clear as much virus as possible. Suturing of the wound should be avoided.

Prevention

We can however prevent the disease from reaching that point by:

Giving postbite prophylaxis: Immediately someone is bitten you should give first aid treatment of the bite with the aim of removing as much virus as possible. This involves immediate flushing of the wounds and scratches preferably with running water and washing the surrounding skin with a lot of soap and water. Puncture wounds should be irrigated with a sterile catheter using methylated spirit and povidone. Iodine is also virucidal and may be used to clean the wound.

Bite wounds should not be sutured immediately to prevent more traumas from the suturing needle, which will increase the areas for viral entry into the body tissue. Suturing may be done 24–48 hours after the bite using very few sutures under the cover of antirabies serum locally.

Antirabies Vaccine

Vaccination against rabies is used in two distinct situations: (1) To protect those who are at risk of exposure to rabies, i.e., pre-exposure vaccination; (2) to prevent the development of clinical rabies after exposure has occurred, usually following the bite of an animal suspected of having rabies, i.e., postexposure prophylaxis.

The vaccines used for pre-exposure and postexposure vaccination are the same, but the immunization schedule differs. Rabies immunoglobulin is used only for post-exposure prophylaxis.

Pre-exposure Vaccination

Pre-exposure vaccination should be offered to people at high-risk of exposure to rabies, such as laboratory staff working with rabies virus, veterinarians, animal handlers and wildlife officers, and other individuals living in or traveling to countries or areas at risk. Travelers with extensive outdoor exposure in rural areas—such as might occur while running, bicycling, hiking, camping, backpacking, etc.—may be at risk, even if the duration of travel is short. Pre-exposure vaccination is advisable for children living in or visiting countries or areas at risk, where they provide an easy target for rabid animals.

Pre-exposure rabies vaccination consists of three full intramuscular (IM) doses of cell-culture or embryonated-egg-based vaccine given on days 0, 7 and 21 or 28 (a few days' variation in the timing is not important). For adults, the vaccine should always be administered in the deltoid area of the arm; for young children (under 1 year of age), the anterolateral area of the thigh is recommended. Rabies vaccine should never be administered in the gluteal area: Administration in this manner will result in lower neutralizing antibody titers.

Postexposure Prophylaxis

In countries or areas at risk of rabies, the circumstances of an animal bite or other contact with an animal suspected to be rabid may require postexposure prophylaxis. In such situations, medical advice should be obtained immediately.

Strict adherence to the WHO-recommended guidelines for optimal postexposure rabies prophylaxis virtually guarantees protection from the disease. The administration of vaccine, and immunoglobulin if required, must be conducted by, or under the direct supervision of, a physician. Postexposure prophylaxis depends on the type of contact with the confirmed or suspect rabid animal, as follows:

Passive Immunization

Human rabies immunoglobulin (HRIG) or equine rabies immunoglobulin (ERIG) or F(ab')2 products should be used for category III exposures as well as for some category II exposures (see table above). Passive immunization should be administered just before or shortly after administration of the first dose of vaccine given in the postexposure prophylaxis regimen. If it is not immediately available, passive immunization can be administered up until the seventh day after initiation of the primary series of postexposure prophylaxis (with cell-culture or embryonated-egg rabies vaccine).

Dosage and administration: The dose for HRIG is 20 IU/kg body weight and for ERIG and F(ab')2 products 40 IU/kg body weight. The full dose of rabies immunoglobulin, or as much as is anatomically feasible, should be administered into and around the wound site. Any remainder should be injected IM at a site distant from the site of active vaccine administration. Multiple needle injections into the wound should be avoided. If the correct dose of rabies immunoglobulin is too small to infiltrate all wounds, as might be true of a severely bitten individual, it can be diluted in physiological buffered saline to ensure greater wound coverage.

Active Immunization

Cell-culture or embryonated-egg-based rabies vaccines should always be used for postexposure prophylaxis. They can be administered either IM or ID.

Intramuscular regimens: Both a five-dose and a four-dose IM regimen are recommended for postexposure vaccination; the five-dose regimen is the more commonly used:

The fivedose regimen is administered on days 0, 3, 7, 14 and 28 into the deltoid muscle.

- The four-dose regimen is administered as two doses on day 0 (one dose in the right and one in the left arm (deltoid muscles), and then one dose on each of days 7 and 21 into the deltoid muscle.

An alternative postexposure regimen for healthy, fully immunocompetent exposed people who receive wound care plus high-quality rabies immunoglobulin plus WHO-prequalified rabies vaccines consists of four doses administered IM on days 0, 3, 7 and 14.

Intradermal regimens: Intradermal administration of cell-culture and embryonated-egg-based rabies vaccines has been successfully used in many developing countries that cannot afford the five- or four-dose IM schedules.

- The two-site ID method: one ID injection at two sites on days 0, 3, 7 and 28.

The volume per intradermal injection should be 0.1 mL with both purified vero cell rabies vaccine, and purified chick embryo rabies vaccine.

PLAGUE

The plague is a bacterial infection that is highly infectious. It was of great public heath concern in the mid-nineteenth century. It occurs in epidemics that may claim a large number of people within a short-time. It is spread by fleas that live on rodents. It is uncommon this days but East Africa continues to be one of the few remaining foci of the plague in the world. Small outbreaks have occurred in Uganda, Kenya, Tanzania, the Democratic Republic of Congo (Zaire) and Namibia. *Y. pestis* involving rodents and fleas.

Epidemiological Determinants

Agent factors: The microorganism is a Gram-negative bacillus called Yesinia pestis (formerly *Pasteurella* pestis).

Reservoir of Infection: Wild rodents (e.g., field mice gerbils, skunks and small animals) are the natural reservoirs of plague.

Host factors: Host factors are explained under some sub-heading described below

- **Age and sex:** Affects all the ages and sex.
- **Human activities:** Hunting, grazing, cultivation, harvesting and construction activities or while engaging in outdoor recreation.
- **Movement of people:** It is associated with movement of people and cargo by sea or land.
- **Immunity:** No natural immunity. Immunity after recovery is relative.

Environment

- **Season:** It is usually season in nature
- **Temperature:** 20 to 25 deg C
- **Humidity:** 60% is favorable
- **Rainfall:** Heavy rainfall especially in the flat fields tend to flood the rat burrows.

Urban and rural areas

Human swelling

Mode of transmission

Five basic types of transmission:

1. Commensal rats - rat fleas - man
2. Wild rodents - wild rodent flea or direct contact - man
3. Wild rodents, peridomestic rodents, commensal rodents, commensal rodent fleas - man
4. Man - human flea - man
5. Man - man

Clinical Presentations

There are three clinical presentations of the plague: Bubonic plague, septicemic plague and pneumonic plague.

Bubonic Plague

Bubonic plague is the commonest form of the plague. It is characterized by swelling of the lymph glands (buboes) which appear within 24 hours of the onset of the disease. The glands most affected are those of the groin, although the armpit and other places may also be affected. The buboes vary in size and may be tender or nontender. Bubonic plague may be complicated by septicemia.

Septicemic Plague

Septicemic plague may be due to an initial infection with highly virulent organisms, or it may be a terminal complication of the bubonic plague. When it is an initial infection, glandular involvement is minimal. The illness is of sudden onset. The patient is prostrated, febrile, weak, pale and apathetic. Stupor, coma and death may follow on the first, second or third day, or later. In the septicemia stage the bacilli are everywhere in the organs, including the lungs. The patient may cough and spread the bacilli to attendants who then develop the pneumonic type of plague.

Pneumonic Plague

Pneumonic plague usually follows or complicates the other two forms of plague. Attendants and visitors are at especially high-risk of infection because of the numerous bacilli the patient coughs out. The illness is characterized by sudden onset of rigors, malaise, intense headache, body aches, fever, and severe prostration. This form of plague is rare in the tropics.

In the early stages it may be difficult to diagnose pneumonic plague, but the extreme illness of the patient in the absence of definite physical signs should raise the suspicion of this type of plague. At first the sputum is watery, but soon it becomes blood stained. Pleural effusion may form, and death usually occurs within 1–2 days.

This is the most infectious and the most fatal form of the plague.

A few people who contract bubonic plague may not appear to be very sick. The fever comes down when the bubo bursts and starts discharging pus. The lesion can be differentiated from lymphogranuloma venereum by making a smear of the pus.

Incubation Period

Bubonic plague: 2 to 7 days
Pneumonic: 1–3 days
Septicemic: 2–7 days.

Laboratory investigations:
- Staining
- Culture
- Serology.

Management

Use of antibiotics has drastically reduced the incidence of the plague as the bacilli are very sensitive to most antibiotics except Penicillin. Early treatment with streptomycin 1 g 12-hourly for 3 days and then 1 g daily for 7 days, or tetracycline or chloramphenicol 500 mg four times a day by mouth for 7 days are all effective. Cotrimoxazole is also effective in doses of 2 tablets twice a day for 7 days.

Prevention and control:
- **Control of cases:**
  - Early diagnosis and notification
  - Isolation
  - Treatment
  - Disinfection.
- **Control of fleas:** Break the chain of transmission.
- **Control of rodents:** Mass destruction of rodents.
- **Vaccination:** Plague vaccine
- **Chemoprophylaxis:**
  - Tetracycline – 500 mg q6h for 5 days
  - Sulfonamide 2–3 g for 5–7 days.
- Surveillance
- Health education.

TETANUS

Tetanus is an acute, often fatal, disease caused by an exotoxin produced by the bacterium *Clostridium tetani*. It is characterized by generalized rigidity and convulsive spasms of skeletal muscles. The muscle stiffness usually involves the jaw (lockjaw) and neck and then becomes generalized which persists throughout illness punctuated by painful paroxysmal spasms of the voluntary muscles.

Public Health Significance and Occurrence

Tetanus occurs worldwide but is now rare in developed countries due to high immunization rates. Infection is most likely in older people who have never been immunized or who have waning and inadequate immunity.

Tetanus is still common in developing countries with low immunization rates and where contact with animal excreta is more common. Tetanus, particularly neonatal tetanus, is a significant cause of death in these settings.

Intravenous drug use is an independent risk factor for tetanus in the absence of acute injuries and may be linked to localized case clusters.

Epidemiological Determinants

Agent factors: Clostridium tetani gram positive organism. *C. tetani* usually enters the body through a wound. In the presence of anaerobic (low oxygen) conditions, the spores germinate. Toxins are produced and disseminated via blood and lymphatics. Toxins act at several sites within the central nervous system, including peripheral motor end plates, spinal cord, and brain, and in the sympathetic nervous system. The typical clinical manifestations of tetanus are caused when tetanus toxin interferes with release of neurotransmitters, blocking inhibitor impulses. This leads to unopposed muscle contraction and spasm. Seizures may occur, and the autonomic nervous system may also be affected.

Clinical Features

Reservoir of infection: Organisms are found primarily in the soil and intestinal tracts of animals and humans so the natural habitat of the organism is soil and dust.

Communicability: Tetanus is not contagious from person to person. It is the only vaccine-preventable disease that is infectious but not contagious.

Host Factors

- **Age:** It is a disease of active age (5 to 40 years).
- **Sex:** Higher incidence is found in males, females are more exposed to the risk.
- **Occupation:** Agricultural work are at special risk.
- **Immunity:** No age immune unless protected by previous immunization.

Environment

It depends upon the man's physical and ecological surroundings.

Mode of Transmission

Infection is acquired by contamination of wounds with tetanus spores. Transmission is primarily by contaminated wounds (apparent and inapparent). The wound may be major or minor. In recent years, however, a higher proportion of patients had minor wounds, probably because severe wounds are more likely to be properly managed. Tetanus may follow elective surgery, burns, deep puncture wounds, crush wounds, otitis media (ear infections), dental infection, animal bites, abortion, and pregnancy.

Incubation period: The incubation period ranges from 3 to 21 days, usually about 8 days. In general the further the injury site is from the central nervous system, the longer is the incubation period. Shorter incubation periods are associated with a higher chance of death.

Clinical features: On the basis of clinical findings, three different forms of tetanus have been described.

Local tetanus: It is an uncommon form of the disease, in which patients have persistent contraction of muscles in the same anatomic area as the injury. These contractions may persist for many weeks before gradually subsiding. Local tetanus may precede the onset of generalized tetanus but is generally milder. Only about 1% of cases are fatal.

Cephalic tetanus: It is a rare form of the disease, occasionally occurring with otitis media (ear infections) in which *C. tetani* is present in the flora of the middle ear, or following injuries to the head. There is involvement of the cranial nerves, especially in the facial area.

Generalized tetanus: The most common type (about 80%) of reported tetanus is generalized tetanus. The disease usually presents with a descending pattern. The first sign is trismus or lockjaw, followed by stiffness of the neck, difficulty in swallowing, and rigidity of abdominal muscles. Other symptoms include elevated temperature, sweating, elevated blood pressure, and episodic rapid heart rate. Spasms may occur frequently and last for several minutes. Spasms continue for 3–4 weeks. Complete recovery may take months. Neonatal tetanus (NT) is a form of generalized tetanus that occurs in newborn infants. Neonatal tetanus occurs in infants born without protective passive immunity, when the mother is not immune. It usually occurs through infection of the unhealed umbilical stump, particularly when the stump is cut with an unsterile instrument.

Prevention

Active immunization: Tetanus is best prevented by active immunization with tetanus toxoid. It stimulates the production of the protective antitoxin. The aim should be to vaccinate the entire community and ensure a protective level of antitoxin approximately 0.01 IU/mL serum throughout life. All persons should be immunized regardless of age.

Two preparations are available for active immunization.

1. Combined vaccine - DPT
2. Monovalent vaccines:
   - Plain or fluid (formal) toxoid
   - Tetanus vaccine, adsorbed (PTAP, APT).

Combined Vaccine

Tetanus vaccine is offered routinely to infants (Expanded Immunization Programme) in combination with diphtheria vaccine and killed *B. pertussis* organisms as DPT vaccine. According to the National Immunization Schedule, the primary course of immunization consists of 3 doses of DPT, at intervals of 4–8 weeks, starting at 6 weeks of age, followed by a booster at 18 months of age, and a second booster (Only DT) at 5–6 years of age and a third booster (Only TT) after 10 years of age.

Monovalent Vaccines

Purified tetanus toxoid (adsorbed) has largely supplanted plain toxoid because it stimulates a higher and longer-lasting immunity response than plain toxoid. However, the latter maybe employed for purposes of booster injection when rapid protection is indicated.

A primary course of immunization consists of two doses of tetanus toxoid adsorbed (each dose 0.5 mL, injected into the arm) given at intervals of 1–2 months. The longer the interval between the two doses, the better is the immune response. The first booster dose (the third in order) should be given a year after the initial two doses. The opinion was expressed that no more than one additional booster does given 5 years after the third does is required in adults (including pregnant women) in developing countries. Frequent boosters must be avoided.

Reactions following the injections of tetanus toxoid are uncommon. They are less likely to occur with a refined and adsorbed toxoid such as purified tetanus toxoid (aluminum phosphate adsorbed). However, in persons giving history of allergy usual precautions should be observed. Purified tetanus toxoid should be stored between 4 and 10° C. It must not be allowed to freeze at any time.

Passive Immunization

Temporary protection against tetanus can be provided by an injection of human tetanus hyper immunoglobulin (TIG) or ATS.

- **Human tetanus hyperimmunoglobulin:** It is the best prophylactic to use. The dose for all ages is 250 IU. It does not cause serum reactions. It gives a longer passive protection up to 30 days or more compared with 7–10 days for horse ATS. Human tetanus Ig is now available in India—it is produced by the Serum Institute of India, Pune.
- **ATS (Equine):** If human antitoxin is not available, equine antitoxin (anti-tetanus serum or ATS) should be used. The standard dose is 1500 IU, injected subcutaneously after sensitivity testing. ATS gives passive protection for about 7–10 days. Being a foreign protein, ATS is rapidly excreted from the body and there may be very little antibody at the end of 2 weeks. Because of this drawback, ATS may not cover the tetanus incubation period in all cases.

ATS has other disadvantages too

- It causes sensitivity reaction in many people because it contains foreign proteins. A person receiving ATS for the first time may tolerate it well, but there is a possibility that subsequent injections of horse serum may lead to allergic reactions varying in severity from rash to anaphylactic shock. It is estimated that the incidence of serious systemic reactions to ATS is 5 to 10% of the persons who receive it. It is well to remember that local tests for sensitivity are unreliable as to general sensitivity to horse serum.
- Another drawback of ATS is that it stimulates the formation of antibodies to it and hence a person who has once received ATS tends to rapidly eliminate subsequent doses. As such the value of second and subsequent doses of ATS becomes questionable. In practice, therefore, ATS becomes less and less reliable as a prophylactic. These drawbacks have been responsible for the growing unpopularity of ATS as an agent for immediate protection against tetanus.

Active and Passive Immunization

Simultaneous active and passive immunization is widely carried out in nonimmune persons. The patient is given 1500 units of ATS or 250 units of Human Ig in one arm, and 0.5 mL of adsorbed tetanus toxoid (PTAP or or glutaral region). This should be followed 6 weeks later by another dose of 0.5 mL of tetanus toxoid, and a third dose one year later. The purpose of antitoxin is for immediate temporary protection, and the purpose of toxoid is for long lasting protection.

Antibiotics

Active immunization with tetanus toxoid is the ideal method of tetanus prophylaxis, but it is of no immediate avail to a person who is nonimmune and has sustained injury. ATS as an agent for immediate protection against tetanus has its drawbacks. For these reasons, antibiotics are indicated in the prophylaxis against tetanus. A single intramuscular injection of 1.2 mega units of a long-acting penicillin (e.g., benzathine penicillin) will provide a sustained concentration of the drug for 3 to 4 weeks, which is sufficient to kill any vegetative forms of tetanus bacilli that may emerge from the sporulating stage. Penicillin has no effect on tetanus spores. For patients who are sensitive to penicillin, a 7-day course of erythromycin estolate 500 mg 6-hourly by mouth will kill vegetative forms of *Cl. tetani* but not spores. Antibiotics should be given as soon as possible after an injury, before a lethal dose of toxin is as possible after an injury, before a lethal dose of toxin is produced in the wound, which may be as soon as 6 hours after injury. Antibiotic prophylaxis should not be relied upon for patients seen later than 6 hours after injury. Moreover, it is not certain whether the antibiotic can reach the bacilli, if there is dead tissue present in the wound. Therefore, antibiotic alone is ineffective in the prevention of tetanus; it is not a substitute to immunization.

Prevention of Neonatal Tetanus

Neonatal tetanus is well controlled in some industrialized countries through clean delivery practices alone. Over the last decade, most programs in developing countries have concentrated on training the traditional birth attendants, providing home delivery kits and educating pregnant women about the 'five cleans' - clean hands, clean delivery surface, clean clothes, clean blade for cutting the cord, clean cord tie for tying the cord and no application on the cord stump. Operational research has shown that training of birth attendants alone can reduce death due to neonatal tetanus by 90%.

Tetanus toxoid will protect both the mother and her child. For unimmunized women during pregnancy two doses of tetanus toxoid should be given, the first as early as possible during pregnancy and the second at least a month later and at least 3 weeks before delivery. According to the National Immunization Schedule these doses may be given between 16 and 36 weeks of pregnancy, allowing an interval of 1–2 months between the 2 doses. In previously immunized pregnant women, a booster dose is considered sufficient. There is no need for a booster at every consecutive pregnancy, because of the risk of hyperimmunization and side-effects.

In areas where the incidence of neonatal tetanus is high, the primary 2-does course can be extended to all women of child-bearing age, particularly if the present coverage of antenatal care is low. In developing countries, the majority of pregnant women are not coming for antenatal checkup. Since a pregnant women coming for an antenatal visit may in fact never return again, immunization should be given regardless of the month of pregnancy as there is no evidence to suggest that tetanus toxoids are dangerous or harmful to the fetus. The golden rule is that no pregnant mother should be denied even one does of tetanus toxoid if she is seen late in pregnancy.

The infants born to the mothers who have not previously received 2-doses of tetanus toxoid are exposed to the risk of neonatal tetanus. They can be protected by injection of antitoxin (heterologous serum, 750 IU), if it is a administered within 6 hours of birth.

LEPROSY

Leprosy is endemic in several states and union territories of India, with the annual case detection rate of 4.56 per 10,000 population. The prevalence rate of leprosy is 0.4 per 10,000 population in the country. Of the new cases detected during 2020–2021, 58.1% were multibacillary, 39% were women, 5.8% were children less than 14 years of age, and 2.41% had visible deformities. The rate of visible deformities was 1.1 per million population.

In March 2021, 79,898 patients were under free MDT treatment for leprosy across the country. Despite COVID-19 disruption of health services during 2020–2021, 65,147 new cases of leprosy were identified, diagnosed and provided free treatment. Continuity of these essential healthcare services during pandemic response ensures that leprosy is cured and disability is prevented

Leprosy (Handsen's disease) is a chronic infectious disease caused by *M. leprae*. It is clinically characterized by one or more of the following cardinal features like Hypopigmented patches, Partial or total loss of cutaneous sensation in the affected areas (the earliest sensation to be affected is usually light touch), Presence of thickened nerves and Presence of acid-fast bacilli in the skin or nasal smears.

Determinants of Leprosy

- **Agent:** Leprosy is caused by *Mycobacterium leprae* intracellular, obligatory parasite. It is a slow growing bacillus and one Leprosy bacillus takes 12–14 days to divide in to two. It is an acid-fast bacillus and is stained red by a dye called carbol fuschin.
- **Source of infection:** Untreated Leprosy affected person (Human beings) is the only known source for *M. leprae*.
- **Portal of exit:** The major sites from which bacilli escape from the body of an infectious patient is respiratory tract

especially nose. Only small proportion of those suffering from Leprosy can transmit infection.

- **Transmission of infection:** Leprosy is transmitted from untreated Leprosy affected person to a susceptible person through droplets, mainly via the respiratory tract.
- **Portal of entry:** Respiratory route appears to be the most probable route of entry for the bacilli.

Incubation period: Incubation period (duration from time of entry of the organism in the body to appearance of first clinical sign and symptom) for Leprosy is variable from few weeks to even 20 years. The average incubation period for the disease is said to be 5–7 years.

Host Factors

Age: Leprosy can occur at any age but is usually seen in people between 20–30 years of age. Increased proportion of affected children in the population indicates the presence of active transmission of the disease in the community. As the disease burden declines, it is seen more in older age groups.

Gender: Disease occurs in both the genders. However, males are affected more as compared to females.

Immunity: Occurrence of the disease depends on susceptibility/immunological status of an individual.

Socioeconomic factors: Leprosy is a disease generally associated with poverty and related factors like overcrowding. However, it may affect persons of any socioeconomic group.

Factors Influencing Susceptibility

- **Age:** Children are more susceptible than adults.
- **Individual immunity:** May be determined by certain genetic factors which influence the susceptibility of an individual
- **Climate:** Leprosy is prevalent in tropical and subtropical climates.

Diagnosis of Leprosy

A case of leprosy is diagnosed by eliciting cardinal signs of leprosy through systematic clinical (and wherever required bacteriological) examination. At least one of the following cardinal (unique and very important) signs must be present to diagnose leprosy.

- Hypopigmented or reddish skin lesion(s) with definite sensory deficit
- Involvement of the peripheral nerves, as demonstrated by definite thickening with loss of sensation and weakness of the corresponding muscles of the hands, feet or eyes
- Demonstration of *M. leprae* in the lesions.

The first two cardinal signs can be identified by clinical examination alone while the third can be identified by examination of the slit skin smear.

A person with cardinal signs of leprosy and yet to complete full course of MDT may be called as "case of leprosy".

After making a diagnosis of leprosy, one should group the patient based on certain characteristics. This is important because it helps in selecting the correct combination of drugs for a given patient **(Table 11.15)**.

Table 11.15: Criteria for grouping.

	Characteristic	*PB (Pauci Bacillary)*	*MB (Multi Bacillary)*
1.	Skin lesions	1–5 lesions	6 and above
2.	Peripheral nerve	No nerve/only one nerve involvement	More than one nerve
3.	Skin smear	Negative at all sites	Positive at any site

Grading of Disabilities

Hands and Feet

- **Grade 0:** No anesthesia, over palm/sole no visible deformity or damage
- **Grade 1:** Anesthesia present, over palm/sole but no visible deformity or damage
- **Grade 2:** Visible deformity or damage present.

Eyes

- **Grade 0:** No eye problem due to leprosy; no evidence of visual loss
- **Grade 2:** Severe visual impairment (vision worse than 6/60; inability to count fingers at six meters), lagophthalmos, iridocyclitis and corneal opacities.

Management of Leprosy

The treatment of leprosy is in the form of Multi Drug Therapy (MDT) which is the combination of two or three of the following drugs:

a. Cap. Rifampicin
b. Tab. Dapsone
c. Cap. Clofazimine

Details treatment regimen the doses has been explained in **Tables 11.16 and 11.17**. MDT kills the bacilli (*M. leprae*) in the body and thus stops the progression of the disease and prevents further complications.

1. As the M. leprae are killed, the patient becomes non-infectious and thus the spread of infection in the body is reduced. Moreover, spread of infection to other persons is also reduced.
2. Using a combination of two or three drugs instead of one drug alone will ensure effective cure and there are no chances of development of resistance to the drugs.

Based on the grouping, the patients can be given any one of the standard MDT regimens mentioned below. In children, the dose may be adjusted suitably.

When the patient has completed the required number of doses (monthly pulses) of standard MDT regimens, she/he is released from Treatment-RFT.

Regarding fitness of patient for MDT, before starting treatment one must look for the following:

- **Jaundice:** If the patient is jaundiced, you will have to wait until jaundice subsides.
- **Anemia:** If the patient is anemic, treat the anemia also simultaneously.

Table 11.16: MDT regimen (Adult).

	Drugs used (adult)	*Dosage*	*Frequency of administration*	*Criteria for RFT*
MB leprosy	Rifampicin Dapsone Clofazimine Clofazimine	600 mg 100 mg 300 mg 50 mg	Once monthly Daily Once monthly Daily	Completion of 12 monthly pulses
PB leprosy	Rifampicin Dapsone	600 mg 100 mg	Once monthly Daily	Completion of 6 monthly pulses

Table 11.17: MDT regimen (Child—10–14 years of age).

	Drugs used (child)	*Dosage*	*Frequency of administration*	*Criteria for RFT*
MB leprosy	Rifampicin Dapsone Clofazimine Clofazimine	450 mg 50 mg 150 mg 50 mg	Once monthly Daily Once monthly Every other day	Completion of 12 monthly pulses
PB leprosy	Rifampicin Dapsone	450 mg 50 mg	Once monthly Daily	Completion of 6 monthly pulses

Table 11.18: Types of Lepra reactions.

Features	*Type 1 (Reversal reaction)*	*Type 2 (ENL reaction)*
Skin	Existing lesions suddenly become red, swollen, warm, and tender. New lesions may appear. Lesions when subsiding may show scales on the surface	Red, painful, tender, subcutaneous nodules (ENL) appear commonly on face, arms and legs. They appear in groups and subside within a few days even without treatment
Nerves	Nerves close to the skin may become enlarged, tender and painful (neuritis) with loss of nerve function	Nerves may be affected but not as common or severe as in Type 1
Other organs	Rarely affected	Other organs like eye, joints, bones, testes, kidney may be affected
General symptoms	Not common	Fever, joint pains, fatigue

- **Tuberculosis:** If the patient is taking Rifampicin, ensure that he continues to take Rifampicin in the dose required for the treatment of tuberculosis along with other drugs required for the treatment of leprosy.
- **Allergy to Sulfa drugs:** If the patient is known to be allergic to sulfa drugs, Dapsone should be avoided. Clofazimine may be used instead.

Leprosy Reaction

It is acute inflammatory response occurring in the course of the disease. It can occur at any time before, during or after treatment. It must be promptly diagnosed and treated to prevent any disability. Patients with the following characteristics are more likely to develop leprosy reactions:

- Multiple lesions
- Lesions close to the peripheral nerve
- Lesions on the face
- Postpartum period.

These patients should be monitored more frequently for early detection of reaction and its prompt management.

There are two principal types of Lepra reactions. Type 1 and Type 2 **(Table 11.18)**.

- Type 1 Lepra Reaction also known as Reversal Reaction may occur both in PB and MB leprosy.
- Type 2 reaction is also known as Erythema Nodosum Leprosum (ENL) and occurs only in MB leprosy.

The patient will need Corticosteroids in addition to rest and analgesics. The drug of choice is Prednisolone. The usual course begins with 40–60 mg daily in single dose preferably in the morning (up to a maximum of 1 mg/kg of body weight), and the reaction is generally controlled within a few days. The dose is then gradually reduced fortnightly and eventually stopped. Proper precaution should be taken in patients with diabetes, peptic ulcer, hypertension, etc. Necessary precautions for administering steroid should be taken.

Type 2 Lepra Reaction (ENL)

Type 2 reaction	*Treatment*
Mild: few nodules, mild fever	Analgesics
Severe: severe pain over nodules, tendency for ulceration, high fever, involvement of internal organs	Steroid-Prednisolone whole course not exceeding 2 to 3 weeks (same dose as for type 1 reaction but faster tapering)
Neuritis	Prednisolone regimen as for neuritis in Type 1 reaction

Clofazimine is also effective for Type 2 reaction but is less potent than corticosteroids and often takes 4–6 weeks to develop its full effects, so it should never be started as the sole agent for the treatment of recurrent Type 2 reaction. However, clofazimine may be extremely useful for reducing or withdrawing corticosteroids in patients who have become dependent on them.

Self-care

Hands and Feet

- Inspect the hands/feet daily for hot, tender spots
- Soak the hands/feet for about half an hour in water.
- Scraping hard skin (if fissures/cracks present) using any stone without sharp edges.
- Apply vaseline or cooking oil when hands/feet are wet.
- Protect hands against heat and friction.
- Walk slowly with short steps. Use footwear for anesthetic feet.
- Clean the wound with soap and water. Dress with clean cloth.
- Consult medical officer if ulcer is foul smelling
- Oil massage and passive movements to keep the joints mobile.

Eyes

- Check eyes daily using mirror.
- Wear protective devices
- Put moistening eye drop
- Red/painful eye, consult doctor.

SEXUALLY TRANSMITTED DISEASES

The sexually transmitted (STD) are a group of communicable disease that are transmitted predominantly by sexual contact and caused by a wide range of bacterial, viral, protozoal and fungal agents and ectoparasites.

Definition: Disease that is produced and spread from person to person by sexual contact is termed as sexually transmitted disease.

Burden of the disease: The incidence of STIs is high among the High-Risk Groups 2.5%. Approximately 3 Crore episodes of STIs/RTIs occur every year in India. Prevalence of symptoms suggestive of STI/RTI in women was in the range of 23–43%, while in men, it is in the range of 4–9% (NACO, 2009).

Common STI

Bacterial:

- Syphilis
- Gonorrhea
- Chancroid
- Nongonococcal urethritis
- Chlamydial infection
- Lymphogranuloma Venereum.

Protozoal: Trichomoniasis.

Viral:

- Herpes
- HIV
- Genital warts
- Anal warts
- Hepatitis.

Not always sexually transmitted:

- Pubic lice infestation
- Vaginitis
- Scabies
- Molluscum contagiosum.

The classification of causative organisms for STIs is depicted in **Table 11.19**.

Table 11.19: Classification of causative organisms for STIs.

Pathogen	*Disease or syndrome*
Neisseria gonorrhea	Gonorrhea, urethritis, PID
Treponema pallidum	Syphilis
Haemophilus ducreyi	Chancroid
Chlamydia trachomatis	Urethritis, cervicitis
Calymmatobacterium granulomatis	Donovanosis
Herpes simplex virus	Genital herpes
Hepatitis B virus	Acute and chronic hepatitis
HIV	AIDS
Candida albicans, Trichomonas vaginalis	Vaginitis

Epidemiological Determinants

Agent Factors: Over 20 pathogens have been found to be spread by sexual contact.

Host Factors

- **Age:** Mostly observed STD incidence rates are 20–24 years olds followed by the 25–29 and 15–19 years of age. The vaginal mucosa and cervical tissue in young women is immature which makes them more vulnerable to STI than older women. Women are especially at risk in cultures where they marry or become sexually active during early adolescence. On average, women become infected at a younger age than men.
- **Gender:** Since the mucosal surface that comes into contact with the infective agent is much greater in women than in men, women can be more easily infected than men.
- **Immune status:** The immune status of the host and virulence of the infective agent affect transmission of STI. Certain STIs increase the risk of transmission of HIV. HIV, in its turn, facilitates the transmission of some STIs, and worsens the complications of STI by weakening the immune system.
- **Marital status:** Frequently of STD infection is higher among single, divorced and separated persons than among married couples.

Social/Cultural Factors

In some societies men's risky behavior of multiple sexual partners is tolerated thus putting them and their partners at risk of infection. Also in cultures where the girl-child is married off to an adult male at a very young age exposes the girl to infection. Further, with growing industrialization and consequent urbanization, there is a large group of single poorly paid and unemployed young people who migrate from rural to urban areas in such for employment. In such circumstances, sexual intercourse for pleasure and gain assumes an important role. This promiscuous sexual behavior is closely associated with the acquisition of STIs.

Socioeconomic status—low socioeconomic groups have higher morbidity rate.

Behavioral Factors

Risky behaviors such as having multiple sexual partners, having sex with commercial sex workers, and having unprotected sexual intercourse makes it more likely for a person to acquire an STI. Indeed, people who have had an STI in the last year are at risk of getting infected again if they have not been able to change their sexual behavior.

Demographic Factors

- Population explosion
- Marked increase in the number of young people
- Migration
- Increasing educational opportunities for women delaying their marriage.

Social Factor

- Prostitution
- Broken homes
- Sexual disharmony
- Marital incompatibility
- Easy money
- Emotional immaturity
- Urbanization and industrialization
- Social disruption
- International travel
- Changing behavioral pattern
- Social stigma
- Alcoholism
- Lack of sexual hygiene
- Poverty.

Males

- Ulcers/sores
- Discharges (urethral)
- Swellings/growths—warts (groin/scrotum)
- Pain/burning when voiding.

Females

- Ulcers/sores
- Vaginal discharge
- Swellings/growths-warts (groin/labia)
- Burning when voiding
- Pain (low abdominal/backache).

The associated features of STI Syndromes are depicted in **Table 11.20**.

Table 11.20: Associated features of STI syndromes.

Syndrome	*Possible etiological agent*	*Clinical presentation*
Vaginal discharge	*Neisseria gonorrhoeae*	Greenish yellow discharge may be massaged from the urethra or seen oozing from the endocervix!
	Chlamydia trachomatis	Scanty mucopurulent or purulent discharge
	Trichomonas vaginalis	Frothy, profuse, greenish yellow, tout smelling discharge
	Candida albicans, or other Candida species	White, curd-like discharge involving the vaginal wall and cervix
	Gardnerella vaginalis (anaerobic bacteria)	Profuse foul smelling and homogenous greyish white discharge. Adherent to vaginal wall.
Urethral discharge	*Neisseria gonorrhoea*	Abundant pus-like discharge dripping from the urethra. Incubation period 3–10 days
	Chlamydia trachomatis	Mucoid or serous discharge scanty, usually seen in the morning. Incubation period 10–14 days. Urethral irritation
Genital ulcer diseases	*Haerpes simplex virus*	Multiple shallow and tender ulcers. May start as vesicles grouped together. Itchy. Incubation period 1 week.
	Treponema pallidum	Single, painless, relatively dean ulcers without pus. Incubation period up to 3 weeks.
	Hemophilus ducreyi	Multiple, soft. Deep, tender ulcers with profuse pus. Incubation period 1 week.
	Lymphogranuloma venereum (LGV)	Single, small and transient ulcers. Incubation period 1–2 weeks.
	Granuloma inguinale, *Calymmatobacterium granulomatis* (Donovan bacilli)	Large and beefy ulcers. Variable incubation period.
Inguinal bubo	*Haemophilus ducreyi, Chlamydia trachomatis* (L1-L3 immunotypes), *Lymphogranuloma venereum*	Several nodes mated together
Genital venereal warts	Condyloma acuminatum, *Human papillomavirus* (HPV)	Cauliflower-like warts, may be single or multiple on vulva, vagina, perineal areas, penis, urethra and sub-prepuce.

Contd...

Contd...

Syndrome	Possible etiological agent	Clinical presentation
	Molluscum contagiosum. Pox group virus	Umbilicated papules multiple with whitish, cheesy material being expressed when squeezed.
Lower abdominal pain	Neisseria gonorrhoea, Chlamydia trachomatis	Cervical-vaginal discharge, which is purulent. Painful with frequent micturition, fever, malaise, lower backache. May fallow menstrual periods.
Ophthalmia neonatorum	Neisseria gonorrhea, Chlamydia trachomatis, and others	Mucoid or purulent discharge within the first month in life.
Source: MOH, National Guidelines for Reproductive Tract Infections Services		

GONORRHEA

Gonorrhea is a fairly common sexually transmitted disease caused by a gram negative intracellular diplococcus bacterium, *Neisseria gonorrheae*. It is an acute or chronic purulent infection characterized by urethral or vaginal discharge. It is often abbreviated as 'gc'. Gonorrhea is by far the commonest of the so called 'classical STDs', that is STDs known before the emergence of HIV all over the world. Gonorrhea can cause sterility in both females and males and accounts for a serious decline in birth rate in some communities. In females, gonorrhea may cause death due to salpingitis and peritonitis or predispose them to ectopic pregnancy. In males it may cause urethral strictures resulting in urine retention, hydronephrosis and uremia, also causing death.

Epidemiology

Gonorrhea is caused by gonococcus, a gram-negative kidney-shaped diplococcus, which can only grow intracellularly. This type of gonococcus is known as *Neisseria gonorrhoeae*. The gonococcus is not able to penetrate intact skin or squamous epithelium. It prefers columnar epithelium, such as in the urethra, endocervix, rectum and conjunctiva. While contact of mucous membranes with gonococcal pus is usually only possible during sexual intercourse, there are exceptions. For instance, in the case of gonococcal ophthalmia neonatorum, the infection is contracted during passage through the birth canal. Another exception is gonococcal vulvovaginitis. The vagina of an adult woman of reproductive age is lined with squamous cells which contain glycogen. Through bacterial action, this glycogen is metabolized into lactic acid, thus producing a low pH. This low pH protects the vaginal wall from invading gonococci. The glycogen content of the cells is determined by estrogen levels and is therefore low before puberty and after menopause. So before puberty and after menopause the vagina is less resistant to gonoccocal infections.

Mainly through sexual contact: Vaginal, anal or oral sex. Bacteria are transmitted through vaginal and seminal fluids and the incubation period is between 2–10 days. Transmission can also occur to the neonate during delivery leading to Ophthalmia Neonatorum.

Risk Factors

- People who do not use condoms during vaginal, anal or oral sex
- Multiple sex partners
- History of sexually transmitted diseases
- Below the age of 30 have an increased risk of being infected with gonorrhea
- Low socioeconomic status.

Clinical Symptoms

Once infected, the symptoms of gonorrhea can take between two and ten days to show up. In males the common symptoms include:
- Irritation at the urethral meatus
- Burning sensation (dysuria) when passing urine
- Purulent profuse yellowish discharge from the urethra
- Occasionally terminal hematuria (blood in the urine) may occur
- Swollen testicles.

In women, about 50% of infected women have no symptoms. The female urethra is short and the urethritis and discharge often go unnoticed. As a result of this, many women are only seen in clinics when they have developed symptoms due to complications. The cervix is usually the first site of infection. From there, the infection moves up into the uterus and into the fallopian tubes. In those cases that develop symptoms, these are likely to include:
- Bleeding after coitus
- Pain or burning sensation when urinating
- Frequency and urgency in micturition
- Vaginal discharge that is yellow or bloody
- Abdominal cramps.

In untreated cases, the infection in the majority of women remains latent for several months or years, during which time they form an important reservoir for the spread of the disease.

Incubation period: Three to four days.

Diagnosis

- History collection about sign and symptom
- Smear examination for detection of the organism
- Urethral smear for men
- High vaginal swab
- Urinalysis for microscopy

- Gram stain showing pus cells and intracellular Gram-negative diplococci is 95% sensitive.

Management

Treat according to guideline. Mainly gonorrhea cases will treated by antibiotic and the drug of choice for antibiotic is ciprofloxacin spectinomycin cefixime, ceftriaxone, etc.
- Treatment of partner within last 3 month
- Condom use should promoted
- Counsel for compliance, safe sex
- Refer to ICTC for diagnosis of HIV.

Complications

If left untreated, gonorrhea can lead to infertility in both men and women. In women, untreated gonorrhea often leads to pelvic inflammatory disease, which increases the risk of ectopic pregnancy and infertility. In men, gonorrhea that is not treated often leads to inflammation of the testicles (epididymitis), which can lead to infertility. The infection can also spread to the rest of the body and cause joint inflammation as well as infect the heart valves and/or the brain.

SYPHILIS

Syphilis is a sexually transmitted disease caused by spirochaete bacteria, *Treponoma pallidum*. It is often called the 'Great Imitator' because syphilis symptoms resemble those of other common diseases. The majority of syphilis sufferers are male, accounting for about 60% of all cases. Syphilis is the 2nd most common genital ulcer disease in Kenya, the first being genital herpes. It is a disease characterized by a primary lesion on the skin or mucous membrane followed by a long period of latency and then late lesions.

Modes of Transmission

- Syphilis is almost always transmitted through sexual contact with an infected person. The syphilis bacteria can easily spread from the ulcers on an infected person to the mucous linings of the mouth, genitals, and anus of an uninfected sexual partner.
- Though unlikely, it is possible to contract the infection by coming into contact with the broken skin of an infected person.
- Syphilis can also be passed from an infected mother to her unborn child (congenital route).
- Through blood transfusion with blood from an infected person.

Risk Factors

- Multiple sex partners are also at risk.
- Healthcare workers may be at risk of contracting the disease, due to increased contact with those infected with the disease.
- Drug users who share needles or pipes are also at risk as are those working and living in a corrections facility.

Symptoms

Syphilis symptoms occur in stages:
- Primary syphilis results in painless firm ulcers or sores called 'chancres.' These usually appear on the external genitalia, inside the vagina and they can also appear on the lips, tongue, and other body parts in cases of oral sex, between 10–90 days (average three weeks) after exposure. These chancres generally disappear within a few weeks, but if left untreated, the disease can progress to chronic stages.
- Secondary syphilis begins with the syphilis rash. This is an infectious brown skin rash that typically occurs on the bottom of the feet and the palms of the hand. The patient may present with constitutional symptoms such as fever, sore throat. Late secondary syphilis presents with condylomatous smooth snail ulcers on the oral cavity with generalized lymphadenopathy and associated alopecia (loss of hair). **The secondary stage** may last one to three months and begins within six weeks to six months after exposure. People with secondary syphilis.
- Tertiary stage of syphilis can last for many years ranging from 2–20 years after secondary stage, and one may suffer from joint and bone damage, increasing blindness, numbness in the extremities, or difficulty in coordinating movements and neurosyphilis. If the infection is not treated, it may then progress to a stage characterized by severe problems with the heart, brain, and nerves that can result in paralysis, blindness, dementia, deafness, impotence, and even death if it is not treated.

Diagnosis

Darkfield examinations and direct fluorescent antibody (DFA) tests of lesion exudate or tissue are the definitive methods for diagnosing early syphilis.

A presumptive diagnosis is possible with the use of two types of serologic tests:
- Venereal Disease Research Laboratory [VDRL] and RPR);
- Treponemal tests (e.g., fluorescent treponemal antibody absorbed [FTA-ABS] and *T. pallidum* particle agglutination [TP-PA]).

Treatment

The duration of suffering with syphilis for less than a year, a single dose of penicillin is usually enough to destroy the infection. For those allergic to penicillin, doxycycline tetracycline, or another antibiotic can be given instead in a later stage of disease, more doses will be needed.

CHLAMYDIA URETHRITIS

Chlamydia is a sexually transmitted disease caused by the bacteria *Chlamydia trachomatis*. Because it is often associated with no symptoms, it is also called 'The Silent Disease.' More than 75% of women and 50% of men exhibit no symptoms when suffering from the disease. Chlamydia is one of the most commonly occurring STDs. Prolonged infection can cause infertility and damage to the reproductive organs.

Symptoms of Chlamydia

Chlamydia symptoms may be mild and can easily go undetected. Women are more likely to experience few symptoms associated with the infection although chlamydia in men can also result in few or no symptoms. Signs of chlamydia usually appear between 1 and 3 weeks after infection, though sometimes they can take longer to manifest. Early chlamydia signs and symptoms tend to be mild and include pain during urination, frequent urination, and low fever. Later symptoms can be more intense and include nausea, fatigue, and abnormal discharge from the vagina or penis. Oral chlamydia, usually passed through oral sex, can result in a sore throat and throat infection. In anal infections, swelling of the rectum can occur. Though rare, males suffering from the disease may experience swelling of the testicles. Other symptoms in women include abdominal pain, lower back pain, irregular menstrual bleeding or spotting, and pain during sex.

Complications of Infection

If left untreated, chlamydia can move through the body causing serious health problems. As the infection travels, it can cause eye and throat infections as well as rectal infections. Long-term infection can lead to damage in the uterus and fallopian tubes in women and, in rare cases, sterility in men. It also leads to an increased risk for developing Pelvic Inflammatory Disease (PID), which can cause fertility problems. Chlamydia infection is dangerous to newborns. If one is pregnant and infected with chlamydia, one can transmit the infection to the child. Chlamydia infection also increases the risk of contracting HIV. Women with chlamydia are up to 5 times more likely to contract HIV, the virus that leads to AIDS. In rare cases, chlamydia can cause Reiter's syndrome, a disease characterized by arthritis, skin lesions, and inflammation of the urethra and eyes.

Diagnosis and Testing

- Physical exam and history.
- In women, chlamydia is best detected through a cervical swab. This procedure is very similar to a pap smear.
- The most common tests look for antigens that the bacteria produce in the body.
- A culture test may also be performed. This test fosters the growth of chlamydia bacteria in a dish so that it can be analyzed under a microscope.

Treatment

The choice antibiotic for chlamydia is Norfloxacin 800 mg stat Doxycycline 100 mg orally twice a day for 7 days OR IM Spectinomycin 2 mg stat and Doxycycline 100 mg BD × 7 days can be administered.

CHANCROID

This is an acute venereal infection that presents as a rugged painful necrotizing ulcer on the genitalia accompanied by inflammatory swelling and suppuration of the regional lymph nodes. It is caused by a gram-negative bacilli called *Haemophilus ducreyi,* which is spread through sexual contact. Chancroid can also be transmitted through direct skin-to-skin contact with an infected person's ulcers.

Clinical Presentation

Primarily there is development of painful, pus-filled ulcers in the genital region 3 to 5 days after sexual contact. The ulcers are painful and soft on palpation and there is swelling and suppuration of the local lymph nodes. Those infected typically notice the appearance of raised, red bumps on the genital region. In men, these bumps usually develop on the penis or perianal region. In women, bumps generally appear on the labia, cervix, vagina, or rectum. Within a few days, these bumps become filled with pus and eventually rupture, leaving rugged, painful, open sores in the genital region. Ulcers can bleed or ooze pus and can take weeks to heal without medication.

Diagnosis

The infection can be diagnosed relatively easily by taking a swab from one of the ulcers and examining it under a microscope for evidence of the chancroid bacteria.

Treatment

Successful treatment for chancroid cures the infection, resolves the clinical symptoms, and prevents transmission to others. In advanced cases, scarring can result, despite successful therapy. The drug of choice are ciprofloxacin, erythromycin, ceftriaxone and azithromycin.

Inguinal Bubo

Inguinal and femoral buboes are localized enlargements of the lymph nodes in the groin area, which are painful and may be fluctuant (soft with a feeling of liquid inside). When buboes rupture, they may appear as ulcers in the inguinal area. As we saw in Chancroid, buboes are frequently associated with *lymphogranuloma venereum* and chancroid. In areas where *granuloma inguinale* is common, it should also considered as a cause of inguinal bubo.

If you come across buboes with a genital ulcer, you should use the genital ulcer flowchart to treat it.

Treatment

The treatment is erythromycin tablet 500 mg qid for 14 days or doxycycline capsules 100 mg bd for 14 days. Some cases may require longer treatment than the 14 days recommended. Buboes might require aspiration through intact skin or incision and drainage to prevent the formation of inguinal/femoral ulcerations.

MOLLUSCUM-CONTAGIOSUM

Molluscum-contagiosum is a skin infection that is caused by a virus called the Poxvirus. It causes a rash of tiny sores that can appear on areas of the skin or on the mucus glands of eyes, mouth, nose, or genitals.

Epidemiology

Affects almost 8% of the world's population, molluscum contagiosum can affect men, women, and children. The highest incidences occur in tropical and warm climates around the world. Overall infection rates are approximately 5 to 8% of the population. Additionally, up to 20% of people with HIV/AIDS have the disease. In individuals coinfected with HIV, the lesions may be severe and more widespread. Molluscum contagiosum is contracted by skin-to-skin contact with an infected person. In adults, this skin-to-skin contact is generally in the form of sexual activity.

Treatment

Molluscum contagiosum usually resolves without any type of treatment. However, it can take a while for the virus to disappear. Treatment usually involves removing the molluscum in order to prevent it from spreading.

BALANITIS

Balanitis is inflammation of the glans penis. Balanitis involving the foreskin and prepuce is termed balanoposthitis. The most common complication of balanitis is phimosis, or inability to retract the foreskin from the glans penis. Patients usually present with the following complaints:

- Penile discharge
- Inability to retract foreskin
- Impotence
- Difficulty in urinating or controlling urine stream;
- Tenderness of the glans penis.

Causes

- Diabetes is the most common underlying condition associated in adult balanitis.
- Other causes include poor personal hygiene; chemical irritants (e.g., soap, petroleum jelly); penile cancer
- Several organisms and viruses cause balanitis, including the following:
  - Candidal species
  - Anaerobic infection
  - Human papilloma virus
  - *Gardnerella vaginalis*
  - Trichomonal species
  - Group B and group A streptococci.

Diagnosis

This may include careful identification of the cause with the aid of a good patient history, swabs and cultures, and pathologic examination of a biopsy.

Treatment

This will depend on the cause and maintenance of good hygiene.

Control of STDs

Primary prevention means protecting a person from becoming infected. It has been shown that most STIs are transmitted from a reservoir of infected individuals and their sexual partners. In you target control measures to this group you intervention will be highly effective, as you have seen, everybody is susceptible to acquiring STIs, however, some behavior exposes some individuals more than others.

The control of STD may be consider under the following headings:

- Initial planning includes:
  - Problem definition
  - Establishing priorities
  - Setting objective
  - Considering strategies.
- Intervention strategies includes:
  - Screening
  - Contact tracing
  - Cluster testing
  - Case holding and treatment
  - Epidemiological treatment
  - Personal prophylaxis
    - Contraceptives
    - Vaccines
  - Health education.
- Support components includes:
  - STD clinic
  - Laboratory services
  - Primary health care
  - Information system
  - Legislation
  - Social welfare measures.
- Monitoring and evaluation.

EPIDEMIOLOGY OF CHRONIC NONCOMMUNICABLE DISEASES AND CONDITIONS

Noncommunicable Disease

A noncommunicable disease, or NCD, is a medical condition or disease which by definition is noninfectious and nontransmissible among people. NCDs may be chronic diseases of long duration and slow progression, or that may result in more rapid death. They include autoimmune diseases, heart disease, stroke, many cancers, asthma, diabetes, chronic kidney disease, osteoporosis, Alzheimer's disease, cataracts, and more. While sometimes (incorrectly) referred to as synonymous with 'chronic diseases', NCDs are distinguished only by their noninfectious cause, not necessarily by their duration. Some chronic diseases of long duration, such as HIV/AIDS, are caused by transmissible infections. Chronic diseases require chronic care management as do all diseases that are slow to develop and of long duration.

The World Health Organization (WHO) reports NCDs to be by far the leading cause of mortality in the world, representing over 60% of all deaths. Out of the 36 million people who died from NCDs in 2005, half were under age 70 and half were women. Of the 57 million global deaths in 2008, 36 million were due to NCDs. That is approximately

63% of total deaths worldwide. Risk factors, such as a person's background, lifestyle and environment are known to increase the likelihood of certain NCDs. Every year, at least 5 million people die because of tobacco use and about 2.8 million die from being overweight. High cholesterol accounts for roughly 2.6 million deaths and 7.5 million die because of high blood pressure. By 2030, deaths due to chronic NCDs are expected to increase to 52 million per year while deaths caused by infectious diseases, maternal and perinatal conditions and nutritional deficiencies are expected to decline by 7 million per year during the same period.

NCDs and Global Health

Referred to as a 'lifestyle' disease, because the majority of these diseases are preventable illnesses, the most common causes for noncommunicable diseases (NCD) include tobacco use (smoking), alcohol abuse, poor diets (high consumption of sugar, salt, saturated fats, and trans fatty acids) and physical inactivity. Currently, NCD kills 36 million people a year, a number that by some estimates is expected to rise by 17 to 24% within the next decade.

Historically, many NCDs were associated with economic development and were so-called a 'diseases of the rich'. However, with an estimated 80% of the four main types of NCDs—cardiovascular diseases, cancers, chronic respiratory diseases and diabetes—now occurring in low- and middle-income countries, and with two-thirds of people who are affected by diabetes now residing in developing nations, NCD can no longer be considered just a problem affecting affluent societies. As previously stated, in 2008 alone, NCD's were the cause of 63% of deaths worldwide; a number that is expected to rise considerably in the near future if measures are not taken.

CARDIOVASCULAR DISEASE

Cardiovascular disease is one of the important public health problem and major cause of death worldwide. It comprise with group of disease, e.g., hypertension, coronary heart disease, rheumatic heart disease, peripheral vascular disease and congenital heart disease.

Coronary Heart Diseases

In 2013 CAD was the most common cause of death globally, resulting in 8.14 million deaths (16.8%) up from 5.74 million deaths (12%) in 1990 CHD is the most common type of heart disease. In the United States, CHD is the #1 cause of death for both men and women. It is responsible for around 73,000 deaths in the UK each year. About 1 in 6 men and 1 in 10 women die from CHD. In the UK, there are an estimated 2.3 million people living with the condition and around 2 million people affected by angina (the most common symptom of coronary heart disease). CHD generally affects more men than women, but from the age of 50 the chances of developing the condition are similar for both men and women. The risk of death from CAD for a given age has decreased between 1980 and 2010 especially in the developed world. The number of cases of CAD for a given age has also decreased between 1990 and 2010 In the United States in 2010 about 20% of those over 65 had CAD, while it was present in 7% of those 45 to 64, and 1.3% of those 18 to 45. Rates are higher among men than women of a given age.

Coronary heart disease (Syn. Ischemic heart disease) has defined as 'impairment of heart function due to inadequate blood flow to the heart compared on its needs, caused by obstructive changes in the coronary circulation to the heart. is a group of diseases that includes: stable angina, unstable angina, myocardial infarction, and sudden coronary death. A narrowing of the coronary arteries that prevents adequate blood supply to the heart muscle. Usually caused by atherosclerosis, it may progress to the point where the heart muscle is damaged due to lack of blood supply. Such damage may result in infarction, arrhythmias, and heart failure.

Manifestations includes:

- Angina pectoris
- Myocardial infraction
- Irregularities of the heart
- Cardiac failure
- Sudden death.

Measurement of burden of diseases: Some of the specific indicator can be used for measuring disease burden:

- **Proportional mortality ratio:** Proportional mortality ratio means number of deaths within a population due to a specific disease or cause (CHD) divided by the total number of deaths in the population during a time period, such as a year. Proportional of all deaths currently attributed to it.
- **CHD incidence rate:** Sum of fatal and nonfatal attack rates.
- Age specific death rates.
- Prevalence rate.
- Case fatality rate.
- Measurement of risk factor levels.

Risk Factors

- **Modifiable Nonmodifiable:** High Serum cholesterol, obesity, lack of physical activity, lack of estrogen in women, diabetes mellitus, hypertension, cigarette smoking and tobacco use.
- **Nonmodifiable:** Type of personality, genetic factors, Race (nonwhite populations), Gender (male), increasing age Smoking.

Prevention of CHD

- **Population strategy:**
  - Prevention in whole population
    - Dietary changes
    - Smoking
    - Blow pressure
    - Physical activity
  - *Primordial prevention:* It aims to controlling or modifying as many risk factors as possible.
- **High-risk strategy:**
  - Identifying risk
  - Specific advice.

- **Secondary prevention:** Revascularization procedures for patients with angina pectoris.

HYPERTENSION

Hypertension is a worldwide epidemic and important risk factor for coronary artery disease, stroke and renal diseases. It is the largest decline in mortality within the last four decades.

Blood pressure is the force exerted by blood against the walls of the blood vessels and is sufficient to maintain tissue perfusion during activity and rest.

Hypertension is sustained elevation of BP. In adults, HTN exists when systolic blood pressure is equal to or greater than 140 mm Hg or diastolic BP is equal to or greater than 90 mm Hg. The diagnosis of HTN requires that elevated BP at least in 3 occasions in several weeks.

Classification of BP for Adults

Category	Systolic	Diastolic
Optimal	<120	<80
Normal	<130	<85
High normal hypertension	130–139	85–89
Stage I	140–159	90–99
Stage II	160–179	100–109
Stage III	>180	>110

Classification of Hypertension

According to the etiology of hypertension it can be classified as:

- **Primary (essential) hypertension:** When BP elevated without any identified cause it is termed as essential hypertension. It accounts 90 to 95% of all HTN. The exact cause is unknown but some contributing factors like increased SNS activity, increased sodium intake, increased sodium retaining hormone, etc.
- **Secondary hypertension:** When BP is elevated due to some identified cause like coarctation of aorta, endocrine disorder like hyperaldosteronism, renal diseases, etc. It accounts 5–10% among adults and 80% among children. Once the causative factor is eliminated/corrected BP become normalized.

Risk Factors

Risk factor for essential hypertension may classified as:

- **Nonmodifiable risk factor:**
  - *Age:* BP rises progressively with age in both sexes. Elevated BP is present in approximately 50% people above 60 year of age.
  - *Gender:* HTN is more prevalent in male in young adulthood and early middle age. After 55 HTN is more prevalent among female.
  - *Ethnicity:* Incidence of HTN is twice high among African American.
  - *Family history:* Risk of HTN is increases for those with a close relative having HTN. Study shows that 3% risk among normotensive parent whereas 45% among children of two hypertensive parent.
- Modifiable risk factor.

RHEUMATIC HEART DISEASE

Rheumatic heart disease is the ultimate, sequelae and crippling stage of Rheumatic Fever, which in turn is the result of streptococcal pharyngitis.

Rheumatic fever is an acute febrile disease, affecting the connective tissues particularly in the heart and joints, which occurs following the infection of throat (pharynx) group A beta-hemolytic streptococci. Thus also Rheumatic fever is a noncommunicable disease, it results from communicable pharyngitis.

Definition

- According to Lewis et al RHD is the chronic condition/disease resulting from rheumatic fever that is characterized by swelling and deformity of valves.
- RHD is an acute, recurrent inflammatory disease that causes damage to the heart as a sequel to group A beta-hemolytic, streptococcal infection, particularly the valves, resulting in valve leakage (insufficiency) and/or obstruction (narrowing or stenosis).
- Rheumatic fever is an inflammatory disease of the heart potentially involving all the layers of the heart, i.e., endocardium, myocardium and pericardium.

Etiology

Streptococcal infections:

- Gram-positive nonmotile spherical bacteria occurring in chains
- Most species are saprophytes and some are pathogenic
- Many pathogenic species are hemolytic they have ability to destroy red blood cells.

Pathophysiology

- Rheumatic fever is a sequel to group A streptococcal infection that occurs in about 30% of untreated infections. (Nettina SM et al. 2006)
- It is a preventable disease through the detection and adequate treatment of streptococcal pharyngitis.
- Connective tissue of the heart, blood vessels, joints and subcutaneous tissues are affected.
- Lesions in connective tissue are known as Aschoff bodies, which are localized area of tissue necrosis surrounded by immune cells.
- Heart valves are affected, resulting in valve leakage and narrowing.
- Compensatory changes in the chamber size and thickness of chamber walls occur.
- Heart involvement (carditis) also includes pericarditis, myocarditis and endocarditis.

Clinical Feature

- **Fever:** Fever is present at the onset of acute illness and may be accompanied by profuse sweating. It may last for about 12 weeks and longer has a tendency to recur.
- **Polyarthritis:** This occurs 90% of cases. Large joints like ankle, knees, elbows and wrists are involved. The pain and swelling come on quickly and also subside spontaneously within 5 to 7 days. There is residual damage to the joint.
- **Carditis:** Occurs only 60 to 70% of cases. It starts early in the course of RF. All layers of the heart—pericardium, myocardium, and the heart valves are involved. The involvement of heart is manifested by tachycardia, cardiac murmur, cardiac enlargement, pericarditis and heart failure. The most common finding is the first degree AV block.
- **Nodule:** Nodule below the skin tend to appear four weeks after the onset of RF. They are small, painless and nontender. They last for a variable period of time and then disappear and leaving no residual damage.
- **Brain involvement:** This manifests as abnormal jerky purposeless movements of the arms, legs and the body. It gradually disappears leaving no residual damage.
- **Skin:** Various types of skin rash are known to occur. It is thus obvious that except carditis all other manifestation of RF do not cause permanent damage.

The presence of two major criteria, or of one major and two minor criteria, indicates a high probability of acute rheumatic fever, if supported by evidence of Group A Streptococcal infection.

Diagnostic Evaluation

- Throat culture to determine presence of streptococcal organisms
- Sedimentation rate, WBC count and differential and CRP increased during acute phase of infection
- Elevated Antistreptolysin O-ASO titer
- ECG prolonged pulse rate interval or heart block.

To diagnose rheumatic fever Jones criteria for guidance can be followed **Table 11.21**.

Table 11.21: Jones criteria (revised) for guidance in the diagnosis of rheumatic fever.

Major manifestation	*Minor manifestation*		*Supporting evidence of streptococcal infection*
	Clinical	**Laboratory**	
Carditis Polyarthritis Chorea Erythema marginatum Subcutaneous nodule	• Previous rheumatic fever or rheumatic heart disease • Arthralgia • Fever	• Acute phase reactant • Erythrocyte sedimentation rate, C-reactive protein, leukocytosis prolonged p-r interval	Increased titer of anti-streptococcal antibodies ASO (ANTI-STREPTOLYSIN O), others Positive throat culture for Group A streptococcus recent Scarlet Fever

Complication

- Heart failure
- Atrial fibrillation
- Infective endocarditis
- Atrial and ventricular arrhythmias.

Problem

- Rheumatic Heart Disease is a major public health problem in India. About 20% of all sore throats among children are due to streptococcal infection and those about 2% result in Rheumatic fever.
- Almost 80% of those who get Rheumatic fever end up with Rh heart disease. Thus RHD is the most common and most widely prevalent heart disease (30 to 50% of all cardiac cases) among children in India.
- Its prevalence is about 6/1000 children in the age group of 5 to 15 years. About 6 million children in India are suffering from RHD and Rh heart disease is the responsible for about 30% of all cardiovascular death.
- It is estimated that about 2 to 3/1000 of all overall population in the country, including people of all age group and both the sexes are suffering from RHD.
  In the last 2 decades, the incidence of Rh fever and the prevalence of RHD have fallen remarkably as the living conditions improved, indicating relation between the prevalence of the disease and the socio-economic factors. Thus it indicates that RHD is one of the most readily preventable chronic disease.
- It occurs more during winter and early spring session.

Epidemiological Factors

1. **Agent Factors:** The onset of RF is usually preceded by a streptococcal sore throat of the streptococci. It is the group A Streptococcus that has been the incriminated as the causative agent.
   It has been suggested that not all strains of group A Streptococcus lead to RF. It is believed that there might be some strains with 'rheumatogenic potential.' The serotype that has attracted special emphasis is M type 5 which is frequently associated with RF.
   All group A Streptococci are sensitive to penicillin.
   Carriers: Carriers of Group A Streptococcus are frequent, e.g., convalescent, transient and chronic carriers. In view of the high carrier rate, their eradication is not even theoretically possible.
2. **Host factors:**
   a. *Age:* RF is typically a disease of childhood and adolescence (5 to 15 years) although it also occurred in adults (20% cases). The initial attack of RF occurs at a young age, progress to valvular lesions faster and is associated with pulmonary arterial hypertension. The cause of 'Juvenile' disease in India is not known.
   b. *Sex:* The disease affects both sexes equally but prognosis is worse for female than in male.

c. *Immunity:* An immunological basis for RF and RHD has been proposed. The most prevalent concept is the toxic immunological hypothesis. According to this theory, group A streptococcal products have certain toxic products and components of the streptococcus and of host tissues have an antigenic cross-relationship, leading to immunological processes that result in attack RF.

3. **Environmental factors**
   a. *Socioeconomic status:* RF is a social disease linked to poverty, overcrowding, poor housing conditions, inadequate health services, inadequate expertise of health care providers and a low level of awareness of the disease in the community. It declines sharply when the standard of living is improved, but even in the most affluent countries, there are areas where the disease still exists.
   b. *High-risk group:* The school age children between 5 and 15 years; slum dwellers; and those living in a closed community (barracks). The direct and indirect results of environmental and health system determinants on rheumatic fever and rheumatic heart disease is depicted in **Table 11.22**.

Prevention of Rheumatic Heart Disease

Primary Prevention

- **Health promotion: Measure prevention of primordial preventions are:**
  - Improvement in the living conditions
  - Improvement in sanitation in and around the house
  - Prevention of overcrowding
  - Prevention of malnutrition among children
  - Health education of the people regarding dangers of sore throat
  - 'Health fair' should be conducted in the schools to make the children health conscious.
- **Specific protection:**
  - No vaccine is available.
  - Chemoprophylaxis of the contacts of case of pharyngitis of scarlet fever with Benzathine penicillin.
  - 'Secondary prophylaxis' is given for all cases of Rheumatic fever to prevent RHD with 1.2 million units of Benzathine penicillin, once in 3 weeks, regularly for 5 years or until the age of 18 years, whichever is later. If they have developed RHD, prophylaxis is continued for life.

Secondary Prevention

Early diagnosis and treatment

- By conducting periodical 'School Health Survey', to detect the case of sore throat.
- By surveillance of 'high- risk' groups, such as slum dwellers.
- Detected case of sore throat (or acute pharyngitis) is treated by 1 dose of 1.2 million units' o Benzathine penicillin, a long acting one. This essential prevents the subsequent development of Rheumatic fever and RHD.

Tertiary Prevention

- **Disability limitation:** Giving intensive treatment with Aspirin for joint pains and prednisolone for carditis, lifelong Benzathine penicillin, 1.2 million units once in 3 weeks and balloon valvotomy or valve replacement.
- **Rehabilitation:** By social, vocational and psychological measures of those who are suffering from RHD.

DIABETES MELLITUS

Diabetes Mellitus is a chronic, progressive disease characterized by the body's inability to metabolize carbohydrates, fats, and proteins leading to hyperglycemia (high blood glucose level). The underlying cause of diabetes is the defective production or action of insulin, a hormone that controls glucose, fat and amino acid metabolism. Chronic hyperglycemia, from whatever cause, leads to a number of complications cardiovascular, renal, neurological, and ocular and others, such as intercurrent infections.

Classification

According to WHO Diabetes Mellitus is divided into three category.

1. **Diabetes Mellitus (DM)**
   - Type 1 or insulin dependent diabetes mellitus
   - Type 2 or Noninsulin dependent diabetes mellitus
   - Malnutrition related diabetes mellitus (MRDM)
   - Other types (Secondary to pancreatic, hormonal, drug induced, genetic and other abnormalities)

Table 11.22: Direct and indirect results of environmental and health system determinants on rheumatic fever and rheumatic heart disease.

Determinants	*Effects*	*Impact on RF and RHD burden*
Socioeconomic and environmental factors: (poverty, under nutrition, overcrowding, poor housing)	Rapid spread of group A streptococcal strains. Difficulties in accessing health care	• Higher incidence of acute streptococcal pharyngitis and suppurative complications • Higher incidence of acute RF • Higher incidence of recurrent attacks
Health system related factors: • Shortage of resources for health care • Inadequate expertise of health care providers • Low level awareness of the disease in the community	Inadequate diagnosis and treatment of Streptococcal pharyngitis Misdiagnosis or late diagnosis of acute RF Inadequate secondary prophylaxis and/or noncompliance with secondary prophylaxis	• Higher incidence of acute RF and its reference. • Patients' awareness of the first RF episode. • More severe evolution of disease. • Untimely initiation or lack of secondary prophylaxis. • Higher rate of recurrent attacks with more frequent and severe heart valve involvement, and higher rate of repeated hospital admissions and expensive surgical interventions.

2. **Impaired glucose tolerance (IGT)**
3. **Gestational diabetes mellitus (GDM)**

1. **(a) Type 1 or insulin dependent diabetes mellitus (IDDM):** IDDM is also called 'Juvenile onset diabetes mellitus', is characterized by destruction of pancreatic beta cells, leading to absolute insulin deficiency. Its onset is typically abrupt and is usually seen in individual less than 30 years of age. It is lethal unless promptly diagnosed and treated. This form of diabetes is immune mediated in over 90% of cases and idiopathic are less than 10% of cases. It occurs mostly in children, the incidence is highest among 10 to 14 years old age group, but occasionally occurs in adults.
   It is catabolic disorder in which circulating insulin is virtually absent, plasma glucagon is elevated, and the pancreatic beta cells fail to respond to all insulinogenic stimuli. Exogenous insulin is therefore required to reverse the catabolic state, prevent ketosis, reduce the hyperglucagonemia, and reduce blood glucose.
1. **(b) Type 2 or Noninsulin dependent diabetes mellitus (NIDDM)**
   Type 2 Diabetes Mellitus, previously called NIDDM or adult onset Diabetes Mellitus is a disorder involving both genetic and environmental factors. Type 2 Diabetes Mellitus is the most common type of Diabetes Mellitus, affecting 90% of all people who have the disease. Type 2 Diabetes Mellitus is usually diagnosed after the age of 40 and it is more common among older adults.
   It is frequently mild, slow to ketosis and is compatible with long survival if given adequate treatment. Its clinical picture is usually complicated by the presence of other disease process.
2. **Impaired glucose tolerance:** Impaired glucose tolerance (IGT) describes a state intermediate-'at risk' group-between diabetes mellitus and normally. It can only be defined as the oral glucose tolerance.
3. **Gestational Diabetes Mellitus:** Gestational Diabetes Mellitus is a type of Diabetes Mellitus diagnosed during pregnancy.

Problem Statement

World: Diabetes is an ICE BERG disease. Although increases in both the prevalence and incidence of type 2 Diabetes have occurred globally, they have been especially dramatic in societies in economic transition.

Currently the number of cases of Diabetes worldwide is estimated to be around 347 million, of these more than 90% are type 2 Diabetes. In 2008, an estimated 1.2 million people died from consequences of High Blood Sugar. More than 80% Diabetes death occur in low and middle income countries.

- The prevalence of Diabetes was highest in the Eastern Mediterranean region and the region of the Americas (11% of both sexes) and lowest in the WHO European and Western Pacific Regions (9% of both sexes).
- Unfavorable modification of lifestyle and dietary habits that are associated with urbanization are believed to be the most important factors for the development of Diabetes. The prevalence of diabetes is approximately twice in urban areas than in rural population.

India

During the year 2004, there were estimated 37.7 million cases of Diabetes in the country, of these 21.4 million were in urban areas and 16.3 million in rural areas. The estimated total mortality due to Diabetes was 1.09 lacs from them 62.5 thousand in urban areas and 46.6 thousand in rural areas. Same year 2.2 million DALYs were lost due to the disease.

Natural History

Epidemiological Determinants

Agent: The underlying cause of Diabetes is insulin deficiency which is absolute in type 1 diabetes and partial in type 2 Diabetes. This may be due to a wide variety of mechanisms:
- Pancreatic disorder: Inflammatory, neoplastic and other disorders, such as cystic fibrosis.
- Defects in the formation of insulin, e.g., synthesis of an abnormal, biologically less active insulin molecule.
- Destruction of beta cells, e.g., viral infections and chemical agents.
- Decreased insulin sensitivity, due to decreased number of adipocyte and monocyte insulin receptors.
- Genetic defects, e.g., mutation of insulin gene.
- Autoimmunity.

Evidence is accumulating that the insulin response to glucose is genetically controlled. The overall effect of these mechanisms is reduced utilization of glucose which leads to hyperglycemia accompanied by glycosuria.

Host factors:
- **Age:** Although diabetes my occur at any age, surveys indicates that prevalence rises steeply with age. Type 2 diabetes usually comes to light in the middle year of life and thereafter begins to rise in frequency.
  - Malnutrition related diabetes affect large number of young people.
  - The prognosis is worse in younger diabetics who tend to develop complications earlier than older diabetics.
- **Sex:** In some countries (e.g., UK) the overall male - female ratio is about equal. In South East Asia, an excess of male diabetics has been observed.
- **Genetic factors**
- **Immune mechanisms:** There is some evidence of both cell mediated and of humoral activity against islet cells. Some people appear to have defective immunological mechanism and under the influence of some environmental 'trigger' attack their own insulin producing cells.
- **Obesity:** Obesity particularly central adiposity has long been accepted as a risk factor for type 2 diabetes and the risk is related to both the duration and degree of obesity.
- **Maternal diabetes:** Offspring of Diabetic pregnancies including gestational diabetes are often large and heavy

at birth, tend to develop obesity in childhood and are at high-risk of developing type 2 diabetes at an early age. Maternal diabetes associated with intrauterine growth retardation and low birth weight, when associated with rapid growth catch-up later on, appears to increase the risk of subsequent diabetes in the child.

Environmental Risk Factors

Susceptibility to diabetes appears to be unmasked by a number of environmental factors acting on genetically susceptible individual. They include:

- **Sedentary lifestyle:** Sedentary lifestyle appears to be important risk factors for the development of type 2 Diabetes. Lack of exercise may alter the interaction between insulin and its receptors and subsequently leads to type 2 Diabetes.
- **Diet:** A high saturated fat intake has been associated with a high-risk of impaired glucose tolerance, and higher fasting glucose and insulin levels.
- **Dietary fibers:** In many controlled experimental studies, high intake of dietary fibers have been shown to result in reduced blood glucose and insulin levels in people with type 2 Diabetes and impaired glucose tolerance. A minimum daily intake of 20 grams of dietary fiber is recommended.
- **Malnutrition:** Malnutrition in early infancy and childhood may result in partial failure of β-cell function. Damage to β-cells may well explain the associated well impaired carbohydrate tolerance in Kwashiorkor.
- **Alcohol:** Excessive intake of alcohol can increase the risk of diabetes may damaging the pancreas and liver and by promoting obesity.
- **Viral infection:** Among the viruses that have been implicated are rubella, mumps and human coxackie virus B4. Viral infection may trigger in immunogenetically susceptible people a sequence of events resulting in β-cell destruction.
- **Chemical agent:** A number of chemical agents are known to be toxic to β-cells, e.g., alloxan, streptozotocin, the rodenticide VALCOR, etc. A high intake of cyanide producing foods (cassava and certain beans) may also have toxic effects on β-cells.
- **Stress:** Surgery, trauma and stress of situations, internal or external may 'bring out' the disease.
- **Other factors:** High and low rates of diabetes have been linked to a number of social factors, such as occupation, marital status, religion, economic status, education, urbanization and changes in lifestyle, etc.

Screening for Diabetes

In the past, the commonest approach to diabetes screening was a preliminary, semiquantitative test for glucose in a urine sample, followed by an oral glucose tolerance test for those found to have glycosuria. The underlying assumption is that early detection and effective control of hyperglycemia in asymptomatic diabetes reduces morbidity.

- **Urine examination:** Urine test for glucose, 2 hours after a meal is commonly used in medical practice for detecting cases of Diabetes.
  - Most studies now confirm that although glucose is found in urine in the most severe cases of diabetes, it is often absent in milder forms of the disease, and such cases are likely to be missed by urine test. This is known as lack of 'sensitivity'. For these reasons, urine testing is not considered an appropriate tool for case finding or epidemiological surveys of the population.
- **Blood sugar testing:** Mass screening programs have used glucose measurements of fasting, postprandial or random blood sample.

Target Population

Screening of the whole population for diabetes is not considered a rewarding exercise. However, screening of 'high-risk' group is considered more appropriate. These groups are:

- Those in age group 40 and over
- Those with a family history of diabetes
- The obese
- Women who have had a baby weighing more than 4.5 kg
- Women who show excess weight gain during pregnancy
- Patients with premature atherosclerosis.

Prevention and Care

- **Primary Prevention:** Two strategies for primary prevention have been suggested:
  a. *Population strategy:* The scope for primary prevention of type 1 Diabetes is limited on the basis of current knowledge and is probably not appropriate. However the development of prevention programs for type 2 Diabetes based on elimination of environmental risk factors is possible. There is pressing need for primordial prevention—that is prevention of the emergence of risk factors in countries in which they have not yet appeared.
     The preventive measures comprise maintenance of normal body weight through adoption of healthy nutritional habits and nutritional exercise. The nutritional habits include an adequate protein intake, a high intake of dietary fiber and avoidance of sweet foods.
  b. *High-risk strategy:* There is no special high-risk strategy for type 1 Diabetes. At present there is no practical justification for genetic counseling as a method of prevention.
     Since NIDDM appears to be linked with sedimentary life style, over nutrition and obesity, correction of these may reduce the risk of diabetes and its complications.
     Since alcohol can indirectly increase the risk of diabetes, it should be avoided.
- **Secondary prevention:** When Diabetes is detected, it must be adequately treated. The aims of treatment are:

- To maintain blood glucose levels as close within the normal limits as is practicable.
- To maintain ideal body weight. Treatment is based on:
  - Diet alone: Small balanced meal more frequently
  - Diet and antidiabetic drug
  - Diet and insulin.

  Good control of Blood glucose protects against the development of complications.
- *Self-care:* A crucial element in secondary prevention is self-care. That is the Diabetic should take a major responsibility for his own care with medical guidance, e.g., adherence to diet and drug regimens, examination of his own urine and where possible blood glucose monitoring, self-administration of insulin, abstinence from alcohol, maintenance of optimum weight, attending periodic checkups, recognition of symptoms associated with glycosuria and hypoglycemia, etc.

  Home blood glucose monitoring: Assessment of control has been greatly aided by the recent facility of immediate, reasonably accurate, capillary blood glucose measurements either by one of the many meters now available or the direct hemoglucotest strips.

  The patient should carry an identification card showing his name, address, telephone number (if any) and the details of treatment he is receiving. In short, he must have a working knowledge of diabetes. All these mean education of patients and their families to optimize the effectiveness of primary health care services.
- **Tertiary prevention:** Diabetes is major cause of disability through its complications, e.g., Blindness, kidney failure, coronary thrombosis, gangrenes of the lower extremities, etc. The main objectives at the tertiary level are to organize specialized clinics (Diabetes clinics) and units capable of providing diagnostic and management skills of a high order.

  There is a great need to establish such clinics in large town and cities. The tertiary level should also be involved in basic clinical and epidemiological research. It is also been recommended that local and national registries for diabetic should be established.

ANEMIAS

Introduction

Anemia is a condition that develops when blood lacks enough healthy redblood cells or hemoglobin. Hemoglobin is a main part of red blood cells and binds oxygen. If you have too few or abnormal red blood cells, or your hemoglobin is abnormal or low, the cells in your body will not get enough oxygen.

Symptoms of anemia like fatigue occur because organs are not getting what they need to function properly.

What Causes Anemia?

There are many types of anemia, which are divided into three groups:

1. Anemia caused by blood loss
2. Anemia caused by decreased or faulty red blood cell production
3. Anemia caused by destruction of red blood cells.

Anemia Caused by Blood Loss

Red blood cells can be lost through bleeding, which can occur slowly over a long period of time, and can often go undetected. This kind of chronic bleeding commonly results from the following:

- Gastrointestinal conditions, such as ulcers, hemorrhoids, gastritis (inflammation of the stomach), and cancer.
- Use of nonsteroidal anti-inflammatory drugs (NSAIDs), such as aspirin or ibuprofen, which can cause ulcers and gastritis.
- Menstruation and childbirth in women, especially if menstrual bleeding is excessive and if there are multiple pregnancies.

Anemia Caused by Decreased or Faulty Red Blood Cell Production

With this type of anemia, the body may produce too few blood cells or the blood cells may not function correctly. In either case, anemia can result. Red blood cells may be faulty or decreased due to abnormal red blood cells or a lack of minerals and vitamins needed for red blood cells to work properly. Conditions associated with these causes of anemia include the following:

Sickle cell anemia is an inherited disorder that affects African-Americans. Red blood cells become crescent-shaped because of a genetic defect. They breakdown rapidly, so oxygen does not get to the body's organs, causing anemia. The crescent-shaped red blood can cells also get stuck in tiny blood vessels, causing pain.

Vitamin deficiency anemia may occur when vitamin B_{12} and folate are deficient. These two vitamins are needed to make red blood cells. Conditions leading to anemia caused by vitamin deficiency include:

- **Megaloblastic anemia:** Vitamin B_{12} or folate or both are deficient.
- **Pernicious anemia:** Poor vitamin B_{12} absorption caused by conditions, such as Crohn's disease, an intestinal parasite infection, surgical removal of part of the stomach or intestine, or infection with HIV.
- **Dietary deficiency:** Eating little or no meat may cause a lack of vitamin B_{12}, while overcooking or eating too few vegetables may cause a folate deficiency.
- **Other causes of vitamin deficiency:** Pregnancy, certain medications, alcohol abuse, intestinal diseases, such as tropical sprue and celiac disease.

  During early pregnancy, sufficient folic acid can help prevent the fetus from developing neural tube defects, such as spina bifida.

Bone marrow and stem cell problems may prevent the body from producing enough red blood cells. Some of the stem cells found in bone marrow develop into red blood

cells. If stem cells, are too few, defective, or replaced by other cells, such as metastatic cancer cells, anemia may result. Anemia resulting from bone marrow or stem cell problems includes:
- Aplastic anemia occurs when there is a marked reduction in the number of stem cells or absence of these cells. Aplastic anemia can be inherited, can occur without apparent cause, or can occur when the bone marrow is injured by medications, radiation, chemotherapy, or infection.
- Thalassemia occurs when the red cells cannot mature and grow properly. Thalassemia is an inherited condition that typically affects people of Mediterranean, African, Middle Eastern, and Southeast Asian descent. This condition can range in severity from mild to life-threatening; the most severe form is called Cooley's anemia.
- Lead exposure is toxic to the bone marrow, leading to fewer red blood cells. Lead poisoning occurs in adults from work-related exposure and in children who eat paint chips, e.g., improperly glazed pottery can also taint food and liquids with lead.

Anemia associated with other conditions usually occurs when there are too few hormones necessary for red blood cell production. Conditions causing this type of anemia include the following:
- Advanced kidney disease
- Hypothyroidism
- Other chronic diseases, such as cancer, infection, lupus, diabetes, and rheumatoid arthritis
- Old age.

Anemia Caused by Destruction of Red Blood Cells

When red blood cells are fragile and cannot withstand the routine stress of the circulatory system, they may rupture prematurely, causing hemolytic anemia. Hemolytic anemia can be present at birth or develop later. Sometimes there is no known cause. Known causes of hemolytic anemia may include:
- Inherited conditions, such as sickle cell anemia and thalassemia.
- Stressors, such as infections, drugs, snake or spider venom, or certain foods.
- Toxins from advanced liver or kidney disease.
- Inappropriate attack by the immune system (called hemolytic disease of the newborn when it occurs in the fetus of a pregnant woman).
- Vascular grafts, prosthetic heart valves, tumors, severe burns, chemical exposure, severe hypertension, and clotting disorders.
- In rare cases, an enlarged spleen can trap red blood cells and destroy them before their circulating time is up.

Red cells may appear abnormal when examined microscopically. Signs and symptoms of anemia relate to the inability of the blood to supply body cells with enough oxygen. It includes:
- **Tachycardia:** The heart rate increases to improve blood supply and speed circulation.
- **Palpitation:** It is caused by the increased effort of the overworked heart muscle.
- **Breathlessness on exertion:** When oxygen requirement increase, respiratory rate and effort rise.

Iron Deficiency Anemia

Iron deficiency anemia occurs because of a lack of the mineral iron in the body. Bone marrow in the center of the bone needs iron to make hemoglobin, the part of the red blood cell that transports oxygen to the body's organs. Without adequate iron, the body cannot produce enough hemoglobin for red blood cells. The result is iron deficiency anemia. This type of anemia can be caused by:
- An iron-poor diet, especially in infants, children, teens, vegans, and vegetarians
- The metabolic demands of pregnancy and breastfeeding that deplete a woman's iron stores
- Menstruation
- Frequent blood donation
- Endurance training
- Digestive conditions, such as Crohn's disease or surgical removal of part of the stomach or small intestine
- Certain drugs, foods, and caffeinated drinks.

Iron deficiency is the most prevalent nutritional deficiency and the most common cause of anemia:
- Iron deficiency anemia is characterized by a defect in hemoglobin synthesis, resulting in red blood cells that are abnormally small (microcytic) and contain a decreased amount of Hemoglobin (hypochromic).
- The capacity of the blood to deliver oxygen to body cells and tissues is thus reduced.

The end result of iron deficiency is nutritional anemia which is not a disease entity. Due to iron deficiency there may be other functional disturbances, such as impaired cell-mediated immunity, reduced resistance to infection, increased morbidity and mortality and diminished work performance.
- Nutritional anemia is a major problem of malnutrition affecting the most vulnerable group (i.e., pregnant and lactating women, children) and very poor population.
- Nutritional anemia pertains to that condition where the hemoglobin level goes down the normal limit because of lack of one or more nutrients in the diet.
- Hemoglobin level is the determinant factor of nutritional anemia.
- In a developing country like India, 70% of total population of women and children are found to be anemic.

Diagnosis of Anemia

Anemia can be detected by the simple measurement of the hemoglobin in the blood.

Hb level of 10–11 g/dL is supposed as early stage of anemia, while Hb level below 10 g/dL is considered anemia. The cut-off points for detection of anemia is depicted in **Table 11.23**.

Table 11.23: Cut-off points for detection of anemia.

Age group	*Hb (venous blood g/dL)*
Male (adult)	13
Female (adult-nonpregnant)	12
Females (adult-pregnant)	11
Children (1/2–6 years)	11
Children (6–14)	12

Causes of Nutritional Anemia

Main causes:
- Lack of Iron
- Low quantity of folates or folic acid
- Lack of Vitamin B_{12}.

Contributing Factors:
- Lack of iron in diet.
- Excessive loss of iron from body. This includes conditions like excessive hemorrhage, menstruation, malaria, parasitic infestation, multiple deliveries and other hematological disorders.
- Protein Energy Malnutrition and Imbalanced diet.
- Lack of vitamins especially folic acid in diet.
- Excessive hemolysis and reduced formation of hemoglobin and red blood cells.

Signs and Hazards of Nutritional Anemia:
Main signs are:
- Exhaustion
- Difficulty in breathing
- Suffocation
- Headache
- Blurring of visions
- Excessive sleep
- Yellow skin
- Anorexia
- Edema
- Cardiac problems.

Besides this, nutritional anemia can lead to infections and loss of working ability. In severe cases, the patient can die.

Anemia and its public health significance: An overview
- Anemia is the most common Nutritional Disorder.
- Iron deficiency Anemia is the most common and widespread form of Anemia accounting for about 95% of anemia cases.
- Other Nutritional factors like Folic Acid, Vitamin B_{12} and others account for another 3–4% of the causes.
- Iron deficiency is the commonest nutritional cause of anemia.
- It may be associated with a Folic Acid deficiency, especially during pregnancy.
- Infants, preschool children, adolescents and women of childbearing age, particularly pregnant women, are at greatest risk of developing iron deficiency anemia.
- However, adult males may also be at risk, especially where there is inadequate food intake or frequent parasitic infestation.

Public health significance of anemia (based on hemoglobin %):
- In normal population, 2.5% of the population would be below the threshold.
- Iron Deficiency anemia would be considered a Public Health Problem if the prevalence of Hb% is below the normal level in >5% of the population.
- Anemia is the most common indicator used to screen for iron deficiency, the term anemia, and Iron deficiency anemia are used interchangeably.

Impact of iron deficiency anemia on society and iron deficiency adversely affects:
- The cognitive performance, behavior, and physical growth of infants, preschool and school-age children
- Reduces immune status, and increases disease burden in the community of all age groups
- Reduces physical capacity to of all age groups
- Increases perinatal risks for mothers and neonates
- Increases overall infant mortality.

Economic impact of iron deficiency depends on:
- The individuals affected in various age and gender categories
- The costs incurred by the public and private sectors
- The societal consequences of increased maternal mortality and loss of productivity
- Long-term consequences of impaired mental development and human productivity.

Prevention and treatment of anemia programs under NACP (National Anaemia Control Programme):
- Pregnant women are regularly screened for anemia during pregnancy.
- Pregnant women are given 100 tablets of 60 mg Elemental Iron and 500 μg Folic Acid as prophylaxis to prevent anemia
- Pregnant Women with Moderate Anemia are given 200 IFA tablets to be taken twice a day.
- Pregnant Women with severe anemia (Hb% <7 gm/dL) are treated with Parenteral Iron
- Lactating Mothers are provided 60 mg of elemental Iron and 500 mcg of Folic Acid tablets for 3 months.

Treatment and preventive measures:
- Treatment of nutritional anemia depends on the hemoglobin level of blood.
- Women suffering from anemia should be given iron tablets 200 mg 3 times a day till anemia is controlled.
- Children should be given 'Iron Syrup'. In severe stage, blood transfusion may be needed.
- For Prevention, 180 mg of ferrous sulphate and 0.5 mg folic acid tablets should be given every day for 2–3 months or till the hemoglobin level returns to normal.
- Nutritional anemia can be effectively controlled by fortification of salt by iron, changes in dietary habits, treatment of intestinal parasites and nutritional education.

OBESITY

Introduction

Obesify may be defined as an abnormal growth of adipose tissue due to an enlargement of fat cell size (hypertrophic obesity) or an increase in fat cell number (hyperplastic obesity) or a combination of both.

However, obese individual differs not only the amount of excess fat that they store, but also in the regional distribution of the fat within the body. According to fat distribution it is also 'abdominal fat distribution' or 'android distribution/ obesity'.

Prevalence

- Worldwide, at least 2–8 million people die each year as a result of being overweight or obese, and estimated 35.8 million (2.3%) of DALYS are caused by overweight or obesity.
- In 2008, 35% of adults aged 20+ were overweight (BMI >/25 kg/m) (34% men and 35% women.)
- The worldwide prevalence of obesity has nearly double between 1980 and 2008.
- As obesity is a key risk factor in natural history if other chronic and noncommunicable disease, a typical time sequence of emergency of chronic disease following the increased prevalence obesity is important in public health planning.

Epidemiological determinants: The etiology of obesity is complex, and is one of multiple causation.

Age: Obesity can occur in any age, and generally increased with age.

- Infants with excessive weight gain have an increased incidence of obesity in later life.
- About 1/3rd of obese adults have been so since childhood.

Sex: Women generally have higher rate of obesity than man:

- Men were found to get more weight between the ages of 29 and 35 years while women gain most in between 45 and 49 years.
- It has been claimed that women BMI increase with successive pregnancy.

Genetic factor: There is a genetic components in the etiology of obesity

Physical inactivity: There is convincing evidence that regular physical activity is protective against unhealthy weight gain:

- Whereas sedentary lifestyle articulacy sedentary occupation and inactivity recreation, such as watching TV.
- Physical activity and physical fitness are important modifier and morbidity related to overweight and obesity.

Socioeconomic status:

- The relationship of obesity to social class has been studied
- There is a clear inverse relationship between socioeconomic status and obesity
- There is found that to be more prevalent in the lower socioeconomic group.

Eating habit: Eating habits (e.g., Eating between meals, preference to sweets, refined food and fats) are established very early in life. The component of diet, the periodicity with which it is eaten and the amount of energy derived from it are all relevant to the etiology of obesity.

Psychosocial Factors

Psychosocial factors (e.g., emotional disturbance) are deeply involved in the etiology of obesity. Overeating may be symptoms of depression, anxiety, frustration and loneliness in child hood as well as it is in adult.

- **Family tendency** obesity frequently runs in families (obese parents frequently have obese children)
  - But this is not necessarily explained solely by inflated of genes.
- **Endocrine factors:** These may be involved in occasional cases, e.g., hyperthyroidism, growth hormones deficiency, etc.
- **Alcohol:** Studied proved that the relationship between alcohol consumption and adiposity was generally positive for men and negative for women.
- **Education:** In most affluent societies there is an inverse relationship between educational level and prevalence of overweight.
- **Ethnicity:** Ethnic groups in many industrialized countries appears to be especially susceptible to development of obesity and its complications.
- **Drugs:** Use of certain drugs, e.g., Corticosteroids, contraceptives, insulin, p-adrenergic blockers, etc. can promote weight gain.

Classification of Obesity

Use of BMI obesity may be classified:

- Body mass index is a simple index of weight for height that is used to classify overweight and obesity in adult
- It is defined as the weight in kilogram divided by square of the square of height in meters (kg/m).

The BMI values are age independent and the same for both sexs. Classification of malnutrition/obesity according to BMI is depicted in **Table 11.24**.

- Although it can generally be consumed that individuals with BMI of 30 or above have an excess fat mass in their body.

Table 11.24: Classification of malnutrition according to BMI.

Classification	*BMI*	*Risk of comorbidities*
Underweight	<18.50	Low (but risk of other clinical problems increase.
Normal range	18.50–24.99	Average
Overweight	>/25.00	
Preobese	25.00–29.99	Increased
Obese class 1	30.00–34.99	Moderate
Obese class 2	35.00–39.99	Severe
Obese class 4	>/40.00	Very severe

- BMI does not distinguish between weight associated with muscle and weight associated with fat.

Assessment of Obesity

Before we consider assessment of obesity, it will be useful to first look at body composition as under:
- Active mass (muscle, liver, heart)
- The fatty mass (fat)
- The extracellular fluid (blood, lymph, etc.)
- The connective tissue (skin, bones, etc.)

Body Weight

Body weight have some formula:
- BMI = weight kg/height 2 (m)
- Brocca index = height cm 100
- Ponderal index = height (cm)/cube root of body weight (kg)
- Corpulence index = Actual weight/Desirable weight.

Skin Fold Thickness

- A large proportion of total body fat is locate just under the skin
- Since it is most accessible, the method most used is the measurement of skinfold thickness
- The measurement may be taken at all the four sites, matrices, biceps, subscapular and suprailiac region.
- The sum of the measurement should be less than 40 mm in boys and 50 mm in girls.

Waist Circumference and Waist Hip Ratio (WHP)

- Waist circumference is measured at mid point between the lower border of rib cage and the iliac crest.
- It is convenient and simple measurement that is unrelated to height, correlates closely with BMI and WHR and is an approximate index of intra-abdominal fat mass and total body fat.
- There is an increased risk of metabolic completion for men with a waist circumference >/88 cm.

Prevention and Control

Weight control is widely defined as approaches to maintaining weight within the 'healthy'(i.e., 'normal' or acceptable) range of BMI of 18.5 kg/m^2–24.9 kg/m^2 throughout adulthood.

It should also include prevention of weight gain of more than 5 kg in all people, in those who are already overweight.

Physical Activity
- Contributes to weight loss
- Helpful for the prevention of overweight and obesity
- Helps maintain weight loss
  - *Occupational work:* Carpentry, construction, waiting tables, farming
  - *Household chores:* Washing floors or windows, gardening, or yard work
  - *Leisure time activities:* Walking, skating, biking, swimming, playing Frisbee, dancing, softball, tennis, football, aerobics.

The Critical Role of Healthy Eating
- Good nutrition leads to a healthier life.
- Many do not eat based on My Pyramid recommendations.
- MyPyramid, which is the newest Food Guide Pyramid, recommends the following for a healthy lifestyle:
  - Make half your grains whole
  - Vary your veggies
  - Focus on fruit
  - Get your calcium rich foods
  - Go lean with protein
  - Find your balance between food and physical activity.

STROKE: CEREBROVASCULAR ACCIDENT

The term 'stroke (syn: apoplexy) is applied to acute severe manifestations of cerebrovascular disease. It causes both physical and mental crippling.

Stroke is a syndrome of rapidly developing signs and symptoms of focal loss of cerebral function due to sudden death of brain cells caused by disturbance in the blood supply to the brain. This vascular disturbances can be due to ischemia caused by blockage (thrombosis or embolism) or by hemorrhage, resulting in infarction of the brain. Therefore stroke is also called as 'cerebrovascular accident'.

A stroke occurs when blood flow to the brain is interrupted by a blocked or burst blood vessel. The term stroke is applied to acute sever manifestation cardiovascular disease. It cause both physical and mental crippling.

Definition

WHO defined stroke as 'rapidly developed clinical signs of focal disturbance of cerebral function; lasting more than 24 hours or leading to death, with no apparent cause other than vascular origin'. The 24 hour threshold in the definition excludes transient ischemic attack (TIA) which is defined to last less than 24 hours, and patients with stroke symptoms caused by subdural hemorrhage, tumors, poisoning or trauma are excluded.

Stroke includes a number of syndromes with differing etiologies, epidemiology, prognosis and treatment. These are as:
- Ischemic stroke (accounts for 83% of total cases)
  - Lacunar infract
  - Carotid circulation obstruction
  - Vertebrobasilar obstruction
- Hemorrhagic stroke (accounts for 17% of total stroke)
  - Spontaneous intracerebral hemorrhage
  - Subarachnoid hemorrhage
  - Intracranial aneurysm
  - Arteriovenous malformation.

Magnitude of the Problem

Stroke is one of the leading causes of disability, morbidity and mortality worldwide.

Global burden:

- Nearly 20 million people suffer from acute strokes every year.
- About 6.1 million people die each year majority of deaths occur in developing areas and 33.72% of the subjects were aged less than 70 years.
- About 15 to 30% of survivors are permanently disabled. The incidents are much lower in India (approximately 2 per 1000 population), higher in USA and Europe (between 6 and 8% per 1000) and very high in Japan (15 per 1000 and even more).
- In demographically developed countries, the average age at which stroke occur is around 73 years
- Stroke is the fourth leading cause of death in the United States
- 795,000 people in the US suffer strokes each year
- 133,000 deaths in the US each year
- The probability of first stroke or first TIA is around 1.6 per 1000 and 0.42 per 1000 respectively.
- Stroke patients are at highest risk of death in the first weeks after the event, and between 20–50% die within first month depending on type, severity, effectiveness of treatment and complication.
- Patients who survive may be left with no disability or with mild, moderate, or severe disability.
- However patients with history of stroke are at risk of a subsequent event of around 10% in the first year and 5% in the year thereafter.

Burden in India:

- Nearly 1.5 million people suffer from acute strokes every year.
- About 0.63 million die each year.
- Prevalence rate is about 2 to 5% of total population.
- About 12% of strokes occur among people below 40 years of age.
- India will report 1.6 million stroke cases during 2015, at least one-third of whom will be disabled.

Epidemiology

Risk factors: As per IHD, hypertension and diabetes mellitus, the risk factors for stroke can be classified as nonmodifiable and modifiable factors.

Nonmodifiable factors:

- **Age:** Risk increases with increasing age, starting from the age of 50 years. The peak risk is after 65 years of age. In India almost 20–25% of strokes may occur before 50 years of age.
- **Sex:** Women in general have lower risk than male.
- **Race:** In western world, risk is higher in black populations. In our country, no such ethnic differential has been noticed.
- **Family history:** Persons with a positive family history of stroke among their first degree blood relatives have a higher risk.

Modifiable factors:

- **Hypertension:** Depending upon the level of BP, the risk may be 2–8 times higher and 1.5–4 times higher for SBP and DBP, respectively
- **Tobacco smoking:** The risk among people who smokes 20 cigarettes per day is 2 times higher as compared to those who smokes less than 5 cigarettes per day.
- **Diabetes mellitus:** The risk of stroke among diabetes is 1.5–3 times higher, especially for the atherothrombotic variety of stroke.
- **Transient ischemic attack (TIA):** It is an acute episode of neurological deficit, which lasts for less than 24 hours and is reversible. History of TIA is a major risk factor for subsequent full-blown stroke.
- **Carotid atherosclerosis:** Stenosis of carotid arteries is an important risk factor of stroke.
- **Pre-existing cardiac disease:** Preexisting IHD, CHF, LVH, AF and valvular disease are important risk factor.
- **Other risk factors:** Dyslipidemias (raised total cholesterol, raised LDL and low HDL), obesity habitual inactivity and sickle cell disease are other risk factors for stroke. In addition there is a slight increase in risk among women who use oral contraceptives.
- Drugs like cocaine, amphetamines and sympathomimetics predispose the risk of strokes.

Signs and Symptom

- It depends upon the area of the brain affected. More the area of the brain affected, more the functions lost.
- Sudden onset of face weakness, arm drift and speech abnormal. It is abbreviated as FAST (F–facial weakness, A–arm drift, S–speech abnormal, T–time to act).
- Depending upon the involvement of spinothalamic, corticospinal and medial lemniscus, there will be hemiplegia, numbness, reduction in sensation, initial flaccidity followed by spasticity and hyper-reflexia.
- If brainstem is affected, symptoms of deficit due to involvement of cranial nerves occur.
- If cerebellum is affected, there will be alerted walking gait, vertigo and disequilibrium.
- Loss of consciousness, headache, vomiting usually occur in hemorrhagic stroke because of increased intracranial pressure from leaking blood compressing the brain.

Diagnosis

- Neurological examination
- CT scan
- MRI
- Doppler/ultrasound of carotid artery
- Arteriography
- Blood test for cholesterol level.

Prevention and Control

Prevention and control at all the three level is important.

Primary Prevention

Actions towards primary prevention should start early, during early adulthood itself. The primary preventive measures are as follows:
- Avoidance of smoking
- Regular brisk physical exercise
- Adopting healthy dietary methods, with low consumption of salt, low consumption of saturated fats and overall fat, reduction of overall dietary energy consumption and including plenty of fruits, fresh vegetables, whole grain and possibly fish in diet.
- Maintaining healthy body weight (BMI <25, preferably <23; waist circumference <90 cm for men and <80 cm for women), by a combination of diet and physical activity.
- Avoiding alcohol consumption.

Secondary Prevention

This will include early detection and management of health problems, which have high potential to cause stroke, by screening of individuals and communities. The following screening is advisable:
- Screening for diabetes through blood sugar and management of those found diabetes
- Screening and treatment for hypertension
- Screening and treatment for lipid abnormalities
- Screening for cardiac abnormalities and treatment (e.g., with anticoagulants, if there is arterial fibrillation).

Tertiary Prevention

This is very important though it needs highly specialized neurological team and adequate facilities. The following steps are undertaken:
- Immediate diagnosis as regards the etiology and the exact location of the lesion, and aggressive management to save life:
- Prevention and management of complication during hospital stay.
- Proper patient and relative education regarding selfcare and prevention before discharge.
- Adequate physiotherapy, provision of aids (such as walking aids, wheel chair, etc.) for rehabilitation at home.
- Follow up treatment and frequent reviews along with dialogues with relatives.

Stroke Control Program

- The aim of a stroke control program is to apply at community level effective measures for the prevention of stroke. The first priority goes to control of arterial hypertension which is a major cause of stroke.
- As TIA may be one of the earliest manifestation of stroke, there early detection and treatment is important for the prevention of stroke
- Control of disease, elimination of smoking, and prevention and management of other risk factors at the population level are new approaches.
- Facilities for the long-term follow-up of patients are essential.
- The education and training of the health personnel and of the public form an integral part of the program.

BLINDNESS

Blindness is strictly defined as the state of being totally sightless in both eyes. A completely blind individual is unable to see at all. The word *blindness*, however, is commonly used as a relative term to signify visual impairment.

Blindness is defined as the state of being sightless. A blind individual is unable to see. In a strict sense the word 'blindness' denotes the inability of a person to distinguish darkness from bright light in either eye. The terms blind and blindness have been modified in our society to include a wide range of visual impairment. Blindness is frequently used today to describe severe visual decline in one or both eyes with maintenance of some residual vision.
- Worldwide, between 300 and 400 million people are visually impaired due to various causes. Of this group, approximately 50 million people are totally blind, unable to see light in either eye. Eighty percent of blindness occurs in people over 50 years old.
- As per Survey in 2001-02, prevalence of blindness is estimated to be 1.1%. Rapid Survey on Avoidable Blindness conducted under NPCB during 2006-07 showed reduction in the prevalence of blindness from 1.1% (2001-02) to 1% (2006-07). Various activities/ initiatives undertaken during the Five Year Plans under NPCB are targeted towards achieving the goal of reducing the prevalence of blindness to 0.3% by the year 2020.

Types

According to extent of blindness, it may be:
- Partial blindness means you have very limited vision.
- Complete blindness means you cannot see anything and do not see light. Most people who use the term 'blindness' mean complete blindness. The categories of vision impairment is depicted in **Table 11.25**.

Other types may be:
- **Color blindness:** It is the inability to perceive differences in various shades of colors, particularly green and red, that others can distinguish. It is most often inherited (genetic) and affects about 8% of males and under 1% of women. People who are color blind usually have normal vision otherwise and can function well visually. This is actually not true blindness.

Table 11.25: Categories of vision impairment.

Categories of visual impairment	*Visual acuity*	
	Maximum less than	*Minimum equal to or better than*
Low vision	6/18 6/60	6/60 3/60
Blindness	3/60 (finger counting at 3 meter) 1/60 (finger counting at 1 meter) No light perception	1/60 (finger counting at 1 meter) Light perception

- **Night blindness:** It is a difficulty in seeing under situations of decreased illumination. It can be genetic or acquired. The majority of people who have night vision difficulties function well under normal lighting conditions; this is not a state of sightlessness.
- **Snow blindness:** It is loss of vision after exposure of the eyes to large amounts of ultraviolet light. Snow blindness is usually temporary and is due to swelling of cells of the corneal surface. Even in the most severe of cases of snow blindness, the individual is still able to see shapes and movement.

Causes

Blindness has many causes. In the developed country, the leading causes are:

- Accidents or injuries to the surface of the eye such as chemical burns or sports injuries.
- Diabetes
- Glaucoma
- Macular degeneration.

The type of partial vision loss may differ, depending on the cause:

- With cataracts, vision may be cloudy or fuzzy, and bright light may cause glare
- With diabetes, vision may be blurred, there may be shadows or missing areas of vision, and difficulty seeing at night
- With glaucoma, there may be tunnel vision and missing areas of vision
- With macular degeneration, the side vision is normal but the central vision is slowly lost.

Other causes of vision loss include:

- Infection like trachoma, leprosy, herpes simplex, etc.
- Vitamin A deficiency
- Ocular inflammatory disease
- Blocked blood vessels
- Complications of premature birth, e.g., retrolental fibroplasia
- Complications of eye surgery
- Optic neuritis
- Blood vessel disease, e.g., stroke
- Retinitis pigmentosa
- Tumors, such as retinoblastoma and optic glioma
- Chemical poisoning from toxic agents, such as methanol.

In India

Main causes of blindness are as follows: Cataract (62.6%), Refractive Error (19.70%), Corneal Blindness (0.90%), Glaucoma (5.80%), Surgical Complication, (1.20%), Posterior Capsular Opacification (0.90%), Posterior Segment Disorder (4.70%), Others (4.19%), estimated national Prevalence of childhood blindness/low vision is 0.80 per thousand.

Changing concept of eye health care

Nowadays eye health care concept has been changed from acute intervention to comprehensive eye health care, which includes:

- **Primary eye care:** Inclusion of eye care in primary health care system. The objective of primary eye care is to increase the coverage and quality eye health care through primary health care approach and thereby improve the utilization of existing resources. This is one of the most important approach for prevention of blindness at community level. The promotion and protection of eye health together with on-the-spot treatment for the commonest eye diseases.
- **Epidemiological approach:** Epidemiological approach focuses on measurement of indices, prevalence of disease and their risk factor. The local epidemiological factor will determine the type of service needed.
- **Team concept:** The gap of trained health personnel can be minimized by use of auxiliary health personnel like village health guide, ophthalmic assistant, multipurpose health worker and involvement of NGO.
- **Establishment of national programs:** Initially national program was started by voluntary agencies by conducting eye camps then focused on single disease like trachoma control program. The goal of national program for control of blindness in India was to reduce the blindness 0.3% by the year 2000.

ACCIDENT AND ITS CONTROL

Introduction

Accident is an unintended injury, death or property damage, occurring in a sequence of events which usually produce unintended injury, death or property damage. Among the many causes of death, accident constitute a critable epidemic in the developed countries. Accidents are part of the price we pay for technological progress and are no longer considered accidental, because majority of them are preventable.

According to WHO, accident is defined as an event, independent of human will, caused by an outside force acting rapidly which results in bodily or mental injury.

Definition

Accident is defined as an accident is that unpremeditated event resulting in recognizable damage.

The Problem in World: Injuries constitute a variable epidemic. During 1990s road traffic injuries ranked ninth among the leading causes of deaths in the world. Injuries are responsible for approximately 9.1% of all causes of deaths in the world and about 16% of the disabilities are reported due to injuries. They are also the major cause of death among persons aged 10–24 years. In the developed regions, 57% of male deaths and 43% of female deaths in this age group are due to injuries, mainly traffic accidents and drowning.

Accidents are not the prerogative of developed nations. In developing countries accidents are shown to be as numerous as in developed countries. It is increasing rapidly as a cause of death in absolute numbers and in terms of proportion.

Injuries due to road traffic, occupational accidents, burns, poisoning, suicides and violence are observed to be major causes of mortality and morbidity in the region. Road traffic injuries are the most common injuries in all the countries of the region, except in DPR Korea and Maldives. With 16–18% annual increase in motorization in the region, the rate of road traffic injuries is higher than in other parts of the world. Persons injured in road traffic accidents occupy nearly 10–30% of beds in hospitals.

India

Accidents are definitely on an increase in India. Increasing mechanization in agriculture and industry, induction of semi skilled and unskilled workers in various operations and rapid increase in vehicular traffic have resulted in an increase in morbidity and mortality due to accidents. Overcrowding, lack of awareness and poor implementation of essential safety precautions result in an increasing number of accidents. Consumption of poisonous substances accidentally or intentionally is also on the rise. Deaths, disabilities and hospitalization due to injuries continue to have impact of socioeconomic loss to individuals, families, society and infrastructure. The traditional view of injury as an accident, has resulted in the neglect of this aspect of public health. Today injuries are low in priority for policy makers, and only few plans are drawn for injury prevention.

Types of Accident

Road Accident

In the 20th century, the epidemic of road accidents has become a great problem. In India the major cities like Mumbai, Bengaluru and Delhi lead in the number of causalities per 1000 vehicles. India has the highest accident rate in the world in spite of the fact that the road traffic density is quite low, there are almost 885000 deaths from road accidents annually in the world. In addition for every death there are as many as 30 to 40 minor injuries and 10–15 serious injuries recurring long periods of expensive care, nursing and treatment.

The peak mortality and morbidity from road accidents are seen in the 15–24 years of age group in males. A large proportion of vehicles involved in accidents were two wheelers. Compared to cares, they are unstable and provide little protection for their riders in accidents. At present in some countries more than one third of all traffic deaths occur users of two wheeled vehicles.

Developing countries are very different from the industrialized countries with regard to the environment and the mix of vehicles in the traffic stream.

The following are the more important differences:

- Large numbers of pedestrians and animals share the roadway with fast moving and slow moving vehicles
- Large number of old, poorly maintained vehicles
- Large number of motor cycles, scooters and mopeds
- Low driving standards
- Large number of buses, often overloaded
- Widespread disregard of traffic rules
- Defective roads, poor street lighting, defective layout of cross roads and speed breakers
- Unusual behavior of men and animal.

Domestic Accident

By domestic accident is meant an accident which takes place in the home or in its immediate surroundings and more generally, all accidents not connected with traffic, vehicles or sport. The most frequent causes of domestic accidents are:

- Drowning, burn, poisoning, falls, injury from sharp and pointed equipment, bite and other injuries from animals.
- Domestic accidents are a frequent cause of death or disability at the extremes of life. They account for about 75% of injury to people over 65 in the industrialized countries. At all ages, people who are subjected to attacks of unconsciousness have an increased risk of domestic accident, e.g., epilepsy, vertigo.

Industrial Accident

Industrial accidents are a class by themselves. Every year, almost a thousand workers die and another 250000 are injured in industries. Industrial accidents impose a heavy burden of national economy.

Industrial accidents have been far more successfully controlled not withstanding rapid development of industrialization. This is because industrial accidents occur in a stable environment in which repetitive tasks are performed so that scientific investigation aimed at prevention is relatively easy.

Railways Accident

Daily over 11000 trains carry over one crore passengers throughout the country, with the increase in number of trains and passengers, the increase in number of accidents and causalities resulting there from is not unexpected. The main factor involved in railway accident is human failure.

Suicide

It is also a type of accidental death. It is more in males than females. Suicides have been increasing at an alarming rate in SEAR countries. Incidence rates of 11 per lakh population in Bangladesh, 36 per lakh population in India, 8 per lakh in Srilanka and 22 per lakh in Thailand per year have been reported. Nearly 70% of suicides in all countries have been reported in the age group of 15–34 years with male-female ratio of 1:1:2 to 1:3 from different countries. Poisoning, hanging, self immolation and drowning are the most commonly reported methods of suicide.

Burn

Over one lakh people are affected by burns and scalds in India annually and 20000 of them die according to rough

Table 11.26: Primary factors in accident.

Human factors	*Environmental factors*
Age: Young people Education: Poor educational status Medical conditions • Sudden illness • Heart attack • Impaired vision	Relating to road • Defective, narrow roads • Defective layout of cross roads and speed breakers • Poor lighting • Lack of familiarity • Relating to vehicle
Fatigue Psychosocial factors • Lack of experience • Risks taking • Impulsiveness • Defective judgment • Delay in decisions • Aggressiveness • Poor perception • Family dysfunction Lack of body protection • Helmets • Safety belts.	• Excessive speed • Old, poorly maintained • Large number of two and three wheelers • Overloaded buses • Low driving standards Bad weather • Inadequate enforcement of existing laws. • Mixed traffic slow and fast moving pedestrians and criminals.

estimates. In 1991, the reported deaths were 22036. Ten percentages of all accidental deaths and seven percent of all suicides in India were caused by fire.

Causes of Accident

Some of the primary factors in accident are explained in **Table 11.26**.

Road accident:
- Excessive speed
- Defective roads
- Poor street lighting
- Defective layouts of cross roads and speed breakers
- Defective vehicles
- Fatigue
- Alcoholism
- Unusual behavior of men and animal.

Domestic accident:
- Keeping the poisons within the reach of children
- Not labeling them properly
- Constructing the platform to the wells
- Lighting the stove on the floor
- Keeping away the sharp or pointed instruments
- Not to play with animals
- Defective floors
- Bad lighting
- To be careful about the persons who are at risk.

Railway accident:
- Faulty railway lines
- Negligence of the personnels
- Becoming a victim of terrorist, etc.

Measurement of the problem:
- **Mortality:** The following epidemiological indices will be useful in assessing the magnitude of the problem:
  - Proportional mortality rate
  - Number of deaths per million populations
  - Death rate per 1000 registered vehicles per year
  - Number of accidents or fatalities as a ratio of the number of vehicles per kilometer or passengers per kilometer
  - Death of vehicles occupants per 1000 vehicles per year, etc.
- **Morbidity:** Morbidity is measured in terms of serious injuries and slight injuries.
  The serious of injury is assessed by a scale known as 'Abbreviated injury scale'. Morbidity rates are generally less reliable because of under reporting and misreporting.
- **Disability:** An important outcome of the accident process is disability, which may be temporary or permanent, partial or total. Measurement of disability in terms of its duration is a limited concept: It does not take into consideration the psychological and social of an accident or injury.

Accidents in Children

An accident is a sudden cause of death or an emergency in children. Accidents are usually related to the growth and development of the children. In urban areas of the developing countries, due to overcrowding, one room may be used for the multipurpose, such as for sleeping, cooking, or playing. Such a room may have electrical appliances and other materials used for day-to-day living. This surrounding, if unprotected, may cause accidents in children.

Children from the age of six months to one year can move from place to place. The mobility increases as children learn to turn from side to side, creep, crawl, cruise, and walk. Gradually, the learn to climb up and down. During the process of progressive mobility children may lack coordination and judgment of space. These sudden changes in their activities may place the children at the risk of accidents.

Some parents or caregivers may not be aware of the changes in the children's development. This lack of knowledge or ignorance may add to the predisposing factors where children are exposed to the accident prone circumstances.

Until the preschool age, children may have an accident in the home or surrounding the home, where they play, explore, or imitate others. School age children move about and develop interest in play away from home, may beat the play ground, river, street, or pool. At later age children may become adventurous and become prone to many more accidents.

Common accidental injuries in the different age group:

Infancy:
- **Fall:** Falls are common infants when they turn from side to side, creep, crawl, and walk. Due to lack of motor coordination and lack of the sense of space, they easily fall from the height. **Precautions**—infants should be never left alone, on the cot, table, or any other unprotected surface, from where they can easily fall.
- **Foreign body aspiration:** Infancy is the oral phase, when infants explore everything by putting them in the mouth. If small objects are put in the mouth, they may

get aspirated. **Precautions**—the care should be taken to leave any small objects in infants hand within their reach. Toys should not have any small removable parts. Infants should never be fed solid foods which are difficult for them to chew, such as groundnuts.

- **Burns:** A stove, cooking gas stove, electrical hot plate, electrical heater, or such appliances should never within the reach of infants. If children get access to these appliances, can get burns. **Precautions**—all heating equipments and electrical appliances should be kept at higher level where children cannot reach.
- **Foreign bodies in ear, nose or trachea:** Infants enjoy putting small things into openings or holes like, nose, ear, mouth. **Precautions**—infants should not have access to any small things such as beads, stones, nuts or button.
- **Drowning:** Infants may move towards the tub, water pool, well, because they enjoy water. They may get into it and being helpless may get drowned. **Precautions**—the precaution is always necessary not to leave children alone near the water tubs, water drums, wells or water. The water drums should be always covered. The door of the house should be always closed so that infants cannot go out.

Common accidents in toddlers and preschool children: After the age of one year, the mobility of the children is increased. Children like to walk, run, climb up and down. They enjoy moving about always. They are interested in the surrounding. They open the doors, drawers, cupboards, tins, or boxes, for investigating. As they are not aware of the danger related to their activity, they are prone to accidents in many circumstances.

Falls, burns, ingestion of foreign bodies, aspiration of foreign bodies, drowning, suffocation and vehicle accidents are common in this age. **Precautions**—toddlers are egocentric. The negative statement, such as do not, should never be used to control their activities. They should be instructed about the expected activities. The proper directions for the activity are recommended. Their activities should be under the supervision. The stairs, gates should be protected. The doors should be shut. Protective screens for windows are advisable. Hot things, stove, electrical appliances should be out of their reach. The harmful objects, such as medications, kerosene, and sharp instruments should be kept beyond their reach.

The caregiver or the older sibling should be given appropriate instruction about the protective care of very young children. The toys should be provided which have fast color, blunt edges, and which do not have small removable parts.

Accidents in school age children: Being more active and adventuresome, school ages children are prone to falls, sports injuries, drowning and vehicle accidents. **Precautions**—schools age children should be explained the use of the toys, safety rules, and protective behavior. They should be encouraged to play in safe place, such as playgrounds, gardens, halls or indoor.

They should be taught the precautions for using match box, fire, electricity, sharp instruments and open water places. In early school age, supervisory games may be encouraged.

Measures to prevent accidents: Since accidents have assumed the proportion of an epidemic, measures appropriate to control an epidemic should be undertaken. The various measures comprise the following:

- **Survey:** Accident do not just happen, they are caused. The causes must be determined by survey which will indicate the appropriate measures needed in a given situation. Detailed environmental data relating to the road, vehicle, weather, etc., must also be collected, without adequate data collection, analysis and interpretation there could be no effective counter measures, evaluations and strategies for prevention.
- **Safety education:** There is widespread belief that accidents are inevitable. This fatalistic attitude must be curbed. It has been aptly said that 'If accident is a disease, education is a vaccine.' Safety education should be part of general education. It should be imparted in schools and factories. The driver need to be trained in proper maintenance of vehicles and safe driving. Young people need to be educated regarding risk factors, traffic rules and safety precautions. They should also be trained in first aid.
- **Promotion of safety measures:** The factors which tend to cause accidents must be sought and eliminated, or measures should be taken.
  - The use of seat belts reduces the number of fatalities and nonfatalities injuries by approximately 50% each. They should be made compulsory for cars, light trucks and similar vehicles.
  - *Safety helmet:* They reduce the risk of head injury by 30% on an average and that of fatalities by 40%. They prevent of the laceration of scalp to a great extent. Recently, the full face integral helmet has become very popular.
  - *Leather clothing and boots:* Leather clothing reduces risk of extensive superficial soft tissue injury.
  - *Children:* Another safety measure is to ensure that children remain seated when they are in a vehicle. They should be prohibited to take the front seats of cars.
  - *Others*: These comprise use of door locks, proper vehicle design, use of laminated high penetration resistance windscreen glass, etc.
- **Alcohol and other drugs:** Alcohol impairs driving ability and increases the risk of an accident as well as the severity of its consequences. Conclusions of surveys carried out in several countries have shown that alcohol is direct cause of 30 to 50 mg/100 mL. Impairment from alcohol can occur at blood alcohol levels s low as 50 mg/100 mL and that accident risk rises significantly between 50 and 80 mg/100 mL.

Drugs, such as barbiturates, amphetamines and cannabis impair one's ability to drive safely. They should be avoided altogether.

- **Primary care:** Planning, organization and management of trauma treatment and emergency care services should be a fundamental element of health services managerial process. Emergency care should begin to the accident site, continue during transportation and conclude in the hospital emergency room. At any of these stages a life may be saved or lost, depending upon the skill of the health care worker and the availability of needed emergency equipment. To achieve these ends, there should be an accident services. Organization and one fully equipped specialized trauma care hospital in all major units.

- **Elimination of factors:** The factor which tend to cause accidents must be sought and eliminated. For example, reduction of electric voltage, improvement of rods, imposition of speed limits, marking a danger point, provision of fire guards, use of safety equipment in industries, improvement of housing, safe storage of drugs, poisons and weapons, etc.
- **Rehabilitation services:** Rehabilitation consists of a number of elements which each injured person should benefit from. These are medical rehabilitation, social rehabilitation, occupational rehabilitation, etc. The aim of rehabilitation is to prevent, reduce or compensate disability and thereby handicap.
- **Enforcement of law:** Legal and regulatory measures are enforced by the state to prevent accidents, such as enforcement of speed limits, compulsory wearing of seat belts and crash helmets, checking of blood alcohol concentration in drivers and regular inspection of vehicles. In addition, there are factory and industrial laws to ensure safety of the people at work.
- **Accident research:** The future of accident is in research, such research will be concerned with gathering precise information about the extent, type and other characteristics of accidents correlating accident experience with personal attributes and the environment in which accident occur, investigating new and better methods of altering human behavior seeking ways to make environment safer and evaluating more precisely the efficiency of control measures.
- **Home and community:** Nurses can help in accident prevention whether they are actively practicing nursing in a hospital or community nursing agency or whether they are not currently practicing professionally. Nurses should be able to point out good sources of general information on the national level, such as the reports of the national safety council. The local or country health department, the local police department the visiting nurse association, the welfare and health council, and similar agencies are all good sources of help.

Groups have a stronger voice than teacher associations various religious and social organizations and many other groups are interested in the problem of accident control. Efforts should be made to work with existing agencies and group phases of accident prevention that should be of community interest includes:

- Teaching of accident prevention in the public school
- Better control and inspection of homes for the aged
- Rigid enforcement of driving regulations
- Improvement of street lighting and traffic signals at busy intersections
- Periodic inspection of all automobiles
- Promotion of laws protecting the public from flammable clothing, potentially harmful toys and similar items.

Accident in and about home cause almost one third of all accidental deaths each year. Fall accounts for about half of the accidents in and the home, and fire, burns and poisoning accounts for most of the reminder. People fall from roof, windows, high ladders and steps and are fatally burned or otherwise injured while using solvent and cleansing agent without proper knowledge of the hazards children are poisoned by substances left in unlocked or easy to reach cupboards or containers, it should be checked in regular intervals.

Hospital

In the hospital the nurse should take an active part in accident prevention. Early ambulation patients and unconscious patients has more prone to accident hazards. An infinite number of improvements that might reduce accident could be made in general hospital. They vary with each situation, for example, hand rail should be installed in the corridors of medical and surgical units where patients walk about each day. Fall out of bed can be prevented by the use of a high lobed and the judicious use of side rails and sedatives. Elderly patients should be placed in low height beds and in location where they will have frequent observation. Side rails are kept raised for unattended infant and unconscious patients. A confused patient may attempt to climb over a side rail and thus have further to fall; therefore, a jacket restraint may be more useful in these situations. Persons who are weak and need to be reminded to call for consistence before getting out of the bed.

The danger of accidental injury or death from fire must be constantly born in mind by all hospital personnel. If smoking is allowed in patient units, the patient who smokes is encouraged to get out of bed. Faulty electrical equipment should not be used. Any signs of smoke or fire are investigated and report immediately and take appropriate action.

Provision of Emergency Care and Role of Nurse

There is great variability in the quality of care given to persons who have been injured outside the hospital. In the past first aid care was often given by poorly trained person with adequate equipment, many communities now prepare specially trained persons to respond the emergency call. Emergency medical technician has preparation beyond basic first aid training and preparation in transportation of injured, but they do not carry-out intrusive procedures. In some communities nurses care part of the rescue teams. Quality emergency care in a community requires community organization with input from health professional as well as other interested citizens.

General principles of management for an accident:

- Remain calm and think before acting

- Identify yourself as a nurse to victim and by standers
- Do a rapid assessment for life-threatening problems
- Carry-out life saving measures as indicated
- Do a systematic assessment before initiating general first aid measures
- Keep victim using down or in the position found (unless orthopnea is present)
- Protect victim from dampness and cold
- If victim is conscious, explain what is occurring, assure that help will be given
- Avoid unnecessary handling or moving, move victim only if danger is present
- Do not give fluid if there is possibility of abdominal injury or if anesthesia will be necessary within a short time
- Do not transport victim until all first aid measures have been carried out and appropriate transportation is available.

CANCER

Cancers are a large family of diseases that involve abnormal cell growth with the potential to invade or spread to other parts of the body. They form a subset of neoplasm. A neoplasm or tumor is a group of cells that have undergone unregulated growth, and will often form a mass or lump, but may be distributed diffusely.

Categories

The major categories are:

a. Carcinomas which arise from epithelial cells lining the internal surface of the various organs.
b. Sarcomas which arise from mesodermal cell constituting the various connective tissues.
c. Lymphomas, myeloma and leukemia's arising from the cells of bone marrow and immune systems.

Risk Factors

Cigarette smoking and tobacco use: Tobacco use is strongly linked to an increased risk for many kinds of cancer. Smoking cigarettes is the leading cause of the different types of cancer like Acute Myelogenous Leukemia (AML). Bladder cancer, Esophageal cancer, Kidney cancer, Lung cancer, Oral cavity cancer and Pancreatic cancer, etc.

Infections

Certain viruses and bacteria are able to cause cancer. Viruses and other infection-causing agents cause more cases of cancer in the developing world (about 1 in 4 cases of cancer) than in developed nations (less than 1 in 10 cases of cancer). Examples of cancer-causing viruses and bacteria include: Human Papilloma Virus (HPV) increases the risk for cancers of the cervix, penis, vagina, anus, and oropharynx. Hepatitis B and hepatitis C viruses increase the risk for liver cancer.

Diet

Diet is being studied as a risk factor for cancer. It is hard to study the effects of diet on cancer because a person's diet includes foods that may protect against cancer and foods that may increase the risk of cancer.

It is difficult for people who take part in the studies to keep track of what they eat over a long period of time. This may explain why studies have different results about how diet affects the risk of cancer.

Some studies show that fruits and nonstarch vegetables may protect against cancers of the mouth, esophagus and stomach. Fruits may also protect against lung cancer.

Some studies have shown that a diet high in fat, proteins, calories, and red meat increases the risk of colorectal cancer, but other studies have not shown this.

Radiation

Radiation exposed is a known cause of cancer. There are two main types of radiation linked with an increased risk for cancer: Ultraviolet radiation from sunlight: This is the main cause of nonmelanoma skin cancers. Second is Ionizing radiation including Medical radiation from tests to diagnose cancer such as X-rays, CT scans, fluoroscopy, and nuclear medicine scans. Scientists believe that ionizing radiation causes leukemia, thyroid cancer, and breast cancer in women. Ionizing radiation may also be linked to myeloma and cancers of the lung, stomach, colon, esophagus, bladder, and ovary. Being exposed to radiation from diagnostic X-rays increases the risk of cancer in patients and X-ray technicians. The growing use of CT scans over the last 20 years has increased exposure to ionizing radiation. The risk of cancer also increases with the number of CT scans a patient has and the radiation dose used each time.

Immunosuppressive Medicines

Immunosuppressive medicines are linked to an increased risk of cancer. These medicines lower the body's ability to stop cancer from forming. For example, immunosuppressive medicines may be used to keep a patient from rejecting an organ transplant.

Obesity

Studies show that obesity is linked to a higher risk of the following types of cancer postmenopausal breast cancer, colorectal cancer, endometrial cancer, esophageal cancer, kidney cancer, and pancreatic cancer. Some studies show that obesity is also a risk factor for cancer of the gallbladder.

Environmental Risk Factors

Being exposed to chemicals and other substances in the environment has been linked to some cancers:

- Links between air pollution and cancer risk have been found. These include links between lung cancer and second hand tobacco smoke, outdoor air pollution, and asbestos.
- Drinking water that contains a large amount of arsenic has been linked to skin, bladder, and lung cancers.

Studies have been done to see if pesticides and other pollutants increase the risk of cancer. The results of those studies have been unclear because other factors can change the results of the studies.

Genetic Factors

Genetic factors are some time responsible for cancer. When a person was born with a genetic mutation, or change, which makes that person more likely than usual to get cancer. This genetic mutation could have come from either the person's mother or father or both. Hereditary cancer may also be called familial cancer or cancer in the family. Approximately 5% to 20% of all cancers are hereditary. This is a relatively small percentage of cancer.

Prevention and Control of Cancer

Primary Prevention

Primary prevention means eliminating or minimizing exposure to the causes of cancer, and includes reducing individual susceptibility to the effect of such causes. This approach offers the greatest public health potential and the most cost-effective long-term method of cancer control. Cancer prevention should be a key element in all national cancer control programmes. Prevention not only focuses on the risks associated with a particular illness or problem but also on protective factors. Among prevention activities, emphasis should be placed on:

- Tobacco control
- Dietary changes
- Physical activities and avoidance of obesity
- Reducing alcohol use
- Reducing carcinogenic occupational and environmental exposures
- Immunization against hepatitis B virus
- Combating schistosomiasis
- Avoidance of prolonged exposure to the sun
- Health education on early detection by identifying warning signs.

1. **Control of tobacco and alcohol consumption:** Tobacco is the single most important modifiable risk factor for cancer. Tobacco smoke contains approximately 4000 chemicals of which at least 438 can cause cancer. Tobacco smoking causes cancer of the lung, larynx and oesophagus. Smoking is also associated with cancers of the pancreas, bladder, and pelvis of the kidneys, ureter and squamous cell carcinoma of the uterine cervix. Tobacco chewing is the most important risk factor for cancer of the oral cavity. Inhalation of secondary smoke, known as "passive smoking" is a unique feature of smoking. It results in increased risk of cancers among nonsmokers exposed to tobacco smoke. Similarly increasing alcohol consumption is associated with cancers of the mouth, pharynx (excluding nasopharynx), larynx, esophagus and liver. The risk relationship between cancer and alcohol is nearly a linear relationship with the risk increasing with increasing amount of alcohol consumed. Co-existence of tobacco habits can have a multiplicative effect on development of cancer. Control of alcohol requires actions similar to those for tobacco control. The actions should be targeted towards individual and community and include taxation, general public education, encouraging highly vulnerable groups.
2. **Dietary change:**
   - **Eat plenty of fruits and vegetables:** Base your diet on fruits, vegetables and other foods from plant sources, such as whole grains and beans.
   - **Limit fat:** Eat lighter and leaner by choosing fewer high-fat foods, particularly those from animal sources. High-fat diets tend to be higher in calories and might increase the risk of overweight or obesity—which can, in turn, increase cancer risk.
   - **Limit red meats (beef, pork, lamb) and avoid processed meats:** Limit red meats to 18 ounces per week, says Collins, who suggests using chicken, seafood, or legumes in place of red meat. Collins is not saying to never eat red meat, just do so in moderation.
   - **Limit consumption of salty foods and foods processed with sodium:** Do not go over 2,400 milligrams per day, and use herbs and spices instead, says Collins. She adds that processed foods account for most sodium intake nowadays—not salt you add when cooking or eating.
3. **Maintain a healthy weight and be physically active:** Obesity increases the risk of postmenopausal breast cancer, and cancers of the endometrium, colorectum, kidney, and esophagus. It is also associated with cardiovascular disease and adult-onset diabetes. The fundamental causes of obesity and overweight are societal, resulting from an environment that promotes sedentary lifestyles and over-consumption of high-calorific food. There is also convincing evidence to show that physical activity has a beneficial influence on the risk of colorectal cancer and probably has a beneficial effect on breast cancer risk, independent of its effect on obesity. So as a community health nurse it is our role to spread message for prevention of obesity. Moderate activities, such as walking for one hour a day is required to maintain normal body weight, especially in sedentary people. In addition, more vigorous activities such as brisk walking several times a week may give additional benefit concerning cancer prevention.
4. **Reducing alcohol use:** The consumption of alcoholic beverages convincingly increases the risk of cancers of the oral cavity, pharynx, larynx, esophagus, liver, and breast (and probably colorectum). The carcinogenic effect of alcohol in relation to oral, pharyngeal, laryngeal and esophageal cancer is exacerbated by tobacco use. Primary liver cancer is strongly associated with cirrhosis of the liver, whether induced by toxic or infectious agents. In developed countries, cirrhosis is related principally to alcohol consumption. The risk relationship between alcohol and cancer is nearly a linear dose response relationship between volume of drinking and risk. The pattern of drinking does not

seem to have an important role. So it is major concern to educate the community about risk of alcohol use and how to reduce it's consumption.

5. **Control of occupational cancer:** The control of occupational cancer calls for the identification and assessment of existing or potential hazards. The preventive measures for occupational cancer include control of carcinogen, protective measures for workers, health check-up of worker and health education. Wherever occupational cancer hazards are found to exist, exposure standards must be set that will minimize the risk to workers. This typically requires the appropriate government, scientific, industrial, and labor organizations to review and discuss relevant data and then to agree on controls.
   Cancer control programs should encourage action at government level to prohibit:
   - The importation of hazardous work practices that involve exposure to known carcinogens;
   - The dumping of hazardous waste in such a manner that drinking-water or air will become contaminated with carcinogens.
6. **Protect yourself from the sun:** Skin cancer is one of the most common kinds of cancer—and one of the most preventable. Try these tips:
   - **Avoid midday sun:** Stay out of the sun between 10 AM and 4 PM, when the sun's rays are strongest.
   - **Stay in the shade.** When you are outdoors, stay in the shade as much as possible. Sunglasses and a broad-rimmed hat help, too.
   - **Cover exposed areas:** Wear tightly woven, loosefitting clothing that covers as much of your skin as possible. Opt for bright or dark colors, which reflect more ultraviolet radiation than pastels or bleached cotton.
   - **Do not skimp on sunscreen:** Use generous amounts of sunscreen when you are outdoors, and reapply often.
   - **Avoid tanning beds and sunlamps:** These are just as damaging as natural sunlight.
7. **Combating schistosomiasis:** Schistosomiasis is one of the most widespread human parasitic infections, responsible for a substantial amount of bladder cancer in Egypt, Iraq, and west and south-eastern Africa. The causative organism, Schistosoma, passes part of its life cycle in snails that inhabit shallow waters, and is then released into the water, infecting humans by penetrating the skin. Passing of urine or feces into the water by infected people then continues the life cycle. Schistosomiasis control focuses on reducing disease through periodic, large-scale population treatment with praziquantel; a more comprehensive approach including potable water, adequate sanitation, and snail control would also reduce transmission.
8. **Get immunized:** Cancer prevention includes protection from certain viral infections. Talk to your doctor about immunization against:
   - **Hepatitis B:** Hepatitis B can increase the risk of developing liver cancer. The hepatitis B vaccine is recommended for certain high-risk adults—such as adults who are sexually active but not in a mutually monogamous relationship, people with sexually transmitted infections, intravenous drug users, men who have sex with men, and health care or public safety workers who might be exposed to infected blood or body fluids.
   - **Human papillomavirus (HPV):** HPV is a sexually transmitted virus that can lead to cervical and other genital cancers as well as squamous cell cancers of the head and neck. The HPV vaccine is available to both men and women age 26 or younger who did not have the vaccine as adolescents.
9. **Avoid risky behaviors:** Another effective cancer prevention tactic is to avoid risky behaviors that can lead to infections that, in turn, might increase the risk of cancer. For example:
   - **Practice safe sex:** Limit your number of sexual partners, and use a condom when you have sex. The more sexual partners you have in your lifetime, the more likely you are to contract a sexually transmitted infection—such as HIV or HPV. People who have HIV or AIDS have a higher risk of cancer of the anus, liver and lung. HPV is most often associated with cervical cancer, but it might also increase the risk of cancer of the anus, penis, throat, vulva and vagina.
   - **Do not share needles:** Sharing needles with an infected drug user can lead to HIV, as well as hepatitis B and hepatitis C—which can increase the risk of liver cancer. If you are concerned about drug abuse or addiction, seek professional help.
10. **Get regular medical care:** Regular self-exams and screenings for various types of cancers—such as cancer of the skin, colon, prostate, cervix and breast—can increase the chances of discovering cancer early, when treatment is most likely to be successful.
11. **Cancer education:** Warning signs (danger signals) of cancer are:
    - C—Change in bowel or bladder habits
    - A—A sore that does not heal
    - U—Unusual bleeding or discharge
    - T—Thickening or lump in the breast or elsewhere
    - I—Indigestion or difficulty in swallowing
    - O—Obvious change in a wart or mole
    - N—Nagging cough or hoarseness
    The education about warning signs are very essential for the public to detect cancer in early stage.
    Cancer can affect any part of our body but some of the common cancer which can be managed by early detection are explained below. They are generally Breast cancer, cervix cancer, colon cancers etc.

BREAST CANCER

Breast cancer is the commonest cancer among women all over the world. In India, it is the second most common cancer among women after cancer of the uterine cervix and is emerging as the commonest cancer in urban centers. Data from Hospital Based Cancer Registry (HBCR) show that only about 15% of patients present in localized stage. Regional Lymph nodes are involved in around 75% at the time of presentation and about 10% have distant metastases at the time of presentation. Breast cancer is the most diagnosed cancer among women worldwide, accounting for 1 in 4 cancer cases. It is the most frequent cancer amongst both sexes and is the leading cause of death from cancer in women. The estimated 2.3 million new cases indicate that one in every 8 cancers diagnosed in 2020 is breast cancer. In 2020, there were an estimated 684,996 deaths from breast cancer, with a disproportionate number of these deaths occurring in low-resource settings. Breast cancer cells usually form a tumor that can often be seen on an X-ray or felt as a lump. If spread outside the breast through blood vessels and lymph vessels, it becomes advanced breast cancer. When breast cancer spreads to other parts of the body (such as the liver, lungs, bones or brain), it is said to have metastasized, and is referred to as metastatic breast cancer.

Risk Factors

Some risk factors can impact on a woman's likelihood of developing breast cancer.

- **Age:** The older woman gets, the higher risk of developing breast cancer.
- **Genetics:** Women who have a close relative who has/had breast or ovarian cancer are more likely to develop breast cancer.
- **History of breast cancer:** Women who have had breast cancer, even noninvasive cancer, are more likely to develop the disease again, compared to women who have no history of the disease.
- **Dense breast tissue:** Women with more dense breast tissue have a greater chance of developing breast cancer.
- **Estrogen exposure:** Women who started having menstruation earlier or entered menopause later than usual have a higher risk of developing breast cancer. This is because their bodies have been exposed to estrogen for longer.
- **Obesity:** Post-menopausal obese and overweight women may have a higher risk of developing breast cancer, because there are higher levels of estrogen in obese menopausal women.
- **Personal history of breast cancer:** A history of breast cancer in one breast increases the risk of developing a new cancer in the other breast or in another part of the same breast by 3 to 4 times.
- **Reproductive history:** Certain reproductive factors slightly increase risk. These include giving birth to a first child after age 30, null parity, starting menstruation before age 12, and entering menopause after age 55.
- **Hormone replacement therapy (HRT):** Using combined hormone therapy after menopause (estrogen and progesterone) increases breast cancer risk for current or recent users, especially if used for longer than 2 to 3 years. The use of estrogen alone after menopause does not appear to increase the risk of developing breast cancer.
- **Alcohol consumption:** Compared with nondrinkers, women who drink alcoholic beverages are at increased risk. The risk increases with the amount of alcohol consumed. Risk for those who consume 2 to 5 drinks daily is increased by about 1½ time normal.
- **Oral contraceptive use:** Using oral contraceptives appears to slightly increase a woman's risk for breast cancer, but only for a limited period of time. Women who stopped using oral contraceptives more than 10 years ago do not appear to have any increased breast cancer.

Diagnosis

- **Breast self-examination:** The first person to detect any lump in the breast is the woman herself. For this, it is essential that every woman be aware of the size, shape and consistency of her breasts, and know when there is an abnormal change in any of these. The details of breast self-examination has been discussed in the Chapter 2, Family Health Nursing.
- **Clinical Breast examination (CBE):** This is to be performed by a physician, trained nurse or a health worker. It is recommended that women may be examined for any lump in the breast when they have come for other reasons.
- **Mammography:** This is an X-ray image of the breast taken with low dose radiation. Two films per breast are taken. This investigation is good for picking up micro calcifications. Mammography is advised once at the age of 40 years to establish the baseline and then every 3 years.
- **Ultrasonography:** For women less than 40 years of age when indicated ultrasound of the breast is usually done as their breasts are dense and mammography is not advisable for them.

Clinical Manifestations of Breast Cancers

- A painless lump in the breast
- Dimpling of the skin in the area of the lump appearing like orange peel—"peaude orange" appearance.
- Watery, yellow, and blood-stained nipple discharge
- Pain in the breast
- Inversion of the nipple
- Presence of a patch of dry flaky skin on the nipple and change in appearance or texture of the breasts—usually seen in Paget's disease
- General symptoms—fever, loss of appetite, fatigue
- A pain in the armpits or breast that does not seem to be related to the woman's menstrual period
- Pitting or redness of the skin of the breast; like the skin of an orange
- A rash around (or on) one of the nipples
- A swelling (lump) in one of the armpits

- An area of thickened tissue in a breast
- The nipple changes in appearance; it may become sunken or inverted
- The size or the shape of the breast changes
- The nipple-skin or breast-skin may have started to peel, scale or flake.

Prevention of Breast Cancer

- **Avoid becoming overweight:** Obesity raises the risk of breast cancer after menopause, the time of life when breast cancer most often occurs. Avoid gaining weight over time, and try to maintain a body-mass index.
- **Eat healthy to avoid tipping the scale:** Embrace a diet high in vegetables and fruit and low in sugared drinks, refined carbohydrates and fatty foods. Eat lean protein such as fish or chicken breast and eat red meat in moderation, if at all. Eat whole grains. Choose vegetable oils over animal fats.
- **Keep physically active:** Research suggests that increased physical activity, even when begun later in life, reduces overall breast-cancer risk by about 10% to 30%. All it takes is moderate exercise like a 30-minute walk five days a week to get this protective effect.
- **Drink little or no alcohol:** Alcohol use is associated with an increased risk of breast cancer. Women should limit intake to no more than one drink per day, regardless of the type of alcohol.
- **Do not smoke:** Research suggests that long-term smoking is associated with increased risk of breast cancer in some women.
- **If you bear children, breastfeed your babies for as long as possible:** Women who breastfeed their babies for at least a year in total have a reduced risk of developing breast cancer later.
- **Avoid hormone replacement therapy:** Menopausal hormone therapy increases risk for breast cancer. If you must take hormones to manage menopausal symptoms, avoid those that contain progesterone and limit their use to less than three years.
- **Get regular breast cancer screenings:** Follow your doctor or health care provider's recommendations to decide what type of screening you need and how often you need it.

CANCER OF THE UTERINE CERVIX

Cervical cancer is the third most common cancer among women in the world and the leading cause of death from cancer among women in developing countries. In India more than 100,000 new cases of cervical cancer occur each year and nearly 75,000 women die annually from this disease. Human Papilloma Virus (HPV) infection, which is a sexually transmitted infection, is the primary cause of this cancer. HPV prevalence increases with multiple sexual partners for both spouse, and poor genital hygiene of both partners. Symptoms of cancer of the uterine cervix: In the early stages, there will be no symptoms. By the time symptoms appear, disease may have already spread. Common symptoms are:

- Post-menopausal bleeding
- Post-coital bleeding
- Intermenstrual bleeding
- Blood stained discharge per vaginum
- Excessive seropurulent discharge
- Backache
- Lower abdominal pain.

Screening for Cervical Cancer

Screening for cervical cancer can be considered in women aged 30 to 59 years, as the chances of detecting pre-cancerous lesions are maximum in this age group. Regular population-based screening using Pap Smear cytology is internationally accepted screening method for cervical cancer. In low resource setting, Visual Inspection with Acetic Acid is a useful alternative to categorize women as "high risk" and "low risk".

Pap Smear

The ectocervix and the endocervix are scraped to collect cells that are spread on a glass slide, stained in the laboratory and examined under microscope. Depending on the features of the cells seen under microscope the cytopathologist (or a trained technologist) can report the smear as 'negative' (normal) or 'positive' (abnormalities suspicious of low-grade or high-grade CIN). Most abnormal Pap tests are caused by viral infections, such as human papilloma virus (HPV) infection, or other types of infection, such as those caused by bacteria, fungi (yeast), or protozoa (*Trichomonas*). Natural cervical cell changes (atrophic vaginitis) related to menopause can also cause an abnormal Pap test. In some cases, untreated cervical cell changes that cause abnormal Pap tests may progress to precancerous or cancerous changes.

Visual Inspection using Acetic Acid (VIA)

Naked-eye visual inspection of the uterine cervix, after application of 5% acetic acid (VIA) provides simple tests for the early detection of cervical precancerous lesions and early invasive cancer. The results of VIA are immediately available and do not require any laboratory support. Acetic acid caused intracellular dehydration and coagulation of protein within abnormal cervical cells. So the abnormal cells will turn white after application of acetic acid.

Instruments and Materials Required

- Examining table
- Light source
- Bivalve speculum (Cusco)
- Instrument tray or container
- Bottles with normal saline
- 5% acetic acid (freshly prepared)
- Cotton-tipped - swab sticks
- Disposable gloves

- 0.5% chlorine solution for decontaminating
- Forms and registers for recording the findings.

Preparation of 5% acetic acid: Acetic acid is to be freshly prepared everyday: Carefully add 5 mL of Glacial acetic acid into 95 mL of distilled water and mix thoroughly.

Storage: Unused acetic acid should be discarded at the end of the day.

Note: It is important to remember to dilute the glacial acetic acid, since the undiluted strength causes a severe chemical burn if applied to the epithelium.

Procedure of VIA Examination

- Explain the screening in detail to the woman.
- The woman should be reassured that the procedure is painless, and every effort should be made to ensure that she is fully relaxed and remains at ease during testing.
- Written informed consent should be obtained before screening.
- The woman is invited to lie down in a modified lithotomy position on a couch with leg rests or knee crutches or stirrups.
- Gently introduce the speculum and open the blades of the speculum to view the cervix in the presence of good light source.
- Identify the external os, columnar epithelium (red in color), squamous epithelium (pink) and the squamocolumnar junction.
- Proceed to identify the transformation zone, the upper limit of which is formed by the squamocolumnar junction. (Cervical neoplasias occur in the transformation zone nearest to the squamocolumnar junction).
- Gently, but firmly, apply 5% acetic acid using a cotton swab soaked in acetic acid. The secretions should be gently wiped off. The swabs after use should be disposed of in the waste bucket.
- The curdy-white discharge associated with candidiasis is particularly sticky, and if particular care is not taken to remove it properly, it may mimic an acetowhite lesion, thus leading to a false-positive result.
- After removing the swab, carefully look at the cervix to see whether any white lesions appear, particularly in the transformation zone close to the squamocolumnar junction, or dense, nonremovable acetowhite areas in the columnar epithelium.
- The results one minute after application of acetic acid should be reported. Note how rapidly the acetowhite lesion appears and then disappears.

Carefully Observe

- The intensity of the white color of the acetowhite lesion: if it is shiny white, cloudy white, pale-white or dull-white.
- The borders and demarcations of the white lesion: distinctly clear and sharp or indistinct diffuse margins; raised or flat margins; regular or irregular margins.
- Whether the lesions are uniformly white in color, or the color intensity varies across the lesion, or if there are areas of erosion within the lesion.
- Location of the lesion: Is it in, near or far away from the transformation zone? Is it abutting (touching) the squamocolumnar junction? Does it extend into the endocervical canal? Does it occupy the entire, or part of, the transformation zone? Does it involve the entire cervix (which usually indicates early preclinical invasive cancer)?
- Size (extent or dimensions) and number of the lesions.

Reporting the Outcome of VIA (Fig. 11.4)

Visual inspection aided (VIA) with acetic-acid is shown in **Figure 11.4**. Acetowhite lesion with punctation—a precancerous condition has been observed.

VIA Negative (–) (Fig. 11.5A)

VIA screening is reported as negative in the case of any of the following observations:

- No acetowhite lesions are observed on the cervix.
- Polyps protrude from the cervix with bluish white acetowhite areas. Nabothian cysts appear as button-like areas, as whitish acne or pimples.
- Dot-like areas are present in the end cervix, which are due to grape-like columnar epithelium staining with acetic acid.
- There are shiny, pinkish-white, cloudy white, bluish-white, faint patchy or doubtful lesions with ill-defined, indefinite margins, blending with the rest of the cervix.
- Angular, irregular, digitating acetowhite lesions, resembling geographical regions, distant (detached) from the squamocolumnar junction (satellite lesions).
- Faint line-like or ill-defined acetowhitening is seen at the squamocolumnar junction.
- Streak-like acetowhitening is visible in the columnar epithelium.
- There are ill-defined, patchy, pale, discontinuous, scattered acetowhite areas.

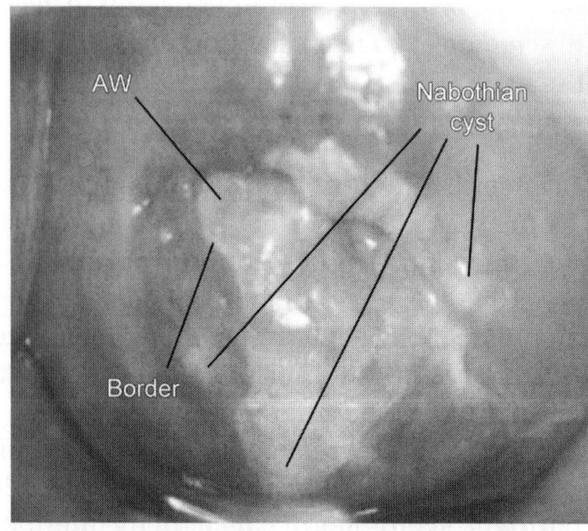

Fig. 11.4: Visual inspection of cervix aided (VIA) with acetic-acid.

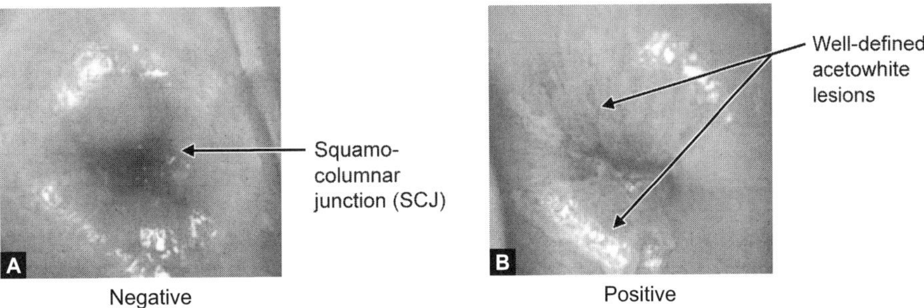

Figs. 11.5A and B: (A) Visual inspection of cervix aided shows negative result; (B) Visual inspection of cervix aided positive result.

VIA Positive (+) (Fig. 11.5B)

The VIA test outcome is reported as positive in any of the following situations: There are distinct, well-defined, dense (opaque, dull- or oyster-white) acetowhite areas with regular or irregular margins, close to or abutting the squamocolumnar junction in the transformation zone or close to the external os if the squamocolumnar junction is not visible.

- Strikingly dense acetowhite areas are seen in the columnar epithelium.
- The entire cervix becomes densely white after the application of acetic acid.
- Condyloma and leukoplakia occur close to the squamocolumnar junction, turning intensely white after application of acetic acid.

ORAL CANCER (FIG. 11.6)

Oral cancer, also known as mouth cancer, is cancer of the lining of the lips, mouth, or upper throat. In the mouth, it most commonly starts as a painless white patch, that thickens, develops red patches, an ulcer, and continues to grow. When on the lips, it commonly looks like a persistent crusting ulcer that does not heal, and slowly grows. Other symptoms may include difficult or painful swallowing, new lumps or bumps in the neck, a swelling in the mouth, or a feeling of numbness in the mouth or lip. It is a heterogeneous group of cancers arising from different parts of the oral cavity, with different predisposing factors, prevalence, and treatment outcomes. Oral cancer includes cancers of the lips, tongue, cheeks, floor of the mouth, hard and soft palate, sinuses, and pharynx.

Definition of Cancer

Uncoordinated and uncontrolled growth of the tissue, resulting from multiplication of its cells and the condition persists even after the stimulus or the initiating factor is removed.

Risk factors for the development of oral cancer: Oral cancer is the sixth most common cancer reported globally with an annual incidence of over 300,000 cases, of which 62% arise in developing countries like India. The common risk factors are:

- **Smoking:** It has been shown that those smoking 40 or more cigarettes/day are 5 to 7 times more at risk of developing cancer than nonsmokers.
- **Smokeless tobacco use:** Users of dip, snuff, or chewing tobacco products are 50 times more likely to develop cancers of the cheek, gums, and lining of the lips.
- **Consumption of alcohol:** Oral cancers are about six times more common in drinkers than in nondrinkers. This possibly acts as irritant or solvent which facilitates penetration of mucosa by other carcinogens like tobacco. It may also suppress efficiency of DNA repair after exposure to carcinogens. Using alcohol and tobacco together increases your chances even more.
- **Poor dental hygiene and constant chronic trauma to mucosa:** Poor oral hygiene can lead to dental cavities and gum disease, and has also been linked to heart disease, cancer, and diabetes. Chronic mucosal trauma resulting from sharp teeth, dentures, faulty restoration, or implants has frequently been associated with the development of oral cancer. Trauma may result in cancer formation by two mechanisms. It has been proposed that persistent mechanical irritation causes DNA damage and may eventually result in cancer formation or chronic mucosal trauma results in inflammation, thereby releasing chemical mediators such as cytokine, prostaglandins, and tumor necrosis factor. Such an inflammation leads to oxidative stress. This could induce genetic and epigenetic changes damaging DNA, inhibiting its repair, altering transcription factors, preventing apoptosis, and stimulating angiogenesis, thus resulting in carcinogenesis.
- **Excessive sun exposure, especially at a young age:** Ultraviolet radiation from the sun can cause lip cancers.
- **Viruses:** Human papillomavirus (HPV) can infect the mouth and throat and cause cancers of the oropharynx (back of the throat, including the base of the tongue and tonsils), i.e., oropharyngeal cancer. HPV is thought to cause 70% of oropharyngeal cancers in the United States. Similarly herpes simplex virus (HSV) may enhance the development of oral carcinoma in individuals who are already at increased risk of the disease because of tobacco consumption and cigarette smoking.
- **Age:** Oral cancers can take years to grow. Most people find they have it after age 55. But more younger men are getting cancers linked to HPV.
- **Gender:** Men are at least twice as likely as women to get oral cancer. It could be because men drink and smoke more than women do.

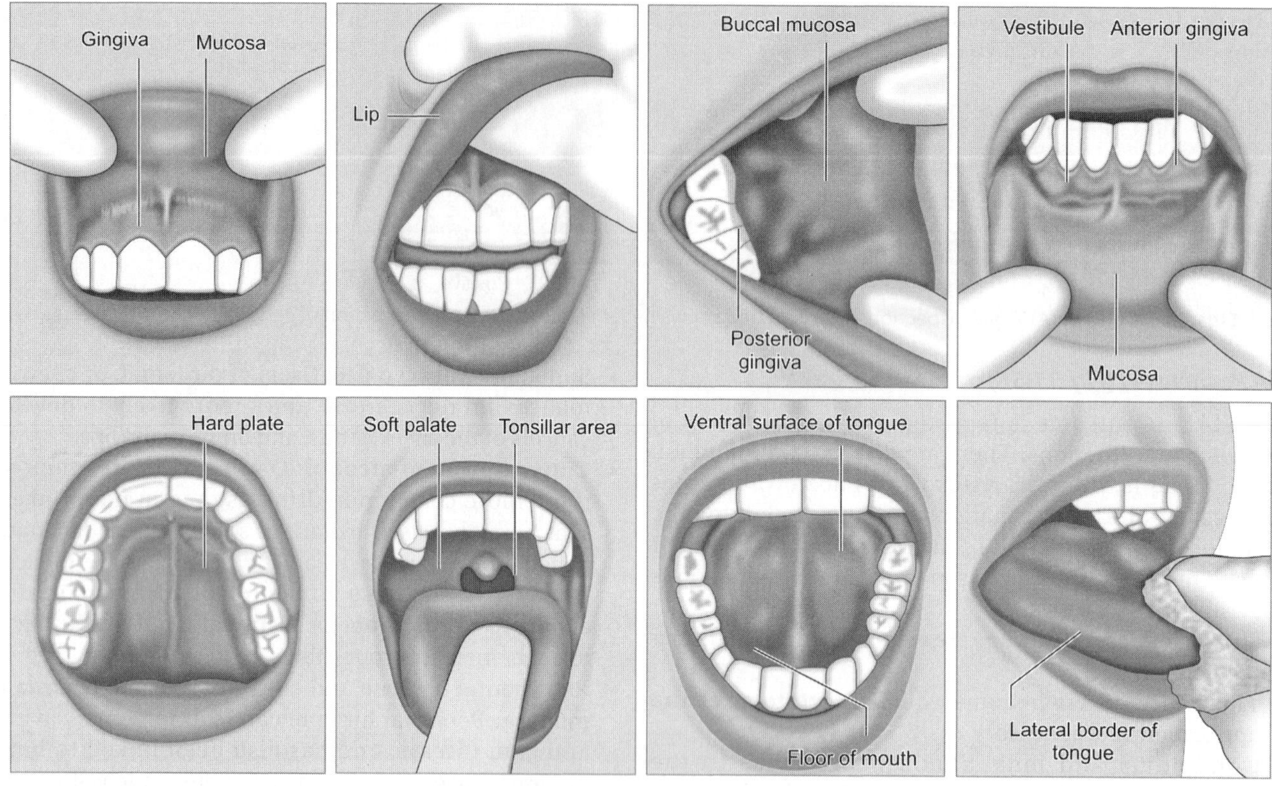

Fig. 11.6: Oral cancer screening.

- **Poor diet:** Studies have found a link between oral cancer and not eating enough vegetables and fruits.

Spread of Squamous Cell Carcinomas of the Oral Cavity

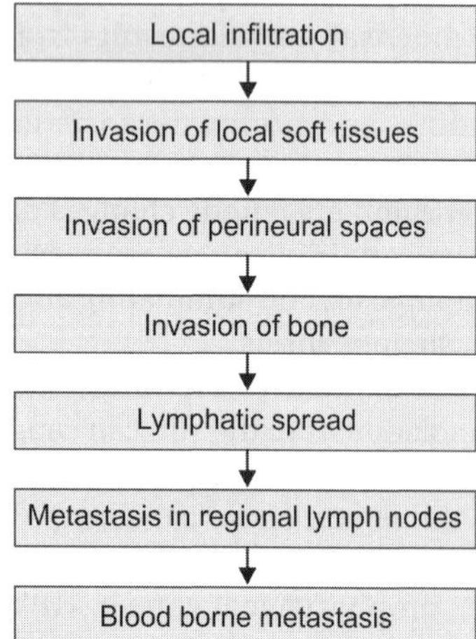

Signs and Symptoms

Warning Signs of Oral Cancer

- Long standing nonhealing ulcer for more than 2 weeks
- A white or red raised patch in the mouth
- Restriction in mouth opening
- A lump or growth in the mouth, lump in the neck.

Other Symptoms

- Reduced mouth opening
- Burning sensation in the mouth
- Change in voice
- Sores on your lip or inside your mouth that bleed easily and do not heal within two weeks.
- Rough spots or crusty areas on your lips, gums or inside of your mouth.
- Areas in your mouth that bleed for no obvious reason.
- Numbness, pain or tenderness on your face and neck or in your mouth that occur without apparent cause.
- Difficulty chewing or swallowing, speaking or moving your jaw or tongue.
- Unintentional weight loss.
- Earache and chronic bad breath.

Diagnosis

Oral cancer tests include:

- **Physical examination:** Your healthcare provider will look at the entire inside of your mouth and might feel around your mouth. They will also examine your head, face and neck for potential signs of pre-cancer or cancer.
- **Brush biopsy also called scrape biopsy or exfoliative cytology:** Healthcare providers use a small brush or spatula to gently scrape the area in question to obtain cells examined for cancer.
- **Incisional biopsy:** Your healthcare provider will remove small pieces of tissue to get cells to be examined for cancer.
- **Indirect laryngoscopy and pharyngoscopy:** Your healthcare provider uses a small mirror on a long thin handle to look at your throat, the base of your tongue and part of your larynx (voice box).

- **Direct (flexible) pharyngoscopy and laryngoscopy:** They may use an endoscope to look at areas of your throat and mouth that can not be seen with mirrors. An endoscope is a thin, flexible tube with an attached light and viewing lens.

Self-examination of Oral Cavity

Method of doing self-examination of oral cavity:

- Self-examination can detect oral lesions at an early stage. All habitual tobacco users should do self-examination of oral cavity on a monthly basis.
- Oral cavity should be examined thoroughly using a mouth mirror and a white light. A torch can be used for proper light.
  - Rinse the mouth with water and stand before a mirror in adequate light
  - Normal oral cavity lining is soft and pink
  - Look in the mirror for any abnormal white or red patch, ulcer or roughened area, granular area or swelling in the mouth
  - If any abnormality—patch (white/red), ulcer, rough area, granular area or swelling in the mouth is found then the individual must visit the health facility for further examination and management by a health professional.

Primary Prevention

Primary prevention means eliminating or minimizing exposure to the causes of cancer, and includes reducing individual susceptibility to the effect of such causes. This approach offers the greatest public health potential and the most cost-effective long-term method of cancer control. Cancer prevention should be a key element in all national cancer control programs. Prevention not only focuses on the risks associated with a particular illness or problem but also on protective factors. Among prevention activities, emphasis should be placed on:

- Tobacco control
- Dietary changes
- Physical activities and avoidance of obesity
- Reducing alcohol use
- Reducing carcinogenic occupational and environmental exposures
- Immunization against hepatitis B virus
- Combating schistosomiasis
- Avoidance of prolonged exposure to the sun
- Health education, relating to sexual and reproductive factors associated with cancer.

Control of Occupational Cancer

The control of occupational cancer calls for the identification and assessment of existing or potential hazards. The preventive measures for occupational cancer include control of carcinogen, protective measures for workers, health check-up of worker and health education. Wherever occupational cancer hazards are found to exist, exposure standards must be set that will minimize the risk to workers. This typically requires the appropriate government, scientific, industrial, and labor organizations to review and discuss relevant data and then to agree on controls.

Cancer control programs should encourage action at government level to prohibit:

- The importation of hazardous work practices that involve exposure to known carcinogens;
- The dumping of hazardous waste in such a manner that drinking-water or air will become contaminated with carcinogens.

Obesity increases the risk of postmenopausal breast cancer, and cancers of the endometrium, colorectum, kidney, and esophagus. It is also associated with cardiovascular disease and adult-onset diabetes. The fundamental causes of obesity and overweight are societal, resulting from an environment that promotes sedentary lifestyles and over-consumption of high-calorific food. There is also convincing evidence to show that physical activity has a beneficial influence on the risk of colorectal cancer and probably has a beneficial effect on breast cancer risk, independent of its effect on obesity. So as a community health nurse it is our role to spread message for prevention of obesity. Moderate activities, such as walking for one hour a day is required to maintain normal body weight, especially in sedentary people. In addition, more vigorous activities such as brisk walking several times a week may give additional benefit concerning cancer prevention.

Reducing Alcohol Use

The consumption of alcoholic beverages convincingly increases the risk of cancers of the oral cavity, pharynx, larynx, esophagus, liver, and breast (and probably colorectum). The carcinogenic effect of alcohol in relation to oral, pharyngeal, laryngeal and esophageal cancer is exacerbated by tobacco use. Primary liver cancer is strongly associated with cirrhosis of the liver, whether induced by toxic or infectious agents. In developed countries, cirrhosis is related principally to alcohol consumption. The risk relationship between alcohol and cancer is nearly a linear dose response relationship between volume of drinking and risk. The pattern of drinking does not seem to have an important role. So it is major concern to educate the community about risk of alcohol use and how to reduce it's consumption.

Combating Schistosomiasis

Schistosomiasis is one of the most widespread human parasitic infections, responsible for a substantial amount of bladder cancer in Egypt, Iraq, and west and south-eastern Africa. The causative organism, *Schistosoma*, passes part of its life cycle in snails that inhabit shallow waters, and is then released into the water, infecting humans by penetrating the skin. Passing of urine or feces into the water by infected people then continues the life cycle. Schistosomiasis control focuses on reducing disease through periodic, large-scale population treatment with praziquantel; a more comprehensive approach including potable water, adequate sanitation, and snail control would also reduce transmission.

PARASITIC ZOONOSES

Taeniasis

A group of cestode infections which are important zoonotic diseases. Two parasites of importance in taeniasis are *Taenia saginata* and *Taenia solium*.

Agent Factors

- ***T. saginata*:** This parasite is virtually global in distribution, wherever beef is eaten.
- ***T. solium*:** It is endemic in many countries of Latin America, Africa and Asia as well as in some parts of Europe and the USSR.

Hosts of Infection

T. saginata and *T. solium* pass their life cycles in two hosts.

The larval stage of *T. saginata* mainly occurs in cattle. The pig is the main host for the larval stage of *T. solium* but man may also be infected. This may lead to muscular, ocular and cerebral cysticercoids.

Mode of transmission: These infections are acquired:

a. Through the ingestion of infective cysticerci in undercooked beef (*T. saginata*) or park (*T. solium*)
b. Through ingestion of food, water or vegetables contaminated with eggs; and
c. Reinfection by the transport of eggs from the bowel to the stomach by retroperistalsis is considered to be rare.

Clinical Ill Health

The impact of tapeworm infection in man is difficult to quantity because in the vast majority of cases, they do not lead to clinical ill health, except occasional abdominal discomfort, anorexia and chronic indigestion.

Straying of proglottids may sporadically cause appendicitis or cholangitis. The most serious risk of *T. solium* infection is cysticercosis.

Human Cysticercosis

Human infection is caused by the ingestion of eggs of *T. solium* in contaminated water or food (hetero-infection) or regurgitated eggs from the small intestine (auto-infection). The eggs disintegrate and the infective stages leave the intestine via the hepatic portal system, and are dispersed throughout the body where they develop to form cysticerci. Cysticerci that develop in the central nervous system (neurocysticercosis), represent a serious threat to the individual and even to the community, if this conditions is prevalent. As a result of mechanical pressure, obstruction or inflammation, a variety of pathological changes are produced, leading to epilepsy intracranial hypertensive syndromes, hydrocephalus, psychiatric diseases or death.

Control Measures

The methods usually employed for control are: (a) treatment of infected persons, (b) meat inspection, (c) health education and (d) adequate sewage treatment and disposal (1, 4). Early detection and early treatment of *T. solium* cases is essential to prevent human cysticercosis. Effective drugs (e.g., praziquantel and niclosamide) are available for the treatment of these infections. Surgical removal of symptom—producing cysts.

Hydatid Disease

Hydatid disease is a group of cestode infections which are important disease in man.

Agent Factors

- *E. granulosus*
- *E. multilocularis*
- *E. oligarthus*
- *E. vogeli*

Host Factors

It is becoming increasingly evident that human behavior especially in relation to dogs and cats, uncontrolled slaughter of food animals, indiscriminate disposal of offal and carcasses, and eating habits of the people play an important part in the epidemiology of the disease. Human infection is acquired usually in childhood through contact with infected dogs. The impact of hydatidosis can be described on in terms of human suffering, cost of medical diagnosis, hospitalization and surgery, man-hours lost, as well as in terms of temporary or permanent incapacity. The retarded growth of animals, and reduction in the quality and yield of meat, milk and wool and condemnation of offal are also very great for hydatid disease in an occupational diseases of certain groups. For example, shepherds and their families in endemic area and shoe-makers.

Mode of Transmission

Human infection occurs by ingestion of the eggs of Echinococcus inadvertently with food, unwashed vegetables or water contaminated with faces from infected dogs.

Incubation Period

Variable from months to years depending upon the number and location of cysts and how rapidly they grow.

Clinical Features

In man, symptoms of hydatid disease are usually manifested several years after exposure. The cysts grow slowly from 5 to 20 years before they are diagnosed. The size of the cyst may vary from a pinhead to that of a small football. It has been estimated that more than 70% of the cysts become located in the right lobe of the liver, and the rest in lungs, brain, peritoneum, long bones and kidney. The cysts are filled with watery fluid and contain a large number of tapeworm heads. Cysts of small size are generally asymptomatic. Large cysts, however, cause pressure symptoms (e.g., jaundice in liver cysts) in vital organs they may cause severed symptoms.

Diagnosis

- **Clinical:** Based on the history of residence in and endemic area close association with dogs and the presence of a slowly growing cystic tumor
- **X-ray:** A plain X-ray permits the location for the cyst. Modern techniques of diagnosis include ultrasonography and CAT scan.
- **Serological:** Serological tests with a high degree of sensitivity and specificity have been introduced such as the indirect immunofluorescent test. ELISA is regarded as a relatively simple method with a high sensitivity superior to that of some other serological procedures.
- The intradermal (Casoni) test is still in wide use, since it is simple to perform. This test often lacks specificity.

Treatment

There is no specific treatment excepting surgical removal of cysts which is not without considerable risk in as much as the accidental penetration of one of the cysts can lead to anaphylactic shock which may prove fatal.

Prevention and control:

- Preventing dogs from gaining access to raw offal at slaughter houses and on farms, and to dead animals, this involves control of slaughter houses, proper meat inspection and destruction of infected viscera.
- *Control of dogs:* This involves elimination of stray dogs, drastic reduction of dog population, an effective dog-registration system; surveillance of dogs based on periodic stool examinations after administration of a taenifuge such as arecoline hydrobromide, followed by the isolation and treatment of infected animals with praziquantel, a single oral dose of 5 mg/kg of body weight will remove all adult worms from the dogs.
- Health education of the public particularly butchers, dog owners, animal breeders and shepherds is the basis of effective prevention.

Leishmaniasis

Leishmaniasis are group of disease caused by parasites of the genus *Leishmania* and transmitted man by phlebotomine sand fly. They are responsible for various syndrome in humans. Kala-azar or visceral leishmaniasis, cutaneous leishmaniasis, anthroponotic leishmaniasis, zoonotic leishmaniasis and post kala- azar dermal leishmaniasis.

Agent Factors

Agents: At least nineteen different leishmaniasis parasites have been associated with human infection.

Disease	*Organism*
Kala-azar or visceral leishmaniasis	*Leishmania donovani*
Cutaneous leishmaniasis	*L. tropica*
Mucocutaneous leishmaniasis	*L. braziliensis*

Host Factors

- **Age:** All Age
- **Sex:** Especially in male
- **Socioeconomic status:** Poor
- **Occupation:** Farm people, forest worker, 'mining workers', etc.

Environmental Factors

- **Attitude:** Occurs in plane area not high attitude.
- **Season:** March and April generally after rain.
- **Area:** Rural area.
- **Developmental project:** Ironically developmental project.

Mode of Transmission

- Person to person by biting of phlebotomine sand fly.
- Incubation period variable generally 1 to 4 month range is 10 days to 1 year.

Clinical Features

- **Kala-azar:** Splenomegaly hepatomegaly, fever anemia, weight loss, darkening of hand, feet, abdomen, etc. Kala-azar—Black sickness.
- **Post kala-azar dermal leishmaniasis:** It appears one to several years after cure of kala-azar. The leason consist of multiple nodular infiltration of the skin without ulceration.
- **Cutaneous leishmaniasis:** Painful ulceration in the body mistaken as leprosy expose to sandfly bite, e.g., legs arms and face.

Mucocutaneous leishmaniasis painful ulceration around the margins of mouth and nose.

Control measure:

1. Active passive case detection and treatment.
   Treatment: Pentavalent antimony compounds are the sheet anchor of the treatment. The recommended schedule is a daily injection of sodium stibogluconate 20 kg per kg of body weight for 20 days. Post Kala- azar dermal leishmaniasis will respond to this treatment well.
   Animal control: Specially dog.
2. **Sandfly control:** Application if residual insecticide such as DDT, sanitation measures, elimination of breeding places (e.g., cracks in mud or stone walls, rodent burrows) location of cattle sheds and poultry as a fare distance from house and improvement of housing and general sanitation.
3. **Personal prophylaxis:** There is no drug for personal prophylaxis. Use of individual protective measure such as avoiding sleeping on floor, using fine mesh net insect repellent for temporary protection and keeping environment clean.

SURFACE INFECTION

Trachoma

Trachoma is a chronic infectious disease caused by chlamydia trachomatis which may progress conjunctival scarring and can cause inward deviation of eye lash.

Epidemiological determinants

- *Agent factors—Chlamydia Trachomatis*
- *Reservoir of Infection—Infected persons*
- *Period of communicability—Low, it is infective as long active infection is present.*

Host factors

- **Age:** It is acquired commonly during infancy and childhood.
- **Sex:** It appears equal in males and in females.
- **Predisposing factors:** Direct sunlight, dust, smoke and irritant.

Environment: Season April and May again July and September (when number of eye seeking fly is more)

Quality of life: Poor.

Customs: Applying kajal in eye.

Mode of transmission:

- *Eye to eye transmission (by contacting with ocular discharge)*
- *Eye seeking flies*

Control of trachoma

- Assessment of the problem
- Chemotherapy (Tetracycline erythromycin or rifampicin)
- **Mass treatment:** Tetracycline ointment application to all children.
- **Surgical correction:** Individual with lid deformities can should be actively sought out.
- **Surveillance:** Ointment Surveillance.
- **Health education:** Environmental control and behavioral pattern change.
- Evaluation of activities.

DISEASE PREVENTION AND CONTROL

The term disease control describes ongoing operations aimed at reducing controlling disease control activity may be focus on primary prevention or secondary prevention or secondary prevention. Most control program combines the two. The concept of tertiary prevention is comparatively loss relevant to control effort.

Concept of Disease Control

Every disease has certain weak points susceptible to attack. The basic approach in controlling disease is to identify these weak points and break the weakest links in the chain of transmission. This requires send epidemiological knowledge of disease that is its magnitude distribution in the time place and person multifactorial causation, source of infection and dynamic of transmission.

Measure to Control Disease

Disease control involves all the measures designed to prevent or reduce as much as possible the incidence prevalence and consequence of disease of diseases. This includes community participation, political support and intrasectoral coordination.

Broadly the measures should taken based on:

- Controlling the reservoir or source of infection
- Interrupting the route of transmission
- Protecting the susceptible host (people at risk).

Controlling the Reservoir

Elimination of the reservoir may be pretty easy with the animal reservoir but it is not possible in humans in whom then get measures of reservoir control comprise early diagnosis, notification, isolation, treatment quarantine surveillance and disinfection all direct reduce the quantity of agent available for dissemination.

Early Diagnosis

- The first step in the control of a communicable disease is its rapid identification. It is the corner stone on which the edifice of disease control is build.
- Early diagnosis is needed for a treatment of patients for epidemiological investigation
- To study time place and person distribution.
- For the institution of prevention and control measures.

Notification

Once an infectious disease had been detected, it should be notified to the local health authority, whose responsibility is to put operation control measure including provision of medical care to the patient, perhaps in a hospital.

Usually the international health regulation certain prescribed diseases are notified by the national health authority to WHO.

Those diseases subject to international health regulation, Third Annotated edition 1983 are cholera plague and yellow fever diseases under surveillance by WHO—Louse-born. Typhus fever, relapsing fever, paralytic polio, malaria, viral influenza etc.

Epidemiological Investigation

An epidemiological investigation is called for whenever there is a disease outbreak the methodology for which is given elsewhere. Broadly the investigation covers the identification of source of infection and the factor influencing spread in the community. These may be include geographical situation, client condition cultural pattern and the actor of agent and environment.

Isolation

It is defined as separation for the period of communicability of infected person or animal from other to prevent direct or indirect transmission of infections agent and those infected to susceptible.

The purpose of isolation to protect the community for preventing transfer of infection from reservoir to susceptible host.

Treatment

Many communicable diseases have been famed by effective drugs. The object of treatment is to kill the infections agent when it is still in the reservoir. If before it is disseminated, treatment reduced the communicability of disease cut short the duration of illness and prevent the developed of secondary cases.

Quarantine

Quarantine has been defined as the limitation of freedom movement of such well persons or domestic animals exposed to communicable disease for a period of time not longer than the longest incubation period of disease. In such a manner as to prevent effective contact with those so exposed. Quarantine measures are also applied by health authority to a ship, an aircraft by health authority to a ship, an aircraft, a train, road vehicle other means of transport or container. To prevent the spread of disease, reservoir of disease or vector of disease.

Interruption of Transmission

A major aspect of communicable disease control relates to 'breaking the chain of transmission' or interruption of transmission. This may mean changing some components of man is environment to prevent the infective agent from a patient or carrier from entering the body of susceptible person.

Protection of the Susceptible Host

The third link initial chain of from mission is the susceptible host or people at risk. They may be protected by one or more of the following strategies.

Active Immunization

One effective was of controlling the spreads to strengthen the host defenses. Under certain circumstances this may be accomplished by active immunization, e.g., polio, TT, diphtheria and measles with booster help to help to maintain adequate level of community. Then there are offered to high-risk groups or restricted to definite geographic areas where the disease in endemic.

Passive Immunization

There are three types of preparations are available for passive immunity.

1. Normal human immunoglobulin
2. Specific human immunoglobin
3. Antiserum or Antitoxin.

Passive immunization is a short-term experiment useful only when exposure to infection has list accrued.

It has a limited value in the mass control of disease.

Combined (passive and active immunization)

In some diseases (e.g., Tetanus, diphtheria) passive immunization is often undertaken in conjunction with inactivated vaccine in products. To provide both immediate passive immunity and slowly developing active immunity.

It the infections are given at spread sites the immune response to the active agent may or may not be impaired by immunoglobulin.

Chemoprophylaxis

Chemoprophylaxis implies the protective from or prevention of disease. This may be achieved by casual prophylaxis or clinical prophylaxis.

Casual Prophylaxis

This implies the complete prevention of infection by early elimination of the invading or migrating casual agent for example. No casual prophylaxis for malaria.

Clinical Prophylaxes

Prevention of clinical symptoms. If does not necessary man elimination of infection.

Nonspecific Measure

Nonspecific measures are interrupting pathways of transmission are of general applicability. Improvements in the quality of life (better housing, water supply, sanitations nutrition education fall into this category. Nonspecific measures will also include legislative measures wherever needed. Another important nonspecific measure is community involvement in disease surveillance, disease control and other public health activities.

Eradication

Eradication means termination of all transmission of infection by extermination of the infectious agent through surveillance and containment. Eradication is an absolute process, an all or nonphenomenon restructured termination of an infection from the whole world. It implies that disease was no longer occurring in a population. To date only diseases has been eradicated that is smallpox.

The term elimination is sometime used to describe 'eradication' of disease from a large geographical region or political justification. In the state of our present the diseases which are amenable to eradication are measles, diphtheria, polio and guinea worm.

SURVEILLANCE

Surveillance must follow control measures. It has been defined as the continuous scrutiny of all aspects of occurrence and spread of diseases that are pertinent to effective control surveillance goes beyond the passive reporting of cases. It includes laboratory confirmation of presumptive diagnose, finding the source of infection, route of transmission, identification of all cases and susceptible contact and still others who are at work in order to finally prevent further spread of diseases.

Definitions of Surveillance

- Surveillance has been defined as the continuous scrutiny of the factors that determine the occurrence and distribution and other condition of ill health
- Surveillance is defined as regular collection and analysis of prevalent mortality as well as morbidity pattern and

other health related important events occurring in a given community setting
- Surveillance also connotes exercise of continuous scrutiny of health indices, nutritional status, environmental hazards, health practice and other factors that may effect health. Thus we have epidemiological surveillance nutritional surveillance demographic surveillance, serological surveillance etc.

Objectives

- To identify and monitor as early a stage as possible, any variation in the health condition of employees which may be related to working environment.
- To provide information about new and changing trends in the health status of a population, e.g., morbidity, mortality, nutritional status or their indicators and environmental hazards, health practices and other factors that may affect health.
- To provide feedback which may be expected to modify the policy and system itself and lead to redefinition of objectives.
- To provide timely warning of public health disasters so that interventions can be mobilized.
- To detect changes in trend or distribution in order to initiate investigative or control measures.
- Characteristics of surveillance.
- It is an ongoing, action-oriented process that continues uninterruptedly.
- It is a process that is distinguished by its applied value rather than by scientific accuracy. It stresses on practicality, uniformity and rapidity rather than on accuracy or completeness.
- It is a process that supports the management cycle in all its phases. It supports the planning phase with baseline information, assists the implementation phase by guiding action in result-oriented directions, and helps the evaluation phase by providing fresh data for periodic assessment.

Types of Surveillance

- **Serological surveillance:** Serological surveillance identifies patterns of current and past information, included in surveillance and systematic collection of pertinent morbidity and mortality data, the orderly consolidation of these data, special field investigations and rapid dissemination of this information to those responsible for control or prevention.
- **Sentinel surveillance:** No routine notification system can identify all cases of infection or disease. A method for identifying the missing cases and thereby supplementing the notified cases is required. This is known as sentinel surveillance. The sentinel data is extrapolated to the entire population to estimate the disease prevalence in the total population. The advantage of such a system are that the reporting biases are minimized, and feedback information to the providers is simplified. Sentinel surveillance agencies could be interested and competent physicians in selected areas to report the cases of disease in their areas.
- **Epidemiological surveillance:** It refers to the investigation of infectious diseases. The sudden growth of bacteriology and smothered the development of epidemiology is require.
- **Nutritional surveillance:** The concept of nutritional surveillance is derived from disease surveillance. Nutritional surveillance has been defined as keeping watch over nutrition, in order to make decisions that will lead to improvement in nutrition in population.
- **Demographic surveillance:** Demography is the scientific study of human population. It focuses its attention on three readily observable human phenomena, i.e.,
  - Changes in population size
  - The composition of the population
  - The distribution of population in space.
  - It deals with five demographic process namely fertility, mortality, marriage, migration and social mobility. These five processes are continuously at work within a population determining size, composition and distribution. The main source of demographic statistics in India are population census.
  - Surveillance may comprise.
  - Individual surveillance: This is surveillance of infected persons until they are no longer of significant risk to other individuals.
  - Local population surveillance, e.g., surveillance of malaria.
  - National population surveillance, e.g., surveillance of smallpox after the disease has been eradicated.
  - International surveillance: At the international level, the WHO maintains surveillance of important diseases, e.g., influenza, malaria, palio, etc., and gives timely warning to all national governments.
  - Surveillance cycle.

A surveillance system operates as a revolving cycle that comprises three phases:
- Phase I–collection of data
- Phase II–analysis of data
- Phase III–dissemination of data.
- Attributes of sound surveillance system
- Validity
- Flexibility
- Acceptability
- Simplicity
- Predictability
- Representativeness
- Differences (surveillances and monitoring).

Surveillance:

- Continuous scrutiny of the factors that determine the occurrence and distribution of a disease and other conditions of ill health.
- Surveillance implies only observation and reporting of findings without intervention.

Monitoring:

- Often used interchangeably with surveillance. But monitoring refers to ongoing measurement of health services or a health program with a view to evaluate the particular program/service or intervention with the constant adjustment of performance in relation to the results.
- Monitoring is the observation of change after there has been an intervention of some sort.

National Surveillance Program

Ministry of health and family welfare has launched the national surveillance program for communicable diseases for detection of early warning signals of outbreaks and rapid response for prevention and control of these outbreaks and diseases. During outbreak of plague—1994, malaria—1995 and dengue hemorrhagic fever 1996 highlighted the urgency for strengthening disease surveillance system are recognized and appropriate follow-up action initiated. In 1997 a model district surveillance plan was drafted. Subsequently in 1998 a concept plan was developed by the National Apical Advisory Committee under Secretary (Health).

Under this program, the surveillance system is strengthened through training of medical and paramedical personnel dessemination of technical information and guidelines, upgradation of laboratories modernization of communication and data processing systems. The program includes to promote community participation in the prevention and control of outbreaks.

Presently the program is in operation in 80 districts of 28 states.

Multidisciplinary rapid response teams (RRTS) have been constituted a state and district levels under the program. These terms have been provided training in surveillance, prevention and control of outbreaks.

CHAPTER 12

Community Mental Health Nursing

INTRODUCTION

The difference between a healthy person and one who is mentally ill is the fact that the healthy one has all the mental illness and the mentally ill person has only one.

—**Robert Musil**

Mental health is an important constituent of optimum health. Mental health is essential for a healthy and successful life. Mental and physical health is interrelated, and that is the reason behind the popularity of saying 'healthy mind in healthy body'.

Burden of mental disorders had risen over last few decades. Mental health is a state of well-being in which the individual realizes his or her own abilities, can cope with the normal stresses of life, can work productively and is able to make a contribution to his or her community. WHO estimated that globally over 450 million people suffer from mental disorders. Currently mental and behavioral disorders account for about 12% of the global burden of diseases. This is likely to increase to 15% by 2020. Major proportions of mental disorders come from low and middle income countries.

Definition

The application of knowledge of psychiatric nursing in preventing, promoting and maintaining mental health of people to help in early diagnosis and care and to rehabilitate the clients after mental illness. —**B. Kapoor**

The process of involving raising the level of mental health among people in a community and reducing the number of cases suffering with mental illness. —**K. Lalitha, 2005**

Concept

The community mental health services were focused to render the health care services in familiar home environment, where the client will be at ease; stress related to hospital environment can be avoided. The client will develop adaptive coping strategies very easily to overcome the stressors related to mental illness.

The services will be provided to total population in a geographical area rather than specific client alone. Following services are provided in consultation with community mental health nurse:

- Education
- Crisis intervention
- Family therapy
- Group therapy
- Psychotherapy
- Interaction skill training
- Promotive, preventive and rehabilitative services
- Follow-up services.

MAGNITUDE OF MENTAL HEALTH PROBLEMS

- Between 1990 and 2019, the global number of disability-adjusted life years (DALYs) due to mental disorders increased from 80.8 million [95% uncertainty interval (UI) 59.5–105.9] to 125.3 million (93.0–163.2).
- The proportion of global DALYs attributed to mental disorders increased from 3.1% (95% UI 2.4–3.9) to 4.9% (3.9–6.1).
- Years lived with disability (YLDs) contributed to most of the mental disorder burden, with 125.3 million YLDs [95% UI 93.0–163.2; 14.6% (12.2–16.8) of global YLDs] in 2019 attributable to mental disorders.
- Globally, the age-standardized DALY rate for mental disorders was 1426.5 (95% UI 1056.4–1869.5) per 1,00,000 population among males and 1703.3 (1261.5–2237.8) per 100,000 population among females.
- A 2017 study estimated that globally 792 million people lived with a mental health disorder of some kind, translating to 10.7% of the global population.
- The most prevalent were anxiety (284 million people, 3.8% of the population) and depression (264 million people, 3.4% of the population).
- Data published in 2015 estimated that mental disorders are attributable to 14.3% of deaths worldwide, or approximately 8 million deaths each year. According to the World Health Organization, depression can lead to suicide, which contributes to over 700,000 deaths every year. Suicide is the fourth leading cause of death in 15–29-year-olds.
- Despite there being effective treatments for mental health disorders, over 75% of people in low- and middle-income countries receive no treatment for them.

India Statistics

In 2017, 197.3 million (95% UI 178.4–216.4) people had mental disorders in India, including 45.7 million (42.4–49.8) with depressive disorders and 44.9 million (41.2–48.9) with anxiety disorders. The contribution of mental disorders to the total DALYs in India increased from 2.5% (2.0–3.1) in 1990 to 4.7% (3.7–5.6) in 2017.

In 2017, depressive disorders contributed the most to the total mental disorders DALYs 33.8%, followed by anxiety disorders 19.0%, idiopathic developmental intellectual disability 10.8%, schizophrenia 9.8%, bipolar disorder 6.9%, conduct disorder 5.9%, autism spectrum disorders 3.2%, and attention-deficit hyperactivity disorder 0.3%, other mental disorders comprised 8.0% of DALYs.

Global burden of diseases (GBD) 2019 showed that mental disorders remained among the top ten leading causes of burden worldwide, with no evidence of global reduction in the burden since 1990. The estimated years of life lost (YLLs) for mental disorders were extremely low and do not reflect premature mortality in individuals with mental disorders.

Mental illness is definitely a burden to India, there remains to be a massive treatment gap. The Economic Time 20 March, 2022 depicted that with 9000 psychiatrists in total in combination with 700 psychiatrists graduating every year, it works out to be 0.75 psychiatrists per 100,000 people in India. This is far below the recommended level of at least 3 psychiatrists per 100,000 people. In terms of availability of beds, as little as 56,600 public psychiatric beds exist for a 130 crore population. Moreover, not only that the vast majority of trained psychiatrists and psychologists are in metros and big cities, where treatment costs are prohibitively high. Approximately 30,000 psychiatric beds and only 43 mental health hospitals are available in India. The vast treatment gap is not about the numbers only; the conditions of existing infrastructure are extremely poor.

The government plans to improve its mental health services network, especially amid the pandemic, Finance Minister Nirmala Sitharaman said while presenting the Union Budget for 2022-23 on Tuesday, February 1. She announced an open platform for the National Digital Health Ecosystem, which will consist of digital registries of health providers and health facilities, unique health identity, consent framework and universal access to health facilities.

Scope of Community Mental Health Nursing

The mental illness will be ranging from severe disabling to less incapacitating and long term in nature. Community mental health nurse will apply systemic, scientific knowledge to adopt nursing process in rendering care to the mentally ill. Varied community facilities are available to provide mental health care for total population.

- **Day care center:** The concept of day care center was introduced by DE Cameren in 1946 where the client will receive treatment in day time only. Patient will learn discipline and routine life.
- **Quarter way home:** Located within the hospital campus, client will carry out their activity. There is no appointment of regular hospital staff.
- **Half way home:** Complete hospitalization is not required but patient are not allowed to perform their activity independently and supervision is required. Before discharge clients are put in half way home. Regular medical services are provided.
- **Group home:** 15–20 recovered clients with similar problem are placed in a home. That may be in hospital or in community setting where moral, emotional or social support are provided to each other.
- **Foster home:** Client will get home like environment. To get home like care social agencies will appoint families to take care of the clients.
- **Sheltered workshop:** To fulfil the individual's vocational goal work oriented vocational rehabilitation are provided but in a controlled environment.
- **Mental health emergency care:** Mental health emergency care can be provided through hotline, emergency clinic or home visits.
- **Self-help group:** The members of self help group will help the individual as well as family member.
- **Suicide prevention center:** Some voluntary agencies are working for prevention of suicide by identifying risky population and provide support, e.g., helping hand in Bangalore, Sahara in Mumbai, etc.

MENTAL HEALTH CARE SERVICES IN INDIA

Trends British Era

Indian mental health is a child born to British parents and bred in Indian culture.

- The Indian Lunacy Act (1912) was based on the British legislation then in force. The history of Indian psychiatry runs parallel to British psychiatry and the basic structure remains the same even to this day.
- **Creation of Asylums:** To keep the dangerous lunatics and severely disturbed cases, or when relatives were unable to manage them, owing to poverty or other constraints.
- European Mental Hospital, later the Hospital for Mental Diseases and the Central Institute of Psychiatry, Ranchi was meant almost entirely for European patients and was staffed by British Army doctors.
- The treatment of lunatics was in the hands of church, which even accorded death as the severest punishment for insanity and faith healers also treated mentally sick.
- In 1943, Dr. Fraser had written an article in the British Medical Journal on ganja psychosis. The UK psychiatrists studied the cultural taboos in India about intoxicating substances and showed great interest in this addiction.
- The birth of the Royal Medico Psychological Association, the precursor of the Royal College of Psychiatrists in the 1960s, marks the beginning of modern scientific psychiatry in England and India.
- The first Indian Psychiatrist to be recognized by the Royal College of Psychiatrists is Professor Narendra Wig.

Mental Health Care in Independent India

- Indian mental health professionals continued to care the mentally sick in asylums and custodial in its outlook, which imposed limits on the number of patients who could receive services.
- Nonspecific psychotherapy and Western models of psychoanalysis were practiced.
- Nursing care for patients was provided by general nurses.
- The research literature focused primarily on in-depth psychological understanding of mental disorders, focusing primarily on the individual.

Mental Health Care in Evolution India

- Enhancing the capacity of the mental health infrastructure to serve a greater number of service seekers.
- Improving the quality of services in custodial institutions and developing innovative approaches in noncustodial settings.
- **Increased the number of mental institutions:** At the time of independence, India had about 30 institutions for the mentally ill, with 10 of them having been built prior to the 20th century.
- The concept of a day hospital is another important innovation in the 1960s. Integrating mental health with general health—1933 the 1st General Hospital Psychiatric Unit (GHPU).
- GHPU began its collaboration with departments of neurology and were often termed as neuropsychiatric clinics.
- In the 20 years that followed independence, 90 GHPU came into existence.
- It was a struggle to get a few beds allotted to psychiatric patients in the general medical wards, psychiatric patients were shifted to OPD.
- GHPUs became more accessible than the custodial institutions. Comprehensive medical care to psychiatric patients became easily available.
- In 1970s, slow and steady reduction of beds in custodial institution, growth in GHPUs and Out-patient services were seen.
- Occupational therapy and recreational facilities were introduced.
- Between 1960–1972, the research focus was on the magnitude and nature of mental health problems in the community.
- Family intervention concept was introduced by Dr. Vidya Sagar at the Amritsar Mental Hospital. At the same time Mental Health Centres, Christian Medical College (CMC) Vellore also introduced family involvement in patient care. It was practiced at NIMHANS in the 1960s and culminated in the opening of the family ward.

Mental Healthcare Services as on Today

- The development of disabilities as a consequence of social isolation and institutional care in remote asylums led to the de-institutionalization movement.
- The focus shifted to community-based care, which became the basis of the National Mental Health Program (NMHP) that was launched in India in 1982.
- At present District Mental Health Program (DMHP) is under implementation in 25 districts, spread across 20 states/Union Territories (UTs).
- Hon'ble Supreme Court orders dated 15 October, 2002 empowered the central government to obtain necessary information from the states to project comprehensive mental health services in the country.
- The Mental Health Act, 1987 and the State Mental Health Rules 1990, appear to have made little impact was identified.
- The Hon'ble Supreme Court in CWP NO. 334 of 2001 forced the state governments to enforce licensing and regulatory supervisions relating to private psychiatric clinics and nursing homes.
- Custodial atmosphere in most mental hospitals has to be changed.
- Mapping of mental health services.
- Mental health resources were examined from all states/UTs between May and July 2002. The findings and suggestions are as follows:
  - Severe manpower shortages in all categories of mental health personnel but are more among clinical psychologists, psychiatric social workers and psychiatric nurses.
  - Uneven distribution of these scarce resources.
- Proposed mental health plan
  - To relocate long-stay patients into the community.
  - Refractory patients (who can not be placed back into their families) may be admitted as paid patients in district/subdivisional hospital/Federal Government hospitals near their hometown and maintenance therapy can be continued by physician.
  - Legal steps under the provisions of the MHA, Sections 79 and 80, may be taken to recover the cost of maintenance.
  - With community-based mental healthcare facilities in place through the DMHPs, early identification and treatment of those suffering from mental disorders.
- Restrategized NMHP (2003) proposes to implement the DMHP in 200 districts across the country, along with strengthening the departments of psychiatry in an equal number of medical colleges and modernization of 37 government mental hospitals.
- It is suggested to start crisis Intervention Units in at least one medical college in each state and the unit will consist of one psychiatrist, one psychiatric social worker, one psychiatric nurse and one psychiatric nursing orderly.
- The National Mental Health Policy (NMHP-2001) and The National Health Policy-2002 (NHP-2002) covers mental health. The observations are (NMHP2001).
  - DMHP covers only 25 out of 593 districts across India.
  - Uneven distribution of psychiatric services.
  - Most of the mental hospitals are physically dilapidated, still gives custodial rather than therapeutic care.

  - Many psychiatric patients are in the hospital for more than 5 year.
- The observations are (NMHP 2001):
  - Teaching of psychiatry at the undergraduate level remains inadequate
  - The average doctors are ill-equipped to deal with mental illness.
  - Postgraduate training in medicine and allied specialties has no psychiatric component taught, although 40% of population attending general hospital OPD suffers from emotional rather than physical problems.
  - Worthwhile research, especially in the field of community psychiatry is limited to a few institutions such as NIMHANS, AIIMS, etc.

  Vision 2020 (NMHP) calls for an urgent, time-bound remedial action plan which would ensure:
  - Accessibility of at least basic psychiatric facilities within the community to as large a section of the population as possible in all parts of the country.
  - Affordability of the services with regard to initial capital cost as well as recurring expenditure (including that on essential drugs) to accord with our limited resources and low-income level of the consumer population.
  - Adaptability to the widely varying geographical, socio-cultural and economic mosaic of our vast country.
  - Acceptability of mental health care by the target population in the context of low levels of literacy, ignorance, superstition, economic backwardness and lack of empowerment of women, adolescents and children.
  - Assessment of performance at the ground level through continuous monitoring.

The government plans to improve its mental health services network, especially amid the pandemic, Finance Minister Nirmala Sitharaman said while presenting the Union Budget for 2022-23 on Tuesday, February 1. She announced an open platform for the National Digital Health Ecosystem, which will consist of digital registries of health providers and health facilities, unique health identity, consent framework and universal access to health facilities.

HISTORY OF PSYCHIATRIC NURSING

Emergence of Discipline of Psychiatric Nursing

- **1860's:** Florence Nightingale found school at Saint Thomas Hospital in London.
- **1882:** The first psychiatric nurse was Linda Richards, an American lady, started school for psychiatric nurses at the McLean Psychiatric Asylum in Waverly, Massachusetts.
- **1890's:** Psychiatric nursing practices is primarily custodial, mechanistic and directed by psychiatrists.
- **1920's:**
  - Nursing mental disease, the first psychiatric nursing test, was written by Harriet Bailey (standard textbook for 20 years)
  - Most textbooks were written by psychiatrists, only few pages address psychiatric nurses.

Movement of Psychiatric Nursing into the Mainstream of Nursing

- **1930's:** National League for Nursing Education recommends that psychiatric nursing context and clinical experience be part of the curriculum in all basic nursing programme.
- **1940's:** New medical surgical procedures—Armstrong and Sheila Rouslin wrote (insulin shock. therapy/ECT) first textbook on group therapy promote the role of psychiatric technique in nursing practice and mentioned as nurses are participants in psychiatric treatment.
- **1946:** Fully developed psychiatric course was started at John Hopkins Hospital USA.
- **1947:** Nursing profession identified specific functions of a psychiatric nurse.
- **1948:** Institute of Mental Health in America started eight postgraduate programme.
- **1950:** Affiliation was granted to psychiatric nursing.

Confirmation of Psychiatric Nursing as a Speciality

- **1950's:** Hildegard Peplau emphasized psychodynamic concepts and counseling techniques; she described the phases of interpersonal relationship.
  - Gwen Tuder demonstrated nursing interventions with a sociopsychiatric base.
  - National League for Nursing introduces the concept of psychiatric nurse specialist, first NIMH grants to integrate mental health concepts into nursing curriculum.

Confirmation of Specialist Role

- **1960's:** Psychological therapies further enlarged the role by the nurse as a counselor and psychotherapist.
  - Psychiatric nursing was made compulsory.
  - The Community Mental Health Centers Act pushes trends in psychiatric nursing toward expanded and specialised roles.
- **1963:** Community Mental Health Act passed in US.
- **1970:** The first master's level certificate programs for advanced psychiatric nursing practice was developed.
- **1973:** Standards of nursing practice established by the ANA.

Period of Decline and Retrenchment

1980's: ANA council of specialists in psychiatric and mental health nursing develop a classification system for psychiatric nursing diagnosis.

- Psychiatric nursing leaders recommend incorporating new psychobiologic knowledge into clinical practice.

The Decade of the Brain

1990's: ANA psychiatric mental health nursing psychopharmacology project published, intended to increase the knowledge.

- Psychiatric nursing leaders urge nurses to use the challenging circumstances.

MENTAL HEALTH NURSING IN INDIA

- **1787:** Lunatic asylum in Kolkata was established.
- **1794:** Lunatic asylum in Madras was established
- **1858:** Bombay asylum was established
- **1912:** Indian Lunacy Act.
- **1917-50:** Psychiatric nursing was carried out by army nurses at the army hospitals.
- **1920:** The term asylum was replaced by "Mental hospital"
- **1925:** The Indian mental hospital was built up in Ranchi.
- **1937:** Madras government organized 3 months psychiatric nursing course at the Mental hospital Madras.
- **1946:** Health survey committee's report recommended preparation of nursing personnel in psychiatric nursing also.
- **1947:**
  - The postgraduate diploma course in Ranchi was planned.
  - The nursing profession started to identify the specific functions of psychiatric nurse.
- **1950:** The Indian Nursing Council included 5 to 8 hours psychiatry in the syllabus (not compulsory)
- **1954:** All India Institute of Mental Health at Bangalore was formed. (Later known as NIMHANS)
- **1956:** One year postgraduate course in psychiatric nursing was started at NIMHANS (Bengaluru).
- **1960:** First world wide Mental Health year was celebrated.
- **1961:** ICN included psychiatric nursing in the basic nursing curriculum.
- **1962:** Mysore Government started a nine month course in psychiatric nursing for male nurses in lieu of midwifery which was reduced to 6 months duration from 1976.
- **1964:** Mudaliar committee recommended psychiatric nurses.
- **1965:** INC included psychiatric nursing as a compulsory course
- **1967:** The TNAI formed a separate committee for psychiatric nursing to improve the perception of psychiatric nursing
- **1975:** Psychiatric nursing was offered as elective subject in MSc nursing.
- **1976:** First postgraduate study in psychiatry at masters level offered by college of nursing, New Delhi.
- **1977-78:** 15 hours of theory in psychiatric nursing was added to the syllabus.
- **1978:** Alma-Ata declaration of Health for All by 2000 AD brought a major challenge to Indian Mental Health professional.
- **1980:** Practical, theory and oral examination were made a requirement of GNM at RAK College of nursing New Delhi (30–35 hours of theory in Psychiatric nursing)
- **1980:** Psychiatric nursing was offered as elective subject in Diploma in nursing.
- **1981:** Community psychiatric model was set up.
- **1982:** National mental Health programme was started.
- **1983:** Diploma in Psychiatric nursing was started.
- **1986:** Recent revision of General nursing and midwifery syllabus included in depth the contents of Psychiatric Nursing.
- **1987:** Mental Health Act came into force.
- **1990:** Government of India formed an 'Action Group' at Delhi to pool the opinion of Mental Health experts about National Mental Health program.
- **1991:** The Indian Society of Psychiatric Nurse (ISPN) was formed at NIMHANS (Bengaluru).
- **2004:** INC revised the GNM syllabus with 70 hours of theory, 216 hours practical and 2 weeks of internship. School level practical exam in mental health nursing was also incorporated.
- **2004:** Post BSc (N) Syllabus also was revised by INC with 60 hours of theory, 240 hours of practical with university practical exam in mental health nursing
- **2004:** INC revised the BSc (N) syllabus with 90 hours of theory, 270 hours of practical and internship of 2 weeks with university practical exam in mental health nursing
- **2005:** The National consortium for PhD in nursing was started by INC in collaboration with WHO and RGUHS, Karnataka. It calls for the nurses to register PhD in nursing in five disciplines including psychiatric nursing.
- **2006:** MSc (N) syllabus was revised by INC with 150 hours of theory and 650 hours practical in first year, 150 hours of theory and 950 hours of practical in second year.
- **2013:** National Mental Health Care Bill was launched.

MODELS OF COMMUNITY-BASED PSYCHIATRIC CARE

The different models of community-based psychiatric care vary according to the target population and range of services offered. Ideally a model should provide a comprehensive system of care coordinating needed service delivery.

Patient-centered Healthcare Homes

It also known as patient-centered medical home. It is not a place but a model of primary care that delivers the care functions of primary health care.

The home is designed to expand available services to include focus on the health, housing, social and personal supports needed to achieve and maintain health for whole person, not just a patient.

These health care homes needed to work close with their community partners, e.g., social service agencies, school, child care centres, family resource centres and public health departments.

The core of home is team-based care that provides integrated care management and supports individuals in their health goal. The elements are:

- Accountability
- Access to care
- Comprehensive (whole person) care
- Continuity
- Coordination and integration
- Person and family-centered care.

Collaborative Care and Care Management

A collaborative care is a structured approach to care based on principle of chronic disease management. It has two key elements.

1. *Systematic care management:* It is most often done by a nurse to facilitate case identification, coordination of a treatment plan, patient education, close follow-up and monitoring progress. It can be done at primary care centres or by telephone.
   - **Consultation:** It occurs among primary care providers, care manager and a mental health specialist. It can be done at varying level of intensity.
2. *Care management:* It is core element of patient centred health care homes and of new approaches designed to improve chronic illness care. It is team-based care that helps individual in their self-management goals.
   - It coordinates care to reduce fragmentation and unnecessary use of services and prevent avoidable conditions and promote independence and self care.
   - Care management includes counseling, pharmacy review, utilization management and specific disease management program.

Function of Care Manager

- Develop and maintain rapport with patient and provider.
- Educate patient and family.
- Monitor symptoms and communicate findings to provider.
- Develop and maintain self-care action plan.
- Maximize adherence to treatment plan.

Case Management Model

It involves linking the service system to the consumer and coordinating the service components, so that the consumer can achieve successful community living. The component of case management includes:

- Patient identification and out reach
- Mental health treatment
- Crisis response services
- Health and dental care
- Housing
- Income support and entitlement
- Peer support
- Family and community support
- Rehabilitation services
- Protection and advocacy.

Focus of Case Management

- Problem-solving to provide continuity of services.
- Overcome problems of rigid systems, fragmented services, poor use of resources and problem of inaccessibility.

Activities of Case Management

- Identification and outreach
- Assessment
- Service planning
- Linkage with needed services
- Monitoring service delivery
- Advocacy.

NATIONAL MENTAL HEALTH PROGRAM

Mental Health Care in Independent India

At the time of independence, the existing mental health infrastructure and specialist manpower was very scanty. The situation can be understood by comparing the 10,000 psychiatric beds in India in 1947 for a population of over 300 million, with that of UK, with one tenth the population of India having over 150,000 psychiatric beds. The first two decades of independent India, were devoted to doubling the mental hospital beds followed by setting up of general hospital psychiatric beds (Wig, 1978). However, the major breakthrough occurred in 1975, when a new initiative to integrate mental health with general health services, also referred to as community psychiatry initiative, was identified as the approach to develop mental health services. Community psychiatry in India is nearly four decades old. Starting as isolated extension psychiatric clinics in primary health clinics, (Srinivasa Murthy, 2000) today the integration of mental health care in general services covers over 127 districts (about 20% population of the country). The National Mental Health Programme (NMHP) was formulated in 1982 to develop a national level initiative for mental health care. During the last 25 years, there are a large number of other community initiatives to address a wide variety of mental health needs of the community like homeless mentally ill, day care centres, half-way homes, long stay homes, rehabilitation facilities, suicide prevention, care of the elderly, substance use persons, and disaster mental health care.

Background to NMHP

The need for setting up of district psychiatric clinics was recognized in the 1960's as part of the Mudaliar Committee Report (Mudaliar, 1962). A few centres did come up following this report. However, the important national level professional initiative is the discussions of the Indian Psychiatric Society at Madurai in the early 1970 are where the need to integrate mental health care with general health care was voiced. Simultaneously, in 1975, the Expert Committee on Mental health of the World Health Organisation published the important document' Organisation of mental health services in developing countries' (WHO, 1975). These professional ideas were put to practical test both at Bengaluru and Chandigarh centres, by taking up pilot programmes to integrate mental health with general health services during the 1975-1981 periods. (Wig et al., 1981, Kapur et al., 1981).

Implementation of NMHP

In the 1980's, the Government of India felt the necessity of evolving a plan of action aimed at the mental health component of the National Health Programe. For this, an expert group was formed in 1980, who met a number of times and discussed the issue with many important people concerned with mental health in India as well as with the Director, Division of Mental Health, WHO, Geneva. Finally, in February 1981, a small drafting committee met in Lucknow and prepared the first draft of the NMHP. This was presented at a workshop of experts (over 60 professionals) on mental health, drawn from all over India at New Delhi on 20–21 July 1981. Following the discussion, the draft was substantially revised and a new one was presented at the second workshop on 2 August 1982 to a group of experts from not only the psychiatry and medical stream but also education, administration, law and social welfare. The final draft was submitted to the Central Council of Health, India's highest health policy-making body at its meeting held on 18–20 August 1982, for its adoption as the NMHP for India (DGHS, 1982).

Aims

- Prevention and treatment of mental and neurological disorder and their associated disabilities.
- Use of mental health technologies to improve general health service.
- Application of mental health principles in the total national development to improve quality of life.

Objectives

- To ensure the availability and accessibility of minimum mental health care for all in the foreseeable future, particularly to the most vulnerable and underprivileged section of the society.
- To encourage application of mental health knowledge, general health care and in social development.
- To promote community participation in the mental health service development and to stimulate efforts towards self help in the community.

Strategies

- Integration of mental health with primary health care through the national mental health programme
- Provision of tertiary care institution for treatment of mental disorders
- Eradication of stigmatization of mentally ill patients and protecting their right through regulatory institution like the central and state mental health authority.

Approaches

- Integration of mental health care services with the existing general health services.
- To utilize the existing infrastructure of health services and also to deliver the minimum mental health care services.
- To provide appropriate task-oriented training to the existing health staff.
- Equitable and balanced distribution of resources.
- Linkage with community development.

A national advisory group of mental health was formed under the chairmanship of secretary, Ministry of health and family welfare for the effective implementation of the national mental health program.

THE SERVICE COMPONENT OF NMHP

The service component comprised of:

- **Village and subcenter level:** Multipurpose workers (MPW) and health supervisors (HS) under the supervision of Medical officers (MO) to be trained for:
  - The management of psychiatric emergencies
  - Administration and supervision of maintenance treatment for chronic psychiatric disorders
  - Diagnosis and management of grand mal epilepsy
  - Liaison with local school teachers and parents regarding mental retardation and behavior problems in children
  - Counseling in problems related to alcohol and drug abuse
- **Primary health centers (PHC):** MO aided by HS to be trained for:
  - Supervision of MPW's performance
  - Elementary diagnosis
  - Treatment of functional psychosis
  - Treatment of uncomplicated cases of psychiatric disorders associated with physical diseases
  - Management of uncomplicated psychosocial problems
  - Epidemiological surveillance of mental morbidity
- **District hospital:** The district hospital must have 30–50 psychiatric beds. There should be at least 1 psychiatrist attached to every district hospital. The psychiatrist is entrusted with the responsibility of clinical care of patients and training and supervision of nonspecialist health workers.
- **Teaching psychiatric unit and mental hospital:** Their main role would be:
  - Providing help for difficult cases
  - Teaching
  - Specialized facilities such as occupational therapy units, psychotherapy, counseling and behavior therapy.

Rehabilitation

The subcomponents of rehabilitation include maintenance treatment of epileptics and psychotics at the community levels and development of rehabilitation centers at both the district level and the higher referral centers.

Prevention

This component was community-based, with the initial focus on the prevention and control of alcohol-related problems and later on other issues like addictions, juvenile delinquency and suicides.

Features of the NMHP

- Decentralized and phased training courses were conducted for all the health personnel of the district so

that they would deliver basic mental healthcare services to the needy.
- The services covered a population of 1.5 million distributed in seven talukas.
- A program officer for mental health was appointed in the district health and family welfare office, who organized a mental health clinic in the premises and also toured the entire district to monitor the program.

A simple recording and reporting system was developed. The district health officer monitored the progress every month during the monthly review meetings along with other health programs.

Five essential drugs were made available for distribution in all the health centres in the district.

During the first three years of the project (1985-88), 1200 patients with psychosis, 3,525 patients with epilepsy, 750 patients with neurosis and 380 mentally retarded (learning disabled) persons were registered. Forty-two percent of patients with psychosis and 53% of those with epilepsy took treatment regularly and showed improvement. Seventy percent of patients came from places within a five-kilometer range of the health center. Thus, distance and availability of free care facilities appear to be important factors in good compliance.

Good performers in the mental health care program of the system were good in all other health programs. Poor performers appeared to have had many personal and psychosocial problems which came in the way of their performance.

As the mental health services became popular, patients reached the centres within a few days/weeks of the onset of the illness and took a short and straight path instead of taking a long path by visiting various faith healers and other agencies.

The district program gave professionals an idea as to how to organize services in a cost-effective manner and maintain a reasonable quality.

The main strength of NMHP document drafted in 1982 was that it envisaged the integration of mental healthcare with the general primary healthcare.

On the other hand there was some inherent weaknesses of this model of care. These were:

The program emphasized more on curative components rather than the preventive and promotive components:
- Role of support of families in the treatment of the patient was not given due importance;
- Short-term goals were given priority over the long-term planning;
- The administrative structure of the programme was not clearly outlined;
- No estimates of budgetary support were made.

After reviewing the progress made during 1982-88, it was concluded that although the developments in this area raised the hopes for beginning a big program in the country, the financial constraints somehow restricted it. In the Ninth five-year plan ₹ 28 crores were allocated to NMHP. In-depth analysis and consultation with the stakeholders led to a major change in NMHP and was launched with certain changes in 2003.

NMHP Tenth five-year plan was launched, with a plan to extend the DMHP to 100 districts. Tenth plan allocated ₹139 crores and emphasized:
- The need to broaden the scope of existing curriculum for undergraduate training in psychiatry and to give more exposure to psychiatry in undergraduate years and internship.
- Need for DMHP to be spread to the entire country in a more effective manner.
- Streamlining/modernizing mental hospitals to overcome their custodial role.
- Strengthening the Central and State mental health authorities with a permanent secretariat.

Appointment of MO at State Headquarters

During the Eleventh five-year plan in NMHP the focus was on establishing centers of excellence in mental health, increasing intake capacity and starting postgraduate courses in psychiatry, modernization of mental hospitals and upgradation of medical college psychiatry departments, focus on nongovernment organizations (NGOs) and public sector partnerships, media campaign to address stigma, a focus on research and several other measures.

The emphasis of NMHP-1982 was primarily on the rural sector. It is being realized that the urban mental health needs should also be addressed under the ambit of NMHP.

The NMHP was restrategied in the year 2003 (10th five year plan) with the following components:
- Extension of DMHP in to 100 districts
- Upgradation of psychiatric wing of medical college/Govt. Hospitals
- Modernization of state mental hospital
- IEC
- Monitoring and evaluation.

Agencies like World Bank and WHO contacted to support various components of the programme. Funds are provided by Govt. of India to the state Govt. and the nodal institutes to meet the expenditure on staff, equipment, medicine, vehicle, stationery, contingency, training, etc. for initial 5 years and thereafter they should manage themselves.
- It provides creation of state mental health authority to carry out the said function.
- The Central Mental Health Authority oversees the implementation of Mental Health Act, 1986.
- The National Human Right Commission also monitors the conditions in the mental hospitals along with the government of India and the states are currently acting on the recommendation of the joint studies conducted to ensure quality in delivering mental care.

Thrust Areas of 10th Five Year Plan

- DMHP is an enlarged and more effective forum covering the entire country.
- Streamlining and modernization of mental hospitals in order to modify their preset custodial role.

- Upgrading department of psychiatry in medical colleges and enhancing the psychiatric content of medical curriculum at the UG and PG level.
- Strengthening the state and central mental health authorities with a permanent secretariat.
- Research and training in the field of community mental health, substance abuse and child psychiatry clinic.

In the 11th Five Year Plan, the NMHP has the following components/schemes:
- District Mental Health Program (DMHP)
- Modernization of state-run mental hospitals
- Upgradation of psychiatric wings of medical colleges/ general hospitals
- Manpower development scheme
- IEC activities
- Training and research
- Monitoring and evaluation.

District Mental Health Program (DMHP)

The main objective of DMHP is to provide community mental health services and integration of mental health with general health services through decentralization of treatment from specialized mental hospital-based care to primary health care services. On the basis of 'Bellary model' District Mental Health Program was launched in 1996 in 4 districts under NMHP and was expanded to 27 districts of the country by the end of 9th Five year plan period. Presently, the DMHP is being implemented in 123 districts of the country.

Objectives

- To provide sustainable basic mental health services to the community and to integrate these services with other health services
- Early detection and treatment of patients within the community itself
- To see that patients and their relatives do not have to travel long distances to go to hospitals or nursing homes in the cities
- To take pressure off the mental hospitals
- To reduce the stigma attached towards mental illness through change of attitude and public education
- To treat and rehabilitate mental patients discharged from the mental hospitals within the community.

The DMHP envisages a community-based approach to the problem, which includes:
- Training of mental health team at identified nodal institutions.
- Increase awareness and reduce stigma related to mental health problems.
- Provide service for early detection and treatment of mental illness in the community (OPD/Indoor and follow-up).
- Provide valuable data and experience at the level of community at the state and center for future planning and improvement in service and research.

Based on the evaluation conducted by an independent agency in 2008 and feedback received from a series of consultations, it was decided by the Government of India that DMHP should be revised and consolidated assistance on new pattern with added components of life skills education and counseling in schools, college counseling services, workplace stress management and suicide prevention services should be provided. These components are in addition to the existing components of clinical services, training of general health care functionaries, and IEC activities in DMHP. The team of workers at the district under the program consists of a psychiatrist, a clinical psychologist, a psychiatric social worker, a psychiatry/ community nurse, a program manager, a program/case registry assistant and a record keeper.

Modernization of State-run Mental Hospitals

Most of the state-run mental hospitals in the country were established long ago and are now in dilapidated state. The infrastructure of these hospitals stands on custodial care pattern. The assistance under this scheme is provided for modernization of state-run mental hospitals from custodial care to comprehensive management. As per the existing scheme to modernize the existing state-run mental hospitals, a one-time grant with a ceiling of ₹ 3.00 crores per hospital is provided. The grant covers activities, such as construction/repair of existing building(s), purchase of cots and equipment, provision of infrastructure, such as water tanks and toilet facilities, etc. It does not cover recurring expenses towards running the mental hospitals and cost towards drugs and consumables. This is the grant for modernization of the mental hospitals only and any increase in the number of beds in the hospital is not permitted.

Upgradation of Psychiatric Wings of Medical Colleges/General Hospitals

Every medical college should ideally have a Department of Psychiatry with minimum of three faculty members and inpatient facilities of about 30 beds as per the norms laid down by the Medical Council of India. Out of the existing medical colleges in the country, approximately 1/3rd of them do not have adequate psychiatric services. This is a scheme for strengthening of the psychiatric wings of government medical colleges/hospitals which provides for a one-time grant of ₹50 lakhs for upgradation of infrastructure and equipment as per the existing norms. The aim of the scheme is to strengthen the training facilities for undergraduates and postgraduates at psychiatry wings of government medical colleges/hospitals. The grant covers construction of new wards, repair of existing wards, procurement of items, like cots, tables and equipment for psychiatric use, such as modified ECTs.

Manpower Development Scheme

In order to improve the training infrastructure in mental health, Government of India has approved the Manpower

Development Components of NMHP for XI Five Year Plan. It has two schemes which are as follows:

Centers of Excellence (Scheme A)

Under Scheme A, at least 11 Centers of Excellence in mental health were to be established in the 9th plan period by upgrading existing mental health institutions/hospitals. A grant of up to ₹ 30 crores is available for each center. The support includes capital work (academic block, library, hostel, lab, supportive departments, lecture theaters etc.), equipment and furnishing, support for faculty induction and retention for the plan period. The commitment to take over the entire funding of the scheme after the 11th five year plan period from the state government is required. The proposal of the State Governments for these centers must include definite plan with timelines for initiating/increasing PG courses in Psychiatry, Clinical Psychology, PSW and Psychiatric Nursing.

Setting Up/Strengthening PG Training Departments of Mental Health Specialties (Scheme B)

To provide further impetus to manpower development in Mental Health, Government Medical Colleges/Hospitals are supported to start PG courses in Mental Health or to increase the intake capacity for PG training in Mental Health. The support involves capital work for establishing/improving mental health departments (Psychiatry, Clinical Psychology, Psychiatric Social Work, and Psychiatric Nursing), equipment, tools and basic infrastructure, support for engaging required/deficient faculty for starting/enhancing the PG courses. The support of up to ₹ 51 lacs to ₹ 1 crore per PG department is available.

IEC Activities

NMHP has dedicated funds for IEC activities for the purpose of increasing awareness and removal of stigma for mental illness. The funds are allocated at central and state levels for IEC activities. An amount of ₹ one crore is allocated for the purpose of IEC activities at the central level.

The team of workers at the central level in the National Mental Health Cell is as follows:

- Two Consultants
- Two Research Associates.

Research

The other major contribution of professionals has been in mental health research. The ICMR, New Delhi, gave a big push to mental health research in the 1980s. This research has not only brought to light the importance of understanding mental disorders, such as schizophrenia in the cultural context, but has also shown the feasibility of developing models involving schools, primary health care and general practitioners, as well as working with families. This new knowledge has continuously supported the development of mental health programs.

Human Resource Development

The other major development is the growth in human resources. At the time of the formulation of the NMHP, the number of psychiatrists was under 1000 and in the past 27 years, it has more than tripled, to about 3500. However, the number of trained clinical psychologists, psychiatric social workers and psychiatric nurses is inadequate and this is unfortunate because they form a vital part of the team. The 11th Five Year Plan specifically addresses this need by funding the setting up of centers of excellence, as mentioned earlier. Another lacuna is the very limited training in psychiatry for undergraduate medical students.

Legislation

Some of the changes mentioned above have been supported by legislation for mental health care, namely the Narcotic Drugs and Psychotropic Substances (NDPS) Act, 1985, the MHA, 1987, and Persons with Disability Act 1995. All these legislations have changed the penal approach to mental healthcare to an approach centering around promotion, prevention and rights. The Persons with Disability Act, 1995 is important because for the first time, mental illness has been included as one of the disabilities. The recent UN Convention on Rights of Persons with Disabilities (UNCRPD), 2006 adds a new dimension to the rights of the mentally ill. It is expected that some of the other existing laws will be changed to bring them in harmony with the current thinking and approach towards the mentally ill in India.

Traditional Systems of Care for Mental Health

Indian psychiatrists have examined and utilized the traditional healthcare systems for the care of mental disorders, using Yoga and Ayurveda, 82–86 Indian philosophy 87–91 and traditional healers, 92–94. Systematic research has been done on yogic practices and their effect in different mental disorders in the past 2–3 decades. There is a resurgence of academic interest in the effects of different types of yogic practices and the mental health relevance of the Bhagavad Gita. In January 2009, the Indian Psychiatric Society published a volume on Spirituality and Mental Health, containing over three dozen articles on various aspects of spiritualism and mental health. Initially, yoga and meditation were used in a wide range of mental disorders. In addition, the special relationship between the patient and the therapist in the Indian context and its advantages were explored. This was followed by a comparison of standard treatment with yoga in psychoneuroses, anxiety, drug addiction and psychogenic headache. There were also a number of studies on various aspects of transcendental meditation and its physiological effects. All this leads one to conclude that there will be further examination of spirituality, in general, and the impact of yoga and meditation, in particular, in the coming years, using a wide variety of physiological and psychological tools.

CHALLENGES FOR MENTAL HEALTH CARE IN INDIA

- Large 'unmet need' for mental health care in the community
- Poor understanding of psychological distress as requiring medical intervention in the general population
- Limited acceptance of modern medical care for mental disorders among the general population
- Limitations in the availability of mental health services (professionals and facilities) in the public health services
- Poor utilization of available services by the ill population and their families
- Problems in recovery and reintegration of persons with mental illnesses
- Lack of institutionalized mechanisms for organization of mental health care.

Barrier

- Poor funding in the initial period
- Limited undergraduate training in psychiatry
- Inadequate mental health of human resources
- Limited number of models and their evaluation
- Uneven distribution of resources across states
- Nonimplementation of the MHA, 1987
- Privatization of health care in the 1990s.

Lacunae

While these efforts have been noteworthy, there have been lacunae in some areas. The NMHP has been criticized for the following reasons: (i) it has a top-down approach; (ii) it is not based on the cultural aspects of the country; (iii) it is not effective; (iv) it is driven by WHO policies; and (v) it does not involve community leaders.

POPULATION AT RISK FOR MENTALLY ILL

Urbanization has an effect on mental health owing to the influence of factors, such as overcrowded, polluted and a fast-paced environment. Research shows that conditions of poverty have a direct relationship with risk of mental illness. The fight for survival with poor living conditions puts immense strain on the mental health of the poor. The urban poor are faced with problems of violence and abuse coupled with increased costs and reduced social support. Urban slums play host to rural migrants who are highly vulnerable to mental illness due to the strenuous city life and difficult living conditions.

One way to view population at risk is to focus on types of crises that individuals experience in their lives. It is grouped into two broad categories:

1. Maturational crises
2. Situational crises.

Maturational Crisis

Crisis is associated with various stages of growth and development.

Adolescent

Task of this stage is identity vs role confusion. So, there is conflict over issues of control and they need independence. In this period, there are rapid physical and hormonal changes occurring, which makes them susceptible for development of psychological problem. Issues in this period include suicide, drug abuse, sexual experimentation, issues related to self-esteem and body image, etc.

Marriage

Marriage is considered as most common maturational crisis as no people can possibly coordinate always. Each one has an inner life structure with its own idiosyncrasies. Depending on what has gone before, each one will alternate differently between times of feeling full of certainty, hope, heightened potential and times of feeling vulnerable, unfocused and scared. Additional conflict arises when marriage is influenced by crossovers in religion, ethnicity, social status, race, etc.

Parenthood

The coming of the child is a crisis, a turning point in the couple's life in which old pattern of living must be changed for new ways of living and new values. This is a type of journey in which there is no return. Because the family operates as a system, the addition of a new member influences all parts of the system as a whole. If it is the first child, then the relationship between the spouses is affected by the care of infant. If there are older children, they may resent the attention showered on the new arrival and show their resentment in variety of creative ways. All these kinds of challenging situations give rise to psychological disorder.

Midlife

During this period, lots of psychological problems arise, such as regressive type of behavior. This may be due to:

- **Alteration in perception of the self:** One's perception of self being middle-aged/old may come slowly or suddenly. (mainly by seeing grey hair, wrinkled skin, decreased muscular tone, weight gain, etc.)
- **Alteration of perception of others:** During this midlife, difficulty arises when parents' values conflict with the relationships and types of lifestyles their children choose. This requires a sensitive shift of caring from both. They must adapt to the new roles of parent and adult child. This involves both financial and emotional commitment.
- **Alteration in perception of time:** This stage is the end of youth and beginning of old age. During this period, a person may think that 'I have not done all I want to do or accomplish all.' Depression or sense of loss may occur when individual realized that some life goal may go unmet.

Retirement

A person has achieved self-esteem through work-related activities, creativity and productivity. Termination of these activities may result in loss of self-worth and, in turn, depression may result.

Situational Crises

Situational crises are acute responses that occur as a result of an external circumstantial stressor. There are unlimited situational crises. Some of these may give rise to mental illness that may include:

Poverty

It has a direct correlation with mental disorder because person may be unable to meet basic amenities, like inadequate and crowded living conditions, nutritional deficiencies, medical neglect, etc.

Environmental Condition

It includes natural calamities, like flood, earthquake, hurricanes, tornadoes, etc.

Trauma

Individual who encountered traumatic experiences (assault, physical/mental torture, rape, kidnap, etc.) in his/her life may develop mental illness.

Certain factors may increase risk of developing mental health problems that include:

- Having a biological (blood) relative, such as a parent or sibling, with a mental illness.
- Experiences in the womb, e.g., having a mother who was exposed to viruses, toxins, drugs or alcohol during pregnancy.
- Stressful life situations, such as financial problems, a loved one's death or divorce.
- A chronic medical condition, such as cancer.
- Brain damage as a result of a serious injury (traumatic brain injury), such as a violent blow to the head.
- Traumatic experiences, such as military combat or being assaulted.
- Use of illegal drugs.
- Being abused or neglected as a child.
- Having few friends or few healthy relationships.
- A previous mental illness.

Level of Prevention

The level of prevention of mental illness in a community mainly depends on assuming the whole community as a client. The community health nurse will assess the whole community and identify the needs of mental health services. The levels of prevention includes prevention of mental retardation by proper antenatal care, proper parenting skill by the parents, addressing and treating of crises (individual. family and community) early identification of mental illness and provide prompt treatment and rehabilitate them where ever necessary.

- Primary prevention
- Secondary prevention
- Tertiary prevention.

Primary Prevention

- **Aim:** Services aimed at reducing the incidence of mental disorder within the population.
- **Targets:** Primary prevention targets both individual and environment.
  It emphasizes on:
  - Assist individual to increase their ability to cope effectively with stress.
  - Diminishing harmful forces present within the environment.

Role of Nurse

Nurse focuses on the target population who are at risk and provide education. Examples include education on:

- Parenting skill and child development to new parents.
- Technique of stress management.
- Physical and psychosocial effects of alcohol to school and college students.
- Ways to cope with changes of different maturational stages and transitional periods.
- Concept of mental health.
- Provide support to unemployed and homeless.

Secondary Prevention

Secondary prevention aimed to reduce the prevalence of psychiatric illness by shortening the course of illness.

—Sadock and Sadock, 2003

Secondary prevention is accomplished through:

- Early identification of problem.
- Prompt initiation of effective treatment.

Role of a Nurse

In secondary prevention, a nurse focuses on recognition of symptom and provision of or referral of treatment, e.g.

- Ongoing assessment of risk group.
- Provision of care for individuals in whom illness symptoms have been assessed (group counseling, provision of medication)
- Referral for treatment among whom illness is detected.

Tertiary Prevention

This service aims at reducing the residual defects that are associated with severe or chronic illness. It can be accomplished through:

- Preventing complication
- Promoting rehabilitation in order to achieve maximum level of functioning.

Tertiary level of care can be provided individually or in a group basis and in a variety of settings.

Role of a Nurse

In tertiary prevention, nurse helps the client to learn socially appropriate behavior so that they can get satisfaction by performing their role, e.g.

- Consider rehabilitation process at the time of diagnosis and treatment planning.
- Teach about ADL and encourage to perform independently up to his maximum capacity.
- Refer to after-care centres like support group, day care center, group home, half-way home, etc.

CRISIS INTERVENTION

Stressful situations are a part of everyday life. Any stressful situation can give rise to crisis. It is a kind of disequilibrium which requires problem-solving approach in order to preserve self-esteem and promote growth. Crisis comes originally from Greek word 'Krises' which means 'separate' or 'divide'. Crisis can occur with any age and to anyone. It does not respect age, socioeconomic or sociocultural difference. Crisis is a term commonly used in own society for instances in which circumstances are suddenly altered.

Due to industrial development and industrial technology, people are more aware of things and computerized technology, due to which lifestyle is also changed. Everywhere we are finding competition through which tension and stress occur to the individual and which create crisis. Sudden death, divorce and separation are other causes of crisis.

Crisis is a turning point resulting from a stressful event or threat to one's well-being.

Definition

Crisis is a sudden event in one's life that disturbs homeostasis, during which usual coping mechanisms cannot resolve the problem. **—Lagerquist, 2001**

Caplan (1964) defines the crisis as psychological disequilibrium in a person who confronts a hazardous circumstance that for him constitutes an important problem which he can for the time being neither escape nor solve with his customary problem-solving resources.

According to Rapport (1965), an essential property of crisis is the potential for promoting growth. Crises present challenges and call for new responses.

Characteristics of Crisis

According to Kaplan and Sadak, the characteristics of crisis may be:

- It is precipitated by specific identifiable events.
- It is personal by nature.
- It is acute and not chronic.
- It has potential for psychological growth or deterioration.

Types of Crisis

Crisis can occur in a person by three ways:

1. Individual crisis
2. Family crisis
3. Community crisis.

Individual Crisis

Maturational Crisis

It is also called the expected crisis. The expected ones are those periods that occur with some degree of predictability as the result of result of maturation, e.g., stage of growth and development of an individual. It occurs during transition from phase of life to the next, such as from childhood to adolescence and from adolescence to adulthood. For example, adolescent issues, such as dating, sexual activity, career choice, etc.

Situational Crisis (Unexpected Crisis)

The unexpected is an accidental occurrence called situational crisis. These crises follow anticipated sudden events over when no control can be exerted. For example divorce, death, etc.

Family Crisis

Maturational Crisis

Duvall and Miller developed a right stage family cycle based on variety of family pattern, age and child family function.

- **Stage I:** Married couples
  - Allocation of responsibilities
  - New residence
  - Learning how to live together on daily basis.
- **Stage II:** Child-bearing
  - New role of the parents
  - Develop a patterning skill which includes money, energy, etc.
- **Stage III:** Families with preschool parents
  - First child between 2½ and 6 years, when second child is born
  - Need demand for adequate space and equipment.
- **Stage IV:** Families with school children
  - Children independence
  - Parents must establish relationship.
- **Stage V:** Families with teenagers
  - Rapid physiological and psychological changes and bring a distinct set of problems
  - Parents should limit and protect adolescents simultaneously allowing freedom.
- **Stage VI:** Families launching young adults
  - Marriage problem
  - Family shrinking to the original pair, parents may become in-laws and grandparents.
- **Stage VII:** Families with middle-aged parents
  - Children may leave the home
  - Placement of members in the larger society
  - Family members establish roots in society through relationships in church, school, political and other organization which will protect the family members from undesirable outside influences
- **Stage VIII:** Families with aging members
  - Retirement or ends with the death of both spouses
  - Children may not meet the needs of elderly couple.

Situational Crisis

Stressful, unanticipated events that may precipitate a family crisis include the birth of a premature infant, death of family members, diagnosis of serious illness.

Community Crisis

Maturational Crisis

Growth demands in health care services through government as education, safe water supply, sewage disposal, utilities, public safety, fire protection, etc.

Situational Crisis

Situational crisis in a community can result from events, such as natural disasters or the sudden influx of a large number of refugees.

Baldwin identified six classes of emotional crisis which progress by degree of severity.

Dispositional Crisis

An acute response to an external situational stressor, e.g., husband bit her wife due to stress at work place.

Crisis of Anticipated Life Transition

Normal life cycle transition that may be anticipated but over which the individual may feel a lack of control.

- Crisis resulting from traumatic stress
- Maturational crisis
- Crisis reflecting psychopathology.

Phases of Crisis

The development of a crisis situation follows a relatively predictable course. Caplan (1964) has outlines four specific phases through which individual progress in response to precipitating stressor and which culminate in the state of acute crisis. During crisis the anxiety increases, coping skill become less available and less effective.

Phase I

The individual is exposed to a precipitating stressor. There is rise in tension. People commonly experience feelings of discomfort and bewilderment from the impact of the stimulus demands the habital solving responses. Previous problems solving technique are employed to a precipitating situation. Anxiety increases, previous problem-solving technique employed.

Phase II

Previous problem-solving technique does not relieve the stress, anxiety further. Coping technique that helped in past are attempted. Individual begins to feel large deal of discomfort and confusion. There is rise in tension produces lack of success and continuation of stimulus due to failure of previous problem-solving technique.

Phase III

All possible resources (Internal/external) are used to resolve the problem and discomfort. Individual tries to view the problem in different perspective and tries new problem-solving technique. The individual may try to view the problem from different perspective or even to overlook certain aspect of new problem resolution may occur at this phase.

Phase IV

If the problem continues and unable to solve because of its tension is beyond a further threshold or its breaking point as a result it converts drastic results. Anxiety reach to panic state, cognitive disorder, labile emotion and psychotic thinking may appear. In this stage the person mobilizes internal and external resources and tries out new problem-solving methods or redefines the threat. So that the old methods can work. Resolution may occur in this phase. If new or old problem-solving methods are put into action and are effective.

Crisis Reflecting Psychopathology

Emotional crisis in which preexisting psychopathology has been instrumental or in which psychopathology significantly impairs or complicates adaptive resolution. Examples of psychopathology that may precipitates crisis include border line personality, severe neuroses, characterological disorder or schizophrenia **—Baldwin, 1978**

Psychiatric Emergencies

Crisis situation in which general functioning has been severely impaired. The individual rendered in competent or unable to assume personal responsibility. Example included actually suicidal individual, drug overdoses, reaction to hallucinogenic drugs, acute psychoses, uncontrollable anger and alcohol intoxication.

Setting for Crisis Intervention

Nurses works in many setting in which they see people in crisis:

- Hospitalization are often stressful for patient and their families and are precipitating causes of crisis
- Nurses in community mental health center
- Department of psychiatry
- Schools
- Occupational health centers.

Precipitating Factors

- The illness, the limitation imposed on activities change in body image due to surgery and losses or threats may precipitate a situational crisis.
- The stress if being dependent on nurses for care can precipitate a crisis for the hospitalized patient.
- Nurses work in obstetric pediatric, geriatric or adolescent setting often observe patients or family members undergoing maturational crisis.
- Community and home health nurses works with patient in their own environment can often spot and intervene in family crisis.

Indication for crisis therapy:

- The anxious mother
- The acting out adolescent

- Newly retired depressed attempt
- People with suicidal attempt
- Psychosomatic patients
- Survivors of sudden cardiac arrest
- Crime
- Accident victims
- Any death occurs in the family
- Persons with marital conflict
- Persons with drug abuse
- Persons with depression and anxiety.

Crisis Intervention

Individual Crisis

- Eliminate hazardous situations which may produces crisis, e.g., ensure that work in a safety guidelines are follows to prevent situational crisis.
- Identify vulnerable groups (Police, members of military) before exposure to stressful situation. Provide anticipatory education about stress reduction and coping strategies.
- Advice those exposed to crisis producing situation about coping alternation and available resources.
- Provide the knowledge about effectiveness of coping strategies through health education.
- Provide additional, physical, social and informational resources to individual under stress.

Family Crisis

Intervention for family crisis are:
- Provide information that is brief, consist and concrete family to record
- Ascertain comprehension by asking family to repeat to you to what information they given
- Provide for or allow ventilation of feeling
- Maintain a constant, nonanxious pressure in the face of family
- Inform family as to range of behaviors within the norm for crisis.

Denial

- Identify what purpose denial is serving for family
- Evaluate appropriateness of use of denial in terms of time
- Do not actively support denial but neither hopes for the future
- If denial is prolonged and dysfunctional in direct and specific factual representation may be essential.

Anger, Hostility, and Distrust

- Allow for ventilation of angry feelings, clarifying thoughts, fears and beliefs
- Do not personalize family's expressions of these strong emotions
- Institute family control within the hospital environment when possible
- Remain available to families during their venturing of these emotions.

Grief and Depression

- Acknowledge family's grief and depression
- Encourage them to be precise about what it is they are grieving about
- Allow the family appropriate link for grief
- Remain sensitive to your own unfinished business and hence, comfort or discomfort with family's grieving.

Hope

- Clarify with families their hopes, individually and with one another
- Clarify with families their worst fear in reference to the situation
- Support realistic hope
- Offer gentle factual information to reframe unrealistic hope
- Assist families in reframing unrealistic hope in some other fashion.

Community Crisis Intervention

Disaster Situations

The community response on disaster characteristically consists of four phases:

Heroic Phase

The heroic phase typically lasts through at least the first week post-disaster. Shock of the disaster pulls people together and emotions are strong. Large amounts of energy are expended in rescue efforts, providing shelter and community emergency stabilization.

Emergency medical teams, neighbors and friends rally around the survivors, offering emotional support and tangible supplied needed for recovery.

Honeymoon Phase (Bowenkamp, 2000)

- Honeymoon phase occurs when the 'commonly pulls together and outside resources are brought in' after initial search and recovery phase. The honeymoon phase typically lasts up to six months post-disaster. During this phase, survivors rely on the fact that different agencies have made promises of aid and they trust that these promises will be fulfilled. Sharing the experience of the trauma with others and tangible evidence of continuing support are crucial.
- Emergency resource may start to withdrawn towards the end of the honeymoon phase and this can increase survivor anxiety.

Disillusionment Phase

- This phase usually appears as the initial emergency response starts to subside. This phase can last up to a year or more post-disaster.
- People start to realize the extent of their losses. Survivors can experience anger, resentment and bitterness at the loss of support, particularly, if it is sudden and complete.

- It can feel like a double loss when, the previously felt sense of community investment in their cause begins to fall apart.
- Kaplan, and Bodwer (2000) suggest that opportunities for psychological debriefing sessions should continue for a period well beyond the initial disaster experience for victims of extreme stress.

Reconstruction Phase

- The final phase reconstruction, occurs with the realization that the survivor will used to bear the primary responsibility for rebuilding his or her life.
- Ongoing support is required as the survivor learns to cope with new roles and responsibilities and to develop new alternatives to living a full life post-trauma.
- This phase can last for several years with the individual gradually getting back to full normal functioning after a disaster.
- Although the disaster experience records in memory, it is never lose and the person never again fully trusts in the continuity of life.

Violence

Violence is a special form of crisis in that it involves the use of physical force and demands and immediate response for the client's protection as well as that of others in the clients path.

—**Cahill et al., 1991**

It is a psychosocial emergency that can be just as critical as a life-threatening medical emergency.

Violence is associated with power and control, usually the perpetrator feels powerless or out control and the behavior is a maladaptive attempt to restore emotional balance.

The cause of violent behavior is organic and the nurse should assure these in an organic component until otherwise indicated, drugs and alcohol often are implicated.

The violent client must be stabilized immediately for the protection of self and others.

These characteristic indications of increasing tension leading to violence. The indicators of potential violence are described in **Table 12.1**.

Treatment of Violence Clients

- Providing a safe, nonstimulating environment.
- The client should be checked thoroughly for potential weapons. Prevention of violent behavior is best.
- The nurse can use simple strategies, such as calling the client by name, using a low, tone of voice, or presenting a show of force if necessary to help the client defuse tension.
- Encouraging the client to physically walk and to vent emotions verbally can be helpful.
- Sometimes the environment is overstimulation and the client clause down if taken to an area that provides less sensory input.

Phases of Crisis Intervention Based on Nursing Process

Guilera and Messick (1982) have described four specific phases in the technique of crisis intervention. These phases are clearly comparable to the step of the nursing process.

Table 12.1: Indicators of potential violence.

Behavioral categories	*Suggested indicators*
Mental status	Confused
	Paranoid ideation
	Evidence of drug involvement
	Organic impairment
Motor behavior	Agitated
	Pacing
Body language	Eyes dazing
	Spitting
	Menacing posture
Speech patterns	Rapid
	Incoherent
	Menacing tones
	Verbal threats

Phase 1: Assessment

In this phase the nurse gathers information regarding the precipitating stressor and the resulting crisis. A nurse in crisis intervention might perform some of the following assessment. In this phase the crisis helper collect data regarding the precipitating factor which causes stress. The crisis helpers:

- Ask the client to explain the event and when it occurred.
- Assess physical and mental status.
- Whether previous coping mechanism tried and what is the result and also new one has tried or not.
- Assess for support system.
- Assess individual's feelings, support system, coping skills, perception, strength, limitation, etc.

Client's Feelings

- The nurse asks clients to describe the feelings they experience.
- By accepting the feelings without judgment, the nurse assists clients to accept their own feelings.
- The nurse naturally will feel some discomfort in the presence of a person in pain.
- The human inclination is to stop the person from crying and to stop talking about what is horrible and upsetting.
- By avoiding the topic of distress, the client at least appears to be in less pain.
- Nevertheless, it is beneficial for the person in crisis to express feelings and experience the pain or frustration.
- Therefore, the nurse must learn to tolerate these feelings of discomfort.
- The nurse must understand cognitively and emotionally that ultimately clients make their own decisions.

Client's Perception of the Event

- The nurse first determines the client's perception of the stressful event.
- How threatened is the client?
- Is the client realistic or distorting the meaning of event?

Client's Support Systems

- After determining the client's perception of the event, the nurse focuses on who will be available to support the client. Questions, such as the following can help identify the client's support systems: 'Whom do you trust?', 'Who is your best friend?', 'Is there a member of your family with whom you are particularly close?'
- The nurse also should inquire to the client's religious beliefs. For many families, God is a source of comfort and strength.
- It is best to have several supportive people involved with the client.
- Because a crisis period lasts for a brief time and the nurse will be involved only temporarily, the client needs others on whom to rely for continued support.

Client's Coping Skills

- The nurse must encourage the client to describe coping methods as specifically as possible.
- Then the nurse should determines whether the client's coping mechanisms are adaptive or maladaptive.

Client's Potential for Self-harm

- Assessment of clients in crisis is not complete without asking if they are having thoughts of hurting themselves.
- Clients who have attempted suicide before or have attempted suicide before or have decided how, when and where to kill themselves need protection.
- The suicidal clients should not be left alone.

Nursing Diagnosis

Information from the comprehensive assessment is then analyzed and appropriate nursing diagnosis reflecting the immediacy of the crisis situation are identified.

Possible nursing diagnosis for the client in crisis may include following:

- Anxiety related to situation and maturational crisis, threat of self-concept, unmet needs, and traumatic event, as evidenced by restlessness, insomnia, verbalizations, of fear of going crazy, feelings of inadequacy, fearlessness and focus on self.
- Ineffective individual coping related to inadequate coping and personal vulnerability as evidenced by inability to problem solves, altered society participation, inappropriate use of defense mechanisms in ability to meet role expectations and anxious mood.
- Altered thought processes related to situational and maturational crisis, threat to self-concept and high anxiety level, as evidenced by inability to problem solve or make decisions, inaccurate interpretation of the environment, easy distractibility and inappropriate affect or thinking.
- Impaired social interaction related to self-concept disturbance and unmet dependency needs as evidenced by verbalized or observed discomfort in social situations, verbalized or observed inability to receive or communicate a satisfying sense of belonging and caring and dysfunctional interaction with peers, family and others.
- Social isolation related to height level of anxiety and possible regression, evidenced by absence of supportive significant others (family, friends, group) uncommunicate and withdrawn behavior and preoccupation with own thoughts.
- Self-esteem disturbance, altered role performance related to perception of overwhelming problem lack of support systems and high anxiety level, as evidenced by self-destructive behavior, lack of responsibility for self-care, verbalization of sense of worthlessness, inability to recognize own accomplishments and lack of appropriate behavior.

Planning

In the planning phase of nursing process, the nurse selected the appropriate nursing activities for the identified nursing diagnosis. In planning intervention the type of crisis as well as the individual strength and available resources for support are taken into consideration. Goals are established for intervention.

Goal

The minimum therapeutic goals of crisis intervention is psychological resolution of the individual's immediate crisis. To reach that end the following goals are set.

- Establishing a working relationship with the client
- Identifying the specific problem
- Reducing the distortion of the clients perception of the event
- Improving the client's self-esteem
- Decreasing the client's anxiety
- Promoting involvement of family and friends
- Reinforcing healthy coping mechanisms
- Validating the client's ability to solve the problem.

Intervention

- Use a realty oriented approach
- Remain with individual who is experiencing panic anxiety
- Establishing a working relationship by showing unconditional acceptance, by active listening or by attending the immediate needs
- Discuss lengthy explanation or rationalization of the situation
- Set firm limits on aggressive destructive behavior
- Clarify the problem that the individual is facing
- Help the individual determine what he or she believes precipitated crisis
- Acknowledge feeling of angry, helplessness or any other
- Nursing intervention may takes places in different level using a variety of technique in a classic model 'shield' described like a hierarchy from the most basic to most complex.

Evaluation

The last phase is evaluation when the nurse evaluate the patient whether the intervention resulted a positive resolution or not. If the goals have not been met she should be return to first step and assessment continue again. It is the phase to evaluate the outcome of crisis intervention, i.e., whether the stated objective has achieved or not. The resolution stage is often neglected as once the level of the crisis is reduced teams often strive to pass people onto other services as quickly as possible. The consequence of doing this is often a fairly rapid return to a crisis situation. Time needs to be dedicated to working on the resolution phase and certain tasks should be completed prior to discharge or transfer to another team. Ongoing evaluation of the interventions carried out is essential to monitor improvement and identify progress in managing the crisis. This can be done either in an informal manner by the named worker, or more formally through multidisciplinary team.

Approaches for Crises Intervention

These includes intervention that directly change the patient's physical or interpersonal situation. These intervention provides situational support or remove stress. **Figure 12.1** shows the approaches for crises intervention and **Figure 12.2** is an example of crises intervention model.

General Support

General support includes interventions that convey the feeling that the nurse is on the patients side and ready to help the person.

Generic Approach

The generic approach is designed to reach rich individuals and large groups as quickly as possible. It applies a specific method to all people faced with a similar type of crisis. The expected course of the particular type of crisis is studied and mapped out. The intervention is set up.

Individual Approach

The individual approach is a type of crisis intervention similar to the diagnosis and treatment of a specific problem in a specific patient. The nurse must understand the specific patient characteristics that lead to the preset crisis and must use the intervention that is most likely to help the patient develop an adaptive response to the crisis. It is particularly useful in combined situational and maturational crisis. The introduced approach is also helpful when symptoms include homicidal and suicidal risk. In these instances the nurse should make a formal safety contract in which the patient agrees not to harm himself/herself or others.

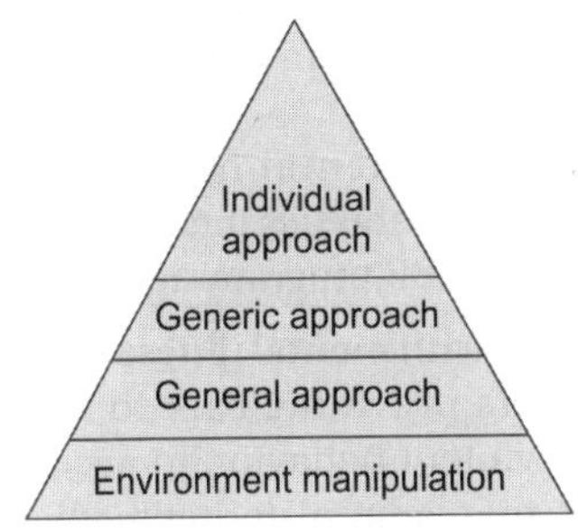

Fig. 12.1: Approaches for crises intervention.

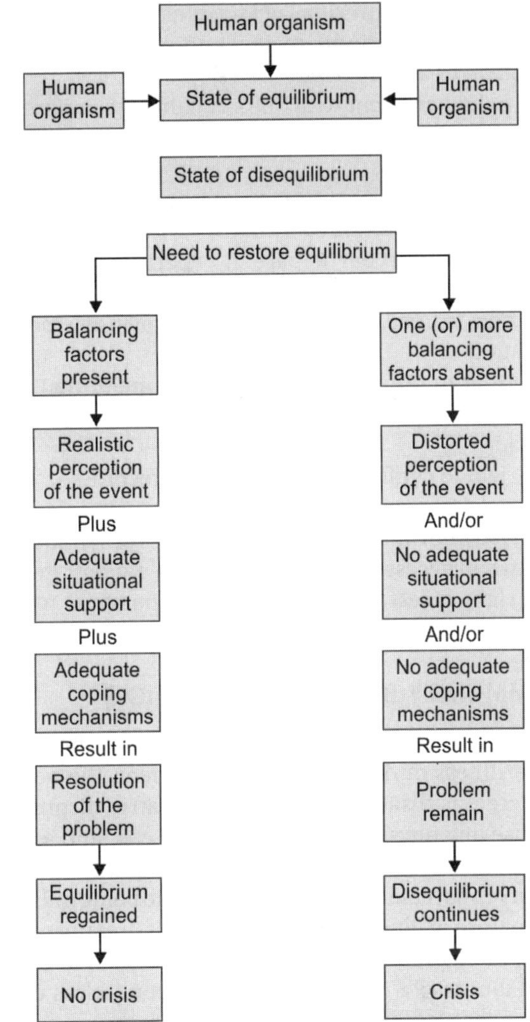

Fig. 12.2: Crises intervention model.

Paradigm: The effect of balancing factors in a stressful event.

HUMAN RIGHTS OF MENTALLY ILL

Persons with disability, especially those suffering from mental illness and other barriers like mental retardation do not get proper attention from the authorities in the matter of access to justice. The result is that they are sidelined and are viewed only from the prism of the paternalistic 'social welfare' which looks upon them as merely as persons who are in need of special protection by the State and the society. India being a signatory to the UN Convention on the Rights of Persons with Disabilities (CRPD) 2008 and since our country has ratified the Convention, it is obligatory for our legal system to ensure the human rights and fundamental freedoms of persons with disability.

- Right to appropriate treatment and related services in the setting that is most supportive and least restrictive to personal freedom.

- The right to an individualized written treatment or service plan, right to periodic review and revision of the plan based on treatment need.
- The right consistent with one's capabilities to participate in and receive a responsible explanation of the care and treatment process.
- The right to refuse treatment except in an emergency situation or as permitted by law.
- The right not to participate in experimentation in the absence of informed voluntary written consent.
- The right to freedom from restraint except in an emergency situation.
- The right to human treatment environment that affords reasonable protection from harm and appropriate privacy.
- The right to confidentiality of medical record.
- The right to access to medical record except information received from third parties under promise of confidentiality and when access will be detrimental to patients health.
- The right access to use of telephone, personal mail and visit.

COMMUNITY-BASED REHABILITATION

If a person is unable to perform an activity because of disease/illness or due to bodily impairment, the person is considered as disabled. Though psychiatric disorders do not cause any physical impairment, they can stop a person from doing many activities that are expected of them. The disability in psychiatric illnesses is dynamic being influenced by the nature of illness, phase of the illness, treatment status and social support network available to them. Patient with mental illness (PWMI) are treated as second-class citizens with no adequate facilities or provision from the government. As a result, they face chronic ill health and the families experience economic and social burden. In certain cases this leads to social destitution. CBR is a strategy within general community development for the rehabilitation, equalization of opportunities and social inclusion of all people with disabilities. The primary objective of CBR is the improvement of the quality of life of people with disability/marginalized persons.

Purpose

To enable development practitioners to include mental health issues in the existing CBR programmes through increased understanding of PWMI, recognizing psychosocial disabilities, appreciating the similarity in approaches, cost effectiveness etc.

CBR and People with Mental Illness

Development and changes in the concept of CBR over the last two decades has influenced the thought of inclusion of mental health in CBR programmes. The CBR strategy shifts rehabilitation interventions to homes and communities of people with disabilities. Basic services are provided or facilitated by CBR workers who are minimally qualified nonprofessionals but who are highly qualified change agents. The main goal of rehabilitation has become broader and focuses beyond the individual, to the family and communities in which people live. CBR recognizes that breaking down barriers to inclusion in society is as important to the mission of the CBR programme as is the functional rehabilitation of individuals with disabilities. Thus the universal mission of CBR is:

- To enhance activities of daily life of disabled persons
- To create awareness in disabled person's environment to achieve barrier free situations around him and help him in meeting all human rights
- To create a situation in which the community of the disabled persons, participates fully and assimilate ownership of their integration in to the society. The ownership lies with the affected persons.

Inclusion of Mental Health into CBR

There are a number of reasons why mental health should be integrated into community-based rehabilitation programmes:

- Community processes, full participation, equal opportunities, social inclusion, gender, diversity and a focus on rights are some of the key common elements of CBR work. Community mental health work is no different so the programmes integrate well together.
- The high prevalence of psychosocial disabilities emerging through mental illness and its impact on communities, societies and economies means that CBR workers are confronted with the issues in their work. CBR programmes can have a positive impact on the lives of PWMI, their families and on the situations in which people live by including people with psychosocial disabilities in their programmes. **—(WHO 2010)**
- There are a limited number of mental health professionals and mental health services in low-income countries, making a CBR strategy which empowers community level stakeholders to take action an important strategy.
- The emerging trend away from vertical health programmes to integrated, multipurpose health programme models favors primary level services and community-based strategies.
- There is an increasing recognition of the importance of early detection and treatment of mental illness in order to prevent chronic conditions.
- The goal of continuity of care and inclusion of people who are mentally ill into the community is more readily achieved when there is an existing community-based strategy.
- The prevalence of mental health problems among people with other disabilities means that a mental health component in the CBR programmes brings added value.

The care for people with mental illness can be provided by:

- Family members providing care to PWMI starts from baring all the violent behavior, to accompanying them for treatment, than administering medicines, helping to engage in gainful productive work.

- Community providing support for the well-being of PWMI. This is seen in the form of not labelling them as mad people, giving opportunities and advocating for the ensuring measures to meet the needs of PWMI.
- Rehabilitation workers providing care for the PWMI and their families. This starts with identification, assessment, follow-up, home-based support and linking them to existing groups and mainstreaming.
- Organization providing support to deal with other associated problems of PWMI and their caregivers. This is seen in the form of conducting camps, integrating them into their existing programmes.
- Provided with the above support, the role of mental health professionals would be more meaningful.

Steps of Rehabilitation

- **Reduction of impairment:** Rehabilitation interventions with psychiatric patients require reduction or elimination of the symptoms and cognitive impairments that interfere with social and vocational performance. These impairment should be reduced and eliminated.
- **Remediation of disabilities through skill training:** Skills training on self-care, interpersonal skill, vocational functioning, recreation, employment pursuits, etc., are used to remediate disabilities in social, family and vocational functioning.
- **Remediating disabilities through supportive intervention:** Help the individual for compensating for handicap by learning skills in living and working environment.
- **Remediation of handicap:** In addition to clinical rehabilitation intervention, the disabled person can helped to overcome their handicaps through social rehabilitation intervention, e.g., community support programmes.

Suggested Activities for Inclusion of People in the Existing CBR Programmes

Promote Community-based Mental Health Services

The community-based services should emphasize on community acceptance, family involvement, social integration and livelihood opportunities as a key component of interventions while rehabilitating people with disabilities. Similar approach is required for PWMI for integrating them into the community. An approach, where in medical inputs are seen as a part of a larger whole including income generation and mainstreaming individuals with mental health problems into the full community.

Work with Disability People's Organizations (DPOs)

Disabled people's organizations are the organization where, people with disabilities have united in and advocates for their own rights to influence decision-makers in governments and all sectors of society. Disabled people's organizations have arisen in response to societal barriers that have prevented the equal participation of people with disabilities, and as a reaction against the control of people with disabilities by others. Service users can advocate for access to treatment with coordination of disabled people's organizations and access to treatment as near as possible.

Involve people with mental illness and their families in livelihood programs for getting appropriate services.

Promote Community Mental Health Services

Mental health professionals in several low-income countries are actively promoting community mental health (CMH) and are attempting to influence their governments to initiate measures to bring mental health into the primary health care system. CBR programmes can work with mental health professionals, local health center staff and users of mental health services to promote community mental health services. Many mental health problems can be effectively resolved by working together with people who experience mental illness in their own homes and communities, using resources and support networks that are available to them. Awareness raising campaigns and large-scale dissemination of knowledge and skills would help in reducing the stigma attached to illness. Building knowledge and awareness among families can make the real difference, in ensuring that PWMI are integral members of the family and community, participating in all social and cultural activities.

- **Street theaters:** Street theaters play a major role in generating awareness in the community. Some organizations also have formed puppet shows troops. Street plays can provide knowledge on causes, treatments and symptoms of mental illness. The purpose is to demystify the subject and to raise the awareness of the public on mental health issues. Street theaters can also highlight the important roles and responsibilities of families and the community, which could go long way in rehabilitating PWMI. The street theater performances can be followed by question and answer sessions, where people can ask specific questions.
- **Self-help groups:** Self-help groups are a common feature of CBR and development work. A self-help group of women were clearly working hard to be strong in the face of personal tragedy and unrelenting poverty. Comprising twelve members, they came together with the support of CBR worker to promote savings of ₹100 per month per person so that individuals can accumulate enough to buy a buffalo. This would then be a source of regular income, the milk being sold to a cooperative at a guaranteed rate per liter. One of the women had lost her husband to snakebite the previous week and so the group was rallied around to support her and her three children.

Seek Out Alliances for Training and Mutual Support

Local community organizations staff like community rehabilitation workers/field staffs, coordinators of self-help/user groups and other programmes, lay volunteers/animators, nurses, and health workers; who are not professionals in mental health or health care provide a variety of services. Many of these informal community-care providers have little or no formal mental health care training, but in many low-income countries they are the main source of community mental health provision. They are usually accessible and generally well accepted in local communities. They can help with the integration of people with mental disorders into community activities and the other developmental activities of their own organizations, and thus play an supportive role in meeting the treatment needs of PWMI.

Some of the important roles of the CBR and the community development workforce are:

- Awareness creation and dissemination of information
- Identification of people with mental health problems and referral to health services
- Crisis support
- Home-based support—supportive care, including basic information and counseling
- Helping in the activities of daily living skills and community reintegration
- Formation of caregivers groups/associations
- Advocating for the rights of PWMI
- Preventive and promotive services
- Organizing affected people to advocate for meeting their needs.

SUBSTANCE ABUSE

Excessive use of alcohol, psychoactive drugs and chemicals like volatile substances causes psychological disorder. In India 20–40% of subjects aged above 15 years are current user of alcohol, and nearly 10% of them are regular or excessive user. Nearly 15–30% of patient are developing alcohol-related problem and seeking admission in psychiatric hospitals.

Abuse

It is a maladaptive pattern of substance use that impairs health. The major dependence producing drugs are:

- Alcohol
- Opioids
- Cannabis
- Cocaine
- Sedative and hypnotics
- Nicotine
- Hallucinogens.

Factor Affecting Substance Abuse

Psychological Factor

- Sense of inferiority
- Low self-esteem
- Inability to cope with pressure of living society
- Loneliness, unmet need
- Sexual immaturity.

Social Factor

- Religious reason
- Peer pressure
- Urbanization
- Extended period of education
- Unemployment
- Over crowding
- **Occupation:** Chef, barmen, army personnel, actor, entertainer, etc.

Easy Availability of Drug

Drug that can be obtained from elicit sources, e.g., street drugs.

Psychiatric Disorder due to Substance Abuse

- Alcohol dependence syndrome
- Opioid disorder
- Cannabis use disorder
- Cocaine use disorder
- LSD use disorder
- Barbiturate use disorder.

Prevention of Substance Abuse

- Provision of recreation and entertainment
- Proper channelization of energies of the adolescents into constructive activities
- Health education
- Inculcation of the dangers of drug abuse students, teacher and the family increasing awareness
- Provision of periodic psychiatric guidance
- Strict implementation of drug control measures
- Measures for deaddiction
- Effective prevention and intervention programs consider cultural context, social resistance skills, and developmental level of the child
- Skills training
- Teaching the problem solving and coping skills in the skills
- Development of proper social and problem solving skills
- Treatment of family problems
- Increased opportunities for prosocial activities with peers.

ALCOHOL DEPENDENCE SYNDROME

Symptom

- **GI:** Gastritis, peptic ulcer, Ca. stomach, pancreatitis, malabsorption syndrome.
- **CVS:** HTN, cardiomyopathy
- **CNS:** Peripheral neuropathy, epilepsy, cerebral degeneration
- **Damage to fetus:** Fetal alcohol syndrome, LBW, still birth.
- **Social:** Marital disharmony, unemployment, financial problem, accident, criminality.

Psychiatric Disorders

- Acute intoxication
- Withdrawal syndrome
- Alcohol induced amnestic disorder
- Alcohol induced psychiatric disorder.

OPIOD DISORDER

- The commonly used narcotics in India are heroin, pethidine, fortwin, etc.

- **Acute intoxication:** Bradycardia, apathy, hypotension, respiratory depression.
- **Withdrawal syndrome:** Watery eye, running nose, loss of appetite, irritability, tremor, sweating, cramps etc.
- **Complications:** Peripheral neuropathy, parkinsonism, criminality, AIDS
- **Treatment:** Detoxification, antidote (naloxone).

CANNABIS USE DISORDER

It is derived from hemp plant *(Cannabis sativa)*. The dried leaves and flower is called as marijuana, Ganja. It is either smoked or taken in liquid form:

- **Acute intoxication:** Impairment of consciousness and orientation, tachycardia, euphoria, dream-like state
- **Withdrawal syndrome:** Mostly found within 72–96 hr. Increased salivation, hyperthermia, insomnia, decreased appetite.
- **Complications:** Hypomania, paranoid psychosis.
- **Treatment:** Supportive and symptomatic.

COCAINE USE DISORDER

The street name is 'crack'. It can be taken orally, smoking or parenterally.

- **Acute intoxication:** Pupillary dilatation, tachycardia, hypertension, sweating.
- **Withdrawal syndrome:** Agitation, depression, anorexia, fatigue and sleepiness.
- **Complications:** Acute anxiety reaction, seizure, respiratory depression, cardiac arrhythmia, etc.
- **Treatment:** Amyl nitrate is an antidote, diazepam also be used.

LSD USE DISORDER

It is a powerful hallucinogen. It effects by acting on 5-HT levels in brain.

- **Acute intoxication:** It is characterized perceptual changes occurring in clear consciousness, illusion, paranoid ideation, automatic hyperactivity, marked anxiety, etc.
- **Withdrawal syndrome:** Flashback (brief experiences of the hallucinogenic).
- **Complications:** Anxiety, depression, visual hallucinosis.
- **Treatment:** Symptomatic treatment with antianxiety, antidepressant.

PREVENTION OF SUBSTANCE USE DISORDER

Primary

- Reduction over prescribing by doctor
- Identification and treatment of family member who may be contributing to drug abuse.
- Make social change: Putting up price of alcohol, controlling advertising about alcohol, controlling sale.
- Increasing individual's personal and social skill, i.e., development of self-esteem.
- Health education to college students and youth about dangers of substance abuse.
- Overall improvement socioeconomic improvement of the population.

Secondary

Early detection and counseling.

WELFARE AGENCIES WORKING FOR MENTALLY CHALLENGED PEOPLE

There are various welfare agencies are working for mentally challenged people at international national and local level.

International Level

At international level World Health Organization (WHO) Integrates mental health concerns to prevent and control mental disorders. One of the objective of WHO in it's Mental health action plan (2013-2020) is to provide comprehensive, integrated and responsive mental health and social care services in community-based settings. The United Nations Educational Scientific and Cultural Organization (UNESCO) also seeks to build peace through international cooperation in Education, the Sciences and Culture. It is associated with young people's mental and physical health as well as on their well-being over the short and long-term.

The World Federation for Mental Health (WFMH) purposes to promote cooperation at international level between governmental, nongovernmental mental health agencies. The Federation has been granted consultative status by both WHO and UNESCO. It assists UN agencies by collecting information on mental health conditions all over world.

The goals of WFMH are as follows:

- To promote mental health and optimal functioning
- To prevent mental, neurological and psychosocial disorders
- To heighten public awareness about the importance of mental health
- To improve the care and treatment of those with mental, neurological and psychosocial disorders.

The International Society for Mental Health Online (ISMHO): It is a nonprofit organization formed in 1997 to promote the understanding, use and development of online communication information and technology for the international mental health community. It serves as a valuable resource for researchers, clinicians and ordinary people interested in the topic of online mental health.

American Academy of Child and Adolescent Psychiatry: The mission is to promote the healthy development of children, adolescents, and families through research, training, prevention, comprehensive diagnosis and treatment.

The JED Foundation: The JED Foundation provides expertise in promoting emotional and mental health and preventing suicide among teens, young adults, and college students. This organization has been founded in 2000 and Focusing on Suicide prevention, and mental illness. They equip teens and young adults with the skills and knowledge to help themselves and each other. They encourage community awareness, understanding and action for young adult mental health.

American Psychiatric Association (APA): The APA is the main professional organization of psychiatrists and trainee psychiatrists in the United States, and the largest psychiatric organization in the world. Its more than 37,000 members are involved in psychiatric practice, research, and academia representing a diverse population of patients in more than 100 countries. The association publishes various journals and pamphlets, as well as the Diagnostic and Statistical Manual of Mental Disorders (DSM). The DSM codifies psychiatric conditions and is used mostly in the United States as a guide for diagnosing mental disorders.

American Psychiatric Nurses Association: It is a professional association of psychiatric-mental health nurses. Founded in 1986, it provides continuing education and a range of professional services to a membership of more than 9000 nurses. It publishes position papers on mental health issues and the care of persons with psychiatric disorders. The Association is committed to the specialty practice of psychiatric-mental health (PMH) nursing and wellness promotion, prevention of mental health problems, and the care and treatment of persons with psychiatric disorders.

Mental Health Agencies in India

The Alzheimer and Related Disorders Society of India (ARDSI): First started in Cochin, and has now spread to more than a dozen centers in India. It works with families who have a member affected by dementia. ARDSI is a registered national, nonprofit voluntary organization engaged in the care, support, training and research of dementia since it's inception in 1992.

Objectives of ARDSI

- To initiate and encourage formation of Day care (morning to evening), Home care (providing care at the homes for people with dementia)
- To secure from Governmental and nongovernmental sources, better facilities for care.
- To undertake and support research into the causes, prevalence, caregiving and other aspects of Alzheimer's and other forms of dementia.
- To encourage training of health personal in geriatric care and dementia.
- To educate the general public about dementia through all available media.

The Richmond Fellowship Society: The Richmond Fellowship (RF) was started in the year 1959 in UK by Ms. Elly Jansen which Provides effective rehabilitation services to people recovering from severe mental health problems

Schizophrenia Research Foundation (SCARF): It is a NGO organization in Chennai founded in 1984 by a group of philanthropists and mental health professionals SCARF is one of the very few NGOs in the world to be named as a Collaborating Center of the World Health Organization (WHO) for Mental Health Research and Training.

Objectives of SCARF:

- Treatment and rehabilitation of people suffering from Schizophrenia
- Community outreach programmes in urban slums and villages to offer treatment and improve awareness.
- Educating the public about schizophrenia, to create awareness and understanding, to facilitate early detection, and to eliminate social stigmatisation.
- Training programmes to various groups of workers on principles of detection and management of mental illnesses.
- Lobbying extensively with the Government and other apex bodies for programmes for the mentally disabled.
- Research into biological, social and psychological aspects of Schizophrenia.

Sangath Society (Goa): It is a NGO working towards increasing access to mental healthcare for 20 years now. Sangath is providing access to rural population in the form of physical, psychological, and social therapies.

Umeed and the Research Society (Mumbai): Umeed provides specialized care for most developmental disabilities and has moved into areas of training, research and advocacy. It is now one of the country leading NGOs, much respected for its work in the field of children with disabilities.

Shraddha Rehabilitation Foundation: Nonprofit organization established by Dr Bharat Vatwani, a Mumbai based Psychiatrist, in 1989. Based in Karjat, Maharashtra, the foundation aims to find, restore and reunite, the mentally ill patients back with their families.

The Banyan: The Banyan is an nongovernmental organization based in Chennai India was founded in 1993. Over the past two decades, has expanded to offer a range of comprehensive mental health solutions for men and women who are either homeless, or living in a state of abject poverty.

The Live Love Laugh Foundation: It is a nonprofit organization that deals with mental health issues. It was founded in 2015 by Deepika Padukone as a nonprofit NGO to bring awareness to mental health in India.

The foundation focuses on the following objectives:

- To create awareness and reduce the stigma around depression
- To fund and support community-based mental health projects that can have a sustainable and a large-scale impact on the society.
- To support research in the area of mental health in India.
- Mental Health Agencies focusing on substance abuse problems are: Parivarthan in Maharashtra, Kripa Foundation, Alcoholics Anonymous and Samaritans. Mental Health Agencies that work on suicide prevention activities are: Sneha (Chennai), Saarthak (Delhi), Suicide Prevention India Foundation (SPIF).

Activities and Programs of Mental Health Agencies

The activities and programs of mental health agencies are classified under four major headings. Those are:

- Treatment, care and rehabilitation
- Community-based activities and prevention
- Research and training
- Advocacy and empowerment

Treatment, Care and Rehabilitation

The programs include a spectrum of activities such as individual and group counseling, vocational rehabilitation and livelihood skills training, cognitive retraining, family support and counseling, self-help groups, recreation and leisure activities

Out-patient clinics, in-patient care, day care programs and long-term residential care like community-based rehabilitations within this spectrum of services, a range of treatments including drug and psychological treatments are offered.

Community-based Activities and Prevention

Primary prevention activities like crises intervention, identification of stressors, telephone helplines for depressed and suicidal persons, educational programs in schools and workplace for prevention of substance abuse. Secondary and tertiary prevention includes screening and prompt treatment. Community-based rehabilitation programs for child and adult mental disabilities, SCARF's vocational support activities and telemedicine to expand access to specialist in rural areas. Comprehensive service for the 'wandering' mentally ill.

Research and Training

SCARF's studies on schizophrenia is the most widely cited research in developing countries. Sangath's studies on the treatment of depression are amongst the largest such studies from India. Ashagram's community program for schizophrenia has generated the first scientific evidence of the use of the community-based approach for rehabilitation of a mental disorder.

Advocacy and Empowerment

Raises awareness in different sectors of community. Documentation and dissemination of relevant facts and research for changes in law, e.g., Inclusion of mental disability in the disability legislation of India. SCARF organized a film festival called the "Frame of Mind" which features several short films on mental health and stigma. Support groups for Alcoholism, Schizophrenia, Alzheimer's disease and Autism.

Strengths of Mental Health Agencies

- **Working in partnerships:** It has ability to strike up collaborations and partnerships with other agencies or individuals with ease.

Most acute treatment (short-term)	• Locked inpatient unit • 24-hour crisis bed
Intensive outpatient treatment (usually short-term)	• Partial hospitalization programme (PHP) • Psychiatric home care • Assertive community treatment (ACT) • Intensive substance abuse programme
Transitional outpatient treatment (usually long-term)	• Psychosocial rehabilitation programme (PRP) • Clinical case management
Ongoing outpatient treatment (long-term)	• Community mental health center (CMHC) • Private therapist office

Fig. 12.3: Types of mental health services.

- **Innovations in practice:** Mental Health Agencies are, typically, closer to the community they serve and hence in a better position to be more sensitive to changing needs and perceptions.
- **Transparency in administration:** The activities of Mental Health Agencies are driven not by profit but by the desire to achieve a basic quality of care for all clients, irrespective of their ability to pay. Different types of mental health services are depicted in **Figure 12.3**.

Limitations of Mental Health Agencies

- **Sustainability:** A key problem facing most is the source of their funding. Staff members have no guarantee of employment beyond a defined project period.
- **Accountability:** There has been considerable public concern regarding the misuse of funds and lack of financial accountability of agency in general.
- **Scope:** The most important limitation is the limited scope of individual in mental health agencies. The world of most mental health agencies is confined to a city or a few villages.

ROLE OF COMMUNITY HEALTH NURSE

Community mental health nursing is the application of specialized knowledge to populations and communities to promote and maintain mental health and to rehabilitate population at risk that continue to have residual effects of mental illness.

Community mental health nursing is differing from hospital set-up. The community settings requires that the psychiatric nurse possess knowledge about a broad array of community resources and be flexible in approaching problems related to individual psychiatric symptoms, family and support symptoms and basic living needs such as housing and financial support.

Attributes

- Awareness of strength and weakness of self
- Nonjudgmental attitude
- Problem solving skill
- Knowledge of community resources
- Understanding the social values, culture and political issues
- Coordinator with different available services.

Carr et al. (1984) have identified the following roles for nurses working in community mental health services:

- **Consultative role:** This means giving advice to other professionals in the community about the type and level of nursing care required for a group.
- **Clinician role:** Providing direct nursing care to the patients in the community.
- **Therapeutic role:** Employing psychotherapeutic and behavioral methods for management of patients.
- **Assessor:** The nurse may assess the care given to the client/group and may also assess the outcome of ongoing care process.
- **Educator:** Creating awareness in the community about mental health and mental illness with special focus on vulnerable groups.
- **Trainer:** Training of paraprofessionals, community leaders, school teachers and other caregiving professionals in the community.
- **Manager/administrator:** Management of resources, planning and coordination.
- **Domiciliary care:** Services are provided to the client by visiting their homes. Services like administration of medication, assessment of level of the functioning, monitoring side effect of medication, counseling of patient and their family member, etc.
- **Liaison role:** Community mental health nurse by liasoning reduces the gap between patient and hospital, client and employers, etc.
- **Preventive role:** The preventive role are primary, secondary and tertiary.

Other areas of community health psychiatric nursing are:

- Social skill training
- Anxiety management and relaxation
- Bereavement counseling
- Group meeting
- Community outreach work services
- Child care services
- Adult and elderly care services.

CHAPTER 13

Geriatric Care

INTRODUCTION TO CONCEPT OF GERIATRIC CARE

Development begins with conception and continues until death. It is gradual and continuous process and involves many complex changes in all dimensions of person through life span. There are various stages in the growth and development of human life. These stages are infant, toddler, preschooler, school age child, adolescent, adulthood, middle age, old age. Society has taught us all kinds of 'things' regarding aging, including the process of aging and 'normal' changes that occur. Most of what we hear from others comes in the form of 'myths' of normal aging. Knowledge of these myths makes aging a fearful, unhappy approaching event for many of us. However, it should be the sight of a new beginning. Understanding the aging process; what, why, and how changes occur; and strategies to prepare ourselves for these changes gives new life and appeal to a very special time in all our lives. There is a growing appreciation that everyone does not age in the same way or at the same rate. Many of the changes that occur from aging result from a gradual loss. These losses often begin in early adulthood, but thanks to the ability of our organs to adjust and maintain health, the actual loss is not experienced until it is fairly extensive. Most organs seem to lose function at about one percent a year, beginning around age 30. Interestingly enough, the majority of these changes are not seen until after age 70. The biggest difference in the rate of aging and organ efficiency lies in the presence of disease and/or the ability of the body to adapt to external stress. Changes that occur with aging fall into three categories: physical, psychological, and social. As changes begin to happen in one area of a person's life, most likely the other two will be affected as well. There is a wide variation among individuals in the rate of aging and, within the same person, different organ systems age at different rates. However, we all experience common changes to some degree. How our age can be a result of our diet, exercise, personal habits, and psychosocial factors. An important fact to remember is that biological age does not equal to chronological age.

The study of the physical and psychological changes which are incident to old age is called gerontology. It is the study of the aging process including clinical, psychological, economical and social problems of older, adults and society. Thus geriatrics is the medical specialty that deals with physiology of aging and with the diagnosis and treatment of diseases affecting the aged. It is the branch of medicine dealing with the problems of aging and the disease of the elderly. The care given to the elderly is called geriatric nursing.

Definition

Geriatrics is the branch of medicine dealing with the physiological and psychological aspects of aging, with diagnosis and treatment of diseases affecting older adult.

Gerontology is the study of all aspects of an aging process and its consequences.

Geriatric nursing is concerned with assessment of health and functional status of older adult, diagnosis, plan and implementation of health care service to meet the identified needs and evaluating the effectiveness of such care. It is the nursing care and the services provided to older adults. The aim of geriatric nursing is 'to safeguard and increase health to the extent possible and to provide comfort and care to the extent necessary'.

SENIOR CITIZEN IN INDIA—AN INDIAN SCENARIO

Population aging is one of the most discussed global phenomena in the present century. Countries with a large population like India have a large number of people now aged 60 years or more. The population over the age of 60 years has tripled in last 50 years in India and will relentlessly increase in the near future. The world is aging rapidly. According to IJRSMS, April–June 2014, In every 8 seconds, a baby boomer turns 60 in the world; by the end of 2015 nearly 15% of our population will be over 65 years of age. People aged 60 and older in World make up over 11%. According to 2011 census of India the elderly age group population are 8% and in Odisha 9.3% of total population. As per WHO health statistics, 2015 At present 95 million people in India are above the age of 60. It's estimated that near about 8 million people are currently above the age of 80 years. The Indian Express, 2012 had published the US census bureau report which states that India's older population is projected to quadruple by mid-century, while that of the world is expected to triple. Although China and India are the world's most populous countries, their older populations do not represent large percentages of their total populations today. Both countries are projected to undergo more rapid aging by 2050; the population of China and India will be around 350 million and 240 million in the age group of 65 and above respectively.

Reasons for Aging Population

The reasons for increase in the size of elderly people are:

Improvement in sanitation, housing, nutrition and medical innovations, including vaccination and the discovery of antibiotics which prevent disease and increases longevity of life. Today many people are living into their 70's and 80's.

Aims of Geriatric Nursing

- Make the client to accept the emergency need
- Need for referral or further treatment
- Help the client to adaptively cope
- Solve the problem of an individual
- Return to normal level of functioning.

Goals of Geriatric Nursing

- Assist older people in achieving optimal health, well-being quality of life.
- Nursing care of the older person is increasingly acknowledged that a nursing specialty requiring specific professional knowledge, skills and carrier structure.
- Nurses need to be prepared to understand aging process, health and nursing needs of elderly.
- Nursing care services need restructuring that will help elderly people in achieving health and longevity and independence.
- Nurses need to take active part in policy making including the allocation of resources within the health and social action.
- Maintain the client physiologic reserves carefully.
- Prevent multi system complication. Teach client and family members what symptoms to report to the health care provider.
- Provide safe and cultured environment with comfortable temperature, good lighting. Teach safety measures in the home.
- Allow the client extra time to carryout activities particularly those require physical coordination.
- Encourage independence, teach the family to allow the client to provide self care independently.
- Beware of stereotype of aging. Treat each client as a unique person.
- The major role of nurse for geriatrics.

THEORIES OF AGING

Aging is a normal process of human development. Patterns of aging is what happens, how and when that present vary greatly among older people. Various theories have been proposed to explain the process of normal aging.

BIOLOGICAL THEORIES

Biological theories attempt to explain physical aging as an involuntary process which leads to cumulative changes in cells, tissues and fluids. Intrinsic biological theories changes arise from internal predetermined causes. Extrinsic biological theories tell that environmental factors lead to structural changes which in turn cause degenerative changes. The important biological theories are as follows.

Telomeric Theory

This is an extension of the 'Hayflick Limit.' Telomeres are specialized DNA sequences at the end of chromosomes protect the ends of chromosomes from becoming frayed or tangled.

They shorten with each cell division. When the telomeres become too short, the cell enters the senescence stage. In the normal process of DNA replication, the end of the chromosome is not copied exactly, which leaves an unreplicated gap. The enzyme, telomerase, fills the gap by attaching bases to the end of the chromosomes **Figure 13.1.** As long as the cells have enough telomerase to do the job, they keep the telomeres long enough to prevent any important information from being lost as they go through each replication. With time, telomerase levels decrease. With decreasing telomerase levels, the telomeres become shorter and shorter.

Shortened telomeres are found in:

- Atherosclerosis
- Heart disease
- Hepatitis
- Cirrhosis.

The Programmed Theory/Biological Clock Theory

The programmed theory proposes that every person has a "Biologic clock" that starts ticking at the time of conception. In this theory each individual has a genetic program specifying an unknown but predetermined number of cell divisions. As the program plays out, the person experiences predictable changes such as atrophy of the thymus, menopause, skin

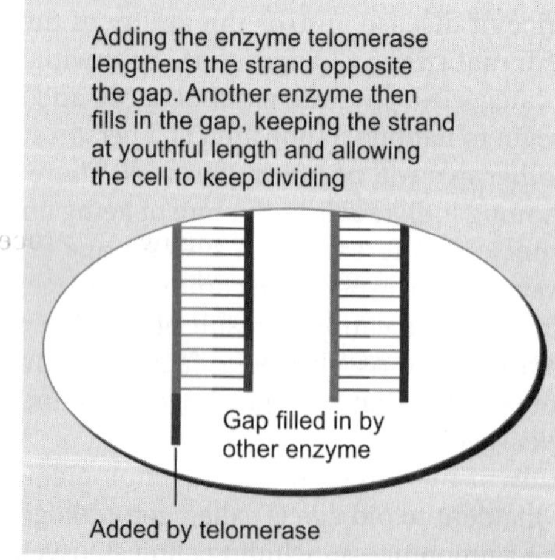

Fig. 13.1: DNA sequences at the end of chromosomes.

changes and graying of the hair. Aging has a biological timetable or internal biological clock.

Genetic Theory

Every person has a limited amount of genetic material that will run out over time. All events are specifically programmed into genome and are sequentially activated. After maturation genes have been activated, there are no more programs to be played and as cells age there may be chance of inactivation of genes. There is also the existence of one or more harmful genes that activate overtime, resulting in the typical changes seen with aging and limiting the life span of the individual. Organism failure occurs in later life because of the presence of imperfect genes activated over lengthy periods of time. Two gene types, one supports growth and vigor, and the other supports senescence and deterioration.

Molecular Theories

The aging is controlled by genetic materials that are encoded to predetermine both growth and decline.
- The error theory
- The somatic mutation theory.

The Error Theory

The error theory proposes that errors in ribonucleic acid protein synthesis cause errors to occur in cells in the body, resulting in a progressive decline in biologic function. Aging is a result of internal or external assaults that damage cells or organs so they can no longer function properly.

The Somatic Mutation Theory

Genetic mutations occur and accumulate with age in the somatic cell causing the cell to deteriorate and malfunction accumulation of mutations result in damage to the DNA. The theory states that aging is an imbalance between DNA's ability to repair itself and accumulating DNA damage. When the damage exceeds the repair, the cell malfunctions and this can lead to senescence. This theory also proposes that aging result from deoxyribonucleic acid (DNA) damage caused by exposure to chemicals or radiation and this damage causes chromosomal abnormalities that lead to disease or loss of function later in life. Exposure to X-ray radiation and or chemicals can induce chromosomal abnormalities.

Cellular Theories

The cellular theories propose that aging is a process that occurs because of cell damage. When enough cells are damaged, overall functioning of the body is decreased. The free radical theory, crosslink or connective tissue theory, Clinker theory and wear and tear theory have been included in this group.

The Free Radical Theory (by Denham Harman 1956)

During aging, damage produced by free radicals cause cells and organs to stop functioning. The term free radical describes any molecule that has a free electron, and this property makes it react with healthy molecules in a destructive way. It states that increased unstable free radicals produce effects harmful to biological systems such as chromosomal changes, pigment accumulation and collagen alteration. The free radicals are derived from environmental pollutants, oxidation of dietary fat, protein, carbohydrate and elements. A free radical is a molecule with an unpaired, highly reactive electron. One type of very reactive free radical is the oxygen free radical, which may be produced during metabolism of fat or as a result of environmental pollution. Free radical molecule creates an extra negative charge. This unbalanced energy makes the free radical bind itself to another balanced molecule as it tries to steal electrons.

The Crosslink or Connective Tissue Theory/ Glycosylation Theory of Aging

In this theory, strong chemical bonding between organic molecules in the body causes increased stiffness, chemical instability, instability of connective tissue and DNA. Organic molecules derived from lipid proteins, carbohydrates and nucleic acids. The accumulation of cross-linked proteins damages cells and tissue, slowing down bodily processes. Example, non-enzymatic glycosylation reactions occur when glucose molecules attach to proteins causing a chain of chemical reactions resulting in a structural change to the proteins, i.e., loss of flexibility of connective tissue and microvascular changes in arteries. Cell molecules from DNA and connective tissue interact with free radicals to cause bonds that decrease the ability of tissue to replace itself. The results in the skin changes typically attributed to aging such as dryness, wrinkles, and loss of elasticity. Fibrous tendons, loosening teeth, diminished elasticity of arterial walls and decreased efficiency of lungs and GI tract. It is the binding of glucose (simple sugars) to protein, (a process that occurs under the presence of oxygen) that causes various problems.

The Clinker Theory

According to this theory some potentially harmful substances accumulate in the body of aging person over the years. One substance that has been identified as *lipofuscin* which is a mixture of chemical waste products from normal cellular activities that becomes concentrated in the cells of the body, e.g., heart and brain. High Lipofuscin concentrations make cells appear darker in color age pigment. Accumulation of glucose has also been implicated in causing age changes—it binds to molecules causing them to stick together. Another substance that accumulates between cells with age is a protein called *amyloid.* In some disease conditions (*amyloidosis*) its concentrations become excessive and interferes with normal organ function. Amyloid is found in high concentrations in the brains of ALZHEIMER'S disease patients. The Clinker theory combines the somatic mutation, free radical and crosslink theories to suggest that chemicals produced by metabolism accumulate in normal cells and cause damage to body organs such as the muscles, heart, nerves and brain.

The Wear and Tear Theory

Body is similar to a machine, which loses function when its parts wear out. Wear and Tear theory says due to repeated injury or over use, internal and external stressors (physical, psychological, social and environmental) including trauma, chemicals and build up of naturally occurring wastes, body cells structures and functions wear out or are over used. Effects from the residual damage accumulate and the body can no longer resist stress. Good health maintenance practices will reduce the rate of wear and tear, resulting in longer and better body function.

The Neuroendocrine Theory

This theory elaborates on wear and tear by focusing on the neuroendocrine system. This system is a complicated network of biochemicals that govern the release of hormones which are altered by hypothalamus. The hypothalamus controls various chain-reactions to instruct other organs and glands to release their hormones, etc. The hypothalamus also responds to the body hormone levels as a guide to the overall hormonal activity. Accordingly, as ages the secretion of many hormones declines and their effectiveness is also reduced due to the receptors down-grading. Hormones effects growth, metabolism, temperature, inflammation and stress. This theory highlights due to hormonal change's there is changing in aging process, e.g., menopause.

Immunological Theory

The immunologic theory proposes that aging is a function of changes in the immune system. An aging immune system is less able to distinguish body cells from foreign cells. The immune system weakens over time, making an aging person more susceptible to disease, increase in autoimmune disease and allergies Over time, cells involved in immune function are less self-regulatory, resulting in cells being misidentified as foreign material and being attacked by the immune system's own defenses. This leads to diseases such as diabetes mellitus, rheumatic heart disease and arthritis. There are several erratic, cellular mechanism capable of precipitating attack on various tissues through auto aggression or immuno-deficiencies. The weight of thymus gland decreases with age.

The Mitochondrial Decline Theory

The power producing organelles are mitochondria. Their primary job is to create Adenosine Triphosphate (ATP) and they do so in the various energy cycles that involve nutrients such as Acetyl-L-Carnitine, CoQ10 (Idebenone), NADH and some B vitamins, etc. Enhancement and protection of the mitochondria is an essential part of preventing and slowing aging.

The Membrane Theory of Aging

This theory has been stated by Professor Imre Zs. It is the age-related changes of the cells ability to transfer chemicals, heat and electrical processes that impair it. As older the cell membrane becomes less lipid (less watery and more solid). This impedes its efficiency to conduct normal function and in particular there is a toxic accumulation.

Rate-of-Living Theory

Rate-of-Living theory says the greater an organism's basal metabolic rate, the shorter the life span. Free radicals or other metabolic by-products play a role in senescence. Example, animals with the most rapid metabolisms tend to have the shortest lifespans, i.e., birds have a shorter lifespan than humans. Studies examining the relationship between metabolic rates and longevity have produced inconsistent results, limiting the usefulness of this theory.

PSYCHOSOCIAL THEORIES

Psychosocial theories of aging attempt to explain changes in behavior, roles and relationship that occur as individual age. This attempt to predict and explain the social interactions and roles that contribute to successful adjustment to old age in older adults.

It tries to explain age-related changes in cognitive function such as intelligence, memory learning and problem solving. Sociological theory attempts to explain changes that affect socialization and life satisfaction.

Disengagement Theory

Cummings and Henry (1961) states that aging people withdraw from customary roles and engage in more introspective, self-focused activities. The disengagement theory was developed to explain why aging process separate from the mainstream of society. This theory proposes that older people are systematically separated, excluded, or disengaged from society because they are not perceived to be of benefit to the society as a whole. This theory further proposes that older adults desire to withdraw from society as they age, so the disengagement is mutually beneficial.

The Activity Theory

This theory proposes that activity is necessary for successful aging. The activity theory occurs when individuals engage in a full day of activities and maintain a level of productivity to age successfully. The activity theory basically says: The more you do, the better you will age. It makes a certain kind of sense, too. People who remain active and engaged tend to be happier, healthier, and more in touch with what is going on around them. Same goes for people of any age. Active participation in physical and mental activities helps maintain functioning well into old age. Purposeful activities and interactions that promote self-esteem improve overall satisfaction with life, even at the older age. The continuation of activities performed during middle age is necessary for successful aging (Lemon, Bengston and Peterson, 1972).

The Continuity Theory

The continuity theory states that individuals who age successfully continue habits, preferences, lifestyle, and relationships through midlife and later. Again, this theory makes a certain kind of intuitive sense. People who are doing well in midlife, who are happy, healthy, and just plain dandy should carry over the habits and ideals that made them that way. Basically, good stuff should be continued because it's good stuff!

This theory state that personality remains the same and the behaviors become more predictable as people ages. Personality and behavior pattern developed during a life time determine the degree of engagement and activity in older adulthood. Personality is a critical factor in determining the relationship between role activity and life satisfaction (Neugarten, 1964).

The Subculture Theory

Rose (1965) theorized that older adults from a unique subculture within society to defend against society's negative attitude toward aging and the accompanying loss of status. Older adults are a subculture with their own norms and beliefs. The subculture occurs as a response to loss of status. In the subculture, individual status is based on health and mobility, instead of on education, occupation and economic achievement.

DEVELOPMENTAL THEORIES

These theories trace personality and personal adjustment throughout a person's life. Many of these theories are specific in identifying life-oriented tasks for the aging person. These theories are Erikson's theory of development, Havighurst's theory, Newman's theory, Peck's theory and Jung's theory.

Erikson's Theory

Erickson's (1963) theory identifies eight stages of developmental tasks that an individual must comfort throughout the life span:

- Trust versus mistrust
- Autonomy versus shame and doubt
- Initiative versus guilt
- Industry versus inferiority
- Identity versus identity confusion
- Intimacy versus isolation
- Generativity versus stagnation
- Integrity versus despair.

The last of these stages is the domain of late adulthood, but failure to achieve success in tasks earlier in life can cause problems later in life. Adulthood is characterized by a struggle between 'Generativity' and Stagnation.

Generativity

Generativity indicates here:

- Giving back to society by raising children
- Being productive at work
- Being involved in the community
- Guiding, parenting, and monitoring the next generation.

Stagnation

Stagnation means being unproductive feeling anger, hurt and self absorption. As one becomes mature, there is a struggle between 'Ego Integrity' and despair 'Ego Integrity' means exploring life as a retired person who is not identified with an occupations contemplating accomplishment and feeling life is successful.

Despair

When anybody not accomplishing life goals feeling guilty about the past. The final pathway dissatisfied which leads to despair and further leads to depression and hopelessness respectively. The stage pertaining to older adults is: Ego integrity versus Despair. The task of this stage is acceptance of one's life as meaningful and that death is part of life, versus despair, which is failure to accept the meaningfulness of one's life, along with fear of death.

Peck's Theory

- Peck expanded Erikson's theory and focused more on later developmental stages. Body transcendence versus body preoccupation is a phase concerned with enjoyment of life in the face of physical discomforts associated with aging.
- Ego transcendence versus ego preoccupation is a phase concerned with the older adult's ability to focus on the welfare of the future generation.

Robert Peck

Robert Peck stated that the elderly go through three developmental stages to reach full psychosocial development.

- **Stage 1:** Ego Differentiation vs. Work Role Preoccupation other than on one's own inevitable death.
- **Stage 2:** Body Transcendence vs. Body Preoccupation
- **Stage 3:** Ego Transcendence vs. Ego Preoccupation.

Ego Differentiation vs. Work Role Preoccupation

As a person matures, that person moves from 'Work Role Preoccupation' which is a concept that describes defining oneself through work or an occupation. A person finds new meaning and value in his or her life. This process is called 'Ego Differentiation. 'Ego Differentiation is concerned with the value a person places on a job and to a certain extent, the family. Need to prevent feelings of uselessness and loss of ego integrity that can occur with retirement. Retirement can disrupt functioning if ego integrity mainly met through work. Activities other than work needed to provide a sense of continued value to self and to society'.

Body Transcendence vs. Body Preoccupation

Body Transcendence vs. Body Preoccupation suggests that a person either accepts the limitations that accompanies the aging process (Body Transcendence) or dwells on diminishing abilities (Body Preoccupation). Here the older person must see beyond physical aging and appreciate satisfaction in other areas. Emphasize other abilities—cognitive and social skills to compensate for physical changes, enjoy life to the fullest despite minor physical limitations.

Ego Transcendence vs. Ego Preoccupation

Ego Transcendence vs. Ego Preoccupation means if a person believes his or her life has worth and 'life contributions' will live on after death, the person experiences 'Ego Transcendence.' Otherwise, the person may feel that he or she has lived a useless life and experience 'Ego Preoccupation.' It is possible if self-examination occurs. The person may be:

- Devote energies to the welfare of future generations
- Avoid being overly concerned with self
- Realizes that death is natural and inevitable
- Remains active and works to make the world a better place in which to live
- Leaves a personal legacy to be admired by others.

Havighurst Theory

- Havighurst's (1968) theory details the process of aging and defines specific task for late life, including adjusting to decreased physical strength and health, adjusting to retirement and decreased income, adjusting to the loss of a spouse, establishing a relationship with one's age group, adapting to social roles in a flexible way, and establishing satisfactory living arrangements.
- Later maturity is Havighurst's term for older adults. The task for later maturity is disengagement. Disengagement from tasks of middle age allows involvement in new roles such as grandparent, citizen, friend.

Jung's Theory

Jung's theory proposes that the development continues throughout life by a process of searching, questioning and setting goals that are consistent with the individual's personality. As individuals age, they go through a reevaluation stage at midlife, at which point they realize there are many things they have not done. At this age they begin to question whether the decision and choices they have made were the right choices for them. This is so called "midlife crisis", which can lead to radical career or lifestyle changes or acceptance of the self as is. As aging continues, Jung proposes that the individual is likely to shift from an outward focus (wit concerns about success and social position) to a more inward focus. Successful aging includes acceptance and valuing of the self without regard to the view of others.

AGING MYTHS AND FACTS

- **Myth:** Most people aged 65 and older have moderate or severe memory impairment.
- **Fact:** Although short-term memory declines, long-term memory remains fairly intact.
- **Myth:** Most people aged 65 and older have a moderate or severe disability.
- **Fact:** The majority of people aged 65 and older are not disabled, and the percentage with a disability has decreased from 24% of Americans in 1982 to 21% by 1994.
- **Myth:** If you live long enough, you will end up in a nursing home.
- **Fact:** Overall, less than 5% of people aged 65 and older live in a nursing home.
- **Myth:** You cannot teach an old dog new tricks.
- **Fact:** Older people can learn if given a bit more time. They are more detail oriented and careful.
- **Myth:** Older people have no interest in or capacity for sex.
- **Fact:** Although sexual capacity declines with age, it does not disappear.
- **Myth:** People aged 65 and older are too old to take part in an exercise or weight lifting program.
- **Fact:** Physical activity at any age can strengthen the heart, lungs, and muscles. Exercise may also lower blood pressure and help slow bone loss.
- **Myth:** If an older person has been a life-long smoker, quitting will not make a difference late in life.
- **Fact:** It is never too late to quit. Breathing should become easier and blood flow to arms and legs increases when a smoker of any age quits.
- **Myth:** The older a person gets, the less sleep he or she needs.
- **Fact:** In later life, the quality of sleep changes, not total sleep time needed. Waking up tired is not normal and can be helped.
- **Myth:** Older drivers have most of the driving accidents.
- **Fact:** Older drivers have fewer accidents per miles driven and tend to avoid speeding and driving at night. However, people aged over 70 are more likely to die from crash injuries and should have their vision and hearing checked regularly.
- **Myth:** Older people do not need to worry about getting AIDS.
- **Fact:** About 10% of all people with AIDS in the United States were 50 when first diagnosed. This means older people need to take the same precautions as younger people.
- **Myth:** Heart disease is a man's disease and osteoporosis is a woman's disease.
- **Fact:** Heart disease is the number one killer of both women and men. Women are at special risk for osteoporosis, but one in five Americans with or at risk of developing the disease are men.
- **Myth:** Older people tend to become slow, grumpy, and set in their ways.
- **Fact:** Personality is one of the constants of life. As they age, people are likely to be have as they have since becoming adults. We all experience sensory losses, including changes in vision, hearing, sense of taste, and sense of smell. These changes are gradual, barring disease, and occur at different rates and degrees from person to person. Age-related changes do not affect the ability to enjoy life. If personality seems to be changing significantly; sensory changes, depression, or reactions to medication may be the cause.

FACTORS WHICH INFLUENCE AGING

Aging proceeds due to number of hereditary and environmental factors.

Hereditary Factors

The possibility of survival into old age is determined by hereditary factors. Some families are more long lived than others, given the same circumstances. A preposition to certain disease and physical strength determines health and vitality and have genetic basis.

Environmental Factors

Three types of environmental factors which can influence rate of aging in human and they are:
- Abiotic factors
- Biotic factors
- Socioeconomic factors.

Abiotic Factors

Those physical and chemical components of environment, such as climatic influences, pollutants and radiation.

Biotic Factors

Which result from the influences of living organism, these organism share man's environment. The aging process is affected by such things like pathogens, parasites and quality or availability of food products.

Socioeconomic Factors

Sometimes responsible for adverse living or working condition which increase wear and tear stressful living conditions are accelerate the process of aging.

NORMAL CHANGES IN AGING

Gradual reduction in the number of normally functioning cells as the aging process continues and the ability to adapt to the environment is decreased. Physical, physiological, psychological and social activities are influenced by aging. Physical and physiological changes:
- Appearance
- Vital signs
- Protective (skin and immune protection)
- Sleep patterns
- Nutrition and metabolism
- Digestion and elimination
- Reproductive function
- Endocrine functions.
- Nervous system.

Appearance

Physical changes of aging are reflected in the appearance of individual. Skin becomes dry and wrinkled because of loss of elasticity and subcutaneous fat tissue is lost. Small skin hemorrhages are noted; these may look like small red dots just about anywhere on your body. A few of these are normal. The sweat glands also shrink, reducing sweating and making it more difficult muscles tend to become weaker is that there is less lean muscle mass and they shrink from lack of use.

For your medical provider to assess dehydration by skin alone. The result of changes in the functioning of critical body organs means that the elderly tend to become more sensitive to drugs.

Changes in Vitals

Vital sign changes are:
- Body temperature
- Respiration
- Pulse rate
- Blood pressure.

Body Temperature

The center of the thermoregulation of the body is in the hypothalamus. Content temperature is maintained in the body by various regulatory mechanisms such as vasoconstriction, vasodilatation and sweating. A number of factors contribute to a failure of efficient temperature regulation in the elderly such as reduced appreciation of cold, environmental factors like poor heating, inadequate clothing, poor nutritional status. Hypothermia is common problem. A temperature of 98.6°F by mouth for a patient whose usual temperature range is 97.8°–98°F by mouth.

Pulse Rate

Some changes in the heart take place as aging progresses. It is capable of hypertrophy in response to increased demand. In old age predisposes to development of a number of pathological lesion, especially in brain, heart and lungs. Changes in pulse rate occur as a result of changes in the blood vessels. In young person blood vessels are elastic and smooth on the inside wall. With age blood vessels work less efficiently because of *atherosclerosis and arteriosclerosis.*

The inability of the blood vessels to dilate or constrict causes the hart to work harder. The pulse may be bounding because heart is working much harder to deliver oxygenated blood to the cells of the body. Because of changes in the blood vessels, pulse may be weak and difficult to count in the extremities. Locating the vessel may be difficult because of the blood vessel stiffness. It shows the difference between feeling a pen (a stiff vessel) and a straw (a soft vessel), it would be easier to feel blood moving through the straw than the pen. It develops a number of pathological lesion, especially in brain, heart and lungs.

Respirations

There is a fall in vital capacity. The older people require to breathe more deeply in order to achieve expansion of lower lobes. Increasing rigidity of chest wall and ribcage becomes more immobile limiting the movement necessary for effective respiration. Changes in the spine and rib cage result from aging or disease can affect how the lungs expand. Respiratory rate is affected by the reduced efficiency of the lungs.

Blood Pressure

Blood pressure may become elevated because the heart is working much harder to pump blood through the blood vessels that are no longer elastic and smooth. Hypertension is a common problem in older adults. A single high measurement indicate a possible problem with heart function.

Changes in Protective Function

Normal aging of the skin is influenced by factors such as:

- Age and heredity
- Diet
- Health status
- Environment.

Skin becomes drier and more fragile with age due to the loss of moisture. Wrinkles and lines appear, the skin may sag. When care for the person it needs gentleness because the skin can tear easily and provide an entrance for harmful microorganism into the body.

Along with the changes hair becomes thinner especially in male. Loss of subcutaneous fat offers insulation against old. Older adult may feel cold than a younger person. They need enough covering to keep them warm and comfortable.

Immune system is less efficient may prone to disease caused by harmful microorganism. Immune system can be protected when the older is protected by taking vaccine against influenza. Practice hand-washing is to prevent the spread of microorganisms.

Changes in the Senses

Vision

Eye becomes less able to focus on object. This condition is called presbyopia. Ability to read book and watch television is decreased. Eye's ability to adopt to change from light to dark decreases with age. Eyes also become sensitive to glare. Glare from sunlight, highly polished floor or mirror may be painful to the elderly person's eyes. Changes in the peripheral vision the range of vision narrows with age, eyes may become dry as part of aging process. To understand peripheral vision, look straight ahead. Using eyes to look first to the right and then to left. Peripheral vision allows us to see danger that may not be directly in front of us.

Hearing

It becomes less acute as person ages high pitched sounds become difficult to hear, 1000 pitched sounds and voices are easier to hear. Use a low pitch when speak to patients.

Older persons lose the ability to tell from which direction a sound is coming. It needs to repeat words until patients can understand.

Accumulation of cerumen in the ear may effect elderly person's ability to hear sounds. Cerumen can be removed by irrigating (washing out) the ear. The doctor or nurse performs the irrigation.

Touch

Sense of touch may also be reduced. Person may be unable to determine the temperature the ability to detect hot or cold may also be impaired. A condition of hypothermia may occur. It needs special awareness of the possibility of an accidental burn.

Taste

The change can be part of normal aging process. Taste buds decrease in number as well as in their ability to recognize normal taste sensations. Smoking also interferes with the ability to taste food.

Smell

A decrease in the sense of smell may affect the way food tastes. The decrease in the ability to smell. The inability to smell smoke from a fire or gas leak in the home lead to tragedy. A smoke detector, low cost safety device used in the home or health care institutions.

Changes in Activity and Mobility

Bone changes depend upon the amount of bone development and type of skeleton an individual has. Women have higher incidence of osteoporosis after menopause and excessive bone loss occurs. When an individual has partial gastrectomy or received administration of corticosteroids. Lack of use of joints leads to loss of function. There is gradual reduction in power of muscles. Physical reactions becomes slower because changes in nervous system. Stamina reduced there is decreased capacity for continuous muscular effort over a period of time. Due to aging progresses, neuromuscular coordination is diminished, reducing the ability to learn new skills. There is limitation in daily routine during old age.

The ability to be active and mobile changes to a different degree in each aging. Bones and muscles change with age result in a shorter stature. Bones can become brittle due to a condition called osteoporosis. Bone becomes thin and brittle from loss of calcium, fractures can occur more easily. Take action to prevent injury to your patient muscle strength and tone are affected by a decrease in activity and mobility. Walking and performing the activities of daily living can cause fatigue. Joint stiffness especially in the early morning. This stiffness may be due to arthritis. Discomfort can limit movement in the affected extremities. It may be difficult and painful for the person to hold a cup of coffee or open a door allow more time for the patient with arthritis to complete task. Some patient require help in morning when the stiffness and pain at their highest level.

Changes in Sleep Pattern

Elderly person may sleep five or six hours per night. Help patients sleep by keeping to bed time routine as much as possible.

Changes in Nutrition and Metabolism

In old age gums recedes, causing difficulty with wearing of dentures, leading to problems of eating and speaking. Teeth are lost. Individuals who are sensitive about their appearance may avoid social contact and activities.

In the older age adequate nutrition need to have an active and healthy life. Many factors alter person's nutritional intake as well as metabolism.

- Person's appetite reduced because of decrease in the sense of taste and smell.
- Amount of saliva produced in the mouth decreases, making chewing and swallowing food more difficult. Patient may choke on food as a result of decreased saliva production.
- Need for calories decrease in the older adult.
- Inability to open packages or poor liquids to prepare meals may result in a weight loss.
- Loose dentures affect chewing ability, patient may not able to chew nutritious food like apples or meats, so intake of calories, minerals and vitamins may decrease.
- Dietary intake may be affected by a person's finances and the inability to get to a store.

Changes in Digestive and Elimination Functions

With age, the passage of food from the esophagus to the stomach may be slowed because the peristalsis that helps move the food along slows down. Changes the lining of stomach, decrease in the secretions necessary for the breakdown of food also reduce the efficiency of digestion. Peristalsis in the intestine changes resulting in constipation because fecal material is moved. Appetite also reduce sensory awareness in relation to taste and smell will contribute to the need for attention to be given to preparation of food for elderly in an attractive manner.

Kidneys atrophy in later years of life. Vascular changes may disturb renal function. Unable to control excretions is associated with age-related changes. Bladder has less capacity for holding urine. In males the prostate gland may enlarge and make emptying the bladder difficult. Constipation is common in elderly and is due to variety causes. Poor bowel function, limited diet, lacking roughage and lack of exercises can contribute to constipation more than the effects of aging. Keep fluid within patient's reach and encourage activity and movement of extremities. Encourage patients to eat the balanced diet provided by institution because it includes food that contain fiber. Fiber increases the bulk of stool and makes it softer. These actions help the stool move faster through the intestinal tract and thus prevent constipation.

Endocrinal Functions

These are affected by a loss of active cells from the gland which occurs in old age, resulting in reduced function and lowered production of hormones. Incidence of diabetes found in between 60 to 70 years of age. Early detection and treatment reduce the severity of illness to maintain health of the individual.

Changes in Nervous System

Aging causes reduction in nerve cells. Nerve conduction becomes slower reflexes are slower causing slower response to stimuli. Due to decrease blood flow to the brain causing dizziness and increased risk for fall. There is progressive loss of brain cells. All these affects the personality and mental function. Memory is shorter and forgetfulness increases. Confusion dizziness and fatigue may occur. Memory of distant past is better than recent past.

Reproductive Functions

Aging brings changes in reproductive function. Gradual decline in sexual vigor, muscle strength and active sperm. In women menstrual cycle ceases as a result of degenerative changes in ovaries, some atrophy of the vagina, uterus and breast occurs. Degenerative changes in tests and prostrate gland in man occur more gradually. Sexual activity may continue for a longer time but men becomes impotent by 75 years of age.

Changes In Psychosocial

It includes *loss of self esteem acceptance or nonacceptance of physical changes coping with personal losses slow process of information and possible depression.* Physical and environmental factor have an important influence on mental abilities. There are personality changes which effect activity and social adjustment. There are also changes in remembering, forgetting, intellectual abilities and learning abilities. The older person may become depressed for a number of reasons.

- Loss of spouse
- Decreased financial resources
- Relocation to a new home or living quarters
- Loss of usefulness to society
- Inability to live alone
- Separation from friends and family
- Inability to accept changes in the body.

Sociological Changes

Society determines the role of elderly person to a greater extent than physical and mental condition associated with aging. Retirement lead to loneliness, deprivation and is often associated with reduce income, deteriorating housing standards and a poor nutritional level. Social isolation from service and activities also changes in lifestyle, widowhood and loss of other family members and friend. Atrophy of nerve mechanism and cells affects hearing and sight and this may limit social contacts also contribute to withdrawal and isolation.

Spiritual Changes

Religious attitudes and feeling tends to increase. Attendance to religious services decrease with increasing age for many reasons.

Changes in Cognitive Function: There is a variety of changes in cognitive function associated with aging. The most common are:

Loss of memory: Changes in the ability to remember events. Short-term memory is lost. Long-term memory is usually keen. The ability to learn remains but learning may take longer because the brain may need more time to process information.

Disorientation: May experience disorientation. A change in routine or environment such as being hospitalized or admitted to nursing home in older adults. Disoriented person may not know their identity, others identity, where they are, the time (year, month, date and hour).

Disorientation is not a normal change due to aging. It may due to a disease such as Alzheimer's disease, an infection or medications. Medications can cause disorientation in following ways:

- The wrong amount was taken by the patient.
- Multiple medications react with each other in the brain.
- A side effect of the medication occurs.
- A build up of the medication occurs.

Why to Pay Attention Towards Aging Population?

Old age can no longer be ignored. Aging in and aging by itself is not a health problem. It is a gradual life long, normal irreversible, physiological process, its process however can be delayed and many of the associated problems can be prevented. It varies with each individual, the various changes takes place during the process of aging.

HEALTH PROBLEMS OF THE AGED

Problems due to the aging process:

Biological age is not identical with chronological age. Aging is an inevitable developmental phenomenon bringing along a number of changes in the physical, psychological, hormonal and the social conditions. The common problems due to aging are as follows:

- Senile cataract
- Glaucoma
- Nerve deafness
- Bony changes affecting mobility
- Emphysema
- Failure of special senses
- Changes in mental outlook.

Problems Associated with Long-term Illness

Chronic diseases are more frequent among the older people. These are:

- Degenerative disease of heart and blood vessel
- Cancer
- Accidents
- Diabetes
- Diseases of locomotor system
- Respiratory illness such as bronchitis, asthma, emphysema
- **Genitourinary system:** Enlargement of prostate, dysuria, nocturia, frequent and urgency of nutrition.

Psychological Problems

- **Mental changes:** Impaired memory, rigidity of outlook and dislike of change.
- Sexual adjustment
- Emotional disorders.

Aging and Chronic Disease

Normal age-related changes often are exacerbated by the presence of chronic disease. Chronic health problems confuse normal aging with aging by disease. The risk of these problems increases with age. Chronic disease is sometimes a fact of life with older people, whereas with younger people acute illness is more prevalent. Some people have long standing chronic illnesses that they bring along with them into older adulthood, such as diabetes, arthritis, and hypertension. These diseases already may have caused deterioration of body organs through their own mechanisms and your noncompliance with medical orders as required by your health care providers. Some of the normal aging changes also make you vulnerable to developing medical problems. Chronic illness itself often can make carrying out activities of daily living difficult, can interfere with your loss of control, and can cause depression and/or social isolation. Expenses for medical care are increased. Multiple medications are prescribed, sometimes creating more problems for the elderly person.

Selected Disruptions of the Aging Process

Alzheimer's Disease

Alzheimer's disease is an irreversible, progressive disease which affects brain function. The messages in the brain become confused and memory fails. The ability to perform ADLS decline. It is incurable can be frightening, frustrating for the patient and family. Quality nursing care is needed. Although Alzheimer's disease seems to be the catchall phrase for anyone who has become disoriented or confused, it really is a disease state in its own right. 'Dementia' is the proper terminology that refers to a group of symptoms, such as confusion, disorientation, memory loss, and behavior changes that characterize certain diseases and conditions. Dementia has a gradual onset involving the loss of brain cells that interfere with a person's intellectual capacity and her ability to function in routine daily activities. Dementia is not normal in later life. When these types of symptoms occur, a complete check-up by your physician is critical. Dementia-like symptoms can be caused by many other problems that are reversible and treatable.

Parkinson's Disease

Parkinson's disease in which muscles lose the ability to move. Disease can be traced to an imbalance in the chemicals of the brain. Patient's body movement slower, tremors appear and muscles become stiff and rigid. The muscles of the mouth are rigid, the patient may droop and difficulty swallowing. Patient may have slurred and slowed speech and develop mask-like expression on the face. Physical changes may affect patients' psychologic functioning. Patient may feel helpless or depressed. They may need counseling to help them deal with their illness.

When caring for patients with this disease keep in mind that their intelligence is not affected.

Cancer

It is a disease in which certain cells of the body change into nonfunctioning. Nonfunctioning cells can spread out to other areas of body and can affect any part or organ in the body. Care varies according to individual needs. Keep the patient comfortable and pain free. The goal of care is to help the patient remain comfortable.

Overweight and Obesity

Being overweight or obese increases your chances of dying from hypertension, type 2 diabetes, coronary heart disease, stroke, gallbladder disease, osteoarthritis, sleep apnea, respiratory problems, dyslipidemia and endometrial, breast, prostate, and colon cancers. In-depth guides and practical advice about obesity are available from the National Heart Lung and Blood Institute of the National Institutes of Health.

Tobacco

Tobacco is the single greatest preventable cause of illness and premature death in the US. Tobacco use is now called 'Tobacco dependence disease.' The Centers for Disease Control and Prevention (CDC) says that smokers who try to quit are more successful when they have the support of their physician.

Substance Abuse

Substance abuse usually means drugs and alcohol. These are two areas we do not often associate with seniors, but seniors, like young people, may self-medicate using legal and illegal drugs and alcohol, which can lead to serious health consequences. In addition, seniors may deliberately or unknowingly mix medications and use alcohol. Because of our stereotypes about senior citizens, many medical people fail to ask seniors about possible substance abuse.

HIV/AIDS

Between 11 and 15% of US AIDS cases occur in seniors over age 50. Between 1991 and 1996, AIDS in adults over 50 rose more than twice as fast as in younger adults. Seniors are unlikely to use condoms, have immune systems that naturally weaken with age, and HIV symptoms (fatigue, weight loss, dementia, skin rashes, swollen lymph nodes) are similar to symptoms that can accompany old age. Again, stereotypes about aging in terms of sexual activity and drug use keep this problem largely unrecognized. That's why seniors are not well represented in research, clinical drug trials, prevention programs and efforts at intervention.

Mental Health

Dementia is not a part of aging. Dementia can be caused by disease, reactions to medications, vision and hearing problems, infections, nutritional imbalances, diabetes, and renal failure. There are many forms of dementia (including Alzheimer's Disease) and some can be temporary. With accurate diagnosis comes management and help. The most common late-in-life mental health condition is depression. If left untreated, depression in the elderly can lead to suicide. Here is a surprising fact: The rate of suicide is higher for elderly white men than for any other age group, including adolescents.

Injury and Violence

Among seniors, falls are the leading cause of injuries, hospital admissions for trauma, and deaths due to injury. One in every three seniors (age 65 and older) will fall each year. Strategies to reduce injury include exercises to improve balance and strength and medication review. Home modifications can help reduce injury. Home security is needed to prevent intrusion. Home-based fire prevention devices should be in place and easy to use. People aged 65 and older are twice as likely to die in a home fire as the general population. Elder abuse is the mistreatment of the elderly person through physical, verbal and psychologic means. Physical abuse may take the form of hurting the person's body, sexual abuse or withholding food, clothing or medical help. Restraining the person in a bed or locking the person in a room is also a form of abuse. Not cleaning and changing a person who has been incontinent in a form of abuse. For a caregiver to abuse an elderly person is a serious offence. There are physical, psychological, exploitation, self neglect, violation of rights, sexual abuse.

GERIATRIC CARE

General Principles of Geriatric Care

- Consider Individuality. Consult his preferences. Their potentialities should be utilized. Do not attempt to alter lifelong character and behavior. Give time to listen, to learn and to adapt. Help him cope with thought of death.
- Be patient, kind and sympathetic. Communicate effectively, demonstrate respect.
- Encourage independence and encourage him to make his choices and decisions.
- Assist elderly to achieve emotional stability. Support him during his periods of anxiety. Give the person time to express his feelings. Praise their even minimal achievement.
- Stimulate mental activity and sensory input and physical activity to uplift their self esteem, self concept and confidence.
- Make elderly's stay at home interesting and lively. Arrange to have small library, indoor games, religious place for worship, celebrate festivals, take them out for some religious lectures or any visit, have pets in the house.
- Provide diversional/occupational therapy. Share your world with the elderly.
- Maintain privacy.
- Handle them gently.

- Make them comfortable by providing comfortable bed, bed linen, etc. Keep bed dry, smooth and unwrinkled.
- Encourage them to maintain body hygiene, thus regulate body temperature. Assist them to protect themselves in changing weather.
- Assist them to take care of visual, auditory and dental aids.
- Protect from injuries, falls and accidents, etc. Make arrangements of night lights or under bed lights to avoid confusion and accidents among elderly.
- Ensure adequate nutrition.
- Facilitate elimination (urine and stool). Encourage them to maintain external genitalia hygiene.
- Encourage them to do active range of motion exercises. Maintain body alignment and posture. Encourage mobility.
- Help elderly to establish good sleep patterns.
- Caution elderly about the use of drugs.
- Have them physically examined annually and whenever needed.
- Observe psychophysical changes which alter their body image and behavior.

HEALTH ASSESSMENT OF GERIATRIC

Introduction

People are very essential for rendering need-based care. The geriatric assessment is a multidimensional, multidisciplinary diagnostic instrument designed to collect data on the medical, psychosocial and functional capabilities and limitations of elderly patients. Various geriatric practitioners use the information generated to develop treatment and long-term follow-up plans, arrange for primary care and rehabilitative services, organize and facilitate the intricate process of case management, determine long-term care requirements and optimal placement, and make the best use of health care resources.

The need for such comprehensive assessment arises because of potential or actual breakdown of independent living due to aging process, vulnerability, multiple pathology, harmful effects of drugs, inadequate or lack of social and economic support.

The purposes of comprehensive assessment of elderlies are:

- To assess health and functional status.
- Identify potential and actual problems.
- Identify strengths and weaknesses
- To determine the health needs and develop program of actions to be implemented to meet their needs.

The objectives of comprehensive assessment of elderlies are:

- To prevent breakdown of independent living.
- To deal with potentials problems of breakdown for independent living.
- To deal with actual problems of independent living
- To support and rehabilitate.

Assessment Levels

The assessment of older adults by primary level, secondary level, and tertiary level. The nature and objectives of assessment may vary at each level depending upon the nature of services rendered at each level.

The Primary Level Assessment

The primary level assessment can be done within the framework of primary health care team comprising of physician community health nurse or health visitor and a social worker. In India there is no organized system of assessment of older population in the primary health care system.

At this level, a detailed first level assessment can be done which would provide base line information about elderlies regarding their health and functional status, cognitive status, factors affecting their health and functional status, social support system and financial supports, etc. Such an assessment can help in planning and providing basic health promotive, preventive and maintenance services that can be given at primary level. Those who need secondary and tertiary level services can be referred to such agencies at secondary and tertiary level.

Methods and Techniques of Assessment

The data for assessment can be gathered using different methods such as direct questioning, observation, examinations and investigations. The techniques which can be used are interviewing, self reporting, making observation, doing systematic examination and investigations. The instruments which can be used include interview schedule, questionnaire, observation check list, various examination and investigational devices, etc. There are certain specific skills, i.e., inspections, auscultation, palpation percussion, etc., are involved while doing systematic examination.

There are some difficulties in interviewing and taking history from an old person due to impaired cognition, auditory or visual sensory loss, fear of the possible consequences of the evaluation or poor physical endurance. For these reasons the elderly clients may fail to give desirable information about themselves. It is therefore useful to have relative or some significant person present at the time of health assessment, so that they can confirm, supplement and give the missing information. If the client is unable to hear, the information can be obtained in writing through questionnaire. In such situation, some of the important information should be obtained because this process is very tiring for them. The interviewer should observe both verbal and nonverbal cues to be correlated with the information obtained. The interviewer should also be alert about the information regarding difficulties expressed by the client as he/she may either minimize them to show to be independent or maximize to seek attention. Simple and direct questions should be asked.

The interview should be held in a quiet, private and comfortable place which is free from distractions. It is necessary for an interview to establish trusting and supportive relationship. The examination couch/table should be fixed at a level that the client can get on and off easily. The backrest and pillow, etc., should be at an appropriate angle to give comfortable posture as many elderly find it difficult to lie flat. While doing examination, privacy is to be maintained, adequate draping should be done, only that area of the body which is to be examined should be exposed.

The Assessment Performa/Instrument

There are a number of standardized instruments available for screening various aspects of elderlies. But it is useful to have well developed proforma to gather and record baseline information, using different methods and techniques. The extent of comprehensiveness of the proforma will depend upon the purpose and objectives of assessment. The instrument can have the various areas on which information are collected either by interview or by questionnaire and by examination. These areas can be organized in two sections. The third section can be for making assessment plan of actions and implementation, evaluation and follow-up. The assessment areas are:

Information by the Interview (i.e., History Taking)

- **General information or biodata:** These information include the name, address, sex, date of birth, marital status, educational status, past and present occupation, height and weight, the name and address of next of kin and any relevant telephone number if the elderly is living alone, hobbies and interest, use of personal devices, e.g., cane, walker, wheelchair, etc.
- **Social aspects:** A complete assessment of social aspects can be done if a social worker is there. Otherwise, when social worker is not there, the assessment can be done by community health nurse in a limited way by obtaining some of the important information as under:
  - When the elderly is living with family, the information that needs to be obtained includes family size, family composition, their general health status, occupation, leisure time activities, status of elderly in the family, his or her involvement in the household activities, family support to the elderly in daily living and functional activities, etc.
  - When the elderly is living alone, the information needs to be obtained includes family background, i.e., number of surviving members, reasons for living alone, duration of living alone, the kind of support from relatives, friends, neighbors; periodicity of contact with them.
  - **Housing condition:** These information include whether the house is rented or owned, number of rooms, facilities available, living facilities available to elderly, etc.
  - Monthly income, source of income, expenditure on various aspects.
- **Nutritional status:** The information which needs to be obtained includes—number of meals and the menu, availability of food items, difficulties faced with regard to money, efforts, availability, etc. Associated health problems interfering with ingestion, digestion and absorption of food, stability of weight, etc.
- **Activities of daily living:** According to William (1989) the activities of daily living include tasks specific to individual which are necessary to maintain personal autonomy, activities which are performed inside the house to maintain domestic equilibrium and activities performed outside the house necessary for sociability with outside the world.
- **Previous medical history:** It includes information on any significant previous illness, injury, operation, etc.
- **Current health problems:** It is advisable to draw out a list of problems to be enquired from the client. It can be related to various systems of the body.
- **Current medical treatment:** Once the problems are identified after inquiry, it is important to obtain information. Whether the client is taking any treatment, duration of treatment, from where the treatment is being taken whether, there is any improvement, how often the follow-up is done, names of prescribed drugs and nonprescribed drugs.
- **Substance abuse:** Information can be obtained regarding use of alcohol, i.e., drinking behavior and its effects. A standarised test, i.e., the Michigan Alcoholism screening Test-Geriatric version developed by Michigan University in 1991, can be used to assess the problem of alcohol use. Information can also be obtained about smoking and use of tobacco.

Cognition: It is very important to determine cognitive function of an elderly individual. Cognitive function refers to individual's ability to absorb, store, integrate and utilize information. The cognitive functions include orientation to person, time and place; memory, i.e., ability to remember three objects after 1 minute; concepts utilization, i.e., ability to understand and explain the concepts compute numbers; judgement, follow commands, write sentences, etc. Standardized instruments are available for screening cognitive functions. The commonly used instruments include Mini Mental Status Examination (MMSE) and short portable Mental Status Questionnaire (SPMSQ).

Information by Observation and Examination

The information obtained by observation and examination is objective information which based on evidence. It is observed and examined by the community health nurse, physician and a social worker. Much of the information which is taken by history taking/asking questions: can also be observed, e.g., whether the client is active, can move around with or without support, sit comfortably on chair/bed, can feed himself/herself. Observation can also be made on the client's diet, such as the type of healthy easily digestible food the client is taking, etc.

Making Assessment and Planning Action

Making assessment: Once the informations are collected, these need to be compiled and analyzed by the team to get the complete picture of health status of elderlies and the problems faced by them. The analysis will reveal the following about each elderly which can be recorded on individual assessment proforma and the elderly community as a whole by compiling the information.

- Health status of elderly
  - Healthy with no threatening problems
  - Exposed to the risk, i.e., having threatening problems
  - Having actual medical problems
  - Functional disabilities
  - Having social problems.
- The risk situation, i.e., problems related to the diet, living arrangement, family support, accident hazards, work or re-employment, finance, etc.
- The health problems as expressed by the elderly.
- The medical disabilities observed by the physician.
- The major functional disabilities.

Planning future actions: The future actions need to be planned for individual elderly and for the entire elderly community on the basis of the findings of assessment. These are:

- General health education of elderlies who are found normal and healthy to maintain their health and to be alter about any risk factors which may come up, take necessary and proper medical help during any emergency.
- Extensive health education of those who are found at risk of death with the risk factors. Health education to be given in group and individually to be more specific.
- Medical services to those who are found having medical problems. These need to include provision for consultation, further investigations and diagnosis, treatment with due consideration of the aging process.
- Follow-up service by the community health nurse. The community health nurse needs to help, guide, supervise elderlies in taking care of themselves, provides direct care and support, helps in getting social services if means and facilities permit, helps in taking help from voluntary and local social welfare agencies; helps in taking the services of specialists. She involves family members in giving care to elderlies. The periodicity and the nature of follow-up services would depend upon the condition and needs of elderlies and working situations.
- It would be better to have a clinic for elderly either independently or as part of health center to be able to give comprehensive services without any inconvenience and difficulties to the elderlies.

The Assessment at the Secondary and Tertiary Levels

At these levels, the assessment is done when the breakdown has already taken place and it requires institutionalization. The assessment consists of nursing medical, social, functional assessment and also of other specialties as indicated. It will involve medical treatment, nursing care and rehabilitation. Future plan must be worked out by the multidisciplinary team and need to be discussed with the family and/or caretaker and client if it is practicable.

Any of these screening tests can be used for Indian population. But these need to be translated and validated. The scoring must take into consideration the background of the Indian population. It is essential to take permission from the concerned authority.

Elderly members of the community make a heavy demand on most health and social service. Preventive services that help to achieve the best possible state of health and independence in old age not only add to the quality of life enjoyed by the elderly, but also reduce the demand for curative services. The identification of nursing needs in the elderly through an adequate assessment system should be done by team members using health need assessment tools. Old person requires positive approach towards health and well-being. Old person also requires promotion of health, prevention of illness, early diagnosis, treatment and rehabilitation. Needs as per changes in old age which require priority care are: monitoring health, physical, social, physiological and social health. Prevention of accidents, malnutrition, diarrhea or constipation, skin dryness or infection, mental, social or emotional problems. Rehabilitation of old age person with regard to physical care, economical and social life, mental activities. It would help to promote health and prevent illness.

Institutionalization

It means to place an individual in the care of an institution. People who live in a nursing home often prefer to be called residents. Their illness makes them unable to care for themselves at home. They do not have family or friends who can help them with ADLs. They may be disoriented and require the constant supervision available in nursing home. They are recovering from an illness or surgery for which they were hospitalized. They need physical therapy.

APPROACHES TO AGING

Medical Approach

Many hospitals now having special units for the care of the aged both in the inpatient and outpatient departments. Training is given to medical nursing and other health professionals. Health promotional and specific preventive measures such as health examination for early diagnosis and treatment are provided.

Family centered approach – family care – many of the aged are reluctant to go to institutions for the care of the aged. Thus family care is encouraged. The family care include:

- An elderly person in the family should be helped to live independently. Family member should help an elderly person to achieve a reasonable quality of life.
- Family member should understand that an elderly person has a slower pace of living. They have high level of depending because of illness and disabilities. Comfort and safety are important in day to day living.

Hence, rehabilitation and socialization has an important place of total care.

- Old person has self respect and dignity as an individual. Family environment should such that the elderly person has the feeling of physical, mental and social independence and has opportunities for mental activity and interest.
- Elderly person requires care by team members. Care of old person accordingly need to be coordinated with the activities of family members and geriatric care.
- Comprehensive assessment should be carried out which influence family environment, personal and social factors which influence needs and problems. It determined by functional ability and dependency level of the aged persons. Based on assessment specific exercise, occupation, clothing and other needs will have to be met.
- These situations will reflect his living, sleeping, cooking, laundering arrangements and facilities. Financial situation of the old age member would reflect his future care arrangement.
- Limitation of physical, mental disabilities does not imply that the individual should be patronized or treated as being incapable of normal human being feelings and responses.
- It is difficult in understanding due to loss of sensory functions and reduced comprehension. They should be encouraged to be out of bed as much as possible to promote ability and mental activity and to reduce the risk of complication such as pressure sore, contractures, dehydration thrombosis and dependency. Cleanliness and personal tidiness are important to health and safety but should not become dominating issues.
- Physical comfort and safety of the elderly is also important. Due to changes special attention should be given to care of skin, movement of joints, exposure to heat and cold and fluid intake should be adequate. Good lighting, correct height of bed, chair and other environmental features should contribute towards the safety of elder person. Infection and over medications are hazards which should kept in mind.
- Promotion of mental activity and interests of elderly may contribute to the feeling of well-being. There should be balance between shared activities and individual activities.

Community Approach

Maintenance of health and independence—health education is directed towards primary, secondary, tertiary education, primary education is provided for the prevention of disease or injury and the promotion of positive health. The elders are encouraged to participate in activities that are beneficial to health and to avoid those that are injurious.

Secondary education is concerned with early detection of signs of ill health and timely intervention and care. Tertiary education is given following disease or injury to encourage the individual return to independent existence. They are encourage to reduce excessive intake of alcohol and to give up smoking. Opportunities for health promotion such as good housing, balanced diet or education to adapt in the home environment to counteract disability. Care and cleanliness will add to a comfortable home. In the community home care services, meals on wheel services, social services and community health nursing are well provided along with other social welfare measures, supplementary persons and national assistance. There is provision for day care center, railway concession, clinics, bank interest and old age allowance, etc.

Multidisciplinary Team Work

Team conferences should be encouraged in institutions and day care centers for elders. Common goal should be shared by all the personnel giving care which avoid confusion and encourage cooperative effort in providing care. A nurse may be the team leader while caring for a technically ill. The team members should respect one another's professional expertise and avoid professional jealousies or superiorities only then the aged person can be served effectively.

There is a rise in the number of elders in 1000 community, planning and providing care for the aging population community health nurses should increase their knowledge and participate in research in aging and age-related physical and mental disorder.

The follow-up of hospitalization and the type of domiciliary care provided by the nurse will enable her to get successful support from the community and thus initiate innovative care programs for the senior citizen.

FUNCTIONS OF GERONTOLOGICAL NURSE

A nurse who has specialization in geriatrics or in the care of old people is called geriatric nurse or gerontological nurse.

- **Guiding:** Giving guidance to people of all ages regarding aging process.
- **Eliminating:** Eliminating ageism or notion of old age as disease.
- **Respecting:** Respecting the rights of old people.
- **Observing:** Observing the facilities provided to old people and improving them.
- **Noticing:** Noticing health hazards that may happen in old age and try to reduce them.
- **Teaching:** Teaching how to take care of old people, for those who are caring for them.
- **Opening Channels :** Opening the channels of developmental activities for the care of the aged.
- **Listening:** Listening attentively to the problems of old people and giving due importance to them.
- **Offering:** Offering positivism—presenting different possibilities of life.
- **Generating:** Generating energy for the participation in the care of aged and researches for new supporting techniques.
- **Implementing:** Implementing activities for rehabilitation and readjustment.

- **Coordinating:** Coordinating different services related to the care of the aged.
- **Assessing:** Assessing the needs and health of the old peoples.
- **Linking:** Linking, contacting services according to need.
- **Nurturing:** Preparing future nurses for the care of the aged.
- **Understanding:** Understanding every old person as an invaluable asset of the society.
- **Recognizing:** Recognizing the moral and religious aspects of old age and giving them recognition.
- **Supporting:** Supporting the old people in accepting realities and preparing them mentally for impending death.
- **Education and encouraging:** Educating and encouraging old people for self care.

NURSES ROLE IN HEALTH CARE OF THE ELDERLY

Nursing care is recognized as the largest single component of services required to care for elderly to contribute to the maintenance of health and prevention of disease.

Health Assessment

A Nurse should have a detailed examination of the old person and then assess his health. This includes assessment of physical, mental, social and economic resources. In the health assessment of the old persons are:

- Daily activities of living.
- Activities related to use of equipment or procedures.
- Health screening
- Laboratory tests.

Arranging/Promoting Good Nutrition

Less financial resources, change in taste, disinterest in food, loss of appetite, trouble of preparing food, non availability of foodstuff, inability to eat, necessity to change food, etc., affect the nutrition of old people.

Hence a complete nutritional assessment of the old person should be done and he should be protected from malnutrition and deficiencies by giving balanced and modified diet.

Promoting Activity and Exercise

Physical exercises and activity are the basic keys to health in old age. Through this in addition to keeping up physical ability, emotional and mental balance also are maintained.

Preventive Care of Elderly

In case of the elderly, their physical and mental safety is very important. Gerontological nurse and caregivers should pay special attention to the following safety measures:

- Protection from unhealthy environment
- Protection from mental tensions
- Special care of personal health
- Protection from physical and mental injuries, threats and fatigue
- Providing rehabilitation services.

Providing Psychological Support

The mental health of old aged person depends upon his mental status in his entire life. Loneliness, neglect, sense of uselessness or being a burden and social inactivity may create imbalance of mind in the old person.

The problem of loneliness of the old people can be solved by family counseling or by encouraging them to participate in cultural and social activities or by forming old age groups. Creating a state to utilize their experience or increasing their religious, spiritual interests and activities are also helpful in providing mental support to the old people.

The role of nurse in dealing with different for geriatrics in different condition

- **For impaired vision:** The role of nurse is to provide bright light for reading and deem light in bed room and bathroom provide safety rails to protect client from fall. Regular eye check-up and correction of eye glasses with appropriate lens and give treatment in early stage of infection.
- **For impaired hearing:** Role of nurse is to talk slowly and distinctly. Simple language and short sentences, low pitched voice and using of nonverbal communication. Periodical checkup and cleaning the auditory canal and teaching the traffic rules to avoid accident.
- **If patient is unable to recognize temperature:** Check temperature of water/liquid before giving to the patient for drinking, bath, enema, hot and cold application of skin. Do not apply hot application and pressure directly over the skin.
- **Alteration in smell and taste:** Create meal time, provide good flavor to increase appetite, create pleasant atmosphere, remove the bedpans, serve food attractively which increases appetite. Maintain good oral hygiene, check gas leaks and cylinders. Supply Vitamin B to the one who takes antibiotics.
- **In impaired skin integrity:** Nurses should give attention to pressure point, frequent change in position, soft smooth unwrinkled bed, avoid prolonged exposure to hot and cold application. Keep the skin dry and clean. Provide well-balanced diet. Intake of adequate fluid and the patient must do active and passive exercises. Avoid the application of drying agent (spirit, detergent).
- **For impaired mobility:** Active and passive exercises and physiotherapy to prevent deformity, avoid slippery surface and provide adequate light.
- **If there is impairment of nervous system:** Check the vital signs provided by hearing aids, take care of the supply of food, adequate treatment of disease condition. Administration of medication. Help the client perform activities of daily living.
- **If there is dyspnea and disease condition of heart:** Nurse is to provide complete bed rest, cardiac position, salt-free diet, TPR and BP, intake output chart. Administer oxygen inhalation, adequate treatment of disease condition.

- **Dyspnea even at rest:** Provide Fowler's position, apply suction, administer O_2, turn client every two hourly to avoid hypostatic pneumonia, steam inhalation and encourage him to drink large amount of fluid, isolate if there is infection, postural drainage to bring out secretion, vital signs check-up and adequate treatment for disease condition.
- **If there is endocrine disorder:** Daily examination of limbs for cuts, blisters, reddened areas. Do not allow the client to walk barefoot, keep the feet clean and dry, control diabetes mellitus through diet in case of noninsulin-dependent diabetes, check urine/blood sugar to evaluate dietary control. Encourage to do exercises which reduce blood glucose and to avoid smoking. In hypoglycemic condition, give sweetened drink. Administer insulin.
- **If there is alteration of GI system:** Nurse always assesses the ability of the client to swallow the food before feeling starts. Position the client in an upright position, keep the suction apparatus ready. Give mouth care before and after feeding. Encourage to take small bites of food. Give small amount in frequent intervals. Encourage large amount of fluid intake. Regular medical checkup to detect disease in early stage.
- **If there is retention of urine:** Always provide privacy, keep silence and use normal position. Keep bed pan and bathroom clean. Open the tap and the water flow which stimulates micturition reflex. Catheterization if ordered. Establish regular voiding schedule.
- **For general problems:** Relieve anxiety, reassure patient, assess the ability of client to do any activity, never leave the client alone, provide comfort, withdrawal of alcohol, provide good recreation facility, build up general health to immunity, supply balanced diet and vitamins, avoid cross-infection, regular medical checkup if there is any disease in early stage.

In the community, the nurse should assess the immediate and long-term needs/problems of the aged and their families always teaching, supportive, advising and guiding. She should plan with the family in providing total care as well as rehabilitation.

Health Teaching

The nurse should assess the immediate need/problem and to provide health teaching:

- Preservation of dignity and individuality
- Education of the patient and family
- Every client needs to educate preventive services
- Regular physical checkup
- Immunization
- Purpose of every treatment and medication
- Safety measures to prevent burn, fall, poisoning
- Good health habit
- Exercise, practice of yoga
- Rehabilitation, recreation
- Certain procedure to carry out at home
- Feeding device when patient unable to feed orally.

OLD-AGE REHABILITATION

Rehabilitation can be defined in a number of ways. Pragmatically, it can be seen as a process that aims to restore the functional capacities of a disabled person. The major goal of rehabilitation programs for older people is to assist them to manage personal activities of daily living without the assistance of another person. If this is not possible, the goal is to minimize the need for external assistance through the use of adaptive techniques and equipment. It is important for medical practitioners who work with older people to be able to recognize both a person's need for rehabilitation and his or her potential to benefit from it.

Older People Who may Benefit from Rehabilitation

Older people who may benefit from rehabilitation typically have a major disability of recent onset. They have had a stroke, hip fracture or other fracture, a fall-related injury, or a major illness (such as severe cardiac failure); or they have ongoing severe osteoarthritis or Parkinson's disease. The disability will have compromised their ability to live independently, or semi-independently.

Most older people with recent significant disability, or deterioration in a pattern of stable disability, have the potential to benefit from rehabilitation. Chronological age per se should not be a factor in determining participation in a rehabilitation program. The major consideration is the ability to benefit from rehabilitation. The prime determinants of this are the severity of the presenting disability and the extent of pre-existing disability. Severe cognitive impairment is a risk factor for a poor response to a rehabilitation program. Older people with more minor disability, as a result of wrist fracture or knee osteoarthritis, can also benefit from rehabilitation programs, often on an outpatient or domiciliary basis.

Assessment

A broad, whole-person view is obviously important when assessing an older person for rehabilitation. After interviewing and examining the patient, it is necessary to speak with family members and the patient's general practitioner. A formal assessment of the person's premorbid functional status is essential, ideally using a standardized instrument, such as the Barthel Index. If the person was not independently mobile before the current illness, a rehabilitation program is unlikely to achieve this after the illness. The present level of disability, which is a strong predictor of outcome, should also be assessed, but should not totally determine the person's suitability for a rehabilitation program.

It is essential that the underlying medical problems are identified and managed. Cardiac failure, anemia and chronic urinary sepsis are examples of conditions that negatively impact on a person's ability to participate in and benefit from a rehabilitation program. Rehabilitation is a 'highly energetic process, and to gain the most benefit, participants need to be as well and as medically stable as possible. Hearing and vision should also be assessed and corrected as far as possible to maximize the older person's ability to participate.

A cognitive assessment should also be performed on all patients being considered for a rehabilitation program. There are a variety of standardized assessment tools, but the Mini-Mental State Examination is the one most widely used in Australia. This is a screening tool rather than a diagnostic test, and the results should be interpreted carefully. For example, major language impairments will be associated with a low score irrespective of underlying cognitive function. Although poor cognitive function is associated with limited rehabilitation benefits in older people, it should not rule out an older person from an inpatient rehabilitation program.

Depression is also common in older people presenting for rehabilitation. A standardized assessment questionnaire, such as the Geriatric Depression Scale (short form) can be used to evaluate the level of mood disturbance and determine whether treatment or further psychiatric assessment is required.

Management

Rehabilitation Process

Rehabilitation for older people should have specific goals. These are most commonly mobility and self-care without the assistance of another person. The goals can be achieved most effectively by a team of health professionals from a variety of professional backgrounds working collaboratively. Key health professionals are nurses, doctors, physiotherapists, occupational therapists, speech pathologists and social workers. Methods of coordination must be in place, and these generally include formal case discussion meetings, and involving the older person and his or her family in goal setting and program design. There is strong evidence that this approach is effective.

The case reports illustrate the process of rehabilitation in older people with major disability. The essence of the process is to work towards defined rehabilitation goals, with specific and coordinated problem-solving as difficulties are encountered. While there are common elements in rehabilitation programs for older people—specifically, retraining of mobility and self-care—each rehabilitation program is individualized to satisfy the person's unique needs and desires.

Comorbid medical conditions are almost universal in older people participating in rehabilitation programs, and these can unpredictably complicate and interrupt rehabilitation. For these reasons, time-specified clinical pathways do not work well with older people. Pain should be treated, and bed rest avoided. Careful attention to care of pressure areas is often required. Half-a-century ago, Asher eloquently summed up the problems of too much bed rest: 'Look at a patient lying long in bed, the blood clotting in his veins, the lime draining from his bones, the scybala stacking up in his colon, the flesh rotting from his seat'.

In reviewing progress with rehabilitation, achievement of specific goals should be monitored. In general, the ability to achieve certain tasks tends to be regained in a defined order. For example, grooming and feeding are generally achieved early in a rehabilitation program after stroke, while stairs-climbing is a much later goal. The use of a functional assessment scale that is rescored regularly during the rehabilitation program assists this process. The Functional Independence Measure and the Barthel Index are those most widely used.

Specialized Rehabilitation Programs for Older People

An example of a specialized program is amputee rehabilitation. Because of the effects of vascular disease, older people have a much higher incidence of amputation than other age groups. Rehabilitation for older people with lower-extremity amputation follows the same principles as for other disabling illnesses.

The mobility of the older person will be much better if the knee joint can be preserved. Management of stump edema with correct bandaging, prevention of contractures and strengthening exercises should begin immediately after surgery. Fitting of a temporary prosthesis occurs as soon as feasible, and will depend on the availability of specialist prosthetic services, which are found at most rehabilitation units catering for older people. Costs of artificial limbs are heavily subsidized for older people receiving government pensions. Discharge from inpatient care occurs when the patient is able to manage semi-independently with a prosthesis or a wheel-chair.

Psychosocial Issues

Rehabilitation programs for older people also have a major psychosocial component. A major advance in recent rehabilitation practice is recognition and resolution of psychosocial issues. Assisting an older person to adapt to the consequences of a disabling illness is an essential component of the rehabilitation program, and counseling, listening and quiet encouragement are important.

Complex intergenerational issues often arise in the family setting, which may relate to the family's concern about the impact of the disability on the wider family. This is a valid concern, as most assistance for people with disability is provided by family members, particularly spouses and daughters. Often family members have been assisting an older person before the current illness and crisis, and feel burdened and fatigued. It may be possible to resolve some of these issues through discussion and provision of appropriate support services, in addition to the rehabilitation program.

Ward Setting for Rehabilitation and the Older Person

Rehabilitation should take place in a setting that is appropriate and supportive of the rehabilitation needs of older people. Wards should be designed with toilets and bathrooms close to the patients' beds and a separate dining room should be available. Ward furniture should encourage independence, with variable bed heights, chairs with arms to aid transfers (and some with variable height), and bathrooms with equipment to assist disabled people (grab rails, raised toilet seats, a chair to sit on when grooming and a mirror placed at an appropriate height). An extensive range of mobility aids should be available, including a variety of walking frames and wheel-chairs (also wheel-chairs that can be operated with one arm).

Communication

Communication with an older person's family, general practitioner and other health professionals outside the rehabilitation setting are fostered by formal meetings, which may be face-to-face or by telephone. The formal family interview is often the key setting to communicate progress with rehabilitation and to update and finalize goals. The general practitioner should be invited to participate in this dialogue, and the case-conferencing provisions of the revised Medicare Benefits Schedule (Primary Care Incentives) should assist this process.

Rehabilitation for Older People in Community Settings

Contemporary rehabilitation practice occurs in the community and other settings outside hospital, as well as in traditional inpatient rehabilitation units. Home rehabilitation is increasingly an option for older people. Studies in patients with stroke or hip fracture, and in groups of patients with a mix of disabilities, suggest that outcomes of home rehabilitation are at least equivalent to those after traditional inpatient rehabilitation. In these programs, multidisciplinary rehabilitation is provided in the home, generally with the general practitioner supervising the patient's medical care.

In patients with less severe disability, rehabilitation may be conducted and supervised mainly by a single health professional, such as a physiotherapist or a speech pathologist, who consults with other health professionals about specific issues. An example may be a nurse assisting an older person to become more independent in self-care who consults a physiotherapist or rehabilitation physician for specific help with the patient's mobility retraining.

Rehabilitation for older people should be provided on an episodic rather than a continuing basis. When goals are achieved or when it is clear that only limited improvement is possible, they should be discharged from rehabilitation. Often older people will have multiple episodes of rehabilitation in association with specific disabling health conditions.

Costs of Rehabilitation for Older People

Among older people assessed for rehabilitation, a large group will require a long period of rehabilitation to recover from their disability, or will not recover sufficiently to return home. In general, these people have severe premorbid disability, or have developed very severe physical or cognitive disability as a result of their recent illness or injury. At least, two important issues flow from this.

Firstly, a decision that a person is unsuitable for rehabilitation may not be accepted by the person or his or her family, or the referring health professionals. It is quite likely that the person has some potential to improve his or her level of functioning, even if remaining dependent. Studies after stroke confirm this, as people with all levels of disability appear to benefit from coordinated care after stroke. A more appropriate approach may be to view the person as being unsuitable for admission to an inpatient rehabilitation program, but to outline rehabilitation goals that can be achieved in other settings, such as a nursing home. These goals commonly relate to mobility, continence and self-care, and are achievable in a suitably supportive residential aged-care setting, with input from a physiotherapist or occupational therapist. Follow-up can be arranged to monitor progress with these limited goals, and to provide feedback and suggestions for further rehabilitation management to aged-care staff, the person's family and the general practitioner.

The second issue is the risk that patients with higher levels of disability will be excluded from rehabilitation services because of the perceived high cost of treatment. It is important that outcomes of rehabilitation programs for older people are monitored carefully. There will always be some patients who will not recover sufficiently to return home or to manage in a low-level residential aged-care facility (hostel), and, therefore, will require nursing home placement. In our opinion, an approximate benchmark for the proportion of older patients discharged from rehabilitation to high-level residential aged-care (nursing home) should be 10–15%. Although these patients have not been able to gain sufficient independence to live in another setting, they may still have made useful gains in mobility, continence or self-care.

Rehabilitation includes all those activities which aim at restoring the person's highest degree of independent living. Family members may require the help of physiotherapist, occupational and social worker and speech therapist. Interdependence of physical, mental and social factors in elderly can make it essential for a social worker to help the old aged in community. Rehabilitation of elderly person has to be a continuing process, which is recommended as soon as any problem arises or is identified. Rehabilitation normally requires functional loss, diseases or specific condition, mental status involving emotional problems and any sensory deprivation which cause defects in hearing, vision, touch or physical balance. Special problems, which arise, are arthritis, stroke, Parkinson's and incontinence. All require expert guidance of the rehabilitation team.

SUCCESSFUL AGING

The terms 'healthy aging' and 'optimal aging' have been proposed as alternatives to successful aging.

Successful aging consists of three components:
- Low probability of disease or disability
- High cognitive and physical function capacity
- Active engagement with life.

Six suggested dimensions of successful aging include:
- Good subjective health assessment (i.e., good self-ratings of one's health)
- Length of abled life

- Good mental health
- Objective social support
- Self-rated life satisfaction in eight domains, namely marriage, income-related work, children, friendship and social contacts, hobbies, community service activities, religion and recreation/sports.

For successful aging, a great deal of care, which includes well-balanced diet, regular exercises and prevention of injuries and infection are essential.

Diet and Feeding Pattern

- Geriatric people are more susceptible to medical problems, such as disability and disease, which can impact appetite, the ability to plan and prepare food, chewing and swallowing, self-feeding, and general nutrient intake. A nutrient-dense, plant-based diet can help prevent or support the healing of a number of disorders that impact the elderly, including macular degeneration and arthritis. The daily energy requirements for old ages are 1,600 to 2,200 calories.
- Intake of energy-rich foods, like sweets, fried or high-fat foods, cereals and starches needs to be reduced while liberal amounts of milk and milk products, fresh fruits, vegetables, particularly green leafy vegetables, should be included to meet the vitamin and mineral needs.
- An adequate intake of calcium, in particular, should be ensured to compensate for its losses.
- Food rich in fats, especially saturated fats, should be avoided and instead oils containing high levels of polyunsaturated fatty acids, such as sunflower oils, soybean oil, etc., should be used to prevent and control the condition of hypertension and other cardiovascular diseases. The foods which should be taken by a geriatric person from different food group have been depicted in **Table 13.1**.
- Intake of simple sugars should be reduced as these provide only empty calories.
- Dietary fiber has a beneficial effect in various conditions associated with aging, such as constipation, diabetes and cardiovascular diseases. Adequate amount of food rich in dietary fiber should be included in the diet.
- With the advancement of age, the capacity to digest and tolerate large meals often decreases. Therefore, the quantity of food given at a time needs to be decreased. Small frequent feeds can be encouraged to meet their nutritional needs.
- Due to the loss of teeth particularly if dentures are not used, modifications in consistency need to be done. The diet should be soft, well-cooked and should include foods that need little or no mastication, such as milk and milk products, soft cooked eggs, tender meats, gruels, soft cooked vegetables, grated salads, fruit juices, soft fruits like banana or stewed fruits.
- An increase in starchy, fiber-providing foods and a reduction in fatty and sugary foods are likely to be beneficial, particularly if individuals are overweight. However, a low-fat, high-fiber diet is not appropriate for all elderly people, especially those with repeated infections, generally poor health or a poor appetite. It is important that older people choose a nutrient rich diet, high in foods providing protein, vitamins and minerals such as milk and dairy products, meat, eggs, fish, bread, cereals, and fruit and vegetables. A varied diet will also help to ensure adequate nutritional intake. Snacks can be an important part of the diet in older age groups, particularly for those unable to cope with large meals at one sitting. The food for the elderly should be colorful, attractive and tasty and should be served in pleasant surroundings so as to arouse their appetite and interest in the food.

Using different colors and shapes in cooking can stimulate the senses and add to eating enjoyment. The addition of herbs and spices can also make food more interesting.

Table 13.1: The principles of a healthy balanced diet.

Food group	*Examples*	*Quantity*
Bread, other cereals and potatoes	Bread, pasta, rice, breakfast cereals and potatoes	These should be the main part of every meal (one third of meal)
Fruit and vegetables (fresh, frozen and canned)	Oranges, apples, bananas, carrots, peas and tomatoes	These should be a main part of every meal and at least five servings should be consumed a day
Milk and dairy foods	Milk, cheese, yogurt	Three servings a day
Meat, fish and alternatives	Chicken, eggs and fish	One or two servings a day
Foods containing fat and foods containing sugar	Crisps, fizzy drinks, sweets, butter, margarine, cakes and biscuits	Should be consumed only in moderation

Exercises

Not only food but also different types of exercises bring successful aging. Because of pain, weakness, illness or hospitalization, the majority of people in the elderly population have decreased daily activity. This inactivity can cause decreased circulation, reduced heart strength and endurance, and a compromised ability to maintain independence in functional activities. Completing daily exercise while seated allows overall health to be improved while increasing independence and decreasing fall risk. High levels of physical activity and physical fitness have been shown to lessen morbidity. A graded, inverse relationship between total physical activity and mortality has been identified. Physical activity initiated in late life continues to improve mortality, having a strong effect on longevity, even when accounting for factors, such as smoking, hypertension, family history and weight gain. Studies have demonstrated benefits for patients with conditions as varied as cardiovascular disease, respiratory disease, dementia and cancer. More recent work has demonstrated that physical activity may also offset disability. Analysis of more than 10,000 older adults participating in the Established Populations for Epidemiologic Studies of the Elderly (EPESE) demonstrated that there was an almost 2-fold increased likelihood of dying without disability among those most physically active compared to those who were sedentary. Exercises like leg exercises, arm and hand exercises, trunk exercises, can also practice by seating in a chair. Practicing of different types of asana and pranayama can also help in maintaining oneself in successful aging.

Asanas

Surya Namaskara

Surya Namaskara is a group of twelve asanas in which various categories of postures are included. Regular practice of Surya Namaskara from the time of youth lessens the trouble of old age to a great extent. Practice of Surya Namaskara may not be easy for people who are already aged but regular practice from the young age enables one to perform the postures even in a very advanced stage of life.

Pavanamuktasana

The series of asanas known by the name Pavanamuktasana are highly beneficial for the management of locomotor disorders and gastrointestinal problems of old age. During practicing, the knees and thighs are pressed against the chest and belly in this asana. The gas trapped in the large intestine gets released in this Asana. Therefore, it is called 'Pavanamuktasana.'

Ardhamatsyendrasana

It is a spinal-twisting asana. This is very beneficial in keeping the body flexible and fighting the musculoskeletal problems of old age.

Bhujangasana

Bhujangasana is a backward-bending asana which helps in fighting the problems of drooping shoulder and many other spinal disorders.

Savasana

There is no better relaxing posture than the Savasana which provides rest not only to the body but also to the mind. Savasana removes fatigue from the body and provides rest to the mind. Savasana is one of the best fighters of psychological problems, like depression and mental stress.

With the counseling of experts, the senior citizen can do other Asanas too according to his requirements and capability for specific problems in the body.

Pranayama

Pranayama is the yogic practice having tremendous preventive and curative potential for geriatric treatment especially for the psychosomatic and emotional problems.

Nadisodhana

Nadisodhana pranayama is one in which air is retained in the lungs for a specific period. As a result, even the remote corners of the capillaries are filled with oxygen. This is highly beneficial for various problems of the lungs. Filling and retention of air in the capillaries maximize the circulation of oxygen to the various parts of the body which relieves the body from complications due to insufficient supply of oxygen. Nadisodhana is highly effective in managing cardiac health problems.

Bhramari

Bhramari pranayama gives a good exercise to the brain cells by the sound vibration. This helps in the management of senile loss of memory and other related problems. It is a good practice to fight depression and is a good device to release tension and mental stress. It not only calms down the mind but also creates feeling of happiness. The pranayama is highly praised for keeping the mind cheerful.

Bhastrika

Bhastrika pranayama is highly beneficial for problems like asthma and other respiratory disorders. The yogis, who practice this Pranayama regularly experience an unspeakable happiness in their mind. While performing **Bhastrika Pranayamma** a person pumps air or prana (life force or breath) vigorously throughout the entire system.

Kriyas

Kapalabhati

Among the Kriyas, Kapalabhati is one of the best practices with multifarious benefit for the young and old alike. It is either a pranayama exercise or one of the six cleansing techniques practiced in certain levels and styles of yoga. It is highly preventive and curative for phlegmatic health problems of the body. In addition to its various health benefits, it is greatly helpful in keeping the blood pressure and blood sugar normal.

Neti

Neti kriya is another beneficial practice for the aged to fight respiratory problems.

Trataka

Trataka is immensely helpful in fighting ophthalmic problems. It is a very good practice to fight senile cataract and glaucoma.

Mudra

Khechari Mudra

Khechari Mudra is an extremely significant practice for fighting the aging process in a human body. According to the perception of a yogi, the decaying process in the body is because of the loss of the invigorating fluid oozing from the head in the body. Khechari Mudra is exclusively designed to check the flow of the fluid at its emanating place in the palate. In Khechari Mudra, one reverses the tongue and obstructs the points from where the fluid leaks out in the palate. Practice of Khechari Mudra regularly from the young age certainly delays the aging process.

Dharana and Dhyana

Dharana is to fix the mind to a particular point for a specific period. Dhyana is an advanced stage of Dharana. These two practices are extremely fruitful in managing many psychological and psychosomatic disorders of the practitioner. These two practices are greatly helpful in fighting depression and stress in old age and keeping the mind composed.

Swadhyaya

Swadhyaya is an important component of Yoga. Swadhyaya has two parts. One is a regular study habit of spiritual books. The second is repetition of sacred Mantras. Swadhyaya is a great helper in culturing spirituality and keeping the mind calm. A strong habit of Swadhyaya fights senile loss of memory and acts as an excellent dispeller of depression.

Ishvarapranidhana

Ishvarapranidhana, another great component of Yoga, is complete surrender to God. Practice of this develops spirituality in a person which provides immense strength to face complications of life with great bravery.

Keeping all the aspects in mind, providing a proper diet to the old will keep them free from most of the diseases and they would be able to lead an active and happy life. A proper diet, exercise with yoga and pranayama and a pleasant environment are important for adding healthy and happy years to the life of our elderly. Also to be borne in mind is the fact that '**Everyone of us has to reach this phenomenon of nature one day or the other, provided we are lucky enough**.'

WELFARE PROGRAMMES FOR THE OLD PEOPLES IN INDIA

Introduction

It is the fundamental obligation of the State in terms of Article 41 of our Constitution to provide assistance to the aged and pension benefits to the employees after their retirement by their employers. In India context, retirement is a symbol of old age. In the retirement process, the person pass through the following phase:

- **Remote phase:** Even when retirement is near or approaching, person does not get ready for it.
- **Near phase:** When retirement is very near, making imaginary plan for it. (Day dreaming)
- **Honeymoon phase:** Just after retirement person wants to do all those things which he could not do so far or was always desirous of doing. But health and financial resources may cause problems in fulfilling his dreams or imaginations.
- **Disenchantment phase:** The problems/realities of retired life may dispirit the person. His excessive dream regarding retired life may result in more disappointments. At this stage, person may begin to come out of false imaginations.
- **Stability phase:** Person understands the realities of retired life. He makes adjustments to his new roles.
- **Termination phase:** This happens either taking up some work again or due to illness or incapacity.

The year of the aged (1990) though celebrated in our country with great pomp and show, our government has done precious little for the upliftment of the status of the aged community.

The determination of old age is naturally linked with the average life expectancy. The United Nations had adopted International Plan of Action at the World Assembly of Aging at Vienna during 1982.

Services Available for Aging Population

Old Age Homes

The old age home is a residential unit for poor destitute aged persons of 60 years and above. Aged persons coming from lower-income groups and middle-income groups of society, in desperate need for shelter, can also be considered for admission in these Homes, subject to thorough inquiry and discretion of the voluntary organizations concerned.

Day Care Centers for the Aged

Assistance to voluntary organizations is given for maintenance of day care centers for at least 50 persons in urban/slum/rural/tribal areas. The aim of these programs is to keep the aged integrated with their respective families and to supplement the activities of family in looking after the needs of the aged.

Mobile Medicare Services for the Aged

Under this programme, grant is provided to voluntary organizations, which have experience and expertise in providing medicare services to the aged in rural/urban/slum/areas.

Noninstitutional Services for the Aged

Under this program, a social worker is appointed to provide for services to the aged like legal counseling assistance for supplying pension, GPF, HRA, Income Tax, Bank Services, etc. The scheme of assistance to Panchayati Raj institutions/voluntary organizations for construction of Old Age Homes was launched during 1996–97.

Pensionary Benefits and other Public Assistance

The aged can be divided into two categories: (i) those who have retired on attaining the age of superannuation from the government or organized sector and are entitled to pensionary benefits and (ii) those who have reached the age of 60+ and are drawing public assistance in their old age for their survival.

Article 309 of the Constitution stipulates that Acts of the appropriate Legislature may regulate the recruitment and conditions of service of persons appointed to public services in connection with the affairs of the Union or any States. The benefits available to government servants at the time of their retirement/superannuation are the pension and is governed by Central Civil Services (Pension) Rule 1952 Scheme (for nonindustrial staff except railways) and the contributory Provident Fund Scheme (for industrial staff and is governed by the Contributory Fund (India) Rules, 1962).

Voluntary Organizations for the Welfare of the Aged

Help Age India

It was established in 1978 for the cause and care of the elderly people with its head office in New Delhi. It sometimes uses the services of NSS volunteers for events like painting competition, debates, etc., and collection of funds to provide facilities to the elders. 'Adopt a Granny' scheme is intended to provide rehabilitation at the doorsteps to the elders living under poverty line.

Age Care India

It is a premier national voluntary organization for the welfare of the aged people in the country registered on 18th November 1980 as nonpolitical, nonprofit, secular, charitable, educational, cultural and social welfare organization under the Societies Registration number XXI of 1860.

It has four types of membership viz. (a) founder members; (b) life-members; (c) associate members; (d) temporary members.

It has been celebrating Elder Day on 18th November every year since '1981 to honor senior citizens above 80 years of age, to give them social recognition and respect.

Government Schemes for the Aged

The Ministry of Social Justice and Empowerment is implementing a Central Scheme of Assistance for the programmes relating to the aged from November 1992. Under the scheme, financial assistance is provided to voluntary organizations for establishing and maintaining of day care centers, old-age homes, and mobile-Medicare units as well as for supporting and strengthening non-institutional services for the aged.

Five-Year Plan and the Aged People

Programs for the Elderly will be taken up in the IX-Plan to ensure well-being and continued participation in the community. Efforts will be made to reach/disseminate information regarding various welfare measures and special concessions being extended to the 'Senior Citizens', so that the rural elderly can also come forward to enjoy these privileges along with their urban counterparts.

In extending housing facilities, the concept of 'Sheltered Homes' for the lonely/destitute Elderly will be explored with the help of private and public agencies as well as the NGOs. Protection will be provided against the dangers of life and property; abuse and exploitation of older persons.

THE NATIONAL POLICY ON OLDER PERSONS

The National Policy on Older Persons was announced by the government in 1999, declared as the International Year of Older Persons by the UN. The year 2000 has been declared as the National Year of Older Persons by the Government of India. The decision to frame a policy for older persons was first mooted in the '80s, following the World Assembly on Aging held at Vienna in 1982. In 1987–88 an Inter Ministerial Committee was constituted by the GOI for this purpose. The process of formulating the policy gathered momentum in the two years preceding 1999. According to ministry officials, the process envisaged active involvement of voluntary organizations, research bodies, schools of social work, and so on. A number of regional consultations were held along with a national level consultation to discuss the draft policy document prepared by the ministry for getting feedback from a broad range of positions and approaches.

Subsequent international efforts made an impact on the implementation of the National Policy on Older Persons. The Madrid Plan of Action and the United Nations Principles for Senior Citizens adopted by the UN General Assembly in 2002, the Proclamation on Aging and the global targets on aging for the Year 2001 adapted by the General Assembly in 1992.

The policy and plans were put in place by central and state governments for the welfare of older persons. The state governments issued their policies and programs for the welfare of older persons. While some States and Union Territories implemented their policies with vigor, most states particularly the big ones were behind perhaps due to financial and operational deficiencies.

Pensions, travel concessions, income tax relief, medical benefit, extra interest on savings, security of older persons through an integrated scheme of the Ministry of Social Justice and Empowerment as well as financial support was provided for Homes, Day Care Centers, Medical Vans, Help Lines, etc., are extended currently. The Ministry of Social Justice and Empowerment coordinates programs to be undertaken by other Ministries in their relevant areas of support to older persons.

The primary objectives of this policy are to:

- Ensure the well-being of the elderly
- Encourage families to take care of their older family members by adopting mechanisms for improving inter generational ties
- Encourage individuals to make adequate provision for their own as well as their spouse's old age.
- Provide protection on various grounds like financial security, health care, shelter and welfare, including protection against abuse and exploitation.
- Enable and support voluntary and non-governmental organizations to supplement the care provided by the family and recognizing the need for expansion of social and community services with universal accessibility.
- Provide care and protection to the vulnerable elderly people by ensuring for the elderly an equitable share in the benefits of development.

- Provide adequate healthcare facility to the elderly.
- Create awareness regarding elderly persons to help them lead productive and independent life.

Concessions and Facilities for Senior Citizens Based on the Policy 1999

Ministry of Social Justice and Empowerment

Ministry of Social Justice and Empowerment is the nodal Ministry responsible for welfare of the Senior Citizens. It has announced the National Policy on Older Persons covering all concerns pertaining to the welfare of older persons. The National Policy on Older Persons recognizes a person aged 60 years and above as a senior citizen. The Ministry is also implementing following schemes for the benefit of Senior Citizens:

- **An Integrated Programme for Older Persons (Plan Scheme):** This Scheme has been formulated by revising the earlier scheme of 'Assistance to Voluntary Organisations for Programmes relating to the Welfare of the Aged'. Under this Scheme, financial assistance up to 90% of the project cost is provided to NGOs for establishing and maintaining Old Age Homes, Day Care Centers, Mobile Medicare Units and to provide noninstitutional services to older persons.
- **The Scheme of Assistance to Panchayati Raj Institutions/Voluntary Organizations/Self-Help Groups for Construction of Old Age Homes/Multi-Service Centers for older persons (Non Plan Scheme):** Under this Scheme, one time construction grant for Old Age Homes/Multi-Service Center is provided to nongovernmental organizations on the recommendation of the State Governments/UT Administrations.

Ministry of Finance

Income tax rebate up to an income of ₹1.85 lakh p.a. Higher rates of interest on saving schemes of senior citizens. A Senior Citizens Savings Scheme offering an interest rate is 9% per annum on the deposits made by the senior citizens in post offices has been introduced by the Government through Post Offices in India doing savings bank work.

Ministry of Road Transport and Highways

Reservation of two seats for senior citizens in front row of the buses of the State Road Transport Undertakings. Some State Governments are giving fare concession to senior citizens in the State Road Transport Undertaking buses and are introducing Bus Models, which are convenient to the elderly.

Ministry of Health and Family Welfare

Separate queues for older persons in hospitals for registration and clinical examination.

Department of Telecommunications

Faults/complaints of senior citizens are given priority by registering them under senior citizens category with VIP flag, which is a priority category. Senior citizens are allowed to register telephone connection under N-OYT Special Category, which is a priority category.

Ministry of Railways

Indian Railways provide 30% fare concession in all Mail/Express including Rajdhani/Shatabdi/Jan Shatabdi trains for senior citizens aged 60 years and above. Indian Railways also have the facility of separate counters for Senior Citizens for purchase/booking/cancellation of tickets. Wheel Chairs for use of older persons are available at all junctions, District Headquarters and other important stations for the convenience of needy persons including the older persons. Ramps for wheel chairs movement are available at the entry to important stations. Specially designed coaches with provisions of space for wheelchairs, hand rail and specially designed toilet for handicapped persons have been introduced.

Ministry of Civil Aviation

Indian Airlines is providing 50 percent Senior Citizen Discount on Normal Economy Class fare for all domestic flights to Indian senior citizens who have completed the age of 65 years in the case of male senior citizens and 63 years in the case of female senior citizens subject to certain conditions. Air India is offering discount to senior citizens of 60 plus on flights to USA, UK and Europe. Further, Air India has now decided to reduce the age of 60 plus for discount on their domestic routes as well with immediate effect. Sahara Airlines is offering 50% discount on basic fare for travel on its domestic flights only to senior citizens who have attained the age of 62 years. Discount is applicable in economy class only.

Ministry of Consumer Affairs, Food and Public Distribution

Under the Antyodaya Scheme, the Below Poverty Line (BPL) families which also include older persons are provided food grains at the rate of 35 kg per family per month. The food grains are issued @ ₹3/kg for rice and ₹2/kg for wheat. The persons aged 60 years above from the BPL category were given priority for identification. Under the Annapoorna Scheme being implemented by the States/ UT Administration, 10 kg of food grains per beneficiary per month are provided free of cost to those senior citizens who remain uncovered under the old age pension scheme. Instructions to State Governments for giving priority to the Ration Card holders who are over 60 years of age in Fair Price Shops for issue of rations.

MCD, Delhi

MCD, Delhi, has opened a separate counter to facilitate the senior citizens for submission of property tax bills. A rebate of 30% of the property tax due on the covered space of a building up to one hundred sq. mtrs. of the covered space has been allowed by the corporation in the case of any self-occupied residential building singly owned by a man who is 65 years or more in age.

Miscellaneous

Courts in the country accord priority to cases involving older persons and ensures their expeditious disposal. Under the Old Age Pension Scheme, monthly pension is given at variable rates to the destitute old by various State Governments/UT Administrations.

THE NATIONAL POLICY OF SENIOR CITIZENS 2011

The foundation of the new policy, known as the 'National Policy for Senior Citizens 2011' is based on several factors. These include the demographic explosion among the elderly, the changing economy and social milieu, advancement in medical research, science and technology and high levels of destitution among the elderly rural poor (51 million elderly live below the poverty line). A higher proportion of elderly women than men experience loneliness and are dependent on children. Social deprivations and exclusion, privatization of health services and changing pattern of morbidity affect the elderly. All those of 60 years and above are senior citizens. This policy addresses issues concerning senior citizens living in urban and rural areas, special needs of the 'oldest old and older women'.

Objectives

- Strengthen integration between generations, facilitate interaction between the old and the young as well as strengthen bonds between different age groups.
- Development of a formal and informal social support system.
- Reach out in particular to the bulk of senior citizens living in rural areas.

The Focus of the New Policy

- Mainstream senior citizens, especially older women, and bring their concerns into the national development.
- Promote the concept of 'aging in place' or aging in own home, housing, income security and homecare services, old age pension and access to health care insurance schemes and other programs and services to facilitate and sustain dignity in old age. The thrust of the policy would be preventive rather than cure.
- The policy will consider institutional care as the last resort. It recognizes that care of senior citizens has to remain vested in the family which would partner the community, government and the private sector.
- Being a signatory to the Madrid Plan of Action and Barrier Free Framework it will work towards an inclusive, barrier-free and age-friendly society.
- Recognize that senior citizens are a valuable resource for the country and create an environment that provides them with equal opportunities, protects their rights and enables their full participation in society.
- Long-term savings instruments and credit activities will be promoted to reach both rural and urban areas. It will be necessary for the contributors to feel.
- Employment in income generating activities after superannuation will be encouraged.
- Support and assist organizations that provide counseling, career guidance and training services.
- States will be advised to implement the Maintenance and Welfare of Parents and Senior Citizens Act, 2007 and set-up Tribunals so that elderly parents unable to maintain themselves are not abandoned and neglected.
- States will set-up homes with assisted living facilities for abandoned senior citizens in every district of the country and there will be adequate budgetary support.

Areas of Intervention of Policy

The concerned ministries at central and state level as mentioned in the 'Implementation Section' would implement the policy and take necessary steps for senior citizens as under:

Income Security in Old Age

A major intervention required in old age relates to financial insecurity as more than two-third of the elderly live below the poverty line. It would increase with age uniformly across the country.

Indira Gandhi National Old Age Pension Scheme

- Old age pension scheme would cover all senior citizens living below the poverty line.
- Rate of monthly pension would be raised to ₹1000 per month per person and revised at intervals to prevent its deflation due to higher cost of purchasing.
- The 'oldest old' would be covered under Indira Gandhi National Old Age Pension Scheme (IGNOAPS). They would be provided additional pension in case of disability, loss of adult children and concomitant responsibility for grand children and women. This would be reviewed every five years.

Public Distribution System

The public distribution system would reach out to cover all senior citizens living below the poverty line.

Income Tax

Taxation policies would reflect sensitivity to the financial problems of senior citizens which accelerate due to very high costs of medical and nursing care, transportation and support services needed at homes.

Microfinance

Loans at reasonable rates of Interest would be offered to senior citizens to start small businesses. Microfinance for senior citizens would be supported through suitable guidelines issued by the Reserve Bank of India.

Health Care

With advancing age, senior citizens have to cope with health and associated problems some of which may be chronic, of a multiple nature, require constant attention and carry the risk of disability and consequent loss of autonomy. Some health problems, especially when accompanied by impaired functional capacity require long-term management of illness and nursing care. Health care needs of senior citizens will be given high priority.

It would have a judicious mix of public health services, health insurance, health services provided by not-for-profit organizations including trusts and charities, and private medical care. While the first of these will need to be promoted by the State, the third category given some assistance, concessions and relief and the fourth encouraged and subjected to some degree of regulation, preferably by an association of providers of private care.

Safety and Security

- Provision would be made for stringent punishment for abuse of the elderly.
- Abuse of the elderly and crimes against senior citizens especially widows and those living alone and disabled would be tackled by community awareness and policing.
- Police would be directed to keep a friendly vigil and monitor programs which will include a comprehensive plan for security of senior citizens whether living alone or as couples. They would also promote mechanisms for interaction of the elderly with neighborhood associations and enrolment in special programs in urban and rural areas.
- Protective services would be established and linked to help lines, legal aid and other measures.

Housing

- Shelter is a basic human need. The stock of housing for different income segments will be increased. Ten percent of housing schemes for urban and rural lower income segments will be earmarked for senior citizens. This will include the Indira Awas Yojana and other schemes of the government.
- Age friendly, barrier-free access will be created in buses and bus stations, railways and railway stations, airports and bus transportation within the airports, banks, hospitals, parks, places of worship, cinema halls, shopping malls and other public places that senior citizens and the disabled frequent.
- Develop housing complexes for single older men and women, and for those with need for specialized care in cities, towns and rural areas.
- Promote age friendly facilities and standards of universal design by Bureau of Indian Standards.
- Since a multi-purpose center is a necessity for social interaction of senior citizens, housing colonies would reserve sites for establishing such centers. Segregation of senior citizens in housing colonies would be discouraged and their integration into the community supported.
- Senior citizens will be given loans for purchase of houses as well as for major repairs, with easy repayment schedules.

Productive Aging

- The policy will promote measures to create avenues for continuity in employment and/or post retirement opportunities.
- Directorate of Employment would be created to enable seniors find reemployment.
- The age of retirement would be reviewed by the Ministry due to increasing longevity.

Welfare

- A welfare fund for senior citizens will be set-up by the government and revenue generated through a social security cess. The revenue generated from this would be allocated to the states in proportion to their share of senior citizens. States may also create similar funds.
- Non-institutional services by voluntary organizations will be promoted and assisted to strengthen the capacity of senior citizens and their families to deal with problems of the aging.
- All senior citizens, especially widows, single women and the 'oldest old' would be eligible for all schemes of government. They would be provided universal identity under the Aadhar scheme on priority.
- Larger budgetary allocations would be earmarked to pay attention to the special needs of rural and urban senior citizens living below the poverty line.

Multigenerational Bonding

- The policy would focus on promoting bonding of generations and multigenerational support by incorporating relevant educational material in school curriculum and promoting value education.
- Value Education modules and textbooks promoting family values of caring for parents would be promoted by NCERT and State Educational Bodies.

Media

Media has an important role to play in highlighting the changing situation of senior citizens and in identifying emerging issues and areas of action. The policy would focus on involving mass media as well as informal and traditional communication channels on aging issues, such as:

- Natural disasters/emergencies.
- Provide equal access to food, shelter, medical care and other services to senior citizens during and after natural disasters and emergencies.
- Enhance financial grants and other relief measures to assist senior citizens to re-establish and reconstruct their communities and rebuild their social fabric following emergencies.

Implementation Mechanism

There will be efforts to provide an identity for senior citizens across the country and the Aadhaar Unique identity number will be offered to them so that implementation of assistance schemes of Government of India and concessions can be offered to them. As part of the policy implementation the Government will strive for:

- **Establishment of Department of Senior Citizens under the Ministry of Social Justice and Empowerment:** The Ministry of Social Justice and Empowerment will establish a 'Department of Senior Citizens' which will be the nodal agency for implementing programs and services for senior citizens and the NPSC 2011. An interministerial committee will pursue matters relating to implementation of the national policy and monitor its progress. Coordination will be by the nodal ministry. Each ministry will prepare action plans to implement aspects that concern them and submit regular reviews.
- **Establishment of Directorates of Senior Citizens in States and Union Territories:** States and union territories will set-up separate Directorates of Senior Citizens for implementing programs and services for senior citizens and the NPSC 2011.
- **National/State Commission for Senior Citizens:** A National Commission for Senior Citizens at the center and similar commissions at the state level will be constituted. The Commissions would be set-up under and of the Parliament with powers of Civil Courts to deal with cases pertaining to violations of rights of senior citizens.

Establishment of National Council for Senior Citizens

A National Council for Senior Citizens, headed by the Minister for Social Justice and Empowerment will be constituted by the Ministry. With tenure of five years, the Council will monitor the implementation of the policy and advise the government on concerns of senior citizens. A similar body would be established in every state with the concerned minister heading the State Council for Senior Citizens.

- The Council would include representatives of relevant central ministries, the Planning Commission and ten states by rotation.
- Representatives of senior citizens associations from every state and Union Territory.
- Representatives of NGOs, academia, media and experts on aging.
- The council would meet once in six months.

Responsibility for Implementation

The Ministries of Home Affairs, Health and Family Welfare, Rural Development, Urban Development, Youth Affairs and Sports, Railways, Science and Technology, Statistics and Programme Implementation, Labour, Panchayati Raj and Departments of Elementary Education and Literacy, Secondary and Higher Education, Road Transport and Highways, Public Enterprises, Revenue, Women and Child Development, Information Technology and Personnel and Training will setup necessary mechanism for implementation of the policy. A five-year perspective Plan and annual plans setting targets and financial allocations will be prepared by each Ministry/Department. The annual report of these Ministries/Departments will indicate progress achieved during the year. This will enable monitoring by the designated authority.

Role of Block Development Offices, Panchayat Raj Institutions and Tribal Councils/Gram Sabhas

Block Development offices would appoint nodal officers to serve as a one point contact for senior citizens to ease access to pensions and handle documentation and physical presence requirements, especially by the elderly women. Panchayat Raj Institutions would be directed to implement the NPSC 2011 and address local issues and needs of the aging population. In rural/tribal areas, the tribal council or gram sabha or the relevant Panchayat Raj institution would be responsible for implementation of the policy. The provisions of the 13th Finance Commission for special funding to them would be made applicable.

Health Care Facilities

A **Health facility** is, in general, any location where health care is provided. Health facilities range from small clinics and doctor's offices to urgent care centers and large hospitals with elaborate emergency rooms and trauma centers. The number and quality of health facilities in a country or region is one common measure of that area's prosperity and quality of life. There are a variety health care facilities also available for geriatric peoples. They are:

- Geriatric clinics
- Special camps/fix day services for aged
- Separate registration and medicine counters
- Free supply of medicine to BPL elderly
- Free diagnosis/X-rays/ECG, etc./reservation of beds
- Medical insurance/mediclaim
- CGHS for some categories
- Ambulance services
- Training to medical/nursing/paramedical for care of elderly.

Legal Support

Maintenance and Welfare of Parents and Senior Citizens Act, 2007 is a legislation enacted in 2007, initiated by Ministry of Social Justice and Empowerment, Government of India to provide more effective provision for maintenance and welfare of parents and senior citizens. This Act make it a legal obligation for children and heirs to provide maintenance to senior citizens and parents, by monthly allowance. This Act also provides simple, speedy and inexpensive mechanism for the protection of life and property of the older persons. After being passed by the parliament of India received the assent of President of India on December 29, 2007 and was published in the Gazette of India on December 31, 2007.

Free legal aid/cells: In different states there are free legal aid cells which can be provide support to the geriatric people.

NGOs and voluntary organizations: In a democratic, socialistic and welfare society, voluntary organizations are indispensable and they perform a number of functions for the welfare of its members, the development of the country and integration and solidarity of the society and nation specially there are a lot of **Voluntary organizations providing service to the geriatrics peoples they are:**

- Help Age India, Delhi
- Rajasthan Voluntary Health Association, Jaipur
- Voluntary Health Association, TTT Institution, Chennai
- Healthy services societies, Hyderabad
- Missionary of Charity (Mother Teresa Center), Kolkata
- Ramakrishna Math and Mission, Belur Math, Howrah, West Bengal
- West Bengal Voluntary Health Association, Kolkata
- Sambandh, Bhubaneswar, Odisha
- Community Aid and Sponsorship programme, ARDSI (Hyderabad), Dignity Foundation (Mumbai) TNAI, International Longevity Center (ILC), etc.

International Year of Older Person

1999 is being observed as the International year of the older persons. The population of older persons 60+ in India ranks the fourth largest in the world and by the end of the present century; it will be second only to China.

NATIONAL PROGRAMME FOR HEALTH CARE OF THE ELDERLY (NPHCE)

National Policy on Older Persons adopted by the Government of India in 1999 and Section 20 of 'The Maintenance and Welfare of Parents and Senior Citizens Act, 2007' dealing with provisions for medical care of Senior Citizen. The National Programme for Health Care of the Elderly (NPHCE) is a program, forms part of the Non-Communicable Division in the Ministry which is monitored by the channel of Section Officer, Under Secretary, Deputy Secretary and Joint Secretary. The program is sponsored by Ministry of Health and Family Welfare, Government of India.

The Vision of the NPHCE

The vision of the NPHCE are:

- To provide accessible, affordable, and high-quality long-term, comprehensive and dedicated care services to an aging population
- Creating a new 'architecture' for Aging
- To build a framework to create an enabling environment for 'a Society for all Ages'
- To promote the concept of Active and Healthy Aging.

Objective of the Program

The basic objective of the NPHCE program is to provide separate, specialized and comprehensive health care to the senior citizens at various level of State health care delivery system including outreach services.

- To provide an easy access to promotional, preventive, curative and rehabilitative services through community based primary health care (PHC) approach
- To identify health problems in the elderly and provide appropriate health interventions in the community with a strong referral backup support
- To build capacity of the medical and paramedical professionals as well as the care takers within the family for providing health care to the senior citizen
- To provide referral services to the elderly patients through district hospital regional medical institutions
- Convergence with National Rural Health Mission (NRHM), Ayush and other line departments like Ministry of Social Justice and Empowerment.

Funding Pattern

The Center will bear 75% of the total budget and the State Government will contribute 25% of the budget. A total amount of ₹1710.13 crore has been approved for XII Five Year Plan for NPHCE. Out of this, an amount of ₹1147.56 crore is earmarked for activities proposed to be undertaken up to district level. An amount of ₹562.57 crore has been earmarked for tertiary level activities. An allocation of ₹150.00 crore has been made for the year 2013-14 out of which ₹50.00 crore relates to National Health Mission NCD Flexi Pool for activities up to district level and ₹100.00 crore relates to Health Sector, i.e., tertiary level activities.

Strategies to Achieve the Objectives of the NPHCE

- Community based PHC approach including domiciliary visits by trained health care workers.
- Dedicated services at PHC/Community Health Center (CHC) level including provision of machinery, equipment, training, additional human resources, Information, Education and Communication (IEC), etc.
- Dedicated facilities at the district hospital with 10 bedded wards, additional human resources, machinery and equipment, consumables and drugs, training and IEC.
- Strengthening of 8 Regional Medical Institutes to provide dedicated tertiary level medical facilities for the elderly, introducing PG courses in geriatric medicine, and in-service training of health personnel at all levels.
- IEC using mass media, folk media and other communication channels to reach out to the target community.
- Continuous monitoring and independent evaluation of the Program and research in geriatrics and implementation of NPHCE.
- Promotion of public private partnerships in geriatric health care.
- Mainstreaming Ayush—revitalizing local health traditions and convergence with programs of Ministry of Social Justice and Empowerment in the field of geriatrics.
- Reorienting medical education to support geriatric issues.

ELDERLY ABUSE

Introduction

Each year hundreds of thousands of older persons are abused, neglected, and exploited. Many victims are people who are older, frail, and vulnerable and cannot help themselves and depend on others to meet their most basic needs. Abusers of older adults are both women and men, and may be family members, friends, or 'trusted others.' Elder abuse tends to take place where the senior lives: most often in the home where abusers are often adult children, other family members such as grandchildren, or spouses/partners of elders. Elder abuse can also occur in institutional settings, especially long-term care facilities.

Definition

Elder abuse is a term referring to any knowing, intentional, or negligent act by a caregiver or any other person that causes harm or a serious risk of harm to a vulnerable adult. Legislatures in all 50 states have passed some form of elder abuse prevention laws.

General Signs of Abuse

The following are warning signs of some kind of elder abuse:

- Frequent arguments or tension between the caregiver and the elderly person
- Changes in personality or behavior in the elder.

If you suspect elderly abuse, but are not sure, look for clusters of the following physical and behavioral signs.

Physical Abuse

Physical elder abuse is nonaccidental use of force against an elderly person that results in physical pain, injury, or impairment. Such abuse includes not only physical assaults such as hitting or shoving but the inappropriate use of drugs, restraints, or confinement. The sign and symptoms are:

- Unexplained signs of injury such as bruises, welts, or scars, especially if they appear symmetrically on two side of the body
- Broken bones, sprains, or dislocations
- Report of drug overdose or apparent failure to take medication regularly (a prescription has more remaining than it should)
- Broken eyeglasses or frames
- Signs of being restrained, such as rope marks on wrists
- Caregiver's refusal to allow you to see the elder alone.

Emotional Abuse

In emotional or psychological abuse, people speak to or treat elderly persons in ways that cause emotional pain or distress. In addition to the general signs of physical abuse. The emotional elder abuse include: verbal forms and nonverbal form:

The verbal of emotional elder abuse include:

- Intimidation through yelling or threats
- Humiliation and ridicule
- Habitual blaming or scapegoating.

Nonverbal psychological elder abuse can take the form of:

- Ignoring the elderly person
- Isolating an elder from friends or activities
- Terrorizing or menacing the elderly person.

Sexual Abuse

Sexual elder abuse is contact with an elderly person without the elder's consent. Such contact can involve physical sex acts, but activities such as showing an elderly person pornographic material, forcing the person to watch sex acts, or forcing the elder to undress are also considered sexual elder abuse. The signs and symptoms of sexual abuse are:

- Bruises around breasts or genitals
- Unexplained venereal disease or genital infections
- Unexplained vaginal or anal bleeding
- Torn, stained, or bloody underclothing.

Neglect by Caregivers or Self-neglect

Neglect or abandonment by caregivers is failure to fulfill a caretaking obligation, constitutes more than half of all reported cases of elder abuse. It can be intentional or unintentional, based on factors such as ignorance or denial that an elderly charge needs as much care as he or she does, self-neglect means older family member, friend, or neighbor living alone is no longer taking care of themselves. The sign and symptoms are as such:

- Unusual weight loss, malnutrition, dehydration
- Untreated physical problems, such as bed sores
- **Unsanitary living conditions:** Dirt, bugs, soiled bedding and clothes
- Being left dirty or unbathed
- Unsuitable clothing or covering for the weather
- Unsafe living conditions (no heat or running water; faulty electrical wiring, other fire hazards)
- Desertion of the elder at a public place.

Financial Exploitation

This involves unauthorized use of an elderly person's funds or property, either by a caregiver or an outside scam artist which can be observed by:

- Significant withdrawals from the elder's accounts
- Sudden changes in the elder's financial condition
- Items or cash missing from the senior's household
- Suspicious changes in wills, power of attorney, titles, and policies
- Addition of names to the senior's signature card
- Unpaid bills or lack of medical care, although the elder has enough money to pay for them
- Financial activity the senior could not have done, such as an ATM withdrawal when the account holder is bedridden
- Unnecessary services, goods, or subscriptions.

Health Care Fraud and Abuse

- Duplicate billings for the same medical service or device
- Evidence of overmedication or under medication
- Evidence of inadequate care when bills are paid in full
- **Problems with the care facility:** Poorly trained, poorly paid, or insufficient staff; crowding; inadequate responses to questions about care.
- Not providing health care, but charging for it

- Overcharging or double-billing for medical care or services
- Getting kickbacks for referrals to other providers or for prescribing certain drugs
- Recommending fraudulent remedies for illnesses or other medical conditions
- Medicaid fraud.

Risk Factors for Elder Abuse

It is difficult to take care of a senior who has many different needs, and it is difficult to be elderly when age brings with it infirmities and dependence. Both the demands of caregiving and the needs of the elder can create situations in which abuse is more likely to occur.

Risk Factors among Caregivers

Many nonprofessional caregivers—spouses, adult children, other relatives and friends—find taking care of an elder to be satisfying and enriching. But the responsibilities and demands of elder caregiving, which escalate as the elder's condition deteriorates, can also be extremely stressful. The stress of elder care can lead to mental and physical health problems that make caregivers burned out, impatient, and unable to keep from lashing out against elders in their care.

Among caregivers, significant risk factors for elder abuse are:

- Inability to cope with stress (lack of resilience)
- Depression, which is common among caregivers
- Lack of support from other potential caregivers
- The caregiver's perception that taking care of the elder is burdensome and without psychological reward
- Substance abuse.

Even caregivers in institutional settings can experience stress at levels that lead to elder abuse. Nursing home staff may be prone to elder abuse if they lack training, have too many responsibilities, are unsuited to caregiving, or work under poor conditions.

Risk Factors from Elders

Several factors concerning elders themselves, while they are at greater risk for abuse:

- The intensity of an elderly person's illness or dementia
- Social isolation;, i.e., the elder and caregiver are alone together almost all the time
- The elder's role, at an earlier time, as an abusive parent or spouse.
- A history of domestic violence in the home
- The elder's own tendency toward verbal or physical aggression.

In many cases, elder abuse, though real, is unintentional. Caregivers pushed beyond their capabilities and ignore the needs of the elders in their care.

Preventing Elder Abuse and Neglect

Preventing elder abuse means doing three things:

1. Listening to seniors and their caregivers
2. Intervening when you suspect elder abuse
3. Educating others about how to recognize and report elder abuse.

Role of Caregiver to Prevent Elder Abuse

If you are overwhelmed by the demands of caring for an elder, do the following:

- Request help, from friends, relatives, or local respite care agencies, so you can take a break, if only for a couple of hours
- Find an adult day care program
- Stay healthy and get medical care for yourself when necessary
- Adopt stress reduction practices
- Seek counseling for depression, which can lead to elder abuse
- Find a support group for caregivers of the elderly
- If you are having problems with drug or alcohol abuse, get help.

And remember, elder abuse helplines offer help for caregivers as well. Call a helpline if you think there is a possibility you might cross the line into elder abuse.

What You can Do as a Concerned Friend or Family Member?

- Watch for warning signs that might indicate elder abuse. If you suspect abuse, report it.
- Take a look at the elder's medications. Does the amount in the vial jive with the date of the prescription?
- Watch for possible financial abuse. Ask the elder if you may scan bank accounts and credit card statements for unauthorized transactions.
- Call and visit as often as you can. Help the elder consider you a trusted confidante.
- Offer to stay with the elder so the caregiver can have a break—on a regular basis, if possible.

Protecting Yourself, as an Elder, against Elder Abuse

- Make sure your financial and legal affairs are in order. If they are not, enlist professional help to get them in order, with the assistance of a trusted friend or relative if necessary.
- Keep in touch with family and friends and avoid becoming isolated.
- If you are unhappy with the care you are receiving, whether it is in your own home or in a care facility, *speak up*. Tell someone you trust and ask that person to report the abuse, neglect, or substandard care to an elder abuse helpline or long-term care ombudsman, or make the call yourself.

Reporting Elder Abuse

If you are an elder who is being abused, neglected, or exploited, tell at least one person. Tell your doctor, a friend, or a family member whom you trust. Or call one of the help lines listed in Resources and References below.

If you see an older adult being abused or neglected, do not hesitate to report the situation. Do not assume that someone else will take care of it or that the person being abused is capable of getting help if he or she really needs it.

Many seniors do not report the abuse they face even if they are able. Some fear retaliation from the abuser, while others believe that if they turn in their abusers, no one else will take care of them. When the caregivers are their children, they may be ashamed that their children are behaving abusively or blame themselves: 'If I had been a better parent when they were younger, this would not be happening.' Or they just may not want children they love to get into trouble with the law.

How to Report Elder Abuse?

There is a list of helplines to call in your country, see the Resources and References section below. In the US, for example, the first agency to respond to a report of elderly abuse is usually Adult Protective Services (APS). Its role is to investigate abuse cases, intervene, and offer services and advice, although the power and scope of APS varies from state-to-state. Wherever you are reporting elder abuse, though, there are some important things to remember to ensure that you are able to communicate effectively in different situations.

Try to be Specific as You can in Your Description

You do not need 'hard evidence' to report abuse. In many situations, abuse can be subtle or happen gradually. However, the more specific details you can provide, the clearer the picture of abuse can become. For example, if you are worried that your neighbor is not taking care of himself, instead of reporting, 'My neighbor is having a hard time taking care of himself', try 'I have noticed that my neighbor wears the same outfit over and over again and it is looking very dirty. When I come to the door, I smell urine and even feces. The house also smells like there is trash accumulating inside.'

Understand the Elder does have the Right to Refuse Services

As painful as it may be, unless the older adult no longer has the mental capacity to make their own decisions, he or she does have the right to refuse help. A senior may refuse to admit they are being abused because they are afraid the caregiver will retaliate, or because they are worried about who will take care of them if their abusive caregiver is removed. Sadly, an elder adult may view having an abusive caretaker as better than having no caretaker and being forced to move out of their own home. In these situations, if it is safe for you to do so, continue to stay in contact and encourage the elder to consider alternatives to home care. For example:

- Taking tours of assisted living or other facilities, without any immediate pressure to move, may help dispel myths or eradicate the older person's fears about moving
- Offering services on a trial basis can help the elder see the positive changes they can have, and make them more open to change. For example, if self-neglect is an issue, encourage them to try housekeeping help for a month, or a meal delivery service for a few weeks.
- Keeping the older adult and caregiver connected to support services can help reduce feelings of isolation and depression, two major risk factors for elder abuse. Also, the more support there is for the elder and the caregiver, the more eyes there will be to watch for any warning signs of abuse.
- If a family caregiver is suspected of abuse, other family members may have the best chance of convincing the older adult to consider alternative care.

Keep Your Eyes and Ears Open

If you see future incidences of abuse, continue to call and report them. Each elder abuse report is a snapshot of what is going on. The more information that you can provide, the better the chance the elder has to get the level of care he or she needs. Older adults can be increasingly isolated from society and, with no school or work to attend, it can be easy for abuse cases to go unnoticed for long periods.

Reporting Abuse in the Home and Self-neglect

Sadly, two of the most common sources of elder abuse are abuse by a primary caregiver—often an adult child—and self-neglect. Here are some tips for handling these situations.

Elder Abuse in the Home

- Try to have different family members or neutral parties involved in the older adult's care to provide checks and balances, including reviewing finances. The greater the cognitive or physical impairment of the elder, the more people need to be involved in their care. While there is no excuse for abuse, caregiving can be extremely taxing, both mentally and physically. If a caregiver is unable to get any respite, has disrupted sleep, or is experiencing his or her own health problems, there is a greater risk for elder abuse.
- Feelings of shame can often keep elder abuse hidden. You may not want to believe a family member could be capable of abusing a loved one, or you may even think that the older adult would be angry at you for speaking up. But remember, everyone deserves to live with dignity and respect. The earlier you intervene in a situation of elder abuse, the better the outcome will be for everyone involved.

Look for Common Risk Factors for Elder Abuse in the Home

- **Substance abuse** can impede a caregiver's ability to provide adequate care. It also increases the risk of financial abuse as the caregiver struggles to finance a substance abuse habit.

- **A history of domestic violence** or other violence can often be a marker for elder abuse later in life.

Self-neglect

You may notice that an older family member, friend, or neighbor living alone is no longer taking care of themselves. They may appear increasingly disheveled, lack basic personal hygiene, or their home may be growing dirtier and dirtier. In many cases of self-neglect, the older person will refuse to get assistance. However, there are still things that you can do to help.

Remember, any older adult deserves dignity and respect. He or she may be in denial, feel ashamed about needing help, or worried about having to leave home. Do not stop checking in with the older adult, even if you are brushed off. Enlist others to express their feelings of concern to the elder. Sometimes a peer or a neutral party, such as a geriatric care manager, may have a better chance of getting through.

Make sure the older adult is connected with medical services. Self-neglect can be a sign of depression, grief, dementia, or other medical causes. If you know the person's doctor, you can share your concerns. While the doctor may not be able to discuss the case with you if you do not have the older adult's permission, you can write a letter or call to make sure that your concerns are heard.

It can be a real challenge to respect an older adult's right to autonomy while at the same time making sure they are properly cared for. If you are concerned that a person's ability to take care of themselves safely is compromised, you can look into legal guardianship or legal conservatorship. If there is not an appropriate family member available, a guardian can be appointed by the court.

Aging is a natural process. Old age is an incurable disease. Sir James Sterling Ross commented you do not heal old age, you protect it, you promote it, you extend it. Old age should be regarded as a normal, inevitable, biological phenomenon. As the global population of elderly increases we all should aware of concept of health and active aging. As a nursing personnel we need to understand the impact of positive approach to aging which would promote meaningful and enjoyable life for older people.

School Health Nursing

CONCEPT OF SCHOOL, SCHOOL HEALTH AND SCHOOL OF NURSING

School is defined as an educational institution where groups of pupils pursue defined studies at defined levels, receive instructions from one or more teachers, frequently interact with other officers and employees, such as principal, various supervisors/instructors, and maintenance staff, etc., usually housed in a single building.

School Health

School health refers to a state of complete physical, mental, social and spiritual well-being and not merely the absence of disease or infirmity among pupils, teachers and other school personnel.

School Health Services

Ideally school health services refer to need-based comprehensive services rendered to pupils, teachers and other personnel in the school to promote and protect their health, prevent and control diseases and maintain their health. But practically, it refers to providing need-based comprehensive services to pupils to promote and protect their health, control diseases and maintain their health.

Objectives of School Health Services

- The promotion of positive health.
- The prevention of disease.
- Early diagnosis, treatment and follow-up of defects.
- Awakening health consciousness in children.
- The provision of healthy living.

Goals of School Health Services

To prepare the younger generation to adopt measures to remain healthy so as to help them to make the best use of educational facilities, to utilize leisure in productive and constructive manner, to enjoy recreation and to develop concern for others to help the younger generation become healthy and useful citizens who will be able to perform their role effectively for the welfare of themselves, their families, and the community at large and country as a whole.

Need of School Health Service

- School children constitute a vital and substantial segment of population.
- School children are vulnerable section of population by virtue of their physical, mental, emotional and social growth and development during this period.
- School children are exposed to various stressful situation.
- Children coming to school belong to different socio-economic and cultural backgrounds which affect their health and nutrition status and require help and guidance in promoting, protecting and maintaining their health and nutritional status.
- Children in school age are prone to get specific health problems.

Philosophy of School Health Services

- A healthy child is mentally alert, receptive, will not miss school due to minor sickness and will have better performance in his/her studies.
- Health is not just freedom from sickness or infirmity but the realization of the full potential of the child which has physical, mental, social and spiritual components.
- Prevention is better than cure; interventions when health breaks down are costly and time consuming.
- School health services will help identify any deviations from normal growth and development, any health problem so that timely, therapeutic, corrective and rehabilitative actions can be taken to improve and maintain health and continue studies.
- While early diagnosis and prompt and adequate treatment is of great importance, follow-up care is equally important for effective school health services.
- Rehabilitation of physically and mentally handicapped children can be done and must receive adequate attention.
- Health knowledge and skills learnt not only will benefit the child but also it will benefit the school, the parents, family and community.
- Emphasize on health education to promote, protect, improve and maintain health of children and staff.
- Emphasize on learning through active and desirable participation.
- Be ongoing and continuous program.
- Have an effective system of record keeping and reporting.

COMPONENTS OF SCHOOL HEALTH SERVICES

Health Promotive and Protective Services

Wholesome School Environment

The physical environment of school buildings and school grounds is a key factor in the overall health and safety of students, staff, and visitors. School buildings and grounds must be designed and maintained to be free of health and safety hazards, and to promote learning. Studies have shown that student achievement can be affected either positively or negatively by the school. The selection of the site for the school should be easily reached by the people and it should be located in calm and quite area away from market, there must be 10–15 m^2/scholars. School building must be damp, fire and rat proof.

Policies and protocols must be in place to ensure food protection, sanitation, safe water supply, healthy air quality, good lighting, safe playgrounds, violence prevention, and emergency response, among other issues that relate to the physical environment of schools. The State Fire Code under RSA 153: 5 and the State Building Code under RSA 155 establish the basic requirements for the construction, operation, and maintenance of school buildings. A number of state agencies including the department of education, department of health and human services, department of environmental services, department of safety, department of labor, and others, enforce numerous statutes and administrative rules that address topics such as alcohol, tobacco, and other drugs, food service hazardous materials such as asbestos, lead, mercury, radon, etc., laboratories and other shops. The school should be far away these types of shops. In addition to this the wholesome school environment require playgrounds, safe drinking water, sanitation and housekeeping. School emergency response plans, standards for school buildings and traffic safety.

Maintenance of Hygiene

Personal Hygiene

In this aspect both School Health Nurse and teacher will educate the child about cleanliness and hygiene. The teacher will in his daily appraisal observe the maintenance of personal hygiene of the students. Personal hygiene include the care of whole body from head to toe which include care and cleanliness of head, mouth, eye, ear, nose each and every part of the body. The teacher always emphasize on proper handwashing technique and teach them the steps of handwashing and when to do it like before and after taking food, after toileting, after touching any infectious or unclean material. Researches show that washing hands properly is the most effective way of preventing transmission of communicable diseases. Other form of personal hygiene are proper oral hygiene, bathing, perineal hygiene for girls and using of clean clothes, etc. Poor personal hygiene leads to scabies, pediculosis, dental carries and other diseases. So it is the duty of teacher to observe the hygiene of school children in daily appraisal.

Environmental Hygiene

The school environment include the surrounding of inside and outside of class room and over all outside school which include class. Environmental hygiene include maintenance of good indoor ventilation. Cleanliness of the school premises including classrooms, kitchen canteen, toilets, bathrooms, and school buses and cleanliness of frequently touched surfaces, such as furniture, toys and commonly shared items (such as computer keyboards) need to be clean at least daily by using appropriate disinfectant then it will be rinsed with water and kept dry. The school premises should be kept clean and decorated a beautiful garden. The public should be educated to keep the outside surrounding clean by avoiding open field defecation and avoiding of dumping of garbage near the school.

Nutritional Services

The school going age is more vulnerable age for different type of nutritional disorder like under nutrition, anemia and other vitamin deficiency disorders. There are a lot of national nutritional program like Mid day Meal Programme, Anemia Control Programme launched in school and the school teachers are taking a major responsibilities for conduction of such types of programs. During providing nutritional service the quality and quantity of food observed properly. The meal should meet the recommended dietary requirement. Food hygiene should be maintained during selection, preparation and preservation of food.

Physical and Recreational Activities

Other physical and recreational activities help the student for their total growth and development. Engaging other physical and recreational activities can help the students to bring out the hidden qualities of the students. Recreational activities help the student for developing their mental health, removing stress and promotes their physical and mental health. Indirectly, it also helps in promoting their studies.

Promotion of Mental Health

Promotion of mental health is an important aspect of school health service. The school is the right place for shaping the child's behavior and promoting mental health. The mental health of the child affects the physical health and learning process. Some of the school children problems are drug addiction, juvenile delinquency and maladjustment. The school teacher plays an important role helping the child to attain positive mental health. Some of the students also having very low IQ and they are consider as mentally retarded children. In such cases have to identify them and can refer them for special treatment or if possible take special care for themselves.

Health Education

Health education is an important part of a comprehensive school health program. Health education builds students' knowledge, skills, and positive attitudes about health. Health education teaches about physical, mental, emotional and social health. It motivates students to improve and maintain their health, prevent disease, and reduce risky behaviors. The goal of the health education program is to help students learn how to make wise decisions that promote their health and well-being. The role of the school nurse in the health education program is to supplement the health instruction given by the classroom teacher. Health education curricula and instruction help students learn skills. They will use to make healthy choices throughout their lifetime. Effective curricula result in positive changes in behavior that lower student risks around alcohol, tobacco, and other drugs, injury prevention, mental and emotional health, nutrition, physical activity, prevention of diseases and sexuality and family life. Health education promotes learning in other subjects. In general, healthy students learn better. Numerous studies have shown that healthier students tend to do better in school. They have higher attendance, have better grades, and perform better on tests.

The school nurse supports health promotion activities and assists teachers in obtaining appropriate materials and resource people. School nurses may coordinate in service education on health-related topics. School nurses may sometimes assist the classroom teacher to enhance a specific health unit in the classroom.

Prevention of Common Communicable Diseases

Schools are gathering places where children learn and play. Some children may be too young to take proper personal care. As such, communicable diseases can easily spread through close person-to-person contact. The source of infection can be children, staff and parents. Person-to-person contact may lead to cross-infection, i.e., the transmission of infective agents from one person to another. There are four factors crucial to the spread of communicable diseases. They include the infective agent, the source of infection, the mode of transmission and the host. Hence, the control of the spread of communicable diseases should focus on controlling all these four factors so as to break the chain of infection. Building up the body immunity by having a balanced diet in accordance with the food pyramid, adequate rest and sleep, regular exercise and avoidance of smoking is vital to the prevention of communicable diseases. Moreover, good personality, food and environmental hygiene should be observed. Vaccination can provide extra protection against some communicable diseases. Personal hygiene of the students and other school personnel also very important aspect in prevention of common communicable diseases. Handwashing of the students, cook, food server, is also important. Teachers must supervise the children to perform proper hand hygiene in schools. Teacher in his daily inspection identify the students having communicable diseases and educate themselves and their parents regarding necessary precaution for prevention of its transmission by following different isolation technique.

Immunization

Immunization is a part of school health service. Immunization should be provided to the students. As per national schedule, it is a fixed day activity for the school health nurse. It should be coupled with education. All the faculty of the school should be cooperative in conducting such programs. A record of all immunization should be maintained as part of school health records when the child leaves the school, the health record should be accompanied with him. Apart from general hygienic practice and vaccination, school/center staff should adopt appropriate preventive measures against communicable diseases.

Therapeutic Services

Health Appraisal

Health appraisal consists of periodic medical examination of school children and also teachers and other school personnel.

- **Periodic medical examination:** In 1961, The School Health Committee of India recommended detail medical examination for the children who are newly entered in the school and there after every 6 months. The physical examination includes screening of general health, assessment of anemia/nutritional status, visual acuity, hearing problems, dental checkup, common skin conditions, heart defects, physical disabilities, learning disorders, behavior problems, etc. Teachers and school personnels are also evaluated for any communicable diseases like pulmonary tuberculosis or any other health problems.
- **Daily morning inspection:** Some of the children help the teachers in detecting those children who need medical attention, they are unusually flushed face, any rash or spots, sore throat, rigid neck, nausea, vomiting, red or water eyes, headache, symptoms of acute cold, chills or fever, diarrhea, body pain, head lice, skin infections like scabies, etc.

Treatment and Follow-up

After periodic medical examination students or other teachers and school personnel should be given appropriate treatment and follow-up. Special clinics should be conducted based on the finding. The school health Nurse identify any deviation in health condition and make referral to nearest health center.

Care of the Handicapped

Children with minor or mild cases of disability can attend regular schools, severe forms (e.g., the deaf, blind, or mentally retarded) can attend special institutes. Handicapping conditions may be congenital or acquired required special attention in school. Some forms of handicapping conditions in regular school are like rheumatic valvular disease, musculoskeletal deformities, mild paralytic, poliomyelitis, healed rickets, impaired vision mainly due to errors of refraction, and may be corneal opacity impaired hearing neglected chronic otitis media, ear injury by foreign body, or any other physical and mental disorders. This type of students should be under constant observation of the teacher. Sometimes the students with mild mental retardation can be studied among the general student, the teacher should provide special attention to them. The teacher can council to their parents regarding special education.

School Health Records

School records are books, documents, diskettes and files in which are embodied information on what goes on in school (e.g., social, academic and non academic activities, important events, etc), the school plant as well as other relevant information focusing on the growth and development of the school. Health records are also important records in all school records. **Each school child should have his own health record, for registration of events and activities related to health.** These records are useful to analyze and evaluate the school health programmes and provide a useful link between the school, home and the community.

Importance of maintenance of school health record in school:

- For future reference, whenever registered health data are needed; e.g., past medical history to assist diagnosis of existing disease.
- Allows follow-up of chronic disease.
- Collecting statistical data and indices of school children for research purpose or future planning implementation and evaluation of health services.

Legal Considerations of Student Health Records

There are legal and regulatory considerations regarding student records and their use. From a legal standpoint, any record relating to a student which is used by school district personnel constitutes a student record. It includes formal records which have been developed for specific purposes. It also includes informal records or notes, if such notations are placed in a student's folder or record. Any record prepared by an outside agency, and transmitted to the school, also becomes part of the student record if it is added to the student's folder and used by school personnel.

There are mainly two types of health records, these are primary or cumulative health record which is specially done in school and supplementary which is done by family members.

Primary Cumulative Health Records

A cumulative health record is maintained for each student during their school years. It includes a place to record information regarding health history, immunization procedures, medical examinations, screening procedures, medical recommendations, medical referrals, teacher observations, a problem list, progress notes, flowsheets, etc.

Supplementary School Health Records

The complete student health record frequently includes supplementary records, such as health history reports from parents, reports of medical examinations by the family physician, dental examination reports, reports from vision and hearing specialists, and medical requests for program adaptation of various kinds.

The cumulative health record and all supplemental records included in the student's folder thus become part of the total health record of each student.

Health Education

Health education curricula and instruction help students learn skills they will use to make healthy choices throughout their lifetime. Effective curricula result in positive changes in behavior that lower student risks around: Alcohol, tobacco, and other drugs, injury prevention, mental and emotional health, nutrition, physical activity, prevention of diseases and sexuality and family life.

Health education promotes learning in other subjects! One study showed that reading and math scores of third and fourth grade students who received comprehensive health education were significantly higher than those who did not. In general, healthy students learn better. Numerous studies have shown that healthier students tend to do better in school. They have higher attendance, have better grades, and perform better on tests.

DISASTER MANAGEMENT

A disaster can be defined as any occurrence that causes damage ecological disruption, loss of human life or deterioration of health and health services on a scale sufficient to warrant an extraordinary response from outside the affected community or area (Please refer chapter 19 to learn more about disaster and it's management).

The role of students are important in disaster management because they are the major mass and act as the best volunteer to save the life of the people if they will be well trained. In their curriculum, their role in disaster management like rescuing the individual and providing first-aid has already been included.

Disaster Management and Role of Students

Disaster management can be defined as the organization and management of resources and responsibilities for dealing with all humanitarian aspects of emergencies.

Aim

To provide prompt and effective medical care to maximum possible to minimize mortality rate and rehabilitate the injured.

Objectives

To prepare the staff and institutional resources for effective performance in disaster situation.

Principles of Disaster Management

- Prevent the disaster occurrence.
- Minimize the casualties.
- Prevent further casualty.
- Evacuate injured to medical facilities.
- Provide definite medical care.
- Rescue the victims.
- Provide first aid.

Role of Students in Disaster

Our educational system has includes the training programs like military training programmes in NCC to the students from school level to have the helping nature in them at times of need and also for nation's safety.

Phases of Disaster Management and Role of Students

- Prevention phase
- Preparedness phase
- Response phase
- Recovery phase.

Disaster Risk Management includes sum total of all activities, programs and measures which can be taken up before, during and after a disaster. Away to think about school's level of preparedness is to measure the 3R's of disaster. That are *Readiness, Response, and Recovery.*

Before a Disaster (Predisaster)

Readiness is the level at which the students are prepared to respond to an emergency if the disaster can happen. *Prevention and preparedness phase* are included in this phase.

Preparedness

Preparedness activities that are taken to build capacity and identify resources that may be used:

- **Develop** crisis and emergency response protocol.
- **Sharing information:** In most incidences, two-way radios are the only reliable form of communications.
- **Awareness:** The basic role of the student, awareness of what to do before, during and after disasters.
- **Rallies:** They can spread awareness through rallies in streets regarding the coming disaster and the readiness.
- **Education:** Educate about some safety tips for some common type of disaster and their readiness.
- **Communication** channels must be in place to allow numerous agencies access to information about detected potential threats.
- **Training:** Students should participated in various training programme like NCC, Fire fighter training, swimming or rescue techniques during flood, rope riding training during gas leaking.
- **Using the mass media to deliver warnings to the public:** Local media agencies should inform people about information on food and water safety, injury and disease prevention through TV and radio.
- **First aid kit** of the school which includes antiseptic lotion, gauge piece, cotton, band aid, spirit, adhesive plaster, etc., should kept ready.
- **Emergency kit** which contains flashlight with extra bulbs and extra batteries, portable battery-operated radio, emergency food and water with purification tablets or chlorine bleaching powder in your kit to purify drinking water from other sources. A supply of non-perishable packaged or canned food, blankets and extra clothing, soap, toilet paper, toothbrushes, and other items to keep you clean, other items in the emergency kit might include: Paper and pens, permanent markers, etc., should kept ready.
- **Disaster corner should prepared** which should have a clear wall to put emergency directions. Your classmates and the teachers put up posters, and post explanations of different types of disasters that happen in your area. Cut out appropriate articles from newspapers for the 'Disaster Corner'.

During a Disaster (Disaster Occurrence)

Response and rescue are included in this phase. Response means activities taken immediately during disaster or emergency occurs. Students should take initiation to ensure that the needs and provisions of victims are met and suffering is minimized. The mobilization of the necessary emergency services and first responders in the disaster area such as:

Health Care Community

- Hospital
- Public health department

Police and Ambulance Nonhealth Care Community

- Fire fighter
- Government officials
- Media, etc.

Saving Life

Immediate evacuation of high-risk groups such as:

- Infants
- Pregnant women
- Nursing mothers
- Sick persons
- Old age people.

Student's Role

- School crisis team is activated depending on the nature of disaster.
- **Contact** school and municipal incident command post to see where you may be needed.

- **Activate** resources for immediate, concrete need of the people.
- **Apply** your training activities to rescue the victims.
- **Survival technique** like swimming to save drowning, fire extinguishing technique in fire hazard, rope riding, etc., can be done by trained students.

In rescue of the injured victims the knowledge regarding TRIAGE is very essential for the students.

TRIAGE/Level of Disaster

The meaning of TRIAGE is 'TO SORT'. It covers 'TRI' means three levels according to the severity of injury and it is indicated by color tags. The three levels are:

- **Emergent:** It means highest priority care.
- **Urgent:** It means higher priority care.
- **Non-urgent:** It means priority of care.

This is a command and control kit for all types of multi-casualty incidents to identify TRIAGE sites from distance.

Contents

1	(Red)	Immediate	Treatment	Area	Flag
1	(Yellow)	Delayed	Treatment	Area	Flag
1	(Green)	Minor	Treatment	Area	Flag
1	(Black)	Morgue	Treatment	Area	Flag

Use of TRIAGE

- The immediate step to be taken by removal of debris with **black tag**, and send to mortuary.
- **For Red tag:**
  - Assess the symptoms of shock-like feeling sick, weak, cold, and dizziness, confused and short of breath.
  - Inspect for signs of external blood loss and apply direct pressure of the affected area.
  - Provide necessary life-saving services such as resuscitation, control of bleeding, immobilization, etc., and arrange for transport.
- **Yellow tag:** Provide first-aid to the victims according to the condition can be shifted to the hospital or home when relations are available.
- **Green tag** is used for minor treatment.

After a Disaster (Postdisaster)

Recovery is the process of restoring the social and emotional equilibrium of the affected people.

Student's Role

- **Reduce anxiety** with education and provide reassurance to the affected people.
- **Help** them to deal with stress and get back to their pre-disaster level of functioning.
- **Educate** them about the facilities available by the government or any other agencies.
- **Advise** about the intake of safe chlorinated drinking water.
- **Assessing** the food supplies after the disaster. Provide the victims the basic needs by distributing relief.
- **Help** the agencies in distribution of HALOGEN tablets for water purification.
- **Prepare plantation** programme inside and outside the school premises.
- **Generate awareness** on water and sanitation among the children in the school and circulate this message to the affected people to prevent epidemics.
- **Educate people** about the occurrence of snake bite in flood.
- **Help the agencies** in vaccination against communicable diseases like cholera, typhoid, etc.
- **Listening** to victims tell and retell their feelings related to the disaster and their current situation.
- **Encouraging victims** to share their feelings with one another. If it seems appropriate to do so.
- **Helping victims** make decisions.
- **Aware** people about snake bite.

General Awareness on Safety Tips

The students must know some safety tips on some selected disaster which are common in their location to save their life and also the life of affected victims.

Cyclone: Safety Tips

Before the Cyclone

- Keep alert about the community warning systems—loudspeakers, bells, drums or any traditional warning.
- Get to know the nearest cyclone shelter/safe houses and the safest route to reach these shelters system.
- Prepare an emergency kit as mentioned before.
- Keep important documents, passbook, etc., in a tight plastic bag and take it along with your emergency kits if you are evacuating.
- In case of warning of serious storm, move with your family to a strong pucca building. Take special care for children, elders, sick, pregnant women and lactating mothers in your family.
- Listen to your transistor radio for updates and advice.
- Beware of the calm `eye'. If the wind suddenly drops, do not assume the cyclone is over; violent winds will soon resume from the opposite direction. Wait for the official 'all clear'.

After the Cyclone

- Do not go outside until officially advised it is safe.
- Listen to local radio for official warnings and advice.
- If you have to evacuate, or did so earlier, do not return until advised.
- Be careful of snake bites and carry a stick or bamboo.

FIRST AID AND EMERGENCY CARE

First aid means the immediate care to sick or injured individual given to prevent further damage. It is the temporary and immediate care given to a person who is injured or suddenly become ill, using facilities or material available at that time before regular medical health is imparted. First aid is often life-saving in nature, school staff is responsible until the parent/guardian or paramedics arrive. The teacher should be well trained to provide first aid during emergencies and treating the minor ailments. First aid can save lives and prevent minor injuries becoming major ones. Under health and safety legislation, employers have to ensure that there are adequate and appropriate equipment and facilities for providing first aid in the workplace.

The minimum first-aid provision is a suitably stocked first-aid container or box, an appointed person to take charge of first-aid arrangements; information for employees on first-aid arrangements. This minimum provision must be supplemented with a risk assessment to determine any additional provision. Not only the person who appointed for giving first aid but also every teacher should have knowledge on first aid during emergency situation. First stay calm, even if faking it then to prioritize injuries. Call for ambulance if needed. Control the crowd. Avoid moving of the client. Only the victim can move when injuries have been evaluated and it is safe to do so. For ALL major events, i.e., accidents, illness, seizures, stings and allergic students, the administration should be notified. The parent/guardian also to be notified. The teacher needs to complete an accident report in the office.

Aims of First Aid

- To preserve life.
- To promote recovery.
- To prevent worsening of the casualty's general condition.
- To arrange for transportation of the casualty to the nearest hospital if required.

Principles of First Aid

- Be in control, both of yourself and the problem.
- Act calmly and logically.
- Be gentle but firm; speak to the casualty kindly but purposefully.
- Build up trust while taking to the casualty through the examination and treatment.
- Explain what you are going to do.
- Answer honestly and say 'no' if you do not know. Avoid misleading information.
- Never leave the casualty alone. Continue to talk to him or her and hold her hands.
- Reassure the casualty.
- Do not separate a child from a parent or guardian, inform relatives.

First Aider

A first aider is just a common person who may have learn a standard method at application of first aid best suited to his skill. He is trained to reach patients, identify the problem, and to provide emergency care and when necessary move patient without causing further injury.

Injuries

Common Sports Injuries

Most major sports injuries can be recognized by their signs and symptoms, and treatment can be provided as required. Head injuries, concussion, lacerations, soft tissue injuries and fractures are recognizable and can be effectively treated by anyone trained in basic first aid. Certain other sports injuries are more common, and may require more specific first aid treatment. These are explained below:

Chest Cramps (or 'Stitch')

Usually caused by cramps of the muscles between the ribs, or the diaphragm high in the abdomen. Brought on by exertion, chest cramps are identified by sharp, spasmodic pain in the chest, difficulty in standing upright, and gasping respirations.

A 'Stitch' will disappear with rest and concentration on deep breathing.

Groin and testicle injuries caused by a blunt injury to the pelvic area. Causes severe pain in the area. The casualty will be unable to stand upright, and will 'guard' the injured area with his hands.

The casualty should be placed on his back with knees slightly bent and have an ice pack applied with caution to the injury site. Seek medical aid.

Muscle Cramps

Caused by over-stretching muscles, or by abnormal muscle contraction. They may also be associated with loss of fluid due to excessive sweating, will have pain, tenderness, loss of power and stiffening or spasms of the muscles. Muscles respond to rest, application of an ice pack, then subsequent gentle stretching.

Do not massage the affected muscles.

Other sports injuries should be treated as they present, and medical aid sought as a matter of course. If these injuries are in the form of sprains and strains, they may require support in the form of strapping or taping.

Head Injuries

Any blow to the head can result in a head injury. Head injuries can cause damage to the:
- **Scalp:** Layer outside the skull bone.
- **Skull:** Bony cage.
- **Brain:** A concussion, a contusion (the brain tissue is bruised), or a hematoma (blood collects in an area of the brain from a broken blood vessel).

Signs and Symptoms

Head injuries that alert the need for medical attention include:
- Loss of consciousness, confusion, drowsiness
- Inability to move any part of the body or weakness in an arm or leg

- Bruise, cut on the scalp
- Severe headache
- Stiff neck
- Vomiting
- Blood or fluid that comes from the mouth, nose or ear
- Loss of vision, blurred or double vision, pupils of unequal size.

Spinal Injuries

Common causes are:
- Accidents—Cars, motorcycles
- Falls
- Diving mishaps—from diving into the water that is too shallow
- A hard blow to back while playing
- Gun shot wound that penetrates the head and neck.

First Aid

- Do the scene survey for safety to self and the casualty.
- Call for the ambulance.

Dental Injuries

- Generally anterior teeth knocked out by direct heat or after tooth extraction, bleeding from tooth socket may occur immediately or after few hours.
- Rinse the mouth with water or saline.
- Place a thick cotton ball in the socket and ask him to bite it.

Ear Injuries

Bleeding from the ears is mainly because of cuts or injury to the external ear as this is very vascular. Bleeding from inside the ear is usually because of fracture skull; injury to the ear drum or ear canal or infection inside.

First Aid

Help the casualty into a half sitting position with his head titled to the injures side to allow blood to drain away. Put on gloves if available. Hold a sterile dressing, non-fluffy pad lightly in place on the ear. Send the casualty to hospital.

Eye Injuries

The eye can bruise or cut by direct blow or by sharp chipped fragments of metal grit and glass.

First Aid

Flood the eye with warm water immediately, use your finger to keep the eye open as wide as possible, hold head under a faucet or pour water into the eye from any clean container for at least 15 mins continuously and gently roll the eyeball as much as possible to wash out.

Loosely bandage both eyes. Seek medical help immediately.

Epistaxis (Bleeding from Nose)

Bleeding occurs from the blood vessel inside the nostril. Bleeding comes from the nose is also a sign of fracture skull.

Causes

- Picking out crusts and hair.
- Blowing the nose.
- High blood pressure.
- Bleeding disorder.
- In summer—usually no cause.
- Injury to the bones of the nose.
- Common cold and other infections.

First Aid

- Sit the casually down with the head well forward and loosen any tight clothing around the neck and chest.
- Advise him to breathe through the mouth and to pinch the soft part of the nose.
- Tell him to split out any blood from the mouth; swallowed blood may cause nausea and vomiting.
- Released the pressure after 10 minutes. If the bleeding has not stopped continue treatment for further 10 minutes. Do not allow the casualty to raise the head.
- While the head is still forward, gently clean around the nose and mouth using a swab or clean dressing soaked in lukewarm water. Do not plug the nose.
- When the bleeding stops, tell the casualty to avoid exertion. Advise the casualty not to blow the nose for at least four hours so as not to disturb the clot.

Severe Bleeding from a Wound

Treatment

- Determine cause of injury.
- Call **for ambulance**.
- Wear gloves, mask, and protective eyewear. Use Standard Precautions (see **Standard Precautions**).
- Control bleeding by placing a clean covering (preferably sterile) over wound and applying direct pressure.
- If injury does not appear to involve broken bone, elevate injured area above the level of the heart.
- If necessary, add more dressings. **Do not** remove previous dressing. Secure dressing in place.
- In case of amputation, see **Amputation.**
- Treat for shock (see **Shock**).
- If necessary, certified personnel should start CPR (see **CPR**).
- Call parent.

FOREIGN BODIES

Foreign Bodies in the Eye

Sand particles, dust, small pieces of glass, coal, and emery stone, metal usually enter the eye as foreign bodies. These particles usually get situated under the eyelid or eyeball.

Signs and Symptoms

- Pain and itching in eye
- Vision may be impaired
- Watering of affected area
- Redness in eye.

Treatment

- Ask the casualty, not to rub the eye.
- Ask him to sit down in a chair, facing the light and lean back.
- Stand behind the casualty, hold the chin in one hand and use the index finger and thumb of your other hand to separate the affected lids. Ask him to look right, left up and down so that every part of the eye can be examined properly.
- If foreign body is visible, wash it with sterile water and on eye irrigator. Eye can be irrigated with tape water, incline the head towards the injured side so that the water will drain out over the check away from the sound eye.
- If this is unsuccessful or water is not available and foreign body is not sticking to the eye, lift the foreign body corner of a clean cloth.
- If the foreign body is under the upper lid, ask the casualty to look down. Grasp the eyelashes and pull the upper lid downward and outward over the lower lid.
- Now foreign body can be removed.
- If foreign body cannot be removed, cover the affected eye with an eye pad. Secure it lightly and consult the doctor.
- Do not try to remove foreign body from eyeball or colored part of the eye.

Foreign Bodies in the Ear

The cases of foreign bodies in the ear occur generally in children.

Solid substance like peas, buttons can enter the ear. Among these, some substance like peas and other seeds absorb moisture, swell up and obstruct the ear and then it become difficult to take things out. Flies, mosquitoes or bed bugs can also enter the ear.

First Aid

Never used pin or piece of wire to take out foreign bodies from the ear because by using them eardrum may get rupture.

Mosquitoes, bed bugs or flies die by putting olive oil or soda bicarbs in lukewarm water into the ear. Then murmuring sound of these insects stops. Now send person to the hospital.

Foreign Bodies in the Nose

Certain foreign bodies like piece of betel nut, grains and peas and other seeds enter the nose. Generally happens mostly in children. By putting olive oil and the oil in the nose either the foreign bodies comes out or the irritation of the nose subside.

Do not sneeze forcefully in effort to take out the foreign body or do not close the unaffected nostril and try to sneeze out with the affected nostril because by doing so there is fear of cessation of respiration. Though there is no immediate risk but the person should be sent to the hospital as soon as possible.

First Aid on Bites and Stings

Animal Bite

Animal bites cause lethal bleeding, but they can produce significant damage. 60–90% of the animal bites in Odisha state come from dogs.

A dog's mouth may carry more than 60 different species of bacteria, some of which are very dangerous to human. Human cat and other animal bites are equally contaminated and dangerous.

First Aid

- If the wound not bleeding heavily, wash it with soap and water.
- Washing should take 5–20 minutes. Scrubbing can traumatize tissues; so avoid it whenever possible.
- Allowing a wound to bleed a little so it will help to remove bacteria left in the tissues.
- Rinse the wound thoroughly with running water.
- Control bleeding with direct pressure and if an extremity is involved and the bleeding continue, use elevation alone with the direct pressure.
- Cover with a sterile, dressing, but do not seal the wound tightly with tape or butterfly bandages.
- Seek medical attention because of the danger of infection, need for further cleaning, the possible for a tetanus shot and stitches to close the wound.

Insect Bites

Insects such as bee, wasps and jelly fish cause stings which are very painful.

Sign and Symptoms

Sharp pain, itching, swelling of the throat if stings in the mouth and throat redness or discoloration at site of the bite.

First Aid

- If the stinger remains in the victim, you may try to remove it carefully with a tweezer or by scraping with the edge of a credit card.
- Be careful not to squeeze the stinger as this will inject more venom. Once a stinger has been removed, the wound should be washed well with soap and water, cold compress will help to relieve pain and swelling, the stung area should be kept lower than heart to slow circulation of the venom.
- Watch for any signs of allergic reactions if they appear, seek medical help without delay.

Snake Bite

Snakes are commonly found in tropical climates. They can be poisonous or nonpoisonous. People who walk in jungles, camp, hike, picnic, or live in snake-inhabited areas should be aware of the potential dangers posed by venomous snakes.

Symptoms of Poisonous Snake Bites

While each individual may experience symptoms differently, the following are the most common symptoms of poisonous snake bites:
- Anxious look
- Fang marks in the skin and redness/swelling at the site of the bite
- Pain localized to site of bite
- Vision disorder—blurred or double vision
- Convulsions
- Fainting
- Dizziness/weakness
- Excessive sweating
- Loss of muscle coordination
- Nausea and vomiting
- Numbness and tingling
- Rapid pulse
- Difficulty in breathing.

First Aid for Snake Bites

- Reassure the casualty to stay calm
- Do not try to capture the snake
- Do not attempt to cut or suck the part to remove the venom
- Immobilize the bitten part
- Maintain the part below the level of the heart
- Wash the wound and dry it with clean cloth
- Lightly compress the limb above the wound
- Monitor vital signs
- Rush to the nearest hospital.

Burn and Scalds

The severity of a burn depends upon its size, depth and location. Burns are most severe when located on the face, neck, hands, feet and genitals. Also, when burns affect large parts of the body, they cause severe fluid loss and infection, and can be life-threatening. Burns result in pain, infection and shock. They are also more serious when the victims are very young or very old.

Burns can cause damage to the body tissues by:
- **Dry heat:** Flames, lighted cigarettes, hot iron
- **Moist heat (scalds):** Boiling water or hot oil
- **Cold:** Liquid nitrogen
- **Chemical:** Acids or alkali
- **Electrical burns:** Electricity or lightning
- **Radiation:** Sunrays or laser

To distinguish a minor burn from a serious burn, the 1st step is to determine the degree and the extent of damage. Burns are classified:

According to the depth
- 1st degree burn
  - Redness
  - Swelling and Pain (such as mild sunburn)
- 2nd degree burn
  - Blisters, redness
  - Very painful
  - Associated with loss of fluid through the damaged skin are the most painful because nerve ending are usually intact, despite severe tissue damage
- 3rd degree burn
  - Deepest
  - Skin is charred and waxy
  - Fat, muscle, even bone may be affected
  - Extremely painful or relatively painless.

Management

Remember 4 C's while managing burns:
- Cool the burnt part by keeping it under running water for at least 10 minutes. Don't put ice on the burn.
- Constrictors should be removed immediately like rings, bracelets, etc., before swelling occurs.
- Cover the burnt part to prevent infection by using any clean cloth for example handkerchief.
- Consult a doctor immediately.

General Care for Burns

- Smother the flames or move the victim away from danger.
- Lay the casualty down on the floor.
- Check the response, airway, breathing and pulse while managing the burn. Resuscitate the casualty if necessary.
- Call for medical help immediately.
- Look and treat for associated injuries or shock.
- Cover all the wounds with clean dressing.

Precautions

- Do not touch or interfere with the burnt area.
- Do not apply toothpaste, hair cream, butter or any ointment.
- Do not cover with cotton.
- Do not remove clothes sticking to the burnt area.
- Do not break the blisters.

Chemical Burns

In case the burns are caused by chemicals, it is important to remove clothing on which chemicals have spilled and flush the affected area with copious amounts of water for 15 to 30 minutes.

Electrical Burns

An electrical burn may appear minor, but the damage can extend deep into the tissues beneath the skin.

Management

- Look first, do not touch.
- Turn off the source of electricity if possible.
- Assess breathing, check pulse.
- Cover the affected area.
- Call for help.

FRACTURES, SPRAINS, STRAINS AND DISLOCATIONS

Fractures, sprains, strains and dislocations may be hard for the nonmedical person to differentiate. Fracture means broken or cracked bones.

Fractures can be caused by:
- **Direct force:** Bones are broken at the point where severe force is applied.
- **Indirect force:** Bones are broken away from the point where severe force is applied.

Types of Fracture

Closed fracture: Skin is intact with broken bone.
Open fracture: Broken bone with open wound.
Skin is broken with evident bleeding.
How to recognize?
- Immobility
- Deformity
- Look for pain
- Look for tenderness
- Look for swelling
- Look for loss of function
- Any unnatural movement
- History of heavy blow or fall.

Complication of Fractures

- Associated injuries may be present
- **Shock:** Hypovolemic or Neurogenic

Management

Aims

- Immobilization and support to the fractured part.
- Minimizing the painful movements.
  - Reassure the casualty and ask not to move.
  - Check circulation and treat for shock.
  - Steady and support the fractured limb.
  - Keep the joints above and below the fractured part immobilized with splint (or any improvised item). Proper splinting may reduce pain.
  - To design a splint, use a rigid material such as wood, plastic or metal.
  - Fasten the splint to the limb with gauze, bandages, and strip of cloth, string or even a belt.
  - Tie bandages firmly.
  - Stop bleeding with direct pressure if possible.
  - If possible elevate the injured part.
  - Transport the casualty to the nearest hospital.
  - Check circulation, breathing, level of consciousness every 10 minutes.

First Aid for Strains, Sprains, Confusions, Dislocations, or Uncomplicated Fractures

RICE (Rest, Ice, Compression, Elevation)

Treatment

Rest

- Stop using injured part
  - Continued activity could cause further injury, delay healing, increase pain, and stimulate bleeding
- Use crutches to avoid bearing weight on injuries of the leg, knee, ankle, or foot
- Use splint for injuries of the arm, elbow, wrist, or hand.

Ice

- Hastens healing time by reducing swelling around injury
  - Sudden cold contracts blood vessels
  - Helps stop internal bleeding from injured capillaries and blood vessels
- Keep damp or dry cloth between skin and ice pack
- Do not apply ice for longer than 15 to 20 minutes at a time
  - Apply at least 3 times throughout the day for 15 to 20 minutes.

Compression

- Hastens healing time by reducing swelling around injury
  - Decreases seeping of fluid into injured area from adjacent tissue
- Use elasticized bandage, compression sleeve, or cloth
  - Wrap injured part firmly
  - Do not impair blood supply
  - Too tight compression may cause more swelling
  - Wrap over ice
  - Loosen the bandage if it gets too tight.

Elevation

Elevate injured part above level of heart
- Decreases swelling and pain
- Use objects and pillows for props, strains, sprains
- What to do?
  - Rest to the injured part
  - Pain killer (analgesic).

SHOCK

Shock is an emergency condition when blood flow to vital organs (brain, heart, kidney) is decreased.

Causes for Shock

- Heart failure
- Severe or sudden blood loss
- Large drop in body fluids (a severe burn or severe vomiting and/or diarrhea)
- Food poisoning
- Exposure to extreme heat or cold for too long.

Other Things that Lead to Shock

- Fracture of a large bone
- Severe allergic reaction
- Severe hypoglycemia

- Excessive of alcohol
- Drug overdose.

Signs and Symptoms of Shock

- Weakness, trembling, restlessness
- Confusion
- Loss of consciousness
- Pale or blue-colored lips, skin and/or fingernails
- Cool and moist skin, sweating
- Weak, but fast pulse
- Rapid, shallow breathing
- Nausea, vomiting
- Extreme thirst.

Management

- Activate emergency medical services.
- Lay the person down, face up
- Elevate the feet about 1 foot with a box or rolled blankets. This causes blood to flow from the legs to the vital organs in the body.

Note: Do not raise the feet or lower the head if you suspect the person has a head, neck, back or leg injury.

- Do not raise feet or move legs if hip or leg bones are broken.
- Loosen tight clothing. Then, cover the person with a coat or blanket to prevent heat loss.
- Monitor for breathing and pulse every 5 minutes.
- Do not give any food or liquids unless person is recovered/alert.
- Reassure the person.
- If the person vomits, roll him or her on the side.

Allergic Reaction

Anaphylactic

Note: An anaphylactic reaction (**shock**) is a severe, and sudden generalized reaction that is potentially life-threatening. Symptoms include respiratory distress or shock.

Signs and Symptoms

- Apprehension
- Rash (particularly on face)
- Swelling of affected areas (particularly on face, tongue, and neck)
- Breathing difficulty, wheezing, gurgling, high-pitched sounds
- Skin is flushed and dry or pale, cool, and clammy
- Increased heart rate, weak pulse.

Treatment

- Call **for ambulance**.
- If individual is known to have allergies, consult the written emergency action plan on file and proceed with physician's recommendations (for example, EpiPen).
- Check individual's pulse and respiration. Be alert for breathing and pulse being slower or faster than usual.
- If necessary, cover with blankets to keep warm.
- If necessary, certified personnel start CPR (see C**PR and Shock**).
- Call parent.

Hives (Rash)/Itching

Note: Hives are eruptions of the skin caused by contact with or ingestion of an allergic substance or food. Hives appear as raised blotches on the skin, pale in the middle, with reddened border, often accompanied by itching. Hives involving mouth, eyelids and tongue are potentially life threatening.

Treatment

- If hives involve eyelids, lips, mouth, or tongue, call for ambulance.
- If individual is known to have allergies, consult the written emergency action plan on file and proceed with physician's recommendations (for example, EpiPen).
- Apply cold compress.
- Give reassurance.
- If individual is too uncomfortable to do school work, send home.
- Call parent.

Swelling

Note: An allergic reaction that causes swelling is potentially life threatening.

Treatment

- If there is face, mouth, and neck swelling, call for ambulance.
- Apply cold compresses.
- Give reassurance.
- Call parent.

Asthma

Note: Asthma is a lung disease that causes repeated episodes of breathing problems. Symptoms of asthma can be mild, severe, or fatal. Asthma is potentially life-threatening.

Signs and Symptoms

- Breathing problems
- Wheezing (high-pitched, whistling sound)
- Coughing
- Tightness in chest
- Shortness of breath.

Treatment

- Place individual in comfortable position, usually sitting, leaning forward.
- Remain calm.
- If individual is known to school personnel as having asthma, refer to the written emergency action plan on file and proceed with physician's recommendations.

- If any of the following conditions exist, call for ambulance:
  - Difficulty breathing (significant use of neck and chest muscles for breathing or poor air movement).
  - Shortness of breath or inability to speak more than 3–5 word sentences.
  - Breathing rate of less than 12 or greater than 30 times a minute.
  - Individual with decreased level of consciousness.
  - Bluish lips or nail beds.
- Call parent.

Bee and Wasp Stings

Note: Individuals with known allergy should have an emergency care plan.

Signs and Symptoms

Local reaction includes intense pain, a whitish bump with a red dot in its center swelling **at the site** of the sting whereas sometime anaphylactic reaction such as rash (particularly on face) swelling of face and tongue, difficulty breathing, wheezing, gurgling, high pitched sounds, skin feels moist and or appears flushed, pale or bluish and rapid, weak pulse may happen.

Treatment

- If necessary, call for ambulance (see **Allergic Reaction**).
- If individual is known to have allergies to bee/wasp stings, consult the written emergency action plan on file and proceed with physician's recommendations.
- If necessary, certified personnel start CPR (see **CPR**).
- Remove stinger as quickly as possible.
- Apply cold compress to reduce pain and swelling.
- If the sting is on the arm or leg, keep extremity below the level of the heart.
- **Call Poison Center** for additional treatment advice.
- Call parent.

ADOLESCENT HEALTH

The adolescence period is most important in the life of an individual and so the child at this stage is to be cautiously guided. This period otherwise known as puberty period when rapid physical growth and psychological changes takes place. It is the most important and sensitive period of one's life. Adolescence is a time of moving from immaturity childhood to maturity adulthood by unfolding a set of transitions that touch upon many aspects of the individual's behavior and development. There are 1.3 billion adolescents in the world on April 2022, more than ever before, making up 16 per cent of the world's population (UNICEF-2022). They are not only in large numbers but are the citizens and workers of tomorrow. The problems of adolescents are multidimensional in nature and require holistic approach. This is also an impressionable period of life. This is also the period of preparation for undertaking greater responsibilities including healthy responsible parenthood. Future of society depends on adolescents and they form a great human resource for the society. Adolescence period is generally extends from 10–19 years in which early adolescence is 10–13 years, middle adolescence is 14–16 years and late adolescence 17–19 years.

Due to the peculiar nature of physical, intellectual, emotional and social development, the adolescent at this stage has peculiar needs and problems. The child/adolescent wants that all his needs should be fulfilled. If fulfillment of need is not possible he faces failures and frustrations and he is emotionally shocked. So, he is unstable and unpredictable. Adjustment becomes a problem to him. If he is left uncared for he turns into either a maladjusted young adult to the society. That is why he is to receive due attention and proper guidance.

Adjustment in home, school and society, adjustment with opposite sex, adjustment to a suitable vacation, freedom from home, development of a sound philosophy of life, health adjustment, financial worries, school failures, conflicts with friends and peer group, unfavorable relation in home, need for social status are some of the sources of the problems of an adolescent.

A large number of adolescents in India are out of school, malnourished, get married early, working in vulnerable situations, and are sexually active. They are exposed to tobacco or alcohol abuse. So adolescent health can be preserved. There are different health issue among adolescents. They are:

Early Pregnancy and Childbirth

Adolescence marks the period between childhood and adulthood when hormonal changes transform boys and girls into young men and women able to have children of their own which leads to curiosity on sex and make them indulged with sex without proper knowledge which leads to teen age pregnancy and other sexual transmitted diseases. Due to the premature development of genital organ the unsafe sex practice make them vulnerable to different complications associated with pregnancy and childbirth and other sexual transmitted disease.

Complications linked to pregnancy and childbirth are the second cause of death for 15–19 year-old girls globally. Some 11% of all births worldwide are to girls aged 15 to 19 years, and the vast majority are in low and middle-income countries.

The 2014 World Health Statistics put the global adolescent birth rate at 49 per 1000 girls this age—country rates range from 1 to 229 births per 1000 girls. One of the Millennium Development Goals, MDG 5, is to achieve universal access to reproductive health, for which one of the indicators is the pregnancy rate among the 15 to 19 age group. Better access to contraceptive information and services can reduce the number of girls becoming pregnant and giving birth at too young an age. Laws that specify a minimum age of marriage at 18 and which are enforced can help. Girls who do become pregnant need access to quality antenatal care. Where permitted by law, adolescents who opt to terminate their pregnancies should have access to safe abortion. More than 2 million adolescents are living with HIV. Although the overall number of HIV-related deaths is down 30% since the peak 8 years ago, estimates suggest that HIV deaths among adolescents are rising. This increase, which has been predominantly in the WHO Africa Region, may reflect the fact that although more children with HIV survive into adolescence, MDG 6 to halt the spread of HIV/AIDS has indicators including the prevalence among 15 to 24 year olds and the proportion of this age group with comprehensive correct knowledge of HIV/AIDS.

Mental Health

Depression is the top cause of illness and disability among adolescents and suicide is the third cause of death. Violence, poverty, humiliation and feeling devalued can increase the risk of developing mental health problems. It is due to maladjustment of adolescents with their transitions. Building life skills in children and adolescents and providing them with psychosocial support in schools and other community settings can help promote good mental health. Program to help strengthen ties between adolescents and their families are also important. If problems arise, they should be detected and managed by competent and caring health workers.

Violence

Violence is a leading cause of death. An estimated 180 adolescents die every day as a result of interpersonal violence. Around 1 of every 3 deaths among adolescent males in the low and middle-income countries in the WHO Americas Region is due to violence. Globally, some 30% of girls aged 15 to 19 experience violence by a partner.

Promoting nurturing relationships between parents and children early in life, providing training in life skills, and reducing access to alcohol and firearms can help to prevent violence. Effective and empathetic care for adolescent survivors of violence and ongoing support can help deal with the physical and the psychological consequences.

Alcohol and Drugs

Harmful drinking among adolescents is a major concern in many countries. It reduces self-control and increases risky behaviors, such as unsafe sex. It is a primary cause of injuries (including those due to road traffic accidents), violence (especially by a partner) and premature deaths. It also can lead to health problems in later life and affect life expectancy. Setting a minimum age for buying and consuming alcohol and regulating how alcoholic drinks are targeted at the younger market are among the strategies for reducing harmful drinking. Drug use among 15 to 19 year olds is also a concern.

Injuries

Unintentional injuries are a leading cause of death and disability among adolescents. In 2012, some 120000 adolescents died as a result of road traffic accidents. Young drivers need advice on driving safely, while laws that prohibit driving under the influence of alcohol and drugs need to be strictly enforced. Blood alcohol levels need to be set lower for teenage drivers. Graduated licences for novice drivers with zero-tolerance for drink-driving are recommended. Drowning is also a major cause of death among adolescents–60000, two-thirds of them boys, drowned in 2012.

Malnutrition and Obesity

Many boys and girls in developing countries enter adolescence undernourished, making them more vulnerable to disease and early death. The number of adolescents who are overweight or obese is increasing in both low and high-income countries. Anemia resulting from a lack of iron affects girls and boys, and is the third cause of years lost to death and disability. Iron and folic acid supplements help to promote health before adolescents become parents. Developing healthy eating and exercise habits at this age are foundations for good health in adulthood. Reducing the marketing of foods high in saturated fats, trans-fatty acids, free sugars, or salt and providing access to healthy foods and opportunities to engage in physical activity are important for all but especially children and adolescents: On average, adolescents consume diets that are inadequate in several vitamins and minerals, including folate, vitamins A and E, iron, zinc, magnesium and calcium. Dietary fiber intake among adolescents is also low. Though anemia control program given importance on adolescent health still majority of them are anemic.

Exercise

Available survey data indicate that fewer than 1 in every 4 adolescents meets the recommended guidelines for physical activity—60 minutes of moderate to vigorous physical activity daily.

Tobacco Use

The vast majority of people using tobacco today began when they were adolescents. Prohibiting the sale of tobacco products to minors and increasing the price of tobacco products through higher taxes, banning tobacco advertising and ensuring smoke-free environments are crucial. Globally, at least 1 in 10 younger adolescents (aged 13 to 15) uses tobacco, although there are areas where this figure is much higher. Cigarette smoking seems to be decreasing among younger adolescents in some high-income countries.

The special aspect of care during this period are:

- Reproductive health care
- Nutrition
- Sex education
- Psychological care
- Hygienic care
- Prevention from substance abuse.

PREVENTIVE STRATEGY

Health Education

The syllabus for adolescent health education should include development of secondary sexual characters and menarche, problems associated with menstrual cycle and menstrual hygiene, Body image, nutritional needs (micronutrients), managing emotional stress, early marriage and its effect, RTI/HIV/AIDS, practicing safe sex, family life including pregnancy, child rearing and responsible parenthood, stress management, substance abuse, counseling for emotional stress, nutritional counseling and early diagnosis and management of medical and behavioral problem. There are a number of standardized case videos created on reproductive health which designed to facilitate discussion about how health professionals or teachers can best interact with adolescent people when providing reproductive and sexual health care. The adolescent videos series focus on the unique communication, counseling, and clinical needs of teen children.

Parent Education

An adolescence is a period of increasing conflict and decreasing closeness occurring in many parent-adolescent relationships. The parent should be properly educated on this. The parent should be educated to develop a sense of consistent positive connection with teenager parent which can help them to identify their problems and help them to cope with transitions. Positive connection can provide back drop against the interaction takes place. If the connection is consistent, positive and characterized by warmth, kindness love and stability, adolescents are more like to flourish socially. Teens with this kind of relationship with parent have higher self-esteems. By behaving adolescents as friend, the parent can monitor their behavior can keep close observation on them without their knowledge. The parent should provide psychological autonomy to the child by encouraging independent thinking and expression of original ideas and beliefs. Avoiding lectureship and spending time with them in recreational activities may be helpful.

Counseling

As the adolescent pass through a series of transitions like that touch upon many aspects of the individual's behavior, development, and relationships biological transition which is due to bodily changes, cognitive transition by which compared to children adolescents think in ways that are more advanced more efficient and generally more complex, social transition make adolescence to increase the amount of time spend with their peers and emotional transition make them vulnerable to different diseases. Counseling on problem solving is very important. A good counselor may be their parent, teacher or a community health Nurse.

Nutrition Counseling

The adolescents are prone to nutritional problems like obesity, eating disorders, extreme dieting, fads and food fetishes. Since chronic diseases often originate with poor eating habits, intervention is often essential to ensure they do not take unhealthy habits into adulthood. Discover stages of change and how you can help address potential nutrient intake problems. For this age group children nutritional counseling is very much essential. Nutrition counseling is an ongoing process in which a health professional, usually a registered dietitian, works with an individual to assess his or her usual dietary intake and identify areas where change is needed. The nutrition counselor provides information, educational materials, support, and follow-up to help the individual make and maintain the needed dietary changes. The goal of nutrition counseling is to help a person make and maintain dietary changes. Healthy Diet: Food intake Carbohydrates, e.g., Rice, Chapati, Protein-based, e.g., Milk, Egg, Dal and Meat. Salads, Vegetables, Fruits Increase fiber, Decrease oily foods, 'No' to soft drink, Unsaturated fat recommended. Proteins Daily requirements, Boys = 0.29–0.32 g/cm height, Girls = 0.27–0.29 g/cm height, 0.8–1.2 g/kg bodyweight, the protein foods included pulses, lentils, soya, dairy products and animal food products for iron and zink food counsel them to take green leafy vegetables, jaggery, wet dates, whole-grain, dried beans, peas and dried fruits, nuts and fortified wheat products, eggs, red meat, etc., for calcium they should take Milk and its products, yogurts, cheese, paneer, banana. Eating is regulated by hunger and satiety, i.e., feeling full Eating should be at regular intervals. Choose healthy snacks and food, Good eating habits. Maintain hygienic habits, Eat slowly, chew properly. Avoid TV viewing or reading while you eat. Take small frequent meals. Never skip meals, specially breakfast. Do not overeat.

Role of Community Health Nurse in Care of Adolescents

As a nurse she should provide friendly health services to the adolescents. She should maintain confidentiality, and she understand the adolescent problems and help them accordingly.

The health providers have a significant role in interacting with the education system and providing support, training and materials in addition to the counseling and services. The Community Health Nurse can organize health education programme for the adolescents in schools for school going adolescents and in community for school drop outs to increase their knowledge on health. They also need to develop effective channels of referral and rehabilitation. The CHN can provide liaison by the adolescents with NGOs and other institutions to which they can assess and utilizes the health services provided to them.

Adolescents confront a number of problems because of the lack of authentic knowledge regarding their process of growing up, particularly, the issues relating to reproductive health which are hided to them.

Therefore it is essential to educate the community members as well as adolescents about the normal physiological changes with special reference to nutrition and health needs of adolescents. A nurse should educate the adolescent about healthy lifestyle and behavior among them.

A nurse should take interest in teaching adolescents. In group, i.e., in community, school, hospital, etc., about their growth, development, nutritional requirement use of dangerous substances like drug and alcohol, risky driving, smoking, unprotected sex relation and pregnancy. She also educate the family members in this regard. She should create a positive and encouraging attitude among parents and family members to interact with adolescents and to give clarifications and correct information on their doubts which will facilitate better relationship of trust and confidence.

Mental Health

Depression is the top cause of illness and disability among adolescents and suicide is the third cause of death. Violence, poverty, humiliation and feeling devalued can increase the risk of developing mental health problems. It is due to maladjustment of adolescents with their transitions. Building life skills in children and adolescents and providing them with psychosocial support in schools and other community settings can help promote good mental health. Program to help strengthen ties between adolescents and their families are also important. If problems arise, they should be detected and managed by competent and caring health workers.

Violence

Violence is a leading cause of death. An estimated 180 adolescents die every day as a result of interpersonal violence. Around 1 of every 3 deaths among adolescent males in the low and middle-income countries in the WHO Americas Region is due to violence. Globally, some 30% of girls aged 15 to 19 experience violence by a partner.

Promoting nurturing relationships between parents and children early in life, providing training in life skills, and reducing access to alcohol and firearms can help to prevent violence. Effective and empathetic care for adolescent survivors of violence and ongoing support can help deal with the physical and the psychological consequences.

Alcohol and Drugs

Harmful drinking among adolescents is a major concern in many countries. It reduces self-control and increases risky behaviors, such as unsafe sex. It is a primary cause of injuries (including those due to road traffic accidents), violence (especially by a partner) and premature deaths. It also can lead to health problems in later life and affect life expectancy. Setting a minimum age for buying and consuming alcohol and regulating how alcoholic drinks are targeted at the younger market are among the strategies for reducing harmful drinking. Drug use among 15 to 19 year olds is also a concern.

Injuries

Unintentional injuries are a leading cause of death and disability among adolescents. In 2012, some 120000 adolescents died as a result of road traffic accidents. Young drivers need advice on driving safely, while laws that prohibit driving under the influence of alcohol and drugs need to be strictly enforced. Blood alcohol levels need to be set lower for teenage drivers. Graduated licences for novice drivers with zero-tolerance for drink-driving are recommended. Drowning is also a major cause of death among adolescents–60000, two-thirds of them boys, drowned in 2012.

Malnutrition and Obesity

Many boys and girls in developing countries enter adolescence undernourished, making them more vulnerable to disease and early death. The number of adolescents who are overweight or obese is increasing in both low and high-income countries. Anemia resulting from a lack of iron affects girls and boys, and is the third cause of years lost to death and disability. Iron and folic acid supplements help to promote health before adolescents become parents. Developing healthy eating and exercise habits at this age are foundations for good health in adulthood. Reducing the marketing of foods high in saturated fats, trans-fatty acids, free sugars, or salt and providing access to healthy foods and opportunities to engage in physical activity are important for all but especially children and adolescents: On average, adolescents consume diets that are inadequate in several vitamins and minerals, including folate, vitamins A and E, iron, zinc, magnesium and calcium. Dietary fiber intake among adolescents is also low. Though anemia control program given importance on adolescent health still majority of them are anemic.

Exercise

Available survey data indicate that fewer than 1 in every 4 adolescents meets the recommended guidelines for physical activity—60 minutes of moderate to vigorous physical activity daily.

Tobacco Use

The vast majority of people using tobacco today began when they were adolescents. Prohibiting the sale of tobacco products to minors and increasing the price of tobacco products through higher taxes, banning tobacco advertising and ensuring smoke-free environments are crucial. Globally, at least 1 in 10 younger adolescents (aged 13 to 15) uses tobacco, although there are areas where this figure is much higher. Cigarette smoking seems to be decreasing among younger adolescents in some high-income countries.

STUDENT COUNSELING

Everyone in the universe do come across some problem or other irrespective of their age, sex, profession or occupation for which man has been taking help of his elders, parents, friends and teachers in solving their problems. School period is a crucial period when the student can pass different transition in their life. The students are like the clay which can provided different shape by proper counseling and guidance. Student counseling is an important aspect of school health. In school most teachers provide a high standards of pupil care, but it is a fact that they have little talent and attitude of counselor because counseling requires special knowledge and attitude to recognize the problem and help an individual pupil or pupils and it emphasize intellectual, social, emotional, cultural and physical, development of the students as well as those services which help to improve instructions.

Definition and Meaning of Counseling

According to Cormier and Hackney in (1987) defined 'Counseling is the helping relationship, that includes someone seeking help, someone willing to give help who is capable or trained to help, in a setting that permits help to be given and received'.

According to Vedanayagam in (1988) defined, 'Counseling is an accepting, trusting and safe relationship in which clients learn to discuss freely what upsets them, to define their goals, to acquire the essential social skills and to develop the courage and self confidence to implement desired new behavior'.

According to Patterson in 1967 pointed out that Counseling is not giving the information, though information may be present and also not giving an advice, and advising refers to academic consultation often given to student by the teacher, who may not be trained counselor. Counseling is not the influencing the attitudes, beliefs and behaviors by persuading, threatening or compelling or not the selection and assignment of individual to jobs.

According to Smith—'Counseling is a process in which the counselor assists the counselee to make interpretation of facts relating to a choice, plan or adjustments, which he needs to make'.

Concept of Counseling

- Counseling is the relationship between two persons in which one of them attempts to assist the other in organizing himself to attain a form of happiness, adjustment to a life situation, i.e., self-actualization.
- An accepted, trusting and safe relationship will be formulated in which client will learn to discuss openly their problems, acquires the social skills, courage, self-confidence to implement desired new behaviors.
- The relationship between two personnel is:
  - *Counselor:* One a professionally trained worker
  - *Counselee:* The person who seeks the services or who cannot cope up alone, who requires help from the skilled personnel to resolve his problem by finding new ways.
- Counseling helps the individual to become aware of himself and the ways in which he is reacting to the behavioral influences to his environment.
- Counseling helps to develop a set of goals for future behavior of an individual.

Principles of Counseling

- Counseling is basically and permissive relationship.
- Counseling emphasized thinking with, not for the individual.
- To avoid dictatorial attitude.
- The counseling relationship is trust and confidence with the client.
- All decision making rests with the client.
- Counseling is centered on the problems of the clients.
- Counseling is a learning situation which eventually results in a behavioral change.
- Everyone participating in the counseling process with comfortable.
- Effectiveness in counseling depends largely on the readiness of the client to make changes and the therapeutic relationship with the counselor.
- The client's family members and significant influencing personnel must be influenced in counseling process.
- Skills of warmth, friendliness, openness and empathy are ingredients of successful counseling process.
- Counselor has to listen attentively, answer questions objectively, reinforce important information.
- To maintain dignity of individuals as individual is primary concern in counseling.

Need of Counseling

The needs of counseling are:

- To help the client to accept actual or impending changes that are resulting from stress. It involves psychological, emotional, intellectual and spiritual support.
- To foster cognitive, behavioral, developmental and emotional growth in clients.
- To encourage the client to examine the available alternatives and to decide or directs which choices are appropriate and useful for problem solution.
- To develop a sense of control for better management of stress. It provides an opportunity for emotional release and to discuss the ways of coping with problems.
- To relieve distress among people who are reacting to difficult circumstances.
- To change the behavior by reducing the stress or risk. It helps the counselee to acquire independence and a sense of responsibility. It helps the client to explore and fully utilize his potentialities and actualize himself.
- To encourage and develop special abilities and right attitude.
- To inspire successful endeavor towards attainment.
- To assist the students in planning for educational and vocational choices.
- To help the student to work out a plan for solving his difficulties.
- To helps in the proper choice of course according to the interest, aptitude and intelligence of the student.

- To help the students to grow, explore and maintain or develop their overall personality.
- To develop readiness for choices and charges to face new challenges.
- To help for efficient use of manpower.
- To motivate the students for self-employment.
- To help the fresher to establish a proper identity.
- To help the students in the period of confusion or turmoil.
- To help the students in checking wastage and stagnation.
- To help the students in need of special help.
- To minimize the incidence of indiscipline, which is leading to destructive activity and social damage.

COUNSELOR

The counseling program cannot just depend upon a counselor alone but has to involve other member of the school like teaching faculty, librarian, hostel warden, physical instructor, medical personnel, etc.

Principal/Vice Principal/Tutor Incharge/ Nursing and Medical Superintendent

For the counseling program to succeed the support of these persons is essential. These persons should recognize the need of the program, provide facilities, finance, give in its rightful place in the school time-table, coordinate with other members of the staff, give publicity to the program and evaluate the counseling program.

Counselor

Although most of the nursing schools/colleges do not have a full time counselor but it is hoped that soon the situation will change and every school will have either fully trained counselor or some tutors who are trained through in-service/distance program to take up the role of a counselor. The NSG Schools may arrange to have visiting counselors from institutions that have them, till they have their own counselors.

Tutors

Tutors are the key professionals in the school setting. Their support and participation is crucial in making the counseling program a success. It is those who have the maximum and important contact with the pupils. They act as a source of referral and appraisal to the Counselor, reinforce the counseling outcomes besides providing conductive environment. They give encouragement and support to the counselor. They also motivate the pupils to utilize the counseling services and help them develop a positive attitude towards counseling.

Parents

As the counseling program extends beyond nursing school parents must be told about the need and scope of counseling program. Pupils life, inspirations, adjustments, personality, the influence of home, etc. So, parents should be made aware of this impact. Parents also provide information about the pupil, i.e., her lifestyle, reading habits, temperament, her interpersonal relationship, style of reaction, her emotional adjustment etc. Parents also act as support to the pupil in the crises situation, academic or emotional disturbance. Thus, in the counseling process they have a two way role. They need to be oriented about their role by the counselor.

Functions of Counselor

Specifically, the functions of a counselor are:

- Pupil appraisal—using appropriate test and non-testing devices.
- Pupil orientation—involving tutors, wardens, librarians, doctors and other resources.
- Helping emotionally disturbed pupil—using counseling techniques.
- Helping pupil overcome academic and social deficiencies.
- Helping pupil overcome their financial, health, sex, residential and messing problems.
- Gaining cooperation from other tutors and helping then in gaining understanding of the pupils.
- Gaining cooperation from parents and other personnel of the counseling process.
- Maintaining up-to-date records of pupils concerning counseling.
- Arranged for referral services for those who need them.
- Evaluating and doing the follow-up work.
- Giving career talks to potential entrants to the nursing profession.
- Disseminating information relating to employment recreational and professional opportunities.

Characteristics of a Good Counselor

In order to provide effective counseling services, the counselor needs to demonstrate certain attributes. Some of these attributes which makes a person a good counselor are as follows:

Self Awareness and Understanding

A person who has awareness of her needs, motivation for helping, feelings, personal strengths and weakness acts as a good counselor.

Good Health

Although no person is totally problem free but a person requires sound physical and mental health. A healthy person can perform his job well, when compared to an unhealthy person.

Sensitivity

A person who is aware of resources limitations and vulnerability of other persons as well as keenly perceptive to other person's feelings and needs are considered to have sensitivity. A person having the understanding of individual will act as a good counselor.

Open Mindedness

A person of open mindedness can receive and accept the other people's values and he will not impose his values on others.

Objectivity

A person with the ability of not getting involved with the other person and at the same time, stand back and see accurately what is happening.

Trust Worthiness

A person who is reliable, honest and does not hurt other persons. He/she keeps the information to herself.

Approachability

It is a must. A student should be able to approach the counselor without any fear. His approach should be pleasant and friendly.

Counseling Services

The counseling services need to be planned and organized within the policy frame work and resources of institution. The services need to be coordinated well with the resources and implemented effectively.

Purposes

- Promotion of normal development of young students.
- Prevent and protect student from developmental problems and turmoils.
- Provide appropriate services when required/felt by the students to deal with any problem/crisis situation.
- Facilitate proper communication within and between the schools, home, the communities and resources.
- Support tutors who help students and who may also need guidance and counseling.

Types of Counseling Services

Orientation Service

It is meant to help the pupils become fully aware of herself and the new environment so that at the beginning of school/college career, they are oriented to the purpose, history, nature and scope of education and practice, besides being helped to acquaint herself with library and other physical and facilities which are available for them in school/college and outside it.

Appraisal Service

It is meant to gather, record, maintain, and use adequate information about each pupil. The purpose of the this service is to help each pupil achieve her optimum potential and for helping her to develop insight as she progresses through school. The information collected about her/his home, education, occupation of parents and another sources, such as pupil's interest, abilities, aptitude, health and general behavior pattern.

Developmental Counseling

It helps individual to achieve personal growth by making them aware of themselves and their environment. Set clear goals for future behavior and methods of achieving these goals. Develop positive attitudes, values, and morals.

Preventive Counseling

It helps an individual to prepare for future specific concerns, such as failures in the examinations, shock of not getting a job or admission, or delay in getting married and specially counseling for abuse of drugs, suicide and truancy.

Facilitative Counseling

It is also as remedial or adjustive counseling which means to correct a fault or an undesirable behavior.

Crisis Counseling

It helps an individual to overcome the effects of crisis situation such as loss of a family member, family conflicts, etc. These situation affects the normal behavior of an individual and she/he may develop a feeling of anxiety, loss, remorse or guilt. The counselor helps the individual understand the situation and develop new pattern of behavior.

Vocational and Placement Services

It is meant to serve the individual and society. Here occupational information is given to the individual. A srrong emphasis is given on placing students in jobs suitable for them. It can be done through coordination with employment exchanges and different employing and placement agencies.

Personal and Social Services

It is meant to help pupils overcome their problems of hostel, mess, and finance, help is also rendered for enabling the foreign students to adjust to new situations. School can organize programs for securing scholarships for students, getting funds from different sources, arranging for different cocurricular activities.

Follow-up Services

The common tools used for conducting follow-up services consist of questionnaires, interviews, letters, and telephone, etc.

THE COUNSELING PROCESS

Counseling process is a problem solving process. Counselor helps students to understand themselves, their potentialities, the assets, the problems they are facing and make decisions to take alternative action to solve their problems. In doing so, the counselor follows certain series of steps or passes through some phases and is referred as counseling processes.

Phases/Steps of Counseling Process

There are 5 different phases/steps of counseling process although it is difficult to divide such a complex process into clearly defined phases. These phases include:

Establishing Relationship

Establishing productive relationship is the core phase in the process of counseling. It affects the progress of the process and acts as a curative agent in itself. It should be recognized that each counselee. Counselor relationship is unique and hence it is not possible to have a generalized relationship. It includes such factors as respect, trust and a sense of psychological comfort which help in formation and sustaining good relationship by which the student can share their feelings.

The relationship is not established in just a single session but may require several sessions before he/she becomes comfortable with you and accepts you into his/her inner world.

Assessment

Making assessment is a phase in which individuals are encouraged to talk about their problems, counselor asks questions, collects information, seeks his/her views, observes and possibly helps the individual to clearly state his/her problems. This is the data collecting phase and involves several specific skills such as observation, enquiry, making associations among facts, recording, making educated guesses, recording of information should be done systematically and promptly.

Setting Goals

Setting goals is a phase based on educated guesses/interpretations made in the previous phase. The major purpose of this phase is to provide direction to the individual and the counselor. It involves making a commitment to a set of conditions, a course of action, or an outcome. Sometimes the individual may find it difficult to set goals or some counselor may resist setting goals. But setting goals help us to know how well counseling is working and when counseling may be concluded. Setting goals may be of two types: Immediate and ultimate.

It should be emphasized that goals are not fixed for all time to come and can be changed whenever new information is received or new insight is developed.

Interventions

It is a phase which is more influenced by the view points, a counselor holds about the counseling process. After setting goals, the question that follows is 'how shall we accomplish these goals'? The intervention used will depend upon the problem area and the nature of specific problem and the individual. Hence, the choice of the intervention is a process of adaptation and the counselor should be prepared to change the intervention when the selected intervention is not working. This is similar to medical treatment. When one treatment does not work, the practitioner tries the alternative treatment. The counseling skills needed are handling the interventions, knowledge of its effects and ability to read client's reactions. Individuals can be asked in the beginning about what interventions they have tried earlier so that other interventions can be used.

Termination and Follow-up

All counseling has its ultimate criterion on successful termination. It must be done without destroying the accomplishments gained and should be done with sensitivity, intention and by phasing. It is not unusual for the individual to have a feeling of a sense of loss; hence termination should be planned over few sessions. Follow-up appointments can also be fixed for sometimes.

Techniques and Tools

It means to achieve our goals and not an end in themselves. The information collected through the use of these tools should be cumulative about the individual as a whole based on a veriety of sources or tools.

Techniques/Methods

Interview

It is the basic tool of getting information from the individual, concerned and his/her significant, others, i.e., parents, siblings, friends, teachers, etc. Interview permits flexibility, clarity and an opportunity for observation to the counselor. At later stage, this understanding forms the basis of therapeutic interview in the process of counseling. Structuring of these interviews help in making the information more reliable and valid.

Observation

It is also a very important method of collecting information by the study of counselors with a specific purpose. Counselor makes the observation either by participating observation, i.e., as a member of the group of counselor (participative) or as an outsider-non-participative observations. Non-participative observations can be made during interview or while doing psychological testing or in the classroom, or in the community/ward. Sometime one-way screens are used to make ties observations. By structuring and using a rating scale/checklist, these observation can be made more reliable and valid.

Record Review

It is another significant method of getting information about counselee from the different records maintained in the school/college. The records are:

Anecdotal records: Anecdotal records consist of recording of important incidents. Anecdote is verbal snapshot of an incident giving actual information about what happened. Decisions should not be made on the basis of single anecdote.

Cumulative record card: Cumulative record card is a method of recording and providing meaningful, significant, comprehensive information about the individual over time. It provide information about student's attendance, achievement, social adjustment in the school, behavior with other students, attitude towards school and teachers. It also contains information regarding estimate of qualifies like hard work, tolerance, sociability and such other attributes which make a portrayal of the student more clear and complete. Cumulative record card can be maintained either in folder form or file form or card form.

Problem/Interest Checklist

It is given pupils to identify their expressed problems or interest.

Rating Scale

Rating scales are used to get the assessment of pupil's characteristics/trait such as initiative, responsibility, truthfulness, attitude of cooperation, honesty, etc., either by others or the pupil herself.

Sociometry

Sociometry is used to measure sociability or social distance amongst the members of a group. Autobiography and diaries maintained by the pupils may also provide useful information. Pupils should be encouraged to keep their diaries in which they can record notes about themselves in relation to courses and certain situations. This self-evaluation will help pupils in developing self-understanding.

Examination and Investigation

It is also useful to gather information about physiological and psychological aspects of an individual. There are variety of specialized devices for doing different examinations and psychological tests to get desired information.

The Tools

The information by using the above-mentioned techniques/methods can be collected by using various non-standardized and standardized tools.

The Nonstandardized Tools

These are developed by the counselors/teachers themselves. The non-standardized tools which are used most commonly include interview schedule (to collect data through interview) observation checklist (to collect information by observation) Record checklist (to collect data by records review) rating scale, etc.

The Standardized Tools

These are the tools which are readymade tools, highly valid and reliable, tested over large population in different areas over time. The tools which are used for testing physiological and psychological aspects are standardized tools which are available for specific purpose.

The psychological tests/tools are the tools which are more often used by the counsel to get information about influence, attitude, aptitudes, interests, personality, sociability, etc. Although a number of psychological tests/tools are available but still not many more testing tools are required in different areas of measurements.

Approaches for Counseling

During the process of counseling by the counselor emphasis the approach. There are three approaches to counseling, i.e.:

Nondirective Approaches to Counseling

In this approach, the individual rendering help does not impose his/her values upon the person being helped. The assumption of this approach is that every individual is capable of solving her/his own problems. According to Rogers, who has developed this approach, the counselee is helped to help herself/himself. The counselor listens and encourages the individual to talk freely on her/his own in an atmosphere of acceptance and in permissive atmosphere, thereby helping him/her tension and express her/his emotions. This approach to counseling is thus more suitable to sort out emotional or personal problems. It is more useful for individuals having anxiety, worry or tension. Talking freely enables an individual to view his/her problem from a new angle and change his/her attitude. This approaches more time consuming as compared to directive counseling.

Directive Approach to the Counseling

This approach to counseling is called as authoritarian or psychoanalytic approach. The counselor is active and directs the individual in making decisions and finding solutions to the problems. The counselor does not force the individual but directs his/her process of thinking. This approach to counseling is based on the assumptions that the training and experience of the counselor makes him/her competent person in helping a person to solve his/her problems. The counseling is a process which includes analysis of the problem, diagnosis or identification of the exact nature of the difficulty, prognosis or making predictions, counseling and follow-up, the process tends to be planned, objective and impersonal and is more suitable to intellectual problems.

Eclectic Approach

This approach is consistent with the modern day life wherein we do not believe in just one set of values but try to harmoniously blend the best values from different culture and these are reflected in the way we eat, dress up and mingle with others. A counselor uses eclectic approach is at times a non-directive counselor, operates on the premises that it is the individual's responsibility to determine his/her own way of life and choose his/her own problems, thus provides him/her with a permissive, accepting environment to talk truly about the problems. At times the counselor is directive when she recognizes that many young people are not ready to assume full responsibility and thus takes the initiative and provides necessary direction. But an eclectic approach counselor is always ready to change his/her plan and is flexible in the approach at every stage of the counseling process.

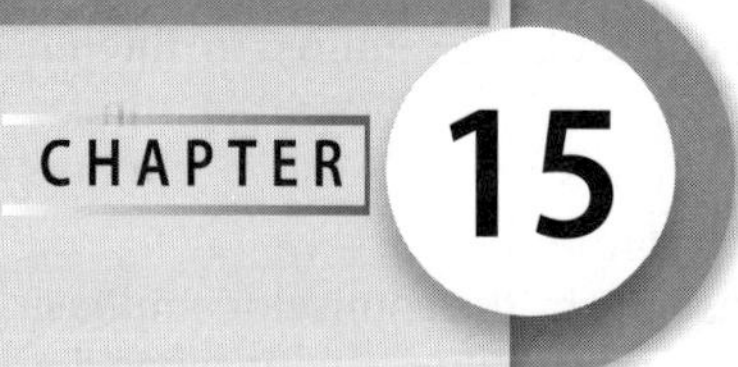

CHAPTER 15 Occupational Health Nursing

INTRODUCTION

The place of work, like home and the school is an important part of man's environment. The health and efficiency of workers working in any organization get influenced in large measures by conditions prevailing in their work environment. The prevailing conditions are related to physical, biological, chemical and social agents. A worker usually exposed to these agents for about 6–8 hours daily. It is, therefore, essential that this environment should be wholesome and free from any kind of harmful agents as far as possible. So the occupational health is to provide a safe occupational environment to promote and preserve the health of workers and to step up their efficiency and productivity.

Definition

The joint ILO/WHO Committee on occupational health, in the course of its first session, held in 1950, gave the following definition:

'Occupational health should aim at the promotion and maintenance of the highest degree of physical, mental and social well-being of workers in all occupations; the prevention among workers of departures from health caused by their working conditions; the protection of workers in their employment from risks resulting from factors adverse to health; the placing and maintenance of the worker in an occupational environment adapted to his physiological and psychological equipment, and to summarize, the adaptation of work to man and of each man to his job.'

Occupational Health Nursing

'The application of nursing principles in conserving the health of worker in all occupations. It involves preventions, recognition and treatment of illness and injury, and requires special skills and knowledge in the fields of health, education and counseling, environmental health, rehabilitation and human relations.'

—American Association of Occupational Health Nurses

Aims and Objectives of Occupational Health

The joint ILO/WHO Committee on Occupational Health, in the course of first session, held in 1950, gave the following general aims:

- Promotion and maintenance of the highest degree of physical, mental and social well-being of workers in all occupations.
- Prevention among workers, of departures from health, caused by their working conditions.
- Protection of workers in their employment from risks resulting from factors adverse to health.
- Placing and maintenance of the worker in an occupational environment adapted to his physiological and psychological equipment, and to summarize, the adaptation of work to man and of each man to his job.

To achieve these general aims it is necessary to serve the following objectives:

- Identify all the hazardous conditions which might be there in work place.
- Plan and implement protective and control measures to deal with identified hazardous conditions in work place.
- Ensure that the physical and psychological demands imposed on workers by their respective jobs are properly matched with their individual anatomical, physical and psychological needs, capabilities and limitations.
- Provide effective services to protect those who are especially vulnerable to adverse working conditions.
- Provide effective services to workers who are incapacitated for any reason to rehabilitate them as soon as possible.
- Using resources effectively and efficiently and protecting the natural environment and creating health supportive environment.
- Improving societal communication and literacy on health, environment and social cohesion.

Basic Principles for the Development of an Occupational Health Service

WHO has identified three basic principles for the development of an occupational health service.

1. It must be ensured that occupational health services are provided through the existing national health services by a process of integration.
2. The service must provide for the total health of the workers and if necessary their families. The primary healthcare approach must be the chosen system for the delivery of such services.

3. The occupational health problems of working women, especially those in the unorganized sector are a matter of urgent concern. There is also a definite need to develop a database on occupational health of women in developing countries. For primary healthcare approach to delivery of occupational health, it is essential to create awareness among the health personnel, NGO's and Women's organizations. It is very important to understand that chronic occupational diseases are only preventable but rarely curable. Even though, in developing countries, health priorities focus more on infectious diseases, improving the health of workers (especially women) will contribute tremendously to national growth and economy.

OCCUPATIONAL ENVIRONMENT

By 'Occupational environment' is meant the sum of external conditions and influences which prevail at the place of work and which have a bearing on the health of the working population. The industrial worker today is placed in a highly complicated environment which is getting more complicated as man is becoming more ingenious. Basically, there are three types of interaction in a working environment.

1. **Man and physical, chemical and biological agents:**
   i. **Physical agents:** The physical factors in the working environment which may be adverse to health are heat, cold, humidity, air movement, heat radiation, light, noise, vibrations, and ionizing radiations. The factors act in different ways on the health and efficiency of the workers, singly or in different combinations. The amount of working and breathing space, toilet, washing and bathing facilities are also important factors in an occupational environment.
   ii. **Chemical agents:** These comprise a large number of chemicals, toxic dusts, vapors, fumes and gases which are potential hazards to the health of the workers. Some chemical agents cause disabling respiratory illnesses, some cause injury to skin, and some may have a deleterious effects on the blood and other organ of the body.
   iii. **Biological agents:** The workers may be exposed to viral, rickettsial, bacterial and parasitic agents which may results from close contact with animals or their products, contaminated water, soil or food.
2. **Man and machine:**
   - An industry or factory implies the use of machines driven by power with emphasis on mass production.
   - The unguarded machines, protruding and moving parts, poor installation of the plant, and lack of safety measures are the cause of accidents which is a major problem in industries.
   - Working for longer hours in unphysiological postures is the cause of fatigue, backache, disease of joints and muscles and impairment of the worker's health and efficiency.
3. **Man and man:** There are numerous psychological factors which operate at the place of work. These are the human relationships amongst workers themselves on the one hand, and those in authority over them on the other.
   Examples of psychological factors include the type and rhythm of work, work stability, service conditions, job satisfaction, leadership style, security, workers participation, communication, system of payment, welfare conditions, degree of responsibility, trade union activities. Incentives and a host of similar other factors, all entering the field of human relationships.
   In modern occupational health, the emphasis is upon the people, the conditions in which they live and work, their fellow-workers and employer.
   The occupational environment and domestic environment both are complementary to each other. The worker takes his worries home, and brings to his work disturbances which arise in his domestic environment. Severe prolonged stress may produce serious physical or mental symptoms which do not allow man to work efficiently.
   According to ecological approach, occupational health represents a dynamic equilibrium or adjustment between the industrial worker and his occupational environment.

OCCUPATIONAL HAZARDS

An industrial worker may be exposed to five types of hazards, depending upon his occupation:

- **Physical hazards:**
  - *Heat and cold:*
    - The common physical hazard in most industries is heat. The direct effects of heat exposure are burns, heat exhaustion, heat stroke, and heat cramps; the indirect effects are decreased efficiency, increased fatigue and enhanced accident rates.
    - Many industries have local 'hot spots'—ovens and furnaces, which radiate heat. Physical work under high temperature is very stressful and impairs the health and efficiency of the workers. For gainful work involving sustained and repeated effort, a reasonable temperature must be maintained in each work room.
    - The Indian Factories Act has not laid down any specific temperature standard. However, the work of Rao (1952, 1953) and Mookerjee et al. (1953) indicate that a corrected effective temperature of 69 to 80°F (20 to 27°C) is the comfort zone in this country and temperature above 80°F (27°C) cause discomfort.

  Important hazards associated with cold work are chilblains, erythrocyanosis, immersion foot and frostbite as a result of cutaneous vasoconstriction. General hypothermia is not unusual.
  - *Light:* The workers may be exposed to the risk of poor illumination or excessive brightness. The acute effects of poor illumination are eye stain, headache, eye pain, lachrymation, congestion around the cornea and eye fatigue. The chronic effects on health include

'miner's nystagmus'. Exposure to excessive brightness or 'glare' is associated with discomfort, annoyance and visual fatigue. Intense direct glare may also result in blurring of vision and lead to accidents. There should be sufficient and suitable lighting, natural or artificial, wherever persons are working.

- *Noise:* Noise is a health hazard in many industries. The effects of noise are of two types: (i) *Auditory effects* which consist of temporary or permanent hearing loss. (ii) *Nonauditory effects* which consist of nervousness, fatigue, interference with communication by speech, decreased efficiency and annoyance. The degree of injury from exposure to noise depends upon a number of factors such as intensity and frequency range, duration of exposure and individual susceptibility.
- *Vibration:* Vibration, especially in the frequency range 10 to 500 Hz, may be encountered in work with pneumatic tools such as drills and hammers. Vibration usually affects the hands and arms. After some months or years of exposure, the fine blood vessels of the fingers may become increasingly sensitive to spasm (white fingers). Exposure to vibration may also produce injuries of the joints of the hands, elbows and shoulders.
- *Ultraviolet radiation:* Occupational exposure to ultraviolet radiation occurs mainly in arc welding. Such radiation mainly affects the eyes, causing intense conjunctivitis and keratitis (welder's flash). Symptoms are redness of the eyes and pain, these usually disappear in a few days with no permanent effect on the vision or on the deeper structures of the eye.
- *Ionizing radiation:* Ionizing radiation is finding increasing application in medicine and industry, e.g., X-rays and radioactive isotopes. Important radioisotopes are cobalt 60 and phosphorus 32. Certain tissues such as bone marrow are more sensitive than others and from a genetic standpoint, there are special hazards when the gonads are exposed. The radiation hazards comprise genetic changes, malformation, cancer, leukemia, depilation, ulceration, sterility and in extreme cases of death. The International Commission of Radiological Protection has set the maximum permissible level of occupational exposure at 5 rem per year to the whole body.

- **Chemical hazards:** The chemical hazards are on the increase with the introduction of newer and complex chemicals. Chemical agents act in three ways: Local action, inhalation and ingestion. The ill-effects produced depend upon the duration of exposure, the quantum of exposure and individual susceptibility.
  - *Local action:* Some chemicals cause dermatitis, eczema, ulcers and even cancer by primary irritant action; some cause dermatitis by an allergic action. Some chemicals, particularly the aromatic nitro and amino compounds such as TNT and aniline are absorbed through the skin and cause systemic effects. Occupational dermatitis is a big problem in industry. Rao and Banerji (1952) were the first to draw attention in India to the prevalence of occupational dermatitis due to machine oil, rubber, X-rays, caustic alkalies and lime.
  - *Inhalation:*
    - **Dusts:**
      - Dusts are finely divided solid particles with size ranging from 0.1 to 150 microns.
      - They are released into the atmosphere during crushing, grinding, abrading, loading and unloading operations. Dusts are produced in a number of industries—mines, foundry, quarry, pottery, textile, wood or stone working industries.
      - Dusts particles larger than 10 microns settle down from the air rapidly, while the smaller one remains suspended indefinitely.
      - Particles smaller than 5 microns are directly inhaled in to the lungs and are retained there. This fraction of the dust is called "respirable dust", and is mainly responsible for pneumoconiosis.
      - Dusts have been classified into inorganic and organic dusts; soluble and insoluble dusts. The inorganic dusts are silica, mica, coal, asbestos dust, etc.; the organic dusts are cotton, jute and the like.
      - The soluble dusts dissolve slowly, enter the systemic circulation and are eventually eliminated by body metabolism.
      - The insoluble dusts remain, more or less, permanently in the lungs. They are mainly the cause of pneumoconiosis. The most common dust diseases in this country are silicosis and anthracosis.
    - **Gases:** Exposure to gases is a common hazard in industries. Gases are sometimes classified as simple gases (e.g., oxygen, hydrogen), asphyxiating gases (e.g., carbon monoxide, cyanide gas, sulfur dioxide, chlorine) and anesthetic gases (e.g., chloroform, ether, trichlorethylene). Carbon monoxide hazard is frequently reported in coal-gas manufacturing plants and steel industry.
    - **Metals and their compounds:**
      - A large number of metals and their compounds are used throughout the industry. The chief mode of entry of some of them is by inhalation as dust or fumes.
      - The ill-effects depend upon the duration of exposure and the dose or concentration of exposure. Unlike the pneumoconiosis, most chemical intoxications respond favorably to cessation, exposure and medical treatment.
    - The industrial physician should be aware of the toxic effects of lead, antimony, arsenic, beryllium, cadmium, cobalt, manganese, mercury, phosphorus, chromium, zinc and others.
  - *Ingestion:* Occupational diseases may also result from ingestion of chemical substances such as lead, mercury, arsenic, zinc, chromium, cadmium, phosphorus, etc. Usually, these substances are swallowed in minute

Table 15.1: Occupational hazard-related disorders.

Hazard	*Undesirable conditions*
Lead	Anemia, hypertension, nephritis, peptic ulcer
Dyes	Asthma; skin, bladder and kidney diseases; precancerous lesions
Solvents	Liver and kidney disease, dermatitis, alcoholism
Silica	Healed or active tuberculosis of lungs, chronic lung disease
Radium and X-rays	Signs of ill-health, especially any blood disease

amounts through contaminated hands, food or cigarettes. Much of the ingested material is excreted through feces and only a small proportion may reach the general blood circulation.

- **Biological hazards:** Workers may be exposed to infective and parasitic agents at the place of work. The occupational diseases in this category are brucellosis, leptospirosis, anthrax, hydatidosis, psittacosis, tetanus, encephalitis, fungal infections, schistosomiasis and a host of others. Persons working among animal products (e.g., hair, wool, hides) and agricultural workers are specially exposed to biological hazards.
- **Mechanical hazards:** The mechanical hazards in industry center round machinery, protruding and moving parts and the like. About 10% of accidents in industry are said to be due to mechanical causes.
- **Psychosocial hazards:**
  - The psychosocial hazards arise from the workers' failure to adapt to an alien psychosocial environment. Frustration, lack of job satisfaction, insecurity, poor human relationships, emotional tension are some of the psychosocial factors which may undermine both physical and mental health of the workers.
  - The capacity to adapt to different working environments is influenced by many factors such as education, cultural background, family life, social habits, and what the worker expects from employment.

The health effects can be classified in two main categories:

1. **Psychological and behavioral changes:** Including hostility, aggressiveness, anxiety, depression, tardiness, alcoholism, drug abuse, sickness, absenteeism.
2. **Psychosomatic ill health:** Including fatigue, headache, pain in the shoulders, neck and back; propensity to peptic ulcer, hypertension, heart disease and rapid aging.

The increasing stress on automation, electronic operations and nuclear energy may introduce newer psychosocial health problems in industry. Psychosocial hazards are therefore, assuming more importance than physical or chemical hazards. There are some occupational diseases which are due to exposure of occupational hazard **(Table 15.1)**.

OCCUPATIONAL DISEASES

Occupational diseases are usually defined as diseases arising out of or in the course of employment by the work or working conditions. This means that the disease must have developed due to exposures in the workplace and that the correlation between the exposures and the disease is well known in medical research. They may be grouped as under:

Diseases due to Physical Agents

- **Heat:** Heat hyperpyrexia, heat exhaustion, heat syncope, heat cramps, burns
- **Cold:** Trench foot, frost bite
- **Noise:** Occupational deafness
- **Light:** Occupational cataract
- **Mechanical factors:** Injury and accidents.

Diseases Caused by Ionizing Radiation

- Acute generalized radiation sickness as a consequence of whole body, or greater part of body, irradiation
- Acute radiation sickness of the type of inflammatory or inflammatory-necrotic changes of skin or subcutaneous tissue
- Chronic dermatitis due to radiation
- Chronic lesion of bone marrow causes leukemia
- Cataract due to radiation
- Malignant neoplasms.

Diseases due to Chemical Agents

A varieties of chemical toxic substance like metal, lead and mercury gases, like carbon monoxide and hydrogen sulfide, organic toxin like chlorinated organic compounds and biological toxin which produced in different factories can enter to the body through different routes and produced different types of diseases.

Dusts of different chemicals can create different diseases:

- **Coal dust:** Anthracosis
- **Silica dust:** Silicosis
- **Asbestos:** Asbestosis
- **Metal dust:** Lung diseases induced by hard metals dust
- **Cane fiber:** Bagassosis
- **Cotton dust:** Byssinosis
- **Hay or grain dust:** Farmer's lung
- **Gases:** Carbon monoxide, hydrogen sulfide, Hydrogen chloride caused gas poisoning.

Skin contact with toxic chemical may be dust or fumes caused:

- Allergic contact dermatitis
- Irritant contact dermatitis
- Oil acne, chloracne, coal tar acne of diffuse nature
- Dermatophyte infections due to contact with biological material from animals
- Occupational photodermatoses.

Chronic Diseases of Locomotor System Related to the Way the Job is Performed

1. Tendovaginitis
2. Bursitis
3. Chronic lesion of meniscus due to the job performed in kneel or squat position

4. Periarticular inflammation of shoulder joint
5. Epicondylitis of shoulder bone
6. Fatigue-induced bone fracture.

Chronic Diseases of Peripheral Nervous System Related to the Way the Job is Performed

1. Carpal tunnel syndrome
2. Groove of ulnar nerve syndrome
3. Guyon tunnel syndrome
4. Common fibular nerve lesion in persons working in squat position.

Diseases due to Biological Agents

Brucellosis, Leptospirosis, anthrax, Tetanus, encephalitis, etc.

Diseases of Visual System Induced by Physical, Chemical or Biological Agents

- Allergic conjunctivitis
- Acute conjunctivitis induced by ultraviolet radiation
- Epidemic viral conjunctivitis or keratitis
- Keratopathy induced by irritant agents, cataract induced by infrared or long-wave ultraviolet radiation central retinal and choroidal degeneration induced by short-wave infrared radiation or visible radiation of blue spectrum.

PNEUMOCONIOSIS

Pneumoconiosis is a disease of lung specially happen due to dusts, the meaning of pneumoconiosis is pneumon = lung, konis = dust, pneumoconiosis = accumulation of inorganic dust in lungs, following non-neoplastic tissue reaction.

Pneumoconiosis is a group of lung diseases caused by inhaled dust particles. They are asbestosis, berylliosis, byssinosis, coal worker's pneumoconiosis, silicosis and bagassosis, etc. Dust within the size range of 0.5 to 3 micron, is a health hazard producing after a variable period of exposure, a lung disease known as pneumoconiosis. It is a disease characterized by fibrosis and caused by the chronic inhalation of mineral dusts, especially silica and asbestos. It is seen in specific occupations such as coal mining and construction industries where the concentration of dust particles is very high. Thus, it can be considered as occupational lung disease.

Pneumoconiosis causes inflammation of the lungs. The lung tissue in normal people is very elastic. This allows it to expand and contract while breathing. In the common types of pneumoconiosis, fibrous tissue gets deposited in the lungs, the condition being called fibrosis. Fibrosis tends to stiffen the lung tissue and restrict its expansion. The affected person may develop breathing problems, cancer and may even die due to the condition. It is important to diagnose the condition early, as the patient must be removed from the environment at the earliest. Also, preventive measures should be taken to protect other workers from the disease.

The hazardous effects of dusts on the lungs depend upon a number of factors such as:

- Chemical composition
- Fineness
- Concentration of dust in the air
- Period of exposure
- Health status of the person exposed.

The important dust diseases are Silicosis, Anthracosis, Byssinosis, Bagassosis, Asbestosis and farmer's lung.

Silicosis

Introduction

Silicosis is an incurable lung disease caused by inhaling large amounts of silica dust, usually over a period of many years.

Silica (silicon dioxide) is a substance naturally found in certain types of stone, rock, sand and clay. Working with these materials can create a very fine dust, known as respirable crystalline silica, which can be easily inhaled.

Once inside the lungs, the dust particles are attacked by the immune system. This causes inflammation (swelling) and gradually leads to areas of hardened and scarred lung tissue (fibrosis). Eventually, the lungs may stop working properly.

What is Silicosis?

Silicosis is a chronic lung disease caused by breathing in tiny bits of silica dust. Silica is the second most common mineral in the earth's crust. It is a major component of sand, rock, and mineral ores like quartz. People who work in jobs where they can be breathing in these tiny silica bits—like sandblasting, mining, construction and many others are at risk for silicosis. When people breathe silica dust, they inhale tiny particles of silica that has crystallized. This silica dust can cause fluid build up and scar tissue in the lungs that cuts down your ability to breathe.

Types of Silicosis

There are three types of silicosis:

1. **Chronic silicosis:** It is the most common type of silicosis, usually occurs after 10 or more years of exposure to crystalline silica at low levels.
2. **Accelerated silicosis:** It occurs 5 to 10 years after exposure and is caused by exposure to higher levels of crystalline silica.
3. **Acute silicosis:** It can occur after only weeks or months of exposure to very high levels of crystalline silica. Acute silicosis progresses rapidly and can be fatal within months.

Silica dust particles act as tiny blades on the lungs. When silica is inhaled through the nose or mouth, particles create small cuts that can scar the lung tissue. Scarred lungs do not open and close as well, making breathing difficult.

People Risk for Silicosis

People who work in the following jobs in the industries are particularly at risk for developing silicosis:

- Highway and bridge construction and repair
- Building construction, demolition, and repair because of exposure to bricks, concrete and mortar

- Abrasive blasting
- Masonry work
- Concrete finishing
- Drywall finishing
- Rock drilling
- Mining and quarrying
- Sand and gravel screening
- Rock crushing (for road base)
- Pottery, ceramics and glass manufacturing
- Sand blasting and stone cutting.

In silicosis, it can take many years for symptoms to appear. However, in 2010 there were 13 deaths due to silicosis and 50 new cases of silicosis were assessed for Industrial Injuries Disability Benefit in 2011.

Most cases of silicosis nowadays are the result of exposure to silica that happened before workplace regulations were introduced.

Symptoms of Silicosis

Symptoms of silicosis may first appear 15 to 20 years after someone's exposure to crystalline silica. As the disease progresses, early symptoms may include:

- Shortness of breath
- Severe cough
- Weakness.

Then, as the disease gets worse, or if silica present in lungs, the body may not be able to fight infections well. This can lead to other illnesses that can cause:

- Weight loss
- Extreme tiredness
- Night sweats
- Chest pains
- Respiratory failure
- Sometimes swollen fingers (finger clubbing).

As the disease progresses over time, these symptoms can become worse.

Acute silicosis caused by short-term exposure to very large amounts of silica is rare. In these cases, the cough and shortness of breath can appear within days or weeks of exposure to silica, with weight loss, tiredness and wheezing developing within a few months or years.

How is Silicosis Treated?

There is no cure for silicosis, as the lung damage cannot be repaired. Treatment aims to relieve symptoms and improve quality of life. The condition will often continue to get worse, leading to further lung damage and serious disability.

It is important to take the following steps, which help limit the risk of complications developing:

- Avoidance of exposed to any more silica
- Stop smoking (if you smoke)
- Have regular skin tests to check for tuberculosis (TB), as silicosis makes you more prone to TB and other infections.

The influenza vaccination and pneumococcal vaccination are also recommended. Your GP can arrange for you to have these. Antibiotics may be prescribed to treat any chest infections that develop.

Anthracosis

A chronic lung disease characterized by the deposit of coal dust in the lungs and by the formation of black nodules on the bronchioles, resulting in focal emphysema. The condition occurs in coal miners and is aggravated by cigarette smoking. There is no specific treatment, most cases are asymptomatic, and preventing further exposure to coal dust may halt progress of the condition. It is also called black lung disease, coal worker's pneumoconiosis, miner's pneumoconiosis. It is a common in coal miners and others who work with coal. It is similar to both silicosis from inhaling silica dust, and to the long-term effects of tobacco smoking. Inhaled coal dust progressively builds up in the lungs and is unable to be removed by the body; this leads to inflammation, fibrosis, and in worse cases, necrosis, asbestosis and other pneumoconioses.

Symptoms of Anthracosis

- Anthracosis in the early stage may be asymptomatic.
- Early symptoms of the disease include shortness of breath, labored breathing, coughing, and production of phlegm.
- At this stage, avoiding exposure to coal dust can stop the progression of disease.

If not treated it may result:

- Progressive lung stiffening
- Impaired lung functions
- Breathing difficulty
- Lung fibrosis
- Breathlessness
- Pneumothorax
- Cardiac failure, low output
- Emphysema
- Pulmonary hypertension.

Treatment of Anthracosis

Treatment of anthracosis is focused on eliminating the symptoms of the disease, reducing oxygen deficiency and preventing infection of the respiratory tract.

Patients are prescribed medicines for the expansion of small airways and steroid agents. Healing properties have physical therapy, for example, coughing with percussion and vibration according to a certain scheme, for the complete removal of sputum.

A mandatory condition for treatment is an increase in fluid intake, up to 2–3 liters per day. If the anthracosis is in the first stage, then conventional therapy is administered for treatment, as with respiratory diseases. But if the disease is in the last stages, then the patient is ventilated or breathed oxygen through the mask.

Asbestosis

Asbestosis is a chronic inflammatory and fibrotic medical condition affecting the parenchymal tissue of the lungs caused by the inhalation and retention of asbestos fibers. It usually occurs after high intensity and/or long-term exposure to asbestos (particularly in those individuals working on the production or end-use of products containing asbestos) and is therefore regarded as an occupational. People with extensive occupational exposure to the mining, manufacturing, handling, or removal of asbestos are at risk of developing asbestosis. Sufferers may experience severe dyspnea (shortness of breath) and are at an increased risk for certain malignancies, including lung cancer and, less commonly, mesothelioma. Asbestosis specifically refers to interstitial (parenchymal) fibrosis from asbestos, and not pleural fibrosis or plaque in.

Symptoms

Symptoms do not show up for 10 to 40 years after initial exposure. The chronic exposure may result in:

- Shortness of breath
- A persistent, dry cough
- Loss of appetite with weight loss
- Fingertips and toes that appear wider and rounder than normal (clubbing), chest tightness or pain, increased risk of developing lung cancer.

Treatment

- There is no cure available for asbestosis
- Supportive treatment of symptoms includes oxygen therapy, respiratory physiotherapy to remove secretions from the lungs by postural drainage, chest percussion, and vibration.
- Nebulized medications may be prescribed in order to loosen secretions or treat underlying chronic obstructive pulmonary disease.
- Immunization against pneumococcal pneumonia and annual influenza vaccination is administered due to increased sensitivity to the diseases.
- Stop smoking as it leads to further damage.

Bagassosis

Bagassosis, an interstitial lung disease, is a type of hypersensitivity pneumonitis, attributed to exposure to moldy molasses (bagasse). Bagassosis was first reported in India by Ganguly and Pal in 1955, in a cardboard manufacturing plant near Kolkata. India has a large sugarcane industry. The sugarcane fiber which, until recently, went to waste, is now utilized in the manufacture of cardboard, paper and rayon.

Cause

Bagassosis is caused by a substance called bagasse which is produced when juice is taken out from sugarcane. This substance is used for making paper. It is believed that a fungus is possibly involved in development of Bagassosis.

Symptoms

Some symptoms and signs of Bagassosis include breathlessness, cough, hemoptysis, slight fever. Acute diffuse bronchiolitis may also occur. An X-ray may show mottling of lungs or a shadow.

Prevention and Management

The following are precautionary measures that can be taken to avoid the spread of bagassosis:

- Dust control—prevention/suppression of dust such as wet process, enclosed apparatus, exhaust ventilation, etc., should be used
- Personal protection—masks/respirators
- Medical control—initial medical examination and periodical checkups of workers
- Bagasse control—keep moisture content above 20% and spray bagasse with 2% propionic acid
- Treatment include adrenal steroids and symptomized management.

Pneumoconiosis Associated with Tuberculosis

This is an occupational lung disease and a restrictive lung disease caused by the inhalation of dust, often in mines, associated with a common, and in many cases lethal, infectious disease caused by various strains of mycobacteria, usually mycobacterium tuberculosis.

Byssinosis

Byssinosis is a rare lung disease. It is caused by inhaling hemp, flax, and cotton particles and is sometimes referred to as brown lung disease. It is a form of occupational asthma.

It occurs almost exclusively in people who work with unprocessed cotton. People who open bales of cotton during the first stage of processing are at the highest risk.

Symptoms

The symptoms of byssinosis in early stage are similar to asthma and include tightness in the chest, wheezing, and coughing. Continuous exposure leads to fever, muscle and joint pain, shivering, tiredness and a dry cough.

Causes and Risk Factors

Byssinosis is most common in textile industry workers. It is caused by the inhalation of raw flax, hemp, cotton dust, and similar materials.

Smoking may increase the risk of developing byssinosis. A history of asthma or allergies may also increase the risk.

Treatment

- Bronchodilators.
- Inhaled corticosteroids
- Supplemental oxygen therapy.
- Nebulizer or other respiratory treatment
- Stop smoking
- Prognosis is good if avoid exposure however, people with long-term and chronic exposure to cotton dust can have an impaired lung function.

Farmer Lung

Farmer's lung is due to inhalatation of mouldy hay or grain dusts. In hay or grain dusts with a moisture contain of over 30% of bacteria grow rapidly. Causing of rising temperature 40 to 50 degree centigrade which encourage the growth of thermophilic actinomycetes of which *Micropolyspora faeni* the main cause of farmer lung.

The technical name for Farmer's Lung is "extrinsic allergic alveolitis", "hypersensitivity alveolitis" or more generally "hypersensitivity pneumonitis". The "-itis" word ending means inflammation, so "alveolitis" means inflammation of the alveoli.

Symptoms

- **Acute stage:** After four to eight hours symptoms such as headache, irritating cough, and shortness of breath upon physical exertion, appear.
- **Subacute stage:** Symptoms persist without further exposure, and increase in severity. Symptoms include: shortness of breath upon exertion, chronic coughing, physical weakness, occasional fever and sweating, decrease in appetite, aches and pains.
- **Chronic stage:** Debilitating effects are now considered long-term. Symptoms include: severe shortness of breath, chronic coughing, physical weakness, occasional fever and sweating at night, decrease in appetite, and general aches and pains.

Cause

Farmer's lung occurs because repeated exposure to antigens, found in the mold spores of hay, crops, and animal feed, triggers an allergic reaction within the farmer's immune system. The defense mechanisms of the body present as cold and flu-like symptoms that occur in individuals who experience either acute or chronic reactions.

These allergens have to be very small—around 5 millionths of a meter (5 microns)—to affect you. Because the particles are so tiny, the normal defenses in your nose and throat miss them, and they go straight to your lung and affect that.

Complications

Complications of farmer's lung include the following: Cor pulmonale, hypoxemic respiratory failure, pulmonary fibrosis.

For people suffering from acute attacks of Farmer's Lung, the first step in treatment is to avoid further contact with moldy dust. For serious cases, bed rest is recommended and oxygen therapy may be needed to relieve shortness of breath.

OCCUPATIONAL DERMATITIS

Occupational dermatitis is a big health problem in many industries. The causes may be; Physical—heat, cold, moisture, friction, pressure, X-rays and other rays; Chemical—acids, alkalies, dyes, solvents, grease, tar, pitch, chlorinated phenols, etc.; Biological—living agents such as viruses, bacteria, fungi and other parasites; Plant products—leaves, vegetables, fruits, flowers, vegetable dust, etc.

The dermatitis producing agents are further classified into: (1) primary irritants, and (2) sensitizing substances. Primary irritants (e.g., acids, alkalies, dyes, solvents, etc.) cause dermatitis in workers exposed in sufficient concentration and for a long enough period of time. On the other hand, allergic dermatitis occurs only in small percentage of cases, due to sensitization of the skin.

Prevention: Occupational dermatitis is largely preventable if proper control measures are adopted: The control measures can be applied before selection also:

1. **Preselection:** The workers should be medically examined before employment, and those with an established or suspected dermatitis or who have a known predisposition to skin disease should be kept away from jobs involving a skin hazard.
2. **Protection:** The worker should be given adequate protection against direct contact by protective clothing, long leather gloves, aprons and boots. The protective clothing should be frequently washed and kept in good order. There are also, what are known as barrier creams which must be used regularly and correctly. There is no barrier cream so far invented which will prevent dermatitis in all occupations.
3. **Personal hygiene:** There should be available a plentiful supply of warm water, soap and towels. The worker should be encouraged and educated to make frequent use of these facilities. Adequate washing facilities in industry are a statutory obligation under the Factories Act.
4. **Periodic inspection:** There should be a periodic medical check-up of all workers for early detection and treatment of occupational dermatitis. If necessary, the affected worker may have to be transferred to a job not exposing him to risk. The worker should be educated to report any skin irritation, no matter how mild or insignificant.

OCCUPATIONAL CANCER

Occupational cancer is caused wholly or partly by exposure to a cancer causing agent (carcinogen) at work, or by a particular set of circumstances at work. Cancer is a leading cause of death worldwide and every tenth lung cancer death is closely related to risks in the workplace. WHO stated that lung cancer, mesothelioma, and bladder cancer are among the most common types of occupational cancers. Most of the exposure risks for occupational cancer are preventable. About 125 million people in the world are exposed to asbestos at the workplace. According to WHO estimates, more than 107,000 people die each year from asbestos-related lung cancer, mesothelioma and asbestosis resulting from occupational exposures. One in three deaths from occupational cancer is caused by asbestos.

Causes of occupational cancer: Occupational cancer is caused by exposure to carcinogens in the workplace. Carcinogens are agents that cause the development or increase the incidence of cancer. There are three different types of occupational carcinogens:

1. **Biological carcinogens:** Some microorganisms such as viruses have been known to cause cancer, either by damaging cells directly or by decreasing the body's ability to control abnormal cells, for example Hepatitis B, HIV viruses and so on.
2. **Chemical carcinogens:** A number of chemicals are known to be carcinogenic. These chemicals may occur naturally, such as asbestos, be manufactured like vinyl chloride, or be by-products of industrial processes, for example, polycyclic aromatic hydrocarbons.
3. **Physical carcinogens:** Agents such as ionizing and ultraviolet (UV) radiation have the potential to cause cancer. Examples of ionizing radiation include X-rays and alpha, beta and gamma radiation. UV radiation can be divided into a number of bands such as UV-B, UV-C, etc., some of which are known to cause skin cancer.

Certain occupational circumstances, such as working as a painter or as a welder are also associated with increased risks of some cancers. In addition, recent studies have started to include analyses of shift work patterns, particularly work at night, and their potential effects on occupational cancer.

Occupational cancer can arise from exposure to many substances or from certain occupational circumstances such as:

- Asbestos fibers (colorectum, larynx, lung, ovary, pharynx, stomach cancers, mesothelioma)
- Wood dusts (nasopharynx, sinonasal cancers)
- UV radiation from sunlight (skin cancers)
- Metalworking fluids and mineral oils (bladder, lung, sinonasal, skin cancers)
- Silica dust (lung cancer)
- Diesel engine exhaust (bladder, lung cancers)
- Coal tars and pitches (nonmelanoma skin cancer)
- Arsenic (bladder, lung, skin cancers)
- Dioxins (lung cancer)
- Environmental tobacco smoke (passive smoke) (lung cancer)
- Naturally occurring radon (lung cancer)
- Tetrachloroethylene (cervix, non-Hodgkin's lymphoma, esophagus cancers)
- Work as a painter (bladder, lung)
- Work as a welder (lung cancer, melanoma of the eye)
- Shift (night) work (breast cancer).

The International Agency for Research on Cancer (IARC) lists over 50 substances which are known or probable causes of workplace cancer, and over 100 other possible substances. The percentage of cancer related to occupational exposure are listed in **Table 15.2**.

Table 15.2: Cancer related to occupational exposure.

Type of cancer	*Related to occupational exposure estimated % (USA)*
Lung	6.3–13%
Bladder	3–19%
Mesothelioma	85–90% (men) 23–90% (women)
Leukemia	0.8–2.8%
Laryngeal	1–20% (men)
Skin cancer (non-melanoma)	1.5–6% (men)
Sinonasal and nasopharyngeal	31–43% (men)
Kidney	0–2.3%
Liver	0.4–1.1 (vinyl chloride only; men)

Prevention and control of occupational cancer: The preventive measures for occupational cancer include control of carcinogen, protective measures for workers, health check-up of worker and health education. The measures should be:

- Every effort should be made to replace carcinogenic substances and agents to which workers may be exposed in the course of their work by non-carcinogenic substances or agents or by less harmful substances or agents; in the choice of substitute substances or agents account should be taken of their carcinogenic, toxic and other properties.
- The number of workers exposed to carcinogenic substances or agents and the duration and degree of such exposure should be reduced to the minimum compatible with safety.
- The competent authority should prescribe the measures to be taken to protect workers against the risks of exposure to carcinogenic substances or agents.
- The competent authority should keep the measures prescribed up to date, taking into account the codes of practices or guides which may be established by the International Labor Office and the conclusions of meetings of experts which may be convened by the International Labor Office, as well as information from other competent bodies.
- Employers should make every effort to use work processes which do not cause the formation, and particularly the emission in the working environment, of carcinogenic substances or agents, as main products, intermediates, by-products, waste products or otherwise.
- Where complete elimination of a carcinogenic substance or agent is not possible, employers should use all appropriate measures, in consultation with the workers and their organizations and in the light of advice from competent sources, including occupational health services, to eliminate exposure or reduce it to a minimum in terms of numbers exposed, duration of exposure and degree of exposure.
- In cases to be determined by the competent authority, the employer should make arrangements for the systematic surveillance of the duration and degree of exposure to carcinogenic substances or agents in the working environment.
- Where carcinogenic substances or agents are transported or stored, all appropriate measures should be taken to prevent leakage or contamination.
- Workers and others involved in occupational situations in which the risk of exposure to carcinogenic substances or

agents may occur should conform to the safety procedures laid down and make proper use of all equipment furnished for their protection or the protection of others.

- The competent authority should periodically determine the carcinogenic substances and agents to which occupational exposure should be prohibited or made subject to authorization or control, and those to which other provisions of this recommendation apply.
- Provision should be made, by laws or regulations or any other method consistent with national practice and conditions, for all workers assigned to work involving exposure to specified carcinogenic substances or agents to undergo as appropriate.
- A preassignment medical examination.
- Periodic medical examinations at suitable intervals.
- Biological or other tests and investigations which may be necessary to evaluate their exposure and supervise their state of health in relation to the occupational hazards.

MEASURES FOR HEALTH PROTECTION OF WORKERS

The aim of occupational health is 'the promotion and maintenance of the highest degree of physical, mental and social well-being of workers in all occupations'. The measures for the general health protection of workers was the subject of discussion by an ILO/WHO Committee on Occupational Health in 1953. The Committee recommended the following:

1. **Nutrition:** Good nutrition is a fundamental requirement for positive health, functional deficiency and productivity. Nutritional status is internationally recognized as an indicator of national development. Nutrition in both input and output of the developmental process: A well nourished healthy work force as a precondition for successful economic and social development such as food security, nutrition health and sanitation are the responsibility of all developed sectors and indeed of all citizen. In many developing countries, malnutrition is an important factor contributing to poor health among workers and low work output. Malnutrition may also affect the metabolism of toxic agents and also the tolerance mechanisms. Under the Indian Factories Act, it is obligatory on the part of the industrial establishments to provide a canteen when the number of employees exceed 250. The aim is to provide balanced diets or snacks at reasonable cost under sanitary control. It is important to combine this action with the education of the workers on the value of a balanced diet. If the worker carries his own lunch to work, provision should be made for a safe and uncontaminated place to store the food before it is eaten to avoid spoilage or contamination. Likewise, some place separate from the workroom should be provided so that the meal may be eaten in sanitary surroundings.
2. **Communicable disease control:** The industry provides an excellent opportunity for early diagnosis, treatment, prevention and rehabilitation. It is a general objective everywhere, to detect cases of communicable disease and to render them noninfectious to others by treatment or removal from the working environment, or both. The communicable diseases of special importance in India are tuberculosis, typhoid fever, viral hepatitis, amebiasis, intestinal parasites, malaria and venereal diseases. Some of the communicable diseases which can be prevented by promotion of environmental sanitation, it includes safe water supply, safe disposal of excreta using sanitary latrine, avoid open field defecation and protection of food from contamination through maintenance of food hygiene, immunization. There should be an adequate immunization program against preventable communicable diseases. Anthrax, undulant fever, and Q fever are examples of communicable diseases which may be of occupational origin. Their control calls for special sanitary measures in the handling of working materials and substances.
3. **Environmental sanitation:** Within the industrial establishment, the following needs attention for the prevention of the spread of communicable diseases by water, food or other means:
   - *Water supply:* A sufficient supply of wholesome drinking water is one of the basic requirements in all industrial establishments. The common glass tumbler for drinking water should be abandoned as it spreads infection. Installation of drinking water fountains, at convenient points should be encouraged.
   - *Food:* If food is sold, its sanitary preparation, storage and handling are essential. Education of food handlers and other measures may be necessary to prevent outbreaks of gastrointestinal disease.
   - *Toilet:* There should be sufficient number of latrines and urinals of the sanitary type, separate for males and females, conveniently situated. It is recommended that there should be at least one sanitary convenience for every 25 employees (males and females separate) for the first 100 employees, and thereafter one for every 50. Garbage and waste disposal should be such as to avoid the breeding of flies and vermin.
   - *General plant cleanliness:* The walls, ceilings and passages should be painted with water washable paint and repainted at least once in 3 years and washed at least once in every 6 months. The dust which settles down on the floor and machinery should be promptly removed by vacuum cleaners or by wetting agents before it is redistributed into the atmosphere by the vibration of the machinery or buildings. A high standard of general cleanliness is one of the fundamentals of accident prevention. It also contributes to the efficiency and high morale of the workers.
   - *Sufficient space:* Sufficient floor space and cubic space are essential to prevent not only respiratory infections but also to ensure a comfortable working environment. The recommended standard is a minimum of 500 cu. ft. of space for every worker; space more than 14 feet above the floor level is not to be taken into consideration.
   - **Lighting:** The results of poor industrial illumination are workers' eye fatigue, increased accidents, decreased production and more rejections of finished products.

Furthermore, defective illumination over a long period of time may result in permanent impairment of vision. There should be sufficient and suitable lighting, natural or artificial or both, in every part of a factory where workers are working or passing through. The standards of illumination for different kinds of work have been set out—precision work for a high degree of accuracy may require 5–75 foot candles; where people work regularly, 6 to 12 foot candles may be sufficient. Illumination in corridors and passages should be at least 0.5 foot candles.

- **Ventilation and temperature:** Poor ventilation not only increases the chances of infection from person to person, but also affects the mental and physical efficiency of the workers. Proper ventilation is also needed for the control of noxious vapors, fumes and dusts and prevention of fatigue and industrial accidents. Effective and suitable provision should be made for maintaining adequate ventilation by circulation of fresh air in every work room; and such a temperature which will secure to workers therein, reasonable conditions of comfort and prevent injury to health.
- **Protection against hazards:** There should be adequate environmental controls designed to protect the workers against exposure to dusts, fumes and other toxic hazards.
- **Housing:** There is usually an acute shortage of housing in industrial areas. Most workers come from rural areas. The housing of workers near a plant must be correlated to essential community amenities and to social and sanitary facilities. Town planning and zoning are highly desirable.
- **Mental health:** The objective of an occupational health service is not only to keep the workers physically healthy, but mentally and psychologically stable. Industrial workers are susceptible to the effects of love, recognition, rejection, job satisfaction, rewards and discipline. The master-servant era is now disappearing from industry. The workers, individually and collectively, like to be recognized, like to have a measure of control over their own affairs, like to have the opportunity to develop skills appropriate to their individual capacity. Over burden of work, lack of job satisfaction, strict rule regulation of the agency, very few leave can cause stress, strain among workers, for good mental health it is important in preventing worker from cumulative fatigue and eliminating such heavy long-time overwork that does not allow workers to recover from fatigue.
  - Reduction of overtime and holiday work hours
  - Observance of 'standard for limit'
  - Proper identification of working hours
  - Promotion of taking annual paid leave
  - Improvement of working time arrangements
  - Thorough implementation of health management measures for workers
  - Establishment of health management system and implementation of health check ups, etc., promote health and happiness
  - Detect signs of emotional stress; identify the cause; treatment; rehabilitation of the ill.

MEASURES FOR WOMEN AND CHILDREN

Occupational Health Problems of Women

Basically hazards posed by physical, chemical and biological agents in work place are similar for male and female workers but the following factors have to be remembered for women workers.

Women on an average, have a smaller stature and have less physical strength; their vital capacity is 11% less; their hemoglobin is app. 20% less; their skin area is larger as compared to circulating volume; they have larger body fat content. They have lower heat tolerance and greater cold tolerance.

Woman's unique reproductive function exposes her unborn child to workplace hazards. Women shoulder the additional burden of household work, care of children and social responsibilities.

Occupational stress is one of the major problems from a gender perspective. Studies from developed countries show that sources of stress in women's lives are more diverse and diffuse than those experienced by men. A number of factors cause stress among working women. These include:

- Multiple overlapping roles as housewives, mothers and workers especially when such roles are physically and mentally demanding with little satisfaction, monetary gain or social rewards.
- Types of job repetitive and monotonous jobs with little control over work place and methods, piece rate system and job insecurity all lead to stress.
- **Sexual harassment:** This is often faced by women in almost all types of occupations except when they occupy top level jobs. It is widely believed that employers show a preference for women only when they are prepared to accept lower wages, are expected to be more docile and submissive.
- **Shift work:** In certain occupations, such as telephone operators who do different shifts including night shifts, interference with family responsibilities causes lot of stress.

Musculoskeletal disorders and ergonomic issues: The heavy manual labor performed by malnourished women often under subhuman working and living conditions, cause a number of health problems of which musculoskeletal problems are one of the commonest problems of women in unorganized sector. Repetitive trauma is often the cause of a variety of musculoskeletal and neurologic disorders in women. Work-related musculoskeletal disorders of the neck and shoulders and upper limbs are also known as cumulative trauma disorders (CTD). Evidences from a number of studies suggest that all these disorders principally result from; constrained working posture, monotonous and repetitive work and psychological stress. Even in mechanical jobs, most of the tools, machines and work stations have been designed for average male and are unsuitable for women from an ergonomic angle.

Reproductive Health Hazards

Many chemicals pose hazards to the embryo especially during organogenesis. This has led to restriction on the employment of women in various hazardous processes under various legislation (e.g., Factories Act, 1984). Exposure to volatile organic solvents, dusts and pesticides and VDT (video display terminal) nonionizing radiation has been found to be associated with increased risk of infertility in women. This could be due to interference with ovulation, fertilization or implantation.

Exposure to solvents increases the risk of spontaneous abortions and there is sufficient evidence of association between exposure to toluene, methylene chloride, tetrachloroethylene, petroleum ether, xylene, formaldehyde, paint thinners and reproductive disorders. Women exposed to toluene have reported a greater frequency of menstrual dysfunction including dysmenorrhea, irregular cycles and spontaneous abortions.

Occupational dust exposures (wood and agriculture based) have also been associated with adverse pregnancy outcome. It is not definite whether it is due to the preservatives such as pesticides or other agents like pentachlorophenol, creosote, formaldehyde, chromium, arsenic, etc. Aflatoxins, one of the commonest mycotoxins found in agricultural grain dusts are known teratogens.

Pesticides: Maternal occupational pesticide exposures has been identified as a risk factor for still birth. Organochlorine pesticides, polyhalogenated biphenyls and chlorophenoxy herbicides such as 2,4-D have been found to be teratogenic. DDT has estrogenic properties. Dioxins, polychlorinated biphenyls have been shown to create a variety of reproductive effects ranging from immune suppression, teratogenicity, hormonal disruptions and even endometriosis.

Need for Special Protection

Women workers require special protection because:

1. The developing embryo may be more susceptible to noxious agents than the exposed mother (e.g., in the case of methylmercury poisoning.
2. Females may be less suited for some work tasks than men; pregnancy may decrease the capacity to cope with many work factors.
3. Women tend to feed themselves less substantially than men and also restrict their nourishment in difficult economic circumstances, the infant mortality is higher amongst children of women employed in industrial work.

Availability of Protection for Women in India

The following types of protection are available for women workers in India:

1. Expectant mothers are given maternity leave for 6 months, of which 6 weeks precede the expected date of confinement; during this period they are allowed 'maternity benefit', which is a cash payment under the Employees State Insurance Act, 1948.
2. Provision of free antenatal, natal and postnatal services.
3. The Factories Act (Section 66) prohibits night work between 7 PM and 6 AM; Section 34 prohibits carrying of excessive weights beyond a certain schedule which has been laid down.
4. The Indian Mines Act (1923) prohibits work underground.
5. The Factories Act, 1976 provides for crèches in factories where more than 30 women workers are employed, and also prohibits the employment of women and children in certain dangerous occupations. Regarding protection of children, the Constitution of India declared: 'No child below the age of fourteen shall be employed to work in any factory or mine or engaged in any other hazardous employment'.
6. **Health education:** Health education is a basic health need. It is an important health promotional measure. Health education in the industrial setting should be envisaged at all levels—the management, the supervisory staff, the worker, the trade union leaders and community. The content varies from matters of personal hygiene and protection to participation of the workers in the planning and operation of the total health service program in industry, implementation of safety and health education at workplaces by displaying posters charts, conducting periodical health awareness program can prevent occupational diseases. For prevention of occupational health hazards, other measure, such as implementation of nationwide Industrial Safety Week and industrial Health Week and establishment of an award system for offices with no industrial accident record can also encourage the workers. For prevention of accidents; publication, dissemination, guidelines on investigation of risks or hazards are also helpful.
7. **Family planning:** Family planning is now recognized a decisive factor for the quality of life, and this applies to industrial workers also. The workers must adopt the small family norm.

OCCUPATIONAL HEALTH TEAM

The purpose of occupational health services is to provide primary, secondary and tertiary prevention facilities to the labor/workers. This also includes protecting workers from being handicaps at the work place. To achieve these aims, we need several people working inside and outside the commercial institution. All such people who are helpful in achieving the aims of occupational health care called members of "occupational health team".

The a healthcare team is made up of the following members:

- Occupational health nurse
- Physiotherapist
- Specialist doctor
- Industrial manager
- Supervisor

- Shift in charge
- Rehabilitation specialist
- Labor welfare officer
- Labor union representative
- Representative of voluntary organization
- Other invited member as per the need.

PREVENTION OF OCCUPATIONAL DISEASES

The various measures for the prevention of occupational diseases may be grouped under three heads; medical, engineering and statutory or legislative.

MEDICAL MEASURES

- **Pre-placement examination:** Pre-placement examination is the foundation of an efficient occupational health service. It is done at the time of employment and includes the worker's medical, family occupational and social history; a thorough physical examination and a battery of biological and radiological examination, e.g., chest X-ray, electrocardiogram, vision testing, urine and blood examination, special tests for endemic disease. A fresh recruit may either be totally rejected or given a job suited to his physical and mental abilities. The purpose of pre-placement examination is to place the right man in the right job, so that the worker can perform his duties efficiently without detriment to his health.
- **Periodical examination:** Many diseases of occupational origin require months or even years for their development. Their slow development, very often, leads to their nonrecognition in the early stages and this is harmful to the worker. This is the reason why a periodical medical checkup of workers is very necessary when they handle toxic or poisonous substances.
  The frequency and content of periodical medical examinations will depend upon the type of occupational exposure. Ordinarily workers are examined once a year. But in certain occupational exposures (e.g., lead, toxic dyes, radium) monthly examinations are indicated. Sometimes, even daily examinations may be needed such as when irritant chemicals like dichromates are handled. The periodical examinations may be supplemented, where necessary by biological and radiological examinations. Particular care should be given to workers returning from medical leave, to assess the nature and degree of any disability and to assess suitability or otherwise of returning to same job.
- **Medical and healthcare services:** The medical care of occupational diseases is a basic function of an occupational health service. In India, the Employees State Insurance Scheme provides medical care not only for the worker but also his family. Within the factory, first aid services should be made available. Properly applied first aid can reduce suffering and disability and hasten recovery. Immunization is another accepted function of an occupational health service.
- **Notification:** National Laws and Regulations (Factories, 1976; Mines Act, 1952; Dock Laborers Act, 1948; etc.) require the notification of cases and suspected cases of occupational disease. In the Factories Act, a list of 22 diseases is included while in the Mines Act 3 diseases and in the Dock Regulations 8 diseases are listed. These diseases are recognized internationally for the purpose of workmen's compensation. The main purpose of notification in industry is to initiate measures for prevention and protection and ensuring their effective application; and to investigate the working conditions and other circumstances which have caused or suspected to have caused occupational diseases.
- **Supervision of working environment:** Periodic inspection of working environment provides information of primary importance in the prevention of occupational disabilities. The physician should pay frequent visits to the factory in order to acquaint himself with the various aspects of the working environment such as temperature, lighting, ventilation, humidity, noise, cubic space, air pollution and sanitation which have an important bearing on the health and welfare of the workers. He should be acquainted with the raw materials, processes and products manufactured. He should also study the various aspects of occupational physiology such as occurrence of fatigue, night-work, shift-work, weight carried by the workers and render advice to the factory management on all matters connected with the health and welfare of the workers. For studies of this kind of physician should enlist the cooperation of safety engineers, industrial hygienists and psychologists.
- **Maintenance and analysis of records:** Proper records are essential for the planning, development and efficient operation of an occupational health service. The worker's health record and occupational disability record must be maintained. Their compilation and review should enable the service to watch over the health of the workers, to assess the hazards inherent in certain types of work and to devise or improve preventive measures.
- **Health education and counseling:** Ideally, health education should start before the worker enters the factory. All the risks involved in the industry in which he is employed and the measures to be taken for personal protection should be explained to him. The correct use of protective devices like masks and gloves should also be explained. Simple rules of hygiene—handwashing, paring the nails, bodily cleanliness and cleanliness of clothes, should be impressed upon him. He should be frequently reminded about the dangers in industry through the media of health education such as charts, posters and hand bills. The purpose of health education is to assist the worker in his process of adjustment to the working, home and community environment.

ENGINEERING MEASURES

- **Design of building:** Measures for the prevention of occupational diseases should commence in the blue-print stage. The type of floor, walls, height, ceiling, roof, doors and windows, cubic space are all matters which should receive attention in the original plan of the building which is put up by the industrial architect. Once the building is constructed, it would be difficult to introduce alternations without much trouble and expense.

- **Good housekeeping:** Good housekeeping is a term often applied to industry, and means much the same as when used domestically. It covers general cleanliness, ventilation, lighting, washing, food arrangements and general maintenance. Good housekeeping is a fundamental requirement for the control or elimination of occupational hazards. It also contributes to efficiency and morale in industry. The walls, ceilings, and passages should be white-washed at least once a year. The dust which settles down on the floor, ledges, beams, machinery and other stationery objects should be promptly removed by vacuum cleaners or by wetting agents. Masks, gloves, aprons and other protective equipment should be kept clean and in a state of good repair. To prevent accidents, the right thing should be in the right place. Not only the inside, but the outside of the plant should also be kept clean and tidy.
- **General ventilation:** There should be good general ventilation in factories. It has been recommended that in every room of a factory, ventilating openings shall be provided in the proportion of 5 sq feet for each worker employed in such room, and the openings shall be such as to admit a continued supply of fresh air. In rooms where dust is generated there should be an efficient exhaust ventilation system. Good general ventilation decreases the airborne hazards to the workers especially hazards from dusts and gases. The Indian Factories Act has prescribed a minimum of 500 cu ft of air space for each worker.
- **Mechanization:** The plant should be mechanized to the fullest possible extent to reduce the hazard of contact with harmful substances. Dermatitis can be prevented if hand-mixing is replaced by mechanical devices. Acids can be conveyed from one place to another through pipes. There may be other similar situations where mechanization can be substituted to hand-operation.
- **Substitution:** By substitution is meant the replacement of a harmful material by a harmless one, or one of lesser toxicity. A classical example is the substitution of white phosphorus by phosphorus sesquisulfide in the match industry, which resulted in the elimination of necrosis of jaw (phossy jaw), zinc or iron paints can blessed in place of harmful lead paints; silver salts can be used in place of mercury salts; acetone can be used in place of benzene. But substitution is not always possible in industry. Where possible, it should be used to the fullest possible extent.
- **Dusts:** Dusts can be controlled at the point of origin by water sprays, e.g., wet drilling of rock. Inclusion of a little moisture in the materials will make the processes of grinding, sieving and mixing comparatively dust-free. Wet methods should be tried to combat dust before more elaborate and expensive methods are adopted.
- **Enclosure:** Enclosing the harmful materials and processes will prevent the escape of dust and fumes into the factory atmosphere. For example, grinding machinery can be completely enclosed. Such enclosed units are generally combined with exhaust ventilation.
- **Isolation:** Sometimes it may be necessary to isolate the offensive process in a separate building so that workers not directly connected with the operation are saved from exposure. Isolation may not be only in space, but also in the fourth dimension of time. Certain operations can be done at night in the absence of the usual staff.
- **Local exhaust ventilation:** By providing local exhaust ventilation of dusts, fumes and other injurious substances can be trapped and extracted 'at source' before they escape into the factory atmosphere. The heart of the local exhaust ventilation is the hood which is placed as near as possible to the point of origin of the dust or fume or other impurity. Dusts, gases and fumes are drawn into the hood by auction and are conveyed through dusts into collecting units. In this way, the breathing zone of workers may be kept free of dangerous dust and poisonous fumes.
- **Protective devices:** Respirators and gas masks are among the oldest devices used to protect workers against airborne contaminants and they are still used for that purpose. There are two classes of respirators. (i) those which remove contaminants from air, (ii) those to which fresh air is supplied. The workers should know what kinds to use, and when and how to use, respiratory devices should not be used as substitute for other control methods. The other protective devices comprise ear plugs, ear muffs, helmets, safety shoes, aprons, gloves, gum boots, barrier creams, screens and goggles. The workers should be instructed in the correct use of protective devices.
- **Environmental monitoring:** An important aspect of occupational health program is environmental monitoring. It is concerned with periodical environmental surveys, especially sampling the factory atmosphere to determine whether the dusts and gases escaping into the atmosphere are within the limits of permissible concentration. The use of 'permissible limits' has played an important part in reducing occupational exposure to toxic substances. Thermal environment, ventilation, lighting would also have to be monitored. Such monitoring should be done by joint collaboration of doctors and engineers.
- **Statistical monitoring:** Statistical monitoring comprises review at regular intervals of collected data on health and environmental exposure of occupational groups. The main objective of these reviews is to evaluate the adequacy of preventive measures and occupational health criteria, including permissible exposure levels.
- **Research:** Research in occupational health offers fertile ground for study which can provide a better understanding of the industrial health problems. There are two kinds of research; pure research and research for the improvement in connection with a manufactured product. Both are important study of the permissible limits of exposure to dusts and toxic fumes, occupational cancer incident

prevention, industrial fatigue and vocational psychology are some aspects of research in occupational health.

LEGISLATIVE MEASURES

Usually legislative measures in occupational health are referred to the acts that will provide occupational health and safety. In order to safeguard the health, safety and welfare of the industrial workers, laws have been framed in every country. The important factory laws in India are:

- Indian Factories Act, 1948
- Employees' State Insurance Act, 1923

Factory Act in India

In India, the First factories Act was passed in 1881. This Act was basically designed to protect children and to provide few measures for health and safety of the workers. This law was applicable to only those factories, which employed 100 or more workers. In 1891 another Factories Act was passed which extended to the factories employee 50 or more workers. International Labor Organization and established in 1919 as a part of league of nations. The Act prescribed working hours, holidays and the employment of young men and women. The amendment in Indian Factories Act 1881 was done in 1911, which made provision for weekly holiday for all the workers and prohibited the employment of women and children below 9 years in the factories. The amendment during 1934 in the factories act made provision for appointment of factory inspectors, prevention of accidents and maintenance of sanitary conditions.

In 1946, Bhore Committee emphasized the need for investigation of occupational diseases and development of departments for teaching and research in occupational health

After independence the rapidly growing industrialization has created a lot of industrial health problems affecting the employer and Government. The Indian Factories Act has been amended 3 times after independence, i.e., in 1948, 1976 and 1987 to improve health, safety and welfare of the workers. The Act extends to whole of India except Jammu and Kashmir. Under the Act the factory refers to any premises including the precincts there of:

- Where in 10 or more workers are working or were working on any day of the preceding 12 months and in any part of which manufacturing process is being carried on with the aid of power or ordinarily so carried on.
- Where in 20 or more workers are working or were working on any day of the preceding 12 months and in any part of which manufacturing process is being carried on without the aid of power or ordinarily so carried on.

The chapter 3rd of this Act deals with the health aspects. It includes sections 11 to 20. The rules under this chapter prescribe the nature and extent of environmental sanitation to promote and protect the health of workers. It gives information about general cleanliness, drainage system, disposal of waste and effluents, ventilation, humidity and temperature, system for control of dust and fumes, adequate space for workers, lighting arrangement, safe drinking water, latrines and urinal facilities, etc.

The chapter 4th of this Act deals with the safety aspects. It includes sections 21 to 40. The rules under this chapter prescribe the precautions for safety against injuries and accidents which are likely to occur in the factory. There is a provision for appointment of safety officer in factories employing 1000 workers.

The Chapter 5th deals with welfare aspects. The various sections in this chapter prescribe specific welfare measures to promote health and provide medical care. These include working facilities, sitting arrangements, first aid equipment and supplies, canteen facility were more than 250 workers are employed, crèche facility where more than 30 women workers are working and employment of welfare officer when there are 500 or more workers.

The chapter 6th deals with work hours, weekly holidays, intervals for rest for adult workers and women workers. The act has prescribed a maximum of 48 working hours per week, not exceeding 9 hours per day; with rest at least for half an hour after 5 hours of continuous work, for adolescents, the hours of work have been reduced from 5–4.5 hours per day.

Besides weekly holidays, every worker will be entitled for live with wages after 1 years of continuous service at the rate as follows: Adult 1 day for every 20 days work, children 1 day for every 15 days work. Leave can be accumulated up to 30 days in case of adults and 40 days in case of children.

The chapter 7th deals with employment of young persons. The Act prohibits employment of children below 14 years of age. The people in the age group of 15–18 years (adolescents) should be duly certified by certifying surgeons regarding their fitness for work. Restrictions have been laid down on employment of women and children in certain dangerous occupations.

Occupational Safety and Health Act (OSHA): The Occupational Safety and Health Act of 1970 is administered by the Occupational Safety and Health Administration to ensure a safe and healthful work environment for employees and preserve human resources. OSHA standards are sets of rules designed to minimize specific on the job risks to employees. These risks include exposure to toxic chemicals, hazardous waste.

This Act created three administrative bodies to carry out its missions:

1. OSHA is primarily responsible for creating and forcing standards and procedures to enhance employee safety and health.
2. National Institute of Occupational Safety Health (NIOSH) engages in safety research and makes recommendations to OSHA.
3. Occupational Safety and Health Review Committee (OSHRC) reviews contested actions made by employers following citations for noncompliance.

OSHA regulation mandate several additional guidelines:

- Development and exposure control plan to eliminate or minimize exposure.

- Make hepatitis B vaccine available to all employees at risk for exposure.
- Store or maintain shares or containment materials in accordance with regulation.
- Provide training program for all employees at the time of initial employment and annually thereafter,.

Statutory Provision Act 1948 for Labor

- **Health:** The Act provides detailed instruction on cleanliness, disposable of waste, ventilation etc. Every employe should protect his employees against health hazards by:
  - Devoting adequate attention to working conditions.
  - Substituting a less toxic substance for the hazardous one.
  - Providing protective clothing.

  Section 11 to 20 of the Act provides detail instruction.
  These are discussed below:
  Sec 11 – cleanliness
  Sec 12 – Disposal of wastes
  Sec 13 – Ventilation and temperature
  Sec 14 – Dust and fume
  Sec 15 – Artificial humidification
  Sec 16 – Over crowding
  Sec 17 – Lighting
  Sec 18 – Drinking water
  Sec 19 – Latrines and urinals
  Sec 20 – Spittoons.
- **Safety:** Section 21 to 41 of the Act provides detail instructions.
  These are discussed below:
  Sec 21 – Fencing of machinery
  Sec 22 – Work on near machinery in motion
  Sec 23 – Employment of young person on dangerous machines
  Sec 24 – Striking gear and devices for cutting off power
  Sec 25 – Self-acting machines
  Sec 26 – Casing of new machinery
  Sec 27 – Prohibition of employment of women and children near cotton-openers
  Sec 28 – Hoists and lifts
  Sec 29 – Lifting machines, chains, ropes and lifting tackles
  Sec 30 – Revolution machinery
  Sec 31 – Pressure plants
  Sec 32 – Floors, stairs and means of access
  Sec 33 – Pits, slump, openings in floor, etc.
  Sec 34 – Excessive weights
  Sec 35 – Production of eyes
  Sec 36 – Precautions against dangerous fumes
  Sec 37 – Precautions against explosive or inflammable dust, gas etc.
  Sec 38 – Precautions in case of fire
  Sec 39 – Power to require specification of defective parts or tests of Stability.
  Sec 40 – Safety of building and machinery
  Sec 40 A – Maintenance of building
  Sec 40 B – Safety officers.
- **Welfare:** Section 42 to 49 of the act provides detail instructions. These are discussed below:
  Sec 42 – Washing facility
  Sec 43 – Facilities for storing and drying clothing
  Sec 44 – Facilities for sitting
  Sec 45 – First aid appliances
  Sec 46 – Canteens
  Sec 47 – Shelters, rest room and lunch rooms
  Sec 48 – Crèches
  Sec 49 – Welfare officer.

Employee State Insurance (1948)

The Employee State Insurance Act, [ESIC] 1948, is a piece of social welfare legislation enacted primarily with the object of providing certain benefits to employees in case of sickness, maternity and employment injury and also to make provision for certain other matters incidental thereto:

- **Medical benefit:** Full medical facilities for self and dependents are admissible from day one of entering insurable employment. Whereas, the primary, outpatient, in patient and specialist services are provided through a network of panel clinics, ESI dispensaries and hospitals, super specialty services are provided through a large number of advanced empanelled medical institutions on referral basis.
- **Eligibility to medical benefit:**
  - From day one of entering insurable employment for self and dependents such as spouse, parents and children own or adopted.
  - For self and spouse on superannuation subject to having completed five years in insurable employment on superannuation or in case of having suffered permanent physical disablement during the course of insurable employment.
  - The rate of contribution for superannuated/disabled is ₹ 1,220 per annum payable in lump sum at the local office for availing full medical care for self and spouse.
- **Sickness benefit (cash):** Sickness benefit is payable to an insured person in cash, in the event of sickness resulting in absence from work and duly certified by an authorized insurable medical officer/practitioner.
  - The benefit becomes admissible only after an insured has paid contribution for at least 78 days in a contribution period of 6 months.
  - Sickness benefit is payable for a maximum of 91 days in two consecutive contribution period. [one year]
  - Payment is to be made by the local office within 7 days of certificate of sickness at a standard rate, which is not less than 50% of the wages.
- **Extended sickness benefit (cash):** Extended sickness benefit is payable to insured persons for the period of certified sickness in case of specified 34 long-term diseases that needs prolonged treatment and absence from work on medical advice.
  - For entitlement to this benefit an insured person should have been in insurable employment for at least 2 years. He/she should also have paid contribution for

a minimum of 156 days in the preceding 4 contribution periods or say 2 years.
  - ESI is payable for a maximum period of 2 years on the basis of proper medical certification and authentication by the designated authority.
  - Amount payable in cash as extended sickness benefit is payable within 7 days following the submission of complete claim papers at the local office concerned.
- **Enhanced sickness benefit (cash):** This cash benefit is payable to insured persons in the productive age group for under going sterilization operation, viz., vasectomy/tubectomy.
  - The contribution is the same as for the normal sickness benefit.
  - Enhanced sickness benefit is payable to the IP's for 14 days for tubectomy and for seven days in case of vasectomy.
  - The amount payable is double the standard sickness benefit rate that is equal to full wages.
- **Maternity benefit (cash):** Maternity benefit is payable to insured women in case of confinement or miscarriage or sickness related thereto.
  - For claiming this insured woman should have paid for at least 70 days in 2 consecutive contribution periods, i.e., 1 year.
  - The benefit is normally payable for 12 weeks, which can be further extended up to 16 weeks on medical grounds.
  - The rate of payment of the benefit is equal to wage or double the standard sickness benefit rate.
  - The benefit is payable within 14 days of duly authenticated claim papers.
- **Disablement benefit (cash):** Disablement benefit is payable to insured employees suffering from physical disablement due to employment injury or occupation disease.
  - An insured person should be an employee on the date of the accident.
  - Temporary disablement benefit at 70% of the wages is payable till temporary disablement lasts and is duly certified by authorized insurance medical officer.
  - In case of permanent disablement, the cash benefit is payable for life. Amount payable is worked out on the basis of earning capacity determined by a medical board.
  - Disablement benefit is payable within one month of submission of the complete claim papers.
- **Dependents benefits (cash):** Dependents benefit [family pension] is payable to dependents of a deceased insured person where death occurs due to employment or occupational disease.
  - A widow can receive this benefit on a monthly basis for life or till remarriage.
  - A son or daughter can receive this benefit till 18 years of age.
  - Other dependents like parents including a widowed mother can also receive the benefit under certain condition.
  - The rate of payment is about 70% of the wages shareable among dependents in a fixed ratio.
  - The first installment is payable within a maximum of 3 months following the death of an insured person and thereafter, on a regular monthly basis.
- **Other benefits:**
  - **Funeral expenses:** On the death of an insured person subject to a maximum of a ₹ 2,500 payable at the local office.
  - **Vocational rehabilitation:** In case of disabled insured persons less than 45 years of age with 40% or more disablement.
  - **Free supply** of physical aids and appliances such as crutches, wheelchairs, spectacles and other such physical aids.
  - **Preventive healthcare** services, such as immunization, family welfare services, HIV/AIDS detection, treatment, etc.
  - **Medical bonus** ₹ 250 is paid to an insured woman or in respect of the wife of an insured person in case she does not avail hospital facilities of the scheme for child delivery.

Americans with Disabilities Act (ADA)

The Americans with Disabilities Act (1990) which becomes effective on July 1992 is designed to eliminate discrimination against disabled persons in employment by enforcing equal access to jobs and accommodations. The ADA broadly defines disabilities as:

- A physical or mental impairment that substantially limits one or more of the major life activities to such individuals.
- A record of having such impairment.

WORKPLACE VIOLENCE

- Workplace violence is any act or threat of physical violence, harassment, intimidation, or other threatening disruptive behavior that occurs at the work site. It ranges from threats and verbal abuse to physical assaults and even homicide. It can affect and involve employees, clients, customers and visitors. Homicide is currently the fourth-leading cause of fatal occupational injuries in the United States. According to the Bureau of Labor Statistics Census of Fatal Occupational Injuries (CFOI), out of the 4,547 fatal workplace injuries that occurred in the United States in 2010, 506 were workplace homicides. Homicide is the leading cause of death for women in the workplace. However it manifests itself, workplace violence is a major concern for employers and employees nationwide.
- **Risk factors for workplace violence:** Certain work factors, processes, and interactions can put people at increased risk from workplace violence. Examples include:
  - Working with the public.
  - Handling money, valuables or prescription drugs (e.g., cashiers, pharmacists).

- Carrying out inspection or enforcement duties (e.g., government employees).
- Providing service, care, advice or education (e.g., healthcare staff, teachers).
- Working with unstable or volatile persons (e.g., social services, or criminal justice system employees).
- Working in premises where alcohol is served (e.g., food and beverage staff).
- Working alone, in small numbers (e.g., store clerks, real estate agents), or in isolated or low traffic areas (e.g., washrooms, storage areas, utility rooms).
- Working in community-based settings (e.g., nurses, social workers and other home visitors).
- Having a mobile workplace (e.g., taxicab).
- Working during periods of intense organizational change (e.g., strikes, downsizing).

Risk of violence may be greater at certain times of the day, night or year; For example:

- Late hours of the night or early hours of the morning
- Tax return season
- Overdue utility bill cut-off dates
- During the holidays
- Pay days
- Report cards or parent interviews
- Performance appraisals.

Risk of violence may increase depending on the geographic location of the workplace; for example:

- Near buildings or businesses that are at risk of violent crime (e.g., bars, banks)
- In areas isolated from other buildings or structures.

Certain occupational groups tend to be more at risk from workplace violence. These occupations include:

- Healthccare employees
- Correctional officers
- Social services employees
- Teachers
- Municipal housing inspectors
- Public works employees
- Retail employees.

Prevention of Work Place Violence

In most workplaces where risk factors can be identified, the risk of assault can be prevented or minimized if employers take appropriate precautions. One of the best protections employers can offer their workers is to establish a zero-tolerance policy toward workplace violence. This policy should cover all workers, patients, clients, visitors, contractors, and anyone else who may come in contact with company personnel. The policy should:

- Be developed by management and employee representatives.
- Apply to management, employee's, clients, independent contractors and anyone who has a relationship with your company.
- Define what you mean by workplace violence in precise, concrete language.
- Provide clear examples of unacceptable behavior and working conditions.
- State in clear terms your organization's view toward workplace violence and its commitment to the prevention of workplace violence.
- Precisely state the consequences of making threats or committing violent acts.
- Outline the process by which preventive measures will be developed.
- Encourage reporting of all incidents of violence.
- Outline the confidential process by which employees can report incidents and to whom.
- Assure no reprisals will be made against reporting employees.
- Outline the procedures for investigating and resolving complaints.
- Describe how information about potential risks of violence will be communicated to employees.
- Make a commitment to provide support services to victims of violence.
- Offer a confidential Employee Assistance Program (EAP) to allow employees with personal problems to seek help.
- Make a commitment to fulfill the violence prevention training needs of different levels of personnel within the organization.
- Make a commitment to monitor and regularly review the policy.
- State applicable regulatory requirements.

CHILD LABOR

Child labor is the practice of having children engage in economic activity, on part or full-time basis. The practice deprives children of their childhood, and is harmful to their physical and mental development. Poverty, lack of good schools and growth of informal economy are considered as the important causes of child labor in India.

Primary causes: International Labor Organization (ILO) suggests poverty is the greatest single cause behind child labor. For impoverished households, income from a child's work is usually crucial for his or her own survival or for that of the household. Income from working children, even if small, may be between 25 to 40% of these household income. Other scholars such as Harsch on African child labor, and Edmonds and Pavcnik on global child labor have reached the same conclusion.

Cultural causes: In European history when child labor was common, as well as in contemporary child labor of modern world, certain cultural beliefs have rationalized child labor and thereby encouraged it. Some view that work is good for the character-building and skill development of children. In many cultures, particular where informal economy and small household businesses thrive, the cultural tradition is that children follow in their parents' footsteps; child labor then is a means to learn and practice that trade from a very early age. Similarly, in many cultures the education of girls is less valued or girls are simply not expected to need formal schooling, and these girls pushed into child labor such as providing domestic services.

Macroeconomic causes: Biggeri and Mehrotra have studied the macroeconomic factors that encourage child labor. They focus their study on five Asian nations including India, Pakistan, Indonesia, Thailand and Philippines. They suggest that child labor is a serious problem in all five, but it is not a new problem. Macroeconomic causes encouraged widespread child labor across the world, over most of human history.

They suggest that the causes for child labor include both the demand and the supply side. While poverty and unavailability of good schools explain the child labor supply side, they suggest that the growth of low paying informal economy rather than higher paying formal economy is amongst the causes of the demand side. Other scholars too suggest that inflexible labor market, size of informal economy, inability of industries to scale up and lack of modern manufacturing technologies are major macroeconomic factors affecting demand and acceptability of child labor.

Consequences of child labor: The presence of a large number of child laborers is regarded as a serious issue in terms of economic welfare. Children who work, fail to get necessary education. They do not get the opportunity to develop physically, intellectually, emotionally and psychologically. In terms of the physical condition of children, children are not ready for long monotonous work because they become exhausted more quickly than adults. This reduces their physical conditions and makes the children more vulnerable to disease. Children in hazardous working conditions are even in worse condition. Children who work, instead of going to school, will remain illiterate which limits their ability to contribute to their own well-being as well as to community they live in. Child labor has long-term adverse effects for India.

Child labor laws and initiatives: After its independence from colonial rule, India has passed a number of constitutional protections and laws on child labor. The Constitution of India in the Fundamental Rights and the Directive of State Policy prohibits child labor below the age of 14 years in any factory or mine or castle or engaged in any other hazardous employment (Article 24). The constitution also envisioned that India shall, by 1960, provide infrastructure and resources for free and compulsory education to all children of the age six to 14 years. (Article 21-A and Article 45).

Legislation for Child Labor in India

The first protective legislation for child labor in India was seen in 1881 in the form if Indian Factories Act which had the provisions prohibiting employment of children below 7 years, limiting the working hours for children to 9 hours a day and providing 4 holidays in a month and rest hours. This was actually made by the ruling British Government to decrease the production in Indian industries through some legal restrictions.

It may be submitted that the labor legislations in India including protective legislation for children have been greatly influenced with the result of various conventions and recommendations adopted by International Labor Organization. Besides Constitutional provisions, there are several legislative enactments which provide legal protection to children in various occupations.

- The Children (Pledging of Labor) Act, 1933
- The Employment of Children Act, 1938

The Minimum Wages Act, 1948 and rules made there under by the government

- The Factories Act, 1948
- The Plantations Labor Act, 1951
- The Mines Act, 1952
- The Merchant Shipping Act, 1958
- The Motor Transport Workers' Act, 1961
- The Apprentices Act, 1961
- The Atomic Energy Act, 1962
- The Beedi and Cigar Workers (Conditions of Employment) Act, 1966
- The Shops and Establishment Act in Various States
- Child Labor (Prohibition and Regulation) Act, 1986

Child Labor (Prohibition and Regulation) Act (1986) was the culmination of efforts and ideas that emerged from the deliberations and recommendations of various committees on child labor. Significant among them were the National Commission on Labor (1966–1969), the Gurupadaswamy Committee on Child Labor (1979) and the Sanat Mehta Committee (1984).

Aims Child Labor (Prohibition and Regulation) Act (1986): The Act aims to prohibit the entry of children into hazardous occupations and to regulate the services of children in nonhazardous occupations. In particular it is aimed at:

- The banning of the employment of children, i.e., those who have not completed their 14th year, in 18 specified occupations and 65 processes
- Laying down a procedure to make additions to the schedule of banned occupations or processes
- Regulating the working conditions of children in occupations where they are not prohibited from working
- Laying down penalties for employment of children in violation of the provisions of this Act and other Acts which forbid the employment of children
- Bringing uniformity in the definition of the child in related laws.

A national policy on child labor was formulated in 1987 to focus on rehabilitating children working in hazardous occupations. The Ministry of Labor and employment had implemented around 100 industry-specific National Child Labor Projects to rehabilitate the child workers since 1988. Initiatives against child labor:

National Child Labor Project Scheme

For rehabilitation of child labor, Government had initiated the National Child Labor Project (NCLP) Scheme in 1988 to rehabilitate working children in 12 child labor endemic districts of the country. Its coverage has increased progressively to cover 271 districts in the country presently. As on date the scheme is in operation in 266 districts.

Under the NCLP scheme, children are withdrawn form work and put into special schools, where they are provided with bridging education, vocational training, mid-day meal, stipend, healthcare facilities, etc., and finally mainstreamed to the formal education system. At present, there are around 7,000 NCLP schools being run in the country with an enrollment of three lakh children. Till date more than 9 lakh working children have already been mainstreamed to regular education under the NCLP.

Non-governmental organizations, many NGOs like Bachpan Bachao Andolan, CARE India, Child Rights and You, Global March Against Child Labor, RIDE India, etc. have been working to eradicate child labor in India. Pratham is India's largest non-governmental organization with the mission 'every child in school and learning well.' Founded in 1994, Pratham has aimed to reduce child labor and offer schooling to children irrespective of their gender, religion and social background. It has grown by introducing low cost education models that are sustainable and reproducible. Child labor has also been a subject of public interest litigations in Indian court.

Elimination of Child Labor in India: Coordination with ILO

The International Labor Organization (ILO) launched the International Programme for Elimination of Child Labor (IPEC) in the year 1991 with the objective to end child labor globally. India was the first country to sign the Memorandum of Understanding (MOU) in the year 1992. During the 11th Plan period, three projects viz., INDUS project, Andhra Pradesh Phase-II and Karnataka Project were implemented in the country under ILO-IPEC. Jointly funded by the Ministry of Labor, Government of India and the Department of Labor, United States of America (USDOL), the INDUS Child Labor Project was implemented in ten hazardous sectors in 21 districts across five states like Delhi, Maharashtra, Madhya Pradesh, Tamil Nadu and Uttar Pradesh. The project adopted a participatory method to identify beneficiaries and enrolling child workers in schools, transitional education centers and vocational training centers were seen as a key strategy for rehabilitation of child and adolescent workers withdrawn from work.

INTERNATIONAL LABOR ORGANIZATION (ILO)

The ILO was founded in 1919, in the wake of a destructive war, to pursue a vision based on the premise that universal, lasting peace can be established only if it is based on social justice. The ILO became the first specialized agency of the UN in 1946.

The unique tripartite structure of the ILO gives an equal voice to workers, employers and governments to ensure that the views of the social partners are closely reflected in labor standards and in shaping policies and programs.

The International Labor Organization (ILO) has four strategic objectives.

1. Promote and realize standards and fundamental principles and rights at work
2. Create greater opportunities for women and men to decent employment and income
3. Enhance the coverage and effectiveness of social protection for all
4. Strengthen tripartism and social dialogue.

In support of its goals, the ILO offers unmatched expertise and knowledge about the world of work, acquired over more than 90 years of responding to the needs of people everywhere for decent work, livelihoods and dignity. It serves its tripartite constituents and society as a whole in a variety of ways, including:

- Formulation of international policies and programs to promote basic human rights, improve working and living conditions, and enhance employment opportunities
- Creation of international labor standards backed by a unique system to supervise their application
- An extensive program of international technical cooperation formulated and implemented in an active partnership with constituents, to help countries put these policies into practice in an effective manner.
- Training, education and research activities to help advance all of these efforts.

Fundamental principles: The fundamental principles of International Labor Organization (ILO) are:

- Labor is not a commodity
- Freedom of expression and association is essential
- Poverty act as a danger for prosperity
- War against want requires to be carried on. Workers and employers should enjoy equal status in free discussion.

Role of International Labor Organization (ILO):

- Full employment, raising standard of living
- Ensure employment, in which workers should get satisfaction
- Facilities for training, transfer of labor-migration for employment, settlement
- Policies with wages, hours and condition of work
- Effective recognition of the right of collective bargaining
- Protection of life and health of workers
- Provision for child welfare, maternity protection
- Provision for adequate nutrition, housing
- Assurance of equality of education and vocational opportunity.

Structure of International Labor Organization (ILO): The structure of ILO consists of three organs to perform effectively. They are: International Labor Conference (ILC), Governing Body and International Labor office.

International Labor Conference (ILC): This organ or wing is also called as policy making/legislative wing of ILO. International Labor Conference holds session once in a year.

It elects governing body. Meetings/sessions are attended by 4 delegates—2 from govt. (Generally Cabinet Ministers)—1 representative of employee—1 representative of employer. Each delegate is accompanied by advisor not exceeding 2 in number. Non-government delegates are chosen by government.

Functions of International Labor Conference (ILC):
- Formulate international standards (Conventions and recommendations)
- Decide expenditure budget
- To make amendments
- Consider labor problems and assist solution
- Select once in 3 years members of governing body
- Elect president.

Governing Body: It is executive wing of International Labor Organization (ILO). Governing Body is a political body implements decisions of ILC with the help of International Labor Office. It consists of 56 titular members—28 government—14 employer—14 employee. Further, it consists of 66 deputy members—28 government—19 employer—19 employee. Governing Body elects director-general after every 5 years. Decides agendas for ILC scrutinize the budget, follow-up recommendations and conventions of ILC.

International Labor Office: It is a focal point for activities of International Labor Organization under the supervision of Governing Body, The International Labor Office is headed by Director-General. Its headquarter is at Geneva. Office employs: 2700 officials from over 150 nations. Office also contains a research documentation center. The International Labor Office is responsible to collect distribute information regarding labor and social problems, ILO Manpower organization, Vocational training, Migrant workers, Women workers, Child workers, Social security, Conditions of work, Health, safety and welfare. Other activities include promotion of handicraft, improvement of small industries, organization of workers education programs.

The International Labor Organization (ILO) is devoted to promoting social justice and internationally recognized human and labor rights, pursuing its founding mission that labor peace is essential to prosperity. Today, the ILO helps advance the creation of decent work and the economic and working conditions that give working people and business people a stake in lasting peace, prosperity and progress. Its tripartite structure provides a unique platform for promoting decent work for all women and men. Its main aims are to promote rights at work, encourage decent employment opportunities, enhance social protection and strengthen dialogue on work-related issues.

ILO in India

India, a founding member of the ILO, has been a permanent member of the ILO governing body since 1922. The first ILO office in India started in 1928. The decades of productive partnership between the ILO and its constituents has mutual trust and respect as underlying principles and is grounded in building sustained institutional capacities and strengthening capacities of partners. It has a two-directional focus for socioeconomic development, overall strategies and ground-level approaches.

The ILO's overarching goal is Decent Work, i.e., promoting opportunities for all women and men to obtain decent and productive work in conditions of freedom, equity, security and dignity. Decent Work is at the heart of ILO's strategies for economic and social progress, central efforts to reduce poverty and a means to achieve equitable, inclusive and sustainable development. India's 11th Plan's vision of faster and inclusive growth through a process which yields broad-based benefits and ensures equality of opportunity for all—with a strong emphasis on decent working and living conditions for all. A number of India's 11th Plan targets are in consonance with the DW agenda.

The Decent Work (DW) concept is translated into Decent Work Country Programmes (DWCPs), prepared and adopted by the tripartite constituents and ILO, at country levels. The DWCP-India (2007–12), aligned to the 11th Plan and the United Nations Development Assistance Framework, focuses on 3 priorities.
- **Priority 1:** Opportunities enhanced for productive work for women and men, particularly for youth and vulnerable groups, especially through skills development
- **Priority 2:** Social protection progressively extended, particularly in the context of informalization
- **Priority 3:** Unacceptable forms of work progressively eliminated.

The cross-cutting issues are special focus while implementing the DWCP under the three priority areas are:
- Social dialogue and strengthening of partners
- Informal economy
- Gender equality.

ILO's current portfolio in India centers around child labor, preventing family indebtedness employment, skills, integrated approaches for local socioeconomic development and livelihoods promotion, green jobs, value-addition into national programs, micro and small enterprises, social security, HIV/AIDS, migration, industrial relations, dealing with the effects of globalization, productivity and competitiveness, etc.

The Decent Work Technical Support Team (DWT) for South Asia stationed in New Delhi, through its team of specialists, provides technical support at policy and operational levels to member states in the sub-region.

Recommendations: The International labor organizations (ILO) has given 203 recommendations from 1919 to 2014 on different aspects for benefits of workers. Some of the recommendation recently from 2000 onwards are:
- **R191:** Maternity Protection Recommendation, 2000 (No. 191)
- **R192:** Safety and Health in Agriculture Recommendation, 2001 (No. 192)
- **R193:** Promotion of Cooperatives Recommendation, 2002 (No. 193)

- **R194:** List of Occupational Diseases Recommendation, 2002 (No. 194)
- **R195:** Human Resources Development Recommendation, 2004 (No. 195)
- **R196:** Work in Fishing Recommendation, 2005 (No. 196)
- **R197:** Promotional Framework for Occupational Safety and Health Recommendation, 2006 (No. 197)
- **R198:** Employment Relationship Recommendation, 2006 (No. 198)
- **R199:** Work in Fishing Recommendation, 2007 (No. 199)
- **R200:** HIV and AIDS Recommendation, 2010 (No. 200)
- **R201:** Domestic Workers Recommendation, 2011 (No. 201)
- **R202:** Social Protection Floors Recommendation, 2012 (No. 202)
- **R203:** Forced Labor (Supplementary Measures) Recommendation, 2014 (No. 203).

THE ROLE OF OCCUPATIONAL HEALTH NURSE

The nurse becomes the first point of contact for Workers. They will readily seek advice from an approachable, accessible healthcare professional that consciously makes the time to talk to them about their concerns. Occupational health nurses are skilled listeners and because of their independent role can often gather information from both management and staff, and help to seek the common ground between both when they are discussing matters related to health, social well-being and quality of working lives.

Workplace surveillance and health risk identification: The Occupational Health Nurse in collaboration with the members of the Safety Office conducts workplace surveillance, a term used to describe activities which determine whether groups of workers may be suffering actual or potential work related injury or illness. Occupational Health Nurse conducts workplace surveillance utilizing methods to detect, appraise, identify and manage health hazards and exposures to physical and chemical hazards at work.

Comprehensive interventions or programs to control all actual and potential health risks to employees and provide the worker with education of potential health risks and strategies to prevent injury and illness. Intervention measures designed to prevent occurrences, monitor exposure and eliminate the problems. Early detection of workplace hazards. Health education for employees to reduce the likelihood of injury/illness. Documentation of health and safety potential risks for each job activity. Utilize statistics to indicate trends and target health risks.

Health surveillance: As part of health surveillance, the Occupational Health Nurse conducts activities which determine whether groups of workers may be suffering an occupational illness as a result of exposure to a particular hazard or group of hazards. Health surveillance is always based on environmental assessments with exposures evaluated and documented. Examples of health risk assessment and medical surveillance include immunization for employees who are exposed to infectious biological agents. This includes those who come into contact with: Animals, human blood or body fluids, certain bacteria and viruses used in research, communicable diseases, etc.

Reduction of workplace injuries/illnesses due to early detection of workplace hazards. Reduction of financial costs associated with exposure to workplace hazards. Increased knowledge of the workplace environment by the worker and employer. Develop statistics to identify significant trends in occupational illness or injuries.

Health promotion and protection: The Occupational Health Nurse is responsible for employee health promotion and protection. This programming focuses on the prevention of illness/injury by promotion of health and well-being using strategies directed towards modifying the behavior of individuals/groups and encouraging them to accept responsibility, in matters which affect their health and over which they have control towards achieving a healthy lifestyle. Anticipatory interventions include strategies for protection from agents causing disease and/or hazards in the work environment and/or university community.

Enhancement of employee well-being by gaining knowledge of risk factors in the workplace. Movement toward a state of optimal health by obtaining management commitment and policies to support development and provision of individual employee and work group programs. Reduction of health risks by programs targeted to meet goals determined by needs assessment of individual workplace. Familiarity with community resources and skill in utilizing community resources such as posters, pamphlets, brochures, fact sheets, newsletters, health programs where applicable. Individual knowledge of risk factors and preventative measures as a foundation for development and provision of health building programs such as smoking cessation, nutrition, hypertension, fitness, which in turn will provide a reduction of financial costs to both the employer and the healthcare system. Reduction of financial, psychological cost to the individual by timely referrals to the Employee Assistance Program when applicable.

Primary care: Primary care is the set of nursing actions that are provided to manage illness or functional challenges in the workplace. The goal is to prevent complications, promote recovery and facilitate rehabilitation of both occupational and non-occupational illness and injury. Primary care is based on the nursing process, on a theoretical base consistent with occupational health nursing practice, on knowledge of the health/illness continuum and on norms and deviations of the continuum.

Appropriate treatment, referral and follow-up so that an early return to work process, where indicated, can be initiated reporting and recording: Confidentiality ensured by utilizing the nursing process. After obtaining an informed consent, investigating and addressing factors which influence progress to optimal functioning. Promoting worker responsibility for self-care which includes: Health education in treatment (where appropriate), collaboration with other health disciplines (where indicated), maintain competence in emergency/primary care.

Counseling: Counseling is the process of helping employees to clarify problems and make informed decisions and choices while giving positive reinforcement. It provides strategic interventions and appropriate referrals to deal with a crisis situation and time for the employee to reflect on impending decisions and evaluate actions taken. Counseling is a broad area that ranges from simple encouragement of clients who are motivated to make positive changes to health behavior to providing direct care for clients in a crisis situation. The type of counseling offered is determined by the level of additional preparation and expertise of the nurse.

- Safety of client and others in the situation is ensured. Confidentiality is ensured. Legal obligation to report criminal or dangerous situations (e.g., child abuse, harm to self or others). Client returns to optimal functioning. Appropriate referral and follow-up are made. Collaborate with internal and external resources. Use contracting and mutual goal setting to promote client's responsibility for self-care. Pursue continuous improvement of counseling ability through education.

Rehabilitation/Case Management: Rehabilitation/Case Management is the process/provision of services necessary to restore an individual to the fullest physical, mental, emotional, social, vocational and economical independence of which they are capable. Rehabilitation cases may be either work or non-work related. Rehabilitation includes preventative processes whereby the Occupational Health Nurse implements knowledge gained from research studies/epidemiological studies within the workplace and work culture.

Return of individual to maximum ability to function in physical, mental, emotional, social, vocational and economical areas by utilizing community resources, referral agencies. Increased individual self-esteem and morale, especially with the modified return to work program when applicable. Participates in facilitated meetings following the RTW principles when workplace stress/issues are prime reason for absence. Reduced WSIB assessments and insurance premiums WSIB penalty avoidance. Improved corporate culture and morale (good corporate citizens). Well established modified work programs by coordinating the return to work to the pre-illness level of the individual through positive communication with all parties involved. Maintain/document statistics to support programs.

The responsibilities of nursing personnel are being stated by WHO's Technical Report series 24 and also by second joint ILO/WHO committee on occupational health convened in Geneva in 1952. These are:

Functions of nursing personnel as stated by WHO's Technical Report series 24:

- Carrying out the therapeutic program designed by physicians for sick patients including personal services aimed at hygiene and comfort.
- Maintenance of the physical and psychological environment conducive to recovery and health.
- Engaging the patient and his family in his recovery and rehabilitation.
- Carrying out measures for the prevention of diseases.
- Instructing people sick or well, in measures promoting total health (physical and mental) in a positive sense.
- Coordinating nursing efforts with other members of community group.

Functions as stated by the joint ILO/WHO committee in 1952:

- Assistance in general administration, maintenance and arrangement of health facilities in the plant.
- Emergency and primary treatment of accidents and illness based on standing order from physicians.
- Assistance in pre-placement and other medical examinations.
- Arranging follow up treatment, where indicated, including health supervision of employees returning to work after illness.
- Assistance in general preventive health measures in the plant.
- Health education and counseling
- Assistance in supervision of factory hygiene and accident prevention.
- Advice on specific health questions to management and workers.
- Maintenance of records and statistics.
- Cooperation with and referral of workers to general community agencies for help as and when necessary.

The precise duties and responsibilities of nurses may vary and would depend upon the general state of development of industrial health services in a plant or region or country.

CHAPTER 16

Rehabilitation

INTRODUCTION

Tertiary prevention means disability limitation and rehabilitation. Tertiary prevention begins early in the period of recovery from illness. It consists of such activities as consistent and appropriate administration of medications to optimize therapeutic effects moving and positioning the patient to prevent complications of immobility and active and passive exercises to prevent disability, minimizing residual disability and helping the client learn to live productively with limitations. Through proper exercise physiotherapy and occupation therapy and corrective, plastic surgery can improve mobility, which is otherwise known as rehabilitation. Rehabilitation may be physical, mental and occupational which makes the individual productive. Occupational therapy can be provided to the client by depending on the nature and extend of disability. By rehabilitation, clients achieve a high level of functioning as possible, despite the limitations caused by illness or impairment. It involves preventing further disability or reduced functioning. In this rehabilitation phase, the client may be staying at home or rehabilitation center.

TERMINOLOGY

Impairment

Any loss or abnormality of psychologic, physical, or anatomic structure or function is known as impairment. It may be physical, cognitive or emotional problem. Any improvement in impairments must be accomplished by medical/mental health professionals. There are some factors responsible for impairment. They are congenital (cerebral palsy), genetic (Down's syndrome), infection (rheumatic heart disease), substances (alcoholic cirrhosis), trauma (burns, spinal cord injuries), autoimmune factors (rheumatoid arthritis), dysfunction of body organs or systems (kidney failure, type I diabetes).

Disability

Any restriction or lack of ability to perform any activity in the manner or within the range is considered normal for a human being. Impairments can result in disabilities. Disabilities involve problems with performing some type of function. Disabilities that remain after impairments have been treated, or may be, addressed by various therapists.

Handicap

A disadvantage for a given individual resulting from an impairment or disability that limits or prevents fulfillment of a role that is normal for that particular individual.

Functional Limitation

Any loss of ability to perform tasks and obligations of usual roles and normal daily life.

Chronic Illness

An irreversible presence, accumulation, or latency of disease states or impairments that involves the total human environment.

CONCEPT OF REHABILITATION

Rehabilitation, commonly known as rehab, is a scientifically developed procedure for ensuring the recovery from any kind of disability, injury or the habit. Rehabilitation is a slow but a steady process. Many of the rehabilitations have ongoing processes involved in them, i.e., some processes in it are continuous. Those are set of special instructions to be followed by the patient in order to ensure that the malfunction does not hit back again.

Definitions

Rehabilitation is defined as the process of restoring the individual to the fullest physical, mental, social, vocational, and economic capacity of which he or she is capable. It is also defined as relearning of former skills, learning new skills necessary to adapt and live fully in an altered lifestyle.

Rehabilitation is the process of maximizing an individual's capabilities or resources to foster optimal independent functioning.

Must begin from the very onset of a traumatic event or diagnosis of a chronic illness.

Every aspect of the individual's needs and care assessed and addressed.

Rehabilitation nursing is directed toward the prevention of complications of disease or trauma and the maintenance or restoration of function.

Objectives

- The basic objective of rehabilitation is to restore the physical, social and psychological potential to a level, so that he can independently function and carry on an independent life.
- Prevent disability and return to normalcy. Maximum level of restoration through different interventions.
- Training in vocational methods to suit working with residual disability and earn lively and independently.

Goals

- Maximize the quality of life of the individual
- Address the individual's specific needs
- Assist the individual with adjusting to an altered lifestyle
- Be directed toward promoting wellness and minimizing complications
- Assist the individual in attaining the highest degree of function and self-sufficiency possible
- Assist the individual to return to home and community.

Basic Aims

The elements of rehabilitation nursing need to be view as a part of basic nursing rather than as specialty. It emphasized on degree and depth of knowledge rather than a matter of completely new body of knowledge.

The three basic aims are:

Prevent Further Impairment

Rehabilitation can occur at any stage of diseases. When a person loses any body part due to any cause, the rehabilitation process first aims to restrict the loss to that limit only. For example, if a person gets paralyzed due to any disease, first we have to treat that disease to prevent further impairment.

Maintain Existing Abilities

Maintaining existing abilities actually entails preventing additional injury or deterioration of uninvolved parts. There also needs to be an emphasis on the maintenance of the ability of noninjured parts. For example, why should someone with fractured hip develop hypostatic pneumonia? Or an amputee develop a hip flex on contracture? So, maintaining existing abilities is continued long after formal rehabilitation program.

Restore as Many Functions as Possible

The nurse works with the health team to help the patient regain strength to relearn activities of daily living. The nurses assist client to achieve their maximum level of health and function by intervening at the primary level to promote health at the secondary level to maintain health or at the tertiary level to restore health. Restorative care settings are those designed to bring the client to the maximal level of health function.

Philosophy

Rehabilitation is a dynamic, health-oriented process that exists an ill or disabled individual to achieve the greatest possible level of physical, mental, spiritual, social and economic functioning.

The rehabilitation process helps the person to achieve an acceptable quality life with dignity, self-respect and independence.

Rehabilitation programs are designed for individuals with physical, mental and emotional disabilities. During rehabilitation, the individual is assisted to adjust to the disability by learning how to use resources and to focus on existing abilities are emphasized.

Every major illness or injury carries with it the threat of disability. The emphasis of rehabilitation is to restore the patient to independent or to preillness or preinjury level of function in as short time as possible. If this is not possible, the aims of rehabilitation are maximal independence and quality of life acceptable to the patient.

Due to advancement of science and technology, the lives of seriously ill, injured and disabled patients recovering from serious illness need rehabilitation.

The economic advantage of rehabilitation is readily apparent. Instead of being unemployed, the person is rehabilitated into employment, and instead of being dependent on society, the person contributes to it.

The greater the number of rehabilitation disciplines working cooperatively with the individual, the greater is the chance of that person reliving the highest potential.

ISSUES IN REHABILITATION

Quality of Life versus Quantity of Life

Rehabilitation focuses on continually improving the quality of the person's life, not merely maintaining life itself. It focus on making the life productive and returning optimum functioning of the body.

Care versus Cure

Rehabilitation gives importance to care and it is provided at the last stage of treatment. When treatment is completed rehabilitation starts. Many conditions remain irreversible; therefore, the focus of care is related to adaptation and acceptance of an altered life rather than to resolving an illness. Rehabilitation generally depends more on care, exercises, like skill training, acceptance of situation rather than on medication.

High Cost of Interdisciplinary Care versus Long-term Care

Rehabilitation is expensive. Success is sometimes seen as a return to productive employment. Patient with chronic illness needs long-term care whereas by rehabilitation may be the individual becomes so sufficiently independent that no caregiver is required.

Ethical Issues

Three moral principles serve as a framework for medical ethic which can be followed during rehabilitation respect for autonomy, beneficence and justice.

Respect for Autonomy

In moral philosophy, autonomy refers to self-governance, or the personal rule of the self. A person must have adequate understanding and not be controlled by others or by personal limitations that prevent choice. When we respect people as autonomous, we recognize their right to hold views, make choices and take actions based on their own set of personal values and beliefs. In rehabilitation also same principles should be followed. They must be accorded the moral right to have their own opinions and act upon them.

Beneficence

The term 'beneficence' means kindness, charity and the doing of good. It refers to a moral obligation to help other people, to avoid harming them, and to try and balance benefits with harms. In the healthcare setting, it means an obligation to promote the health and well-being of the patient and to prevent disease, injury, pain and suffering.

Justice

People are treated according to the principle of justice if they are treated according to what is fair, due or owed to. The principle of justice concerns the question of what is due to whom, and how to distribute the costs and benefits of living in a society.

Ethical Dilemmas

Ethical and moral decisions are made on a daily basis in the field of rehabilitation. Keeping in mind the ethical principles just mentioned, ethical issues in three settings commonly encountered in rehabilitation will be discussed under resource allocation and patient selection, the ethics of team care and ethical issues in goal-setting.

Patient Selection and Resource Allocation

The selection of patients who are to be selected for rehabilitation in any setting is generally made by the physiatrist. Because in many centers demand for admission exceeds the number of available beds, difficult decisions often have to be made. In some cases there may be a clearly defined set of guidelines available, but selection is often more subjective. Patient selection requires consideration of both medical and nonmedical factors. Medical factors include diagnosis, prognosis, secondary complications, functional performance and prognosis and ability to learn. Nonmedical factors can be social, vocational, personal and financial.

Ethical Issues in Teamwork

Because of its emphasis on maximizing a patient's physical, emotional and psychosocial well-being and independence, rehabilitation medicine places a premium on teamwork to help a patient achieve his or her goals. The emphasis within rehabilitation is to try and develop interdisciplinary or transdisciplinary rather than multidisciplinary teams, which means that each person functions within the context of the team, rather than as an isolated individual. The team generally consists of a physiatrist, nurses specialized in care of the rehabilitation patient, a social worker and multiple therapists, although team make-up may vary depending on the rehabilitation center and the focus of the team. The patient should also be included as a member of the team, and whenever possible, should be involved in discussions and decision-making.

Ethical Issues in Goal Setting

When examining teamwork in rehabilitation, the role of the patient within the team must also be considered important in goal setting. Goals are the functional outcomes that the patient and team strive to achieve, and, as such, help to define and focus the team's entire rehabilitative treatment plan. Thus, goals can be used as outcome criteria for evaluating the efficacy of care. In fact, systems of goal setting have become so widely accepted in the rehabilitation industry that quality assurance examiners sometimes use them as indicators. The goal setting must be done by the decision of patient, team members and family members of the patients. The patients themselves want to make their own decisions in societies that respect self-determination and individual rights. They know which goals and outcomes would be most meaningful to them and how much energy and time they wish to expand on therapy and retraining. The members of the rehabilitation team want to provide the patient with the highest possible level of functioning. They may assume and expect that patients will seek and generally follow their advice. So, they are also important in goal setting. Family members often wish to be involved in the design of the treatment program. This expectation is quite reasonable, as family members often assume the burden of providing ongoing care for patients and should be involved in decision-making that affects their own future. That is why, during goal setting, the opinion of patient, family members and team members will be given the same importance.

Cornerstones of Rehabilitation

The cornerstones of rehabilitation may be seen as stepping stones on the 'road to recovery':

- Individually centered
- Community reentry
- Independence
- Functional ability
- Team approach
- Quality of life
- Prevention and wellness

- Change process
- Adaptation
- Patient/family education.

TYPES AND METHODS OF REHABILITATION

Commonly there are four phases involved in the rehabilitation procedure, namely Phase 1, Phase 2, Phase 3 and Phase 4. There are different types of rehabilitations available for different types of disabilities.

Neurological Rehabilitation

In this type of rehabilitation, patients suffering from stroke, neuromuscular disease, certain types of head trauma and spinal cord injury are treated. It aims at making the patient self-dependent and helps to create a positive thinking in the patient. The patient is treated so that he leads an improved life physically, emotionally, and socially.

Cardiac Rehabilitation

Cardiac rehabilitation program is designed to help those people who have heart problem. Heart patients are educated to live a healthy life and reduce stress for the proper functioning of the heart, cardiac rehabilitation, educating people about the various risk factors that contribute to developing a heart disease. These risk factors include high blood pressure, obesity, smoking, drinking, drug abuse, lack of physical activity, etc. Recovery programs from heart disease/surgery, educating people about improving their quality of life.

Drug Rehabilitation

Drug rehabilitation means to make an addict free from the addiction of alcohol, prescription drug and street drugs (cocaine, heroin, etc.) which include counseling programs designed to know the underlined cause behind a person becoming an addict. Educating the person about the various side effects of drug abuse and how it impacts one's social, professional, physical and personal life. Designing programs that will prevent the relapse of the drug addiction.

Alcohol Rehabilitation

Alcohol rehabilitation is to make an alcoholic free from the addiction. It involves programs that will teach people the various bad effects of consuming excess alcohol. Effective detoxification programs cleanse the body from the various toxins of alcohol.

Physical Rehabilitation

Physical rehabilitation is for those people whose lifestyle has changed after they have gone through a serious illness, surgery or accident. Here the therapist introduces programs to improve the mobility and functioning of the injured body part of the patient. It includes appropriate exercise therapy for joint movements.

- Restoring the function of affected part by physiotraining
- Provision of external appliances and splints
- Relief of pain by application of hot and cold fomentation. Bladder and bowel exercise to control incontinence
- Training in daily activities to restore lost function
- Education of patients to maintain the physical status and returning to normal life.

Medical Rehabilitation

Medical rehabilitation includes treatment programs that help a person perform better in all his daily physical and mental activities. Medical rehabilitation is a follow-up treatment after any kind of treatment program. Medical Rehabilitation Programs focus on improving major and minor skills that are required in the basic life, assessing patient in every step to improve the activities of basic living.

Psychosocial Rehabilitation

It is the process of rehabilitation which is not complete without psychosocial intervention.

- To raise the morals of the patient, counseling, positive attitude and support
- Sympathetic attitude of doctors, family members and community support
- Psychotherapy for depression, anxiety, personality changes and suicidal tendency
- Financial support, workplace support to raise the morale and take away depression.

Vocational Rehabilitation

Vocational rehabilitation means to help those people who find it difficult to get employment or retain it after they have gone through a certain situation that caused mental or physical disability in them. Vocational Rehabilitation Program provides physiological and medical assessment, job placement, and on the job training.

Vestibular Rehabilitation

It helps in improving the ear deficit by working on the central nervous system. Also deals in improving eye and head coordination.

Stroke Rehabilitation

This treatment type helps to restore damage that is caused after a stroke, which is the 3rd leading cause for death worldwide. Stroke rehabilitation aims at helping people gain maximum normal functioning after the occurrence of a stroke. Help the person get back to normal lifestyle and be independent in daily activities.

Educational Rehabilitation

Efforts to be made to continue the education:

- Integrated education for disabled child in normal school.
- Preschool training, parents' counseling
- Special training in speech and language
- Orientation and mobility training for blinds

- Day-to-day living and practice training and skill development.

REHABILITATION TEAM AND THEIR ROLES

Rehabilitation usually encompasses a number of special health services that may be made available to the individual patient on the basis of particular need. Personnel representing these special services include the physician and the nurse and may also include a physical therapist, social worker, vocational counselor, or other professional personnel when indicated. Because rehabilitation is a complex process involving the patient and a number of professional personnel, a team relationship usually provides the structure through which each member can make special knowledge and skills available for the greatest benefit to the patient. The team evaluates the patient's need for rehabilitation and develops a plan to give maximum assistance in achieving rehabilitation goals. The patient is key member of the team and that the degree of determination to be rehabilitated may be the deciding factor in the success of the plan. The rehabilitation team promotes independence, self-respect and an acceptable quality of life. The patient's family is incorporated into the team. The family provides ongoing support, participates in problem-solving and learns to provide necessary ongoing care.

The rehabilitation nurse develops a therapeutic and supportive relationship with the patient and the family. She always emphasizes on patient's strengths. Here the nurse assumes role of caregiver, teacher, counselor, patient's advocate and consultant. Frequently, the nurse is called a manager.

Types of Rehabilitation Team

Team composition will vary dramatically depending on the phase of rehabilitation, the rehabilitation setting, the rehabilitation context for rehabilitation with the roles often dependent on the specific health system set up and resources available locally. Every team will not necessarily include all team members but rather the team composition and the clinical role of each rehabilitation team member as health providers are hugely diverse across various healthcare settings. The terms "intradisciplinary", "multidisciplinary," "interdisciplinary," and "transdisciplinary" are increasingly being used interchangeably to define teams within healthcare and outline the various degrees of involvement of the multiple disciplines within the team environment, but there is a huge differences between these different approaches to care. For rehabilitation, there are different types of models of team functioning. These are:

Intradisciplinary

Rehabilitation Team

Intradisciplinary or unidisciplinary teams are composed of professionals from one single discipline and from a single background. Interdisciplinary team may consists of all team members share the same professional skills and training, speak a common language of healthcare, and function in the same role within the group such as a team of public health nurses providing home care. In an intradisciplinary team all professionals belong to the same area of expertise and work towards the achievement of a common goal, individuals can support each other with specific tasks, which may improve the quality of performance.

Multidisciplinary Rehabilitation Team

Characterized by discipline-specific goals, clear boundaries between disciplines, and outcomes that are the sum of each discipline's efforts.

According to Jefferies and Chan (2004), multidisciplinary team working is described as the main mechanism to ensure truly holistic care for patients and a seamless service for patients throughout their disease trajectory and across the boundaries of primary, secondary and tertiary care. The multidisciplinary team (MDT) is a team of professionals that includes representatives of different disciplines, e.g., physiotherapy, occupational therapy, etc., who coordinate the contribution of each discipline with little overlap to assess and treat the patient separately with discipline-specific goals.

Interdisciplinary Rehabilitation Team

Collaborates to identify individuals' goals and is characterized by a combination of expanded problem-solving beyond discipline boundaries and discipline-specific work toward goal attainment.

Interdisciplinary teams differ from multidisciplinary teams in that they overlap practice with shared goals coordinated into a unified management plan, rather than working individually, allowing for group decision-making and group responsibility, with the patient considered an active member of the team. Each team member in an interdisciplinary team builds on each other's expertise to achieve the common, shared goals.

Transdisciplinary Rehabilitation Team

Characterized by the blurring of boundaries between disciplines, as well as by cross-training and flexibility to minimize duplication of effort toward individual goal attainment.

Flexible boundaries and interchangeable roles and responsibilities encourage the exchange of information, knowledge and skills. The interwoven nature of transdisciplinary teams broaden the skill sets of each therapist due to their exposure and substantial interaction with others outside their discipline, but it also allows the team of professionals to work together to reinforce and maintain goals not normally monitored.

Members of the rehabilitation team include:

- **Patients and their families:** Patients and their family members are important members of the healthcare team as the goals and ideas of patients are critically important for determining their ideal model of care.

- **Psychiatrists** (rehabilitation doctors) direct therapies and services provided by the rehabilitation team and coordinate care provided by other specialists.
- **Rehabilitation psychologists** provide psychological testing and individualized and family counseling, if needed.
- **Rehabilitation care coordinators** are registered nurses with special training, who coordinate the care from admission to discharge.
- **Rehabilitation nurses** encourage and help to practice the skills learned in therapy sessions.
- **Physical therapists** develop treatment programs to help the patient improve mobility through exercise and training.
- **Occupational therapists** help to develop the skills needed for the activities of day-to-day life.
- **Recreational therapists** assess the leisure needs and interests and develop treatments to help in return to a satisfying lifestyle.
- **Speech-language pathologists** work to improve speech and language, conversation skills and the thinking skills necessary for communication.
- **Registered dietitians** advise about healthy diet choices and special dietary needs.
- **Respiratory therapists** help the people with breathing disorders, including training in use of ventilators.
- **Medical social workers** provide emotional support, identify economic resources and community agencies and help for making arrangements to leave the hospital and find follow-up care.
- **Vocational case coordinators** help develop a plan to return to work in your community.
- **Child life specialists** help children and their families prepare for, adjust to, and benefit from hospital experiences.
- **Chaplains** support the spiritual, religious and emotional needs of you and your family.

PSYCHOSOCIAL REHABILITATION (PSR)

Psychiatric rehabilitation, also known as psychosocial rehabilitation, and sometimes simplified to psych rehab by providers, is the process of restoration of community functioning and well-being of an individual diagnosed in mental health or mental or emotional disorder and who may be considered to have a psychiatric disability. Psychiatric rehabilitation work is undertaken by rehabilitation counsellors (especially the individuals educated in psychiatric rehabilitation), licensed professional counsellors (who work in the mental health field), psych rehab consultants or specialist psychiatrist, social worker psychologists, occupational therapists and community support or allied health workers.

Definitions

Psychosocial rehabilitation can be defined as a process initiated by a health or mental health professional in collaboration with the patient's family and community, and supported by the policy planner implementing an individualized intervention program that seeks to maximize the patient's assets and minimize his abilities in the area of socio-occupational functioning, centering around the philosophy of mobilizing and utilizing resources available to the community, with the final objective of mainstreaming the client.

A revised definition: Psychosocial rehabilitation is a process initiated by the family of a person with severe mental disorder, in collaboration with the community's natural support system which includes the health professional, that seeks to maximize their socio-occupational functioning of the patient with the final stated objective of preventing marginalization.

It is a process that facilitates the opportunity for individuals—who are impaired, disabled or handicapped by a mental disorder—to reach their optimal level of independent functioning in the community.

The goal of psychosocial rehabilitation is returning the individual to community working and living condition as much independently as possible.

Objectives

- To enable patients to achieve their optimal functioning.
- To enable patients to live independently.
- To empower patients to understand and manage their illness effectively.
- To encourage involvement of families in care.

Ten essential elements that characterize the PSR approach:

1. **Individualization:** Services must be custom tailored to the individual. This means that program delivery must be very flexible and driven by individual choice.
2. **Hope:** Belief in the potential to change and grow of even the most severely disabled individual. Within everyone is an untapped, underutilized human capacity that should be developed.
3. **Client-directed:** People have the right and responsibility for self-determination. This means the consumer makes the decisions including how long they receive the service.
4. **Focus on skills:** The core of rehabilitation is increased competencies through skill acquisition.
5. **Strengths and abilities:** An emphasis on current strengths and abilities and not on symptom reduction or problems from the past.
6. **Environmentally specific:** Strengths and abilities must be assessed in relation to a specific environment. Skills must also be taught in relation to the environment in which they will be used.
7. **Environmental supports:** Modifying the environment and building external supports are equally as important as skill teaching. This includes social change (changing attitudes, rights, laws, etc.)
8. **Partnership approach:** The creation of an intimate environment with no professional authoritative barriers is essential.

9. **Ongoing support:** Programs should not be time-limited but geared to the individual. Program delivery must be very flexible and by individual choice. History has shown us that many seriously mentally ill people succeed as long as support is provided on an ongoing basis.
10. **Skills and supports in balance:** A person can only concentrate on improving/learning 1–2 skills at a time. Supports must be provided in any other deficit areas to enable the person to function until they master the current skills and can move on to learning or improving 1 or 2 more skills. Therefore, skills and supports are always in balance with one another.

Principles

- Psychosocial rehabilitation practitioners convey hope and respect, and believe that all individuals have the capacity for learning and growth.
- Psychosocial rehabilitation practitioners recognize that culture and diversity are central to recovery, and strive to ensure that all services and supports are culturally relevant to individuals receiving services and supports.
- Psychosocial rehabilitation practitioners engage in the processes of informed and shared decision-making and facilitate partnerships with other persons identified by the individual receiving services and supports.
- Psychosocial rehabilitation practices build on strengths and capacities of individuals receiving services and supports.
- Psychosocial rehabilitation practices are person-centered; they are designed to address the distinct needs of individuals, consistent with their values, hopes and aspirations.
- Psychosocial rehabilitation practices support full integration of people in recovery into their communities, where they can exercise their rights of citizenship, accept the responsibilities and explore the opportunities that come with being a member of a community and a larger society.
- Psychosocial rehabilitation practices promote self-determination and empowerment. All individuals have the right to make their own decisions, including decisions about the types of services and supports they receive.
- Psychosocial rehabilitation practices facilitate the development of personal support networks by utilizing natural supports within communities, family members as defined by the individual, peer support initiatives, and self- and mutual-help groups.
- Psychosocial rehabilitation practices strive to help individuals improve the quality of all aspects of their lives, including social, occupational, educational, residential, intellectual, spiritual and financial.
- Psychosocial rehabilitation practices promote health and wellness, encouraging individuals to develop and use individualized wellness plans.
- Psychosocial rehabilitation services and supports emphasize evidence-based, promising, and emerging best practices that produce outcomes congruent with personal recovery.
- Psychosocial rehabilitation programs include program evaluation and continuous quality improvement that actively involve persons receiving services and supports.
- Psychosocial rehabilitation services and supports must be readily accessible to all individuals whenever they need them; these services and supports should be well-coordinated and integrated as needed with other psychiatric, medical, and holistic treatments and practices.

Psychiatric rehabilitation promotes recovery, full community integration, and improved quality of life for persons who have been diagnosed with any mental health condition that seriously impairs their ability to lead meaningful lives. Psychiatric rehabilitation services are collaborative, person-directed and individualized. These services are an essential element of the healthcare and human services spectrum, and should be evidence-based. They focus on helping individuals develop skills and access resources needed to increase their capacity to be successful and satisfied in the living, working, learning, and social environments of their choice.

Psychosocial services, in contrast, have been associated with the term 'mental health' as part of community support movement nationwide since the 1970s. These services, which have roots in education, psychology and mental health (and community services) administration, were basic funded services of new community mental health agencies offering community living and professionalized community support since the 1970s.

Psychiatric rehabilitation services may include: workplace accommodations, supported employment or education, social firms, assertive community (or outreach) teams assisting with social service agencies, medication management, housing, employment, family issues, coping skills and activities of daily living and socializing. Traditionally, '24-hour' service programs (supervised and regulated options) were based upon the concept of instrumental and daily living skills as formulated in the World Health Organization (WHO) definition.

Psychiatric rehabilitation (what services are delivered) consists of eight main areas:

1. Psychiatric (symptom management)
2. Health and medical (maintaining consistency of care)
3. Housing (safe environments)
4. Basic living skills (hygiene, meals, safety, planning, chores)
5. Social (relationships, family, boundaries, communications and community integration)
6. Vocational and/or educational (coping skills, motivation)
7. Financial (personal budget)
8. Community and legal (resources).

Psychosocial Issues

A wide variety of psychosocial issues may be pertinent to any mentally ill client. A list of potential issues is provided herewith.

Although many of these issues will have been apparent from the outset of treatment, it is usually best to try to achieve stability with regard to medication, drug use and the client's social situation before taking them on. Of course, an urgent need with respect to any of these issues would be a priority of the stabilization phase. Psychosocial rehabilitation issue does not only adhere to mental illness, it can also happen in any long-term disability or illness which can affect their mental health.

Potential Psychosocial Rehabilitation Issues

- Vocational planning
- Leisure counseling
- Enhancing social support systems
- Improving family relationships
- Addressing legal problems
- Parenting and child welfare issues
- Budgeting and financial planning
- Social skills training
- Stress management
- Relapse prevention
- Pain management
- Polysubstance use
- Harm reduction
- Anger management
- Eating disorders
- Depression
- Anxiety and phobic disorders
- Trauma issues
- Grieving issues
- Sexual and gender identity issues
- Sexual dysfunction
- Adjustment to chronic illness.

The rehabilitation issues of the action/maintenance phase are aimed primarily at social and psychological adjustment. Vocational enhancements can be a crucial dimension of this process. Vocational goals may involve getting a job or improving vocational opportunities, but they may also address more fundamental impediments to employment, such as literacy and learning disabilities.

Strengthening the client's social support system is another important aspect of social adjustment. Family relationships and peer networks are often the main focus of these efforts. Also, improvement in a variety of social or coping skills may be critical to social adjustment.

Finally, legal issues may be ongoing, as the process of dealing with custody issues or criminal charges can be lengthy. Helping clients obtain legal assistance, and developing objective indicators of progress to present in court are among the strategies to consider.

Other aspects of the rehabilitation process will be more concerned with psychological adjustment. Although increases in the client's self-efficacy and self-esteem are fundamental to an improved attitude and optimism about the future, there may be a wide range of psychological or psychiatric issues to address. These will be easier to diagnose if the client's drug use has stabilized. If concerns about concurrent disorders persist to the action/maintenance phase, it may be desirable to obtain a psychiatric consultation.

Health issues can also be a priority of the action/maintenance phase. These may include pregnancy, dental needs or issues related to chronic diseases, such as HIV infection and chronic viral hepatitis.

In general, how psychosocial rehabilitation issues are addressed is not unique to mentally ill. However, additional practical information is corcened with issues related to polysubstance use, concurrent disorders, infectious diseases and pregnancy.

Some of the identified psychosocial issues may be addressed within the framework of the ongoing individual counseling. In multifunctional settings, specialized individual or group interventions may be provided by other counseling staff (e.g., vocational counseling, family treatment or relapse prevention counseling). If you are not working in a multifunctional setting, referrals to other community agencies may be necessary to obtain appropriate services.

Methods of Psychosocial Rehabilitation

Psychosocial Therapy

Emphasizes the desirability of moving from a secure psychosocial stage of development to a higher one in the manner that is suitable for the individual situations, the research recommended the sufferer to read books and poetry, see film and listen to song associated with his childhood. Material need to be selected according to personal taste and sociocultural environment.

Two main areas as of group development may be identified in professional experience:

1. Milieu therapy use of total living experience to achieve therapeutic objectives, possibly use nonprofessionals such as volunteers, neighbors and friends, (use people as facilitators rather than drugs)
2. The therapeutic community organizes itself democratically with decision-making being undertaken by patient and all level staff, to increase self-esteem and insight through the media of the interpersonal contact experienced in group living and meeting.

Behavior Modification

These groups are under degree of criticism in recent years because frailer rehabilitate suffering from schizophrenia but in London have different picture. It is an attempt to increase level of performance for:

- The therapist needs some skills such as assessment, goal-setting, realistic program to achieve goal and learning suitable techniques.
- Therapy has developed its own specific therapeutic formats:
    - The problem-oriented medical record
    - Social skills training.

Problem-oriented Medical Record

Problem-oriented medical record (POMR) is a method of recording data about the health status of a patient in a problem-solving system, in an easily accessible way that encourages ongoing assessment and revision of the healthcare plan in the heath care team. It is a comprehensive approach to provide treatment. It can also applicable in psychological rehabilitation. When there are a large number of problems, in that case among all problems, the major problems have been identified and treated. The POMR will help the care provider in prioritizing the health problems. For example a 16-yr-old boy has the problems like sexual preoccupations, educational deprivation, poor eye contact, poor self-esteem and difficulties in getting along with his aunt. In that case, when there are a large number of problems with boys some priority for action has to determine. For example, lack of educational attainment may be achieved by improving his level of literacy, which leads to improve self-esteem. Introduction to suitable youth group could reduce his sense of isolation and sexual preoccupations reduce by sport and outlet of energy.

Social Skills Training

Social skills training aims at improving social skill of client. (Liberman et al., 1985:399) identify three areas of skill training:

1. Making suitable international exchanges, e.g., eye contact, smile, propionate voice volume and appropriate length of speech
2. Conversational skill, e.g., asking suitable questions and making appropriate rejoinder
3. **Problem-solving skills:** Covering areas of job interviewing, money management, management of medication and coping with difficult social circumstances, e.g., a hostile landlord.

Social skill training can be assisted by using video replay equipment which allow participants to review their own progress. Possibly use TV program to simulate role play and skill improvement.

Cognitive Therapy

Cognitive therapy (CT) is a type of psychotherapy developed by American psychiatrist Aaron T. Beck. It is based on the cognitive model, which states that thoughts, feelings and behavior are all connected, and that individuals can move toward overcoming difficulties and meeting their goals by identifying and changing unhelpful or inaccurate thinking, problematic behavior, and distressing emotional responses. This approach is use to identify and change dysfunctional thinking, behavior, and emotional responses. In this approach, the therapist takes a more assertive role in listing the client's assumptions about life and his experience and also the individual client can work collaboratively with the therapist to develop skills for testing and modifying beliefs, identifying distorted thinking, relating to others in different ways, and changing behaviors. This method can be applicable in cases of depression, academic achievement, anxiety disorders, addictions and schizophrenia etc. by expressing their feelings.

Social Empowerment

Social empowerment is a broad area of practice drawing upon social work and community development principles. Social empowerment is typically implemented at the four following levels: (1) the individual level—where the person values him/herself and actively wants to participate in life, (2) family level, (3) community level and (4) social policies level impacting local and national level actions to promote social equity and inclusion of all persons. Social empowerment is indispensable to achieving quality of life for people with disabilities. To implement this type of approach, it is necessary to enable clients to have some form of control in their environment so that they have a base from which to start the rehabilitation process. Therefore, clients need a place to which to meet others where he gets training, education, work opportunities and leisure pursuits by which they realize the values, dignity and meaning of life. Social empowerment helps the client to adjust in the society positively and it is most approachable method of social rehabilitation.

Pragmatic Approaches

Rehabilitation needs to be supported by tangible social services. UK has been centered around the work of psychiatric day-centers as focal point of spectrum of required services.

MODELS IN REHABILITATION

The prevailing wisdom about the causes of disability has changed in the last several decades. In the 1950s, impairment of a given severity was viewed as sufficient to result in disability in all circumstances which has been shown in **Figure 16.1**; in contrast, the absence of impairment of that severity was thought to be sufficient grounds to deny disability benefits. Thus, the American Medical Association's Committee on Medical Rating of Physical Impairments stated that 'competent evaluation of permanent impairment requires adequate and complete medical examination, accurate objective measure of function, and avoidance of subjective impressions and nonmedical factors, such as the patient's age, sex and occupation' (American Medical Association, Committee on Medical Rating of Physical Impairment, 1958).

By the mid-1970s, Nagi (1976) outlined a process by which a pathology (e.g., arthritis) gave rise to an impairment (e.g., a limited range of motion in a joint), which may then result in a limitation in function (e.g., an inability to type), which, finally, may result in a disability (inability to work as a secretary). While outlining a process that would seem to move inexorably from pathology to loss of a job, Nagi noted that correlations among impairments, functional limitations,

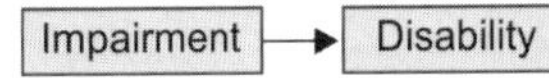

Fig. 16.1: Impairment only leads to disability.

and work loss were poor, and he speculated that the extent to which the environment accommodated limitations largely determined whether disability would result from the onset of a medical condition. In the interim, at least three others have developed models or modifications: the WHO (International Classification of Impairments, Disabilities and Handicaps, 1980), the IOM (*Disability in America,* 1991), and the NCMRR (1993). All of these models attempt to facilitate and improve understanding by describing the concepts and relationships among medical conditions, impairments, functional limitations, and the effects of the interaction of the person with the environment (i.e., handicap, disability, societal limitation) although each uses different nomenclatures for the components.

Nagi's model of disability: Nagi's model of disability explicitly brought the environment into the conceptualization. His model initiated a search for the factors in family, community, and society that affect disability as an outcome. With respect to disability in the work setting, for example, research has focused on the social and demographic characteristics of the individual and family, the individual's prior occupation and the industry in which the individual was previously employed, the flexibility of the workplace with respect to the physical tasks of work and hours of work, the nature of the local economy, customs and laws governing employment, and the extent of income transfer programs (Yelin, 1992).

Although the Nagi model included the environment, it was limited in how it conceived of the environment. In his model, the environment impinges on individuals only when activity limitation interacts with the demands placed on those individuals; the process that gives rise to disability is still inherently a function of the characteristics of medical conditions and attendant impairments **(Fig. 16.2)**.

IOM model: The IOM model was derived directly from Nagi, defining disability as 'a function of the interaction of the person with the environment' and beginning to describe certain subsets of environmental factors that could potentially affect the development of and movement within a disabling process. In this model, physical and social environmental risk factors (as well as biological and lifestyle risk factors) were described as independent variables that exist at all stages of the process. These factors affect progression within the model, and their control, therefore, affects (prevents) disability.

NCMRR model: The NCMRR model adds emphasis to the importance of environment by adding a category called societal limitations to account for restrictions that society places on individuals and that limit their ability to participate independently in tasks, activities, and roles. The unwillingness of employers to provide accommodations and the lack of ramps that deny access to public buildings to persons with disabilities are given as examples.

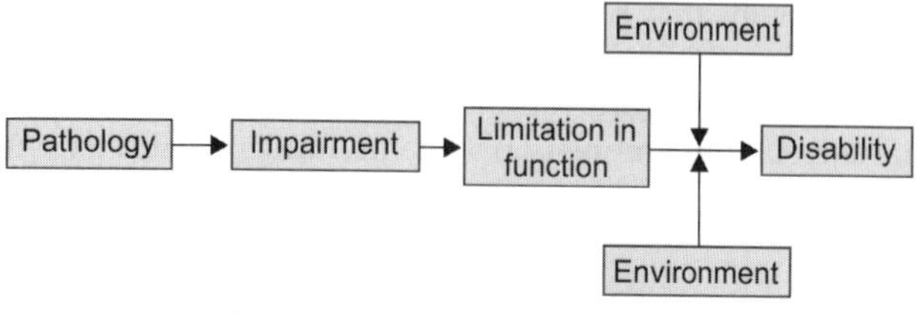

Fig. 16.2: Nagi's model of disability.

New Model for the Enabling-Disabling Process

A common understanding of such terms as injury, impairment, handicap, functional limitation, disabling conditions, and disability is essential to building effective, coherent programs in rehabilitation. As described above, several frameworks have been advanced to describe disability-related concepts, but none of these has been universally adopted. The lack of a uniformly accepted conceptual foundation is an obstacle for proper new set of models, based primarily on the previous IOM model (1991), designed to enhance the robustness of the previous models with respect to reversing the disabling process, i.e., rehabilitation. This section presents an overview of 'the enabling-disabling process explains its stages, and describes the nature of disability.

Overview of the Enabling-disabling Process

An overview of how disabling conditions affect a person's access to the environment is shown in **Figure 16.3**. Access to the environment, depicted as a square, represents both physical space and social structures (family, community, society). The person's degree of physical access to and social integration into the generalized environment is shown as degree of overlap of the symbolic person and the environmental square. (a) A person who does not manifest disability is fully integrated into the society and, therefore, has full access to both: (i) social opportunities (employment, education, parenthood, leadership roles, etc., and (ii) physical space (i.e., space access equivalent to persons without disabling conditions). (b) A person with potentially disabling conditions has increased needs (expressed by the size of the individual) and is dislocated from their prior integration into the environment.

(c) The rehabilitative process attempts to rectify this displacement, either by restoring function in the individual or (d) by expanding access to the environment (e.g., building ramps). The most effective rehabilitation programs include both. The model separates the two only to illustrate that disability is the interaction between the potentially disabling **(Fig. 16.4)**.

New IOM Model

Looking at the enabling-disabling process with more scrutiny requires greater detail in the model. To this end, this report adopts the IOM model (1991) and makes some modifications designed to both improve the model and to adapt it more towards rehabilitation. The original IOM model was conceived with prevention in mind, and the need for identifying risk factors whose control would

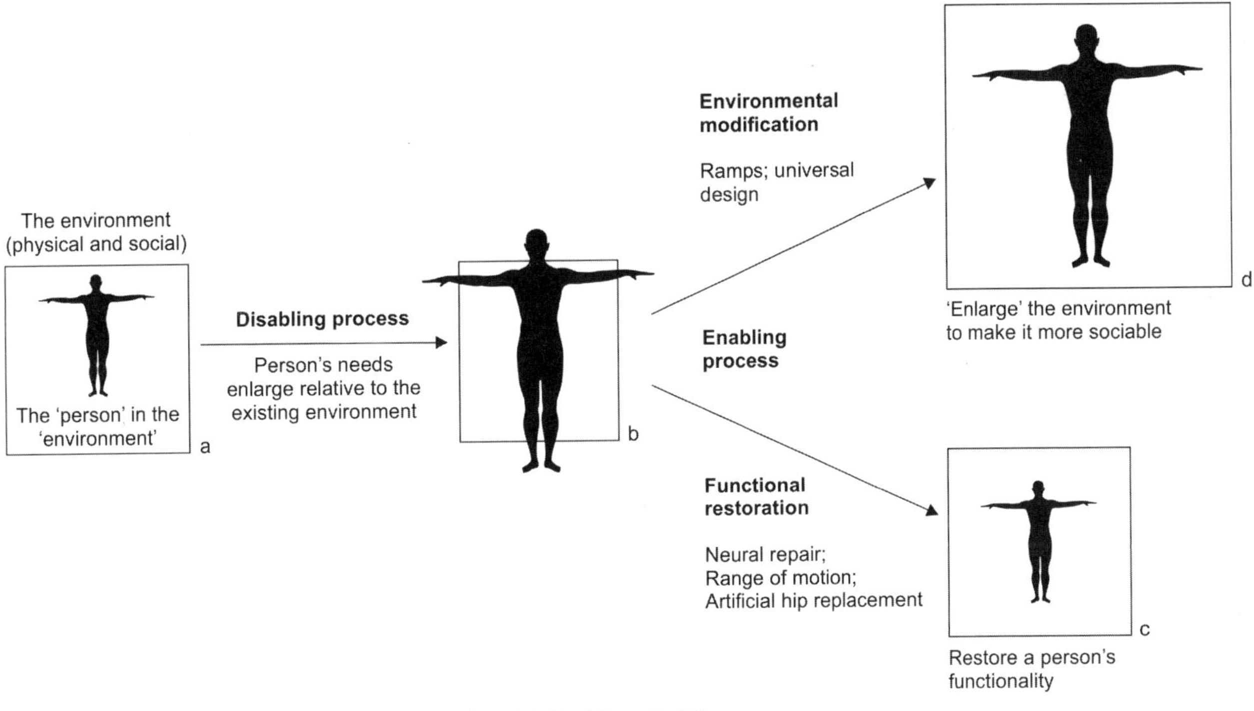

Fig. 16.3: Enabling-disabling process.

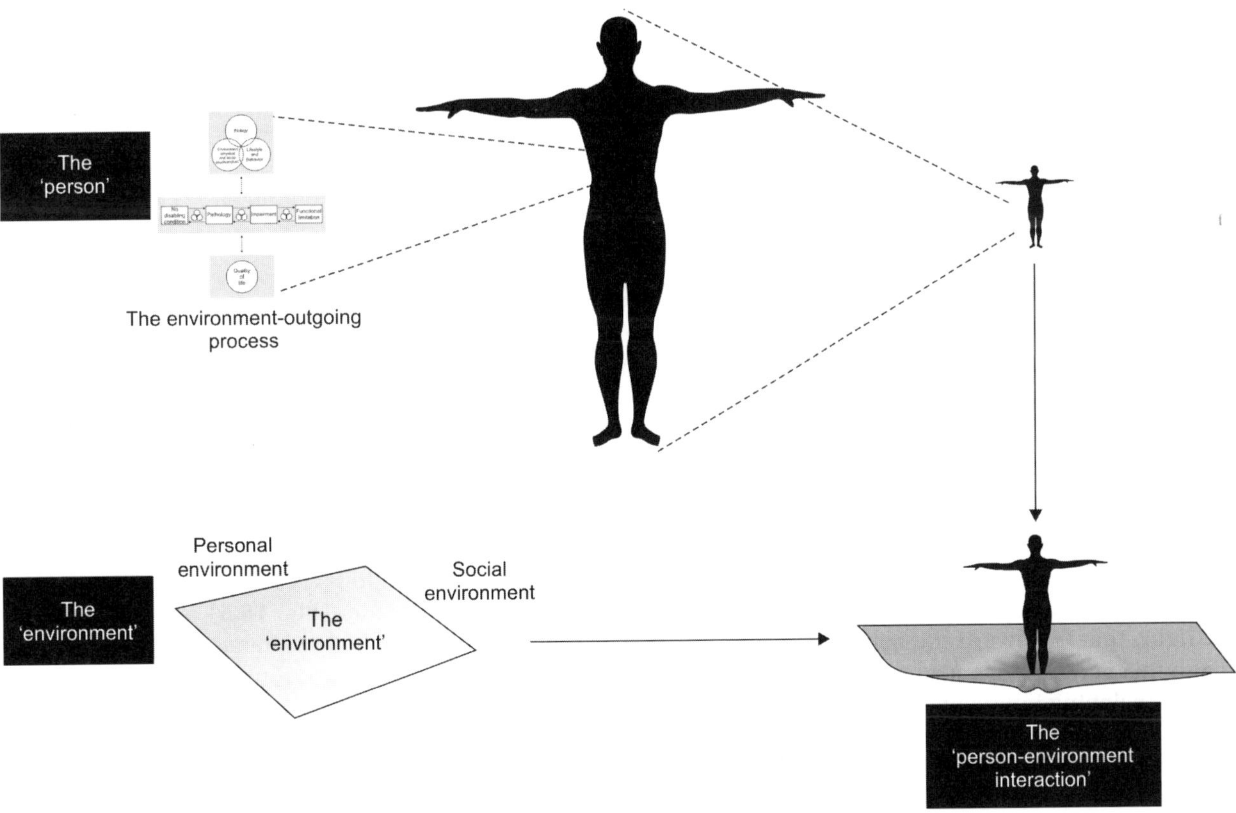

Fig. 16.4: The person-environment interaction.

facilitate the prevention of disability. The 1991 IOM model (IOM, 1991) established a new conceptual foundation in the field of disability in that it analyzed and described the components of the disabling process in such a way as to allow for the identification of potential points for preventive intervention. Identifying and describing the importance of the different types of risk factors that affect the disabling process as well as the interaction and integral nature

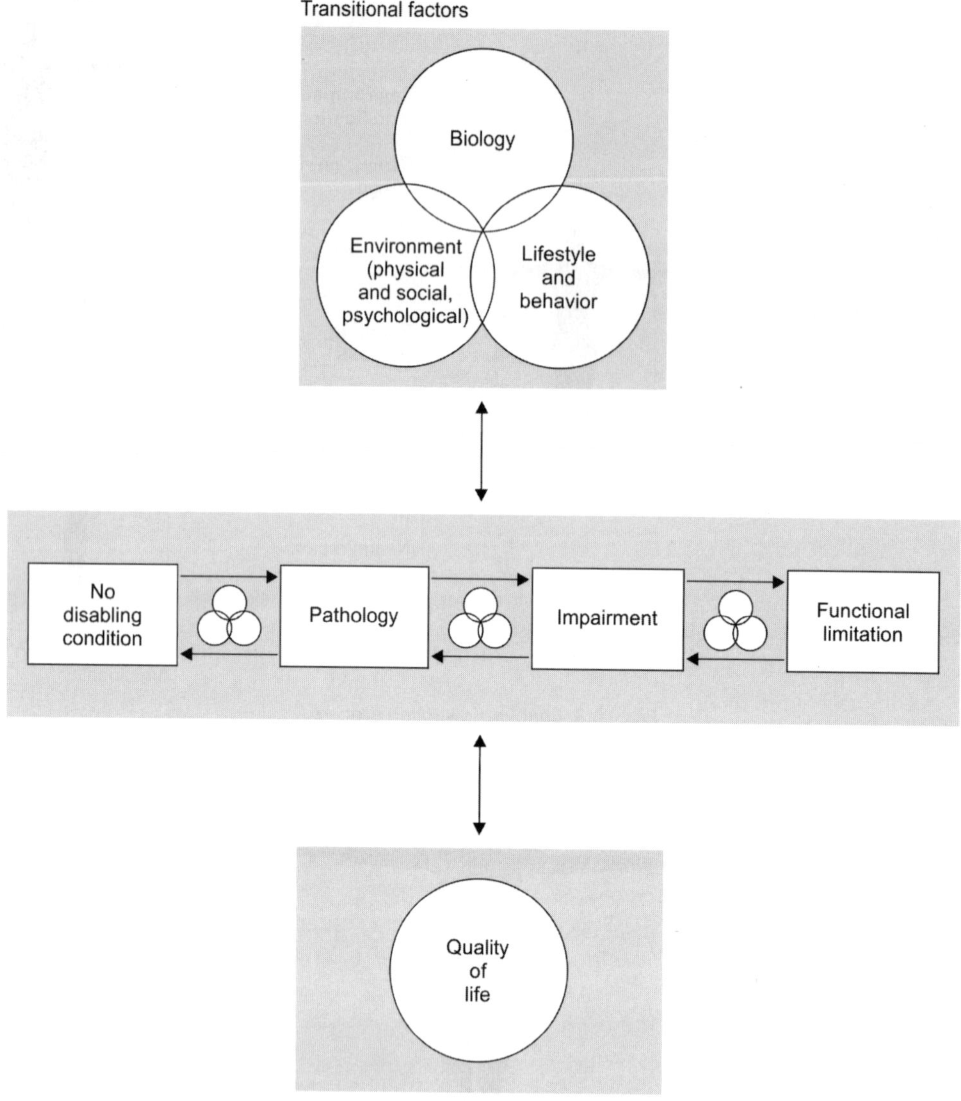

Fig. 16.5: New IOM model.

of quality of life were fundamental contributions to the emerging field of disability prevention. Over time, however, some shortcomings in the 1991 IOM model have emerged, including the implication that the disabling process is unidirectional, progressing inexorably toward disability without the possibility of reversal. The unidirectionality was implied by the arrows in the model that pointed only to the right, that is, toward the condition of disability. Although this may have been a result of that committee's focus on developing interventions to prevent progression in the disabling process rather than reversal, that is, rehabilitation, it is a shortcoming in the original model that needs correction and clarification, especially in the context of rehabilitation.

A second apparent shortcoming in the 1991 IOM model is its limited characterization of the environment and the interaction of the individual with the environment. Although the importance of the environment is discussed in the text in some detail, it is not clearly represented in the model except as a category of risk factors involved in the transition between the various categories of the disabling process.

The third apparent shortcoming in the 1991 IOM model that the committee identified as needing improvement is the representation of societal limitation. Some enhancements to the original model address these shortcomings.

The new IOM model **(Fig. 16.5)** is designed to show disability more clearly as the interaction of the person with the environment.

Person

Arrows pointing left were added to represent the potential effects of rehabilitation and the 'enabling process' (risk factors and enabling factors are now combined into 'transitional factors'). In addition, the new model includes the designation 'no disabling conditions' to indicate that there is a beginning and an end to the disabling process when a pathology impairment, functional limitation, or disability does not exist.

Environment

The 'environment', including the physical, social, and psychological components of the environment, and is represented as a three-dimensional mat that supports and interacts with the person and the disabling process, serving to highlight the importance of the person-environment interaction.

Disability

Disability means lack of ability to perform any activity. It is the end result of disabling process when there is functional limitation

Transitional Factors

In the new model, the committee defines the converse of risk factor as 'enabling factor'. Risk factors are phenomena that are associated with an increase in the likelihood that an individual will move from left to right in the new model, that is, from no disabling condition toward functional limitation. In contrast, enabling factors are phenomena that are associated with an increase in the likelihood that an individual will move from right to left in the new model, that is, toward less limitation.

The general types of enabling factors are the same as the general types of risk factors, that is, environmental (social, psychological, and physical) along with lifestyle and behavioral. So, for example, access to appropriate care and assistive technology would be an enabling factor (social environment), but lack of access would be a risk factor, or a disabling factor; curb cuts and universal design would be enabling factors (physical environment), but a lack of these would be disabling factors; the age of the person is a biological factor that can be either enabling or disabling; and compliance with pharmaceutical prescription regimens would be enabling, whereas drug abuse would be a disabling (behavioral and lifestyle) factor.

Thus, since both disabling and enabling factors affect transitions between the stages of the model, the committee groups them together as 'transitional factors'.

Environment

The environment is represented as a flexible three-dimensional mat in the new model. The strength and resilience of this mat are proportional to the quantity and quality of accessible support systems and the existence of various barriers. Stronger mats equate with more supportive environment, for example, access to appropriate health care, the availability of assistive technology and social support networks, and receptive cultures. Weaker mats equate with nonsupportive environments. For example, physical barriers, discrimination, lack of accessible and affordable assistive technology, and lack of appropriate healthcare result in greater displacement of the mat and, therefore, cause greater disability.

Thus, a person with a given level of impairment or functional limitation (i.e., potential disability) will experience greater disability (more displacement of the mat) in a less supportive environment than he or she would experience in a more supportive environment (indicated by a stronger mat and less resulting displacement) **(Fig. 16.6)**. The amount of disability is proportional to the amount of displacement in the mat that represents the environment. The environment is represented as having two general categories—the social-psychological and the physical.

Examples of the types of things that might be included in each category include:

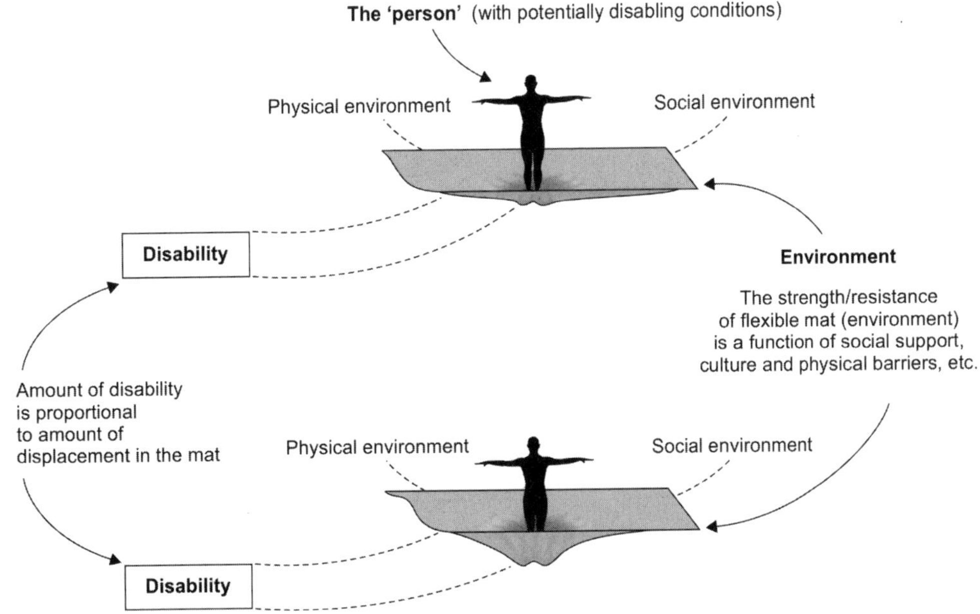

Fig. 16.6: Disability as displacement of the environment mat.

Theoretical Quantification and Mathematical Model of Disability

As a relational concept, disability lends itself to mathematical modeling. At present, this can be done only on a conceptual basis, since quantification of the variables is not yet reliable and reproducible. Nonetheless, a mathematical model is useful in further clarifying the relationship that exists between the person and the environment and how they interact to create disability **(Table 16.1)**.

Beginning with the variables of pathology (*P*), impairment (*I*), and functional limitation (*FL*), the first assumption is that the sum of these variables represents a quantity known as an individual's potential disability, or *PD*: $P + I + FL = PD$. Potential disability is referred to as 'potential' because it is only the interaction of potential disability with the environment that creates true disability. In addition, some (or all) of these variables may be equal to zero. If all are equal to zero, then there is no potential disability.

Environment (*E*) is the denominator in the mathematical model because it is the influence of the environment that creates disability from any given potential. The environment is the variable factor against which the other factors, are measured and that determines the existence of disability. Without environmental factors, there would be no disability. Thus, disability (*D*) can be represented mathematically as the relationship of potential disability (*PD, or* $P + I + FL$) to environment (*E*): $(P + I + FL)/E = D$ *or* $PD/E = D$.

Take the following example. If the range of *PD* (i.e., the sum of $P + I + FL$) is 0 to 10 (where 10 is the maximum potential for experiencing disability) and the range of E is 0.1 to 10 (where 1.0 is a neutral environment, 10 is a very accessible and supportive environment, and 0.1 is a very inaccessible and nonsupportive environment), then the resultant quantity of *D* would range from 0 to 100 (where 100 is maximum disability).

So, for example, if PD were 5 and the environment were a very 'good' one (e.g., $E = 10$), then the level of disability would be 0.5. However, with the same PD (i.e., $PD = 5$) but a less supportive environment (e.g., $E = 1$), then the level of disability would increase from 0.5 to 5. (When *E* is equal to 1, the effect of the environment is neutral and *PD* is equal to *D*).

Mathematically, to allow the environment to exert a truly negative effect in the model, the range of quantities for the denominator (i.e., the environment) should be less than 1.0 but greater than zero; thus, the range would be from 0.1 to 10. Using the example above, if *E* is equal to 0.5 instead of 1, then the level of disability would increase from 5 to 10. If the environment was at its worst (i.e., $E = 0.1$), then the amount of disability would increase to 50 in this example.

Patterns and Facilities for Continuing Rehabilitative Care

Ambulatory Care

The term 'ambulatory care' is used interchangeably with the term 'outpatient care'. Increased use of outpatient emergency service has replaced the family physician in large cities.

Home Care

Well-to-do persons rarely think of going into a hospital. They receive services of a private physician in their own home. The family is responsible for the day-to-day care. Patients who do not require around-the-clock services of a hospital and yet may be too ill to go to outpatient department and can often be taken care at home.

Home Health Aid Services

Home health aid services developed with the increased use of home care plans and particularly after Medicare plans came into existence. Home health aids are being trained in many states and are aligned to home care through a control office that coordinates plan of care often in collaboration with community health nursing agencies.

Table 16.1: Estimating the effects of the environment on disability.

Functional capacity (Qualitative)	*Potential disability (Qualitative)*	*Potential disability (Range: 1–10)*	*Environmental support (Range: 0.1–10)*	*Disability score (Range: 0.1–100)*
High	Low	1	10 (good)	0.1
		1	1 (neutral)	1
		1	0.5 (bad)	2
		1	0.1 (worst)	10
Moderate	Moderate	5	10 (good)	0.5
		5	1 (neutral)	5
		5	0.5 (bad)	10
		5	0.1 (worst)	50
Low	High	10	10 (good)	1
		10	1 (neutral)	10
		10	0.5 (bad)	20
		10	0.1 (worst)	100

Home-maker Services

Also it developed with the increased use of home care plans welfare agency that employs personnel to furnish home-maker service to families with children and to the person who is convalescing, aged or acutely or chronically ill.

Institutional Resources

Many patients and families have to resort to institutional care for the patient because their own facilities are not suitable, nor member of the family can be in attendance during the day, or the kind of care needed by the patient requires close professional supervision.

Foster Homes

Carefully selected families volunteer to take chronically ill persons into their own homes and provide the nonprofessional care that is needed plan is for patients who have no family and who cannot live alone.

REHABILITATION COUNCIL OF INDIA

The Rehabilitation Council of India (RCI) is the apex government body set up under an Act of Parliament to regulate training programs and courses targeted at disabled, disadvantaged, and special education requirement communities. It is the only statutory council in India that is required to maintain the Central Rehabilitation Register which mainly documents details of all qualified professionals who operate and deliver training and educational programs for the targeted communities enacted by Parliament and it became a Statutory Body on 22 June, 1993. The Act was amended by Parliament in 2000 to make it more broadbased. The mandate given to RCI is to regulate and monitor services given to persons with disability, to standardize syllabi and to maintain a Central Rehabilitation Register of all qualified professionals and personnel working in the field of Rehabilitation and Special Education. The Act also prescribes punitive action against unqualified persons delivering services to persons with disability. The amendment brought definitions and discussions provided within the earlier Rehabilitation Council of India Act, 1992, under the ambit of a larger Act, namely Persons with Disabilities (Equal Opportunities, Protection of Rights and Full Participation) Act, 1995.

Objectives of Rehabilitation Council of India

- To regulate the training policies and programs in the field of rehabilitation of persons with disabilities
- To bring about standardization of training courses for professionals dealing with persons with disabilities
- To prescribe minimum standards of education and training of various categories of professionals/personnel dealing with people with disabilities
- To regulate these standards in all training institutions uniformly throughout the country
- To recognize institutions/organizations/universities running masters degree/bachelors degree/PG Diploma/Diploma/Certificate courses in the field of rehabilitation of persons with disabilities
- To recognize degree/diploma/certificate awarded by foreign universities/institutions on reciprocal basis
- To promote research in Rehabilitation and Special Education
- To maintain Central Rehabilitation Register for registration of professionals/personnel
- To collect information on a regular basis on education and training in the field of rehabilitation of people with disabilities from institutions in India and abroad
- To encourage continuing education in the field of rehabilitation and special education by way of collaboration with organizations working in the field of disability
- To recognize Vocational Rehabilitation Centers as manpower development centers
- To register vocational instructors and other personnel working in the Vocational Rehabilitation Centers
- To recognize the national institutes and apex institutions on disability as manpower development centers
- To register personnel working in national institutes and apex institutions on disability under the Ministry of Social Justice and Empowerment.

Specific Role of the Rehabilitation Council of India

The Rehabilitation Council of India's specific role is to develop, standardize and regulate training programs/courses at various levels in the field of Rehabilitation and Special Education. It also maintains the Central Rehabilitation Register for qualified Professionals/Personnel in the area of Rehabilitation and Special Education and promotes Research in Special Education.

As per provisions of RCI Act, prior approval of RCI is a must for all universities/institutions/organizations—government and non-government, etc., to start any training course in the field of Rehabilitation and Special Education. Prescribed norms for each training program have to be fulfilled to be eligible to run a course are as follows:

- To obtain approval of Rehabilitation Council of India/Government of India, the organization/institute/center/university desirous of starting the Masters Degree/Degree/PG Diploma/Diploma/Certificate course should approach RCI through the respective State Government/Union Territory to assess the infrastructural facilities before starting the course.
- The competent authority of State Government/Union Territory Administration must indicate in clear terms whether they are or not in favor of starting a college or institution managed by a nongovernmental organization.
- The institute should adopt the standards of staff, space and equipment, etc., as recommended by the Rehabilitation Council of India and give an undertaking for their phased implementation within the stipulated period.
- The institute must submit in writing the willingness of University/Board who can grant affiliation, if the

Rehabilitation Council of India permits the Masters Degree/Degree/PG Diploma/Diploma course to be started.
- The institute must satisfy Rehabilitation Council of India about possessing enough training facilities to undertake the Masters Degree/Degree/PG Diploma/Diploma course.
- The management must provide adequate facilities to administrative and teaching staff required for Masters Degree/Degree/PG Diploma/Diploma courses as per the recommendation of the Council.
- The management of the institute must submit a plan for the construction of full-fledged division and appoint competent personnel to man the same.

16 categories of professionals/personnel have been covered under the RCI Act as given below:
- Audiologists and speech therapists
- Clinical psychologists
- Hearing and ear-mould technicians
- Rehabilitation engineers and technicians
- Special teachers for educating and training the handicapped
- Vocational counselors, employment officers and placement officers
- Multipurpose rehabilitation therapists, technicians
- Speech pathologists
- Rehabilitation psychologists
- Rehabilitation social workers
- Rehabilitation practitioners in mental retardation
- Orientation and mobility specialists
- Community-based rehabilitation professionals
- Rehabilitation counsellors, administrators
- Prosthetists and orthotists
- Rehabilitation workshop managers.

However, professionals like physiotherapists and occupational therapists are not covered under the RCI Act. RCI trains master trainers, rehabilitation professionals and personnel for creating better service delivery facilities for the persons with disability. However, it does not offer any direct benefit, financial or material help to the persons with disability. RCI does not provide any help to the persons with disabilities for their employment. Nor does it perform any intermediary role between various organizations offering employment to the disabled. The Council is also not responsible to maintain any employment register or coordination with various special employment exchanges. The RCI is facilitating a National Bridge Course through a network of selected institutions (list given on RCI website) for persons not possessing any recognized rehabilitation qualification who have been working in the field of disability and rehabilitation of the disabled before June 1993, i.e., before the RCI came into existence. Such persons must be 10th pass or above in qualification and must produce conclusive proof of working in the field of disability and rehabilitation of the disabled prior to June 1993, in order to be trained under the Bridge Course. All persons trained under the Bridge Course are registered by the Council as Rehabilitation Personnel. The RCI has launched a National Programme on Orientation of Medical Officers Working in Primary Health Centers since July 1999. This has been done with the prime objective of creating awareness and sensitization in the rural areas for creating better service facilities in the much-neglected rural areas of the country. So far, around 8000 medical officers have been trained under this program and 21,000 more are to be trained in the next one year.

Rehabilitation Services in India

A large number of Government departments, NGOs, institutions, voluntary agencies are functioning for disabled/handicapped for their rehabilitation and care. Some of them are enlisted here:
- Ministry of Social Justice and Empowerment.
- Ministry of Health and Family Welfare, Human Resource Development, Labour, Information and Broadcasting.
- Regional and District Rehabilitation Centers.
- Rehabilitation Council of India.
- Occupational Therapy School (Mumbai, Nagpur, etc.)
- All India Institute of Physical Medicine and Rehabilitation (Mumbai, CMC Vellore).
- Occupational Therapy College, Mumbai.
- National Institute of Mentally Handicapped (NIMH) Secunderabad (Regional branches at Mumbai, New Delhi, Kolkata).
- Ali Yavar Jung National Institute for the Hearing Handicapped, Mumbai (Regional branches at Delhi, Kolkata, Secunderabad).
- National Institute for Visually Handicapped, Dehradun.
- National Institute for the Orthopaedically Handicapped, Kolkata, etc.

COMMUNITY-BASED REHABILITATION (CBR)

It is a strategy within general community development for the rehabilitation, equalization of opportunities and social inclusion of all people with disabilities. The primary objective of CBR is the improvement of the quality of life of people with disability/marginalized persons. Key principles relating to CBR are equality, social justice, solidarity, integration and dignity. CBR is not an approach that only focuses on the physical or medical needs of a person or delivering care to disabled people as passive recipients. It is not outreach from a center. It is not determined by the needs of an institution or groups of professionals, neither it is segregated and separate from services for other people.

Institutional rehabilitation provides excellent services to address the problems of individual disabled persons and is often available only for a small number at a very high cost. Moreover, the endeavor in an institution is often out of context to the felt needs of the disabled person, and thus falls short of their expectations. In an institutional rehabilitation program, the community is not linked with the process. Hence, when the disabled person returns home, it may become difficult for them to integrate into their community.

Disability often requires life-long management. Therefore, activities aimed at enabling people with disability should be community-based as much as possible. Sustainability is the ability of project or program to continue to address needs as long as needs exist. The most basic rehabilitation activities can be carried out in the person's own community. A multisectoral/multidisciplinary concept of CBR is to be adopted. This concept emphasizes working with and through the community in response to this conceptual change.

CBR is a systematized approach within general community development, whereby persons with disabilities are enabled to live a fulfilling life within their own community, making maximum use of local resources and helping the community become aware of its responsibility in ensuring the inclusion and equal participation of PWDs. In the process, PWDs are also made aware of their own role and responsibility, as they are part of the community.

CBR is now defined as a community development program that has seven different components:

- Creation of a positive attitude towards people with disabilities
- Provision of rehabilitation services
- Provision of education and training opportunities
- Creation of micro and macro income-generation opportunities
- Provision of long-term care facilities
- Prevention of causes of disabilities
- Monitoring and evaluation.

Principles of CBR

Inclusion

Community-based rehabilitation works to remove all kinds of barriers which block people with disabilities from access to the mainstream of society. Inclusion means placing disability issues and people with disabilities in the mainstream of activities.

Participation

Participation focuses on abilities, not disabilities. It depends on the participation and support of people with disability, family members and local communities. It also means the involvement of people with disabilities as active contributors to the CBR program, from policy-making to implementation and evaluation, for the simple reason that they know what their needs are.

Empowerment of Local People

Empowerment of local people is important for starting any Community Development Program. Local people specifically people with disabilities and their families, should make the program decisions and control the resources. This requires people with disability taking leadership roles within programs. The CBR workers, service providers and facilitators include people with disabilities in planning and organizing the program.

Equity

Principle equity means equality of opportunities and rights. Community-based rehabilitation emphasizes equality of opportunities and rights for all without discrimination. The service will be equally shared among all.

Raising Awareness

Raising awareness about CBR addresses attitudes and behavior within the community, developing understanding and support for people with disabilities and ensuring sustainable benefits. It also promotes the need for and benefit of inclusion of disability in all developmental initiatives.

Primary Health Care and Rehabilitation

Health is defined as a state of complete physical, mental and social well-being and not merely the absence of disease or infirmity. Primary health care is essential health care based on practical scientifically sound and socially acceptable methods and technology made universally accessible to individuals and families in the community through their full participation and at a cost that the community and country can afford to maintain at every stage of their development in the spirit of self-reliance and self-determination. It forms an integral part both of the country's health system, of which it is the central function and main focus, and of all the overall social and economic development of the community. It is the first level of contact of individuals, the family and the community with the national health system bringing health care as close as possible to where people live and work, and constitutes the first element of a continuing healthcare process. Community-based rehabilitation is fully consonant with the concept of Primary Health Care. This approach promotes awareness, self-reliance and responsibility for rehabilitation within the community. It builds on manpower resources in the community, including the disabled themselves, their families and other community members. CBR encourages the use of simple methods and techniques that are acceptable, affordable, effective and appropriate to the local setting.

ROLE AND FUNCTIONS OF A COMMUNITY HEALTH NURSE IN REHABILITATION

Rehabilitative nursing is not a specialty limited to the particular agencies or settings. It is a vital part of nursing in the patient's home, the hospital emergency room, nursing home, clinic and all healthcare settings. The nurse may stimulate development of motivation through an attitude of respect for the patient and confidence in his or her ability to return to his highest level of independence possible. Helping the family to help themselves is an integral part of nursing care.

In any type of disease or condition like cancer arthritis, mental illness stroke, spinal cord injury or a burn, it is the role of a nurse to apply the appropriate technique to provide care during rehabilitation period. The nurse can play different role when providing care in different setting which have been described bellow.

Home Care

The home care rehabilitation nurse acts as an advocate for clients and their families during the re-entry process from the hospital into the home and the community. The home care rehabilitation nurse coordinates the services provided by the interdisciplinary team and enacts the plan of care that has been developed by the client, the physician, and the rehabilitation team. In this role, the home care rehabilitation nurse functions as a clinical resource, a care coordinator, an advocate, a primary care provider, a teacher, a consultant, and a team member. The home care nurse, using rehabilitation expertise, develops an individualized program for the client and the client's family or caregiver. The rehabilitation nurse in the home setting provides client-driven care as part of a continuum between other healthcare settings and the client's home. The goals are to implement the client's self-management skills in the home-setting and to restore the client's relationships with family members and others in the community. The Association of Rehabilitation Nurses believes that the role of the rehabilitation nurse in the home care setting is an essential one in the continuum of care. The value of the rehabilitation nurse can be demonstrated by improved cost-effectiveness of client care, specialized rehabilitation nursing clinical knowledge and skill, reduction in the frequency of complications experienced by rehabilitation clients, increased quality of nursing care, and reduced costs because of the presence of a resident expert to provide consultation services.

Rehabilitation nursing in home care is highly specialized. However, rehabilitation nurses in this setting serve a diverse population. Infants, children, adolescents, young adults, middle-aged adults, and older adults with disabling conditions may receive specialized home care nursing support from rehabilitation nurses in settings that include alternative living situations and their own home. The nurse plays different roles in rehabilitation center.

Practitioner

- Serves as a clinical resource for those involved in rehabilitation nursing practice
- Serves as a clinical resource in the care of clients with a complex chronic illness, disabling condition, or both
- Acts as a resource during a crisis that is aggravated by a chronic illness or a disabling condition
- Assesses the appropriateness of a client's admission to, and the delivery of rehabilitation services in, the home environment
- Provides assistance with discharge planning to ensure a smooth transition into the community or, when appropriate, to help clients who are hiring private attendants
- Collaborates with the interdisciplinary team in the management of the team function in the home environment; is responsible for ensuring that the client is involved as a significant member of the team
- Helps the client and the client's family adapt to changes in lifestyle necessitated by the disabling condition
- Implements rehabilitation nursing care based on scientific knowledge, home care standards, and rehabilitation principles that are appropriate to the home care environment.

Care Coordinator

- Acts as a member of the interdisciplinary health care team and promotes the coordination of client care
- Coordinates the activities of rehabilitation professionals; integrates the knowledge and skills of various rehabilitation disciplines into a comprehensive continuum of care
- Facilitates the design and implementation of the plan of care for clients who are chronically ill or who have disabling conditions.

Advocate

- Advocates for clients and their families or caregivers
- Teaches clients and their families or caregivers to advocate for themselves
- Facilitates the client's transition from the hospital to the home and the community
- Furthers an understanding of home care-based rehabilitation issues among people in the community and among those in government who are in a position to deal with issues related to this patient population.

Educator

- Provides education for clients and their families
- Provides staff orientation and guides staff development, both at the professional and the paraprofessional levels, in the area of rehabilitation home care
- Provides rehabilitation-focused continuing education programs
- Develops policies and procedures that are specific to rehabilitation home care
- Develops educational materials designed to help clients and their family members become knowledgeable consumers in the healthcare arena.

Consultant

- Identifies clients and families who could benefit from rehabilitation home care services
- Provides case management expertise within the home care environment
- Serves as a liaison with third-party payers and justifies the use of funds for rehabilitation home care
- Serves as a resource for rehabilitation nurses and as a process consultant to staff in the home care setting
- Promotes rehabilitation nursing services to community health professionals and to the community at large.

Researcher

- Participates in research involving home care clients and their families

- Participates in the analysis and dissemination of evaluative data that may have an impact on clients and their families
- Incorporates evaluative data into nursing practice.

Functions of the Home Care Rehabilitation Nurse

The home care rehabilitation nurse uses the principles of rehabilitation nursing as defined within the established scope of rehabilitation nursing practice and standards developed by the Association of Rehabilitation Nurses and the American Nurses Association. The functions of the home care rehabilitation nurse can be divided into several categories, which are outlined below.

Assessment

- Reviews and analyzes referral information in consultation with the client, as well as with the client's rehabilitation team members, employers, the family's legal representative, and claims or insurance personnel, as appropriate
- Assesses the client's current personal and functional health status, diagnosis, prognosis, and treatment plan, as well as the caregiver's level of expertise
- Identifies the client's learning needs, vocational rehabilitation requirements, and potential related to his or her functional impairment, medical diagnosis and prognosis, treatment providers, treatment options, financial resources, psychosocial adjustment, and coping mechanisms.

Data Analysis and Formulation of a Nursing Diagnosis

- Identifies temporary or permanent alterations in function that have resulted from the client's injury or illness
- Identifies potential challenges or complications in the client's physiological and/or psychosocial functioning that may have an impact on the client's successful functioning in the home or community
- Identifies potential difficulties that the client may have in being reintegrated into the community
- Identifies the learning needs of the client and the client's family related to successful reintegration into the home or the community.

Establishment of Goals and Plan of Care

- Works with the client to establish realistic goals for achieving optimal outcomes by collaborating with the client and the client's family and by using available resources
- Helps the client and the client's family identify the variables that can influence the achievement of goals
- Develops a comprehensive plan that includes treatment measures to prevent disability; identifies alternatives for the client's treatments when appropriate
- Establishes target dates for achieving goals
- Integrates rehabilitation goals consistent with the realities of the client's family system and home environment.

Implementation

- Uses rehabilitation principles to promote optimal outcomes for the client
- Provides ongoing assessment of the client, the family, and other caregivers
- Coordinates access to accelerated care options, alternative care options, or both, when appropriate
- Coordinates the client's access to appropriate government and community programs and resources
- Coordinates and evaluates in a quality-conscious, cost-effective manner the client's and the family's use of medical equipment, supplies, medications, and other available services
- Provides instruction, based on identified learning needs, to the client and the client's family
- Coordinates referrals for instruction or counseling that are agreeable to the client and the client's family and that are based on identified learning needs
- Intervenes promptly, when necessary, to promote optimal functioning and to prevent complications
- Facilitates and collaborates with the healthcare team and the client for timely discharge planning from the hospital to an alternative level of care, when appropriate
- Coordinates the discharge plan with the client, the healthcare team, and the client's care providers.

Collaboration

- Collaborates with the healthcare team, payers, community agencies, providers, and legal representatives to ensure the client's care throughout the healthcare continuum
- Promotes effective communication between the client, the client's family, and payers
- Participates in team meetings when appropriate
- Incorporates the interdisciplinary team's recommendations and services into the plan of care.

Roles and Functions of the Nurse at Rehabilitation Center

Teacher

- Shares information about the disease processes underlying disabilities and teaches nursing techniques to help clients and their families develop the self-care skills necessary to move toward wellness on the illness-wellness continuum
- Prepares clients and their families for future self-management and decision-making responsibilities by fostering clients' independence and goal achievement
- Reinforces the teaching done by specialists in rehabilitation and other healthcare disciplines and provides resource materials for clients' changing needs
- Provides in-service education for healthcare team members and members of the community regarding the prevention of disabilities.

Caregiver

- Assesses the physical, psychological, sociocultural, and spiritual dimensions of clients and their families, as well as their educational and discharge needs in order to formulate nursing diagnoses
- Plans nursing care while acknowledging that rehabilitation nursing is practiced within a dynamic, therapeutic, and supportive relationship that is constantly changing, as nurses and clients influence one another
- Implements a plan of care by providing nursing care and education directly or through ancillary personnel, as needed, to maintain and restore function and prevent complications and further loss
- Evaluates the nursing care that is being provided and modifies the plan, as needed, to achieve measurable goals and objectives.

Collaborator

- Develops goals, in collaboration with clients, their families, and the rehabilitation team, that are oriented to wellness behavior and are reality-based and that encourage socialization with others
- Participates in the interdisciplinary team process at team conferences and other team meetings and offers input into team decision-making
- Intervenes with team members and other healthcare professionals to ensure that the optimal opportunity for recovery is made available to the client, the most significant member of the rehabilitation team
- Collaborates with team members to achieve cost-effective care by utilizing appropriate clinical measures to meet emergent physical, psychosocial, and spiritual situations.

Client Advocate

- Actively listens, reflects, and guides clients and their families through the stages of the grieving process to mourn the loss of abilities and roles
- Advocates for policies and services that promote the quality of life for individuals with disabilities and participates in activities that will positively influence the community's awareness of disabilities
- Contributes to a safe and therapeutic environment and supports activities that promote the clients' return of function and prevent complications or chronic illness
- Intervenes on behalf of clients to ensure that medical professionals and nonmedical professionals work to maximize clients' success when they return to work or school.

CHAPTER 17

International Health

INTRODUCTION

Health and disease have no geographical or political boundaries. The global community does not only face the problems of known diseases. New diseases can also crop up, with the rapid movement of people and goods around the world and spread very quickly as well. Disease in one part of the world can constant threat to other parts. Disease like plague, cholera spread through trade routes from one to another nation and disease like SARS (COVID-19), Tuberculosis and HIV/AIDS increases the global burden disease.

Disease has economic and social effects that are almost impossible to calculate. Treatment and care for those who are ill places huge burdens on families and communities. It prevents in developing a healthy community and leads to poverty. The prevention and treatment of these diseases should be among the highest priorities of governments of the whole world and the whole world needs to focus on fighting this problem. Global health is the health of the populations in the worldwide context. It has been defined as "the area of study, research and practice that places a priority on improving health and achieving equity in health for all people worldwide. It is about worldwide health improvement (including mental health), reduction of disparities, and protection against global threats that disregard national borders. The global burden of disease is the collective disease burden produced by all diseases around the world. The year 2020 was a devastating year for global health. A previously unknown virus raced around the world, rapidly emerging as one of its top killers, laying bare the inadequacies of health systems. Health services in whole world have struggled to tackle COVID-19, and provide people with vital care. Till 2022, countries around the world continue battle COVID-19 and even vaccines have developed in 2020, India began administration of COVID-19 vaccines on 16 January 2021. The global burden of disease (GBD) was assessed through Global Burden of Disease Study which is a comprehensive regional and global assessment of mortality and disability from major diseases, injuries, and risk factors. It is generally done by the collaborative effort of world health organization, Harvard School of Public Health, the Institute for Health Metrics and Evaluation (IHME), and the World Bank. The GBD project was work out in 1992.

ABOUT GLOBAL BURDEN OF DISEASE PROJECT

The GBD project was commissioned in year 1990 but work out in 1992 and is a collaborative effort between hundreds of experts worldwide, including researchers at the World Health Organization (WHO), Harvard School of Public Health, the Institute for Health Metrics and Evaluation (IHME), and the World Bank. The original project estimated health gaps using disability-adjusted life years (DALYs) for eight regions of the world in 1990. It provided a standardized approach to epidemiological assessment and uses a standard unit, the disability-adjusted life year (DALY), to aid comparisons.

The first GBD 1990 study quantified the health effects of more than 100 diseases and injuries for eight regions of the world in 1990. It generated comprehensive and internally consistent estimates of mortality and morbidity by age, sex and region. The study also introduced a new metric—the disability-adjusted life-year (DALY)—as a single measure to quantify the burden of diseases, injuries and risk factors. The DALY is based on years of life lost from premature death and years of life lived in less than full health. This study was updated for the year 2000–2002 and included a more extensive analysis of the mortality and burden of disease attributable to 26 global risk factors using a consistent analytic framework known as Comparative Risk Factor Assessment (CRA). These estimates were most recently updated for the year 2004.

The Institute for Health Metrics and Evaluation and other academic partners have collaborated on a new GBD 2010, published on 14 December 2012, which provides regional estimates of deaths and DALYs (using a new method for calculation of DALYs) for the years 1990, 2005 and 2010. These estimates contributed to WHO global health estimates which were published in 2013.

The results from GBD 2010 show that 'Infectious diseases, maternal and child illness, and malnutrition now cause fewer deaths and less illness than they did twenty years ago. As a result, fewer children are dying every year, but more young and middle-aged adults are dying and suffering from disease and injury, as noncommunicable diseases (NCDs), such as cancer and heart disease, becoming the dominant causes of death.

Chronic diseases now account for the leading cause of adult deaths globally. It has been expected that by 2020, the number of deaths caused by NCDs in developing countries will equal the deaths caused by communicable diseases. Unfortunately, chronic disease is a neglected global health issue. Much of the developed world has undergone efforts at addressing this issue; however, the developing world still focuses a lot of their attention on infectious diseases. However, even TB, HIV and malaria combined only account for 10% of the deaths in the world.

In 2017, global adult mortality rates decreases plateaued, and, in some cases, mortality rates increased. Alarmingly, conflict and terrorism have become two of the fastest growing causes of death globally (increasing by 118% between 2007 and 2017). Alongside this alarming growth in violence, our era is characterized by epidemics such as opioid dependence, noncommunicable diseases, depression, and dengue fever. Opioid dependence has grown to an unprecedented scale, with 4 million new cases in 2017 and 110000 deaths. Noncommunicable diseases accounted for 73% of all global deaths in 2017, with over half of all deaths (28.8 million) attributable to just four risk factors: high blood pressure, smoking, high blood glucose, and high body-mass index. Obesity prevalence has risen in almost every country in the world—leading to more than a million deaths from type 2 diabetes, half a million deaths from diabetes-related chronic kidney disease, and 180000 deaths related to nonalcoholic steatohepatitis.

In 2017, depressive disorders were the third leading cause of years lived with disability after low back pain and headache disorders, and deaths from dengue fever, a disease often associated with struggling development and urbanization, increased substantially in most tropical and subtropical countries, rising from 24500 deaths globally in 2007 to 40500 in 2017. Sex-specific disaggregation of the data in GBD 2017 uncovers areas where the gendered aspects of health—too often overlooked—can be acted upon. For the first time in the history of the GBD, estimates of health worker density were included. These show that the global shortage and unequal distribution of health workers requires urgent attention in order not to undermine attainment of the Sustainable Development Goals (SDGs). Crucially, GBD 2017 estimates that no country is on track to meet all of WHO's health-related SDGs by 2030. Under-five mortality, neonatal mortality, maternal mortality, and malaria indicators had the most countries with at least 95% probability of success. However, for many other targets—including child malnutrition and violence reduction goals—no country in the world has attained the pace of change that is required for these goals to be met.

GBD 2017 is a reminder that, without vigilance and constant effort, progress can easily be reversed. But the GBD is also an encouragement to think differently in this time of crisis. By cataloguing inequalities in health-care delivery and patterns of disease geography, this iteration of the GBD presents an opportunity to move away from the generic application of UHC and towards a more tailored precision approach to UHC.

The Global Burden of Disease Study 2019 (GBD 2019), coordinated by the Institute for Health Metrics and Evaluation (IHME), estimated the burden of diseases, injuries, and risk factors for 204 countries and territories and selected subnational locations.

A GBD 2019 analysis also produced estimates for health workforce densities for 204 countries and territories from 1990–2019. Data used come from WHO's Global Health Observatory and cross-sectional surveys and censuses that sampled general working-age populations (defined as ages 15–69) in which respondents self-reported employment status and current occupation. Employment and occupation data were mapped to the International Standard Classification of Occupations (ISCO). This dataset includes annual estimates by location for health workforce densities per 10,000 employed individuals for 23 health worker cadres.

The largest declines in risk exposure from 2010 to 2019 were among a set of risks that are strongly linked to social and economic development, including household air pollution; unsafe water, sanitation, and handwashing; and child growth failure. Global declines also occurred for tobacco smoking and lead exposure. The largest increases in risk exposure were for ambient particulate matter pollution, drug use, high fasting plasma glucose, and high body-mass index. In 2019, the leading Level 2 risk factor globally for attributable deaths was high systolic blood pressure, which accounted for 10.8 million (95% uncertainty interval [UI] 9.51–12.1) deaths (19.2% [16.9–21.3] of all deaths in 2019), followed by tobacco (smoked, second-hand, and chewing), which accounted for 8.71 million (8.12–9.31) deaths (15.4% [14.6–16.2] of all deaths in 2019). The leading Level 2 risk factor for attributable DALYs globally in 2019 was child and maternal malnutrition, which largely affects health in the youngest age groups and accounted for 295 million (253–350) DALYs of all global DALYs that year).

COVID-19; SARS-CoV-2 is the major public health burden in the world from 2020 onwards. The morbidity and mortality of global community is dramatically increasing from time to time during 2020-21.

Aims

The GBD has three specific aims:

- To systematically incorporate information on nonfatal outcomes into the assessment of the health status (using a time-based measure of healthy years of life lost due either to premature mortality or to years lived with a disability, weighted by the severity of that disability).
- To ensure that all estimates and projections were derived on the basis of objective epidemiological and demographic methods, which were not influenced by advocates.
- To measure the burden of disease using a metric that could also be used to assess the cost-effectiveness of interventions. The metric chosen was the DALY.

DIFFERENT INDICATORS TO MEASURE GLOBAL HEALTH

There are different indicators to measure the global health are: disability-adjusted life year (DALY), quality-adjusted life years (QALYs), and mortality rate.

Disability-adjusted Life Year (DALY)

The DALY is a summary measure that combines the impact of illness disability and mortality by measuring the time lived with disability and the time lost due to premature mortality. One DALY can be thought of as one lost year of 'healthy' life. The DALY for a disease is the sum of the years of life lost due to premature mortality and the years lost due to disability for incident cases of the health condition.

Quality-adjusted Life Year (QALY)

QALYs combine expected survival with expected quality of life into a single number: if an additional year of healthy life is worth a value of one (year), then a year of less healthy life is worth less than one (year). QALY calculations are based on measurements of the value that individuals place on expected years of survival. Measurements can be made in several ways: by techniques that simulate gambles about preferences for alternative states of health, with surveys or analyses that infer willingness to pay for alternative states of health, or through instruments that are based on trading off some or all likely survival time that a medical intervention might provide in order to gain less survival time of higher quality.

Infant and Child Mortality

Infant mortality and child mortality for children under age 5 are more specific than DALYs or QALYs in representing the health in the poorest sections of a population, and are thus especially useful when focusing on health equity.

Morbidity

Morbidity measures include incidence rate, prevalence, and cumulative incidence, with incidence rate referring to the risk of developing a new health condition within a specified period of time. Although sometimes loosely expressed simply as the number of new cases during a time period, morbidity is better expressed as a proportion or a rate.

The burden of disease can be viewed as the gap between current health status and an ideal situation in which everyone lives into old age free of disease and disability. Causes of the gap are premature mortality, disability and exposure to certain risk factors that contribute to illness.

DEATHS ACROSS THE GLOBE: AN OVERVIEW

Imagine a diverse international group of 1000 individuals representative of the women, men and children from all over the world who died in 2004. Of those 1000 people, 138 would have come from high-income countries, 415 from middle-income countries and 447 from low-income countries.

The Top 10 Causes of Their Deaths

In high-income countries more than two-thirds of all people live beyond the age of 70 and predominantly die of chronic diseases: cardiovascular disease, chronic obstructive lung disease, cancers, diabetes or dementia. Lung infection remains the only leading infectious cause of death.

In middle-income countries, nearly half of all people live to the age of 70 and chronic diseases are the major killers, just as they are in high-income countries. Unlike in high-income countries, however, tuberculosis and road traffic accidents also are leading causes of death.

In low-income countries less than a quarter of all people reach the age of 70, and over a third of all deaths are among children under 14. People predominantly die of infectious diseases: lung infections, diarrheal diseases, HIV/AIDS, tuberculosis, and malaria. Complications of pregnancy and childbirth together continue to be leading causes of death, claiming the lives of both infants and mothers.

RISK FACTORS FOR GLOBAL PROBLEMS

Globalization

Globalization is making moving across the globe at extraordinary speed. The habits and lifestyles of the 'West' are now being imported and adopted by developing nations. It is the increasing interconnectedness of countries and the openness of borders to ideas, people, commerce, and financial capital. (Lancet, 2003) Refers to every aspect of life: cultural, social, psychological, and political which creates both negative and positive impacts on society and its health.

Obesity

Globally, there are more than 1 billion overweight adults, at least 300 million of them obese. Approximately 22 million children under five are estimated to be overweight worldwide. It is stated that 66% Americans Overweight, 30% Americans Obese.

Wealth is also increasing in developing countries as a result of international trade. As people become wealthier, oftentimes unhealthy lifestyles result which raises the likelihood of diseases related to tobacco use, alcohol abuse, physical inactivity, and obesity.

Tobacco use: Tobacco use is a risk factor for 6 of the 8 primary causes of death in the world. By 2020 tobacco is expected to kill more people than any single disease, even HIV/AIDS. The single largest cause of preventable death in the world today. More than ¾ of CVD results from its use. Over 100 million people died from use in 20th century, may kill more than 1 billion in 21st century. Currently 70% of tobacco use is in LIC.

Hypertension: Responsible for 13% of deaths world-wide. Over 26% of adults in the world had hypertension in 2000—expected to jump to 30% by 2025. 2/3 with HTN live in developing world. Treating hypertension can result in a 40%

decrease in risk of stroke and a 15% reduction in risk of MI. Hypertension can be control but due to lack of knowledge and awareness regarding HTN can lead to increase this disease more faster. In Pakistan more than 40% of doctors prescribed sedatives for HTN! In Africa control rates as low as 2% and in Saudi Arabia more than 60% of physicians and nurses in large teaching hospital had poor knowledge of basic techniques of BP measurement. Researchers in Canada have estimated that reducing salt intake by less than 1 tsp per day would reduce the incidence of HBP by 30% and save up to $430 million per year due to a reduced need for physician visits, lab tests and medications.

Lifestyle modifications do work. A study published in the American Journal of Cardiology concluded that many patients with conventional risk factors for CHD can reduce their risk without medications within 12 weeks of starting a TLC program.

Alcohol consumption: Over 125 million people in the world have alcohol use disorders. It is a major cause of disability of males in the world and accounts for one-third of the male neuropsychiatric disease burden. Globally in 2003, the prevalence of alcohol use disorders was estimated at 1.7% which contributes to 4% of Global Burden of Disease. In United States 18.5% of the population age 18 and older suffer from alcohol abuse or dependence. It is third leading cause of death in the US in 2003. Harmful alcohol use was estimated to be responsible for 3.7% of the global mortality in 2002. Clearly this is a widespread problem that needs to be addressed at a global level. It is fundamental and good medical practice to ask our patients about alcohol use. Alcohol use can complicate the management of other health problems, interact with medications, and puts our patients at risk for traffic related accidents.

Physical Inactivity

Physical inactivity is estimated to cause 2 million deaths worldwide annually. Globally it is a causal factor in 10–16% of cases each of breast cancer, colon cancers, and diabetes and 22% of ischemic heart disease. Appropriate regular physical activity is a major component in preventing the growing global burden of chronic disease. It is the risk of getting a cardiovascular disease increases by 1.5 times in people who do not follow minimum physical activity recommendations. Increasing physical activity is a societal, not just an individual problem, It demands a population-based, multisectoral, multidisciplinary, and culturally relevant approach.

Cholesterol

Suboptimal levels of cholesterol contribute to ~2/3 of the global CVD risk. In world level 4.4 million deaths in world related to hyperlipidemia. Cholesterol is responsible for 32% of ischemic stroke and 56% of IHD. Interventions include health education to community people, cooking classes, development of kitchen gardens, community physical activity events can help the people to control the cholesterol level.

Illness: Chronic disease is seen across the globe. Poorer nations are being greatly taxed in caring for these diseases. There are not enough well trained healthcare workers and primary health care clinics in these LMIC have been traditionally focusing on acute and communicable diseases.

Top 4 causes of illness worldwide include:

1. Diarrheal disease
2. Pneumonia and other lower respiratory tract infections
   - Except in Africa which has high levels of malaria
3. Injuries
4. Complications of pregnancy.

Disability

More individuals have iron-deficiency anemia than any other health problem in the world. Other very common conditions, with varying levels of severity, include asthma, arthritis, vision and hearing problems, migraine, major depressive episodes and intestinal worms, etc.

Neglected Tropical Disease (NTD)

Neglected Tropical Disease comprise 13 parasitic and bacterial infections. The global burden of the neglected tropical diseases is equivalent to at least half of the combined global burden of HIV/AIDS, TB and malaria. Over 1.4 billion people affected most of whom live on less than $1.25 per day. NTDs stigmatize, disable, and inhibit individuals from being able to care for themselves or their families—all of which promote poverty. ~90% of the total NTD disease burden are found in Africa, Asia and Latin America. Around half of the world's population is at risk of NTD infections. The NTDs are diseases of poverty, afflicting the world's poorest and trapping them in a cycle of poverty. Research indicates that the control of NTDs would greatly reduce both malaria morbidity and mortality, as well as HIV/AIDS transmission. NTDs are controllable and possibly eradicable by safe and effective drugs already in existence, many of which are donated by pharmaceutical companies (Merck, GlaxoSmithKline, Johnson and Johnson and Pfizer). With public-private partnerships, the integrated control of NTDs can be implemented at marginal costs—approximately 50 cents per person per year.

In one of the world's largest public-health collaborations, 155 experts from 50 countries have a plan to tackle the world's deadliest diseases. They identify top 20 priorities in chronic noncommunicable diseases—things like heart disease, stroke, diabetes, and most cancers—which account for 60% of all deaths worldwide. It is 'a road-map' for action, says lead researcher Abdallah Daar at the McLaughlin-Rotman Center for Global Health in Toronto. It is also the first systematic attempt to prioritize these diseases globally. 'With concerted action, we can avert at least 36 million premature deaths by 2015,' the paper reports. Without, these largely lifestyle-driven diseases will kill some 388 million people in the next ten years, 80% of them in the developing world.

GLOBAL STATUS REPORT ON NCDS 2014

NCDs were responsible for 38 million (68%) of the world's 56 million deaths in 2012. More than 40% of them (16 million) were premature deaths under age 70 years. Almost three quarters of all NCD deaths (28 million), and the majority of premature deaths (82%), occur in low- and middle-income countries. In September 2011, world leaders agreed on a roadmap of concrete commitments to address the global burden of NCDs, including a commitment to establish multi-sectoral action plans and policies for the prevention and control of NCDs. To accelerate national efforts to address NCDs, in 2013 the World Health Assembly adopted a comprehensive global monitoring framework with 25 indicators and nine voluntary global targets for 2025. The World Health Assembly also endorsed a set of actions organized around the World Health Organization (WHO), Global action plan for the prevention and control of noncommunicable diseases 2013–2020. On 10–11 July 2014, the set of actions is organized around six objectives aimed at strengthening national capacity, multisectoral action and boosting international cooperation to reduce exposure to risk factors, strengthen health systems, and monitor progress in attaining the global NCD targets. The objectives are:

- Integrate NCDs into health planning and national development plans
- By 2015, set national NCD targets for 2025, consistent with voluntary global targets
- By 2015, develop national NCD multisectoral plans to achieve the national targets
- By 2016, implement policies and interventions to reduce NCD risk factors and underlying social determinants
- By 2016, strengthen and orient health systems to address NCDs, through people-centered primary health care and universal health coverage.

The target formulated and action plan developed are described bellow.

Global Target 1

A 25% relative reduction in overall mortality from cardiovascular diseases, cancer, diabetes or chronic respiratory diseases: The comprehensive, multisectoral policy actions, interventions and country capacity, including civil/vital registration and surveillance systems, required to attain this target. The shortage of resources in many countries means that implementation of the very cost-effective policy options and interventions ('best buys') would have to be accorded the highest priority.

Global Target 2

At least 10% relative reduction in the harmful use of alcohol as appropriate, within the national context: In 2012, an estimated 5.9% (3.3 million) of all deaths worldwide and 5.1% of disability-adjusted life years (DALYs) were attributable to alcohol consumption. More than half of these deaths resulted from NCDs. The level of alcohol consumption worldwide in 2010 was estimated at 6.2 liters of pure alcohol per person aged 15 years and over (equivalent to 13.5 g of pure alcohol per day). The prevalence of heavy episodic drinking is associated with the overall levels of alcohol consumption and is highest in the WHO European Region and the Region of the Americas.

There are cost-effective policy options to reduce the harmful use of alcohol. They include pricing policies, reduced availability and marketing of alcohol, improved response by health services, and drink-driving policies and countermeasures. Individual interventions such as screening for harmful drinking and treatment of alcohol dependence are also effective, although they are more costly to implement than population-based measures.

Global Target 3

A 10% relative reduction in the prevalence of insufficient physical activity: Insufficient physical activity contributes to 3.2 million deaths and 69.3 million DALYs each year. Adults who are insufficiently physically active have a higher risk of all-cause mortality compared with those who do at least 150 minutes of moderate-intensity physical activity per week, or equivalent, as recommended by WHO. Regular physical activity reduces the risk of ischemic heart disease, stroke, diabetes, and breast and colon cancer. In 2010, 23% of adults aged 18 years and over were insufficiently physically active. Women were less active than men and older people were less active than younger people. Globally, 81% of adolescents aged 11–17 years were insufficiently physically active in 2010. Adolescent girls were less active than adolescent boys, with 84% versus 78% not meeting the WHO recommendation of 60 minutes of physical activity per day. Several high-income countries have reported increased physical activity over the past decade as a result of national policies and programs to improve physical activity. In recent years, more low- and middle-income countries have also set up initiatives to address physical inactivity. Reaching the physical activity target requires multisectoral collaboration between transport, urban planning, recreation, and sports and education departments, to create safe environments that are conducive to physical activity for all age groups.

Global Target 4

A 30% relative reduction in the mean population intake of salt/sodium: Excess consumption of dietary sodium is associated with increased risk of hypertension and cardiovascular disease. Globally, 1.7 million annual deaths from cardiovascular causes have been attributed to excess sodium intake. Current estimates suggest that the global mean intake of salt is around 10 g daily (4 g/day of sodium). WHO recommends a reduction in salt intake to less than 5 g/day (2 g/day of sodium), to reduce blood pressure and the risk of coronary heart disease and stroke. The main source of salt in many countries is processed foods and ready-made meals, while salt added during the preparation of food at home and at the table is significant in others. With the greater availability of processed foods in low- and middle-income countries, sources of sodium are shifting rapidly towards these foods. Establishing a baseline of salt intake is key to setting national targets and devising effective consumer campaigns. Sodium-reduction targets need to be established for each category of food, prioritizing the ones that contribute most to population intake. Policies aimed at reducing population-wide salt consumption should be intersectoral and multidisciplinary and include the participation of all relevant stakeholders. They should be applicable to diverse settings and make use of all available tools, including labeling, legislation, product reformulation, fiscal incentives that encourage the production and consumption of foods with reduced sodium content, and consumer education to ensure their effective implementation.

Global Target 5

A 30% relative reduction in prevalence of current tobacco use in persons aged 15+ years: It is estimated that currently around 6 million people die annually from tobacco use, with over 600,000 deaths due to exposure to second-hand smoke. Measures to ensure reduction in tobacco use include: protecting people from second-hand smoke through national '100% smoke-free' legislation; offering help in quitting tobacco use, warning people about the dangers of tobacco use; enforcing bans on tobacco advertising, promotion and sponsorship; and raising tobacco taxes **(Table 17.1)**. Considerable progress has been made in global tobacco control in recent years, in both the number of countries protecting their population and the number of people worldwide protected by effective tobacco-control measures. In 2013, 95 countries had implemented at least one of the four tobacco control 'best-buy' interventions, at the highest level of achievement, and two countries had all four 'best-buys' in place at the highest level. Many of the countries making progress in implementing 'best-buy' measures were low- or middle-income countries.

Global Target 6

A 25% relative reduction in the prevalence of raised blood pressure, or contain the prevalence of raised blood pressure, according to national circumstances: Raised blood pressure is estimated to have caused 9.4 million deaths and 7% of disease burden—as measured in DALYs—in 2010. If left uncontrolled, hypertension causes stroke, myocardial infarction, cardiac failure, dementia, renal failure and blindness. There is strong scientific evidence of the health benefits of lowering blood pressure through population-wide and individual (behavioral and pharmacological) interventions. The global prevalence of raised blood pressure (defined as systolic and/or diastolic blood pressure equal to or above 140/90 mm Hg) in adults aged 18 years and over was around 22% in 2014. Many modifiable factors contribute to the high prevalence rates of hypertension. They include eating food containing too much salt and fat, inadequate intake of fruits and vegetables, overweight and obesity, harmful use of alcohol, physical inactivity, psychological stress, socioeconomic determinants, and inadequate access to health care. Worldwide, detection, treatment and control of hypertension are inadequate, owing to weaknesses in health systems, particularly at the primary care level. In order to achieve this target, population-wide these modifiable risk factors. In addition, integrated programs need to be established at the primary care level, to improve the efficiency and effectiveness of detection and management of hypertension and other cardiovascular risk factors through a total-risk approach, as recommended by WHO.

Table 17.1: Recommended 'Best Buys'.

Risk factor	*Interventions*
Tobacco use	• Raise taxes on tobacco • Protect people from tobacco smoke • Warn about the dangers of tobacco • Enforce bans on tobacco advertising
Harmful use of alcohol	• Raise taxes on alcohol • Restrict access to retailed alcohol • Enforce bans on alcohol advertising
Unhealthy diet and physical inactivity	• Reduce salt intake in food • Replace trans fat with polyunsaturated fat • Promote public awareness about diet and physical activity (via mass media)

Global Target 7

Halt the rise in diabetes and obesity: Obesity increases the likelihood of diabetes, hypertension, coronary heart disease, stroke and certain types of cancer. Worldwide, the prevalence of obesity has nearly doubled since 1980. In 2014, 11% of men and 15% of women aged 18 years and older were obese. More than 42 million children under the age of 5 years were overweight in 2013. The global prevalence of diabetes in 2014 was estimated to be 9%. Obesity and diabetes can be prevented through multisectoral action that simultaneously addresses different sectors that contribute to the production, distribution and marketing of food, while concurrently shaping an environment that facilitates and promotes adequate levels of physical activity. Diabetes risk can be reduced by moderate weight loss and moderate daily physical activity.

Global Target 8

At least 50% of eligible people receive drug therapy and counseling (including glycemic control) to prevent heart attacks and strokes: Cardiovascular disease was the leading cause of NCD deaths in 2012 and was responsible for 17.5 million deaths, or 46% of NCD deaths. Of these deaths, an estimated 7.4 million were due to heart attacks (ischemic heart disease) and 6.7 million were due to strokes.

This target to reduce heart attacks and strokes is aimed at improving the coverage of drug treatment and counseling in people with raised cardiovascular risk and established disease. It is an affordable intervention that can be delivered through a primary health care approach, even in resource-constrained settings. There are major gaps in the coverage of this intervention to prevent heart attacks and strokes, particularly in low- and middle-income countries. Poor access to basic services in primary care, lack of affordability of laboratory tests and medicines, inappropriate patterns of clinical practice, and poor adherence to treatment are some of the main reasons for these treatment gaps. This intervention to prevent heart attacks and strokes needs to be part of the basic benefits package for moving towards universal health coverage. In addition, context-specific strategies will be required to address multiple gaps in health systems related to access to basic technologies and medicines, the health workforce, service delivery, health information, and referral, with a special focus on primary care.

Global Target 9

Eighty percentage (80) availability of the affordable basic technologies and essential medicines, including generics, required to treat major noncommunicable diseases in both public and private facilities: This target includes the basic requirement of technologies and medicines for implementing cost-effective primary care interventions to address cardiovascular disease, diabetes and asthma. The essential medicines include aspirin, a statin, an angiotensin-converting enzyme inhibitor, a thiazide diuretic, a long-acting calcium channel-blocker, a beta-blocker, metformin, insulin, a bronchodilator and a steroid inhalant. The basic technologies include, at least, a blood pressure measurement device, a weighing scale, height measuring equipment, blood sugar and blood cholesterol measurement devices with strips, and urine strips for albumin assay. These are minimum requirements, without which even basic NCD interventions cannot be implemented in primary care. Currently, there are major gaps in the affordability and availability of basic health technologies and essential medicines, particularly in low- and middle-income countries. The national policies that encourage the availability of basic health technologies and essential medicines should be central to efforts focused on achieving universal health coverage. Drugs must also be used appropriately, so there must be adherence to evidence-based guidelines and education in rational use for both health care professionals and patients. Policies and interventions to attain the nine targets should be given high priority and budgeted in national multisectoral NCD action plans. The nine voluntary global targets should be attained by 2025.

Key Messages of the Global Status Report on Noncommunicable Diseases 2014

Message 1: Noncommunicable diseases act as key barriers to poverty alleviation and sustainable development
Message 2: While some countries are making progress, the majority are off course to meet the global NCD targets
Message 3: Countries can move from political commitment to action by prioritizing high-impact, affordable interventions
Message 4: All countries need to set national NCD targets and be accountable for attaining them
Message 5: Structures and processes for multisectoral and intersectoral collaboration need to be established
Message 6: Investment in health systems is critical for improving NCD outcomes
Message 7: Institutional and human resource capacities and financial resources for NCD prevention and control.

GLOBAL HEALTH PRIORITIES

Health has gained importance on the global agenda. It has become recognized in forums where it was once not addressed. Infectious diseases have gained ground as global health priorities, while noncommunicable diseases and the broader issues of health systems development have been neglected. Approaches to tackling the health problems are increasingly influenced by trade and industrial interests with the emphasis on technological solutions.

Global health refers to health problems that transcend national borders—problems such as infectious and insect-borne diseases that can spread from one country to another. It also includes health problems that are of such magnitude that they have a global political and economic impact.

Global health refers to health problems that are best addressed by cooperative actions and solutions—solutions that involve more than one country. Because global health problems can move across national borders, countries can learn from one another's experiences, both in how diseases spread and in how they can be treated and controlled. Cooperation across countries is essential to addressing those health problems that transcend borders. This includes helping other countries address their particular health care crises.

Global health priorities and the means of addressing the identified health priorities: Global health priorities have in recent years been defined through several processes and by several actors and at various forums. In 2000 and 2001, HIV/AIDS, tuberculosis and malaria came to be discussed in a variety of forums at the UN as well as outside the UN, and commitments to address the three diseases were made.

Millennium Development Goals (MDGs) are a product of consultations between international agencies, but were also adopted by the United Nations (UN) General Assembly in September 2001 as part of the road map for implementing the substantially broader Millennium Declaration, which it had adopted in September 2000. The MDGs have eight goals, three of which are health-focused, namely those on child mortality, maternal health, and HIV/AIDS, malaria and other diseases.

The UN-led Millennium Project, directed by the economist Jeffrey Sachs, has the objective of ensuring that all developing countries meet the MDGs. The whole UN system has since been requested to adapt to addressing the MDGs, and to report to the Secretary General on their achievements in that direction. For health policies, this has meant, for example, pressures from some of the member states, such as the UK, for the WHO to refocus its work on the MDGs, most notably to the goal concerning HIV/

AIDS, malaria and tuberculosis, while its wider mandate as the normative health organization that sets norms and standards and promotes the building up a wider health systems would not be so emphasized. The MDGs have become an important tool to steer both the UN system towards a narrower agenda with more emphasis on selected interventions and country presences, but more recently increased attention has been placed on the need for addressing development—including health policy issues and systems—more comprehensively.

Largely the same priorities for health emerged from the report of the Commission of Macroeconomics and Health (CMH) in December 2001, which concluded that public health resources should be directed to the following priorities: communicable diseases; malnutrition, which exacerbates childhood infections; and maternal and perinatal mortality.

Development aid for health is also largely steered towards tackling communicable infections. USAID has financed population programs, including family planning, for three decades, while its emphasis on health issues is more recent. In 2002, the USAID population, health, and nutrition funding covered HIV/AIDS, family planning/ reproductive health, child survival/maternal health, and infectious diseases. The BMGF has provided strategic funding for the founding of new structures for global health policy making—such as GAVI and GAIN—and for the implementation of the recommendations derived from the CMH. Its Global Health program focuses on infectious disease prevention, vaccine research and development, and reproductive and child health, with emphasis on the development and implementation of technologies, though recurrent costs or chronic conditions are not financed. In GAVI, the substantial BMGF funding is targeted at new vaccines. Efforts have also been made to tackle health challenges through new health technology research and development funding under the Bill and Melinda Gates Foundation funded Grand Challenges in Global Health initiative.

According to global mortality and burden-of-disease calculations, the above-set priorities indeed represent the majority of deaths and ill-health in sub-Saharan Africa, but do not represent the majority of ill-health in any other region. They cover less than a third of the global ill-health. Today, noncommunicable diseases are a cause of the majority of ill-health in developing countries, and their importance is increasing rapidly. They affect all socioeconomic groups and in many cases the risks are biggest in the poorest sections of the populations.

The lists of the current global health priorities can be seen as reflecting health-related problems in the developing countries that are perceived to threaten the vital interests of industrialized countries. Linking national interests to development aid is by no means new. In the 1970s, such concerns were central in, for example, the argumentations for population program implementation. Nevertheless, it is noteworthy that since the mid-1990s the arguments for a greater US engagement in global health have been expressed increasingly in terms of national interests or enlightened self-interest.

GLOBAL HEALTH CONDITIONS

The diseases and health conditions targeted by global health initiatives are sometimes grouped under 'diseases of poverty' versus 'diseases of affluence', although the impact of globalization is increasingly blurring the lines between the two. The global health condition depict both emerging communicable and noncommunicable diseases prevalence. Nowadays noncommunicable diseases highly prevalent both in developed and developing countries but some communicable diseases are still major causes of morbidity and mortality worldwide specially in developing countries which can be addressed. Communicable diseases are also given more importance in global health as it is transmittable.

Respiratory Infections

Infections of the respiratory tract and middle ear are major causes of morbidity and mortality worldwide. Some respiratory infections of global significance include tuberculosis, measles, influenza, and pneumonias caused by pneumococci and *Haemophilus influenzae*. The spread of respiratory infections is exacerbated by crowded conditions, and poverty is associated with more than a 20-fold increase in the relative burden of lung infections.

Diarrheal Diseases

Diarrhea is the second most common cause of child mortality worldwide, responsible for 17% of deaths of children under age 5. Poor sanitation can increase transmission of bacteria and viruses through water, food, utensils, hands, and flies. Dehydration due to diarrhea can be effectively treated through oral rehydration therapy with dramatic reductions in mortality. Important nutritional measures include the promotion of breastfeeding and zinc supplementation. While hygienic measures alone may be insufficient for the prevention of rotavirus diarrhea, it can be prevented by a safe and potentially cost-effective vaccine.

Maternal Health

Complications of pregnancy and childbirth are the leading causes of death among women of reproductive age in many developing countries: a woman dies from complications from childbirth approximately every minute. According to the World Health Organization's 2005 World Health Report, poor maternal conditions are the fourth leading cause of death for women worldwide, after HIV/AIDS, malaria, and tuberculosis. Most maternal deaths and injuries can be prevented, and such deaths have been largely eradicated in the developed world. Targets for improving maternal health include increasing the number of deliveries accompanied by skilled birth attendants.

68 low-income countries tracked by the WHO- and UNICEF-led collaboration. *Countdown to 2015* are estimated to hold for 97% of worldwide maternal and child deaths.

HIV/AIDS

Human immunodeficiency virus (HIV) is transmitted through unprotected sex, unclean needles, blood transfusions, and from mother to child during birth or lactation. Globally, HIV is primarily spread through sexual intercourse. The infection damages the immune system, leading to acquired immunodeficiency syndrome (AIDS) and eventually, death. Antiretroviral drugs prolong life and delay the onset of AIDS by minimizing the amount of HIV in the body.

Malaria

Malaria is a mosquito-borne infectious disease caused by the parasites of the genus *Plasmodium*. Symptoms may include fever, headaches, chills, and nausea. Each year, there are approximately 500 million cases of malaria worldwide, most commonly among children and pregnant women in developing countries. The use of insecticide-treated bednets is a cost-effective way to reduce deaths from malaria, as is prompt artemisinin-based combination therapy, supported by intermittent preventive therapy in pregnancy.

Nutrition

In 2010, about 104 million children were underweight, and undernutrition contributes to about one third of child deaths around the world. Undernutrition is not to be confused with *malnutrition*, which refers to poor *proportion* of food intake and can thus refer to obesity. Undernutrition impairs the immune system, increasing the frequency, severity, and duration of infections (including measles, pneumonia, and diarrhea). Infection can further contribute to malnutrition. Deficiencies of micronutrient, such as vitamin A, iron, iodine, and zinc, are common worldwide and can compromise intellectual potential, growth, development, and adult productivity.

Violence against women has been defined as 'physical, sexual and psychological violence occurring in the family and in the general community, including battering, sexual abuse of children, dowry-related violence, rape, female genital mutilation and other traditional practices harmful to women, nonspousal violence and violence related to exploitation, sexual harassment and intimidation at work, in educational institutions and elsewhere, trafficking in women, forced prostitution and violence perpetrated or condoned by the state'.

Chronic Disease

Approximately 80% of deaths linked to noncommunicable diseases occur in developing countries. Increases in refugee urbanization, has led to a growing number of people diagnosed with chronic noncommunicable diseases. In September 2011, the United Nations is hosting its first General Assembly Special Summit on the issue of noncommunicable diseases. Noting that noncommunicable diseases are the cause of some 35 million deaths each year, the international community is being increasingly called to take measures for the prevention and control of chronic diseases and mitigate their impacts on the world population, especially on women, who are usually the primary caregivers.

For example, the rate of type 2 diabetes, associated with obesity, has been on the rise in countries previously plagued by hunger. In low-income countries, the number of individuals with diabetes is expected to increase from 84 million to 228 million by 2030. Obesity, a preventable condition, is associated with numerous chronic diseases, including cardiovascular conditions, stroke, certain cancers, and respiratory disease. About 16% of the global burden of disease, measured as DALYs, has been accounted for by obesity.

TOP 20 GRAND CHALLENGES TO CONTROL NONCOMMUNICABLE DISEASES

The experts' 20 'grand challenges' to address 'Study and address how poverty increases risk actors'; and 'Move health professional training and practice towards prevention'. The key to success may lie in relatively minor interventions. 'It may look very comprehensive and complicated, but very small changes, if you apply them on a population scale, will have really huge effects,' says Stig Pramming, a UK-based coauthor and executive director of the Oxford Health Alliance. An obese person can cut the risk of diabetes dramatically by losing just 10 lbs (5 kg). The problem is getting more people involved in health decisions. Tackling obesity, for example, will take more than telling people to eat less. 'We all want to lose weight and exercise more,' he says. 'The environment needs to help.' People who want to exercise need safe streets to walk on. People who want fresh fruits and vegetables need somewhere to buy them.

The Top 20, as printed in Nature, have been grouped into six clusters:

Raise Public Awareness

1. **Raise the political priority of noncommunicable disease:** Political priority *is* the degree to which international and national political leaders actively give attention to an issue and back up that attention with the provision of financial, technical, and human resources that are commensurate with the severity of the issues. NCDs are rooted in the social determinants of health and cannot be stopped through individual action alone. By way of example, current global marketing activities are driving the transition towards diets that are high in sugar and saturated fat, thus increasing the risk of developing one or more NCDs. If the political priority against noncommunicable disease can rise then noncommunicable diseases can be prevented.

2. **Promote healthy lifestyle and consumption choices through effective education and public engagement:** Lifestyle is the major risk factor which indulge the individual to have a smoke or alcohol. A healthy lifestyle make the individual fit, energetic and at reduced risk for disease. It is the daily good habits like good nutrition, daily exercise and adequate sleep. Managing stress in positive ways, instead of through smoking or drinking alcohol, are the foundations for continuing good health.
3. **Health education package:** Raise public awareness by providing effective health education package which contain compelling and valid information on different aspects of health to foster widespread, sustained and accurate media coverage and thereby improve awareness of economic, social and public health impacts.

Enhance Economic, Legal and Environmental Policies

4. **Study and address the impact of government spending and taxation on health:** The Government spend a lot on smoking-related health conditions. These disease conditions increased mortality rates for smokers of working age which has great impact on GDP. Research has demonstrated a strong links between increased tobacco consumption, free trade, and foreign direct investment. Recognizing the need for a collective response, is more essential.
5. **Develop and implement local, national and international policies:** Develop and implement local, national and international policies and trade agreements, including regulatory restraints, to discourage the consumption of alcohol, tobacco and unhealthy foods. Changing policy interventions can prevent and treat NCDs. These policies include tax increases to curb tobacco use; restrictions on the marketing of alcohol; replacement of trans fats to promote healthier diets; hepatitis B immunization to prevent liver cancer; and multidrug therapy to prevent heart attacks and stroke.
6. **Study and address the impacts of poor health on economic output and productivity:** The individuals suffering from illness may be weak, unable to work or study and generally unable to provide for children and other dependents. At a more aggregated level, however, it seems likely that a high disease burden may have an adverse impact on a country's productivity, growth and, ultimately, economic development. So for controlling disease minimizing risk factors are more essential.

Modify Risk Factors

7. **Deploy universally measures proven to reduce tobacco use and boost resources to implement the WHO Framework Convention on Tobacco Control:** Multifaceted school-based education programs that are performed in conjunction with community-based campaigns have met with substantial success. The management of nicotine addiction in persons who already smoke has the benefit of clinical tools, that is, systems for weaning persons from nicotine, the efficacy of which is clearly demonstrated. Product regulation, enforcement of clean indoor air standards, and protecting young people from the supposed attractiveness of cigarettes all promise substantial impact. The WHO Framework Convention on Tobacco Control (WHO FCTC) is the first treaty negotiated under the auspices of the World Health Organization. The WHO FCTC is an evidence-based treaty that reaffirms the right of all people to the highest standard of health. The WHO FCTC represents a paradigm shift in developing a regulatory strategy to address addictive substances; in contrast to previous drug control treaties, the WHO FCTC asserts the importance of demand reduction strategies as well as supply issues which should be implemented.
8. **Increase the availability and consumption of healthy food:** Promoting healthy diets and lifestyles to reduce the global burden of noncommunicable diseases requires a multisectoral approach involving the various relevant sectors in societies. The agriculture and food sector figures prominently in this enterprise and must be given due importance in any consideration of the promotion of healthy diets for individuals and population groups. Food strategies must not merely be directed at ensuring food security for all, but must also achieve the consumption of adequate quantities of safe and good quality foods that together make up a healthy diet.
9. **Promote lifelong physical activity:** Physical inactivity has become a serious problem in overall world. There is no debate about the value of physical exertion. Regular physical activity has significant health benefits, and even modest increases in energy expenditure can have health-enhancing effects, including reduction in chronic disease risk—hypertension, type 2 diabetes, high blood lipids, cardiovascular disease, and obesity. Even among children and adolescents, physical activity can prevent or delay the development of hypertension and can reduce blood pressure in those young people who already have hypertension. It also lowered risk of colon cancer, increase in bone density, reduction of anxiety and improvement in body image and mood. So Promote lifelong physical activity is important to prevent common communicable diseases.
10. **Better understand environmental and cultural factors that change behavior:** Health is determined by several factors including genetic inheritance, personal behaviors, access to quality health care, and the general external environment (such as the quality of air, water, and housing conditions). In addition, a growing body of research has documented associations between social and cultural factors and health. Better understanding of environmental and cultural factors that change behavior is importance to avoid such circumstances.

Engage Business and Community

11. **Make businesses a key partner in promoting health and preventing disease:** Generally our businesses

make our life first and full of stress. For a healthy life the individual should make his businesses as a key partner of health. The working environment or businesses field should be conducive for health. The environment should be free from stress, strain and with recreational facilities. In every institution there should be provision of mental health. The business environment will help in promoting health and preventing disease.

12. **Develop and monitor codes of responsible conduct with the food, beverage and restaurant industries:** The **Food Code** is a model for safeguarding public health and ensuring **food** is unadulterated and honestly presented when offered to the consumer. It represents FDA's best advice for a uniform system of provisions that address the safety and protection of **food** offered at retail and in **food** service. It is the organic body and systematized basic standards relating to food, condiments, stimulants and drink and beverages, their concerned raw materials, utensils and equipment use and domestic consumption. In order to make a positive impact on food borne illness, retail and food service operators can use food code. They must achieve active managerial control of the risk factors contributing to food borne illness. Combined with basic sanitation, employee training, and other prerequisite programs.
13. **Empower community resources such as voluntary and faith-based organizations:** Spiritual health has a great impact on human being. Researches also prove that spirituality can help the individual and family to cope with crises situation and improve mental health. In chronic noncommunicable diseases the individual gain acceptance through spirituality. For improving moral and spiritual health the faith-based organizations voluntary organizations should be improved.

Mitigate Health Impacts of Poverty and Urbanization

14. **Study and address how poverty increases risk factors:** Health is determined by several factors including personal behaviors, access to quality health care, and the general external environment (such as the quality of air, water, and housing conditions), poor socioeconomic status or poverty. Poverty creates ill-health because it not only forces people to live in environments that make them sick, without decent shelter, clean water or adequate sanitation but also, deprived of the information, money or access to health services that would help them prevent and treat disease. For achieving global health is necessary to find out and address the poverty increases risk factors that make the individual vulnerable to ill health.
15. **Study and address the links between the built environment, urbanization and chronic noncommunicable disease:** Generally rapid and unplanned urbanization, which has led to different lifestyles characterized by unhealthy nutrition, reduced physical activity and tobacco consumption. These unhealthy lifestyles are associated with common modifiable risk factors for chronic diseases such as hypertension, diabetes mellitus, dyslipidemia and obesity. If these above factors will addressed than surely the chronic noncommunicable disease can be prevented.

Reorientate Health Systems

16. **Allocate resources within health systems based on burden of disease: Disease burden** is the impact of a health problem as measured by financial cost, mortality, morbidity, or other indicators. It is often quantified in terms of quality-adjusted life years (QALYs) or disability-adjusted life years (DALYs), both of which quantify the number of years lost due to **disease** (YLDs). The resource allocation in the health care system should be based on the prioritization of the disease burden.
17. **Move health professional training and practice towards prevention:** The health professional should be trained on prevention of chronic communicable diseases. The in-service education for health professional should be preventive because the chronic noncommunicable diseases can be prevented by adopting healthy lifestyle. The health professional can educate the people regarding adoption of healthy lifestyle.
18. **Increase number and skills of professionals:** Increase number and skills of professionals who prevent, treat and manage chronic noncommunicable diseases, especially in developing countries. The number of public health worker should be increase and public health worker should have IPR skill by which they can motivate the people to prevent chronic noncommunicable diseases and how to manage in home (Exdiabetic patient self-care).
19. **Build health systems that integrate screening and prevention within health delivery:** Importance should be given on primary health care which focus on preventive care with curative care. Mass screening for any suspected diseases can be advisable.
20. **Increase access to medications to prevent complications of chronic noncommunicable disease:** The chronic noncommunicable disease like diabetes mellitus or hypertension can managed lifelong with proper medication. These diseases have various life-threatening complications which can be managed with proper medications. Increase access to medications to the people with chronic noncommunicable diseases is very essential.

Life-saving Progress in Health through the Global Health Program

The global health program aims to harness advances in science and technology to save lives in developing countries.

During much of the last century, major health advances occurred primarily in wealthy countries. Diseases that have been defeated in wealthy nations, however, continue to sicken and kill people in the developing world.

In recent years, global health has begun to receive the attention it deserves. Due to major new investments from governments, private companies, charities, and concerned individuals, the health of those in the developing world is now receiving more funding and attention than at any other point in history. USAID, GFATM, GAIN are playing major role in global health program.

New investments in global health are achieving extraordinary results:

- Programs to deliver childhood vaccines have pushed basic immunization rates to all-time highs.
- Polio cases have declined 99% in the past 20 years—and the world now has the opportunity to get rid of the disease completely.
- The number of people receiving treatment for HIV infection has increased tenfold in just five years.
- Since 2000, aggressive control has helped reduce malaria cases and related deaths by up to half in 25 countries.
- The number of children who die before age 5—a crucial indicator of a society's overall health—has fallen every year for the past few decades and is now less than 9 million worldwide, about half of what it was in 1960.

Research focused on the needs of countries in the developing world has also increased substantially after decades of neglect. For example, new vaccines against meningitis, cholera, and typhoid could soon become available for use. Other important new vaccines are entering late-stage clinical trials.

Science and technology offer incredible potential to improve health in developing countries. The number one global health priority is creating and delivering vaccines for infectious diseases. Millions of lives can be saved in developing countries by ensuring access to effective vaccines that already exist and by developing new vaccines for use.

Initiatives Taken

Priorities Diseases and Conditions

Global health strategy focuses on diseases and health conditions that account for a significant share of illness and death in developing countries. The historically neglected or underfunded health problems were addressed with these considerations in mind, the following areas was focused like infectious diseases including diarrheal diseases, HIV/AIDS, malaria, neglected diseases, pneumonia, polio and other vaccine-preventable diseases, and tuberculosis. The family health including the leading causes of illness and death for mothers and newborns during and immediately after childbirth; nutrition, especially during the first two years of life and family planning are also given importance.

Building Partnerships

Achieving lasting change in health requires bringing together diverse groups, each with a critical role to play, including governments, private companies, research institutes, and international and community organizations. Much of the work involves building and strengthening partnerships with organizations around the world.

Public–Private Partnerships

Many of our grants support partnerships between the public and private sectors to collaborate on critical health goals. For example, we support the efforts of the Global Alliance for Improved Nutrition (GAIN) to produce and deliver nutritious food. We also support a number of product-development partnerships that bring together the unique.

AGENCIES TO TACKLE GLOBAL PROBLEMS

The Global Fund to Fight Aids, Tuberculosis and Malaria (GFATM)

The Global Fund to Fight AIDS, Tuberculosis and Malaria (GFATM) is an international financing organization that aims to attract and disburse additional resources to prevent AIDS, tuberculosis and malaria. A public–private partnership, the organization has its secretariat in Geneva, Switzerland. The organization began operations in January 2002. Microsoft founder Bill Gates was one of the first private foundations among many bilateral donors to provide seed money for the project.

The Global Fund is the world's largest financier of anti-AIDS, TB and malaria programs and by mid-2012 has approved funding of USD 22.9 billion that supports more than 1,000 programs in 151 countries. According to the organization, it has financed the distribution of 270 million insecticide-treated nets to combat malaria, provided anti-tuberculosis treatment for 9.3 million people, and provided AIDS treatment for some 3.6 million people. In 2009, the Fund accounted for around 20% of international public funding for HIV, 65% for tuberculosis, and 65% for malaria.

United States Agency for International Development

The United States Agency for International Development (USAID) is the United States Government agency primarily responsible for administering civilian foreign aid. The US Agency for International Development's (USAID's) programs in global health represent the commitment and determination of the US Government to prevent suffering, save lives, and create a brighter future for families in the developing world. USAID's commitment to improving global health includes confronting global health challenges through improving the quality, availability, and use of essential health services. USAID's objective is to improve global health, including child, maternal, and reproductive health, and reduce abortion and disease, especially HIV/AIDS, malaria, and tuberculosis.

USAID's Bureau for Global Health supports field health programs, advances research and innovation in selected areas relevant to overall Agency health objectives, and transfers new technologies to the field through its own staff's work, coordination with other donors, and a portfolio of grants. Global health issues have global consequences that not only affect the people of developing nations but also directly affect the interests of American citizens.

Global Alliance for Improved Nutrition

The Global Alliance for Improved Nutrition (GAIN) is an independent nonprofit foundation based in Geneva, Switzerland. GAIN was developed at the UN 2002 Special Session of the General Assembly on Children. GAIN is an organization driven by the vision of a world without malnutrition. The alliance's mission is to reduce malnutrition through sustainable market-based strategies aimed at improving the health and nutrition of populations at risk. GAIN's overall target is to improve the nutrition of one billion people. To achieve its goal, GAIN works to reduce malnutrition by improving the efficiency and effectiveness of markets to reach the base of the pyramid. GAIN mobilises public private partnerships to implement innovative and sustainable market-based solutions at scale. GAIN works with diverse partners—governments, international organization partners, nongovernmental organizations, and over 600 companies worldwide. Programs are reaching more than 500 million people in over 30 countries with nutritious foods, up from 400 million in 2009–2010 and 200 million in 2008–2009. Half of those reached are women and children. Sixty-seven percent of beneficiaries are in Africa and 31% in Asia. GAIN has launched public-private partnerships to support market-based nutrition solutions in nutrition interventions areas including: large scale food fortification; maternal, infant and young child feeding; and agriculture and nutrition.

International Health

International health, also called geographic medicine or global health, is a field of health care, usually with a public health emphasis, dealing with health across regional or national boundaries. One subset of international medicine, travel medicine, prepares travelers with immunizations, prophylactic medications, preventive techniques such as bednets and residual pesticides, in-transit care, and post-travel care for exotic illnesses. International health, however, more often refers to health personnel or organizations from one area or nation providing direct health care, or health sector development, in another area or nation. It is this sense of the term that is explained here. More recently, public health experts have become interested in global processes that impact on human health. Globalization and health, for example, illustrates the complex and changing sociological environment within which the determinants of health and disease express themselves.

THE ROLE OF NGOs

Much work in international health is performed by nongovernmental organizations, or NGOs. Services provided by international health NGOs include direct health care, community potable water, vitamin supplementation, and mitigation of endemic and epidemic infectious diseases and malnutrition. Examples of NGOs dedicated to international health include:

- Pakistan Heart Foundation
- CARE
- Médecins Sans Frontières (Doctors Without Borders)
- The International Committee of the Red Cross
- International Medical Corps
- Oxfam
- Partners in Health
- Project HOPE
- Save the Children.

The Role of International Health NGOs in International Development

Health-related NGOs also provide capacity development in areas of need; that is, helping nations develop sustainable domestic health solutions through training programs. An example of this type of aid is the Center for International Rehabilitation, which has provided rehabilitation training for Iraqi physical therapists, physicians, and rehabilitation clinic managers in Tuzla, Bosnia and Amman, Jordan. These trainees then care for amputees, spinal and head injury patients in their home country. The purpose of the NGO Code of Conduct for Health Systems Strengthening is to offer guidance on how international NGOs can work in host countries in a way that respects and supports the primacy of the government's responsibility for organizing health system delivery. The code serves as a guide to encourage NGO practices that contribute to building public health systems and discourage those that are harmful.

Nongovernmental Organizations Working in Global Health

Nongovernmental Organizations (NGOs), such as those listed below, provide valuable resources, tools and funding in the field of global health.

International Organizations

- **The Global Fund to Fight AIDS, Tuberculosis and Malaria:** An international financing institution that invests the world's money to save lives.
- **Joint United Nations Programme on HIV/AIDS (UNAIDS):** An innovative partnership that leads and inspires the world in achieving universal access to HIV prevention, treatment, care and support.
- **World Bank:** A vital source of financial and technical assistance to developing countries around the world to fight poverty, including making investments to improve health.
- **World Health Organization (WHO):** The directing and coordinating authority for health within the United Nations system, responsible for providing leadership on global health matters, including shaping the health research agenda.

- **American Association for the Advancement of Science (AAAS):** An international nonprofit organization dedicated to advancing science around the world by serving as an educator, leader, spokesperson and professional association.
- **American Society for Microbiology (ASM):** A membership organization for microbiologists working to advance the microbiological sciences as a vehicle for understanding life processes and to apply and communicate this knowledge for the improvement of health and environmental and economic well-being worldwide.
- **American Society of Tropical Medicine and Hygiene (ASTMH):** A worldwide community of researchers, clinicians and professionals dedicated to advancing global health through collaboration, education and career advancement in tropical medicine.
- **American Thoracic Society (ATS):** An international society committed to improving global health—particularly regarding tuberculosis diagnosis, treatment and control and is a forceful advocate for tobacco control and smoking cessation.
- **Consortium of Universities for Global Health (CUGH):** A consortium of colleges and universities that builds collaborations and exchange of knowledge and experience among interdisciplinary university global health programs working across education, research and service. It is dedicated to creating equity and reducing health disparities, everywhere.
- **The Global Health Network:** A collection of websites and online communities supporting global health researchers by facilitating collaboration and resource sharing.
- **Infectious Diseases Society of America (IDSA):** Represents physicians, scientists and other health care professionals who specialize in infectious diseases. IDSA's purpose is to improve the health of individuals, communities, and society by promoting excellence in patient care, education, research, public health, and prevention relating to infectious diseases.
- **International Diabetes Federation (IDF):** An umbrella organization of over 200 national diabetes associations in over 160 countries.
- **GBC Health:** A coalition of companies and organizations serving as a hub for business engagement on the world's most pressing global health issues.
- **The Earth Institute:** Columbia University's resource that brings together the people and tools needed to address some of the world's most difficult problems, from climate change and environmental degradation, to poverty, disease and the sustainable use of resources.
- **Global Alliance for Chronic Diseases (GACD):** An alliance of research funders to support clear priorities for a coordinated research effort that will address this growing global health crisis.
- **Global Health Council:** The leading membership organization supporting and connecting advocates, implementers and stakeholders around global health priorities worldwide.
- **Global Health Technologies Coalition (GHTC):** A group of more than 30 nonprofit organizations working to increase awareness of the urgent need for technologies that save lives in the developing world.

INTERNATIONAL HEALTH REGULATIONS (IHR)

We all are living in a global 'village'. International travel and trade are commonplace and increasing. Diseases can travel at the speed of jetliners. In order to prevent the spread, many attempts by individual ruler have been adopted, e.g., Barriers against infection by detection and isolation of travelers quarantine. The classical way to stop the international spread of infectious disease is to erect border controls—for people as well as for goods. At the middle of the 19th century, such quarantine laws in the different European states had become so disparate—and seemed so inept at stopping the spread of cholera—that the First International Sanitary Conference was called in Paris in 1851 by the Foreign Ministers of 14 European countries. It demonstrates the appreciation that the issue of international infection control is connected to the issue of traffic. That is: (i) the free movement of people and goods will increase the risk of cross-border transmission; (ii) quarantine is an impediment to free trade; and (iii) public health arguments can therefore be used to justify trade barriers.

History of the IHR

The cholera epidemics that overran Europe between 1830 and 1847 were catalysts for intensive infectious disease diplomacy and multilateral cooperation in public health. This led to the first International Sanitary Conference in Paris in 1851. In 1948, the WHO Constitution entered into force and in 1951 WHO Member States adopted the International Sanitary Regulations, which were replaced by and renamed the International Health Regulations in 1969. The 1969 Regulations were subject to minor modifications in 1973 and 1981. The 1969 IHR were primarily intended to monitor and control six serious infectious diseases: cholera, plague, yellow fever, smallpox, relapsing fever and typhus. Under the IHR (1969), only cholera, plague and yellow fever remain notifiable, meaning that States are required to notify WHO if and when these diseases occur on their territory. In the early 1990s, the resurgence of some well-known epidemic diseases, such as cholera in parts of South America, plague in India and the emergence of new infectious agents such as Ebola hemorrhagic fever, resulted in a resolution at the 48th World Health Assembly in 1995 calling for the revision of the Regulations. In May 2001, the World Health Assembly adopted resolution WHA 54.14, Global health security: epidemic alert and response, in which WHO was called upon to support its Member States in strengthening their capacity to detect and respond rapidly to communicable disease threats and emergencies. In May 2003, resolution WHA56.28 on Revision of the International Health Regulations, established an intergovernmental working group (IGWG) open to all Member States to review and recommend a draft revision of the International Health Regulations for consideration by the World Health Assembly. The IGWG held two sessions in November 2004 and February/May 2005 with a view to endorsing a final text for consideration by the World Health Assembly at its 58th meeting. The World Health Assembly adopted the IHR (2005) on 23 May 2005 by way of resolution WHA58.3. The IHR (2005) entered into force on 15 June 2007.

The Purposes of the IHR

The purpose of the International Health Regulations is to ensure the maximum security against the international spread of diseases with a minimum interference with world traffic. Following the increasing emphasis on epidemiological surveillance for communicable disease recognition and control, the new regulations are intended to strengthen the use of epidemiological principles as applied internationally, to detect, reduce or eliminate the sources from which infection spreads, to improve sanitation in and around ports and airports, to prevent the dissemination of vectors and, in general, to encourage epidemiological activities on the national level so that there is little risk of outside infection establishing itself.

The International Health Regulations (1969)

The International Health Regulations (1969) were first introduced to help monitor and control four serious diseases that had significant potential to spread between countries, and involve:

Notification of Cases

WHO Member States are obliged to notify WHO for a single case of cholera, plague or yellow fever, occurring in humans in their territories, and give further notification when an area is free from infection. These notifications are reported in WHO's *Weekly Epidemiological Record*.

- **Health-related rules for international trade and travel:** Health-related rules for international trade and travel has been developed specially to restrict the travel under different articles of IHR 1969.
- **Health organization:** Measures for deratting, disinfecting, and disinsecting international conveyances (ships, aircraft, etc.) are to be implemented at points of arrival and departure (ports, airports and frontier posts). The health measures called for are the maximum measures that a state may apply for the protection of its territory against cholera, plague and yellow fever.
- **Health documents required:** Requirements are included for health and vaccination certificates for travelers from infected to noninfected areas; deratting/deratting exemption certificates; health declarations—Maritime Declaration of Health; Aircraft General Declaration.

The International Health Regulations (2005)

The International Health Regulations (2005) or 'IHR (2005)' are an international law which helps countries work together to save lives and livelihoods caused by the international spread of diseases and other health risks. They entered into force on 15 June 2007 and are binding on 194 countries across the globe, including all WHO Member States. The IHR (2005) establish a set of rules to support the global outbreak alert and response system and to require countries to improve international surveillance and reporting mechanisms for public health events and to strengthen their national surveillance and response capacities.

In January 2018, a group of WHO bureaucrats published an article in the British Medical Journal on Global Health entitled "Strengthening global health security by embedding the International Health Regulations requirements into national health systems", in which the authors argued that "the 2014 Ebola and 2016 Zika outbreaks, and the findings of a number of high-level assessments of the global response to these crises, that there is a need for more joined-up thinking between health system strengthening activities and health security efforts for prevention, alert and response. On 19 January 2022 the tenth Emergency Committee meeting was convened by the WHO Director-General under the International Health Regulations (2005) (IHR) regarding the coronavirus disease (COVID-19) pandemic took place on Thursday 13 January 2022 from 12:00 to 17:00 Geneva.

Aims of the IHR 2005

The IHR (2005) aim to prevent, protect against, control and respond to the international spread of disease while avoiding unnecessary interference with international traffic and trade.

The IHR (2005) are also designed to reduce the risk of disease spread at international airports, ports and ground crossings.

The Cause of IHR Revision

The dynamics of communicable disease spread in the world have changed greatly since 1969. The limitations of the IHR (1969), which led to their revision, related to their narrow scope (three diseases), their dependence on official country notification, and their lack of a formal internationally coordinated mechanism to contain international disease spread. In recent decades, cross-border travel and trade have increased and communication technology has developed markedly. News now spreads rapidly via a multitude of formal and informal channels. New challenges have arisen in the public health control of emerging and re-emerging infectious diseases. With its focus on just three diseases (cholera, plague and yellow fever), the IHR (1969) were not equipped to address the growing and varied public health risks that resulted from increased travel and trade in the last quarter of the 20th century. Severe acute respiratory syndrome (SARS) was the first disease of the 21st century to expose vulnerabilities more. In addition, some countries were reluctant to promptly report outbreaks of these diseases for fear of unwarranted and damaging travel and trade restrictions. A way needed to be found to increase the confidence of countries in reporting significant and/or unusual disease events, by linking early disclosure to prompt support and accurate information dissemination about the nature of the event.

To meet these challenges, the IHR (2005) have a much broader scope. They apply to any diseases (including those from new or unknown causes), irrespective of origin or source, that could present significant harm to humans. They address weaknesses learnt in past decades in detecting and responding to disease outbreaks. The IHR (2005) aim at protecting against international disease spread while avoiding unnecessary interference with global travel and trade. By adopting the IHR (2005) the global community has agreed that it will work together to meet these challenges. These are firmly grounded in practical experience, broaden the scope of the 1969 Regulations to cover existing, new and re-emerging diseases, including emergencies caused by noninfectious disease agents. Through a new legal framework, the IHR (2005) ensure a rapid gathering of information, a common understanding of what may constitute a public health emergency of international concern and the availability of international assistance to countries.

The IHR (2005)'s reporting procedures are aimed at expediting the flow of timely and accurate information to WHO about potential public health emergencies of international concern. Under these rules, WHO, as a neutral authority, with critical technical expertise and resources, and an extensive communications network can assess information, recommend actions and facilitate or help coordinate technical assistance, when needed, that is tailored to events as they unfold.

The IHR (2005) provide a framework for mobilizing support from governments, donors and other international partners Adopted at the Fifty-eight World Health Assembly in Geneva in May 2005, the IHR (2005) are binding obligations upon 194 countries under international law.

The Functions of the IHR (2005)

Notification: The IHR (2005) require States to notify WHO of all events that may constitute a public health emergency of international concern and to respond to requests for verification of information regarding such events. This enables WHO to ensure appropriate technical collaboration for effective prevention of such emergencies or containment of outbreaks and, under certain defined circumstances, inform other States of the public health risks where action is necessary on their part. These notification requirements, together with WHO's mandate to seek verification from countries with respect to unofficial reports of events with potential international implications is intended to promote and facilitate information sharing between WHO and States Parties to the IHR (2005).

Key Obligations for States Parties

- Designate or establish a National IHR Focal Point.
- Strengthen and maintain the capacity to detect, report and respond rapidly to public health risks and public health emergencies of international concern.
- Respond to requests for verification of information regarding potential public health emergencies of international concern.
- Assess public health events by using the decision instrument and notify WHO, within 24 hours, of all events that may constitute a public health emergency of international concern.
- Provide routine facilities, services, inspections and control activities at international airports, ports and ground crossings to prevent the international spread of disease.
- Implement appropriate measures recommended by WHO.
- Collaborate with other States Parties and with WHO on IHR (2005) implementation.

National IHR Focal Points and WHO IHR Contact Points

Under the IHR (2005) countries are required to notify and report events and other information through their National IHR Focal Points to a regional WHO IHR Contact Points. Focal points and Contact points must be available on a 24 hour-a-day basis, seven days a week. There are currently 193 National IHR Focal Points and six corresponding WHO IHR Contact Points.

The National IHR Focal Point

- Accessible at all times, 24 hours a day
- Communicate with WHO concerning
- Consultations, notifications, verification and assessments of public health events and public health response
- Ensure coordination with other ministries/sectors within the country; and notify WHO of all events that may constitute a public health emergency of international concern, within 24 hours of assessment, by using a decision instrument—a flowchart that goes through the criteria for assessment and notifications.

Requirements for National Core Capacities Under the IHR (2005)

Each State Party is required to develop, strengthen and maintain core public health capacities for surveillance and response by using existing national resources, such as the national plans for influenza pandemic preparedness. Key sanitary and health services and facilities are also to be developed at international airports, ports and ground crossings designated for this purpose by States Parties.

Recommended Measures

WHO's response to a public health emergency of international concern will include temporary recommendations concerning appropriate public health responses, and may include recommended measures for application by the State affected by such an emergency, as well as by other states and by operators of international transport. These temporary recommendations are made by WHO on a time-limited, risk-specific basis, as a result of a public health emergency of international concern. Standing recommendations indicate the appropriate measures for routine application for specific ongoing public health risks, and are of routine or periodic application. Recommended measures could be directed towards persons, baggage, cargo, containers, ships, aircraft, road vehicles, goods or postal parcels. External advice regarding the IHR (2005). The IHR (2005) include procedures for obtaining independent technical advice concerning IHR implementation. One context is the process for the establishment of an Emergency Committee to advise the Director-General of WHO in determining whether a particular event is, in fact, a public health emergency of international concern and to provide advice on any appropriate temporary recommendations. An IHR Review Committee is tasked with advising the Director-General on technical matters relating to standing recommendations, the functioning of the Regulations and amendments thereto.

Public Health Emergency of International Concern

According to the IHR (2005) a public health emergency of international concern refers to an extraordinary public health event which is determined, under specific procedures. These are:

- To constitute a public health risk to other states through the international spread of disease
- To potentially require a coordinated international response.

To ensure adequate and early communications with WHO about potential international public health emergencies, the IHR (2005) include a decision instrument (Annex 2 of the Regulations) which sets the parameters for notification to WHO of all events which may constitute a public health emergency of international concern (PHEIC) based on the following criteria:

- Seriousness of the public health impact of the event
- Unusual or unexpected nature of the event
- Potential for the event to spread internationally; and/or
- The risk that restrictions to travel or trade may result because of the event.
- Timely and transparent notification of events combined with a collaborative assessment of the risks by the concerned State and WHO, along with effective risk communication will reduce the potential for international disease spread and the likelihood of unilateral imposition of trade or travel restrictions by other countries.

The Emergency Committee

The Emergency Committee is made up of international experts to provide technical advice to the WHO Director-General in the context of a 'public health emergency of international concern' (PHEIC). It provides its views on whether the event constitutes a public health emergency of international concern"

- The temporary recommendations that should be taken by the country
- Experiencing an emergency of international concern, or by other countries
- Prevent or reduce the international spread of disease and avoid unnecessary interference with international trade and travel
- The termination of a public health emergency of international concern.

The Members of the Emergency Committee

WHO maintains an IHR Expert Roster composed of international experts in such fields as disease control, virology, vaccine development or infectious disease epidemiology. WHO's Director-General selects members of the Emergency Committee from this roster and, where appropriate, from other WHO expert advisory panels and committees. Members can be selected on the basis of expertise required for any particular session. At least one member of the Emergency Committee should be an expert nominated by a State Party within whose territory the event arises, and such States Parties are invited to present their views to the Emergency Committee.

The Director-General may also appoint one or more technical experts to advise the committee, on his or her own initiative or at the request of the Committee.

Selection Procedure

Selection of members is based primarily on their technical ability and experience in the relevant fields of expertise. The Director-General aims to ensure that members of the IHR Emergency Committee have the broadest possible geographical representation, and reflect diverse knowledge, practical experience and approaches. Achieving gender balance is also a desirable aim. Members of WHO advisory panels and committees do not receive any remuneration from the Organization. Their names, job titles and any other information that could be determined to be a potential conflict of interest are published on WHO's website.

The Emergency Committee's Job Responsibilities

The Emergency Committee will provide its view to the Director General on:

- Whether the event constitutes a public health emergency of international concern.
- The temporary recommendations that should be taken by countries on areas including travel, surveillance, clinical management, infection control.
- The termination of a public health emergency of international concern.
- All decisions.

WHO's Responsibilities

WHO also has increased responsibilities under the IHR (2005) and will continue to strengthen its ability to fulfill these broadened obligation.

WHO's major tasks include:

- Designating WHO IHR Contact Points
- Coordinating global surveillance and assessment of significant public health risks, and disseminating public health information to States Parties
- Supporting States Parties to assess their existing national public health structures and resources, as well as to build and strengthen their core public health
- Capacities for surveillance and response, and at designated points of entry. The difference between IHR 1969 and IHR 2005 has been given in **Table 17.2.**
- Determining whether particular events constitute a public health emergency of international concern, with advice from external experts
- Developing and recommending measures for use by Member States during a public health emergency of international concern (after consultation with external experts)
- Providing technical assistance to Member States in their response to public
- Health emergencies of international concern; and monitoring and evaluation of IHR (2005) implementation and adapting technical guidelines to reflect the evolving needs.

INTERNATIONAL COOPERATION AND ASSISTANCE

Introduction

The problem of access to medicines unduly burdens for the developing countries around the world. It has been estimated that 'infectious diseases kill over 14 million people each year, nine out of ten of whom live in the developing world.' Children, young adults in Africa Southeast Asia bear a heavy burden in infectious diseases, where half of the deaths among this group are due to six treatable diseases—HIV/AIDS (14% of deaths), acute respiratory syndrome (11%), diarrheal diseases (11%), malaria (8%), measles (6%), TB (2%). Despite the existence of effective medicines, millions of people will continue to suffer die needlessly from these other life-threatening conditions because they cannot access the necessary treatments. It has been estimated that as many as two billion people (one-third of the world's population) lacks access to such essential medicines.

Table 17.2: Difference between IHR 1969 and IHR 2005.

	IHR (1969)	*IHR (2005)*
Scope	Cholera, plague, yellow fever	Any potential public health emergency of international concern (PHEIC)
Risk assessment	Identify specific infectious diseases	Decision instrument to evaluate the risks and potential impact of the public health event
Communications	Health ministry's wire or fax reports to WHO	WHO sends and receives information via designated National Focal Points
Notifications	WHO dependent on official notifications	WHO can initiate requests for information, consider unofficial sources
Actions allowed	Predetermined, disease-specific	Flexible, temporary recommendations
International responses	No mechanism for coordination	Coordinated assistance in response/recommended measure
National capacities	Provide inspections and disease control at points of entry	Provide inspections and disease control at points of entry AND develop minimum core capacities to detect, assess, report, and respond to any potential PHEIC at the local, intermediate, and national levels

Notably those suffering from HIV/AIDS have highlighted the acute need for support of their plight. Novel institutions have been established to provide funds, such as UNAIDS; the Global Fund to Fight AIDS, Tuberculosis, Malaria; the US President's Emergency Plan for AIDS Relief (PEPFAR). Bold declarations have emerged in a variety of policy, for example, World Trade Organization (WTO) member states issued a formal declaration affirming that it's Agreement on Trade-Related Aspects of Intellectual Property Rights (TRIPS) 'can be interpreted, implemented in a manner supportive of WTO members' right to protect public in particular, to promote access to medicines for all'. This includes the government option to use TRIPS 'flexibilities', such as compulsory licensing parallel importation, to address public concerns.

In what manner should developed countries assist and cooperate? To address this question, the tripartite classification of obligations (that is, to respect, to protect, to fulfill) has been used to elaborate on the developed country duty of in greater detail. The duty to respect, which has been called a 'classic' human rights obligation, refers to the requirement that states 'avoid measures that hinder or prevent the enjoyment of rights in another state'. Such measures would include a state's foreign policies any aspects that might interfere with the realization of rights outside of the state. The duty to protect requires that states take account of human rights in their actions as members of organizations, as well as when entering into bilateral multilateral agreements. It also calls upon states to take measures to prevent nonstate entities under their jurisdiction from interfering with the enjoyment of the rights abroad. Such nonstate entities include private corporations that reside within their national jurisdiction but operate internationally or have an impact on other states; measures to prevent them can take the form of domestic legislation to regulate their activities. The duty to fulfill has been defined as the obligation of the state to take positive steps by facilitating, providing, promoting human rights in other states. This particular duty has been considered controversial, given its emphasis on positive state action in other countries, but is gaining acceptance in the human rights community as a 'secondary or subsidiary obligation [that] applies if the domestic state for reasons beyond its control fails to fulfill economic, social, cultural rights' when 'measures taken to respect protect are not sufficient.'

Meaning and Definition

The literal meaning of the word cooperation is work together. International cooperation means cooperation between the nations for any reasons like: health, political affairs, tourism, etc. Here our main focus on cooperation for the improvement of health status of the people around the world.

Importance

- Capitalizing on migration to benefit development can best succeed through cooperative efforts.
- Effective management of migration can only begin to be achieved if there is a clear understanding of the trends and flows in migration movement (based on the collection, sharing, and analysis of migration data between States).
- International cooperation makes a difference in managing labor migration.
- In order to address trafficking in persons, States need to share law enforcement information to understand and follow patterns, and to break up organized crime networks.
- The global commitment to work towards a world with enhanced social equity and reduced poverty that informs the Millennium Development Goals (MDGs) can be achieved.
- Effective migration management requires cooperation and dialogue, not only among States, but also among all interested stakeholders, including international organizations, nongovernmental organizations, and the private sector.
- Effective migration management is achieved through balanced consideration of economic, social, political, humanitarian, developmental, and environmental factors, taking into account the root causes of migratory flows.
- Migration management requires partnerships and responsibility sharing. Cooperation may develop where:
  - There are similar problems to resolve
  - There are similar challenges to manage
  - There are different migration-related interests and goals, but it is in a State's political interest to find a cooperative solution
  - There are some common interests and other conflicting interests.

International cooperation can be bilateral, regional, inter-regional, or international, and that it may occur between or among States, between States and organizations, or between organizations. There are many sectors where international cooperation exists like trade, labor, development, health, data, trafficking, smuggling, and irregular migration are the examples of areas of cooperation. International cooperation can take a variety of forms from informal discussion and the sharing of policy and program information, to more formal operational and activity-based cooperation, including joint management, technical cooperation, and other forms of responsibility sharing.

Bilateral Cooperation

For many years, cooperation between governments in the management of migration has taken place through bilateral agreements. Cooperation is defined as bilateral when originating in an agreement between two countries and their respective official financial or technical agencies. Government agencies channeling funding to developing countries are known as bilateral agencies. Early agreements were primarily in the area of labor migration between States facing labor shortages and those with a labor surplus. In recent years, there has been increasing focus on bilateral agreements dealing with the return and readmission of persons without authorization to stay, sometimes including other forms of cooperation or assistance. Other bilateral cooperation arrangements have included management of a common border.

Multilateral Cooperation

Cooperation is defined as multilateral when the relationship is between a country and multilateral international organizations (e.g., development banks, United Nations agencies) or when the relationship is exists more than two countries.

Regional Cooperation

Regional arrangements for international cooperation have existed for decades. During the 1990s, and continuing into this century, multilateral Regional Consultative Processes (RCPs) are emerging as an effective mechanism to carry forward cooperative efforts in regional or international migration management, offering the participating States the opportunity to share experiences with other States of the same geographic region. Participation is informal and nonbinding. There is a growing convergence of ideas among most Regional Consultative Processes regarding many of the key elements and principles that can guide international migration management, including safeguarding migrant rights, refugee protection, border management, and addressing root causes of migration. Currently, Regional Consultative Processes exist in most regions of the world, and an increasing number of governments participate in one or more of these processes. Trends towards regional economic integration and political cooperation in many parts of the world increasingly include consideration of migration.

Important Points to be Remembered for International Cooperation

- Agreements should be balanced and will normally require some give-and-take by all parties.
- The benefits of the agreement for each party should be meaningful, but realistic and financially feasible.
- Cooperative approaches should include regular evaluation.
- Cooperative agreements should address long-term needs, and not be limited to short- and medium-term goals.

- New policies that result from cooperative agreements should be tested and assessed.
- Interstate cooperation may include the provision of assistance to some States by other States.
- Parties to an agreement should strive for transparent and focused dialogue and exchange of information, particularly where countries share an interest in specific migratory patterns in order to facilitate possible responsibility-sharing arrangements.
- Consideration should be given to developing equitable and effective responsibility-sharing arrangements that reduce the burdens on countries hosting large numbers of refugees and countries of first asylum.

National Policies and International Cooperation

Effective national migration policy is challenged to find, and maintain, a **balance** between measures that address a number of migration-related areas, and to avoid favoring one area over other equally important areas. Effective national-level policy should include the policies that do not consider regular migration and irregular migration in isolation from each other. Consideration of the impact that national migration policy could have on a number of related areas like:

- Economic growth
- Public services
- Social cohesion
- Public protection and national security
- Support for human rights
- International development
- Coordination between responsible authorities at all stages in the migration process and, where appropriate, consideration for centralized migration management functions in a dedicated ministry.

INTERNATIONAL QUARANTINE

The international quarantine has been written in a separate file to be written here.

Federal Law

The federal government derives its authority for isolation and quarantine from the Commerce Clause of the US Constitution.

Federal isolation and quarantine are authorized for these communicable diseases:

- Cholera
- Diphtheria
- Infectious tuberculosis
- Plague
- Smallpox
- Yellow fever
- Viral hemorrhagic fevers
- Severe acute respiratory syndromes
- Flu that can cause a pandemic.

Federal isolation and quarantine are authorized by Executive Order of the President. The President can revise this list by Executive Order. Under section 361 of the Public Health Service Act (42 US Code § 264), the US Secretary of Health and Human Services is authorized to take measures to prevent the entry and spread of communicable diseases from foreign countries into the United States and between states. The authority for carrying out these functions on a daily basis has been delegated to the Centers for Disease Control and Prevention (CDC).

CDC's Role

Under 42 Code of Federal Regulations parts 70 and 71, CDC is authorized to detain, medically examine, and release persons arriving into the United States and traveling between states who are suspected of carrying these communicable diseases. As part of its federal authority, CDC routinely monitors persons arriving at US land border crossings and passengers and crew arriving at US ports of entry for signs or symptoms of communicable diseases. When alerted about an ill passenger or crew member by the pilot of a plane or captain of a ship, CDC may detain passengers and crew as necessary to investigate whether the cause of the illness on board is a communicable disease.

State, Local, and Tribal Law

States have police power functions to protect the health, safety, and welfare of persons within their borders. To control the spread of disease within their borders, states have laws to enforce the use of isolation and quarantine. These laws can vary from state to state and can be specific or broad. In some states, local health authorities implement state law. In most states, breaking a quarantine order is a criminal misdemeanor. Tribes also have police power authority to take actions that promote the health, safety, and welfare of their own tribal members. Tribal health authorities may enforce their own isolation and quarantine laws within tribal lands, if such laws exist.

Who is In Charge?

The federal government:

- Acts to prevent the entry of communicable diseases into the United States. Quarantine and isolation may be used at US ports of entry.
- It is authorized to take measures to prevent the spread of communicable diseases between states.
- May accept state and local assistance in enforcing federal quarantine.
- May assist state and local authorities in preventing the spread of communicable diseases.

State, local, and tribal authorities:

- Enforce isolation and quarantine within their borders.

It is possible for federal, state, local, and tribal health authorities to have and use all at the same time separate but coexisting legal quarantine power in certain events. In the event of a conflict, federal law is supreme.

Enforcement

- If a quarantinable disease is suspected or identified, CDC may issue a federal isolation or quarantine order.
- Public health authorities at the federal, state, local, and tribal levels may sometimes seek help from police or other law enforcement officers to enforce a public health order.
- US Customs and Border Protection and US Coast Guard officers are authorized to help enforce federal quarantine orders.
- Breaking a federal quarantine order is punishable by fines and imprisonment.
- Federal law allows the conditional release of persons from quarantine if they comply with medical monitoring and surveillance.

Criteria for Requesting Federal Travel Restrictions for Public Health Purposes

The Centers for Disease Control and Prevention (CDC) in the Department of Health and Human Services (HHS) is publishing this Notice to inform the public of the criteria CDC considers for requesting federal travel restrictions for public health purposes, including for use of the Do Not Board (DNB) list and Public Health Border Lookout records. Individuals with communicable diseases that pose a public health threat to travelers can be placed on this list to restrict them from boarding commercial aircraft arriving into, departing from, or traveling within the United States. This notice further describes the factors that HHS/CDC will consider in evaluating whether to request that an individual who may have been exposed to a hemorrhagic fever virus be placed on the DNB list, which is administered by the Department of Homeland Security (DHS). It also contains information for individuals who have been placed on this list to respond to this decision in writing.

Signals and Flags used in Quarantine Purpose

Plain yellow, green, and even black flags have been used to symbolize disease in both ships and ports, with the color yellow having a longer historical precedent, as a color of marking for houses of infection, previous to its use as a maritime marking color for disease. The present flag used for the purpose is the 'Lima' (L) flag, which is a mixture of yellow and black flags previously used. It is sometimes called the 'yellow jack' but this was also a name for yellow fever, which probably derives its common name from the flag, not the color of the victims (cholera ships also used a yellow flag). The plain yellow flag ('Quebec' or Q in international maritime signal flags), probably derives its letter symbol for its initial use in quarantine, but this flag in modern times indicates the opposite—a ship that declares itself free of quarantinable disease, and requests boarding and routine port inspection.

Quarantine Laws of Some Nation

Australia

Australia has perhaps the world's strictest quarantine laws on products imported from other countries. As Australia has been geographically isolated from other major continents for millions of years, there is an endemically unique ecosystem free of pests and diseases. If other products are brought inside along with pests and diseases, it would damage the ecosystem seriously and add millions of costs in the local agricultural businesses.

The Australian Quarantine and Inspection Service is responsible for border-inspection of any products which are brought into Australia, and assess the potential risks the products might harm Australian environment. Visitors are required to fill in the information card truthfully before arriving in Australia, and declare what food and any products made of wood and other natural materials they have processed. If the visitor fails to do so, usually a quarantine fine of 220 Australian dollars are to be paid as quarantine infringement notice, and if not, the visitor may face criminal convictions of fining 100,000 Australian dollars and 10 years imprisonment.

Canada

There are three quarantine Acts of Parliament in Canada: Quarantine Act (humans) and Health of Animals Act (animals) and Plant Protection Act (vegetations). The first legislation is enforced by the Canada Border Services Agency after a complete rewrite in 2005. The second and third legislations are enforced by the Canadian Food Inspection Agency. If a health emergency exists, the Governor in Council can prohibit importation of anything that it deems necessary under the Quarantine Act.

Under the Quarantine Act, all travelers must submit to screening and if they believe they might have come into contact with communicable disease or vectors, they must disclose their whereabouts to a Border Services Officer. If the officer has reasonable grounds that the traveler is or might have been infected with a communicable disease or refused to provide answers, a quarantine officer (QO) must be called and the person is to be isolated. If a person refused to be isolated, any peace officer may arrest without warrant.

A QO who has reasonable grounds to believe that the traveler has or might have a communicable disease or is infested with vectors, after the medical examination of a traveler, can order him/her into treatment or measures to prevent the person from spreading the disease. QO can detain any traveler who refused to comply with his/her order or undergo health assessments as required by law.

Under the Health of Animals Act and Plant Protection Act, inspectors can prohibit access to an infected area, dispose or treat any infected or suspected to be infected animals or plants. The Minister can order for compensation to be given if animals/plants were destroyed pursuant to these acts.

Each province also enacts its own quarantine/environmental health legislations.

Hong Kong

Under the Prevention and Control of Disease Ordinance (HK Laws, Chap 599), a health officer may seize articles he/she believes to be infectious or contains infectious agents. All travelers, if requested, must submit themselves to a health officer. Failure to do so is against the law and is subject to arrest and prosecution.

The law allows for a health officer who has reasonable grounds to detain, isolate, and quarantine anyone or anything believed to be infected and to restrict any articles from leaving a designated quarantine area. He/she may also order the Civil Aviation Department to prohibit the landing or leaving, embarking or disembarking of an aircraft. This power also extends to land, sea or air crossings.

Under the same ordinance, any police officer, health officer, members of the Civil Aid Service or Auxiliary Medical Service can arrest a person who obstructs or escape from detention.

United Kingdom

To reduce the risk of introducing rabies from continental Europe, the United Kingdom used to require that dogs, and most other animals introduced to the country spend six months in quarantine at an HM Customs and Excise pound; this policy was abolished in 2000 in favor of a scheme generally known as Pet Passports, where animals can avoid quarantine if they have documentation showing they are up to date on their appropriate vaccinations.

United States

Quarantine law began in Colonial America in 1663, when in an attempt to curb an outbreak of smallpox, the city of New York established a quarantine. In the 1730s, the city built a quarantine station on the Bedloe's Island. The Philadelphia Lazaretto was the first quarantine hospital in the United States, built in 1799, in Tinicum Township, Delaware County, Pennsylvania. There are similar national landmarks such as Swinburne Island and Angel Island (a much more famous historic site, Ellis Island, is often mistakenly assumed to have been a quarantine station, however its marine hospital only qualified as a contagious disease facility to handle less virulent diseases like measles, trachoma and less advanced stages of tuberculosis and diphtheria; persons afflicted with smallpox, yellow fever, cholera, leprosy or typhoid fever, could neither be received nor treated there). During the 1918 flu pandemic, people were also quarantined. The last person to be quarantined in the United States was a woman in 1963 for smallpox.

In the summer of 2007, Atlanta attorney Andrew Speaker made headlines when, while traveling in Italy on his honeymoon, he was diagnosed by the US Centers for Disease Control and Prevention (CDC) with extremely drug-resistant tuberculosis (XDR-TB), a contagious, untreatable and potentially-lethal condition. Against the instructions of US public health authorities, Speaker re-entered the US only to be served by the CDC with a federal order of quarantine at a hospital in New York, the first such order to be issued in nearly half a century. Speaker challenged the CDC's diagnosis of XDR-TB, resulting in an eventual downgrade of his condition and the lifting of restrictions on his movements. The Speaker case generated significant public attention and Congress conducted formal hearings regarding the incident. Speaker's case highlights a crucial issue in public health law, the circumstances, if any, under which public officials may detain individuals against their will in order to protect the public from communicable diseases. In other words, when do utilitarian principles of social good trump the guarantees of individual rights afforded by the United States Constitution.

INTERNATIONAL TRADE IN INDIA

International trade is exchange of capital, goods, and services across international borders or territories. In most countries, it represents a significant share of gross domestic product (GDP). While international trade has been present throughout much of history (see Silk Road, Amber Road), its economic, social, and political importance has been on the rise in recent centuries.

Importance of International Trade

International trade is the backbone of our modern, commercial world, as producers in various nations try to profit from an expanded market, rather than be limited to selling within their own borders. There are many reasons that trade across national borders occurs, including lower production costs in one region versus another, specialized industries, lack or surplus of natural resources and consumer tastes. Without international trade, nations would be limited to the goods and services produced within their own borders.

Risks in International Trade

- War and other uncontrollable events. In addition, international trade also faces the risk of unfavorable exchange rate movements
- Political risk (change in leadership interfering with transactions or prices)
- Intervention (governmental action to prevent a transaction being completed)
- Regulatory risk (e.g., a change in rules that prevents the transaction)
- Credit risk (allowing the buyer to take possession of goods prior to payment)
- Nonacceptance (buyer rejects goods as different from the agreed upon specifications)
- Buyer insolvency (purchaser cannot pay).

Health Risk

International travel can pose various risks to health, depending on the characteristics of both the traveler and the travel. Travelers may encounter sudden and significant changes in altitude, humidity, microbes, and temperature, which can result in ill-health. In addition, serious health risks may arise in areas where accommodation is of poor quality, hygiene and sanitation are inadequate, medical services are not well developed and clean water is unavailable.

The elimination of spatial and temporal barriers, especially by long-distance air transport, means that humans can reach almost any part of the Earth. The contact between microbes, humans, and animals may result in infection, which may be expressed in disease or death. Another potential consequence of the movement of species, such as arthropods, mammals and other animals, and plants may cause major changes in the existing ecosystem, including marine ecosystems. Many examples exist of the harmful effects of invasive species, though many species of well-regarded plants and animals in the Americas were not native to the Americas.

Animals have been the origin of many of the recently identified emerging infectious diseases, including HIV/AIDS, H5N1 avian influenza, severe acute respiratory syndrome (SARS) and swine-origin H1N1 influenza. Populations of animals have expanded rapidly, in large part to accommodate the desire for more animal protein in the diet, which has coincided with the economic resources to buy it. Human travelers can easily carry person-to-person transmitted infections to any part of the world. An example is the human immunodeficiency virus (HIV), which was introduced to all areas of the world almost exclusively by travelers. Recently, swine-origin H1N1 has spread globally, its movement hastened by global air travel. Although drug-resistant forms of tuberculosis can emerge in settings with inadequate and inappropriate treatment regimens, humans also transport and transmit tuberculosis, including multidrug resistant (MDR) and now extensively resistant (XDR) forms of tuberculosis, in geographic areas far from the point of acquisition.

MIGRATION

The movement by people from one place to another with the intention of settling in the new location. The movement is typically over long distances and from one country to another, but internal migration is also possible. Migration may be individuals, family units or in large groups.

Push Factors

- Not enough jobs
- Few opportunities
- Inadequate conditions
- Desertification
- Famine or drought
- Political fear or persecution
- Slavery or forced labor
- Poor medical care
- Loss of wealth
- Natural disasters
- Death threats
- Desire for more political or religious freedom
- Pollution
- Poor housing
- Landlord/tenant issues
- Bullying
- Discrimination
- Poor chances of marrying
- Condemned housing (radon gas, etc.)
- War

Pull Factors

- Job opportunities
- Better living conditions
- The feeling of having more political and/or religious freedom
- Enjoyment
- Education
- Better medical care
- Attractive climates
- Security
- Family links
- Industry
- Better chances of marrying

Human migration is movement by humans from one place to another, sometimes over long distances or in large groups. Historically this movement was nomadic, often causing significant conflict with the indigenous population and their displacement or cultural assimilation. Only a few nomadic people have retained this form of lifestyle in modern times. Migration has continued under the form of both voluntary migration within one's region, country, or beyond and involuntary migration (which includes the slave trade, trafficking in human beings and ethnic cleansing). People who migrate into a territory are called immigrants, while at the departure point they are called emigrants. Small populations migrating to develop a territory considered void of settlement depending on historical setting, circumstances and perspective are referred to as settlers or colonists, while populations displaced by immigration and colonization are called refugees. The rest of this article will cover migration in the sense of a 'change of residence', rather than the temporary migrations of travel, tourism, pilgrimages, or the commute.

Migration Statistics

According to the International Organization for Migration's World Migration Report 2010, the number of international migrants was estimated at 220 million in 2013. If this number continues to grow at the same pace as during the last 20 years, it could reach 405 million by 2050. While some modern migration is a by-product of, political conflicts and natural disasters (for example, emigration from Montserrat to the UK following the eruption of the island's volcano), contemporary migration is predominantly economically motivated. In particular, there are wide disparities in the incomes that can be earned for similar work in different countries of the world. There are also, at any given time, some jobs in some high-wage countries for which there is a shortage of appropriately skilled or qualified citizens. Some countries (e.g., UK and Australia) operate points systems that give some lawful immigration visas to some noncitizens who are qualified for such shortage jobs. Noncitizens, therefore, have an economic incentive to obtain the necessary skills and qualifications in their own countries and then apply for, and migrate to take up these job vacancies. International migration similarly motivated by economic disparities and opportunities occurs within the EU, where legal barriers to migration between member countries have been wholly or partially lifted. Countries with higher prevailing wage levels, such as France, Germany, Italy and the UK are net recipients of immigration from lower-wage member countries such as Greece, Hungary, Lithuania, Poland and Romania.

Some contemporary economic migration occurs even where the migrant becomes illegally resident in their destination country and therefore at major disadvantage in the employment market. Illegal immigrants are, for example, known to cross in significant numbers, typically at night, from Mexico into the US, from Mozambique into South Africa, from Bulgaria and Turkey into Greece, from North Africa into Spain and Italy and from Bangladesh into India.

The pressures of human migrations, whether as outright conquest or by slow cultural infiltration and resettlement, have affected the grand epochs in history and in land (for example, the decline of the Roman Empire); under the form of colonization, migration has transformed the world (such as the prehistoric and historic settlements of Australia and the Americas). Population genetics studied in traditionally settled modern populations have opened a window into the historical patterns of migrations, a technique pioneered by Luigi Luca Cavalli-Sforza.

Forced migration has been a means of social control under authoritarian regimes, yet free-initiative migration is a powerful factor in social adjustment and the growth of urban populations.

In December 2003, The Global Commission on International Migration (GCIM) was launched with the support of Secretary-General of the United Nations Kofi Annan and several countries, with an independent 19-member commission, a threefold mandate and a finite lifespan ending December 2005. Its report, based on regional consultation meetings with stakeholders and scientific reports from leading international migration experts, was published and presented to Kofi Annan on 5 October 2005.

International migration challenges at the global level are addressed through the Global Migration Group, established in 2006.

Different Types of Migration Include

- Seasonal human migration mainly related to agriculture and tourism to urban places
- Rural to urban, more common in developing countries as industrialization takes effect (urbanization)
- Urban to rural, more common in developed countries due to a higher cost of urban living (suburbanization)
- International migration.

Premodern Migrations

Historical migration of human populations begins with the movement of *Homo erectus* out of Africa across Eurasia about a million years ago. *Homo sapiens* appear to have occupied all of Africa about 150,000 years ago, moved out of Africa 70,000 years ago, and had spread across Australia, Asia and Europe by 40,000 years BC. Migration to the Americas took place 20,000 to 15,000 years ago, and by 2,000 years ago, most of the Pacific Islands were colonized. Later population movements notably include the Neolithic Revolution, Indo-European expansion, and the Early Medieval Great Migrations including Turkic expansion. In some places, substantial cultural transformation occurred following the migration of relatively small elite populations, Turkey and Azerbaijan being such examples. In Britain, it is considered that the Roman and Norman conquests were similar examples, while 'the most hotly debated of all the British cultural transitions is the role of migration in the relatively sudden and drastic change from Romano-Britain to Anglo-Saxon Britain,' which may be explained by a possible 'substantial migration of Anglo-Saxon Y chromosomes into Central England (contributing 50–100% to the gene pool at that time).'

Early humans migrated due to many factors such as changing climate and landscape and inadequate food supply. The evidence indicates that the ancestors of the Austronesian peoples spread from the South Chinese mainland to Taiwan at sometime around 8,000 years ago. Evidence from historical linguistics suggests that it is from this island that seafaring peoples migrated, perhaps in distinct waves separated by millennia, to the entire region encompassed by the Austronesian languages. It is believed that this migration began around 6,000 years ago. Indo-Aryan migration from the Indus Valley to the plain of the River Ganges in Northern India is presumed to have taken place in the Middle to Late Bronze Age, contemporary to the Late Harappan phase in India (ca. 1700 to 1300 BC). From 180 BC, a series of invasions from Central Asia followed, including those led by the Indo-Greeks, Indo-Scythians, Indo-Parthians and Kushans in the northwestern Indian subcontinent.

From 728 BC, the Greeks began 250 years of expansion, settling colonies in several places, including Sicily and Marseille. In Europe, two waves of migrations dominate demographic distributions, that of the Celtic people and that of the later Migration Period from the North and East, both being possible examples of general cultural change sparked by primarily elite and warrior migration. Other examples are small movements like that of the Magyars into Pannonia (modern-day Hungary). Turkic peoples spread from their homeland in modern Turkestan across most of Central Asia into Europe and the Middle East between the 6th and 11th centuries. Recent research suggests that Madagascar was uninhabited until Austronesian seafarers from Indonesia arrived during the 5th and 6th centuries AD. Subsequent migrations from both the Pacific and Africa further consolidated this original mixture, and Malagasy people emerged.

Modern Migrations

Industrialization and the rise of nationalism/imperialism. While the pace of migration had accelerated since the 18th century already (including the involuntary slave trade), it would increase further in the 19th century. Manning distinguishes three major types of migration: labor migration, refugee migrations, and urbanization. Millions of agricultural workers left the countryside and moved to the cities causing unprecedented levels of urbanization. This phenomenon began in Britain in the late 18th century and spread around the world and continues to this day in many areas.

Industrialization encouraged migration wherever it appeared. The increasingly global economy globalized the labor market. The Atlantic slave trade diminished sharply after 1820, which gave rise to self-bound contract labor migration from Europe and Asia to plantations. Over population, open agricultural frontiers, and rising industrial centers attracted voluntary migrants. Moreover, migration was significantly made easier by improved transportation techniques.

Romantic nationalism also rose in the 19th century, and, with it, ethnocentrism. The great European industrial empires also rose. Both factors contributed to migration, as some countries favored their own ethnicities over outsiders and other countries appeared to be considerably more welcoming. For example, the Russian Empire identified with Eastern Orthodoxy, and confined Jews, who were not Eastern Orthodox, to the Pale of Settlement and imposed restrictions. Violence was also a problem. The United States was promoted as a better location, a 'golden land' where Jews could live more openly. Another effect of imperialism, colonialism, led to the migration of some colonizing parties from 'home countries' to 'the colonies', and eventually the migration of people from 'colonies' to 'home countries'.

Transnational labor migration reached a peak of three million migrants per year in the early twentieth century. Italy, Norway, Ireland and the Guangdong region of China were regions with especially high emigration rates during these years. These large migration flows influenced the process of nation state formation in many ways. Immigration restrictions have been developed, as well as diaspora cultures and myths that reflect the importance of migration to the foundation of certain nations, like the American melting pot. The transnational labor migration fell to a lower level from 1930s to the 1960s and then rebounded.

The United States experienced considerable internal migration related to industrialization, including its African American population. From 1910–1970, approximately 7 million African Americans migrated from the rural Southern United States, where blacks faced both poor economic opportunities and considerable political and social prejudice, to the industrial cities of the Northeast, Midwest and West, where relatively well-paid jobs were available. This phenomenon came to be known in the United States as its own Great Migration. With the demise of legalized segregation in the 1960s and greatly improved economic opportunities in the South in the subsequent decades, millions of blacks have returned to the South from other parts of the country since 1980 in what has been called the New Great Migration.

International Organization for Migration (IOM)

IOM's Vision on Migration Health

Migrants and mobile populations benefit from an improved standard of physical, mental and social wellbeing, which enables them to substantially contribute towards the social and economic development of their home communities and host societies. The public health approaches for benefits of migrants health has been given in **Figure 17.1**.

IOM's Strategic Objectives on Migration Health

IOM's strategic objectives on migration health are derived from the 2008 World Health Assembly Resolution on the Health of Migrants (61.17) that recommends action along four pillars. These four pillars have been further operationalized and agreed during the Global Consultation on the Health of Migrants organized by WHO, IOM and the Government of Spain (Madrid, 2010):

- Monitoring migrant health
- Enable conducive policy and legal frameworks on migrant health
- Strengthen migrant friendly health systems
- Facilitate partnerships, networks and multi-country frameworks on migrant health.

These strategic objectives are in line with the four basic principles for a public health approach to address the health of migrants and host communities (WHO, 2008):

- To avoid disparities in health status and access to health services between migrants and the host population.
- To ensure migrants' health rights. This entails limiting discrimination or stigmatization, and removing impediments to migrants' access to preventive and curative interventions, which are the basic health entitlements of the host population.
- To put in place lifesaving interventions so as to reduce excess mortality and morbidity among migrant populations. This is of particular relevance in situations of forced migration resulting from disasters or conflict.
- To minimize the negative health outcomes of the migration process on migrants' health outcomes. Migration generally renders migrants more vulnerable to health risks and exposes them to potential hazards and greater stress arising from displacement, and adaptation to new environments.

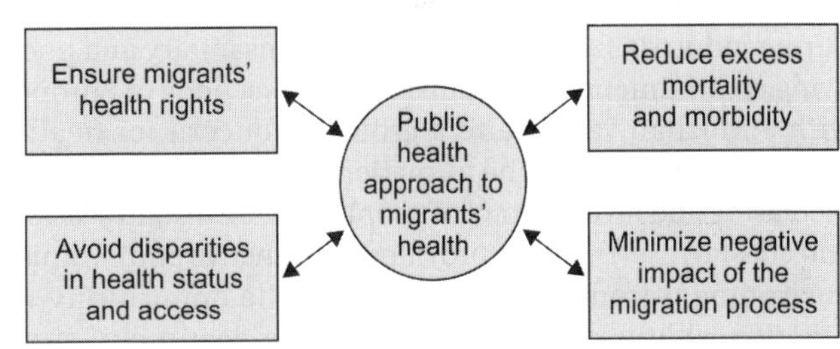

Fig. 17.1: Public health approach to migrant health.

HEALTH TOURISM

Medical tourism refers to the travel of people to another country for the purpose of obtaining medical treatment in that country. Traditionally, people would travel from less-developed countries to major medical centers in highly developed countries for medical treatment that was unavailable in their own communities.

Health tourism is a wider term for travels that focus on medical treatments and the utilization of health care services. It spans a wide field of health-oriented tourism ranging from preventive and health-conductive to rehabilitational and curative forms of travel; the latter being commonly referred to as Medical tourism.

Factors Responsible for Health Tourism

Factors that have led to the increasing popularity of medical travel include the high cost of health care, long wait times for certain procedures, the ease and affordability of international travel, and improvements in both technology and standards of care in many countries. The avoidance of waiting times is the leading factor for medical tourism from the UK, whereas in the US, the main reason is cheaper prices abroad.

Many surgery procedures performed in medical tourism destinations cost a fraction of the price they do in other countries. For example, a liver transplant that costs US $300,000 in America costs about 91,000 USD in Taiwan. A large draw to medical travel is convenience and speed. Countries that operate public health care systems often have long wait times for certain operations.

History of Health Tourism

Health tourism, with a focus on good health, general well-being and its pursuit, is not a new phenomenon. In Ancient time in Italy and throughout the Roman provinces, the Ancient Romans constructed resorts with thermal health spas, and the Ancient Greeks would travel 'to Epidauria to visit the sanctuary of the healing god, Asklepios, who revealed remedies to them in their dreams. From the 15th to 17th centuries, the poor sanitary conditions in Europe prompted an interest by the rich in medicinal spas, mineral springs and the seaside for health purposes. These wealthy individuals would also travel to renowned medical schools for medical assistance. This continued into the 18th and 19th centuries where spa towns, particularly in the south of France, became popular for health cures, the sun, and escaping the cold climatic conditions in the north of Europe. The rapid urbanization and social change experienced during industrialization aggravated the unsanitary and poor living environments in Britain and some sections of Europe, with antiurban values and a growing concern for health developing as a result. The formation of the railways allowed increasing and diverse flows of people to more distant seaside and coastal resorts, which provided a distinctive and escapist environment from urbanization, and the opportunity to practice what was viewed as a healthy pastime of sun-seeking. At the same time, escaping to spas and seaside resorts for 'taking the waters', was not simply about health, as it became fashionable and sociable activity. Spa tourism and sun-seeking persisted into the 20th century. Medicinal springs, spas, beaches and resorts, particularly in warm and dry climates, continued to be considered therapeutic through long exposures to the sun, fresh air and water. In today's climate, health care has become a global market, with emerging, developing and developed nations competing for health tourists.

The types of health and medical interventions on offer have considerably diversified, ranging from superficial treatments (such as facials and massages) to highly invasive and risky surgical procedures (such as open heart surgery) and, in some cases, a combination of both (for example cosmetic tourism, which encompasses cosmetic and reconstructive surgery and some forms of dentistry). Another important development in health and medical tourism appears in the emphasis placed on marketing, and the varied priority placed on health. While health concerns may have been a primary motivator for health tourists prior to the 19th century and in particular the 20th century, today the 'tourist experience' appears to take precedence over health. Health care and beauty treatments may form part of a tourist package in international resorts or on cruises, which often include site-seeing to major destinations. In addition, the focus on the 'tourist experience' over the 'health experience' means health-related tourism can occur in expensive locations, such as the United States. Promotions of health and medical tourism from emerging or developing nations, on the other hand, often attempt to alleviate patient fears by highlighting physician training undertaken at Western locations, the high quality of advanced medical facilities, the absence of waiting times, affordability, and both the quality and quantity of care (such as one-on-one nursing). At the same time, health may remain the primary—or only—motivator for travel. This can be influenced by delays in or the unavailability of medical treatment/s at home. Transplant tourism, for example, occurs because of the long waiting lists for kidney transplants in the developed world that may lead to death before the individual can receive a transplant, and medical tourism (also called medical travel, health tourism or global health care) is a term initially coined by travel agencies and the mass media to describe the rapidly-growing practice of traveling across international borders to obtain health care. It also refers pejoratively to the practice of health care providers traveling internationally to deliver health care.

Services typically sought by travelers include elective procedures as well as complex specialized surgeries such as joint replacement (knee/hip), cardiac surgery, dental surgery, and cosmetic surgeries. However, virtually every type of health care, including psychiatry, alternative treatments, convalescent care and even burial services are available.

Medical Tourism Process

The typical process is as follows:

- The person seeking medical treatment abroad contacts a medical tourism provider, who is commonly referred to as a 'facilitator'.

- The facilitator usually requires the patient to provide a medical report, including the nature of ailment, local doctor's opinion, medical history, and diagnosis, and may request additional information, such as X-rays or diagnostic testing results.
- Certified physicians or consultants may advise on the medical treatment or recommend an initial consultation with a specialist.
- The approximate cost of treatment, the choice of doctor and hospital, expected duration of stay, and logistical information, such as accommodation, ground transportation, and flights are discussed as well.
- A patient may be asked to pay an upfront deposit for treatment. For those destinations which require a visa, the patient will be given recommendation letters for a medical visa for the relevant embassy.
- The patient travels to the destination country, where the medical tourism provider may assign a case executive, who takes care of on the ground experience, including translation, accommodation, and arranging aftercare.
- In the cases where patients self-pay for medical treatment, a final treatment bill will be presented upon completion of treatment.
- If the patient underwent surgery, there may be additional postoperative checks to discharge the patient and deem him or her 'fit for flight' for the return home trip.

Risks

Medical tourism carries some risks that locally provided medical care does not. Some countries, such as South Africa, or Thailand have very different infectious disease-related epidemiology in compare to Europe and North America. Exposure to diseases without having natural immunity can be a hazard for weakened individuals, specifically with respect to gastrointestinal diseases (e.g., Hepatitis A, amebic dysentery, paratyphoid).

The patient with lower immunity can easily get mosquito-transmitted diseases, influenza, and tuberculosis. However in poor tropical nations diseases run the gamut, doctors seem to be more open to the possibility of considering any infectious disease, including HIV, TB, and typhoid, while there are cases in the West where patients were consistently misdiagnosed for years because such diseases are perceived to be 'rare' in the West.

The quality of postoperative care can also vary dramatically, depending on the hospital and country, and may be different from US or European standards. Also, traveling long distances soon after surgery can increase the risk of complications.

Long flights and decreased mobility associated with window seats can predispose one towards developing deep vein thrombosis and potentially a pulmonary embolism.

Other vacation activities can be problematic as well—for example, scars may become darker and more noticeable if they sunburn while healing.

Also, health facilities treating medical tourists may lack an adequate complaints policy to deal appropriately and fairly with complaints made by dissatisfied patients.

Differences in health care provider standards around the world have been recognized by the World Health Organization, and in 2004 it launched the World Alliance for Patient Safety. This body assists hospitals and government around the world in setting patient safety policy and practices that can become particularly relevant when providing medical tourism services.

If there are complications, the patient may need to stay in the foreign country for longer than planned or if they have returned home, will not have easy access for follow-up care.

Legal Issues

Receiving medical care abroad may subject medical tourists to unfamiliar legal issues. The limited nature of litigation in various countries is one reason for the lower cost of care overseas. While some countries currently presenting themselves as attractive medical tourism destinations provide some form of legal remedies for medical malpractice, these legal avenues may be unappealing to the medical tourist. Should problems arise, patients might not be covered by adequate personal insurance or might be unable to seek compensation via malpractice lawsuits. Hospitals and/or doctors in some countries may be unable to pay the financial damages awarded by a court to a patient who has sued them, owing to the hospital and/or the doctor not possessing appropriate insurance cover and/or medical indemnity. Issues can also arise for patients who seek out services that are illegal in their home country. In this case, some countries have the jurisdiction to prosecute their citizen once they have returned home, or in extreme cases extraterritorially arrest and prosecute. In Ireland, especially, in the 1980s–90s there were cases of young rape victims who were banned from traveling to Europe to get legal abortions. Ultimately, Ireland's Supreme Court overturned the ban; they and many other countries have since created 'right to travel' amendments.

Ethical Issues

There can be major ethical issues around medical tourism. For example, the illegal purchase of organs and tissues for transplantation had been methodically documented and studied in countries such as India, China, Colombia and the Philippines. The Declaration of Istanbul distinguishes between ethically problematic 'transplant tourism' and 'travel for transplantation'. Medical tourism may raise broader ethical issues for the countries in which it is promoted. For example, in India, some argue that a policy of 'medical tourism for the classes and health missions for the masses' will lead to a deepening of the inequities' already embedded in the health care system. In Thailand, in 2008 it was stated that, 'Doctors in Thailand have become so busy with foreigners that Thai patients are having trouble getting care'. Medical tourism centered on new technologies, such as stem cell treatments, is often criticized on grounds of fraud, blatant lack of scientific rationale and patient safety. However, when pioneering advanced technologies, such as providing 'unproven' therapies to patients outside of regular clinical trials, it is often challenging to differentiate between acceptable medical innovation and unacceptable patient exploitation.

DESTINATIONS FOR MEDICAL TOURISM

Africa and the Middle East

Jordan

Jordan through their Private Hospitals Association, managed to attract 250,000 international patients accompanied by more than 500,000 companions in 2012, with a total revenues exceeding 1B US$. Jordan won the Medical Destination of the year award in 2014 in the IMTJ Medical Travel Awards.

Israel

Israel is a popular destination for medical tourism. In 2010, Israel treated 30,000 medical tourists, mostly from the former Soviet Union. There are reports that these medical tourists obtain preferential treatment, to the detriment of local patients. Some people come to Israel to visit health resorts at the Dead Sea, and on Lake Kinneret.

Iran

In 2012, 30,000 people came to Iran to receive medical treatment. In 2015, It is estimated that between 150,000 to 200,000 health tourists come to Iran, and this figure is expected to rise to 500,000 a year.

South Africa

South Africa is the first country in Africa to emerge as a medical tourism destination. It offers medical and dental care.

Americas

Brazil

In Brazil, Albert Einstein Hospital in São Paulo was the first JCI-accredited facility outside of the US, and more than a dozen Brazilian medical facilities have since been similarly accredited. Brazil requires visas for US citizens based on a reciprocal arrangement since Brazilians are required to obtain a visa to visit the US.

Canada

Canada has entered the medical tourism field. In comparison to US health costs, medical tourism patients can save 30 to 60% on health costs in Canada.

Costa Rica

In Costa Rica, there are two Joint Commission International accredited (JCI) Hospitals. Both are in San Jose, Costa Rica. When the World Health Organization (WHO) ranked the world's health systems in the year 2000, Costa Rica was ranked as no. 36, which was higher than the US, and together with Dominica it dominated the list amongst the Central American countries. The Council for International Promotion of Costa Rica Medicine-PROMED (www.promedcostarica.org) is the official agency regulating the quality and promoting the country as medical tourism destination. The Deloitte Center for Health Solutions reported a cost savings average of between 30–70% of US prices.

Ecuador

Ecuador is becoming more recognized as a Medical Tourism destination and a top retirement destination worldwide. Ecuador has been declared by International Living Magazine, 'No. 1 out of the 22 best countries on its Annual Retirement Index for five years running.' The World Health Organization (WHO) ranked Ecuador as the 6th most improved health care system in the world.

Mexico

US doctors point out that the Mexican legal system makes it almost impossible to sue Mexican doctors for malpractice. Some clinics may also offer alternative medicine therapies that have been proven ineffective or are banned in the United States. The Mexican government has shut down some of these in recent times, in response to controversial cases like that of Coretta Scott King.

United States

A McKinsey and Co. report from 2008 found that between 60,000 to 85,000 medical tourists were traveling to the United States for the purpose of receiving in-patient medical care. The same McKinsey study estimated that 750,000 American medical tourists traveled from the United States to other countries in 2007 (up from 500,000 in 2006). The availability of advanced medical technology and sophisticated training of physicians are cited as driving motivators for growth in foreigners traveling to the US for medical care, whereas the low costs for hospital stays and major/complex procedures at Western accredited medical facilities abroad are cited as major motivators for American travelers. Also, the decline in value of the US dollar between 2007 and 2013 used to offer additional incentives for foreign travel to the US, although cost differences between the US and many locations in Asia are larger than any currency fluctuations. Several major medical centers and teaching hospitals offer international patient centers that cater to patients from foreign countries who seek medical treatment in the US. Many of these organizations offer service coordinators to assist international patients with arrangements for medical care, accommodations, finances and transportation including air ambulance services. Many locations in the US that offer medical care comparable in price to foreign medical facilities are not Joint Commission Accredited.

Asia and the Pacific Islands

China

Investigations into organ harvesting have been carried out. Investigative journalist Ethan Gutmann estimates that the 'organs of 65,000 Falun Gong and 'two to four thousand' Uyghurs, Tibetans or House Christians were 'harvested' in the 2000–2008 period alone'. It is very likely that 'each person who travels to China for an organ causes the death of another human'. Furthermore, in their announcements to end organ harvesting from prisoners, China only speaks of executed prisoners, but has not acknowledged the organ procurement from non-consenting prisoners of conscience. State-sanctioned organ harvesting continues to this day, according to Doctors Against Forced Organ Harvesting representative Dr. Chen.

Hong Kong

All 12 of Hong Kong's private hospitals have been surveyed and accredited by the UK's Trent Accreditation Scheme since early 2001.

New Zealand

In 2008, it was estimated that on average New Zealand's surgical costs are around 15 to 20% the cost of the same surgical procedure in the USA.

Singapore

Singapore has a dozen hospitals and health centers with JCI accreditation. In 1997 (published 2000), the World Health Organization ranked Singapore's health care system sixth best in the world and the highest ranked system in Asia.

South Korea

The Korea Times reported in a series of articles that Korean hospitals have adopted a discriminatory pricing policy, charging foreigners two to three times more than the full-fee for locals. The paper revealed that the price disparity in medical fees for foreign patients is extremely high, considering that the difference between the lowest and highest fees for the most-sought-after procedures exceeds more than 10 times on average. It claims the government is overlooking soaring medical fees on foreign patients, who are unprotected from malpractice, discriminatory charging, overpricing and patient privacy rights under the Korean Medical Law. The Korea International Medical Association has been set up to encourage medical tourism.

Thailand

Thailand has 37 JCI-accredited hospitals. In 1994 The Thai Dental Council was established and is the premier governing body of dental practices in Thailand, and has now formulated uniform competency requirements for dental practitioners, thus directly influencing the medical and dental teaching programs. The Ministry of Public Health plays an important role in developing health care to promote scientific based education. In addition, the Thai government has placed a more important role in public health programs for its citizens.

Europe

In 2006, it was ruled that under the conditions of the E112 European health scheme, UK health authorities had to pay the bill if one of their patients could establish urgent medical reasons for seeking quicker treatment in another European union country. The European directive on the application of patients' rights to cross-border health care was agreed in 2011.

Armenia

Armenia has become a destination for those seeking medical tourism options.

Finland

On December 9, 2013 the City of Helsinki decided that all minors under the age of 18 and all pregnant mothers living in Helsinki without a valid visa or residence permit, are granted the right to the same health care and at the same price as all citizens of the city. This service will be available sometime early year 2014. Volunteer doctors of Global Clinic have tried to help these people, for whom only acute care has been available. This means that the Finnish health care system is open for all people coming outside of the European Union. The service covers special child health care, maternity clinics and specialist medical care, etc., practically for free. It is still unclear if this will increase so called health care tourism, because all you have to do is come to Helsinki as a tourist and let the visa expire. The Global Clinic in Turku offers health care for all undocumented immigrants for free. While the address of is not widely publicized, the health care officials know where it can be found.

France

British NHS patients have been offered treatment in France to reduce waiting lists for hip, knee and cataract surgery since 2002. France is a popular tourist destination but also ranked the world's leading health care system. This ranking reflects the expertise offered by doctors and surgeons to patients cared for in France. The French National Authority for Health (HAS) issues high-level quality requirements for French health care, with which clinics and hospitals must comply in order to be accredited. European Court of Justice said that National Health Service (England) has to pay back British patients.

Germany

Costs for medical treatment in Germany are commonly 50% of those in the USA.

Turkey

The cost of medical treatments in Turkey is quite affordable compared to Western European countries. Therefore, thousands of people each year travel Turkey for their medical treatments. Turkey is especially becoming a hub for hair transplant surgery.

United Kingdom

National Health Service (England) is public but some private hospitals and clinics in the United Kingdom are medical tourism destinations, especially London. Nevertheless, as at the present time very few UK private hospitals have gone through independent international accreditation (they only have the mandatory registration with the UK's watchdog, the Care Quality Commission), so they have not as yet measured themselves against the best clinics and hospitals elsewhere in the world. It is alleged that health tourists in the UK often target the NHS for its free-at-the-point-of-care treatment, allegedly costing the NHS up to £200 million. A study in 2013 concluded that the UK was a net exporter of medical tourists, with 63,000 UK residents traveling abroad for treatment and about 52,000 patients getting treatment in UK. Medical tourists treated as private patients by NHS trusts are more profitable than UK private patients, yielding close to a quarter of the revenue from only 7% of volume of cases. UK dental patients largely go to Hungary and Poland. Fertility tourists mostly travel to Eastern Europe, Cyprus and Spain.

India

Medical tourism is a growing sector in India. India is becoming the 2nd medical tourism destination after Thailand. India's medical tourism sector is expected to experience an annual growth rate of 30%, making it a $2 billion industry by 2015. As medical treatment costs in the developed world balloon—with the United States leading the way—more and more Westerners are finding the prospect of international travel for medical care increasingly appealing. An estimated 150,000 of these travel to India for low-priced health care procedures every year. Cosmetic surgery, bariatric surgery, knee cap replacements, liver transplants, and cancer treatments are some of the most sought out medical tourism procedures opted by foreigners. Some of the leading hospitals for medical tourism are Apollo Hospitals, Global Hospitals, Bombay Hospital, Hinduja Hospital, Hiranandani Hospital, Akruti Institute of Plastic and Cosmetic Surgery, Columbia Asia, and Fortis Health Care. Medical Tourism in India offers cost effective medical treatments with no waiting lists and accessibility of skilled and experienced doctors so medical tourists around the globe are flocking like never before. Nowadays, India is considered among the best in international medical tourism destinations. Patients get excellent health care services in India. Many foreign nationals worry about the quality of facilities and care they will receive out of the country. There are many well qualified doctors and hospitals in India. Medical procedures often cost half as much (or less) in India as compared to the US Even including the cost of travel and a hotel stay, it can be cheaper to have procedures done out of the motherland than to have them done at home. Low cost treatment does not necessarily mean lower health care standards.

The most well-known medical services that are growing at a faster rate in India and are also included as a part of medical tourism advantages. These treatments are:

- Eye surgery
- Spine surgery
- All types of bone and joints treatments
- Cosmetic surgeries
- Blood vessel treatments
- Stomach-related treatments
- Heat-related treatments and surgeries
- Ayurveda treatments and therapies
- Dental treatments
- Ear, nose and throat (ENT)
- Laser hair removal treatments
- Hair implants and treatments
- Spa and beauty treatments
- Infertility Treatments.

India also offers traditional methods of alternative treatments that include:

- Meditation and yoga
- Ayurveda
- Music therapy
- Homeopathy
- Aroma therapy
- Naturopathy
- Pranic healing
- Reiki.

Ayurveda is mostly practiced in Southern India as a traditional form of alternative treatment which includes the use of natural herbs as medicines.

Major features of medical tourism in India:

- 100% trustworthy
- Top quality healthcare services at low cost
- Expert team of professional doctors
- High-end health care and medical facilities.

Clearly, as health and medical tourism expose, tourism is not necessarily a passive and escapist leisurely activity that is restricted to places that are 'other'. Significantly, tourism can involve an increased engagement with, and be motivated by, current everyday experiences of embodiment. Furthermore, as health and medical tourism involve direct intervention with and on the body, it can be hard work that involves pain, recovery and recuperation. This means that the ultimate benefit might be gained after the tourist arrives home. As a result, health and medical tourism are timeless and spatially dislocated, as the tourist experience is not restricted by time and place. Perhaps these considerations reveal that health and medical tourism are not tourism at all. However, this would ignore that tourism can take many forms, and each of these are at the intersection of various competing interests and forces. Furthermore, due to developments such as health tourism, it appears that answering what tourism and more specifically, what health and medical tourism are seems to be irrelevant. This is not to subsume the importance of tourism and the growing political, economic and social interest in health and medical tourism. Rather, it appears more relevant and important to examine and understand these phenomena subjectively and socioculturally, including the political tensions arising between competing interests.

International Conventions

Since 1852 several conferences were held involving European powers, with a view to uniform action in keeping out infection from the East and preventing its spread within Europe. All but that of 1897 were concerned with cholera. No result came of those at Paris (1852), Constantinople (1866), Vienna (1874), and Rome (1885), but each of the subsequent ones doctrine of constructive infection of a ship as coming from a scheduled port, and an approximation to the principles advocated by Great Britain for many years. The principal countries which retained the old system at the time were Spain, Portugal, Turkey, Greece and Russia (the British possessions at the time, Gibraltar, Malta and Cyprus, being under the same influence). The aim of each international sanitary convention had been to bind the governments to a uniform minimum of preventive action, with further restrictions permissible to individual countries. The minimum specified by international conventions were very nearly the same as the British practice, which had been in turn adapted to continental opinion in the matter of the importation of rags.

Isolating a village in Romania whose inhabitants believe that doctors poison those suspected of cholera. The Venice convention of 30 January 1892 dealt with cholera by the Suez Canal route; that of Dresden of 15 April 1893, with cholera within European countries; that of Paris of 3 April 1894, with cholera by the pilgrim traffic; and that of Venice, on 19 March 1897, was in connection with the outbreak of plague in the East, and the conference met to settle on an international basis the steps to be taken to prevent, if possible, its spread into Europe. An additional convention was signed in Paris on 3 December 1903.

A multilateral international sanitary convention was concluded at Paris on 17 January 1912. This convention was most comprehensive and was designated to replace all previous conventions on that matter. It was signed by 40 countries, and consisted of 160 articles. Ratifications by 16 of the signatories were exchanged in Paris on 7 October 1920. Another multilateral convention was signed in Paris on 21 June 1926, to replace that of 1912. It was signed by 58 countries worldwide, and consisted of 172 articles.

In Latin America, a series of regional sanitary conventions were concluded. Such a convention was concluded in Rio de Janeiro on 12 June 1904. A sanitary convention between the governments of Argentina, Brazil, Paraguay and Uruguay was concluded in Montevideo on 21 April 1914. The convention covers cases of Asiatic cholera, oriental plague and yellow fever. It was ratified by the Uruguayan government on 13 October 1914, by the Paraguayan government on 27 September 1917 and by the Brazilian government on 18 January 1921.

Sanitary conventions were also concluded between European states. A Soviet-Latvian sanitary convention was signed on 24 June 1922, for which ratifications were exchanged on 18 October 1923. A bilateral sanitary convention was concluded between the governments of Latvia and Poland on 7 July 1922, for which ratifications were exchanged on 7 April 1925. Another was concluded between the governments of Germany and Poland in Dresden on 18 December 1922, and entered into effect on 15 February 1923. Another one was signed between the governments of Poland and Romania on 20 December 1922. Ratifications were exchanged on 11 July 1923. The Polish government also concluded such a convention with the Soviet government on 7 February 1923, for which ratifications were exchanged on 8 January 1924. A sanitary convention was also concluded between the governments of Poland and Czechoslovakia on 5 September 1925, for which ratifications were exchanged on 22 October 1926. A convention was signed between the governments of Germany and Latvia on 9 July 1926, for which ratifications were exchanged on 6 July 1927.

One of the first points to be dealt with in 1897 was to settle the incubation period for this disease, and the period to be adopted for administrative purposes. It was admitted that the incubation period was, as a rule, a comparatively short one, namely, of some three or four days. After much discussion ten days was accepted by a very large majority. The principle of disease notification was unanimously adopted. Each government had to notify to other governments on the existence of plague within their several jurisdictions, and at the same time state the measures of prevention which are being carried out to prevent its diffusion. The area deemed to be infected was limited to the actual district or village where the disease prevailed, and no locality was deemed to be infected merely because of the importation into it of a few cases of plague while there has been no diffusion of the malady. As regards the precautions to be taken on land frontiers, it was decided that during the prevalence of plague every country had the inherent right to close its land frontiers against traffic. As regards the Red Sea, it was decided after discussion that a healthy vessel could pass through the Suez Canal, and continue its voyage in the Mediterranean during the period of incubation of the disease the prevention of which is in question. It was also agreed that vessels passing through the Canal in quarantine might, subject to the use of the electric light, coal in quarantine at Port Said by night as well as by day, and that passengers might embark in quarantine at that port. Infected vessels, if these carry a doctor and are provided with a disinfecting stove, have a right to navigate the Canal, in quarantine, subject only to the landing of those who were suffering from plague.

ISOLATION

It refers to various measures taken to prevent contagious diseases from being spread from a patient to other patients, health care workers, and visitors, or from others to a particular patient. Various forms of isolation exist, some of which contact procedures are modified, and others in which the patient is kept away from all others.

Isolation is most commonly used when a patient has a viral illness. Special equipment is used in the treatment of patients on the various forms of isolation. These most commonly include gowns, masks, and gloves.

Forms of Isolation

Strict isolation is used for diseases spread through the air and in some cases by contact. Patients must be placed in isolation to prevent the spread of infectious diseases. Those who are kept in strict isolation are often kept in a special room at the facility designed for that purpose. Such rooms are equipped with a special lavatory and caregiving equipment, and a sink and waste disposal are provided for workers upon leaving the area.

Contact Isolation

Contact isolation is used to prevent the spread of diseases that can be spread through contact with open wounds. Health care workers making contact with a patient on contact isolation are required to wear gloves, and in some cases, a gown.

Respiratory Isolation

Respiratory isolation is used for diseases that are spread through particles that are exhaled. Those having contact with or exposure to such a patient are required to wear a mask.

Blood and Body Fluids Precautions

This method is used when there is concern about communicable diseases found in a patient's body fluid. Health care workers making contact with the patient when body fluids are involved must wear gloves.

Reverse Isolation

Reverse isolation is a method to prevent a patient in a compromised health situation from being contaminated by other people or objects.

Effects of isolation: Isolation can have the following effects on patients:

- Patient may not be able to receive visitors, and in turn, become lonely.
- Patient may be anxious.
- Small children may feel their isolation is a punishment.
- Staff may need to spend more time with patients.
- Patients may not be able to receive certain types of care due to the risk that other patients may become contaminated. This includes forms of care that involve use of equipment common to all patients at the facility, or that involve transporting the patient to an area of the facility common to all patients.

Diseased Workers

Health care workers who become infected with certain contagious illnesses are not permitted in many places to work with patients. While facility rules and laws vary, a common guideline that has been set is 48 hours.

Health Quarantine Regulation in India

Health Regulation enforced by Bureau of Immigration functioning under Ministry of home affairs, Govt of India.

For Entry into India

Any person, Foreigner or Indian, (excluding infants below six months) arriving by air or sea without a vaccination certificate of yellow fever will be kept in quarantine isolation for a period up to 6 days if:

- He arrives in India within 6 days of departure/transit from a yellow fever endemic area.
- Has come on a ship which has started from or transited at any port in a yellow fever endemic country within 30 days of its arrival in India provided such ship has not been disinfected in accordance with the procedure laid down by WHO.

For Leaving India

There is no health check requirement by Indian Government on passengers leaving India.

Persons leaving for a yellow fever infected area are advised in their own interest to get themselves vaccinated and to be possession of valid yellow fever vaccination certificates before they leave the country.

An administrative arrangement for the health control of sea, air and land traffic exists between the Government of India and the Government of Bangladesh. It implies that, if any aircraft or ship or land traffic from a third country arrives first at any airport or port or border check post in either of the agreement countries and then directly (without touching any other third country enroute) reaches the second country of the agreement, all health checks will be completed in the country of first arrival and the travelers will be exempted from any further health check on arrival in the second country.

Persons exempted from production of vaccination certificate: The under mentioned persons are exempted from production yellow fever vaccination certificate:

- Infants below the age of six months.
- Any person suffering from some chronic illness and has poor resistance and is thereby exempted from being vaccinated.
- Crew and passengers of an aircraft transiting through an airport located in yellow fever infected area provided the Health Officer is satisfied that such persons remained within the airport premises during the period of stay.

Countries regarded as yellow fever infected: The following countries are regarded as yellow fever endemic:

Africa: Angola, Benin, Burkina Faso, Burundi, Cameroon, Central African Republic, Chad, Congo, Cote d'Ivoire, Democratic Republic of Congo, Equatorial Guinea, Ethiopia, Gabon, Gambia, Ghana, Guinea, Guinea Bissau, Kenya, Liberia, Mali, Mauritania, Niger, Nigeria, Rwanda, Senegal, Sierra Leone, Sudan, South Sudan, Togo, Uganda.

South America: Argentina, Bolivia, Brazil, Colombia, Ecuador, French Guyana, Guyana, Suriname, Trinidad (Trinidad only), Venezuela, Panama, Paraguay, Peru.

- A Yellow fever vaccination certificate is valid only if it conforms to the model. The validity period of international certificate of vaccination or re-vaccination against yellow fever is 10 years, beginning 10 days after vaccination.
- Foreign nationals residing or who have passed through the Yellow fever endemic countries during the preceding

six days, are granted visas only after the production of vaccination certificate of Yellow Fever. After checking the vaccination certificate an entry reads as 'Valid Yellow Fever Vaccination Certificate Checked' is made in the passport of the foreigner.

INTERNATIONAL HEALTH DAYS AND THEIR SIGNIFICANCE

World Health Day (7 April)

The **World Health Day** is a global health awareness day celebrated every year on 7 April, under the sponsorship of the World Health Organization (WHO). In 1948, the WHO held the First World Health Assembly. The Assembly decided to celebrate 7 April of each year, with effect from 1950, as the World Health Day. The World Health Day is held to mark WHO's founding, and is seen as an opportunity by the organization to draw worldwide attention to a subject of major importance to global health each year. The WHO organizes international, regional and local events on the Day related to a particular theme. World Health Day is acknowledged by various governmental and nongovernmental organizations with interests in public health issues, who also organize activities and highlight their support in media reports, such as the Global Health Council.

World Tuberculosis Day

World Tuberculosis (TB) day is one of eight official global public health campaigns marked by the World Health Organization (WHO), along with World Health Day, World Blood Donor Day, World Immunization Week, World Malaria Day, World No Tobacco Day, World Hepatitis Day and World AIDS Day. It is falling on March 24 of each year and is designed to build public awareness about the global epidemic of tuberculosis (TB) and efforts to eliminate the disease. In 2012, 8.6 million people fell ill with TB, and 1.3 million died from the disease, mostly in the Third World. March 24 commemorates as the World TB Day because in this day, in 1882 Dr Robert Koch astounded the scientific community by announcing to a small group of scientists at the University of Berlin's Institute of Hygiene that he had discovered the cause of tuberculosis, the TB bacillus by which the prevention and cure of tuberculosis is possible. To control Tuberculosis March 24 of each year is considered as World Tuberculosis Day with a specific theme on Tuberculosis.

World Malaria Day

World Malaria Day (WMD) is an international observance commemorated every year on 25 April and recognizes global efforts to control malaria. Globally, 3.3 billion people in 106 countries are at risk of malaria. World Malaria Day was established in May 2007 by the 60th session of the World Health Assembly, WHO's decision-making body. The day was established to provide 'education and understanding of malaria' and spread information on year-long intensified implementation of national malaria-control strategies, including community-based activities for malaria prevention and treatment in endemic areas. April 25 was designated as *Malaria Awareness Day* in 2007 by President George W. Bush, who called on Americans to join in on the goal to eradicate malaria on the African continent. President Bush described it as a day when we focus our attention on all who suffer from this terrible disease. World Malaria Day sprung out of the efforts taking place across the African continent to commemorate Africa Malaria began in 2001.

World Immunization Week (April Last Week)

World Immunization Week is a global public health campaign to raise awareness and increase rates of immunization against vaccine-preventable diseases around the world. It takes place each year during last week of April. Immunization can protect against 25 different infectious agents or diseases, from infancy to old age, including diphtheria, measles, pertussis, polio and tetanus. The World Health Organization (WHO) estimates active immunization currently averts 2 to 3 million deaths every year. However 22.6 million infants worldwide are still missing out on basic vaccines, mostly in developing countries. Inadequate immunization coverage rates often result from limited resources, competing health priorities, poor management of health systems and inadequate surveillance. The goal of World Immunization Week is to raise public awareness of how immunization saves lives, and support people everywhere to get the vaccinations needed against deadly diseases for themselves and their children. World Immunization Week sprung out of the efforts taking place across different countries and regions for a week-long immunization awareness commemoration.

World Leprosy Day

World Leprosy Day is observed internationally on January 30 or its nearest Sunday to increase the public awareness of the Leprosy. It was begun in 1954 by French philanthropist and writer, Raoul Follereau, as a way to raise awareness of this deadly ancient disease. This day was chosen in commemoration of the death of Gandhi, the leader of India who understood the importance of leprosy. Leprosy is one of the oldest recorded diseases in the world. It is an infectious chronic disease that targets the nervous system, especially the nerves in the cooler parts of the body—the hands, feet, and face.

World Cancer Day

World Cancer Day is an international day marked on February 4 to raise awareness of cancer and to encourage its prevention, detection, and treatment. World cancer day was founded by the Union for International Cancer Control (UICC) to support the goals of the World Cancer Declaration, written in 2008. The primary goal of the World Cancer Day is to significantly reduce illness and death caused by cancer by 2020. World Cancer Day targets misinformation, raises awareness, and reduces stigma. Multiple initiatives run on World Cancer Day to show support for those affected by cancer. World Cancer Day unites the world's population in the fight against cancer. It aims to save millions of preventable deaths each year by raising awareness and education about the disease, pressing governments and individuals across the world to take action. Currently, 8.2 million people die from cancer worldwide every year, out of which, 4 million people die prematurely (aged 30 to 69 years) World Cancer Day is the ideal opportunity to spread the word and raise the profile of cancer in people's minds and in the world's media

World AIDS Day

Designated on December 1 every year since 1988, is dedicated to raising awareness of the AIDS pandemic caused by the spread of HIV infection, and mourning those who have died of the disease. Government and health officials, nongovernmental organizations and individuals around the world observe the day, often with education on AIDS prevention and control. World AIDS day was first conceived in August 1987 by James W. Bunn and Thomas Netter, two public information officers for the Global Programme on AIDS at the World Health Organization in Geneva, Switzerland.

World Thalassemia Day

World Thalassemia Day is observed every year on 8th of May to spread awareness amongst people about this deadly disease and to focus on its prevention to avoid its transmission. Thalassemia is a disease of the blood causing destruction (hemolysis) of the red blood cells resulting in deficiency of hemoglobin by which the oxygen supply becomes affected and results in anemic condition. It is a genetic disease, which is inherited or passed on from parents to children. For control of such diseases awareness regarding its cause is very essential.

World Environment Day

World Environment Day (WED) is the United Nations' principal vehicle for encouraging worldwide awareness and action for the environment. It is an annual event that is aimed at being the biggest and most widely celebrated global day for positive environmental action. This day activities take place all year round but climax on 5 June every year, involving everyone from everywhere. This World Environment Day celebration began in 1972 and has grown to become the one of the main vehicles through which the UN stimulates worldwide awareness of the environment and encourages political attention and action. This day, personalize environmental issues and enable everyone to realize not only their responsibility, but also their power to become agents for change in support of sustainable and equitable development. It is also a day for people from all walks of life to come together to ensure a cleaner, greener and brighter outlook for themselves and future generations.

World Blood Donor Day (WBDD)

Every year on 14 June, countries around the world celebrate World Blood Donor Day (WBDD). The event, established in 2004, serves to raise awareness of the need for safe blood and blood products, and to thank blood donors for their voluntary, life-saving gifts of blood. World Blood Donor Day is one of eight official global public health campaigns marked by the World Health Organization.

The National Nutrition Week

The National Nutrition Week (NNW) is an annual nutrition event is observed from 1 to 7 September every year. It was conceived by the Food and Nutrition Board in the year 1982 as an annual event. The basic objective is to intensify awareness generation on the importance of nutrition for health which has an impact on development, productivity, economic growth and ultimately National development. Nutrition is an issue of survival, health and development for current and succeeding generations. Children born underweight have impaired immune function and increased risk of diseases such as diabetes and heart diseases in their later life. Malnourished children tend to have lower IQ and impaired cognitive ability, thus affecting their school performance and productivity in later life. The NNW aims to create a movement to improve nutrition at individual levels. Thus, a series of convergent and well-coordinated actions in different sectors is required to be undertaken in a mission mode to address this gigantic problem of malnutrition.

World Iodine Deficiency Day

World Iodine Deficiency Day is otherwise known as Global Iodine Deficiency Disorders (IDD) Prevention Day which is observed every year on 21st October. The aim behind this day is to generate awareness of adequate use of iodine and to highlight the consequences of iodine deficiency. The iodine deficiency disorders have become a major public health problem worldwide. In today's scenario one third of the world population is at the risk of iodine deficiency disorders. According to the WHO around 54 countries are still iodine deficient. Iodine is a micronutrient which is required for the human growth and development.

World Arthritis Day

On 12 October 2015, World Arthritis Day will be celebrated around the globe. The day was first observed in 1996 by Arthritis Rheumatism International and is now a worldwide event, bringing arthritis sufferers together to get their voices heard. World Arthritis Day aims to raise awareness of the condition and make sure that sufferers and caregivers know all the support and help that is available to them. The day is run in partnership with the European League Against Rheumatism, who represent patients, health professionals and rheumatology researchers from around the EU. They aim to reduce the burden of this condition on individuals and society.

Anti-Obesity Day

Anti-obesity Day (AOD) is observed in various parts of the world on November 26, with several health care organizations and leading Media primarily in India and the Gulf Cooperation Council (GCC) countries marking the day with activities to highlight how Obesity is a public health hazard. In 2001, the Indian Wellness brand VLCC, founded by Mrs. Vandana Luthra, took the first step towards creating awareness about Obesity and its ill-effects through the creation of an anti-obesity initiative to address the global pandemic.

World Hemophilia Day

World Hemophilia Day is an international observance held annually on April 17 by the WFH. It is an awareness day for hemophilia and other bleeding disorders, which also serves to raise funds and attract volunteers for the WFH. The World Hemophilia Day was started in 1989 by the World Federation of Hemophilia (WFH) which chose to bring the community together on April 17 in honor of WFH founder Frank Schnabel's birthday. Every April 17, World Hemophilia Day is recognized worldwide to increase awareness of hemophilia and other inherited bleeding disorders. This is a critical effort since with increased awareness comes better diagnosis and access to care for the millions who remain without treatment.

International Day of Persons with Disabilities

United Nations' (UN) International Day of Persons with Disabilities is annually held on December 3 to focus on issues that affect people with disabilities worldwide.This day is an international observance promoted by the United Nations since 1992. The observance of the Day aims to promote an understanding of disability issues and mobilize support for the dignity, rights and well-being of persons with disabilities. It also seeks to increase awareness of gains to be derived from the integration of persons with disabilities in every aspect of political, social, economic and cultural life. It was originally called 'International Day of Disabled Persons'. The International Day of Persons with Disabilities is coordinated by United Nations Enable, which works to support and promote the rights and dignity of persons with disabilities.

World Rabies Day

World Rabies Day is an international campaign coordinated by the Global Alliance for Rabies Control, a nonprofit organization with headquarters in the United States and the United Kingdom. It is a United Nations Observance and has been endorsed by international human and veterinary health organizations such as the World Health Organization, the Pan American Health Organization, the World Organisation for Animal Health (OIE), the US Centers for Disease Control and Prevention, the World Veterinary Association, and the American Veterinary Medical Association. World Rabies Day takes place each year on September 28, the anniversary of the death of Louis Pasteur who, with the collaboration of his colleagues, developed the first efficacious rabies vaccine. The first World Rabies Day campaign took place in September 2007. World Rabies Day aims to raise awareness about the impact of rabies on humans and animals, provide information and advice on how to prevent the disease, and how individuals and organizations can help eliminate the main global sources. The World Rabies Day campaign is organized through a system of global partnerships from government to local level, and a worldwide community of volunteers.

World Diabetes Day

World Diabetes Day is celebrated worldwide by the over 230 member associations of the International Diabetes Federation in more than 160 countries and territories, all Member States of the United Nations, as well as by other associations and organizations, companies, health care professionals and people living with diabetes and their families. It is the primary global awareness campaign of the diabetes world and is held on November 14 each year. It was first celebrated in 1991 by the International Diabetes Federation and the World Health Organization in response to the alarming rise of diabetes around the world. It is a significant date in the **diabetes** calendar because it marks the birthday of the man who co-discovered insulin 'Frederick Banting'. Banting discovered insulin in 1922, alongside Charles Best. World Diabetes Day is a campaign that features a new theme chosen by the International Diabetes Federation each year to address issues facing the global diabetes community. The global diabetes community including International Diabetes Federation member associations, diabetes organizations, NGOs, health departments, civil society, individuals and companies develop an extensive range of activities, tailored to a variety of groups.

International Day of Older Persons

The International Day of Older Persons is observed on October 1 each year. On December 14, 1990 the United Nations General Assembly voted to establish October 1 as the International Day of Older Persons as recorded in Resolution 45/106. The holiday was observed for the first time on October 1, 1991. The holiday is celebrated by raising awareness about issues affecting the elderly, such as senescence and elder abuse. It is also a day to appreciate the contributions that older people make to society. This holiday is similar to National Grandparents Day in the United States and Canada as well as Double Ninth Festival in China and Respect for the Aged Day in Japan. The observance is a focus of ageing organizations and the United Nations Programme on Ageing.

World Heart Day

World Heart Day, which used to take place every year on the last Sunday in September, is organized by the World Heart Federation, and has been celebrated annually since 2000. As of 2011, World Heart Day is celebrated every 29 September and no longer on the last Sunday of September. Together with its members, the World Heart Federation spreads the news that at least 80% of premature deaths from heart disease and stroke could be avoided if the main risk factors, tobacco, unhealthy diet and physical inactivity, are controlled. Collaborators of the World Heart Federation include several major international nonprofits such as the Indian Heart Association. National activities such as public talks and screenings, walks and runs, concerts or sporting events are organized worldwide by members and partners of the World Heart Federation. It is a chance for people across the globe to take part in the world's biggest intervention against cardiovascular disease (CVD). This year's theme for WHD is Creating healthy, heart choices for everyone everywhere.

International Day for the Eradication of Poverty

The International Day for the Eradication of Poverty is celebrated every year on October 17 throughout the world. It was officially recognized by the United Nations, but the first commemoration of the event took place in Paris, France, in 1987 when 100,000 people gathered on the Human Rights and Liberties Plaza at the Trocadéro to honor victims of poverty, hunger, violence and fear. This call was made by Joseph Wresinski (1917–1988) founder of the International Movement ATD Fourth World. One of the main aims of the day is to make the voice of the poor heard. To this end, commemorations often include testimonies from people living in poverty, describing their own experiences or those of people they know.

CHAPTER 18

Community Health Administration

QUALITY ASSURANCE

As a result of advancement in healthcare technology, increased competition, privatization and awareness among the clients, healthcare system has become well aware of the need to ensure quality. Evolution of nursing as a scientific discipline has accountability toward the patient care, keeping in mind the patient's rights, cost of health services demands quality assurance in nursing.

Defining and attempting to measure quality of care is not new. In fact, the quality of health care is an idea generally attributed to Ernest Codman, a physician who first proposed the end result idea in 1869. Quality of care can be evaluated from the perceptive if individuals, populations or communities. The main aim of quality assurance us to achieved desired outcomes. As now a days we are giving more importance to achieve health for all so quality standard is not only applied to tertiary level of hospital but also in primary care setting like PHC and CHC, etc.

Concept of Quality

Quality is a matter of perception, and like beauty, lies in the eyes of the beholders. It refers to excellence of a product or a service, including its attractiveness, lack of defects, reliability, and long-term durability and the capability to fulfil its intended purpose, produced with least possible cost. It is also defined 'as the degree to which a set of inherent characteristics fulfills requirement'.

'Juran developed a three-part (Trilogy) approach to quality: Quality planning, quality control and quality improvement' **(Fig. 18.1)**.

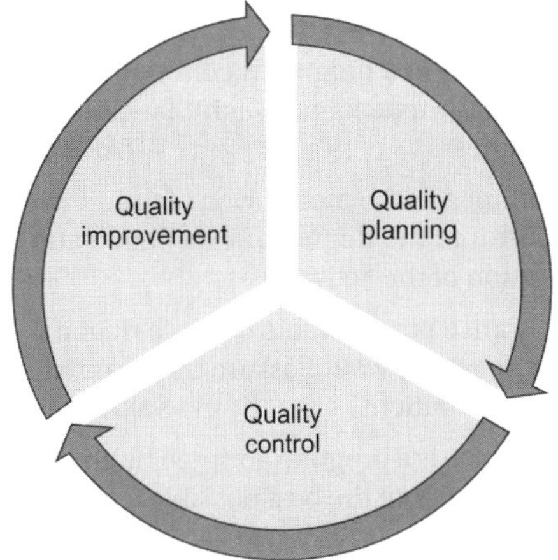

Fig. 18.1: Trilogy approach to quality.

Quality planning: It involves determining who the customers are and what their needs are, then developing products based on those needs and designing processes to those products.'

Quality control: It is the evaluation of performance to identify discrepancies between actual performance and goals.

Quality improvement: It establishes an infrastructure and the project teams to carry out process improvement.

Definitions of Quality in Healthcare Settings

'The quality is described as levels of excellence produced and document in the process of patient care, based on the best knowledge available and achievable at a particular facility.'

—The National Association of Quality Assurance Professionals

The quality defined as 'the degree to which the patient care services increase the probability of desired outcomes and reduce the probability of undesired outcomes given the current state of knowledge.'

—Joint Commission for Accreditation of Health Care Organization

'Quality is doing the right thing right the first time and doing it betters the next.' **—Al-Assaf, 1993**

Quality care is the term used to describe care and services that allow recipients to attain and maintain their highest level of physical and psychological health.

Quality of nursing practice is achieved when organization's processes and activities are designed and implemented to meet the needs and expectations of the receiver on a competent, consistent and continuous basis. **—INC, 2006**

Concept of Quality Assurance

Quality assurance (QA) is the process of assuring compliance to specification, requirements or standards and implementing methods for conformance. It includes planning and design for quality, setting and communicating indications for performance monitoring and compliance of standards. It also includes monitoring of activities of patient care to determine the degree of excellence attained in the implementation of activities. QA may also viewed as a measure of competence demonstrated by efficiency in performance. It also includes evaluation of process, outcome.

In nursing, quality assurance has focused on nursing care delivery structure, process and outcomes. Problem identification, analysis and corrective action has gradually evolved to systematic monitoring of nursing services. It can be a program for formal guarantee for provision of quality nursing care against set standards. The standards of nursing care for patient outcomes and for nurse performance are the basic components of quality management approach.

Definition of Quality Assurance

Quality assurance is a judgment concerning the process of care, based on the extents to which that care contributes to valued outcomes. **—Donabedian, 1982**

Quality assurance as the monitoring of the activities of client care to determine the degree of excellence attained to the implementation of the activities. **—Bull, 1985**

Quality assurance is achievable through ongoing evaluation of patient care which would assure the hospital that all that was done for the patient. **—Sakharkar B.M, 1999**

Quality Assurance is a program adopted by an institution that is designed to promote the best possible care.
—Deloughery, 1995

Quality assurance is program used by providers and managed care plans to evaluate the care provided to plan members and identify and correct care delivery problems.
—Cesta GT, 2002

Quality assurance is the nursing practice through well written nursing standards and the use of those standards as a basis for evaluation on improvement of client care.
—Marker, 1998

Quality assurance, as making sure that the services provided by the hospital are the best possible in a given existing resources and current medical knowledge. **—WHO, 1992**

History of Quality Assurance

- In 1842, Dr Edwin Chadwick, a public health activist and a pioneer, published a report describing the unacceptable sanitary conditions associated with urban and rural communities in Britain and recommended the structural elements of public health 'sanitary police' to monitor the sanitary condition.
- In 1854, Florence nightingale, a leading nurse during the European Crimean war, was the first to notice the positive correlation between the introductions of adequate nursing care to wounded soldiers and decrease in mortality rate among the group. Keeping in mind this concept, she studied the relationship between the quality of care and positive outcomes. She documented the fact in several studies that looked at other components of quality. She also looked at the extent of services and resource utilization and their impact on quality outcomes, and was instrumented in writing up several quality criteria in nursing care. These criteria are considered to be the first nursing care standards in history.
- In 1918, the American College of Surgeon to create the Hospital Standardization Program that provided the criteria and standards for accreditation, which were later adopted by the Joint Commission on Accreditation of Hospital (JCAH).
- Prior to this, in 1910, Abraham Flexor in his report pointed out that education of physician was directly related to the quality of care the patient received and that needed education needed substantial reforms, education, certification and licensure became very important in qualifying a healthcare professional and an educational organization.
- In 1952, JCAH later changed to Joint Commission on Accreditation of Health Care Organization (JCAHO), published its first list of accreditation standard with which hospitals, had to comply in order to receive their accreditation certificate.
- In 1966, Dr Avedes Donabedian, a university physician professor and physician, introduced his famous three measures of quality: structure, process and outcome. He urged healthcare organization to look at all the three measures when monitoring and assessing the quality of care.
- Thereafter in US, introduced:
  - Professional Standards Review Organizations (PSROs) in 1972
  - Health Maintenance Organization in 1974
  - Diagnosis Related Grouping and Prospective Payment System in 1983
  - Peer Review Organization in 1984
  - National Health Quality Improvement Act in 1986.
- In India, a Consumers Protection Act was implemented in 1986.
- The European region of WHO sponsored QA activities related to laboratories, blood banks and radiology among many others.
- In new Millennium, for accreditation of healthcare organization WHO has taken the lead.

Objectives of Quality Assurance

Quality assurance whether in health or education have the main the objectives are:

- To provide technical assistance in designing and implementing effective strategies for monitoring quality and correcting systemic deficiencies
- To refine existing methods for ensuring optimal quality health care through an applied research program.

Purpose of Quality Assurance

- Help patients and potential patients by improving quality of care.
- Assess competence of medical staff, serve as an impetus to keep up to date and prevent future mistakes.

- Bring to notice of hospital administration the deficiencies and in correcting the causative factors.
- Help to exercise a regulatory function.
- Restricting undesirable procedures.

Areas of Improvement in Quality Assurance

In an organization there are several areas for quality improvement. The areas are classified under three broad headings, those are professional, economic and social. Identification of such areas for improvement and selective attention to the development of new techniques in areas of greatest need is essential.

Elements/Components of Quality Assurance

According to Donabedian

- **Structure element:** Structure element denotes the physical, financial and organizational resources provided for health care. It includes infrastructure, equipments in proper workable condition, well qualified and experienced staffing pattern, budget allocation, etc.
- **Process element:** Process means how the work is going on. Organizational structure, the activities of a health system or healthcare personnel in the provision of care, real practice by the means of patient satisfaction are included in process element.
- **Outcome element:** Outcome is the changes in the health status of the patient, a change in the patient's current or future health that results from nursing interventions and cure rate.

According to Manwell, show and Beurri, there are 3A's and 3E's.

- Access to health care
- Acceptability
- Appropriateness and relevance to need
- Effectiveness
- Efficiency
- Equity

Quality Assurance Involves

- Identifying standards for excellence. The areas of improvement in quality assurance has been explained in **Figure 18.2**.
- Evaluating care against those standards
- Taking action to correct deficiencies and to reach these standards.

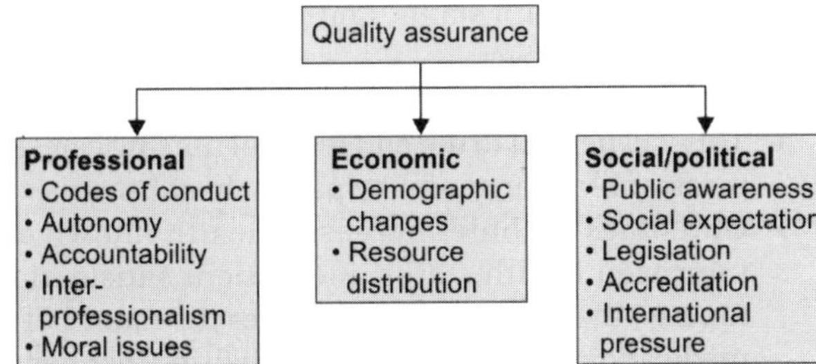

Fig. 18.2: Areas of improvement in quality assurance.

Principles of Quality Assurance

- Quality assurance is a never-ending process of creative destruction, with rapid advances in science and technology and reduced half life of medical knowledge continuous updating is essential.
- The emphasis is on establishing professional excellence patient satisfaction at a reasonable cost.
- Quality is not proportionate to the use of sophisticated technology or to be expense incurred.
- Motto of fees for service should not be pregnant with the comedy of needless services for a fee and tragedy of no services if no fee.
- Technical imperative should not insist on prolonging life at any lost with no consideration to quality of life.
- Managers need to be committed to quality management and all employees must be involved in quality improvement.
- The goal of quality management is to provide a system in which workers can function effectively.
- The focus of quality management is on improving the system, not on assigning blame.
- Every agency has internal and external customers and customers will define quality of the products.

Methods of Quality Assurance

A quality assurance program can be either concurrent or retrospective.

Concurrent Quality Assurance

A hospital administrator uses this method routinely so far as no clinical aspects of hospital care concerned, in the form of daily and periodical administrative rounds. Concurrent evaluation provides opportunity for simultaneous corrective action. Nevertheless, this can also profitably form part of the ward round of clinicians and consultants, because it is done while the patient is still in the ward, oversees things as they happen from day-to-day.

The Retrospective Quality Assurance

Retrospective evaluation acts as a continuous and ongoing self, improvement process. In many instances where people are keen to carryout such an evaluation, the whole process has been gone through with no preparation and in the most haphazard manner. Needless to add, any quality assurance program requires a step by step approach to derive the desired result.

Prerequisites: There are three fundamental prerequisites that need to be fulfilled before the program is instituted:

1. Good medical records
2. Establishment of criteria for diagnosis, investigations and treatment and
3. Cooperation and involvement of medical staff.

Types of Quality Assurance

There are two types of quality assurance:

1. External quality assurance
2. Internal quality assurance

External Quality Assurance

Quality assurance can be evaluated by independent assessors (or) people from outside the institution/hospital.

Internal Quality Assurance

Quality assurance can be evaluated by local assessors (or) senior person from the same institution/hospital.

Process of Quality Assurance

At a basic level, quality assurance process incorporate the following stages/steps (Lang, 1984):

- Setting actual achievements
- Appraising actual achievements
- Planning for improvement
- Taking action when required.

These are referred to as the quality wheel **(Fig. 18.3)**.

- **Setting standards:** Involves writing statements that describe achievable and desirable levels of quality care.
- **Appraising actual achievement:** Appraising actual achievement involves comparing practice with the defined standards through measurement criteria.
- **Planning for improvement:** It is necessary when after appraisal many gap between provision and expectation is identified.

Taking action when required: If quality of care is below the stated accepted levels, the action is taken to raise quality until standards.

MODELS OF QUALITY ASSURANCE AND QUALITY MANAGEMENT

American Nurses' Association (ANA) Model

- **Quality assurance model:** Quality assurance model in nursing is developed by Lang and adapted by the American Nurses Association. The evaluation model is open and circular, indicating a cyclical process that can be entered at any point **(Fig. 18.4)**.
- **Identification of values:** Emphasizes the need to clarify the social, institutional, professional and individual values, along with the advances in scientific knowledge which influence nursing practice. Examination of these beliefs offers insight into what clients, nurses and others think is important in nursing care. Consensus among all interested parties regarding what constitutes good nursing care is needed in order to determine the standards and criteria used to judge quality.

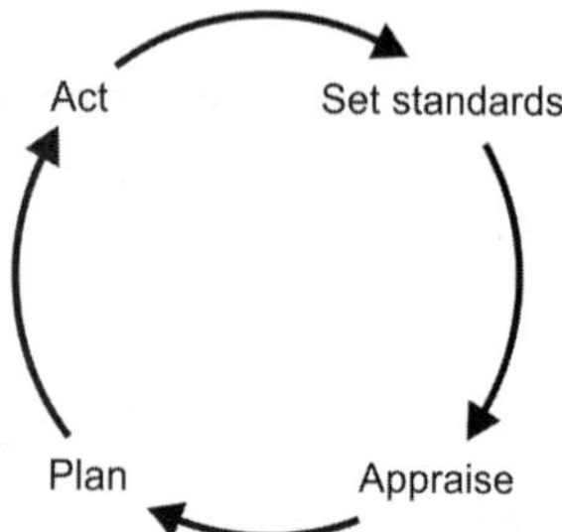

Fig. 18.3: Quality wheel.

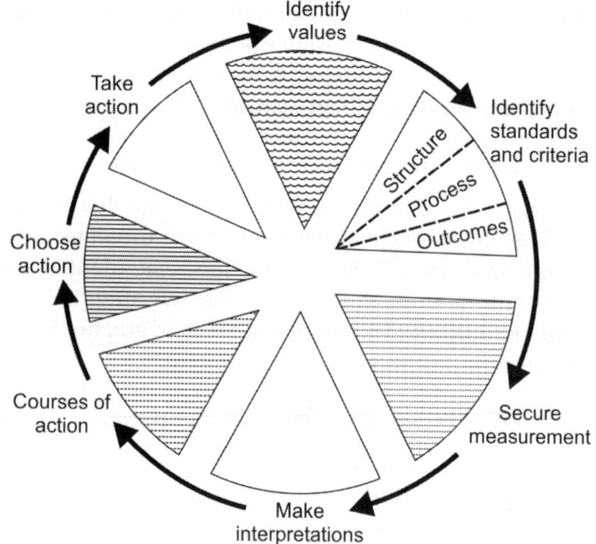

Fig. 18.4: ANA quality assurance model.

- **Identify standards and criteria:** The standards and criteria derived from the values describe the level of nursing care considered acceptable. These standards may range from minimal to achievable, excellent or comprehensive. Standards represent the agreed upon level of excellence, whereas criteria are specific, measurable statements which reflect the intent of the standard and can be compared to actual nursing practice.

  There are three types of standards and criteria in general use—structure, process and outcome.

  1. *Structure standards:* Describe organizational, financial and physical attributes if an agency or service and provider characteristics. For example, patient classification system used to determine staffing needs and all registered nurses must have a minimum of a baccalaureate degree in nursing.
  2. *Process standards:* Focus on the nature of activities and interventions according events in delivery of nursing care. Process includes nurse performance, the nurse patient relationship, continuity and timeliness of care and interactions with other healthcare professional. For example, the nurse will systematically collect data about the patient's health status, and the nurse will treat all patients with respect.
  3. *Outcome standards:*
     - This will pertain to the end result of nursing care and measurable changes in the patient health status.
     - Outcomes include increased health knowledge improved health status and patient satisfaction, for, e.g., the patient correctly states the names of all medications, and the patient verbalizes that pain is controlled.

All three types of standards and criteria can be used alone or in combination to evaluate the quality of nursing practice. However, experts agree that no one type is sufficient to describe the quality of care.

- **Secure measurement:** The next component involves the measurement of current nursing practice against the established standards and criteria. There are many methods which could be used to perform the comparison including concurrent and retrospective audit, direct observation of nurse or patient performance, questionnaire, patient or nurse interview and knowledge testing. The method selected is dependent upon the purpose of the evaluation study and the available instruments and resources. Strengths and weakness of nursing practice should be revealed through this comparison.
- **Make interpretations:** Analysis and interpretation of the data follow as the next component of the model. The purpose here is the identification of discrepancies between the established criteria and current practice. If no variations are discovered, then the remainder of the model is by passed and one begins again with value clarification. It is unlikely, however, that no discrepancies will be found. Judgments are made about strengths, deficiencies and other problems in quality.
- **Course of action:** Suitable courses of action are then considered. Alternatives intended to resolve discrepancies and reward strengths are identified and examined. Decisions may range from simple actions to complex plans entailing many changes.
- **Choose action:** The last two components of the model consist of the selection and implementation of the best actions. Judgments are made about strengths, deficiencies and other problems in quality; it may be positive or negative.
- **Take action:** Some actions may need to be performed immediately while others take longer to initiate. The decisions as to which action to choose are influenced by the organization context and available resources. At this point the cycle is repeated and the actions are reassessed to determine if the expected improvements in practice actually occurred or have been maintained.

Donabedian Model

Donabedian quality framework is recognized as a method of measuring quality as structure, process and outcome in the mid of 1960s.

According to model, 'structure' include the adequacy of healthcare facilities, the qualifications of practitioners and the financial aspects of care. The 'process' were the aspects of care and 'outcomes' are the precise and concrete measurements of effectiveness of care **(Fig. 18.5)**.

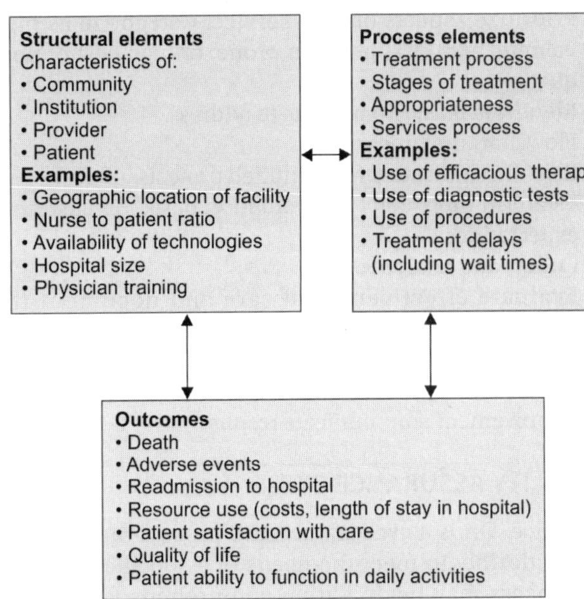

Fig. 18.5: Donabedian model of measuring healthcare system performance.

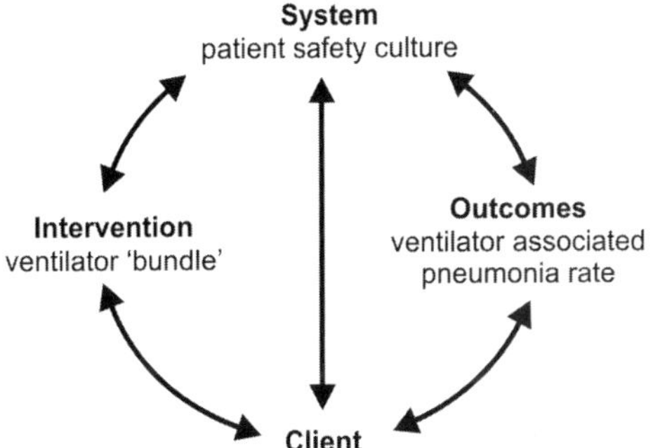

Fig. 18.6: Quality health outcome model.

Wilson's Model

Wilson (1987) in the late 1980's tried to operationalize Donabedian model into a tangible and practical form. He redefined it as inputs, methods or procedures and outcomes. He described 'inputs' as people (personnel), equipment and environment, i.e., the resources needs to attain a defined level of care. 'Methods' or procedures became the everyday practice that is required, i.e., the professional or technical skill or expertise. 'Outcomes' are the target of care or services as measured by productivity, quality and client satisfaction.

Quality Health Outcome Model

Mitchell and his coworkers proposed this model. According to this model, there are dynamic relationships with indicators that not only act upon, but also reciprocally affect the various components as shown in **Figure 18.6**.

Joint Commission 10-Step Process Model

This model includes 10 steps for quality assessment/quality improvement/quality management. These steps provide a systematic methodology for quality management. This model is used for monitoring and evaluation of services. The steps are as follows with suggested:

Joint Commission 10-Step Process:

1. Assign responsibilities.
2. Delineate scope of care/service

3. Prioritize aspects of care/service. Categorize as high volume, high risk, problem prone, or high cost of poor quality
4. Identify at least two projects to address.
5. Flowchart the process.
6. Establish indicators for identified projects
7. Establish thresholds for evaluation based on customer expectations
8. Collect and analyze data
9. Evaluate effectiveness of care and document the level of improvement and determine and implement appropriate actions.
10. Evaluate effectiveness of action and document the level of improvement communicate results.

QUALITY ASSURANCE CYCLE

In practice, QA is a cyclical, iterative process that must be applied flexibly to meet the needs of a specific program. The process may begin with a comprehensive effort to define standards and norms as described in steps 1–3, or it may start with small-scale quality improvement activities (steps 5–10). Alternatively, the process may begin with monitoring (step 4). The ten steps in the QA process are discussed **(Fig. 18.7)**.

Planning for Quality Assurance

This first step prepares an organization to carry out QA activities. Planning begins with a review of the organizations scope of care to determine which services should be addressed.

Setting Standards and Specifications

To provide consistently high-quality services, an organization must translate its programmatic goals and objectives into operational procedures. In its widest sense, a standard is a statement of the quality that is expected. Under the broad rubric of standards there are practice guidelines or clinical protocols, administrative procedures or standards operating procedures, product specifications, and performance standards.

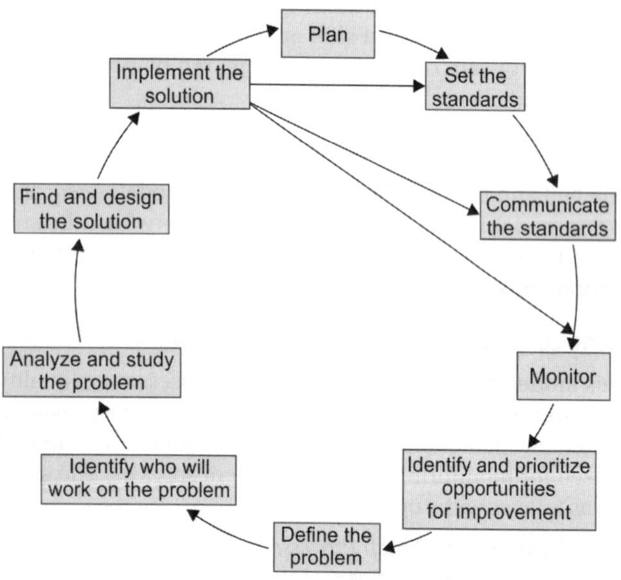

Fig. 18.7: Quality assurance cycle.

Communicating Guidelines and Standard

Once practice guidelines, standard operation procedures, and performance standards have been defined; it is essential that staff members communicate and promote their use. This will ensure that each health worker, supervisor, manager and support person understands what is expected of him or her. This is particularly important if ongoing training and supervision have been weak or if guidelines and procedures have recently changed. Assessing quality before communicating expectations can lead to erroneously blaming individuals for performance when fault actually lies with systemic deficiencies.

Monitoring Quality

Monitoring is the routine collection and review of data that helps to assess whether program norms are being followed of whether outcomes are improves. By monitoring key indicators, managers and supervisors can determine whether the services delivered follow the prescribed practices and achieve the desired results.

Identifying Problems and Opportunities for Improvement

Program managers can identify quality improvement opportunities by monitoring and evaluating activities. Other means include soliciting suggestions from health workers, performing system process analyses, reviewing patient feedback or complaints, and generating ideas through brainstorming or other group techniques. Once a health facility team has identified several problems, it should set quality improvement priorities by choosing one or two problem areas on which to focus. Selection criteria will vary from program to program.

Defining the Problem

Having selected a problem, the team must define it operationally as a gap between actual performance and performance as prescribed by guidelines and standards. The problem statement should identify the problem and how it manifests itself. It should clearly where the problem begins and ends, and how to recognize when the problem is solves.

Choosing a Team

Once health facility staffs have employed a participatory approach to selecting and defining a problem, it should assign a small team to address the specific problem. The team will analyze the problem, develop a quality improvement plan, and implement and evaluate the quality improvement effort. The team should comprise those who are involved with, contribute inputs or resources to, and/or benefit from the activity or activities in which the problem occurs.

Analyzing and Studying the Problem to Identify the Root Cause

Achieving meaningful and sustainable quality improvement efforts depends on understanding the problem and its root cause. Given the complexity of health service delivery, clearly identifying root causes requires systematic, in-depth analysis. Analytical tools such as system modelling, flow charting, and cause-and-effect diagrams can be used to analyze a process or problem. Such studies can be based on clinical record reviews, health center register data, staff or patient interviews, service delivery observations.

Developing Solutions and Actions for Quality Improvement

The problem-solving team should now be ready develop and evaluate potential solutions. Unless the procedure in question is the sole responsibility of an individual, developing solutions should be a team effort. It may be necessary to involve personnel responsible for processes related to the root cause.

Implementing and Evaluating Quality Improvement Efforts

The team must determine the necessary resources and time frame and decide who will be responsible for implementation. In-depth monitoring should begin when the quality improvement plan is implemented. It should continue until either the solution is proven effective and sustainable, or the solution is proven ineffective and is abandoned or modified. When a solution is effective, the teams should continue limited monitoring.

QUALITY ASSURANCE PROGRAM

It is an ongoing program through which we can examine attributes of service. The program is directed towards evaluating the pattern of care that is received by group of patients against the criteria that have been developed to measure the effects of nursing care.

Beneficiaries of Quality Assurance Program

The recipients of care who receive safe effective satisfying services.

The care providers because evaluation offers opportunity to promote personal and professional growth.

The agencies which obtain data for planning cost containment and legal protection.

The profession quality assurance program promotes development of standards and protocol and generations of new knowledge.

Quality Assurance Committee (QAC): A QAC is a committee of suitably qualified and experience people that has been established for the purpose of improving the safety and quality of health services. It is a team of people who meet together to undertake quality assurance activities. Each hospital needs a quality assurance committee to establish criteria and a process for quality assurance and to evaluate care make recommendations and to follow-up work.

The committee should consist of the following.

- Medical administrator
- Two senior clinicians
- Pathologist
- Radiologist
- Nurse administrator
- Medical records officer–secretary
- Additional personnel such as super specialist and consultants can be co-opted on the committee as and when required.

Functions of Quality Assurance Committee

The major functions of quality assurance committee can be broadly classified under some major headings.

- **Coordination:**
    - Collecting information
    - Consider activities that should be related, e.g., quality appraisal and continuing education
    - Communication across patient care disciplines
    - Coordinate actions of hospital authority groups.
- **Information:**
    - Provide a centralized source of reports to the board.
    - Suggest head for intervention to hospital authority groups.
- **Planning:**
    - Helps the achieving the standards
    - Actively participated in planning any program
    - Establish priorities, developing and modifying the standards and criteria.
- **Prodding:** Stimulate or persuade to all the workers to achieve the standards. Insist on effective, productive quality appraisal efforts from all hospital components
- **Consultation:** Provide specific assistance, usually through the coordinator. Act as consultants for all the healthcare providers how to achieve quality.
- **Response:**
    - Internally, acknowledge issues of importance to individuals and departments when suggesting high priority areas for immediate attention.
    - Externally, provide the organization home for responding to quality requirement of external agencies of any, e.g., medical companies.
- **Search for expertise:** Operate openly, not behind closed doors, seek out the specific clinical and or management expertise necessary to reach sound conclusions.
- **Follow-up:**
    - Insist on reports if the impact if implemented changes.
    - Committee members must recognize that their major functions are:
        - To coordinate not to control
        - To inform, not to scold

- To plan and suggests priorities not to do detailed studies in committee and
- To recommend report, not to intervene directly.

Quality assurance committee have to choose the criteria, which are both the best indictors of the achievement of standards, and the easiest to use one way to check criteria is to apply the 'AMBOUR' principles, these are:

A—Attainable/achievable
M—Measurable
B—Behaviorally stated
O—Observable
U—Understandable
R—Relevant/reasonable

- A chairperson with enthusiasm and attention to details helps ensure a successful program.
- Members also need to be interested in quality assurance and knowledgeous about channels of communication, hospital resources, patient population and nursing needs.
- Representation of staff nurse, head nurses and in service instructors from various nursing unit which help to develop and implement a quality assurance program actively.

Steps are to be Followed on Quality Assurance Program

- Approval of the program.
- Task force or committee to be appointed
- Orientation programs to be arranged for the committee member to familiarize with the purpose, principles, methods, etc.
- Examine their belief and behavior concerning quality control through workshop.
- Explore the difference is nursing value through open confrontation.
- Identify institutional supports and constraints to be within measuring and improving nursing quality.

Principles of Quality Assurance Program

- Accurate assessment and successful documenting of patient care.
- Ensure that resource expenditure for QA is appropriate.
- Requires collaborative efforts to measure and improve care.
- Must be focused on client need.
- Manipulate input variables to improve quality.
- Effective QA must be linked with decision-making.
- Effective monitoring
- Feedback to practitioner.

Indicators of Quality Assurance in Hospitals

- Waiting time for different services in the hospital.
- Medical errors in judgment, diagnosis, laboratory reporting, medical treatment or surgical procedures, etc.
- Hospital infections including hospital-acquired infections, cross infections.
- Quality of services in key areas like blood bank, laboratories, X-ray department, central sterilization services, pharmacy and nursing.

Quality Evaluation System in Health Care

The following are the examples of different approaches to quality evaluation that are used in different countries:

Approach

General Approach

It involves large governing or official bodies evaluating a person or agencies' ability to meet established criteria or standard during a given time.

Credentialing

It is a means of achieving a unified, coordinated comprehensive system for nursing. It is a voluntary form of self-regulation seen in healthcare disciplines. It is the formal recognition of professional or technical competence and attainment of minimum standards by a person and agency. This process has four functional components:

- To produce a quality product
- To confirm a unique identity
- To protect the provider and public
- To control the profession.

Licensure

It is a process by which an agency of state government grants permission to individuals accountable for the practice of a profession to engage in that profession and prohibits all other form legally doing so. It is a contact between the profession and the state in which the profession is granted control over entry into an exit from the profession and over quality of professional practice.

Accreditation

It is the process by which a voluntary nongovernmental agency or organization approves and grants accredited status to institutions programs or services which need predetermined structure process and outcome criteria. Its application to nursing indicates a need for all nursing educations programs and all organized nursing services to be accredited. It is a process in which certification of competency, authority, or credibility is presented to an organization with necessary standards.

Recognition

It is defined as a process whereby one agency accepts the credentialing states of and the credential confined by another. The committee recommended that all nursing agencies with credentialing function seek to be recognized by the appropriate bodies.

Certification

It is a process by which a nongovernmental agency or association certifies that an individual licensed to practice a profession has to met certain predetermined standard nursing means that a name has achieved competence in a field of specially within the profession. It is a voluntary, governmental or nongovernmental approach to grant recognition to individuals and organizations that have met high standards in specialized areas.

Specific Approaches

Quality assurance is methods to evaluate identified instances of providers and client interaction, the specific approaches are as follows:

Audit System

Audits are being done through retrospective review of documentation and records against a set of predetermined criteria.

Quality Awards

There are various awards that are given to that organization who maintain quality in many countries, e.g., the European Foundation for Quality Management (EFQM), the Baldrige awards in the United States, and the quality awards are developed within many countries.

Peer Assessment

It is a process, whereby one healthcare practitioner, usually a physician, will evaluate the care of a peer and assist change towards better outcome. These are designed to monitor client specific aspects of care appropriate for certain levels of care. The audit has been the major tool used by peer review committee to ascertain quality of care.

Utilization Review

These activities are directed towards assuring that care is actually needed and that cost appropriate for the level of care provided.

There are three types of utilization review: prospective: assessment of the necessity of care before giving the service; concurrent: a review of the necessity of care while the care being given; and retrospective: analysis of the necessity of services received by the client after the care has being given.

Evaluation Studies

Evaluation studies can be conducted by using various quality assurance models. The main models are: Donabedian, structure-process-outcome model; the Tracer model; the Sentinel model. Donabedian model has already been discussed in previous section. The Tracer mode is a measure of both process and outcome of care. This method provides nurses with data to show the differences in outcome as a result of nursing care standards. The Sentinel method is an outcome measure for examining specific instances of client care.

Clients' Satisfaction

Client satisfaction can be assessed using person or telephone interviews and mailed questionnaire. Date from client satisfaction surveys are used to measure structure; process and outcome of care given.

Incident Review

During a patient's hospitalization several incidents may occur which has a bearing on the treatment and patients' final recovery. The critical incidents may be: delayed attendance by a physician/nurse, wrong administration medication, and negligence in carrying out procedures. The report should contain the name, age exact time and place. Description of how it occurred any precaution taken conditions of patient before e and after the incident, etc. Since these reports are of legal value it should be written carefully.

Decisions for changing anything in the system must be based on facts.

Steps in the Quality Improvement Process in Nursing

- **Select a nursing activity for improvement:** During daily assessment the members of quality control group identified any lacuna which needs to be revise.
- **Assemble a multidisciplinary team to review and revise the nursing activity:** Next steps is they have to call for a meeting to all multidisciplinary groups like all the HODS of hospital, chief matron, the members working infection control unit and other administrators and managers.
- **Delineate all components of the activity using a flow chart:** Here all should plan what to do, how to do. All components of the activity what is wrong and should be modified will be described by using flow chart to save the time.
- **Collect data to measure the current status of the activity:** Here thorough assessment will be done what is present and need to be modified.
- **Set a measurable standard for the activity:** Some time the standards are approved by the accrediatory bodies which needs to be follow or some time the experts will be set their standards.
- **Discuss various plans to meet the standard:** Like problem solving approach the different planning strategies will be develop to meet the standards. Which plan will be most effective in achieving the result in a cost effective way will be adopted.
- Select and implement one plan to meet the standard. The select plan by the committee will be implement to modify the status.
- Collect data to evaluate the implementation of the plan and revise an needed.

Constraints in Rendering Quality Care

- Inadequate resources
- Poor maintenance
- Medical supply—inadequate, interrupted
- Delays
- Poor work culture
- Attitudes of patients and public.

Inadequate Resources

- Space—shortage, wastage, unplanned growth empire building by
- Certain individuals
- Infrastructure—inadequate, improper, irrelevant
- Funds—inadequate, improper, lop sided priorities wastage.
- Equipment—not available, not functioning overused, misused, abused
- Staff—inadequate, poorly motivated, poorly trained, dishonest.

Maintenance

- Building—poorly maintained, leakages, peeled off paint, hanging wires.
- Premises—unclean, no sin ages, poor housekeeping
- Equipments—non function, idle, poor functioning
- Installations—poor safety precautions
- Hazardous practices—improper waste disposal and improper sterilization.

Medical Supplies

- Faulty procedures for procurement, storage and distribution.
- Shortages
- Supply—inadequate, interrupted
- Substandard items
- Adulterated items
- Pilferage
- Unfair practices and kick back.

Work Culture

- Poor discipline
- Too much job security
- Too much job insecurity
- Frequent transfers
- Poor leadership
- Disruptive conflicts
- Poor intersectional cooperation and coordination
- Corruption
- Interference from outside agencies, e.g., politicians

Attitudes of Patients and Public

- Prejudiced about hospital and staff.
- Ignorance about disease
- Ignorance about management of the disease
- Ignorance about likely outcome
- Too much or unreasonable expectations
- Uncooperative behavior
- Crisis of confidence—poor doctor patient relationship
- Resigned acceptance giving no feedback.

QUALITY ASSURANCE IN NURSING EDUCATION

In the era of quality orientation, human rights and a consumer-driven society, the quest is for the best quality of nursing education **(Fig. 18.8)**.

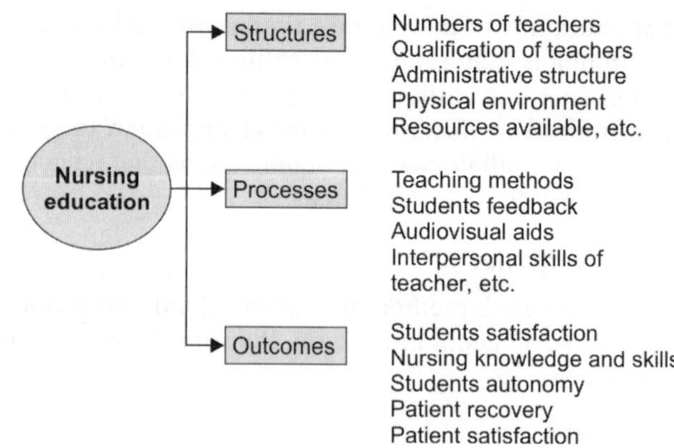

Fig. 18.8: Donabedian triad for quality assurance in nurse education.

Role of INC

The Indian Nursing Council (INC) prescribes the syllabus, including detailed plan and hours of each subject, scheme of examination and admission criteria.

Minimum standards are also set for the physical facility, teaching facility and clinical facility to start a nursing program.

The INC conducts periodic inspections of the institutions to ensure that the set standards are implemented. NMEI should establish a quality assurance system.

In order to improve the quality of nursing care, INC initiated the project of quality assurance by selecting one ward in Dr RML Hospital in New Delhi and one ward in PGI, Chandigarh; continuous and continuing education were planned to all category of nursing personnel for three months in these wards. A nursing audit was conducted and it was found that quality of nursing care improved in these wards and medical personnel appreciated the INC initiative. During this process Teaching Material was developed. We are in the process of finalizing quality assurance model which many of the corporate hospitals would be interested to adopt. There is an urgent need to adopt such a quality assurance models in nursing education to improve the quality of nursing education.

Factors Affecting Quality Assurance

- Lack of resource—infrastructure equipment
- Personnel problems—lack of trained skilled and motivated employee staff in-disciplines, etc.
- Improper maintenance—the building especially sport of leakage of roofs, cleaning of bath rooms, latrines, etc.
- Absence of well informed populace to improve quality-nursing care it is necessary that the people became knowledge to quality care.
- Absence of accreditation laws:
  - Inspect hospitals and ensure that basic requirements are met.
  - Enquire into major incidents of negligence.
  - Take action against health professionals involved in mal practices.

- Lack of good hospital information system.
  - Work load, statistics, admission, bed occupancy procedures, length of stay
  - Activity, audit scheduling of procedure.
  - Absence of conducting patient satisfaction survey.
  - Delay in attendance by doctors and nurse.
  - Discourtesy shown to patient during the course of hospitalization.
- Lack of proper maintenance of nursing care records
- Miscellaneous factors.
  - Lack of good supervision, policy, evaluation tools, and techniques
  - Written job descriptions
  - Continuing educational programs.

Role of Nurse Administrator in Developing Quality Assurance System

Nurse administrator plays a vital role in developing a quality assurance program in her hospital. She participates in the following steps as suggested for ensuring quality of nursing care.

- Deciding upon the philosophy
- Make certain that she as well as her nurses known that she wish to evaluate and why.
- Formulate objectives
- Set standards
- Enlist expert guidance
- Plan carefully and select the evaluation tool suitable to the unit
- Work cooperatively
- Publish the report of the results of evaluation of care.

NURSING AUDIT

Introduction

Nursing audit is an evaluation of nursing service. It was introduced by industrial concern. The report of nursing audit of the hospital, published in 1955, related to the planning, delivery and evaluation of care. It determines its effectiveness, and any area needing improvement and whether the planned care was given.

Definition

Audit is a systematic examination of books and records of business or other organization in order to ascertain or verify and report upon the fact regarding the financial operation.

Nursing audit refers to assessment of the quality of clinical nursing.

Purpose

- Evaluating nursing care given
- Achieves deserved quality of nursing care
- Stimulates to better health.
- Contribute to research
- Focuses on care provides.

History of Nursing Audit

Nursing audit is an evaluation of Nursing service before 1995, very little was known about the concept. It was introduced by the industrial concern and the year was the beginning of medical audit.

Concept of Nursing Audit

A nursing audit is a thorough investigation made to evaluate the overall nursing care received by a patient. An audit is generally done by experienced nurses and audit committee who do not actually work in the ward where the audit is being carried out.

The concept of nursing audit is based on debit and credit system.

Debit System

- Death of the patient which have been prevented.
- Complication of disease due to neglect of nursing care.
- Left against medical advice.
- Hospital born infection.
- Error in treatment
- Absence of total patient care
- Lack of application of nursing process.
- Nursing care learners.

Credit System

- Number of recovered patient.
- Expansion of health knowledge in patient's population.
- Short stay in the hospital
- Regular follow-up in the community
- Research or problem oriented care approach
- Measures for improving public image
- Good nurses record.

Debit system is negative in nature. Its emphases on illness where as credit system is positive in nature and it emphases on health.

Objectives

- To justify the cost increased on human and material resources.
- To study the quality of patient care against defined criteria.
- To take remedial action towards cost effectiveness.
- To assess the competence of nursing staff and serve to keep up to date knowledge and prevent repeated mistakes.

Guideline for Nursing Audit

- **Objective or aim:** Involvement of the health care and fact-finding mission.
- **Standards:** Should be set by participating clinicians.
- **Control:** Should be by participating clinicians and by voluntary participation.
- **Method:** Should be no threatening interesting objective and repeatable.
- **Records:** Should have adequate clinical materials.

- **Types of audit:** There are two types:
  - *Internal audit:* It is carried out continuously by hospital staff and which consists of process of separating and classifying clinical records and evaluating the nursing care given.
  - *External audit:* An outside agency periodically tests the completeness and accuracy of internal audit.

Methods of Nursing Audit

There are two methods:

- **Retrospectives view:** This refers to an in depth assessment of the quality after the patient has been discharged, and patient chart is the sources of data. Retrospective audit is method for evaluating the quality of nursing care by examining the nursing care as it is reflected in the patient care records for discharged patients. In this type of audit specific behaviors are described then they are converted into questions and the examiner looks for answers in the records.

  For example the examiner looks through the patient records and asks:
  - Was the problem solving process used in planning nursing care?
  - Whether patient data collected in a systematic manner?
  - Was a description of patient's pre-hospital routines included?
  - Laboratory test results used in planning care.
  - Did the nurse perform physical assessment?
  - Were nursing diagnosis stated?
  - Did nurse write nursing orders? and so on.
- **Concurrent view:** This refers to the evaluation conducted on behalf of the patients who are still underlying care. It includes assessing the patient at the bedside in relation to predetermined criteria, interviewing the staff responsible for his care and reviewing the patient records and care plan.

Audit Committee

Before carrying out an audit, on audit committee should be found. Comprising of a minimum of five members, who are interested in quality assurance, are clinically competent and able to work together in a group. It is recommended that each member should review not more than 10 patients each month and that the auditor should have the ability to carry out an audit in about 15 minutes. If there are less than 50 discharges per month, then all the records may be audited. If there are large numbers of records to be audited, then an auditor may select 10% discharge.

Nursing Auditors

The choice of nursing auditors depends upon whether the type of nursing audit to be under taken is internal and external accordingly.

- **Internal auditors:** The nursing experts from within the hospital are deputed for internal audit and the auditing is done within agency or hospital.
- **External auditors:** The nursing and medical administration from the ministry, other agency or professional association like TNAI undertake the nursing audit in desired agency of a hospital.

Audit Cycle (Fig. 18.9)

Steps to problem solving process in planning care:

- Collects patient data in a systematic manner:
  - Includes description of patients prehospital routines
  - Has information about the severity of illness
  - Has information regarding lab tests
  - Has information regarding vital signs
  - Has information from physical assessment, etc.
- States nurses diagnosis
- Writes nursing orders
- Suggests immediate and long-term goals
- Implements the nursing care plan
- Plans health teaching for patients
- Evaluates the plan of care.

Advantages

- Can be used as a method of measurement in all areas of nursing.
- Scoring system is fairly simple
- Results easily understand
- Assess the work of all those involved in recording care
- May be useful tool as a part of a quality assurance program in areas where accurate records of care are kept.

Disadvantages

- Appraises the outcomes of the nursing process. So, it is not useful in areas where the nursing process has not been implemented
- Many of the components overlap making analysis difficult.
- It is time consuming.
- Requires a team of trained auditors
- Deals with a large amount of information.
- Only evaluate record keeping. It only serves to improve documentation not nursing care.

Hospital Accreditation System of India

- Indian Hospitals Association—IHA, 1993
- Bureau of Indian Standards—BIS, 1988
- National Accreditation Board for Hospitals and Healthcare Providers—NABH

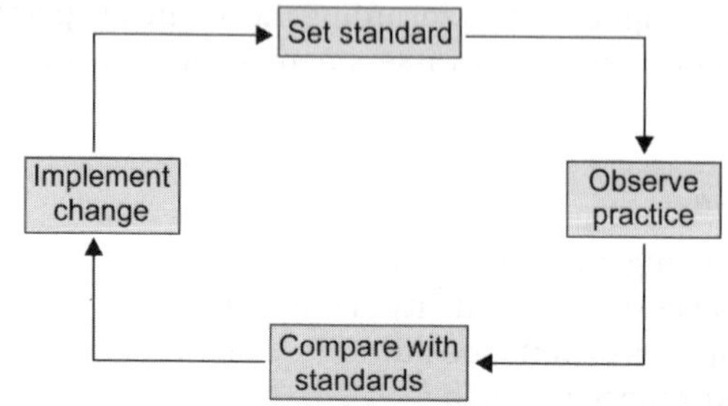

Fig. 18.9: Audit cycle.

STANDARD

Standard can be defined as a benchmark of achievement, which is based on desired level of excellence. As such standards become model to be initiated and may serve, in turn, as basis of comparisons.

—The Oxford Dictionary, 1964

Standard is a established rules or basis of comparison in measuring or judging capacity quantify contest and value of objects in the same category.

Nursing Standard

It is descriptive statement of desired quality against which to evaluate nursing care.

Purpose of Standard

- Give direction and provide guidelines for performance of nursing staff.
- Provide a base for evaluating quality of nursing care, ranging from excellent care of usage care.
- Help to improve quality of nursing care increases effectiveness of care and improves efficiency.
- Help to improve documentation and record of care.
- Help to determine the degree to which standards of nursing care maintained and take necessary corrective action in time.
- Help supervisor to guide nursing staff to improve performance.
- Help to improve basis for decision making and desire alternative system for delivering nursing care.
- Justify demands or resource association.
- Helps to clarify nurses area of accountability.
- Help nurses to define clearly different level of care.

Characteristics of Standards

- Statement must be broad enough to apply to a wide variety of setting.
- Must be realistic, acceptable and attainable.
- Standards of nursing care must be developed by member of nursing profession.
- Should be phased in positive terms and indicated, acceptable performance that in good excellent etc.
- It must express what is desirable.
- It must be understandable and stated in unambiguous terms.
- It is based on current knowledge on scientific practice.
- It must be reviewed and revised periodically.

Sources

The standard can be established, developed, reviewed or enforced by variety of sources as follows:

- Professional organization, e.g., TNAI
- Licensing bodies, e.g., INC, MCI and DCI etc.
- Institution/healthcare agencies, e.g., university Hospital, Health centers.
- Department of institution, e.g., Department of nursing
- Patient care unit, e.g., Specific patient unit
- Government unit at national, state local units
- Individual, e.g., personal standard.

Classification of Standard

There are various types of standards. The classification of standards has been depicted in **Figure 18.10.**

Normatic standard: Normatic standard describes practice considered 'good' or 'ideal' by some authoretive group, professional organization formulate normative standard.

Empirical standard: Describes practice actually observed in large number of patient care setting. It is formulated by regulatory bodies like INC, MCI.

End and means standard: The end standards are patient oriented; they describe the change as desired in a patient physical status or behaviors.

Means standards: The means standards are nursing oriented. They describe the activities and behaviors designed to achieve the end standard.

It includes the information about nurses performances.

- **Structure standard:** A structure standard involves the set up of institution the philosophy goals, objective and structure of the organization, facilities, equipments and qualification of employees the recommended relationship between the nursing department and other department in a health agency.
- **Process standard:** Process standard describes the behavior of the nurse at desired care of performance a process standard involves of performance a process standard involves the activities concerned with delivering patient care. This focuses on what was planned, what was done and what was communicated and recorded.
- **Outcome standard:** Descriptive statements of desired patient care result are outcome standard. An outcome standard measure change in patient health status. The change may be due to nursing care, medical care or as a result of variety of service offered to the patient. Structural standards are agency or group oriented process standard are nurses oriented and outcome standards are patient oriented.

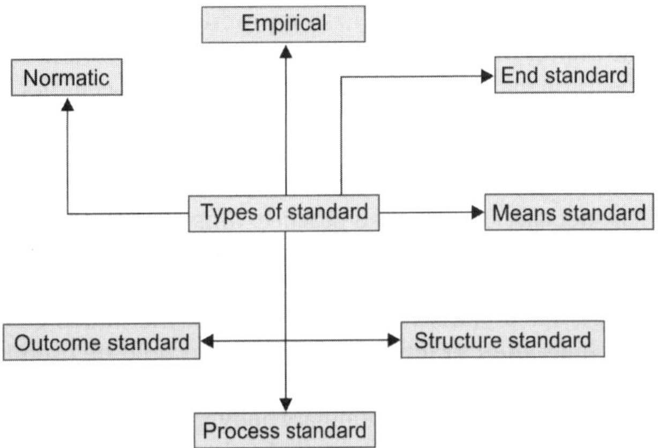

Fig 18.10: Classification of standard.

Standard and Practice Developed by International Council of Nurses, 1949

The Indian Nursing Council Act is the only national legislation directly related to nursing practice.

- The right to refuse to treat a patient except in an emergency situation.
- The right to issue for fees
- The right to add a little or description to ones name
- Unregistered practitioners are not allowed to hold position or appointments in public and local hospitals.

Fundamental Duties

- To exercise a reasonable degree of skill and knowledge in treating patient.
- Owns a relationship to a patient has been established, there is an obligation to attend the patient as long as necessary.
- A practitioner must give personal attention to his case and answer calls with reasonable promptness
- Children must be protected from harming themselves.
- Special precaution must be taken in case of adults who are incapable taking care of themselves.
- The Indian penal code demands that poisonous drugs to be kept in separate containers, properly labeled and marked.
- There is a duty of secrecy to the patients.
- Dangerous diseases must be reported
- Nurses are considered solely responsible for their own professional act irrespective of their employing authority.

STANDARD BY THE INDIAN NURSING COUNCIL

The INC has approved a framework for the endorsement of practice standards. It has been developed in response to increasing requests from professional groups and other organizations for endorsement of their standards by Nursing Council.

- The council has in the framework for post-registration nursing practice education (May 2001) provided the 'framework on which particular competencies for a defined especifically area or a scope pf practice can be developed and demonstrated.'
- The scope of the specially or standards of nursing is defined as specially nursing practice is the exercise of higher. Levels of nursing judgment, discretion and decision making in an area of practice with a specific focus and body of knowledge and practice.
- Practice standards, that have the purpose of improving the quality of professional services and recognize nurse in specialty or advanced practice, must be developed by current experts. Standards must be evidence based.
- The standards allow for audit/monitoring. Individuals or groups of nurses must be able to use the standards to evaluate their practice. The standards could be used in a situation of evaluation or monitoring of professional competence by the disciplinary body.
- The Indian Nursing Council Act is the only national legislation directly related to nursing practice. It provides a basis from which rules for nursing practice can be developed.
  - The right to refuse to treat a patient, except in an emergency situation.
  - The right to sue for fees. (Applicable only to private duty nurses or private practitioners; other nurses are salaried)
  - Unregistered practitioners are not allowed to hold positions or appointments in public and local hospitals.
  - There is a duty of secrecy to the patients. Records must be treated as confidential unless the practitioner is called upon to give evidence in court.
  - Dangerous diseases must be reported.
  - Nursed are considered solely responsible for their own professional acts irrespective of the employing authority.

STANDARD BY THE STATE NURSING COUNCIL (SNC)

The state government controls nursing practice through the state nurse's registration Acts. The state nurses registration councils have authority to prescribe rules of conduct, to take disciplinary action and to maintain registers of nurses, midwives and others.

The TNMC have acts that prevent registration or justify removal from the register for the following offenses

- Conviction for a nonbailable offense.
- Being found guilty of conduct indicating that the individual is not fit to be registered.
- Possessing defects in character.

Unethical practices prohibited the TNMC are:

- The dishonest use of certificates
- Procuring registration by false means.
- Falsification of the register
- Representation of the registration by an unrecognized person.
- Representation of registration as a medical practitioner.
- A fine is the usual penalty imposed for disobeying the law stated by TNC.

Infection control; Standard safety measures

Standard Infection Control Precautions (SICP) are designed to prevent cross transmission from recognized and unrecognized sources of infection. These sources of (potential) infection include blood and other body fluid secretions or excretions (excluding sweat, non-intact skin or mucous membranes) and any equipment or items in the care environment which are likely to become contaminated. Every hospital has an infection control unit which will be handled by an infection control team who will observe the standard precautions followed by each staff members.

Responsibilities of Workers Regarding Standard Infection Control Precautions

All staff providing direct care in a healthcare setting including a patient's/client's own home must apply the principles of SICPs.

All staff have a responsibility to ensure that they comply with the principles of standard infection control precautions.

All staff have a responsibility to encourage patients/clients/residents, carers and visitors and other staff to comply with the principles of standard infection control precautions.

Report to the nurse in-charge when on an assignment, or the client relations Team, any deficits in knowledge or other factors in relation to SICPs, including facilities/equipment or incidents, that may have resulted in cross contamination.

Attend induction and mandatory/update infection prevention and control education sessions and complete online infection control training modules as required.

Report any illness which may be as a result of occupational exposure to the NHS Professionals Flexible Worker Human Resources Department

Not provide direct patient/client/resident care while infectious as this could cause harm. If in any doubt consult the Client Relations Team or Nurse in-charge of the ward where they are on assignment.

Consider the elements of SICPs such as hand hygiene as an objective within staff continuing professional development ensuring continuous updating of knowledge and skills.

Be aware of local and national policies, procedures and campaigns regarding standard infection control precautions.

Infection Control Measures

Apart from general hygienic practices and vaccination, staff of institutions should also adopt specific infection control measures against communicable diseases. The measures fall under two main categories:

1. Standard precautions
2. Transmission-based precautions

In addition, isolating people with specific communicable diseases, urging visitors to observe infection control rules and nursing high-risk person with greater caution, can minimize the risk of communicable disease outbreak in an institution.

Standard Precautions

Standard precautions are based on the concepts that all blood, urine, feces, excreta, saliva, sputum, vomitus, secretions from nonintact skin, wounds and mucous membrane should be treated as potentially infectious.

Everyone should take appropriate protective measures when coming into contact with them. These include:

- Hand hygiene
- Respiratory hygiene and cough manners
- Use of personal protective equipment
- Proper cleansing and disinfection of used or exposed articles
- Prevention of sharps injury
- Waste management
- Isolation of infected patients (infectious unit)
- Barrier nursing
- Safe disposal of infective materials of the infective patients.
- Special treatment of reusable infective materials of the patient

Specific Protections of the staff include:

- Immunization
- Periodical health examinations of the employee

Each hospital has the policy protocol for infection control like hand hygiene BMW managements which each staff members should be followed.

STAFFING RECRUITMENT AND PERFORMANCES APPRAISAL

Staffing is the function by which manager build an organization through the recruitment, selection and development of individuals as capable employees. Staffing involves manning the organization. Structure through proper and effective selection, appraisal and development of personnel to fill the roles designed into the structure.

Activities involved in staffing

Staffing is a function which involves the following activities

- Determine the sources of recruitment of employees.
- Select the capable employees.
- Train the employees according to need.
- Evaluate the performance of employees.
- Arrange for the transfers and promotions of employees.

Importance of staffing

Staffing is one of the most essential functions for every organization. In fact, in the absence of a good staffing system no organization can exist for a long duration. Because in every organization all the resources like, money, material, machine, etc., are utilized properly through man power. Hence, it is too important that all the personnel (employees) in organization should appoint at the job according to their ability, talent, aptitude and specializations which can only be possible through a good staffing system. Thus, it is clear that staffing is too important for every organization.

For filling organizational positions: Good efficient productive staffs are required for not only filling organizational positions but also running of an organization effectively but when observing structure standards the positions should be filled.

- **Maximum and efficient utilization of resources:** Staffing plays an important role in maximum and efficient utilization of resources. Because in every organization all the resources like, money, material and machine, etc., are utilized efficiently through specialized manpower and specialized man power can only appoint in an organization through a good staffing system. Thus, we can say that it helps in maximum and efficient utilization of resources.
- **Reduces cost of production:** Staffing also plays an important role in reducing cost of production. Because it helps in appointing right person at the right job, at the right, time so that no wastage and mistakes can be made by efficient personnel during the production of products. Hence, it is clear that it assists in reducing cost of production.

- **For job satisfaction:** Staffing is an important source for employee's job satisfaction. Because by means of this system jobs are allocated among the personnel according to their ability, talent, aptitude and specializations which give employees more satisfaction regarding their jobs. As a result of that they give their hundred percent efforts behind their jobs.
- **For meeting present and future needs of employees:** Staffing is very important for fulfilling present as well as future needs of employees. Because it gives a clear picture to organization that in coming year how much positions will be vacant and new positions will be established. So that organization can fulfill those vacant and new positions by appointing the deserved candidates. Thus, it is clear that staffing fulfills present and future needs of employees in organization.
- **For maintaining coordination among the employees:** Staffing plays a prominent role in establishing unity and coordination among the employees. Because it assigns their jobs according to their ability, talent, aptitude and specializations which makes them involved in their tasks and ensure healthy and cooperative relationship among the employees.

  For developing competencies: The more experienced person are more competent then less experienced person even if having more educational qualification. Working in the same area getting training and retraining make the personnel more competent.

Staffing Functions

The staffing functions include process of acquiring, training, developing, promoting and retaining employees within the organization. The step of process are depicted in **Figure 18.11**.

Manpower Planning

Manpower planning may be regarded as the quantitative and qualitative measurement of labor force required in an enterprise. It involves in creating and evaluating the manpower inventory and to develop required talents among the employees selected for promotion advancement.

Recruitment

Recruitment is a positive process of searching for prospective employees and stimulating them to apply for the jobs in the organization. In other words, recruitment stands for discovering the source from where potential employees will be selected. The scientific recruitment leads to greater productivity, better wages, higher morale, reduction in labor turnover and better reputation of the concern.

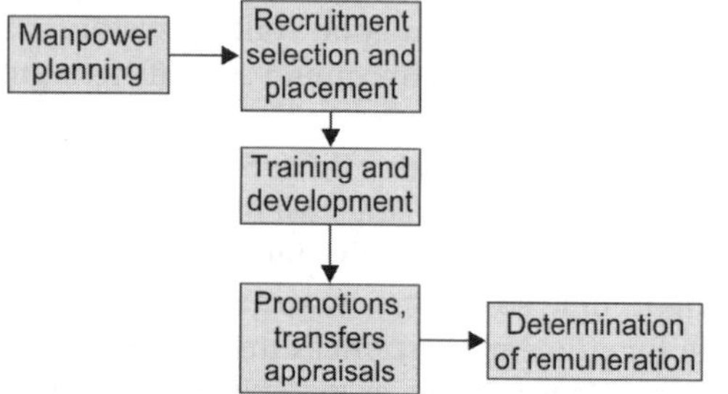

Fig. 18.11: Staffing functions.

Selection

Selection is process of eliminating (among all the candidates considered for possible employment) those who appear unpromising. The purpose of selection process is to determine whether a candidate is suitable for employment in the organization or not.

The chief aim of the process of selection is choosing right type of candidates to fill in various positions in the organization. Selection process requires exactness. A well planned selection procedure is of utmost importance for every enterprise.

Placement

Placement means putting the person on the job for which he is selected. It includes the introduction of the employee with the job.

Training

After selection an employee, the most important and established part of the personnel program is to impart training to the new comer. With the rapid technological changes, the need for training employees is being increasing recognized so as to keep the employees in touch with the new developments.

Every concern must have a systematic training program otherwise employees will try to learn the job by trial and error which can prove to be a very costly method.

Development

A sound staffing policy calls for the introduction of a system of planned promotion in every organization. If employees are not at all having suitable opportunities for their development and promotion, they get frustrated.

Each and every employee should be given to understand the various promotion routes/possibilities and the attendant facilities that are made available in the form of training programs, orientation schemes, etc. to achieve the same.

Promotion

Promotion implies upgrading of an employee to a higher post involving increase in rank, prestige or status and responsibilities. Generally increase in pay accompanies promotion but it is not essential ingredient.

Transfer

Transfer implies movement of an employee from one job to another without any increase in pay, status or responsibilities. Usually transfer takes place between jobs paying approximately the same salaries.

Appraisal

Appraisal of employees reveals as to how efficiently the subordinate is performing his job and also to know his aptitudes and other qualities necessary for performing the job assigned to him. The qualities of employees that are apprised through performance appraisal are ability to do work, spirit of cooperation, managerial ability, self confidence, initiative, intelligence etc.

The main objective of performance appraisal is to improve the efficiency of a concern by attempting to mobilize the best possible efforts from individuals employed in it.

Determination of Remuneration

Fixation of remuneration is the most difficult and complex function of the personnel department because there are no definite or exact means to determine the correct wages.

Job evaluation is the only systematic technique to determine the worth of the job but much remains to be done in this regard. As wages constitute major part of the cost of production, every concern must consider this aspect very seriously.

RECRUITMENT

Recruitment is the process of searching for prospective employees and stimulation them to apply for jobs in the organization. It is a positive process because it increased the selection ratio by attracting a large number of applicants for the advertised jobs. It is otherwise called as hiring. It is the first step towards creating the competitive strength and the strategic advantage for the organization. Recruitment of candidates is the function preceding the selection, which helps create a pool of prospective employees for the organization so that the management can select the right candidate for the right job from this pool. It may be temporary or permanent basis. It is the organizational function that deals with issues related to people such as compensation, hiring, performance management, organization development, safety, wellness, benefit, employees motivation, communication and training. It also determines whether the required will be available at the work spot when a job is actually to be undertaken.

Definition

1. "Recruitment is the development and maintenance of adequate manpower resources. It involves the creation of a pool of available labour upon whom the organization can depend when it needs additional employees".
2. "Recruitment is the process of searching for prospective employees and Stimulating them to apply for jobs in the organization". **—Flippo Edwin, B, 2003**
3. It is the process of seeking out and attracting individuals from the labour market who are capable and interesting in filling the employment vacancies. **—Taylor and Bergmann**

Objectives

The major objective of recruitment is to prescribe the procedures for recruitment and selection of faculty, administrative, professional and technical personnel. Other objectives are:

- To attract people with multidimensional skills and experiences that suit the present and future organizational strategies
- To induct outsiders with new perspective to lead the company
- To infuse fresh blood at all levels of organization
- To develop an organizational culture that attracts competent people to the organization.

Purpose

- Attract and encourage candidates to apply for the post in the organization
- Determine present and future requirements of the organization
- Create a pool of candidates to enable the selection of best candidates for the organization at low cost
- Begin identifying and preparing potential applicants who will be appropriate candidates.

Principles

- It should be done from a central place like administrative officer/nursing service administration
- Termination and creation of any post should be done by responsible officers, e.g., regarding nursing staff the nursing superintendent has to take the decision and not the medical superintendent
- Only the vacant positions should be filled and neither less nor more should be employed
- Job description should be made before recruitment
- Recruitment procedure should be developed by an experienced person
- Recruitment should be done on the basis of definite qualifications and set standards
- A recruitment policy should be followed
- Chances of promotion should be clearly stated
- Policy should be clear and changeable according to the need.

Recruitment Process

It involves a systematic procedure from searching the candidates for arranging and conducting the interview.

- **Identifying vacancies:** It begins with the human resource department receiving requisitions for recruitment from different departments in the organization. It includes the post to be filled, number of vacancies, duties to perform and qualification with experience.
- **Job specification and person specification:** Job specification is helpful to think of the job under categories like training, background of the job, main responsibilities and job boundaries, expectation of job holder, resources

and constraints affecting the job. Hence it is important to look at nature of job and its requirements.

Whereas personal specification includes following:

- *Physical specification:* It includes physical abilities and skills required for particular job. These are physiological variables like vision, age, motor coordination etc.
- *Mental specification:* It includes IQ, memory, judgement, ability to plan, estimate to read, to write, etc.
- *Emotional and social specification:* It includes the personal characteristics, manner, emotional maturity and stability, aggressiveness or submission, extroversion, introversion, initiation, skills in dealing with others, social adaptability.
- *Behavioral specification:* These types of specifications are mostly required at higher levels of management.

- **Advertising vacancies:** This is the method by which the candidate will be located it is either through internal sources or external sources and also decided the method of advertising for the post.
- **Managing response:** This step is to the way adopted to receive the applications and scrutinized each application as per the requirement by the scrutiny committee.
- Short listing and identifying the prospective candidates- after the scrutiny the eligible candidates are shortlisted and a list is prepared for prospective candidates.
- **Arranged interviews:** Interviews dates are finalized. Criteria for the merit list are prepared by the committee and candidates are informed. The selection committee is formulated.
- **Conducting interviews:** Interview is conducted on the scheduled date by the selection committee; then and there the candidates are selected.

Sources of Recruitment

It can be grouped into two categories. These are internal sources and external sources.

- **Internal sources:** It is done within the organization. It includes the candidates who are already on pay roll of the organization and also who were on the pay roll and plan to return or whom organization would like to retire. These includes:
  - *Transfers:* It involves shifting from one department to other or from one hospital to other or from one shift to other. It does not involve any drastic change in the responsibilities, pay and status of employee.
  - *Promotion:* It leads to shifting of nurse employee to a higher position, carrying higher responsibilities, facilities, status and pay.
- **External sources:** These sources lie outside the organization. Various posts are filled from outside by present employees. The methods of this are;
  - *Advertisement:* It is the most effective means to search potential nurse managers or administers from outside the health organization. Advertisement in leading newspaper or in journal is generally given search qualified personnel for vacant posts.
  - *Employment agencies:* This run by the Government are regarded as a good source of recruitment for bedside nurses. It brings employees in contact with the job seekers. It may be public or private.
  - *Deputation:* This method is very common. The employees of one organization are selected on deputation from other organization for filling the vacancies.
  - *On the campus recruitment:* In this method a preliminary search of prospective employees is done by conducting interviews at the campus of various institutions, universities and colleges on the predetermined dates and candidates found suitable are called for further interviews at specified places.
  - *Online recruitment:* The hiring manager can look at the candidates profile online. More details can be built up about candidates with online tests. The candidates is interviewed and if successful clicks into offer zone.
  - *Telecasting:* the practice of telecasting of vacant posts over TV is gaining importance these days. Special program like Youth plus, job watch and employment news etc.
  - *Recommendations:* When present employees or a business friend recommends a person, a type of preliminary screening takes place.
  - *Labor contractors:* Workers are recruited through labour contractors who are themselves employees of the organization.

Method of Recruitment

Recruitment Procedures

- **Advertising:** By giving advertisements in newspapers of local, regional, national and international levels and journal advertisements.
- **Career day programs:** In some places nursing schools and colleges hold, annual career day programs during which recruiting officers from local health agencies, inform senior students about employment opportunities in those organizations.
- **Open house:** It is showcase of the opening of a new service or educational program. If health agency is well organized of their setting will be attractive to idealistic, service-oriented nurses. Invitation to an open house may sent to individual nurses, group of speciality nurses, professional organizations final year students nurses schools/colleges to attend open house for recruitment.
- **Employee referrals:** It is the procedure in which the present staff recruitment their nurse acquaintance, i.e., recruiter who wishes to fill positions in a particular nursing unit should ask employees in the unit to recruit nurses with whom they have worked comfortably in other settings.

Vacancy Announcement Procedures

The appropriate chief executive campus officer shall review the recruitment sources. All pertinent aspects of the position must be advertised.

- **Recruitment period:**
  - *Administrative, professional and technical vacancies:* All above positions must be advertised at least prior to ten working days of the closing date
  - *Faculty positions:* At the community colleges and temporary/non-tenurial faculty positions at four year campuses may be filled through local recruitment only, unless the applicant pool is inadequate. Such positions must be advertised in a newspaper with state wide distribution at least 10 working days prior to the closing date.
  - *National faculty:* Faculty positions to be filled through national recruitment must be advertised at least fifteen (15) working days prior to the closing date.
  - *Closing dates*: Vacancy announcements with specific closing dates should have the same date in all advertising venues.
- **Guidelines, apply to advertisements:**
  - Faculty positions filled only through local recruitment must be advertised in a newspaper with local wide distribution.
  - Faculty positions filled through national, recruitment may be advertised in a newspaper for appointment in the absence distribution.
  - No applicant from outside the university APT workforce shall be approved for appointment in the absence of state-wide recruitment.
- **National advertising:**
  - All tenure—track positions on four-year campuses
  - Temporary faculty appointments of the year campuses when the local applicant pool may be inadequate.
- **Closing dates:**
  - All APT vacancy announcements shall have closing dates and the closing dates should be the same for all advertising venues.
  - Faculty vacancy announcements may have closing dates or may have continuous recruitments for hand to fill positions.
- After the announcement has been approved for publication, the hiring unit is responsible for funding and placing the advertisement in newspapers, journals or other appropriate media.
- All Advertisements will include the phrase "Equal opportunity/Affirmative action institution".

PERFORMANCE APPRAISAL

A performance appraisal is a systematic and periodic process that assesses an individual employee's job performance and productivity in relation to certain pre-established criteria and organizational objectives. Other aspects of individual employees are considered as well, such as organizational citizenship behavior, accomplishments, potential for future improvement, strengths and weaknesses, etc. In short performance appraisal is a method of evaluating an employee's job performance by comparing actual results to expected outcomes.

Criteria of Performance Appraisal

- **Quality:** The degree to which the process or result of carrying out an activity approaches perfection.
- **Quantity:** The amount produced, expressed in monetary terms, number of units, or number of completed activity cycles.
- **Time lines:** The degree to which an activity or a result produced.
- **Cost effectiveness:** The degree to which the use of the organization's resources (e.g., Human, monetary, technological, material) is maximized in the senses of getting the highest gain.
- **Need for supervision:** The degree to which a job performer can carryout a job function without supervisory assistance.
- **Interpersonal impact:** The degree to which a performer promotes feelings of self-esteem, good will and cooperation among coworkers and subordinates.
- **Training:** Need for training for improving his skills knowledge.

Objectives of Performance Appraisal

Work-related Objectives

- To provide a control for work done
- To improve efficiency
- To help in assessing work and plan future work assignment
- To carryout job evaluation.

Career Development Objectives

- To identify strong and weak points and encourage finding remedies for weak points through training
- To determine career potential
- To plan developmental (promotional or lateral) assignments
- To plan career goals.

Objectives of Communication

- To provide adequate feed back on performance.
- To clearly establish goals, i.e., what is expected of the staff member in terms of performance and future work assignments.
- To provide counseling and job satisfaction through open discussion on performance.
- To let employees assess where they stand within the organization in terms of their performance.

Administrative Objectives

- To serve as a basis for promotion or demotion
- To serve as a basis for allocating incentives
- To serve as a basis for determining transfers, and
- To serve as a basis for termination in case of reduction of staff.

Methods of Performance Appraisal

Traditional Methods

- **Straight ranking method:** This is one of the oldest and simplest techniques of performance appraisal. In this method, the appraiser ranks the employees from the best to the poorest on the basis of their overall performance. It is quite useful for a comparative evaluation.

- **Man-to-man comparison method:** In this method the employer compares each employee with all others in the group, one at a time. After all the comparisons on the basis of the overall comparisons, the employees are given the final rankings.
- **Forced distribution method:** To eliminate the element of bias from the rater's ratings, the evaluator is asked to distribute the employees in some fixed categories of ratings. The rater chooses the appropriate fit for the categories on his own discretion.
- **Free essay method:** This traditional form of appraisal, also known as *"Free Form method"* involves a description of the performance of an employee by his superior. The description is an evaluation of the performance of any individual based on the facts and often includes examples and evidences to support the information. A major drawback of the method is the inseparability of the bias of the evaluator.
- **Critical incident method:** In this method of performance appraisal, the evaluator rates the employee on the basis of critical events and how the employee behaved during those incidents. It includes both negative and positive points. The drawback of this method is that the supervisor has to note down the critical incidents and the employee behavior as and when they occur.
- **Field review method:** In this method, a senior member of the HR department or a training officer discusses and interviews the supervisors to evaluate and rate their respective subordinates. A major drawback of this method is that it is a very time consuming method. But this method helps to reduce the superiors' personal bias.
- **Checklist method:** The rater is given a checklist of the descriptions of the behavior of the employees on job. The checklist contains a list of statements on the basis of which the rater describes the on the job performance of the employees.
- **Graphic rating scale:** In this method, an employee's quality and quantity of work is assessed in a graphic scale indicating different degrees of a particular trait. The factors taken into consideration include both the personal characteristics and characteristics related to the on the job performance of the employees. For example a trait like job knowledge may be judged on the range of average, above average, outstanding or unsatisfactory.

Modern Methods

- **Assessment center method:** The purpose of this method was and is to test candidates in a social situation, using a number of assessors and a variety of procedures.
- **Appraisal by results or management by objectives (MBO):** This method has been evolved by peter Drucker. MBO is potentially a powerful philosophy of managing and an effective way for operationalizing the evaluation process.
- **Human asset accounting method:** The human asset accounting method refers to activity devoted to attaching money estimates the value of form's International human organization and its external customer good will.
- **Behavioral anchored rating scales (BARS):** This is a new appraisal technique which has recently been developed. Its supporter claim that it provides better, more equitable appraisals as compared to other techniques.

Using the Performance Appraisal to Motivate Employees

Systematic employee appraisals have been used in management, since the 1920's using the appraisal as a tool to promote employee growth did not begin until the 1950's. Most formal appraisals focus on the professional worker rather than the hourly paid worker. The evaluation of performance appraisals is reflected in its changing terminology. More recently, it was termed performance evaluation but because the term evaluation implies that personal values are being placed on the performance review. The employee must believe that the appraisal is based in a standard to which other employees in the service classification are held accountable and he should have some input into developing the standards or goals on which his or her performance is judged.

The employee must know how information will be obtained to determine performance. Sources could include peers, coworkers, nursing care plans, patients and personal observations. The appraiser should be one of the employee's direct supervisors, e.g., the charge nurse who works directly with the staff nurse should be involved in the appraisal process and interview.

The performance appraisal is more likely to have a positive outcome, if the appraisal is viewed with trust and professional respect.

Performance Appraisal Tools

Trait Rating Scales

A rating scale is a method of rating a person against a set standard which may be the Job description, desired behaviors. The rating scale is probably the must widely used of the many available appraisal methods.

Job Dimension Scales

This technique requires that a rating scale be constructed for each job classification. The rating factors are taken from the contract of the written job description.

Behaviorally Anchored Rating Scales

BARS sometimes called behavioral expectation scales, overcome some of the weakness inherent in other rating systems. As in the job dimension method. The BARS technique requires that a separate rating form be developed for each job classification. Then as in the job dimension rating scales, employees in specific positions work with management to delineate key areas of responsibility. However, in BARS, may specific examples are defined for each area of responsibility. These examples gives various degrees of importance by ranking example of a job dimension is being met. It is less important that a lower ranked example is not. The greatest disadvantage in using this tool with large numbers of employees is the time and expenses. It is an effective tool because it focuses on specific behaviors, allows employees to know exactly what is expected to them and reduces rating errors.

Checklists

There are several types of checklist appraisal tools. The weighted scale, the most frequently used checklist is composed of many behavioral statements that represent desirable job behaviors. Employees receive an overall performance appraisal score based on behaviors or attributes.

Another type of checklist, the forced checklist, required that the supervisor select on undesirable and a desirable behavior for each employee.

Essays

The essay appraisal method is often referred to as the free form review. The appraiser describes in narrative form as employees, strengths and areas where improvement it growth is needed.

Self Appraisals

Employees are increasingly being asked to submit written summaries or port folios of their work-related accomplishment and productivity as part of the self-appraisal process.

Performance Appraisal Process

The performance appraisal process may be defined as a structured formal interaction between an employee and a manager; in which the employees work performance is examined and discussed with a goal of identifying weaknesses and strengths as well as identifying opportunities for improvement and skills development.

From the employee viewpoint the purpose of performance appraisal is fourfold:

- Tell me what you want me to do
- Tell me how well I've done it
- Help me improve my performance
- Reward me for doing well.

In most healthcare facilities, the results of such performance appraisal are used to determine which employees deserve pay increases, bonuses or promotions.

Components of Performance Appraisal

The performance appraisal process gives an employee recognition for his work efforts. Great power rests in such recognition and, in fact, it's well known that human beings prefer even negative recognition to no recognition at all. The performance appraisal process typically consists of four inter-related steps.

Step 1: Clear Expectations

The first step occurs well before an evaluation is ever done. A new employee must be told and must understand exactly what the job expectations are, how performance will be measured, who will 'judge' the work, and how often.

Step 2: Regular Feedback

An employee should also be aware that the performance appraisal process is just that, a process and not a once-a-year drill. Ongoing assessment of performance and the progress in meeting job expectations is vital. It isn't good management style to wait until an evaluation to tell and an employee that he's consistently failing to meeting expectations

Step 3: Documented Progress

Through documentation of the employees performance using the facility's policies, procedures, and forms in the next step. If the facility was a self appraisal, peer review, or 360 degree, make sure the employee clearly understands how he's to be rated before the actual meeting.

Step 4: Future Direction

Finally, set up a time to conduct the performance appraisal interview with the employee. Allow time, and have all documents ready make sure you have coverage for phone calls or other managerial duties so your time with the employee is uninterrupted. Be prepared to end the review with a discussion of a job related development plan that's tailored to that employee.

Ethics of Appraisal

Do not appraise without knowing why the appraisal is needed.

- Appraise on the basis of representative information
- Appraise on the basis of sufficient information
- Appraise on the basis of relevant information
- Be honest in your assessment of all the facts you have obtained.
- Do not write one thing and say another
- In offering an appraisal, make it plan that this is only your personal opinion of the facts as you see them.
- Pass on appraisal information only to those who have good reason to want it.
- Do not imply the existence of an appraisal that has not been made
- Do not accept another's appraisal without knowing the basis on which it was made.

Performance Appraisal in Nursing Management

The best performance review lets a manager an employee communicate—share ideas, opinions and information with the ultimate goal of higher performance and success.

The well orchestrated performance appraisal helps foster the professional growth of an employee and improves the facility's performance.

The performance appraisal process is an ongoing process that prevails the employees from being surprised by anything that's said when the formal interview occurs.

Progressive discipline should be instituted with the goal of turning a poor performance around. If this doesn't work, then termination may be the best solution. JCAHO (Joint Commission in Accreditation of Health Care Organizations) Standards require health care facilities to define their mission and purpose define the qualifications of employees to meet that mission, recruit and retain competent staff and, finally, assess and improve the ongoing competency of the staff the performance appraisal process.

LEGAL STANDARDS OF PRACTICE

Legal standards of practice nursing in a safe, efficient, competent manner, you must understand both the legal regulation of nursing practice and voluntary professional regulation of nursing practice. There are several types of laws that direct nursing practice.

Nurse Practice Acts

In all status in the United States, nurse practice Acts regulate the licensure and practice of nursing, each state or province defines for itself the scope of nursing practice, but most have similar practice acts. The definition of nursing practice published by the ANA is in some ways representative of the scope of nursing practice as defined in most states. In the last decade, how ever, many states have revised their nurse practice acts to reflect nursing growing autonomy and the expanded roles of nurses in practice.

Licensure and Certification

Licensure

In the United States, RN candidates must pass the NCLEX-RN, which is administered by the individual state boards of nursing. Regardless of educational preparation, the examination for RN licensure is exactly the same in every state in the United States. This provides a standardized minimum knowledge base for the client population nurse serve.

Certification

Beyond the NCLEX-RN, the nurse may choose to work toward certification in a specific area of nursing practice. Minimum practice requirements are set, based on the certification the nurse is seeking.

Occupational Safety and Health Act

The occupational safety and health Act of 1970, known as OSHA, established legal standards that define safe helpful working conditions. OSHA is periodically updated and expanded, and it affects you as a nurse in two ways—

- First, it sets standards for your working conditions.
- Second, some of the requirements of the law dictate how you manage clients.

Controlled Substance Acts

Several laws have been enacted that address standards for drug development and marketing. These laws affect the process by which new drugs become available to clients. Most significant for you is the comprehensive drug abuse prevention and control Act of 1970. This law was enacted to regulate the distribution and use of drugs with the potential for abuse.

Health Care Quality Improvement Act

One of the difficult issues in attempting to protect the public from unsafe and incompetent healthcare providers has been the tracking of information related to adverse licensure actions, malpractice payments and adverse professional actions.

Americans with Disabilities Act

The Americans with Disabilities Act (ADA), passed in 1990, was enacted to protect persons with disabilities from discrimination in such areas as housing, employment, education and health services. The act uses a broad definition of disability that includes persons with AIDS or infected with the human immunodeficiency virus (HIV) and persons recovering from drugs or alcohol addition. Many of year clients may be disabled. As a result, you may be assisting your clients to assert their rights under this law, particularly if you work in an out patient or community health setting.

LEGAL ISSUES IN COMMUNITY HEALTH NURSING

A number of legal issues are related to nursing practice, including licensing, nurse practice act, and standards of care. However in these litigious times, the issues that most concern there considering a career in nursing are negligence and malpractice which is more common in community health nursing. Malpractice is the negligence by a professional. Four elements are needed to prove malpractice.

1. Duty
2. Breach
3. Causation
4. Damages.

Duty

Duty stands for a legal obligation owed by one person to another person. When nurses care for clients they assume the duty to care for them in a competent and diligent manner. Nurses are expected to provide the degree of care ordinarily exercised by other nurses participating in the same nursing specialty. Therefore nurses are expected to adheres to standards of care- those imposed by nurses state board of nursing practice act, the national nursing specialty stands of care and scope of practice, and the nurses hospital, or other agency or protocols.

Breach

A breach of duty takes place when there is failure to fulfil the duties established as being the responsibility of nurses. In other words, nurses breach their duties when they do not meet the appropriate standards of care.

Causation

Causation is the most difficult element to prove because it is the factual connection between what the nurse did and the injury to the client. Causation means that the nurses' breach of duty, or failure to meet the appropriate standard of care, caused the client injury or adverse outcome.

Damages

Damages are monetary payment designed to compensate the client for the injury or adverse outcome, and are intended to restore the plaintiff to the condition he or she was in prior to the injury. To recover damages, the clients must establish that she/he suffered physical, financial or emotional injury caused by the nurses' violation of the standard of care. Damages are usually compensatory or punitive.

Community health nursing is the combination of nursing practice and public health practice. The community health nurse is subject to the law relating to nursing practice and public health. The duties of all nurses become legally binding responsibilities for which the nurse is accountable. In addition, the community health nurse have many responsibilities that are unique to public health focused practice, despite the broad nature and varies roles of community health nursing practice, two legal aspects apply to most practice situation such as:

1. Professional negligence or malpractice.
2. Scope of practice.

The issue of scope of practice involves differencing between the practices of physicians, nurses and others healthcare providers. Scope of practice is assessed by, examining the usual and customary practice and profession and taking into account how legislation defines the practice of profession in a jurisdiction.

The usual and customary practices of CHN can be determined through a variety sources which include:

- Contents of CHN education profession are general and special.
- Experiences of other practicing nurses.
- Activities and statements, including and standards of CHN professional organizations.
- Policies and procedures of agency employing nurses.
- Needs and interest of the community
- Literature, including books, text and journal.

Legal aspects of the roles and functions of the CHN especially scope of practice and negligence will prove to be useful information for nurses' in community health. Every community health nurse must consider legal implication of practice in each clinical encounter, i.e., health education, nutrition education, maintaining sanitation and supply of portable water, maternal and childbirth including family planning, communicable diseases control, school health, occupational health and mental healthy, etc., because the community health nurse may be agent of the Govt. When implanting a particular health program, consideration must be given to the power of the state or the relationship of this power to individual right. In each clinical encounter, before treating the client, the community health nurse should know what a standard of care applies to the situations. Standards of care can be learned from expert nurse witness can be found in agency policies and procedures, nursing and heathcare literature.

Roles and Functions of Nurse Manager in Legal Issues

The following are the leadership's roles and managerial functions of a nurse manager in ethical and legal issues, i.e.:

- Serve as a role model by providing nursing care that meets or exceeds accepted standards of care.
- Reports standard nursing care to appropriate authorities.
- Fosters nurse patients' relationships that are respectful, caring and honest, thus reducing the possibility of future lawsuits.
- Joins and actively support professional organization to strengthen the lobbying efforts of nurses' in healthcare legislation.
- Practices nursing with in the area of individual competence.
- Priorities patients' rights and welfare first in decision making.
- Demonstrate vision, risk taking and energy in determining appropriate legal boundaries for nursing practices, thus defining what nursing is and should be in the future.
- Should be knowledgeable responding sources of law and legal doctrines that affect nursing practice.
- Delegate to subordinates wisely, looking at the manager scope of practice and that of those they supervise.
- Understands and adhere to institutional policies and procedures.
- Practices nursing within the scope of the state nurse practice act.
- Monitor subordinates to ensure that they have a valid, current and appropriate license to practice nursing.
- Use forcibility of harm in delegation ad staffing decisions.
- Increase staff awareness of intentional torts and assists them in developing strategies to reduce their liability in these area.
- Provides educational and training opportunities for staff on legal issues affecting nursing practice.

JCAHO STANDARD OF NURSING PRACTICE

JCAHO Standard of Case Management

- In 1975 the JCAHO urged the use of outcome criteria to evaluate nursing.
- Today the JCAHO continuous to recommend the use of
- Outcome criteria using a collaborative approach to patient focused care.
- This collaborative effort by the interdisciplinary work group begins before admission and continuous until discharge.

JCAHO Standards for Quality Improvement

- The JCAHO (1996) is an external review board that establish standards for institutions to ensure that the institution functions within specifies guidelines.
- The hospital standards for nursing care are applicable to all clients in every setting where nursing care is provided.
- Recent changes in the JCAHO guidelines require the continuous monitoring and evaluation of the quality of nursing care provided by the department of nursing.

JCAHO Standards for Client Education

According to the JCAHO (2003), the goal of client and family education is to promote healthy behavior and encourage the clients involvement both in the delivery of health care and in healthcare decisions, to improve outcomes. Educational efforts must take into consideration the clients psychosocial, spiritual and cultural values, as well as his or he desire to actively participate in the educational process.

JCAHO Standard for Medical Mistakes

In January 2003, the JCAHO established National Patient Safety goals in an effort to reduce the risk of medical errors. These evidence-based recommendations require healthcare facilities to focus their attention on a series of specific actions. Data on the achievement of the goals will be made public each year. New goals are announced each year in July. The national patient safety goals for 2004 include:

- Improving the accuracy of patient identification
- Improving the effectiveness of communication among care givers
- Improving the safety after using high alert medications.
- Eliminating wrong site, wrong client, wrong procedure surgery
- Improving the effectiveness of clinical alarm system and reducing risk of nosocomial.

JCAHO Standard for Nursing Practice

Standards of care are the legal guidelines for nursing practice. The JCAHO requires that accredited hospitals have written nursing policies and procedures. The written policies and procedures of the employing institution detail how nurses are to perform their duties. These internal standards of care are quite specific and should be accessible on all nursing units. For example, a policy/procedure outlining the steps that should be taken when changing a dressing or administering medication provides specific information about how nurses are to perform these tasks. The institutional policies and procedures must conform to state and federal laws, as well as community standards and cannot conflict with legal guidelines that define acceptable standards of care. The nurse is obligated to behave honestly and truthfully with regard to the client.

INDIAN PUBLIC HEALTH STANDARDS

National Rural Health Mission (NHM) was launched in the year 2005 to strengthen the Rural Public Health System and has since met many hopes and expectations. The Mission seeks to provide effective health care to the rural populace throughout the country with special focus on the States and Union Territories (UTs), which have weak public health indicators and/or weak infrastructure. Towards this end, the Indian Public Health Standards (IPHS) centers, Primary Health Centers (PHCs), Community Health Centers (CHCs), Sub-district and District Hospitals were published in January/February, 2007 and have been used as the reference point for public healthcare infrastructure planning and upgradation in the States and UTs. IPHS are a set of uniform standards envisaged to improve the quality of healthcare delivery in the country. The IPHS documents have been revised keeping in view the changing protocols of the existing programs and introduction of new programs especially for noncommunicable diseases. Flexibility is allowed to suit the diverse needs of the states and regions. These IPHS guidelines will act as the main driver for continuous improvement in quality and serve as the bench mark for assessing the functional status of health facilities. States and UTs should adopt these IPHS guidelines for strengthening the Public Health Care Institutions and put in their best efforts to achieve high quality of health care across the country.

THE DESIGN OF PRIMARY HEALTH CENTER FOLLOWING IPHS GUIDELINES

From service delivery angle, PHCs may be of two types, depending upon the delivery case load—**Type A and Type B.**

Type A PHC: PHC with delivery load of less than 20 deliveries in a month,

Type B PHC: PHC with delivery load of 20 or more deliveries in a month

The PHC should have a building of its own. The surroundings should be clean. The details are as follows:

PHC Building

Location

It should be centrally located in an easily accessible area. The area chosen should have facilities for electricity, all weather road communication, adequate water supply and telephone. At a place, where a PHC is already located, another health center/SC should not be established to avoid the wastage of human resources. PHC should be away from garbage collection, cattle shed, water logging area, etc. PHC shall have proper boundary wall and gate.

Area

It should be well planned with the entire necessary infrastructure. It should be well lit and ventilated with as much use of natural light and ventilation as possible The plinth area would vary from 375 to 450 sq. meters

Signage

The building should have a prominent board displaying the name of the center in the local language at the gate and on the building. PHC should have pictorial, bilingual directional and layout signage of all the departments and public utilities (toilets, drinking water). Prominent display boards in local language providing information regarding the services available/user charges/fee and the timings of the center. Relevant IEC material shall be displayed at strategic locations.

Entrance with Barrier Free Access

Barrier free access environment for easy access to non ambulant (wheel-chair, stretcher), semiambulant, visually disabled and elderly persons as per guidelines of GOI. Ramp as per specification, Hand-railing, proper lightning, etc., must be provided in all health facilities and retrofitted in older one which lack the same. The doorway leading to the entrance should also have a ramp facilitating easy access for old and physically challenged patients.

Disaster Prevention Measures

For all new upcoming facilities in seismic 5 zone or other disaster prone areas. Building and the internal structure should be made disaster proof especially earthquake proof, flood proof and equipped with fire protection measures. Earthquake proof measures—structural and nonstructural should be built in to withstand quake as per geographical/state govt. guidelines.

Fire fighting equipment—fire extinguishers, sand buckets, etc., should be available and maintained to be readily available when needed. Staff should be trained in using fire fighting equipment. All PHCs should have Disaster Management Plan in line with the District Disaster management Plan. All health staff should be trained and well conversant with disaster prevention and management aspects. Surprise mock drills should be conducted at regular intervals.

Waiting Area

- This should have adequate space and seating arrangements
- The walls should carry posters imparting health education.
- Booklets/leaflets in local language may be provided in the waiting area for the same purpose.
- Toilets with adequate water supply separate for males and females should be available. Waiting area should have adequate number of fans, coolers, benches or chairs.
- Safe drinking water should be available.

Outpatient Department

- The outpatient room should have separate areas for consultation and examination and should have sufficient privacy.
- In PHCs with AYUSH doctor, necessary infrastructure such as consultation room for AYUSH doctor and AYUSH drug dispensing area should be made available.
- OPD rooms shall have provision for ample natural light, and air. Windows shall open directly to the external air or into an open verandah.
- Adequate measures should be taken for crowd management
- One room for immunization/family planning/counseling.

Wards 5.5 m × 3.5 m each

- There should be 4–6 beds in a Primary Health Center. Separate wards/areas should be earmarked for males and females with the necessary furniture.
- There should be facilities for drinking water and separate clean toilets for men and women.
- The ward should be easily accessible from the OPD so as to obviate the need for a separate nursing staff in the ward and OPD during OPD hours.
- Nursing station should be located in such a way that health staff can be easily accessible to OT and labor room after regular clinic timings.
- Cleaning of the wards, etc. should be carried out at regular intervals without interfere with the work during peak hours and also during times of eating.

Operation Theater (Optional)

- To facilitate conducting selected surgical procedures (e.g., vasectomy, tubectomy, hydrocelectomy, etc.). It should have a changing room, sterilization area operating area and washing area.
- Separate facilities for storing of sterile and unsterile equipment/instruments should be available in the OT.
- The OT should be well-equipped with all the necessary accessories and equipment.
- OT shall be fumigated at regular intervals and PHC shall have standard operative procedure for autoclaving.
- OT shall have power back up (generator/invertor/UPS). OT should have restricted entry. Separate foot wear should be used.

Labor Room (3.8 m × 4.2 m)

Newborn care corner: It is a space within the labor room, 20-30 sq ft in size, with well equipped like radiant warmer, oxygen cylinder, suction machine and other equipment for resuscitation. All equipments must be well functioning.

Proper infection control technique must be part of the delivery room.

There should be separate areas for septic and aseptic deliveries.

The labor room should be well-lit and ventilated with an attached toilet and drinking water facilities. Facilities for hot water shall be available.

Separate areas for dirty linen, baby wash, toilet, sterilization.

Standard treatment protocols for common problems during labor and for newborns with all the essential drugs to be provided in the labor room.

Cleanliness shall always be maintained in labor room by regular washing and mopping with disinfectants.

Minor OT/Dressing Room/Injection Room/Emergency

- This should be located close to the OPD to cater to patients for minor surgeries and emergencies after OPD hours.
- It should be well equipped with all the emergency drugs and instruments.
- Privacy of the patients should be ensured.

Laboratory (3.8 m × 2.7 m)

- Sufficient space with workbenches and separate area for collection and screening should be available.
- Should have marble/stone table top for platform and wash basins.

General Store

Separate area for storage of sterile and common linen and other materials/drugs/consumable, etc. should be provided with adequate storage space.

The area should be well-lit and ventilated and rodent/pest free.

Sufficient number of racks shall be provided and drugs shall be stored properly in safe and dry environment.

Inflammable and hazardous material shall be secured and stored separately near expiry drugs shall be segregated and stored separately.

Sufficient space with the storage cabins separately for AYUSH drugs be provided.

Dispensing cum Store Area: 3 m × 3 m

Infrastructure for AYUSH doctor: Based on the system of medicine being practiced, appropriate arrangements should be made for the provision of a doctor's room and a dispensing room cum drug storage.

- Waste disposal pit—As per GOI/central pollution
- Control board (CPCB) guidelines.
- Cold chain room—Size: 3 m × 4 m
- Logistics room—Size: 3 m × 4 m
- Generator room—Size: 3 m × 4 m
- Office room—3.5 m × 3.0 m
- Dirty utility room for dirty linen and used items
- Residential accommodation.

Essential

Decent accommodation with all the amenities likes 24-hours. water supply, electricity, etc., should be available for medical officer, nursing staff, pharmacist, laboratory technician and other staff. If the accommodation cannot be provided due to any reason, then the staff may be paid house rent allowance, but in that case they should be staying in near vicinity of PHC so that they are available 24 × 7, in case of need.

Other Amenities

Adequate water supply and water storage facility (over head tank) with pipe water should be made available.

Computer

Computer with internet connection should be provided for Management Information System (MIS) purpose.

Lecture Hall/Auditorium Desirable

For training purposes, a lecture hall or a small auditorium for 30 person should be available. Public address system and a black board should also be provided.

The staffing pattern and functions of PHC according to IPHS guideline already explained in the chapter 9 and chapter name is healthcare delivery system in India.

THE DESIGN OF COMMUNITY HEALTH CENTER FOLLOWING IPHS GUIDELINES

Physical Infrastructure

The CHC should have 30 indoor beds with one operation theater, labor room, X-ray, ECG and laboratory facility. In order to provide these facilities, following are the guidelines.

Location of the center: All the guidelines as below under this subhead may be applicable only to centers that are to be newly established and priority is to be given to operationalize the existing CHCs. To the extent possible, the center should be located at the center of the block headquarter in order to improve access to the patients. Facility for electricity, all weather road communication, adequate water supply, telephone CHC should be away from garbage collection, cattle shed, water logging area entrance zone

- **Signage:** Prominent display boards in local language providing information regarding the services available and the timings of the institute. Directional and layout signages for all the departments and utilities (toilets, drinking water etc.) shall be appropriately displayed for easy access. All the signages shall be bilingual and pictorial.
- **Barrier free access environment:** For easy access to non-ambulant (wheel-chair stretcher), semiambulant, visually disabled and elderly persons as per 'guidelines and space standards for barrier-free built environment for disabled and elderly persons' of government of India. Ramp as per specification, hand-railing, proper lightning, etc., must be provided in all health facilities and retrofitted in older one which lack the same. Registration cum Inquiry counters. Pharmacy for drug dispensing and storage.
- **Outpatient department:** The facility shall be planned keeping in mind the maximum peak hour load and shall have scope for future expansion. Name of department and doctor, timings and user fees/charges shall be displayed. Layout of the out patient department shall follow the functional flow of the patients:
  - E.g. → Registration → Waiting → Sub waiting → Clinic → Dressing room/Injection Room → Billing → Diagnostics (lab/X-ray) → Pharmacy → Exit
- **Clinics for various medical disciplines:** These clinics include general medicine, general surgery, dental,

obstetric and gynecology, pediatrics and family welfare. Separate cubicles for general medicine and surgery with separate area for internal examination (privacy) can be provided if there are no separate rooms for each. The cubicles for consultation and examination in all clinics should provide for doctor's table, chair, patient's stool, follower's seat, wash basin with hand washing facilities, examination couch and equipment for examination. The pharmacy should be located in an area conveniently accessible from all clinics.

- **Emergency room/casualty:** At the moment, the emergency cases are being attended in OPD during OPD hours and in inpatient units afterwards. It is recommended to have a separate earmarked emergency area to be located near the entrance of hospital.
- **Nursing station:** The nursing station shall be centerd such that it serves all the clinics from that place. The nursing station should be spacious enough to accommodate a medicine chest/a work counter (for preparing dressings, medicines), hand washing facilities, sinks, dressing tables with screen in between and color coded bins (as per IMEP guidelines for community health centers). It should have provision for Hub cutters and needle destroyers.
- **Operation theater/labor room:** In operation theaters or Labor room the following provisions must be assembled.
    - Patient waiting area.
    - Preoperative and postoperative (recovery) room.
    - Staff area.
    - Changing room separate for males and females.
    - Storage area for sterile supplies.
    - Operating room/labor room.
    - Scrub area.
    - Instrument sterilization area.
    - Disposal area.
    - Newborn care corner and Newborn Care Stabilization Unit.

Physical infrastructure for support services: Physical infrastructure for support services must be include the followings:

- **Central sterilization supply department (CSSD):** Sterilization and sterile storage.
- **Laundry:** Storage should be separate for dirty linen and clean linen.
- Outsourcing is recommended after appropriate training of washer man regarding.
- Segregation and separate treatment for infected and noninfected linen.

Engineering services: Electricity/telephones/water/civil engineering may be outsourced.

Maintenance of proper sanitation in toilets and other public utilities should be given utmost attention. Sufficient funding for this purpose must be kept and the services may be outsourced.

Water supply: Arrangements shall be made to supply 10,000 liters of potable water per day to meet all the requirements (including laundry) except fire fighting.

Emergency lighting: Emergency portable/fixed light units should also be provided in the wards and departments.

Telephone: Minimum two direct lines with intercom facility should be available.

Residential Zone

- Minimum 8 quarters for doctors.
- Minimum 8 quarters for staff nurses/paramedical staff.
- Minimum 2 quarters for ward boys.
- Minimum 1 quarter for driver.

If the accommodation cannot be provided due to any reason, then the staff may be paid house rent allowance, but in that case they should be staying in near vicinity of CHC so that they are available for 24 × 7 in case of need.

Function and space requirement for community health center.

It is suggested considering the land cost and availability of land, CHC building may be constructed in two floors.

- Quality assurance in service delivery
- Quality of service should be maintained at all levels
- **Standard Treatment Protocol** is the 'Heart' of quality and cost of care. Standard treatment protocol for all national programs and locally common diseases should be made available at all CHCs. All the efforts that are being made to improve 'hardware, i.e., infrastructure' and 'software, i.e., human resource' are necessary but not sufficient. These need to be guided by standard treatment protocols. Some of the states have already prepared these guidelines. For all ailments covered by national health programs an agreed treatment/case management protocol need to be adhered to voluntarily by the physicians.
- **Diet:** Diet may either be outsourced or adequate space for cooking should be provided in a separate space. The diet within the budget/funds and affordability should be healthy food, nutritious and full of minerals and vitamins.
- **CSSD:** Adequate space and standard procedures for sterilization and sterile storage should be available. A practical protocol for quality assurance of CSSD may be developed in coordination with district hospital lab and implemented to ensure sterilization quality.

Laundry

- **Storage:** Separate for dirty linen and clean linen. Outsourcing is recommended after appropriate training of washer man regarding separate treatment for infected and noninfected linen.
- **Services:** Maintenance of electricity/telephones/water supply/civil engineering, etc., may be outsourced.
- **Waste disposal:** 'Guidelines for health care workers for waste management and infection control in community health centers' are to be followed. A central storage point should be made for biomedical waste collected from all points of CHC which should be located away from OPD and IPD.
- **Charter of patient rights:** It is mandatory for every CHC to have the charter of patient rights prominently displayed at the entrance.

- **Quality control:** The quality can be monitored by the following procedures
  - Internal monitoring
  - Routine monitoring by District Health Authority at least once in a month.
  - *Social audit:* Through Rogi Kalyan Samitis/Panchayati Raj Institution, etc.
  - Medical audit
  - Others like death audit, technical audit, economic audit, disaster preparedness audit, etc.
  - Patient satisfaction surveys.

Patient Safety and Infection Control

Essential

- Hand washing facilities in all OPD clinics, wards, emergency and OT areas.
- Safe clinical practices as per standard protocols to prevent health care associated infections and other harms to patients.
- There shall be proper written handing over system between healthcare staff.
- Safe injection administration practices as per the prescribed protocol.
- Safe blood transfusion practices need to be implemented by the hospital administrators.
- Ensuring safe disposal of biomedical waste as per rules (national guidelines to be followed).
- Regular training of health care workers in patient safety, infection control and biomedical waste management.

The staffing pattern and functions of the community health center had discussed in the chapter 9 and the chapter name is healthcare delivery system in India.

SUBCENTER STANDARD FOLLOWING IPHS GUIDELINES

In the public sector, a subhealth center (subcenter) is the most peripheral and first point of contact between the primary healthcare system and the community. The minimum needs program (MNP) was introduced in the country in the first year of the Fifth Five Year Plan (1974–78) with the objective to provide certain basic minimum needs and thereby improve the living standards of the people. In the field of rural health, the objective was to establish: one subcenter for a population. A subcenter provides interface with the community at the grass-root level, providing all the primary health care services. As subcenters are the first contact point with the community, the success of any nation wide program would depend largely on the well functioning subcenters providing services of acceptable standard to the people. The current level of functioning of the subcenters is much below the expectations. In order to provide quality care in these subcenters, Indian Public Health Standards (IPHS) are being prescribed to provide basic primary health care services to the community and achieve and maintain an acceptable standard of quality of care. Currently the IPHS for subcenters has been prepared keeping in view the resources available with respect to functional requirement for subcenters with minimum standards, such as building, manpower, instruments and equipment, drugs and other facilities and desirable standards which represent the ideal situation.

In view of the current highly variable situation of subcenters have been categorized into two types—Type A and Type B.

Type A Subcenter

It will provide all recommended services except that the facilities for conducting delivery will not be available here. However, the ANMs have been trained in midwifery, they may conduct normal delivery in case of need. If the requirement for this goes up, like not having adequate space and physical infrastructure for conducting deliveries the subcenter may be considered for up gradation to *Type B*.

Staff Recommended

Two ANM (Essential) One Health Worker (Male): (Essential) One Staff Nurse or ANM (if Staff Nurse not available) (Desirable, if number of deliveries at the subcenter is 20 or more in a month) Sanitation services should be provided through outsourcing on full time basis.

Service Provided

Subcenters are expected to provide promotive, preventive and few curative primary healthcare services. Keeping in view the changing epidemiological situation in the country, both types of subcenters should lay emphasis on Noncommunicable diseases related services. Given the understanding of the health subcenter as mainly providing outreach facilities, where most services are not delivered in the subcenter building itself, the site of service delivery may be at village itself.

The major areas for health services are:

- Maternal and Child Health
- Family Planning and Contraception
- Safe Abortion Services (MTP)
- Curative Services
- Adolescent Health Care
- School Health Services
- Control of Local Endemic Diseases
- Disease Surveillance, Integrated Disease Surveillance Project (IDSP)
- Water and Sanitation
- Out reach/Field Services Village Health and Nutrition Day (VHND)
- Home Visits
- House-to-House Surveys
- Community Level Interactions
- Coordination and Monitoring
- National Health Programs.

Physical Infrastructure

A subcenter should have its own building. If that is not possible immediately, the premises with adequate space should be rented in a central location with easy access to population. The states should also explore options of getting funds for space from other Health Programs and other funding sources.

- **Location of the center:** For all new upcoming subcenters, following may be ensured: Subcenter to be located within the village for providing easy access to the people and safety of the ANM. As far as possible no person has to travel more than 3 km to reach the subcenter. The subcenter village has some communication net work (road communication/public transport/post office/ telephone). subcenter should be away from garbage collection, cattle shed, water logging area, etc. While finalizing the location of the subcenter, the concerned Panchayat should also be consulted.
- **Building and lay out:** Boundary wall/fencing: Boundary wall/fencing with gate should be provided for safety and security. In the typical layout of the subcenter, the residential facility for ANM is included
- **Residential facility:** Residential facility for health worker (Male), if need is felt, may be provided by expanding the subcenter building to the first floor. The entrance to the subcenter should be well lit and easy to locate. It should have provision for easy access for disabled and elderly. The minimum covered area of a subcenter along with residential quarter for ANM will vary depending on land availability, type of subcenter and resources. Separate entrance for the subcenter and for the ANM quarter may be ensured.

Type B Subcenter

It should have, about 4–5 rooms with facilities of Waiting Room, one labor room with one labor table and Newborn corner, one room with two to four beds (in case the no. of deliveries at the subcenter is 20 or more, four beds will be provided), one room for store, one room for clinic/office and one toilet facility each in labor room ward room and in waiting area (essential) residential accommodation: This should be made available to the health workers with each one having 2 rooms, kitchen, bathroom and water closet (WC). Residential facility for one ANM is as follows which is contiguous with the main subcenter area.

- Room—1 (3.3 m × 2.7 m)
- Room—2 (3.3 m × 2.7 m
- Kitchen—1 (1.8 m × 2.5 m) y W.C (1.2 m × 9.0 m) y

Bathroom (1.5 m × 1.2 m) residential facility for a minimum of 2 staff and desirably for 3 staff should be provided at type B (MCH) subcenters. A typical layout plan for type A subcenter with ANM residence having area of 85 square meters and type B subcenter having an additional area of 65 square meters on ground floor and 125 square meters on first floor, with area/space specifications.

Signage

The building should have a prominent board displaying the name of the center in the local language at the gate and on the building.

The essential measures at the subcenter by following IPHS guidelines are:

- Disaster prevention measures against earthquake, flood and fire
- Environment friendly features
- Adequate furniture that is sturdy and easy to maintain
- The equipment provided to the subcenters should be adequate to provide all the assured services in the subcenters
- Laboratory facilities minimum for urine pregnancy testing, estimation of hemoglobin by hemoglobinometer uninterrupted power supply has to be ensured
- Potable water for patients and staff and water for other use should be in adequate quantity
- Type B subcenters, landline telephone facility should be provided
- Assured referral linkages
- Toilet facility for use of patients/attendants and subcenter staff must be provided
- Infection Management and Environment Plan 'Guidelines for Health Care Workers for Waste Management and Infection Control in subcenters' of Ministry of Health and Family Welfare, Government of India are to be followed
- Proper maintenance of records of services provided at the subcenters and the morbidity/mortality data is necessary for assessing the health situation in the subcenter area.

STANDARD FOR COMMUNITY HEALTH NURSING PRACTICE

Some standards developed by United Arab Emirates which define community nursing practice and set out the professional expectations for community nurses in the Emirate of Dubai, which are designed to support community nurses who may practice in a variety of settings. They had developed five standards and having a verity of verification criteria

Standard 1: Facilitating Access and Equity

The Community Nurse

- Facilitates equitable access to available healthcare services and promotes comprehensive and holistic care.
- Adopts a wide range of strategies such as home visits, outreach, follow-up and case findings to ensure equity of access to services.
- Promotes client centered health outcomes.
- Advocates for appropriate resource allocation to improve health outcomes.
- Adapts practice in response to the changing health needs of the individual and community. Is proactive in addressing service gaps, health inequalities and accessibility issues, especially for those most vulnerable and uses culturally appropriate and gender sensitive strategies to address them.
- Monitors and evaluates access to appropriate community services on behalf of client.

Standard 2: Promoting Health

A. Health Promotion

The Community Nurse:

- Will apply a 'wellness focus' when promoting health.
- Promotes health and the maintenance of wellbeing in the community and evaluates the impact of nurse interventions.
- Assesses individual and community needs in partnership with clients and stakeholders.
- Identifies which determinants of health require action or change to promote health.
- Integrates health promotion into all aspects of community nursing.
- Ensures that Dubai Health Policies and Regulations are taken into account in the implementation of programs.

B. Prevention and Health Protection

- Collaborates with individuals and communities to make informed choices about protective and preventive health measures and identify potential risks.
- Applies epidemiological principles, such as screening, surveillance, immunization, communicable disease response, outbreak management, and education for health prevention activities.
- Engages in collaborative, interdisciplinary and inter sectoral partnerships to address risks to individual, family, community, using follow-up and referral systems where appropriate.

C. Health Maintenance, Restoration and Palliation

- Links people to community resources and coordinate or facilitate other care needs and supports. .
- Provides education and counseling to clients as appropriate, respecting individual choices.
- Identifies short and long-term health related interventions appropriate to the cultural setting. This standard incorporates strategies from the frameworks of primary health care (World Health Organization, 1978), the Ottawa Charter for Health Promotion (World Health Organization, 1986) and the Population Health Promotion Model (Health Canada, 2000).
- Maximizes the ability of an individual, family or community to take responsibility for and manage their health needs according to resources and personal skills available.
- Responds to health emergencies where appropriate that impact on health outcomes.
- Evaluates outcomes of practice in collaboration with individuals, families, significant others, community partners and other health practitioners.

Standard 3: Building Individual and Community Capacity

The Community Nurse

- Actively involves and collaborates with individuals, groups, organizations and communities in all phases of planned change to increase their skills, knowledge and willingness to promote health outcomes.
- Coordinates with the individual and community to participate in the resolution of their issues and to gather available resources to support taking action on their health issues.
- Supports the individual, family, community or population to develop skills for self-advocacy and apply the principles of social justice to support those who are not yet able to take action for them.
- Supports community action to influence policy change in support of health.
- Actively works with health professionals and community partners to build capacity for health promotion.

Standard 4: Building Relationships

The Community Nurse

- Establishes and maintains nurse-client therapeutic interactions and relationships.
- Establishes a supportive environment which also promotes maximum participation and self determination.
- Respects the ability of the individual or community to know the issue they are addressing and solve their own problems.
- Promotes and supports linkages with relevant community resources where appropriate.
- Maintains a professional and ethical practice in the community.

Standard 5: Demonstrating Professional Responsibility and Accountability

The Community Nurse

- Strives for excellence and is professionally competent and ensures that knowledge, practice and interventions are evidence based.
- Is accountable to a variety of authorities and stakeholders as well as to the individual and community they serve.
- Will take preventive or corrective action to protect individuals and communities from unsafe or unethical circumstances/practices.
- Will ensure that all nursing activities/interventions are documented.
- Where applicable participate in research activities which strengthen health outcomes and community nursing practice.
- Participates in the advancement and profile of community health nursing.
- Provides leadership in community health and takes action on factors which affect autonomy of practice and quality of care.
- Incorporates quality improvement principles in nursing practice.
- Works within the principles of infection control in all activities.
- Acts upon legal obligations to report to appropriate authorities any situations of unsafe or unethical care.

- Assumes responsibility for ongoing educational activities to enhance nursing practice.

POLICIES

Policies and standards are corelate with each other. Policy is A formal, brief, and high-level statement or plan that embraces an organization's general beliefs, goals, objectives, and acceptable procedures for a specified subject area. Policies always state required actions, and may include pointers to standards. Policy attributes include, required compliance (mandatory), failure to comply results in disciplinary action, focus on desired results, not on means of implementation and further defined by standards and guidelines whereas the standard is a mandatory action or rule designed to support and conform to a policy. A standard can make a policy more meaningful and effective.

Definition

Policies are simply guides to decision-making that in turn governs a planned course of action to solve a problem.

—**Rastogi**

Decisions about what kinds of activities are appropriate and when, how, and by whom those activities will be done; may be formal or informal, although those that are written have more legitimacy. —**Jeanette Lancaster**

A policy guides the process of implementation and evaluation of the usefulness of a program. —**Patton and Sawicki**

Types of Policy

Private Policy

A purposive course of action deal with concerns in the family in the family and in private sector voluntary organizations and businesses. Such polices provide guidelines for spending money. For lines of communication, and in organizations providing service and employee conduct.

Public Policy

A purposive course of action deal with concerns at all levels of government, educational system, and publicity owned corporations. Public policy comprises legislation, statutes, regulations, court actions, and institutional guidelines, including provider licensure, medicare agency conditions of participation, annual academic sessions, and profit sharing in corporations.

Health Policy

Actions developed by the public sector or private sector and related to the how, when, where, why, and to whom health care is delivered, how much money is spent, and who is considered a healthcare provider, including scope of practice.

Healthy Policy

Public or private sector actions developed by consumers in collaboration with others through a collective approach to improve the health of the patient (individual, group or community). This approach to developing policy assists consumers to take interest in their own health of others.

Six Step Process to Analyze a Policy Issue (Fig. 18.12)

Step 1: Verifying, defining and detailing the problem: At step one the problems concrete terms are defined, based on the values of the person or persons affected. These persons are the key actors. Their motivations to have the problem solved and their beliefs are important. The boundaries of the problem are also defined. A fact sheet is a useful aid in discussions with others, and the use of numbers is helpful to justify the problem is stated in measurable terms and the problem is stated in measurable terms and goals and objectives are listed for resolving the problem.

Step 2: Establishing evaluation criteria: Will help to develop outcomes for each objective to be met by a policy and to compare alternatives to determine which will be acceptable to the key actors, including the decision makers. Rules will need to evaluate alternatives to avoid choosing a favorite option. Criteria may include evaluation of costs, risks, legalities, effectiveness, political viability, administrative case, equity and timing. It is important to attempt to determine whether the alternatives will meet the meet the objectives defined in step 1.

Step 3: Identifying alternatives: In step 3, the process resolves around choice. Many options should be considered. One option that should be included in this step is no action. Taking suggestions from talking with others is a good, and organizational reactions to alternatives and find out how past problems were solved.

Step 4: Evaluate alternative polices: Step 4 determines whether any polices will work to solve the problem. One can look at what has happened in the past when the options identified have been chosen; look at the links between the variables that may affect the desired outcomes; social,

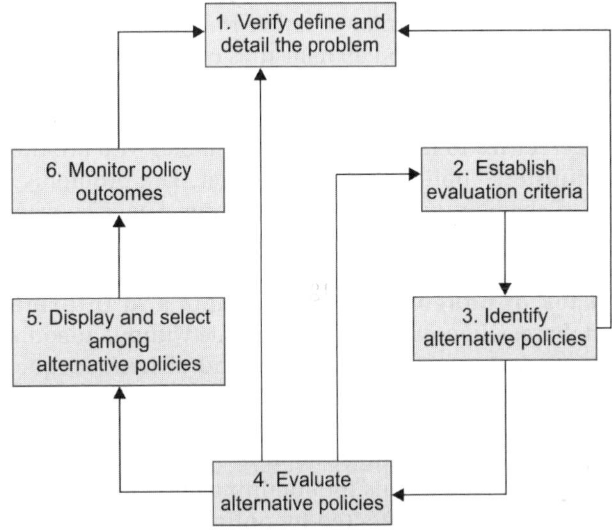

Fig. 18.12: Six step process to analyze a policy issues. (*Source:* Patton C, Sawicki D. 1983)

political, economic, ethical, and environmental; talk with key actors to determine what may happen; describe what outcome is desired; and find data in the literature or through a survey to predict what will happen. It necessary to consider the time, resources, and cost to important each alternative.

Step 5: Displaying alternatives and selecting among them: It involves ranking the alternatives and comparing them with each other based on the criteria in step 2. It is necessary to determine which of the criteria established in step 2 are the most important for each of the one alternative that meet the most criteria.

Step 6: Monitoring and evaluating policy outcomes: It is very important because it allows a comparison of the problem situation before and after the policy implementation. This step answers the question of whether the target goal was met. These comparisons can be made by looking at a situation where the policy was changed.

Weaknesses in India's public policy making

a. **Excessive fragmentation in thinking and action:** One of the main problems with policy-making in India is extreme fragmentation in the structure. For example, the transport sector is dealt with by five departments/ Ministries in the government of India whereas in the US and UK it is a part of one department (Department of Transport and Public Works in the US and Department of Environment, Transport and Regions in the UK). Similar examples exist in the energy, industry and social welfare sectors as well. Such fragmentation fails to recognize that actions taken in one sector have serious implications on another and may work at cross purposes with the policies of the other sector. Besides, it becomes very difficult, even for closely related sectors, to align their policies in accordance with a common overall agenda.
b. **Excessive overlap between policy making and implementation:** Another problem is the excessive overlap between implementation, program formulation and policy making which creates a tendency to focus on operational convenience rather than on public needs. Policy-making in Indian ministries occurs at the levels of Director and above, but the most important level (crucial for consideration of cross-cutting impacts) is that of the Secretaries to the Government of India, who are their Ministers' 'policy advisers-in-chief'. The problems of parliamentary will result that sub-optimal policies, where adequate attention has not been paid to citizen needs, tend to emerge.
c. **Lack of nongovernmental inputs and informed debate:** Often public policy is made without adequate input from outside government and without adequate debate on the issues involved. The best expertise in many sectors lies outside the Government. Yet the policy processes and structures of Government have no systematic means for obtaining outside inputs, for involving those affected by policies or for debating alternatives and their impacts on different groups. Most developed countries have a system of widespread public debate before a policy is approved. For example, in the US, the legislature subjects a new policy initiative to extensive debate not only in Committees but also in the Senate and House.
d. **Lack of systematic analysis and integration prior to policy-making:** Policy decisions are often made without adequate analysis of costs, benefits, trade-offs and consequences. There are several underlying causes for this:
   - *Excessive fragmentation:* This has already been referred to. Fragmentation has led to a widespread prevalence of the 'blind men and the elephant' syndrome in policy-making.
   - *Inadequate time spent on policy-making:* Mainly due to excessive overlap of policy-making and implementation and to overgeneralization of implementation authority.
   - *Inadequate professionalism of policy-makers and advisers:* Involvement of poorly informed generalists is the main cause of poor policy-making and implementation. However, when it comes to the realm of policy-making and the making of trade-offs, experience in government and the private sector suggests that this is usually best handled by an intelligent, well-informed person who has a wide rather than narrow perspective.
   - *Inadequate consultation of in-house specialists:* Even conceding that public policy-making might not be improved by insisting on specialists becoming the policy-makers, it is nevertheless crucial that specialist knowledge be fully consulted and utilized in arriving at policy. For reasons ranging from 'generalist arrogance' to inter service rivalries between groups of specialists, the available expertise of specialists within the Government is often under-utilized.
   - *Mediocrity of in-house specialists:* While there are many outstanding specialists working for the Government, there is a widespread feeling that many in-house specialists are not on top of their specialists. This perception of mediocrity vis-à-vis outside experts tends to worsen the problem of inadequate consultation of even the good in-house specialists who get tarred with the same brush. It also promotes an undue respect for outside specialists and the error of accepting poorly formulated prescriptions from outsiders simply because they have a more professional or expert image.

Reforming the Policy-making Process

The problems highlighted in the analysis can broadly be divided into two types. The first of these is *structural*—too much fragmentation, too much implementation work load on policy-makers, poor structure and process for involving outside experts and stakeholders. The second kind of problem lies with the *competence of the people who man the structure*—inadequate professionalism of the policy-making staff, and inadequate competence of the specialists.

Improving the Competence and Skills of Policy-making

The key requirement is the design of a career path which

- Creates incentives to learn, and to acquire and apply the right skills
- Strengthens links between academic and the administration
- Identifies and weeds out poor performers
- Ensures that only those with the requisite knowledge and intelligence make it to the top policy levels.

Role of Nurses in Public Policy Issues

There is now a growing concern that care expenditure is rising at an alarmingly uncontrolled rate. The changes in economic policies of the nation's globalization, liberalization and privatization under the presiding triad the World Bank, the International Monetary Fund and the World Trade Organization—has no doubt contributed to the sweeping changes that we see today.

Nursing's Responsibility in Cost Containment

Nurses are responsible for the major portion of the work force in the healthcare field. Although nurses and the work forces supervise a major component of the healthcare work force, the decision making about the role of nursing in healthcare delivery is in the hands of others such as the physicians and hospital administrators. As a result of this external control of nursing by others and the internal divisions within nursing, energies become tied of debates related to the profession, rather than to a more constructive approach to addressing the key role of nursing in the provision of affordable health care.

Hospitals have become the center of high technology and expensive treatments. An overwhelmingly large percent of nurses are employed by hospitals. Within this context, nurses get caught in the technology of health care, remaining in many instances mere technicians or adjuncts to this techno centric health service, rather than nursing itself with high employment opportunities, nursing is becoming a mere 'job oriented' profession and within a somewhat protected environment, the implications of high-technology costly care for the few are not overtly troublesome. Responsibility for decision making in the economic, political and ethical realm is not assumed to be part of the practicing nurses' role. The fact that the privileged few receive high-technology quality care while the poor, unemployed and elderly receive little or no medical or health care is not the concern of the practicing nurse within the hospital setting. Nurses are caught up in the competition between institution's control over health care rather than collaborative working in developing comprehensive coordinate health services.

Given this fragmented picture of nursing today, it may be argued that nursing is part of the problem contributing to escalating healthcare costs. Continued conflicts within the profession and control of nursing lead to inappropriate and under-utilization of nursing resources throughout the healthcare system. Given the number of nurses employed in the health care, the number of persons who are supervised by nurses, the capacity of nurses to provide health in contrast to disease care, the placement of nurses in hospitals and community settings, and the type of care needed to prevent expensive institutional care, nursing has the potential for becoming part of the solution. For this to happen, however a number of changes need to occur.

First, there is a critical need to settle our internal divisions. Instead of continuing the unending debate over the value of various categories of certification, i.e., the different levels of qualifications in nursing, the diversified needs of healthcare delivery need to provide the context for defining the multifaceted team of nursing personnel that are needed to provide a high quality health care. The current preoccupation with professionalism is a fruitless quest without considering the total gamut of services for which nursing is responsible. To divide one segment of the profession as 'professional' and not to be concerned about the 'whole' is fatal. Nursing does have the potential to settle these internal divisions. The nursing 'professionals' and organizations should meet regularly to reach common agreement on the educational preparation needed for the levels. If these key internal issues can be worked out, nursing can address broader health delivery issues from a unified position.

The mechanism for continued dialogue between hospital associations and medical associations need to be established. This is also consistent with the changes that are occurring in the nursing field. Increased career orientation, engagement in educational programs to provide career mobility, increasing involvement in broader healthcare issues, aligning themselves with the consumer of healthcare services, in continuing care extending outside the boundaries of hospitals, are all becoming role of nurses. Public policy issues in health care, as the high healthcare expenditure, are an issue of challenge to the nurses, nursing organizations and to nursing profession itself in the years to come.

PROTOCOL

There are two meanings of the word *protocol*. In the legal sense, it is defined as an international agreement that supplements or amends a treaty. In the diplomatic sense, the term refers to the set of rules, procedures, conventions and ceremonies that relate to relations between states. In general, protocol represents the recognized and generally accepted system of international courtesy.

The term *protocol* is derived from the Greek word *protokollan* (first glue). This comes from the act of gluing a sheet of paper to the front of a document to preserve it when it was sealed, which imparted additional authenticity to it. In the beginning, the term protocol related to the various forms of interaction observed in official correspondence between states, which were often elaborate in nature. In course of time, however, it has come to cover a much wider range of international relation.

Definitions

Protocol has several different meanings, all connected to the idea of guidelines or procedures to follow. It is used mostly in formal or academic language.

The most common meaning of protocol is 'a system of rules that explain the correct conduct and procedures to be followed in formal situations.

A protocol defines a set of operational procedures to ensure that there is a well-defined way of doing a particular task.

This is most important when the task is executed over a period of time when different people will be performing the task. For example, there may be a protocol for the treatment and on-going monitoring of a patient with high blood pressure who has undergone major surgery. It should ensure the correct treatment regardless of shift changes, etc. Protocol means you do something a certain way because it has been deemed the 'most effective way' through cumulative past experience.

It is important to know that adhering to the protocol associated with the completion of a task is very important to arrive at a desired solution. Swerving from following a protocol leads to commotion and misunderstandings or sometimes miscommunications too. Protocol consists in doing something in a particular fashion based on some kind of previous experience. Protocol is considered an effective way too based on the past experience derived by somebody by following the laid procedures. These are the differences between policy and protocol. They are indeed different words.

MATERIAL MANAGEMENT

Concept

Materials are an essential resource to achieve the objectives of a healthcare organization. While about 60% of the of funds of health sector are consumed to provide manpower health care being a labor intensive activity, almost 40% of the funds are used up for providing materials. In the absence of materials required for healthcare activities, the manpower deployed is rendered nonfunctional. Therefore, it is of great importance that materials of right quality are supplied to the consumers in right time and at right place of use. All activities involved in the achievement of above stated objectives, i.e., planning for materials, their demand, estimation, procurement, stocking and use.

Definition

Material management is a service function affecting the flow of materials in a manner in which its helps in conserving the materials, cost, best utilization of materials and maintaining the quality of both incoming and outgoing materials. **—Varma**

Functions of Material Management

- Planning and sourcing
- Budgeting
- Researching and analysis
- Indenting, and procuring
- Receiving, storing and preserving
- Accounting and controlling
- Issuing and dispatching
- Disposing.

Areas of Material Management

- Material planning and programming
- Purchasing and inventory control
- Receiving, store housing
- Transportation and material handling.

Elements of Material Management System

Material planning and management is a system having numerous elements. Proper functioning of each of the elements (subsystems) coupled with interdependence of all the subsystems to achieve the primary objectives are the classical characteristics of the material planning and management system. The major subsystem of material planning and management system are:

- Demand estimation
- Procurement
- Receipt and inspection
- Storage
- Issue and use
- Maintenance and repair
- Disposal
- Accounting and information system.

Demand Estimation

A large variety and number of materials are used in hospitals and other healthcare institutions. The advisory committee for development of surgical instrument, equipments and appliances (1963) identified 3200 items of instruments and equipments, being used in a hospital. This is just to illustrate the variety and diversity of storage used for patient care in a hospital situation. There is need for variety reduction of the materials as less the number of materials less will be problems of planning and management of the same. Along with variety reduction there is need for laying down proper specification of the materials. In this area, the Indian standard institute has been and is playing a very important role by standardizing a large number and variety of instrument and equipments. The ISI has setup a number of technical committees to work out the details of standards of surgical instrument, glassware, anesthesia equipments, dental machine, artificial limbs, surgical dressing, utensils, electro medical instruments, rubber goods, etc., Along with standardization, variety reduction, and proper classification of materials a major area of activity of material planning and material supply is demand estimation of each category of material. This should always be done keeping in view the trends in consumption pattern over the last 2-3 years, objectives of the organization, changing emphasis on various programs and activities in the health field. In this field a 'sound data base' and use of advance projection techniques are of great use. These techniques are relatively simple and medical administrator should use term frequently to streamline of material planning and material supply system.

Procurement

Having drawn up the list of requirements, the next step in material planning and supply is the process of procurement of the materials. Most of the states and other organizations have laid down detailed set of rules and regulation regarding the procedure of ordering for materials. The financial authority is also vested in various levels of administrative hierarchy. The basic sprit behind all these rules, regulations, procedure, etc., is to maximize the value of money invested in the purchase of stores. Organization like Directorate General of supplies and Disposals play costs. Many states have medical stores depots which are centralized agencies of procurement and stocking of medical stores. There is also a system of fixed contract (or) running rate contract which is followed in large organization and some state government limited tender rate enquires local spot, and emergent purchase from a part of the complex sub system of procurement. It would neither be appropriate nor feasible to go into the details of these procedures as they are specific to different states/organization. However, the role of DGSD needs special mentioning in the subsystem of procurement of bulk materials.

Receipt and Inspection

The stores ordered are received in the store. A reasonable sound policy and methodology of inspection of incoming stores is an essential element of material planning and supplies. The inspection policy should enumerate the sampling procedure for inspection. Basic facilities for such examination be created in the organization upon the size of stores turn over, governmental and commercial chemical laboratories should also be made use of for analysis of chemical composition of drugs, etc.

Storage

The medical storage should be situated near the other stores of the hospital. It should be easily accessible to suppliers as well as well as indenters. Location of the store will therefore, be guided by the flow activity of the stores. The store should be of adequate size to accommodate all the drugs, instruments, appliances, etc., required for use in form of steel rakes with shelves. Refrigeration should be provided for storage of thermo labile items.

Inventory Control

Inventory control means stocking materials are available whenever required and where ever required. This has to be done at an optimum outlay of financial and human resources. High inventory level leads to high cost of inventories by:

- Locking the finance
- Large storage space
- Large handling and administration changes
- Obsolescence
- Spoilage etc.

Low inventories may lead to frequent stock outstand and high storage cost. Balancing the cost of carrying high inventories and the cost of shortages is done through a system of scientific inventory control.

ABC Analysis

Is the analysis of store items on cost criteria. It has been that a large number of items consume only a small percentage of resources and vice versa. A-items represent high cost center, B- items intermediate cost centers, and C-items are low cost centers.

'A' Items

- Tight controls
- Rigid estimates
- Strict and close watch
- Safety stocks should be low
- Management of items should be done at top management level.

'B' Items

- Moderate controls
- Purchase based on rigid requirements
- Reasonably strict watch and control
- Safety stocks moderate
- Management be done at middle level.

'C' Items

- Ordinary control measure
- Purchase based on usage estimates
- Controls exercises by store keeper
- Safety stocks high
- Management be done at lower level.

Organization for Material Management

Organization is a process of dividing and combining efforts more productive, effective and fruitful. The organization as a body of professionals allocates duties to the managerial staff. It adds certainty and prompties to the work to be done. It avoids gaps and overlapping functions. It establishes a neat pattern of relationships among efforts to be put in, jobs to be done and the work to be performed.

Organization brings together the basic resources. so as to unite people in the interrelated tasks with the intention of accomplishing certain given specific goals.

An organization aims at the:

- Division of work
- Assignment of work
- Creation of an atmosphere under which the work is to be accomplished
- Establishment of relationship among the personal and the units.

Conventional Approach

One of the most important requirements of the organization in material management is an integration of various function assigned to the department. The conventional approach with regard to the material organization is concerned with the integration of all functions of material management under manager who is responsible for achieving the authority from the chief executive of the organization conventional approach, there fore, refers to centralization of all materials function into 'one' powerful authority who becomes the real source of all, which flows downwards in the material management wing of the enterprise.

Under the conventional dispensation all the problems of the materials department are health with at the appear. Here purchasing, inventory control, transportation, distribution, disposal and other allied functions of the department are grouped together and placed under material department headed by the material manager, such a dispensation may be depicted in **Figures 18.13 and 18.14**.

There is no denying the fact that the purchase department under taking is primarily involved in material management. In fact the management of material begins with the purchasing process. Conventionally, the purchasing department is placed under the material management department and the purchase executive is made responsible to the material manager. In many manufacturing units material management is directly linked with the purchase and production planning departments. In order to maintain an effective control over inventories, it is also necessary that the material manager should have a close link with stores department.

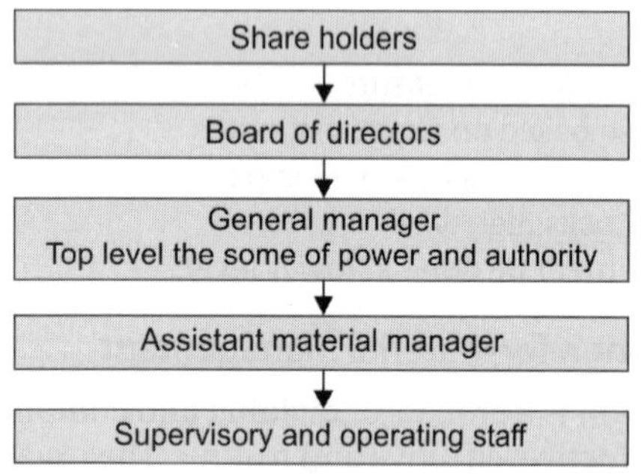

Fig. 18.13: Conventional approach to material management organization at the top level organization chart.

Problems of material management

- Problems relating to material planning
- Problems relating to design and specification
- Problems relating to obsolescence
- Problems relating to procurement.

Problems Relating to Material Planning

An industrial house plans its material requirement well in advance. So, as to avoid eleventh hour arrangements and adjustments. But there are forces and factors which often upset planning.

Problems Relating to Design and Specification

- Close tolerances and precise workmanship
- Ambiguity in drawings
- Purchases inadequate specification to supplies.

Problems Relation to Obsolescence

- Problems of inefficiency
- Less production
- Partial or nonutilization of our installed capacity
- Waste
- Improper utilization of raw material
- High cost of production
- Other allied problems to which we are not able to offer adequate solution.

Problems Relating to Procurement

- Inadequate staff
- Terms of payment
- Management in general.

Evaluation of Material Management

Evaluation of material management is directly linked with the success of the organization. If the organization succeeds the material management has done its job satisfactorily.

Forms of Evaluation

1. **Mere reporting:** Periodic reports by the operating staff to the middle order and top management, analysis of

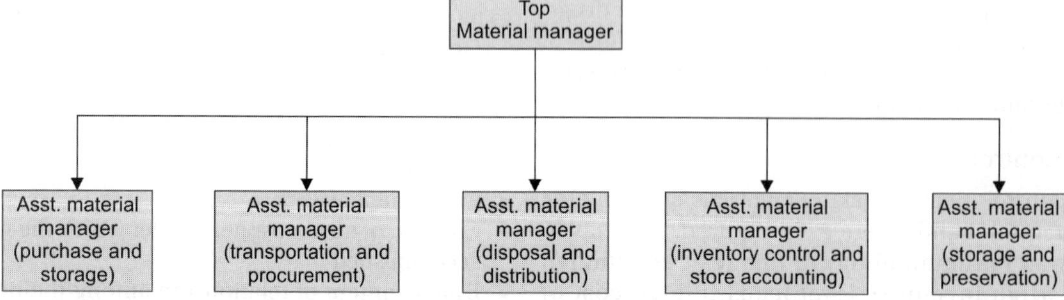

Fig. 18.14: A conventional approach to material management organization at the middle level organization chart.

the same and consequent actions are the accepted form of evaluation of the performance of the materials departments.

While preparing a report the reporting official should take care of the following important points.

- The report should be written in simple language.
- It should be clear
- It should be brief
- It should be related to frequency, i.e., periodicity should be maintained.

2. **Questionnaire:** A separate or combined questionnaire may be prepared to evaluate the performance of the material department. The question include in the list may related to staff delegation training and education of the personnel at work, economic indicators of the nation as well as the organization. Financial procedure and methods, inventory policy, material objectives and allied matters.
3. **Policy decisions:** Under policy decision as a form of performance evaluation, the material department may fix certain procedure and lay down specific criteria for the evaluation of the performance of the materials management.

   The policy decision in respect of procedure and criteria can be the following four forms:
   1. Comparisons may be on the basis of past performance over a given period of time, say one or two or three calendar or financial fear.
   2. Comparisons may be on the basis of similarity between companies of similar nature, size and having similar objectives.
   3. Comparisons may also be on inter- firm basis.
   4. Norms may be prescribed before hand for each of the characteristics and material actions and then a comparison may be made between the norms set and the actual performance.

BUDGET AND BUDGETING

Concept of Budget

One of the primary objectives of management accounting is to provide information to management for planning and control. A widely used device for managerial control is the budget. Because the amount and quality of nursing services depended on budgetary plans, nurses should become proficiency will provide the resources necessary for the safe and effective nursing care.

Definitions

A budget is an estimate of future needs arranged to an orderly basis covering some or all the activities of an enterprise for a definite period of time. **—TN Chhabra**

Budgeting is the formulation of plans for a given period in numerical terms. **—Harold Koortz**

A budget is a plan that uses numerical data to predict that activities of an organization over a period of time. **—Bessie**

Purposes

- Budget supplies the mechanism for translating fiscal objectives into project monthly spending pattern.
- Budget enhances fiscal planning and decision-making.
- Budget clearly recognizes controllable and un-controllable cost areas.
- Budget offers a useful format for communication fiscal objectives.
- Budget allows feed back of utilization of budget.
- Budget helps to identify problem areas and facilitates effective solution.
- Budget provides means for measuring and recording financial success within the objectives of the organization.

Features of Budget

- It should be flexible.
- It should be synthesis of past, present, future.
- It should be product of joint venture for cooperation of executives department heads or different level of management.
- It should be in the form of statistical laid down in specific numerical terms.
- It should have support of top management throughout the period of its planning and implementation.

Importance of Budget

- Budget is needs for planning for future course of action and to have a control over all activities in the organization.
- Budget facilitates coordinating operation of various departments and section for realizing organizational objectives.
- Budget serves as a guide for action in the organization.
- Budget helps one to weight the value and to make decision when necessary or whether one is of a greater value in the program that the order.

Principle of Budget

- Budget should provide sound financial management by focusing on requirement of the organization.
- Budget should focus on objectives and policies of the organization. It must flow from objectives and give realistic expression to the way of realistic such objective.
- Budget should ensure the most effective use of scarce financial and nonfinancial resources.
- Budget requires that program activities planned in advance.
- Budgetary process requires consistent delegation for which fixed duties and responsibilities are required to be allocated to managers at different level for framing and executing budget.
- Budget should include coordinating efforts of various departments establishing a frame of reference for managerial decision and providing certain criteria for evaluating managerial performance.

- Selling budget target requires an adequate checks and balance against the adoption of too high or too low estimate, almost care is a must for fixing targets.
- Budget period must be appropriate to the nature of business or service and to type of budget.
- Budget is prepared under the direction on the supervision of the administration or financial officer.
- Budget are to be prepared and interpreted consistently throughout the organization in the communication in the planning process.

Classification of Budget

Since budget express plans and an organization may have different types of plans, there may be different types of budgets. These may classified on the basis of:

- Coverage of functions—master and functional budget.
- Natured and activity covered—capital and Revenue budget.
- Period of Budget—long-term and short-term budgets.
- Flexibility adopted—fixed and flexible budget.

Master and Functional Budget

A mastered budget is prepared for the entire organization incorporating the budget of different functions. For example, when we refer to the annual budget of Govt. of India. It incorporates the budget out lays of different ministries.

A functional budget is prepared incorporating a major function and its sub functions since an organization may have a number of functions, numerous functional budgets are prepared. For example, production budget, cash budget in an organization.

Capital and Revenue Budget

An organization activities involve two process. Creating facilities for carrying out activities and actual performance activities. Creating facilities for carrying out activities include capital expenditure whole returns accrue over a number of years. For such activities, capital budget is prepared which is essentially a list of what management believes to be worth while projects for acquisition of new assets together with the estimated cost of each project.

Revenue budget involves the formation of target for a year or so in respect of various organizational activities such as production, marketing, finance, etc. Thus a revenue budget includes expenditure and earning for a specific period like one year.

Long-term and Short-term Budget

Many organization integrate their yearly budgets with long-term projection of business activities and along with yearly budget; they prepare budgets for a longer period of 2–3 years. When one budget period is over budgets are prepared for the next year and subsequent 2–3 years.

The short-term budget is for a year and is divided into a number of periods for effective implementation. For example, cash budgets are prepared on yearly basis as well as on monthly or quarterly basis to facilitate better cash management.

Fixed and Flexible Budgets

Generally, organizations prepare budgets which pertain to only certain projected fixed volume of operations for a year or so such budget are known as fixed or static budgets. When an organizations volume of business can be predicted with fair amount of precision, the fixed budget is satisfactory.

A budget which is designed to change in accordance with the activities of the organization is known as flexible budget. It considers several level of activity and assures that labor, material or facilities used in production and hence cost vary with a known relationship to the actual volume of activity.

Types of Budgeting

There are mainly two types of budgeting.

1. Performance budgeting
2. Zero base budgeting.

Performance Budgeting

A performance budgeting is an input/output budget or costs and results budget. It shows costs matching with operations. Performance budget emphasis on nonfinancial measures of performance which can be related to financial measures in explaining changes and deviation from planned performance. Performance measurement are useful for evaluating past performance and for planning future activities. Performance budgeting, results into the following.

- It correlates the financial and physical aspects of every program or activity.
- It improves budget formulation, review and decision-making at all levels of the organization.
- It facilitates better appreciation and review of organizational activities by the top management.
- It makes possible move effective performance audit.
- It measures progress towards long-term objectives.

Zero Base Budgeting

This was applied for the first time in preparing the divisional budgets of Texas instruments of the USA in 1971.

Zero base budget is based on a system where each function, irrespective of the fact whether it is old or new, must be justified in its entirely each time a new budget is formulated. It requires each managed to justify his entire budget in detail from scratch that zero base.

The process of zero base involves four basic steps.

- Identification of decision units that is cluster of activities or assignments within a manager's operation for which he is accountable.
- Analysis of each decision unit in the context of total decision package.

- Evaluation and ranking of all decision units to develop the budget request.
- Allocation of resources to each unit based upon.

Benefits of Zero Base Budgeting

- Effective allocation of resources.
- Improvement in productivity and cost effectiveness.
- Effective means to control costs.
- Eliminator of unnecessary activities.
- Better focus or organizational objectives.
- Saving time of top management.

Budget Process

Annual method, i.e., annual budget will be made in India.
- **Month:** Starts from Sep/Oct of current years.
- **Made by:** Directorate of health and family welfare.

The nursing budget follows three stages of development.
1. Formulation
2. Review and enactment
3. Execution

Formulation Stage

It is usually a set of number of month before the beginning of the fiscal year for the budget. One of the first steps in writing a budget is gathering data for accurate prediction of expenses and revenues (income). Primary sources of data are the objectives for the division of nursing and each cost center. Other data include programs from other departments that will require use or expansion of nursing resources, expansion of nursing clinics and client teaching programs, incentive awards, library requirements, clinical and office supplies and equipments, etc.

Review and Enactment Stage

Review and enactment stage are budget development process that pull all the pieces together for approved of a final budget. Once the cost center managers present their budgets to the budget council, the chief nurse executive will consolidate the nursing budget. The chief executive officer of the organization and the governing broad will then give their approval. Throughout this process, conferences will be held at which budget adjustments are made.

Execution Stage

Execution of the budget involves directing, executing, and evaluating activities. The nurse administrator and managers who planned the budget execute it. Revisions in execution of the budgets are scheduled at stated intervals, frequently once or twice during fiscal year. Certain procedures are followed for evaluating the budget at cost center levels.

Function of Budget in Nursing

- Identifies the importance of and develops short a long range fiscal plans that reflects unit needs.
- Articulate and documents units needs effectively to higher administrative levels.
- Assess the internal and external environment of the organization in forecasting to identify driving forces and barriers of fiscal planning.
- Demonstrate knowledge of budgeting and uses appropriate technique.
- Provide opportunities for subordinates to participate in relevant fiscal planning.
- Coordinates unit level fiscal planning to be congruent with organizational goals and objective.
- Accurately assesses personal needs using predetermined standards or an established patient classification system.
- Coordinates the monitoring aspects of budget control.
- Ensure that documentation of clients need for services in clear and complete for facilitate organizational reimbursement.

Role of Nurse Administrator in Budgeting

- Is visionary in identifying of forecasting short and long-term unit needs, thus inspiring proactive rather than reactive fiscal planning.
- Is knowledgeable about political, social and economic factors that shape fiscal planning in health care today.
- Demonstrate flexibility in fiscal goals setting in a rapidly changing system.
- Anticipates recognized and actively problems solve budgetary constraints.
- Influences and inspires group members to become active in short and large range fiscal planning.
- Recognizes when fiscal constraints have resulted in an ability to meet organizational or unit goals and communicate this insight effectively, allowing the chain of command.
- Ensure that client safely is not jeopardized by cost constraints.

Limitation of Budgeting

Planning, budgeting or forecasting is not an exact science; it uses appropriately and judgment which may not be 100% accurate. At best a budget is an estimate no one knows precisely what will happen in the future.

The success and utility of budgeting depends on the cooperation and participating of all members of management. All person should direct their effort according to the plan. Many time budgeting has paid only lip services to its executing.

A budget is only a tool and neither eliminates nor takes over the place of management. A budget cannot be substituted for management but should only be used by management for accomplishing managerial functions.

The establishment of a budgeting process takes time. Also sometime too much is expected from a budget and in case expectation are not fulfilled the blame is put on the budget. An efficient budgeting program requires that responsible person should understand the philosophy, objective and essential of budgeting.

PUBLIC RELATION

In democratic state public relations are very significant, today the concept of police state has been replaced by the welfare state, state activities have been expanded. The government undertakes multifarious activities for the public welfare. But for this successful accomplishment, public cooperation is essential. The public only cooperates when it has a confidence in the government.

Definitions

Public relations in government is the composite of all, the primary an secondary contacts between the bureaucracy and all the interactions of influences and attitudes established in these contacts. **—According to McCany**

The simplest way of describing the function of public relations and publicity in modern administration is to say that they are concerned with the study of the human factors in industry and, to an increasing degree in government. **—According to JH Brebner**

Need for Public Relations

There are the following factors which go to make public relations for administration.

Expansion of State Activities

Modern state is a welfare state, public administration caters to the need of the society, and it undertakes activities which are meant to promote public goods.

Safeguard Against Public Criticism

The basic difference between private and public administration is that even the smallest error of the public administration soon comes to light; on the other hand even the greatest scandals take place in private sectors, and the public does not learn about them.

Change in Public Policies

Today the public policies have undergone a change they do not have to confine themselves to the execution of laws. Today the public servants have to advertise the policies of the government, and the public should be informed regarding the nature and scope of the available services.

Role of a Salesman

Today the public relations is like salesmanship. As a salesman sells his commodities by advertising them, in the same way modern administrators have to sell government policies and programs. They in other words present their programs before the people in such an attractive package.

Functions of Public Relations Department

The main functions of the public relations officer may be summarized as follows:

Release of Departmental News

Press is very influential organ of public opinion the government has, therefore to maintain good relations with it by providing it full information regarding the departmental policy as well as program.

Explanations

Legislative statues as well as government rules and regulations are made by legal law years; thus through public relations the department provides explanation and illustrations of these rules and regulations.

Background Information

For all its social activities the department has to depends upon the understanding and cooperation of the people, the background information of the administrative decisions is provided to the people to gain their confidence.

Persuasion

At the time of war and other crisis, the government needs more public cooperation. Sometimes people needs more public cooperation. Sometimes people are called upon to come forward to help the government at the cost of their personal interest. For instance the people can be and property.

Direct Sale

Today the government has also become a merchant. It has stepped in to business like private individuals.

Methods and Techniques of Public Relations

Public administration has borrowed methods and technique of public relations from business organizations where they have been developed in systematic and scientific way. They are:

- Communication
- Press and publications
- Radio
- Films and other audiovisual aids
- Advertising
- Public speaking
- Researching
- Research and opinion surveys.

Communication

'Communication is the process of transmitting cues, mainly written and verbal, in order to modify human behaviors'.

Press and Publications

Publicity is an important tool of public relations. Government publishers book, booklets, pamphlets, etc., giving detailed information about the policies, programs and activities of its administrative agencies.

Radio

Radio and television have now become very important and effective media of mass contact and communication. They reach the people more rapidly and have a far wider appeal.

Films and other Audiovisual Aids

Films are another means of effective mass communication they are being widely made use of by governments at national and local levels. For this they maintain studies and prepare documentary films and news streds for free display.

Advertising

No other means of publicity has provoked so much public controversy as advertising. Most people criticize the government advertisement as a cheap sales propaganda, unworthy of a government to indulge in.

Public Speaking

In spite of all written and visual means of mass contact, public speaking has its own charm and importance as a technique of public relations. What the speech imparts enthusiasm and the human feeling of attachment and closeness delivered in a local tone and temper lacks totally in the written statement.

Research and Opinion Surveys

Public relations are two way traffic. It, on the open hand informs people of the public policies and programs, but also, on the other hand, tries to let the government know the public relations to their activities. Hence, research into human behavior and environmental factors is very essential for the successful completion of administrative programs. There is an Indian program evaluation organization attached to the planning commission for examining the result of various operations, undertaken by administration and for recommending the best possible method of work.

Media of Public Relations in India

In India, the work of publicity has been entrusted to an executive department of the government of India, i.e., the ministry information and broadcasting.

The ministry is responsible for:

- Government publicity including publication and advertisement.
- Broadcasting.
- Sanctioning of cinematographic films for exhibition.
- Production and distribution of documentary films and news reels, etc.
- Registration and statistics of newspaper.

The Ministry Performs its Functions of Publicity Through the Following Offices

- Director General of all India radio, New Delhi.
- Director General of television.
- Press information bureau.
- Directorate of advertising and visual publicity (DAVP).
- Publication division.
- Films division, Bombay.
- Central board of films censors.
- Office of the registrar of newspapers for India.
- Five year plan publicity division.
- Indian institute of public relations.

All India radio: In modern age, the radio is the most important media of publicity. All India radio provides special programs for rural people, school children, industrial workers and arm forces.

Television: Although the television started in India from September 15, 1963, its network expanded in the year 1980. From 1982 Asian games, its colored services were inaugurated. Now it is most effective means of mass communication and publicity.

Press information bureau: Its primary function is to inform the public through the press about government activities and keep the government in touch with the main trends of public opinion as reported in the press. It provides required publicity material for both central and state government it has a network of offices throughout India.

Publication division: It is responsible for the production, distribution and sale of popular pamphlets, books, journals, etc., through which information is provided to the people about the activities of government, places of tourist interest and the progress of the various development programs in the country.

Directorate of advertising and visual publicity (DAVP): Its functions include release of display advertisements classified advertisements, production and distribution of posters, folders, pamphlets, etc., it selects newspapers for government advertisements.

Films division: An important machine of publicity for Indian masses is cinematographic films. They have a great importance for masses. Through them people are acquainted with great events happening in the country and abroad. The government publicity department makes full use of these films.

Central board of films censors: It was established in 1952, it consists of one chairman and other members are chosen from the people associated with cultural and social activities. The censor board decides the type of pictures to be shown to the people. It examines all the films and can censor any films or part of it. It issues 'U' and 'A' certificates on their merits.

Research and reference division: Research and reference division undertakes research regarding publicity. This department provides information of its conclusions and achievements to other government departments. These principles serve as guidelines for future programming of the government.

Office of the registrar of newspaper for India: This office maintains statistics of all the newspapers published in the country, their publication, price and ownership. Through these statistics, it evaluates the achievement of publicity.

Five year plan publicity division: Its duty is to make available all information regarding different aspects of five year plans. The all-sided development of the country depends upon these plans.

Indian institute of public relations: It was established on august 17, 1965 at New Delhi. The Indian institute of public relations is run and governed by an executive board subordinate to the information and broadcasting ministry.

Essential Conditions for Successful Public Relation

The following conditions must be created to make public relations successful:

- The public relation officer must be a competent man, who posses all the techniques and media of the science of public relations.
- The first step of success in public relations is the purity of character and conduct. {Prof. Edward burns}
- The use of methods of public relations corresponding to the standard of living and linking of the people.
- According to Dr PD Sharma, 'to succeed, the public relations should be from the inspiration to the people, corresponding to the people, and in confidence of the people.
- The impartial, true and factual information should be placed before the people to take them into confidence.
- Public relations should be established not only with one but all sections of society, for if some specific class is neglected, it shall feel neglected and offended.
- According to Prof. Rox Harls, the interest of the administration lies in the fact that their acts of public relation should be true, clear, certified and responsible.
- During public relations, while making a personal contact, the public official should not display bureautic attitude, normally it is the short coming of the public officials. That they detest common people.
- For powerful and effective public relation, it is essential to receive public grievances and redress them.
- In every government department there should be an enquiry office to provide directions to the newcomers. Public official should fix a time for daily public contact and should strictly adhere to it.
- For good public relations the medium of correspondence is considered to be more effective. Every public letter must invariably be answered.
- The personal behaviors of the officials should courteous. They should be considerate to the public complaints. They should leave no stone unturned in expressing their sympathy and good will to the people.

Role of Nurse in Developing Public Relations

- Nurse develops a skilled communication of ideas to the various public with the objective of producing a desired result in public health.
- Nurse find out what people like and doing more of it and finding out what they do not like and doing less of it.
- Nurse establish management function which evaluates public attitudes and public health.
- Nurse identifies the policies and procedures of an individual or organization with the public interest and executes acceptance.
- Nurse recognize and cultivate within an organization of those virtues and values which become visible externally in the standing of a institute or hospital with it's worker.
- Nurse develop all activities and attitudes intended to judge, influence or control opinion of any groups of person in the interest of any individual, group or institution.
- Nurse applies policies and acts for an organization as they touch the public and either build or destroy good will and good understanding that as so vital to the life of profession in this competitive age.
- Nurse carefully complied analysis of cause and effect used as a guide to conduct.
- Nurse should be specialists in his field, an should possess both theoretical and practical knowledge of his subject.
- Nurse should have purity of character and conduct from this point of view the ideal nurse is one who has the capacity to deliberate impartially in all circumstances.
- Nurse should use of methods of public relations corresponding to the standard of living and likings of the people.
- Nurse should form the inspiration to the people, corresponding to the people and in confidence of the people.
- Nurse established the public relations not only with one but all sections of society.
- The personal behavior of nurse should be courteous, should be considerate to the public complaints.

JOB DESCRIPTION OF DIFFERENT NURSING PERSONNEL

At the state level the Director Nursing is the head of the Nursing Directorate and Controlling Officers of all the Nursing Training Institutions and Nursing cadre in the state. In India, Odisha is the only state having separate Nursing directorate.

Job Descriptions of the Director Nursing under the Hand FW Department

At the state level the Director Nursing is the head of the Nursing Directorate and Controlling Officers of all the Nursing Training Institutions and Nursing cadre in the state.

She/he is responsible to the Secretary, Health and Family Welfare Department and State Government.

Educational qualification: Nursing director at directorate level must have MSc or PhD nursing with at least 10–15 years of administrative experience with adequate amount of teaching or clinical experience.

General Administrative Functions

- The Director of Nursing is the administrative head of the Nursing Directorate and all subordinate offices in the state.

- Develop, maintain and implement nursing policies and procedures with conformity with current standards of nursing practice and philosophy while maintaining compliance with state/INC/University and other statutory body rules.
- She/he will be responsible for planning, budgeting and expenditure of all activities related to the nursing services, institutions and Directorate.
- Communicates and interprets policies and procedures to nursing staff, and monitors staff practices.
- She/he will frame the rules and regulations regarding the Unified nursing cadre with due approval of the Government.
- Evaluates work performance of all nursing personnel and assists in the determination of wage increases as per the policies of the government.
- She/he will be the reporting authority of the Joint Directors, Deputy Directors and Asst. Directors and supervise their work. She/he discharge all responsibilities associated as the reporting authority including leave, travel, etc.
- Responsible for all matters of establishment related to the nursing cadre in the state.
- Liasioning with other Directorates, Directors, Departments, Government, District level officers and development partners, as required to improve the nursing services and training in the state.
- She/he will liaise with Indian Nursing Council/ Universities/Boards for quality nursing care, education and syllabus, etc.

Monitoring and Supervision

- Supervise the work of the Nursing Officers working under the administrative control of the Directorate of Nursing.
- Periodically review the activities of all nursing services.
- Review nursing Management Information System (MIS) reports related to Human Resource (HR), infrastructure, quality of care, finance, etc., for better improvement.
- Conduct periodic visit to ensure required facilities at district and peripheral level to improve training of nurses as well as patient care service delivery system.
- She/he will responsible for proper functioning of the state Nursing Council and Nursing Board.
- She/he will monitor the activities of the private nursing training institutions and ensure teaching standards as per guidelines issued by the Indian Nursing Council and Govt. from time to time.

Financial

- She/he will be responsible for allocation of funds/ departmental resources in an economic and efficient manner in collaboration with related departments.
- She/he will discharge all duties and responsibilities as vested to him/her by Government.

Human Resources

- She/he will coordinate Govt. to frame rules regarding recruitment, promotion, transfer and posting of all cadres of nurses
- Ensure timely submission of Performance appraisal report of the Nursing officers to concerned Departments.
- She/he will assign duties to Officers/nursing personnel as and when required.

Functional Responsibilities

- The Director Nursing will be overall in-charge of all functions related to clinical nursing, public health nursing and nursing education in the state.
- Any other functions as may be assigned by the department from time to time.

Job Descriptions for Joint Director Nursing (Clinical Nursing and Public Health)

The Joint Director Nursing Clinical Nursing and public health, will assist, coordinate the Director Nursing, for proper management of the clinical nursing personnel in the state.

She/he is responsible to the Director Nursing and Health and F.W Department of government.

Educational Qualification

Same as director of nursing.

General Administrative Functions

- She/he is the in-charge of the Clinical Nursing and Public Health Nursing wings of the Nursing directorate.
- She/he will coordinate the Director Nursing in planning, budgeting and implementing of the Clinical Nursing and Public Health Nursing wing of the directorate.
- She/he will discharge all the duties and responsibilities as vested to him/her from time to time as per Government instructions
- She/he will ensure timely submission of Performance Appraisal Report furnished by the Nursing Officers (Clinical wing) of the Directorate before the Director Nursing in time.
- Helps in developing standards for effective care and public health practice by following INC guideline in his state.

Monitoring and Supervision

- She/he will coordinate the work and supervise the Nursing Officers (Clinical wing) of the Directorate.
- She/he will Undertake periodic visit to different clinical nursing and public health nursing set-up in the state as and when required or as directed by the superior authority in order to streamline clinical nursing practices and community health nursing in the state.
- Ensure that the standards should be followed at the clinical 7 public health setting and suggest for modifications
- She/he will ensure proper coordination with the education wing of the directorate to bring current learning into practice.
- She/he will coordinate different authorities for setting up, design and implementation of the Human Resource information system for the clinical and public health nurses.

- She/he will coordinate and assist the Director Nursing for recruitment, deployment of staff for proper implementation of nursing services in the state.

Financial

She/he will discharge all financial power/responsibilities as delegated/vested to him/her by the Director/State Government, delegation of financial power rules and other instructions issued from time to time.

Human Resources

- She/he will ensure for proper supervision and implementation of Job Descriptions assigned to the Clinical Nursing and Public health nursing cadres in the state.
- She/he will coordinate, advice and assists the Director, in framing rules for the recruitment, promotion, transfer and posting, etc., with regards to Clinical and Public Health nurses.

Functional

- To ensure quality in nursing service delivery through verification clinical nursing protocols in hospital and public health facilities.
- Supervise in implementation of the capacity building and training plan for clinical and public health nurses.
- Ensure all clinical nurses are trained in appropriate skills/area and adopt the updated nursing practices while delivering nursing and patient care.
- She/he will coordinate with different authorities to develop infrastructure in order to enable quality nursing services in different healthcare system.

Job Descriptions for Joint Director Nursing (Education)

The Joint Director Nursing (Education), will assist, coordinate the Director Nursing, for proper management of the nursing education and its overall improvement in the state.

She/he is responsible to the Director Nursing, and Health and Family Welfare, Department of state Government.

Educational Qualification

Same as director of nursing.

General Administrative Functions

- She/he will coordinate the Director Nursing for smooth functioning of the Nursing education wing of the Nursing directorate.
- She/he will be responsible and coordinate for the planning, budgeting and implementation of the Nursing education wing of the directorate.
- She/he will assist and coordinate to frame rules for the nursing educators/trainers/faculties and Nursing officers (education wing) of the Nursing directorate
- She/he will ensure that INC standards should be followed at the educational institutions.
- She/he will ensure timely submission of Performance Appraisal Report furnished by the Nursing Officers (Education wing) of the Directorate before the Director Nursing, in time.

Monitoring and Supervision

- She/he will coordinate the work and supervise the Nursing Officers (Education wing) of the Directorate and report compliance
- She/he will undertake periodic visits to the Nursing Schools/Colleges/training institutions or as and when directed by Director/Govt. in order to streamline nursing education system in the state.
- She/he will ensure proper coordination with the clinical wing of the directorate to bring current learning into practice.
- She/he will coordinate for setting up, design and implementation of the Human Resource information system for the nursing institutions in the state.
- Coordinate to take appropriate measures for recruitment, deployment of staff to ensure better nursing education in the state.

Financial

She/he will discharge the administrative and financial powers as vested/delegated to him/her from time to time by the Director/Government financial power rules, and other instructions issued from time to time.

Human Resources

- Coordinate and assist for proper implementation of Job Descriptions/responsibilities of the Nursing faculties/trainers in the state
- Coordinate and assist the Director, in framing rules for the recruitment, promotion and transfer of the Nursing faculties/trainers.

Functional

- She/he will coordinate and assist for the preparation, submission of requirements of all nursing training institutions and ensure timely submission before the Director Nursing.
- Ensure timely submission of institutional visit report and advice suitably to develop nursing education systems in Nursing Schools/Colleges/Training institutions.
- She/he will coordinate with the Director for smooth functioning of the state Nursing Board and Nursing Council.
- She/he will coordinate for selection and admission of students in different nursing training institutions/programs as well as implementation of new courses as per INC and concerned University guidelines.
- Coordinate the Director for Supervision and implementation of the capacity building and training plan in different nursing institutions.
- Maintain and develop the Professional Development framework.

- Manage the educational contracts ensuring best value, quality and flexibility in design and delivery and coordinate performance review activities.
- Promote a culture where individuals and teams are encourage to develop personal and professional knowledge and skills.

Job Descriptions for Deputy Director Nursing (Clinical and Public Health)

The Deputy Director, Clinical Nursing will assist the Director Nursing and Joint Director Nursing (Clinical) for smooth functioning of Clinical wing of the Directorate. He/She is responsible to the Director Nursing, and Health and family welfare department of Government.

Educational Qualification

MSc or PhD Nursing at least 10 years of administrative experience with adequate clinical and/or teaching experience.

Administrative Functions

- She/he will assist the superior authorities of Nursing Directorate (Clinical wing) to plan and prepare budget of the Clinical Nursing and public health nursing wings of the directorate.
- She/he will support Director/Joint Director to frame rules, procedures for the nursing personnel who are under the clinical nursing wing and public health nursing of the Nursing directorate.
- She/he will discharge all the financial and administrative responsibilities as vested to him/her by the superior authorities from time to time.
- She/he will ensure timely submission of Performance Appraisal Report (PAR) of the Assistant Director, Clinical before the Director, Nursing.
- She/he will be in-charge of allocation and maintenance of vehicles for the directorate.

Monitoring and Supervision

- She/he will coordinate the superior authorities to supervise the work of assistant director nursing clinical.
- He/she will ensure periodic visit to different clinical nursing set up 7 monitors the practice of nursing as and when necessary and directed by the competent authority in order to streamline clinical and public health nursing service.
- He/she will ensure proper coordination with the education wing of the directorate to bring current learnings into practice.
- He/she will support in setting up, design and implementation of the HR information system for the clinical and public health nurses.
- He/she will assist the authorities for recruitment, deployment of staff to enable better nursing service delivery system.
- Manage the educational contracts ensuring best value, quality and flexibility in design and delivery and coordinate performance review activities.
- Develop and evaluate models of clinical supervision and reflection in order to support professional practice and improvements in patient care.

Financial

He/she will discharge the administrative and financial powers as vested/delegated to him/her from time to time by the Director/Govt., delegation of financial power Rules, and other instructions issued from time to time.

Human Resources

- Coordinate and assist for proper implementation of job descriptions/responsibilities of the Nursing personnel in different clinical set up in the state.
- Coordinate and assist the Director, in framing rules for the recruitment, promotion and transfer of the clinical and public health nurses.
- He/she will be coordinate and assist for preparation, submission and updation of the gradation list of all the clinical nursing/public health nursing personnel in the state (clinical wing).

Functional

- He/she will coordinate for planning, forecasting, and fulfilling the requirements in different clinical nursing set-up in the state
- He/she will ensure for timely receipt of C.C.Rs/PARs of the clinical nursing personnel and public health nursing personnel
- He/she will assist the superior authorities for preparation of training plan of the clinical nursing cadre.
- He/she will coordinate for implementation of capacity building plan including training, exposure visits, continuing education for the nursing education in clinical nursing Cadre.
- Supervise in implementation of the capacity building and training plan.

Job Descriptions for Deputy Director Nursing (Education)

Educational Qualification

Same as Deputy Director Nursing Clinicals.

The Deputy Director Nursing (Education) will assist the Director Nursing and Joint Director Nursing (Education) for smooth management of Nursing Education wing of the directorate.

He/she is responsible to the Director Nursing and state Health and Family welfare Department .

General Administrative Functions

He/she will assist the superior authorities of Nursing Directorate (Education wing) to plan and prepare budget of the Nursing training institutions .

He/she will support Director/Joint Director to frame rules, procedures for the nursing faculties/trainers who are under the Education wing of the Nursing directorate.

He/she will discharge all the financial and administrative responsibilities as vested to him/her by the superior authorities from time to time.

He/she ensure timely submission of Performance Appraisal Report (PAR) of the Assistant Director, Education before the Director, Nursing.

Monitoring and Supervision

- He/she will coordinate the superior authorities to supervise the work of Assistant Director Nursing Education.
- He/she will ensure periodic visit to different nursing training institutions as and when necessary and directed by the competent authority in order to streamline nursing education in the state.
- He/she will ensure proper coordination with the clinical wing of the directorate to bring current learning into practice of the clinical and Public health nurses.
- He/she will support in setting up, design and implementation of the HR information system for nursing institutions in the state.
- He/she will assist the authorities for recruitment, deployment of staff to enable better nursing education in the state.

Financial

He/she will discharge the administrative and financial powers as vested/delegated to him/her from time to time by the Director and delegation of financial power Rules, Odisha and other instructions issued from time to time.

Human Resources

- Coordinate and assist for proper implementation of Job Descriptions/responsibilities of the nursing faculties/trainers in different nursing training institutions in the state.
- Coordinate and assist the Director, in framing rules for the recruitment, promotion and transfer of the nursing faculties working at different training institutions.
- He/she will coordinate and assist for preparation, submission and updation of the gradation list of all the nursing faculties (education wing).

Functional

- He/she will coordinate for planning, forecasting, and fulfilling the requirements in different nursing training institutions in the state
- He/she will ensure for timely receipt of C.C.Rs/PARs of the nursing faculties/trainers working under the Govt.
- He/she will assist the superior authorities for preparation of training plan of the nursing faculties/trainers.
- He/she will coordinate for implementation of capacity building plan including training, exposure visits, continuing education for nursing cadre.
- Supervise in implementation of the capacity building and training plan.

Job Descriptions for Assistant Director Nursing (Clinical and Public Health)

The Assistant Director Nursing (Clinical and public health) will assist the Director Nursing and Joint Director Nursing (Clinical and Public Health) and Deputy Director Nursing (Clinical and Public Health) for smooth functioning of Clinical wing of the Directorate.

He/she is responsible to the Director Nursing, and Health and Family Welfare Department of Government.

Administrative Functions

- He/she will assist the superior authorities of Nursing Directorate (Clinical and Public Health wing) to plan and prepare budget of the Clinical Nursing and Public Health nursing wings of the directorate.
- He/she will support Director/Joint Director/Deputy Director to frame rules, procedures for the nursing personnel who are under the clinical nursing wing and public health nursing of the Nursing Directorate.
- He/she will discharge all the financial and administrative responsibilities as vested to him/her by the superior authorities from time to time.

Monitoring and Supervision

- He/she will coordinate the superior authorities to supervise the work of nursing services in the state.
- He/she will ensure periodic visit to different clinical nursing set up as and when necessary and directed by the competent authority in order to streamline clinical and public health nursing service.
- Discusses and exchanges views with nursing Superintendent to identify and recognize staff and unit/ward needs.
- He/she will ensure the maintenance of standards at the clinical settings by periodic visits to the clinicals.
- He/she will ensure proper coordination with the education wing of the directorate to bring current learnings into practice.
- He/she will assist the authorities for recruitment, deployment of staff to enable better nursing service delivery system.

Financial

He/she will discharge the administrative and financial powers as vested delegated to him/her from time to time by the Director Nursing delegation of financial power Rules and other instructions issued from time to time.

Human Resources

- Coordinate and assist for proper implementation of job descriptions/responsibilities of the nursing personnel in different clinical set up in the state.

- Coordinate and assist the superior authorities in framing rules for the recruitment, promotion and transfer of the clinical and Public Health Nurses.

Functional

- He/she will coordinate for planning, forecasting, and fulfilling the requirements in different clinical nursing set-up in the state.
- He/she will assist the superior authorities for preparation of training plan of the clinical nursing cadre.
- He/she will coordinate for implementation of capacity building plan including training, exposure visits, continuing education for the nursing education in clinical nursing cadre.
- Performs appropriate committee functions as assigned by DON.
- Participates in Nursing Continuous Quality Improvement initiatives, in service education programs and committee functions as assigned.
- Acts as a professional role model and resource person.
- Supervise in implementation of the capacity building and training plan.

Job Descriptions for Assistant Director Nursing (Education)

The Assistant Director Nursing (Education) will assist the Director Nursing, Joint Director Nursing (Education) and Deputy Director Nursing(Education) for smooth management of Nursing Education wing of the directorate. He/She is responsible to the Director Nursing, and state Health and Family welfare Department.

Administrative Functions

- He/she will assist the superior authorities of Nursing Directorate (Education wing) to plan and prepare budget of the Nursing training institutions .
- He/she will support Director/Joint Director/Deputy Director to frame rules, procedures for the nursing faculties/trainers who are under the education wing of the nursing directorate.
- He/she will discharge all the financial and administrative responsibilities as vested to him/her by the superior authorities from time to time.

Monitoring and Supervision

- He/she will ensure periodic visit to different nursing training institutions as and when directed by the competent authority in order to streamline nursing education in the state.
- He/she will monitor standards in the quality of nursing education at different nursing school and colleges.
- He/she will ensure proper coordination with the clinical wing of the directorate to bring current learning into practice of the clinical and public health nurses.
- He/she will support in setting up, design and implementation of the HR information system for nursing institutions in the state.
- He/she will assist the authorities for recruitment, deployment of staff to enable better nursing education in the state.

Financial

He/she will discharge the administrative and financial powers as vested/delegated to him/her from time to time by the Director and delegation of financial power rules and other instructions issued from time to time.

Human Resources

- Coordinate and assist for proper implementation of Job Descriptions/responsibilities of the nursing faculties/trainers in different nursing training institutions in the state.
- Coordinate and assist the Director, in framing rules for the recruitment, promotion and transfer of the nursing faculties working at different training institutions.

Functional

- He/she will coordinate for planning, forecasting, and fulfilling the requirements in different nursing training institutions in the state.
- Helps in developing and sustaining standards in nursing educations
- He/she will assist the superior authorities planning and programming of continuing education for the nursing faculties/trainers.
- He/she will coordinate for implementation of capacity building plan including training, exposure visits, continuing education for nursing cadre.
- Supervise in implementation of the capacity building and training plan.

Job Description of Principal, College of Nursing

The principal directs the educational and nonteaching staff of the college in conducting program in coordination with the faculties.

Educational Qualification

As per Indian Nursing Council the principal college of nursing should have Masters Degree in Nursing (PhD desirable) within 14 years experience after MSc (N) in College of Nursing and 3 years experience in administration (years of experience is relaxable if suitable candidate is not available) (If a candidate is not available, minimum 5 years of experience in college of nursing, with an aggregate of 14 years teaching experience).

Duties, Task and Responsibilities

Financial

- Plans and prepare budget for the college.

- Acts as drawing and disbursing officer of the establishment.
- Monitors all college expenditure.

Administration

- Principal is responsible for overall administration of the College of nursing establishment.
- Acts as appointing authority of all the nonteaching Gr. C and D posts of the establishment.

Educational

- Teaching and monitoring educational programs of the college.
- Coordinates with faculties in the planning, implementation and evaluation of the programs.
- Planning implementation and evaluation of continuing educational programs.
- Identifies professional development needs of faculty members and facilities staff development program in coordination with the heads of departments/coordinators.

Acts as

- Chairman of committee of course, college council and staff body.
- Member of academic council, science faculty, etc.
- Coordinate with the University and INC for proper implementation of curriculum and examination.
- Act as a role model in teaching to the students.

Supervisory

- Responsible for supervision of all personnel teaching faculties and nonteaching staffs in the college.
- Coordinates and collaborates with faculties in preparing academic staff assignment.
- Plans staff assignments in consultation with faculties and administrative staff.
- Facilitates orientation of new employees to the job responsibilities and other official procedures.
- Facilitates and provides assistance to staff in conducting their activities.
- Writes staff performance reports and reviews the confidential reports of staff.
- Monitors student welfare activities (e.g., Mess, Hostel, health, sports, SNA, etc.
- Facilitates administration of college library.
- Monitors all leave privileges of the faculty, student and nonteaching staffs.

Human Relation and Communication to the Higher Authority

- The principal college of Nursing has to inform staff on matters related to educational program conducted at the college and the staff on matters related to personal and work policies.
- Identifies conflict among staff members and initiates solution.
- Informs students on changes in college policies, procedures standards and curriculum.
- Facilitates student and staff guidance services.
- Informs parents about student status and reviews reports of student performance.
- Facilitates communication interpersonal relationship both inter and intra departmental and with other institutions at state, national and international levels with due approval of the Director Nursing.

Job Description of Vice Principal/Professor

Overview

The Vice Principal/Professor in nursing in directing the staff (teaching) of the college in conducting teaching programs. She assists principal and in assessing, planning, implementing, and evaluating educational programs.

Educational Qualification

According to INC norms the vice principal of college of Nursing should have masters Degree in Nursing with 14 years experience after MSc (N) in College of Nursing. Three years experience in administration (Years of experience is relaxable if suitable candidate is not available) (If a candidate is not available, minimum 5 years of experience in college of nursing, with an aggregate of 14 years teaching experience).

Duties, Task and Responsibilities

Educational

- Assists principal in monitoring the educational programs of the college.
- Assists principal in planning implementation and evaluation of the programs.
- Assists principal in identifying needs for professional development of faculty and facilitates conducts staff development program.
- Participates in teaching various educational programs.

Acts as

- In the absence of principal, chairs the assigned committee meetings.
- Assists in conduct of admission procedures and final university examination.
- Role model in teaching.
- Supervises clinical experience of all educational programs in coordination with coordinators.
- Guides faculty in day to day academic activities of all educational programs.
- Guides and monitors students cumulative record for all educational programs, maintained by respective program coordinators.
- Reviews student progress reports and activities and offers academic guidance.
- Guides the students in conducting seminars, discussions and presentations, etc.

Supervisory

Shares responsibility with principal in supervision of teaching and non teaching staff.

- Plans academic staff assignments in consultation with principal.
- Participates in conduct of orientation program for new faculty members.
- Supervises and guides staff in conducting their activities.
- Assists principal in monitoring student's welfare activities, e.g., (mess, hostel, health, sports, SNA), etc.
- Assists principal in administration and supervision of library.
- Assists principal in maintaining discipline in the college.

Interpersonal

- Assists principal informing:
  - Staff on matters related to educational programs conducted at the college.
  - Staff on matters related to personal and work policies.
- Identifies conflict among staff members, initiates solution and reports to principal when necessary.
- Informs students of changes in college policies, procedures and standards.
- Facilitates guidance and counseling students and staff as per need.
- Any other responsibility assigned by the principal.

Job Description of Readers/Associate Professors

Educational Qualification

According to Indian Nursing Council, the associate professor should have Master Degree in Nursing with 10 years experience after MSc (N) in College of Nursing. (If a candidate is not available, 5 years of experience in College of Nursing with an aggregates of 10 years teaching experience).

- Responsible for planning and implementation of teaching programs.
- Teaching subjects in the curriculum.
- Supervision of clinical teaching program of subjects in hospital/public health field.
- Assisting in the administration of the college of nursing.
- Guides the students in conducting seminars, discussions and presentations, etc.
- Supervision of student's health, welfare and security.
- Assisting in the selection of students and admission.
- Assisting in conducting examinations, tests (sessional and terminals).
- Preparation of reports on student's progress.
- Assisting in maintenance of students records.
- Participation in student guidance activities.
- Guiding-student's extracurricular programs.
- Any other duty assigned.

Job Description of Lecturers/Assistant Professors

Educational Qualification

According to INC norms the lecturers/assistant professors of college of Nursing should have Master Degree in Nursing with 3 years teaching experience after MSc (N).

- Teach and supervise in the courses in clinical nursing/education/administration.
- Assist in curriculum development and evaluation.
- Coordinates with external lecturer for various courses as assigned
- Assist in practice of teaching.
- Guides the students in conducting seminars, discussions and presentations, etc.
- Assist in research projects.
- Acts as counselors.
- Assist in student and staff evaluation.
- Maintain records.
- Any other duties assigned by the principal.

Job Description of Principal, School of Nursing

Professional Qualification

According to INC norms the principal school of nursing should have MSc Nursing with 6 Years of teaching experience or BSc Nursing (Basic)/Post Basic with 8 of Teaching experiences. The job description of the principal school of nursing are as follows:

Administrative

- Participation in all the planning by the controlling authority which relates to the school of nursing.
- Preparation of school budget and making recommendations in these regards to the controlling authority.
- Formulation and implementation of policies in relation to staff students and program.
- Determining the staff requirement and recruitment in accordance with the policies of the institution keeping in mind the minimum requirement laid down by INC.
- Recruitment and selection of students in accordance with the policies of the institution.
- Writing annual confidential reports of the staff.
- Holding staff meeting/conferences with the office staff, students and with different departments.
- Organization and implementation of the curriculum as laid down by the Indian Nursing Council for GNM students.
- Places indents/claims with the higher authorities for uniform, stipend and other grants.
- Prepare job description for all members of the school.
- Planning in service education for all staff.
- To maintain all records pertaining to students, staff and general record of the school.
- General administration of a school of nursing.
- Administration and overall supervision of teaching programs.
- Supervision and guidance of teaching staff including organization of in-service education of staff.

Education

- Works out the syllabus and curriculum keeping with in the frame work as laid down by INC.

- Arranges theory and practical work for each group, with the help of tutors and clinical tutors and clinical tutors so as to meet the laid down objectives.
- Active participation in the teaching program.
- Supervises the clinical training of the students.
- Visit wards/departments regularly where practical training is being carried out.
- Maintains class schedule, rotation plan of clinical experience.
- Maintains records of student's examination, test and assignments.
- Periodic evaluation of the total program.
- Responsibility for conduct of examinations.

Discipline

- To ensure maintenance of good order and discipline both in the school and hostel.
- She will be responsible for welfare of students and staff, i.e., accommodation, health and recreation.

Job Description of Vice-Principal, School of Nursing

According to INC norms the vice principal school of nursing should have MSc Nursing with 4 Years of teaching experience or BSc Nursing (Basic)/Post Basic with 6 years of teaching

Vice-principal of school of nursing is directly responsible to the principal tutor He/she will officiate in the absence of principal tutor and will carry out any other duties assigned to her by the principal tutor.

Common Work Activities of Vice-Principal Include

- Working closely with the principal on a daily basis to ensure the smooth overall operation of the school.
- Supporting committees of staff and parent that function to improve the learning and social environment of the school for the students.
- Teaching classes, developing rapport with the students, handling discipline issues and filling in for the principal when required.
- Resolving conflicts between students, teachers, parents or combinations of conflicts between various individuals.
- Assisting in yearly teacher evaluations, assisting in providing guidance to staff and students, and encouraging a positive climate in the school.
- Directing assemblies and other special gatherings of students for events throughout the year.
- Developing emergency response plans for schools as required by state and federal education agencies. Filing reports and updating as required.
- Record keeping as required through the use of various logs, tracking records, computer programs, inter or intranet software or other programs.

Job Description of Clinical Instructors/Tutors

According to INC norms the clinical instructors/tutors of college/school of nursing should have MSc Nursing or BSc Nursing (Basic/Post Basic). The role and responsibilities are described under some following headings.

As a Teacher

- Carries out all instructions given by the higher authorities.
- Teach students and clarify their duty.
- Gives proper assignment and makes necessary corrections.
- Directs the students to different aspect of study materials.
- Gives frequent test papers and makes them understand their weak points.
- Checks that all necessary things are ready for the students at the time of their admission and starting of each semester.
- Conduct's seminar, group discussion, presentation, debates, etc., for upgrading the student's knowledge.
- Attend regular staff meetings.
- Carries out examination duties and other modalities of examination.
- Responsible for maintaining attendance register and other records of the student's up-to-date.
- Ensures that students maintain proper discipline in the college and clinics.

As a Supervisor

- Makes rotation plan and posts students to various clinical area.
- Supervises the students in clinical area, i.e., community and hospital.
- Acts as liaison between students, college and higher authorities of hospital.
- Give frequent assignments, points out their mistakes and correct it.
- Demonstrates various nursing procedure and have to take care of different categories of patients.
- Conducts, bedside clinics, clinical presentation, ward teaching, nursing rounds for the students.

As a Guide and Counselor

- Guide the students in all activities of the college.
- Encourages and guide in various committees of the college like magazine committee, entertainment committees, curriculum committee, sports committee, library committee.
- Guide and counsel the students in condition of their crisis.
- Guide the students in various extracurricular activities.
- Guide the students in conducting community camps, seminar, etc.

An Incharge of Different Laboratories

- Takes the charge of different laboratories of college like nursing arts laboratory, microbiology, biochemistry, community, etc.
- Responsible for equal physical verification of inventories.
- Issues articles to the students in time of partials.
- Ensure to the cleanliness and maintenance of laboratory and its premises.

Job Descriptions of Nursing Superintendent Grade

As prescribed for Staff-Nurse and should have experience as Nursing Superintendent Grade II.

Nursing Services

- Participates in the formulation of the hospital in general and those specific to the nursing service.
- Determines goals, aims, objectives and policies of the nursing services.
- Implements hospital polices and rules through various NSG units.
- Decides and recommends personnel and material requirement for running various nursing services departments of the hospital.
- Interviews and recruits nursing staff.
- Assistant students selection and recruitment other auxiliary staff.
- Ensure the safe and efficient care rendered in the various NSG departments of the hospital.
- Makes regular visits in hospitals and words.
- Take hospitals rounds with medical superintendent.
- Prepare budgets for NSG services departments.
- Prepare duty roster, plans staff leave, and disburses salary.
- Give counseling and guidance to the subordinate staff .
- Enforces implementation of the hospital rules regulation and policies.
- Participate in hospitals and inter hospital meeting/ conference.
- Investigate complaints and takes necessary steps.
- Supervision, guidance and control of group 'D' employees of the hospital.es of the hospital.
- Inspects hospitals, kitchen and dietary service.
- General and office duties.
- Attendance to general correspondence.
- Maintain necessary records concerning the nursing staff, students, confidential reports and health records, etc.
- Submits annual reports of the nursing service departments to medical superintendent, Indian Nursing Council and Nurses Registration Council.
- Participate in professional and community activities.
- Maintains cordial relations with public and voluntary workers.

Job Descriptions of Nursing Superintendent Grade-II

Educational Qualification

As prescribed for staff-nurse.

Experience

Should have experience as senior staff-nurse.

Duties and Responsibilities

It is the second level nursing supervisory role, it needs at least the Nursing Superintendent Gr-II for three senior staff-nurse.

Patient Care and Ward/Unit Management

- Organizes and plans nursing care activities of the department according to the hospital policies and service needs.
- Plans staffing pattern and the other necessary requirements of her/his department.
- Complies and submits nursing statistics to the concerned authorities.
- Conducts and attends to the departmental and interdepartmental meetings/conferences from time to time.
- Makes regular rounds of her department.
- Ensures to the safety and general dealing of the department.
- Looks into general comforts of the patient and his/her relatives.
- Receives reports from the night supervisor of her department.
- Evaluates nature and quantum of care required in each ward.
- Supervises the proper use and care of the equipment and supplies in the department.
- Officiates in the absence of nursing superintendent Gr-I.

Educational Function

- Arranges classes and clinical teaching of nursing student in the department.
- Implements the ward teaching program and clinical experience of the students with the help of doctors and nurses.
- Does counseling and guidance of staff and students.
- Arranges and conducts staff development programs of his/her department.

Job Responsibility of Ward Sister

Educational Qualification

Registered Nurse and Registered Midwife. Diploma in Nursing Education and Administration/BSc/Post-Basic BSc Nursing and having experience as staff nurse.

Duties and Responsibilities of Ward Sister

The ward sister is the first level supervisor and team leader of the unit. She is directly accountable to the Nursing Superintendent through Deputy Nursing Superintendent for ward management and patient care.

Duties and Responsibility in Relation to Patient Care

She will be responsible:

- To organize and make plan of all nursing activities of her unit for patient care according to hospital policy and rules.
- To establish and reinforce the prepared standard protocol for patient care.
- To take the report of her unit from the on duty staff nurse and will read and sign the report book.
- To make bed to bed round of the department with Staff and students.

- To supervise direct patient care of the unit and provide direct care to seriously ill patients as and when situation arises.
- To assign staff nurses, student nurses for nursing care, specially for acute ill, dangerously ill patient and post operative cases.
- To coordinate with other department for patient care and for smooth running of the unit.
- To supervise dietary arrangement, serving of diet and feeding of the helpless patient.
- To supervise, guide and direct the staff nurses and students to carry out treatment of the patients as prescribed by the physician/surgeon of the unit.
- To check all the records of the patient related to diagnosis, condition and treatment and ensure proper maintenance of records.

Duties and Responsibilities Related to Ward Management and Supervision

- She will take active part to maintain cleanliness of the ward with the help of Assistant Superintendent and Ward Master.
- She will ensure safety and comfort of the patient of the unit.
- She will make duty roster of the staff nurses, student nurses and work assignment.
- She will check the attendance of all nurses posted in her unit and report to the office of Nursing Superintendent.
- She will indent and procure the ward supplies, equipment and drugs.
- She will check the inventory regularly and keep the stock register up to date.
- She will maintain the records of nonserviceable articles and make arrangement for condemnation.
- She will maintain stock register and it will be countersigned by Nursing Superintendent.
- She will face the audit (Internal and External) periodically.
- She will establish and reinforce the standard of nursing procedure as prescribed.
- She will ensure the maintenance of waste management and infection control of the ward.
- She will ensure prevention of wastage and misuse of supplies and drugs.
- She will act as a liaison officer between ward and administration.
- She will maintain good public relation in her unit.
- She will maintain ward statistics and submit to concern authority regularly.
- She will deal with adverse situation and report to the concerned authority.
- She will report any theft or loss to the higher authority through Nursing Superintendent.
- She will report any medico legal cases in the ward to the concern authority.
- She will write and submit performance report of the staff and send to the office of the Nursing Superintendent.
- She will make arrangement for keeping the patients belongings in safe custody as per laid down policy of the hospital.
- She will maintain daily patient's census of the unit and report about the critically ill patients to the Nursing Superintendent.
- She will perform any other duty allotted to her by the Nursing Superintendent/Dy. Nursing Superintendent in the interest of the public and when necessary.
- She will perform morning, evening and night duty in the interest of the Hospital.

Duties and Responsibilities in Relation to Nursing Education

She will be responsible:

- To organize and oversee the orientation program of staff and student.
- To encourage and participate in staff development program in her unit.
- To implement the practical part of the Nursing Educational Program.
- To guide the student for formulation of nursing care pan, nursing care studies for the patient.
- To evaluate the students performance in the ward and report accordingly.
- To assist and supervise the student for incidental teaching, health education program (formal and informal) for the patients and their relatives.
- To help in Medical and Nursing Research.

Job Responsibility of Senior Staff-Nurse

Educational Qualification

As for Staff-Nurse.

Experience

Should have experience as staff-nurse of not less than 5 years.

Duties and Responsibilities

Senior staff nurse is a first level nursing supervisor who is accountable for nursing care management of a ward or a unit.

Direct Patient Care

- Ensure proper admission, discharge of patients.
- Plans nursing care and makes patient assignments as per their NSG needs.
- Assists in the direct care/provides direct care to patients as and when required.
- She see that total health needs of his/her patients are met.
- Ensures safety, comfort and good personal hygiene of his/her patients.
- Assists in planning and administration of the therapeutic diet to his/her patient.
- Ensures the helpless patients are regularly fed as per direction.

- Takes nursing round with staff and students.
- Makes rounds with doctors, assisting them in diagnosis and treatment of patients.
- Coordinates patient care with other departments.

Supervision and Administration

- Ensures safe and clean environment for the ward and other department.
- Makes duty and work assignments.
- Indenting and procurement of ward supplies and equipments and keeps records.
- Does regular inventory checking of her ward/unit.
- Makes list for condemnation of articles and submits it to all the concerned.
- Assists in making ward requirement.
- Ensures that ward statistics are regularly submitted.
- Maintains discipline among the personnel working in the particular ward/unit.
- Deals appropriately with any adverse situation.
- Reports about any medico legal cases.
- Writes and submits confidential reports of the staff.

Educational Function

- Organizes orientation programs for new staff.
- Organizes formal and informal ward teaching, conducts bedside clinics and demonstration, etc.
- Conducts ward conferences/meetings.
- Guides in formulation of nursing care studies, and nursing care plan, etc.
- Evaluates the students performances and submits reports to the school authorities.
- Helps in medical and nursing research.
- Encourages staff development program in her ward.

Responsibility Regarding Teaching of Students

- She will assign patient to student nurse keeping in mind the level of knowledge of the student, the learning objective and need of the patients.
- She will provide direct supervision over patient care by the students in her ward.
- She will teach, supervise and guide nursing procedure performed by student nurses.
- She will guide and help the students in giving health education to the patient of her ward.
- She will participate in clinical teaching program of the students nurse.
- She will assist and participate in any in-service education program.

Job Responsibility of Staff-Nurse

Qualification

General nursing and Midwifery Diploma/Certificate, recognized by Indian Nursing Council or Basic BSc Nursing from a Recognized University according to INC norms. Registered with the Indian Nursing Council.

Duties and Responsibilities

- Carry out the procedures of admission and discharge of the patient.
- Makes bed of serious patients and helps or guides students.
- Maintains personal hygiene and comforts of the patient.
- Attends to the nutritional needs of the patient and feeds the helpless patients.
- Maintains clean and safe environment for the patient.
- Implements and maintains ward policies and routines.
- Coordinates patient care with other team members.
- Take rounds with the doctors when called to list new orders and see that they are carried out.
- Performs various technical tasks related to nursing care.

LEADERSHIP

Introduction

Leadership has been described as the behavior of an individual when directing the activities of a group toward a shared goal. The key aspects of the leadership role involves influencing group activities and coping with change. Thus leader's are people who can influence the behaviors of other's without having to rely on force and whom others accept as a leader. Leadership is an important aspect of managing not only in healthcare setting but also in every organization. The ability to lead effectively is one of the Key's to being effective manager. The essence of the leadership is followership. In other word's it is the willingness of people to follow that makes a person a leader. Moreover, people tend to follow those whom they see as providing a means of achieving their own desires, wants and needs.

Definitions

Leadership refers to the relation between an individual and group around some common interest and behaving in a manner directed or determined by leader.

—Encyclopedia of Social Sciences

Leadership is defined as influence, that is the are a process of influencing people so that they will strive willingly and enthusiastically toward the achievement of group goals.

Leadership is the ability to persuade others to seek defined objectives enthusiastically. It is human factor that binds a group together and motivated it toward goal.

—Keith Davis

Leadership is an ability of a leader/manager to induce subordinates (followers) to work with confidence and zeal.

—Koontz and O Connell, 2004

Features of Leadership

- Leadership is a continuous process of behaviors, it is not one-shot activity.
- Leadership may be in terms of relations between a leader and his followers which arise out of their functioning for common goals.

- By exercising his leadership, the leader tries to influence the behavior of individuals or group of individuals around him to achieve common goals.
- The followers work willingly and enthusiastically to achieve these goals.

Importance of Leadership in Healthcare Setting

Leadership is an important factor for making delivery of health service successful. The importance of good leadership can be discussed as follow:

Motivating Employees

Motivation is necessary for work performance, higher the motivation, better the performance. A good leader, by exercising his leadership, motivates the employees for high performance. Generally during delivery of nursing care A nurse supervisor can motivate the nurses to provide high quality care.

Creating Confidence

A good leader may create confidence in his followers by directing them, giving them advice and getting through them good results in the organization.

Building Morale

Morale is expressed as attitude of employees towards organization, management and voluntary cooperation to offer their ability to the organization. High morale leads to high productivity and organization stability.

Leadership in Healthcare Settings

Clinical leadership is essential healthcare settings and requires clinicians visibly enacting espoused values and plans. The Clinical Excellence Commission (2007:2) of New South Wales suggests that Clinical Leadership occurs at all levels of patient care and refers to the Process of leading a set of activities that improve the delivery of safe clinical care the set of attributes required to lead a team, unit stream or cluster

Here the leadership is a multifaceted process of:
- Identifying a goal or target
- Organizing services
- Motivating other people to act
- Providing support and motivation to achieve mutually negotiated goals

Added to these more generic features of leadership is the responsibility for:
- Care and safety of patients
- Monitoring of both service and individual outcomes.

Hence effective clinical leaders need to be able to:
- Focus on promoting health
- Have the capacity to build effective teams
- Articulate and demonstrate what others cannot see
- Address immediate challenges
- Demonstrate expert clinical skills
- Have a patient focus
- Show selflessness
- Be assertive and able to collaborate with others
- Have the vision to lead their team into a future which is often unknown.

Strategies for Promoting Clinical Leadership

Balding (2005) asserts that although senior management can provide the foundation framework for the clinical governance program, it is the clinical managers who play a critical role in the day to day processes related to patient care. She advocates that attention be provided to develop the capacity of line managers to relate organizational policies into practice, with the provision of resources and supports to empower them. Hence a more systematic and structured delegation of accountability to all levels of the health service organization is achieved.

Balding (2005) advises senior managers that clinical leadership is encouraged by:
- Defining the organization's vision and values for safety and quality care
- Defining the strategic direction consistent with achieving the vision and values
- Collaborating with staff to identify clear achievable goals, roles, resources and processes
- Providing information, skills and resources to staff to enable them to fulfil responsibilities
- Providing support to managers and all staff to enact processes contributing to high quality care
- Facilitating and rewarding a collaborative approach to safety and quality improvement between clinical and non-clinical managers and their teams
- Evaluating the status of quality and leadership in the organization
- Reviewing incentives by increasing those rewarding engagement and removing others not contributing to quality care
- Modeling commitment to safety and quality.
- Embedding improvements in policy and practices

Davidson et al (2006) list the following factors as critical in the development of transformational clinical leadership:
- Available effective role models
- Mechanisms for mentoring and clinical supervision
- Career pathways
- Intentional succession planning
- Other strategies, e.g., Clinical doctorates, collegiality of professional associations, collaborative initiatives with academic institutions or other professions.

Leadership Approaches in Healthcare Setting

Leadership has been described as the behavior of an individual when directing the activities of a group toward a shared goal. The key aspects of the leadership role involves influencing group activities and coping with change. Leadership styles are the approaches or the ways how a leader will lead the groups.

Healthcare systems are composed of numerous professional groups, departments, and specialties with intricate, nonlinear interactions between them; the complexity of such systems is often unparalleled as a result of constraints relating to different disease areas, multidirectional goals, and multidisciplinary staff. Within large organizations such as healthcare systems, the numerous groups with associated subcultures might support or be in conflict with each other. Leadership needs to capitalize on the diversity within the organization as a whole and efficiently utilize resources when designing management processes, while encouraging personnel to work towards common goals. The leadership approaches can be adapted to the healthcare setting to optimize management in this highly complex environment are mainly classified as:

Transactional Leadership Approach

Also known as managerial leadership, is a leadership style where the executive relies on rewards and punishments to achieve optimal job performance from his or her subordinates. As such, transactional leadership is based on an exchange, or transaction: The leader rewards workers who perform their tasks to the specified levels and punishes workers who do not perform to those set standards. The theory also postulates that workers will perform their tasks as the transactional leader wants them to do in exchange for the leader's offering something that the workers want, such as pay.

Transformational Leadership Approach

The transformational theory goes beyond the more traditional style of transactional leadership (which focuses on supervision, organization and group performance) and emphasizes that people work more effectively if they have a sense of mission. The transformational theory requires leaders to communicate their vision in a manner that is meaningful, exciting, and creates unity and collective purpose; the manager who is committed, has vision, and is able to empower others can be described as a transformational leader. Transformational leaders are able to motivate performance beyond expectations through their ability to influence attitudes.

Collaborative Leadership

Collaboration is an assertive and cooperative process that occurs when individuals work together towards mutual benefit, in a form of organizational symbiosis. Collaborative leadership involves communicating information to coworkers and associated organizations, to allow them to make their own informed decisions. Such collaborative communication strategies enhance healthcare management by: encouraging dialogue between multiple stakeholders; sharing knowledge and experiences; and reducing the level of complexity within healthcare organizations. Individuals with different levels of responsibility need to engage with the leadership process, so that they are actively involved in validating and communicating needs and identifying modifications in practices that may be required to address changing demands. Collaborative healthcare leadership requires a synergistic work environment, wherein multiple parties are encouraged to work together toward the implementation of effective practices and processes.

- **Shared leadership:** It results in individual staff members adopting leadership behaviors, greater autonomy, and improved client care outcomes.
- **Distributed leadership:** Here the work is distributed amongst staff members. The advantage is that individuals complement one another's strengths and offset one another's weaknesses.
- **Ethical leadership:** A good leader must have intentions, values, and behaviors that intend no harm and respect the rights of all stakeholders.

Role of Nurse Leader in Organizing Health Camps

Health camps or outreach clinics are the effective strategies adopted by both government and nongovernment organizations, associations, and societies with various interests and scope. A well organized health camp with a concentration on the various principles of planning, coordination, collaboration, tools, and techniques will not only make the health camp successful but also aids in improving the health status of the unreached community who are often deprived of basic to advance.

Planning

Planning is the primary phase of conducting a health camp. This phase Nurse manager must do mapping off overall aspect of health camp including venue, manpower planning, financial planning, resource allocation, logistic and transportation planning with proper planning monitoring and supervision in between the camp. Health camp should always be conducted during holidays or weekends so as to allow maximum number of participants in the camp. Venue should be accessible from the area where there is dense population, preferably in school, local health post, colleges where there are adequate waiting area and examination space. Organizers/leaders need to collaborate with the interested stakeholder so as to ensure adequate budget for conducting the camp. Medicine and consumable supplies can be obtained from prior request to various pharmaceutical companies.

- **Knowledge of health statistics:** Adequate knowledge of recent prevalence of the disease in the targeted community will be very much helpful in planning a health camp scientifically. It would also help in choosing the medicines and specialists for the camp. Availability of proper statistics of certain disease can help in conducting periodic camp in the targeted area so as to decrease the disease prevalence rate through the camp. It can be collected through the proper government or private health authority of the area where camp is going to be conducted. This is the role of nurse to collect valid resent health statistics before starting program.

- **Permission from relevant authority:** After having initial planning for the camp, the nurse manager should also seek permission from the relevant authority to conduct the camp in the desired area. The relevant authority may be a single body or multiple bodies and may include both government, community and private organizations. Depending upon the objectives and modalities of the camp, the permission granting authority ranges from Health Ministry, public health office, municipality, ward office, local committee and concerned authority of the camp venue like school, orphanage, old age care home, etc. The main purpose of this step is to ensure that the organizer will conduct the camp in ethical manner providing a quality care without any profit motive and self-interest.
- **Choosing the date and timing for the camp:** The success of the health camp depends upon the number of persons turning up for it. Choosing a day which is suitable for most of the local residents is vital for the effectiveness of the camp. The health camp should preferably take place on a holiday.
- **Site of the camp:** The venue of health camp should ideally be situated in the center of the village or town. It should be readily accessible by public transport. There has been instances where despite the publicity the health camps had poor attendance just because it was located at some ground which was far from the center of the village where villagers had difficulty in commuting.
- **Camp information dissemination:** Organizer should create a hype for the camp at least few days prior to the event. The camp information can be disseminated by pamphlets with catchy headlines and short sentence mentioning free medicine if applicable, loud speaker announcement in the community, placing a camp banner in the decent visible height and broadcasting through local TV, radio and newspaper.
- **Camp inauguration:** The community heath nurse should always have small opening of the camp in presence of local leaders involving mayor, police personnel, social workers, local health authority personnel. This will help addressing the local authorities commitment to improve the quality of health of the community as well as improving the current health statistics. The inauguration program should not be too long and it should not overshadow the program itself.
- **Multidisciplinary approach:** Health camp should always be led by multidisciplinary manpower ranging from helper, health assistant to different categories of consultants. Even a specific camp should have multidisciplinary approach as those health camps in unreached area tend to have a multiple disease specific service seekers.
- **Technology transfer:** It is the most important aspect during the camp conduction. Technology transfer is the process of sharing the knowledge and technology related to the disease and its management from a competent health professional to the local health professionals residing in health camp area. This will allow the local health professional for early diagnosis of disease even after the camp and refer the case to the preferred treatment destination whenever needed. This allows the general capacity building of the local health professionals so as he/she can manage the patients who come for follow-up after the camp.
- **Community participation:** Local students, members of local clubs, societies, health professionals should be encouraged to volunteer in the camp as well as to help in registration process and crowd management. It also provides them a bond of community participation and a learning opportunity. A multisectoral stake holder's participation is required from the individual level to any organizational level in the community. Unless the local leaders of the society take interest, medical camps will not be able to achieve its objective. The active participation of the community also makes a health camp more fruitful. The overall community participation also helps in making the camp harmonious.
- **Health promotion and awareness:** Medical camps should be encouraged to provide health education to the people attending the camp. There should be volunteers in the camp who can help in health promotion of the local community and providing awareness in various types of diseases and illness prevalent in the community. This will help in sharing the preventive, promotive part of the disease so as to make them aware before the disease process starts.
- **Behavior and manner of volunteers:** All the health volunteers involved in camp should communicate to the community people in local dialects as much as possible. They should also follow the local customs and traditions, rules and mannerisms. The volunteers should act courteously and also guide the patients as per the patient's requirements.
- **Legal and ethical aspect:** Health camp should be strictly conducted under proper ethics. The provision of unauthorized personnel treating the patient, prescribing and distributing drugs may lead to unsuccess of the health camp. There may be the lack of monitoring and supervision by competent authority in these issues but it is sole responsibility of the organizers to follow the legal and ethical aspect. The health volunteers should always be careful about the use of appropriate medicines, especially in regards to antibiotics and should refrain themselves from using third generation drugs which may cause more harm than good.
- **Reporting the data:** The morbidity profile recorded during the camp should be submitted to the local health authority with proper recommendation and photographs if possible. Similarly the morbidity profile of the community can be disseminated by scientific publications so as to deliver it to public health personals working in improving the health status of the people in community.

SUPERVISION

Concept

Supervision is the act of guiding, directing and overseeing the works of employees and other resources to accomplish stated expected output. It refers to monitor the progress of routine work of one's subordinates and guiding them properly. Supervision is an important element of the directing function of management because it converts plans into action. Supervision has an important feature which includes face-to-face interaction between the supervisor and his subordinates. It is an element of direction which consists of "Day-to-day relationship between an executive and his immediate assistant and it also covers different training, workshops, direction, motivation, coordination, maintenance of discipline, etc.," Supervision denotes the functions performed by the supervisors.

Supervision is defined as a two way dynamic and social process undertaken for a specific purpose of fulfillment of organizational goals by striving to maintain the required quality of performance through constantly supporting and assisting the worker to perform the best. Supervision has been defined as a cooperative relationship between the leader and one or more person to accomplish a particular job.

Definitions

- Supervision has been defined as a cooperative relationship between the leader and one or more person to accomplish a particular job. ¢ According to Jean Barret, supervision is kind of teaching which involves advising, helping, inspiring, leading and liberating.
- Terry and Franklin meant supervision as "guiding and directing efforts of the employees and other resources to accomplish stated work outputs".
- According to Margaret Williamson—supervision is process by which workers are helped by designated staff member to learn according to the needs to make the best use of their knowledge and skills and to improve their abilities so that they do their job more effectively and increase satisfaction to themselves and to the agency.
- John D. Millett rightly observed—supervision is more than a process, it is a spirit which animates relationship between levels of organization and which includes maximum accomplishment, or when unsuccessful generates administrative paralysis. Effective management is concerned to realize the first and to avoid the second.

Goals of Supervision

- To bring personal and professional growth of employees (nurses) in order to achieve quality in healthcare system.
- It is the key to maintain standards.
- To persist in the delivery of high quality of healthcare services.
- To assist and to help in the development of staff to their highest potential.
- To interpret policies, objectives and need, etc., of the organization.
- To plan services cooperatively and to develop coordination to avoid overlapping.
- To assist in the problem solving of the matters concerning personal, administrative and operation of services.
- To develop standards of service and methods of evaluation of a personnel and services.
- To evaluate the services given, personal performance, progress made and to suggest changes for improving the work effectively and outcome of the personnel.

Basic Tenets of Supervision

- Supervision is ongoing process invariably interwoven with motivation, performance appraisal, staff development and leadership
- Supervisors are always accountable for the performance of their subordinates working under them/his span of control.
- Supervisors are to help the workers to improve, develop and reinforce knowledge and skill according to their individual needs.
- Supervisors are required to help their workers to develop right attitude.
- Another essential tenet of supervision includes assisting the worker to perform in the best possible way to yield the best results in terms of realization of the organizational goals.

Principles of Supervision

- Supervision should encourage self-expression so as to draw out potential abilities of a worker
- Supervision should provide initiative to individual to take more responsibility.
- Supervision should provide full opportunity to do work in cooperation to develop the team spirit. And develop good interpersonal relationship.
- Supervision should give autonomy to the workers depending from personality, competence and characteristics.
- Supervision interprets policies and give creative instructions
- Supervision should meet the individual needs.
- Supervisor should always think herself as a leader so as to give guidance help and encouragement.
- Supervision should be democratic.
- Supervision should be well planned and adopted to good planning.
- It calls for good planning and organization. Good supervision respects the personality of an individual (employee).

The functions of supervision:

- **Administrative:** Assigning duties or preparing duty roster, providing materials and supplies to facilitate the staff's performance, etc., are administrative functions.
- **Teaching:** By sharing knowledge, providing technical guidance a supervisor plays the role of a teacher.
- **Helping:** The supervisor offers help by solving problems faced by the staff and to complete her work particularly in emergency.
- **Linking:** The supervisor acts as a communication link between the staff and higher authorities and other members of the team. For example a ward sister or sister in-charge is the linking person between the nursing staff and Assistant Nursing Superintendent, Deputy Nursing Superintendent, doctors treating the patients, etc.

- **Evaluation:** Each supervisor is supposed to carry out performance appraisal of all the staff working under her in a unit and provide feedback for improving their efficiency. As a supervisor, therefore, the upward responsibilities to superiors are to:
  - Identify the activities the hospital authorities or the district health authorities want to be done.
  - Arrange to carry out these activities.
  - Keep your higher authorities posted on what is being done.
  - Suggest measures for improving efficiency of workers (in your case, nursing staff) and efficacy of performance.
  - Act as a liaison between your higher authorities in the health management and the nursing personnel, interpreting the requirements of the district health authorities and the hospital authorities to your workforce and vice-versa.
  - Refer matters to your supervisors for their timely.

Types of Supervision

Supervision can be done directly or indirectly. Direct method is based on observation on the spot, which is mostly used in hospital. Indirect methods are based on perusal of records maintained by staff ('patients' records in the hospital), individual conferences or talks, staff meetings and performance during some training sessions; patient's physicians and patients' relatives opinion is also used by a supervisor in a hospital. In community nursing, field visits are scheduled for direct on the spot supervision; indirect methods of observation as mentioned above are also used in the fields as well as in the health centers. Here the community's opinion towards the performance of a worker also serves as an indirect method of supervision.

Styles of Supervision

There are two main styles of functioning which are observe. These are:

Task-centered

When the supervisor emphasizes the task more than the performer whom she/he supervised. This type of supervisors probably believe that 'Ends' are more important than the 'Means': Since her/his concern for the task is high, he/she often neglects the human aspects in dealing with the staff. The staff may view her as a tough task master.

Employee-centered Supervisor

Such supervisors are people oriented. They believe that concern for workers/staff, their needs and welfare is very important. Therefore, if employees are well taken care of, they will be able to work well and be capable of taking on responsibilities. However, such a supervisory style at an extreme can also lead to inefficiency if the subordinates take them as lenient persons. The effectiveness of a style depends on various factors like nature of the task, the nature of the employee and the situation. There are three other supervisory styles which may be seen being practiced by different supervisors. According to the style adopted, the supervisor may become:

- **An autocratic or critical supervisor** who can not tolerate any deviation from norms, lack of quality in work, lack of discipline, etc., the decisions are always made by her self/himself and such supervisors demand subordinates only to follow their directions as given.
- **A benevolent supervisor** who is very protective of her subordinates, keeps telling them what they should do and what they should not, thus providing constant direction. Such supervisors are usually liked by workers but are effective as long as they are physically present as they tend to develop the subordinates as dependent followers.
- **A democratic supervisor** who believes in a style of "Let us agree on what we are to do" in dealing with the subordinates. Such supervisor provides guidance only when requested by the subordinates. The subordinates with this type of supervisor tend to develop confidence in their work. They are quite independent and cooperate with one another and work together.

Stages of Supervision

This whole process is based mainly on three stages.

Stage One: Preparation for Supervision

As a nursing supervisor or Community health nursing officer, she/he have to make the necessary preparation for successful supervision.

- **Study of documents:** You have to study all the documents related to hospital policy, routine, rules, guidelines, procedure manuals, job description of each category of personnel, standard norms, targets, etc., in details.
- **Identification of priorities for supervision:** Prioritise areas, activities and tasks related to nursing care services in a hospital or in a community which should be supervised. This will make your supervision most effective. This is the time when a CHN must identify the priority area to focus based on the need or emergency.
- **Preparation of a supervision schedule:** It is essential that you prepare checklists for observation in the wards in the institutional settings and for field visits in the community settings. You have to prepare plan and schedule of visits on the basis of the priority needs and content supervision as set out in the checklist or any other tool required.

Stage Two: Supervision

- **Establish contacts:** In hospital or community a supervisor has to establish contact with the staffs along with other family members and patients during supervision and also have to know about other members of the team providing comprehensive care to the patients in the wards or people in the community.
- Review of the Objectives, Targets and Norms with the subordinates/supervisees
- As a supervisor you should also review the job descriptions especially the description of the duties, activities and tasks, the duty roster and weekly timetable, to ensure that

Table 18.1: Comparison of traditional and supportive supervision.

Action	*Traditional supervision*	*Supportive supervision*
Who performs supervision	External supervisors	• External supervisors • Staff from other facilities • Colleagues from the same facility (Internal supervision) • Community health committees • Staff themselves through self-assessment
When supervision happens	During periodic visits by external supervisors	• Continuously: During routine work team meetings • Visits by external supervisors
How do supervisors prepare	Little or no preparation	• Supervisors review previous supervisory reports • Supervisors review reported achievements • Supervisors decide before the supervision visit on what they need to focus on
What happens during supervision	• Inspection of facility • Review of records and supplies • Supervisor makes most of the decisions • Reactive problem-solving by supervisor • Little feedback or discussion of supervisor observations	• Observation of performance and comparison to standards • Provision of corrective and supportive feedback on performance • Discussion with clients • Provision of technical updates or guidelines • On site training • Use of data and client input to identify opportunities for improvement • Joint problem-solving • Follow-up on previously identified • Problems
What happens after supervision	No or irregular follow-up	• Actions and decisions recorded • Ongoing monitoring of weak areas and improvements • Follow-up on prior visits and problems

each member of nursing staff knows, understands and accepts them.

- You, as the nursing supervisor along with the nursing staff are to examine how much time i e is at present spent on each of the duties mentioned in the job description
- Observe the nursing staff's motivation about the actual use of work time and its effects on performance of activities through her actual performance.
- As a supervisor you have to observe individual nursing staff carry out his/her tasks.

Observe the performance of all tasks with particular regard to:

- The skills (technical, managerial, conceptual)
- The attitude (towards patients, relatives, colleagues, community leaders, families under supervision, other members of the team, etc.)
- The organization of resources (of equipment, materials including stationery, etc.)
- The utilization of resources (supplies, time other supportive staff, etc., for cost effectiveness)
- You have to identify gaps and needs for follow-up action based on your feedback data attained through your observation. Jointly identify particular needs of staff or improve the staff's knowledge, attitudes and practical skill with regard to activities under priority supervision.
- Ask each staff to suggest specific ways in which the necessary leaning can be accomplished.
- Note the needs for logistic support, supplies or other factors relevant to the proper performance of the tasks.
- Consult with other members of the team in the ward or health team providing' community services.

Stage Three: Follow-up of Supervision

The role of a supervisor does not end in performing the activities involved in supervision. Each supervisor must prepare a report on the observations made during supervision. This report is used as a tool for taking follow up actions which may include:

- Organizing in-service training programs/continuing education programs for the nursing personnel.
- Reorganization of time table/work plan/duty roster.
- Initiating changes in logistic support or supply system.
- Initiating actions for organizing staff welfare activates.
- Counseling and guidance regarding career development and professional growth.

Supportive supervision: Supportive supervision is a process of helping staff to improve their own work performance at their workplace. It is differ from traditional supervision as it is corrective in nature **(Table 18.1)**. It is carried out in a respectful and nonauthoritarian way with a focus on using supervisory visits as an opportunity to improve knowledge and skills of health staff. Supportive supervision is a process that promotes quality at all levels of the health system by strengthening relationships within the system, focusing on the identification and resolution of problems, optimizing the allocation of resources, promoting high standards, teamwork and better two-way communication. Supportive supervision involves directing and supporting healthcare workers in order to enhance their skills, knowledge and abilities with the goal of improving health outcomes for the population they manage. It is an ongoing relationship between healthcare workers and their supervisors. Supportive supervision is recognized as critical part of human resource management for the delivery of quality healthcare services.

CHAPTER 19

Disaster Management

INTRODUCTION

Throughout history, people have been subjected to nature's unexpected attacks that cause destruction, death and injury. Almost every day of the week the news media covers some kind of disaster somewhere in the world. Disasters are not confined to a particular part of the world. They can occur anywhere and anytime. It not only affect the health and wellbeing of people but also large number of people are displaced, killed or injured subjected to greater risks of epidemics. Economic harm is also common in all over world. It causes great harm to the existing infrastructure and threaten the future. Disaster occurrence is a global phenomenon. It can occur at anywhere at any time. Disaster occurrence in any countries affects its health and economic conditions. Most types of natural disaster are suitable to reoccur in the same areas or countries. Furthermore, with the changing ecosystem, deforestation, misuse of land we have every reason to believe that frequency of disasters, such as floods, droughts will increase in the coming decades. Throughout the history, people have been subjected to nature's unexpected attacks that cause destruction, death and injury. Almost every day of the week the news media covers some kind of disaster somewhere in the world. They can occur anywhere and anytime. It not only affect the health and well-being of the people but also large number of people are displaced, killed or injured subjected to greater risk of epidemics.

A disaster can be defined as any occurrence that causes damage ecological disruption, loss of human life or deterioration of health and health services on a scale sufficient to warrantee an extraordinary response from outside the affected community or area. **—WHO**

In world most of the people are killed by earthquake. Percentage of reported people killed by disaster type Earthquake: 34.8%, Epidemic: 10.8%, Ext. temp.: 8%, Flood: 28%, Storm: 16.2%. In India, 59% of the land mass is susceptible to seismic hazard; 5% of the total geographical area is prone to floods; 8% of the total landmass is prone to cyclones; 70% of the total cultivable area is vulnerable to drought. In Odisha altogether 49,736 people were killed and property worth ₹ 8814 crore was lost due to natural disasters and epidemic in a span of 38 years from 1970 to 2007. Cyclones are highly endemic in Odisha. Odisha's vulnerability to disasters includes, about 480 km long coastline, five cyclones in Bay of Bengal each year, situated in Zone-3 in Earthquake Hazard Map, floods in Mahanadi river system and other major rivers, western parts suffer from persisting drought conditions.

Disaster is a result of vast ecological breakdown in the relationship between humans and their environment, as serious or sudden event on such scale that the stricken community needs extraordinary efforts to cope with outside help or international aid. Disasters are sudden catastrophic event that disrupt pattern of life and in which there is possible loss of life and property and edition to multiple injuries. No community is immune to emergencies caused by disasters. The disaster events result in number of death, injury among the community and require immediate assistance to overcome its effects.

DEFINITIONS

- WHO defines disaster as "any occurrence that causes damage, ecological disruption, loss of human life, deterioration of health and health services, on a scale sufficient to warrant an extraordinary response from outside the affected community or area."
- The American Red Cross defines disaster as "An occurrence, either natural or man-made that causes human suffering and creates human that victim's cannot alleviate without assistance"
- UNDP (2004) defines "Disaster is a serious disruption triggered by a hazard, causing human, material, economic or (and) environmental losses, which exceed the ability of those affected to cope."
- Disaster can be defined as "Any catastrophic situation in which the normal patterns of life (or ecosystems) have been disrupted and extraordinary, emergency interventions are required to save and preserve human lives and/or the environment."

Disaster Alphabetically Mean

D: Destruction.

I: Incidence.

S: Suffering.

A: Adminstrative and financial failure.

S: Sentiment.

T: Tragidies

E: Eruption of communicable disease.

R: Research program and its implementation.

Disasters have been the integral parts of the human experience since the beginning of time, causing premature death, impaired quality of life, and altered health status. On average, one disaster per week that requires international assistance, occurs somewhere in the world. Global warming, shifts in climates, sea-level rise, and societal factors may cause to create future calamities. Finally, war, acts of aggression, and the incidence of terrorist attacks are reminder of the potentially deadly consequences of man's inhumanity toward man.

We do not expect disaster, but they happen with living as natural calamities, the individual and technological advances, come from expedient, socioeconomic and political stagnation and war, etc., disaster either man-made or natural, may be inevitable, but there are methods to prevent or manage the way, people and their communities respond to disaster. So, nurses have an important role to play during a disaster to save the lives and to provide healthcare to the victims.

Etymology

The word derives from French "désastre" and that from Old Italian "disastro", which in turn comes from the Greek pejorative prefix dus = "bad" + aster = "star". The ancient people believed that the disaster is occurred due to the unfavorable position of the "planets" or "Act of God". Gradually they understand the mysteries of nature.

Types of Disaster

Disasters are classified in various ways, on the basis of its origin/cause. **Table 19.1** depicts the India's deadliest disaster (in the last century).

Natural Disasters

A serious disruption triggered by a natural hazard (hydro-metrological, geological or biological in origin) causing human, material, economic or environmental losses, which exceed the ability of those affected to cope. Natural hazards can be classified as:

- **Water and climate-related disaster (Hydro-meterological):** Water and climate-related disasters include floods and drainage management, cyclones, tornadoes and hurricanes, hailstorm, cloud burst heat wave and cold wave, snow avalanches. droughts. sea erosion, thunder and lightening, tsunami, etc.
- **Geological-related disaster** includes landslides and mudflows, earthquakes, dam failures/dam bursts and mine fires, etc.
- **Biological-related disaster** includes, biological disasters and epidemics, pest attacks, cattle epidemics and food poisoning.

Earthquake

Earthquake is one of the most destructive natural hazards. An earthquake (also known as a quake, tremor or temblor) is the result of a sudden release of energy in the Earth's crust that creates seismic waves. Earthquake magnitude or amount of energy released is determined by the use of a seismograph which is an instrument that continuously records ground vibration.

Cyclone

Cyclone is a region of low atmospheric pressure surrounded by high atmospheric pressure resulting in atmospheric disturbance accompanied by powerful winds blow fast accompanying with thunder and lightning. In 5th May 2019, the cyclone Fani made landfall near Puri, Odisha. Approximately 72 people have been killed by Fani in India and 64 in Odisha.

Flood

A flood is an overflow of water that submerges land which is normally dry. Flooding is the most common type of disaster worldwide, accounting for an estimated 40% of all natural disasters. High tide cause floods in coastal areas and constant rains extending over a longer period. Deforestation of hills and mountains are the reasons of floods. People in these areas are faced with dangerous of losing lives and property, loss of shelter, displacement, lack of food and clothing epidemics, etc.

Tsunami

A tsunami is a series of waves in a water body caused by the displacement of a large volume of water, generally in an ocean or a large lake. Sea water is displaced with a violent motion and swells up, ultimately surging over land with great destructive power. An underwater earthquake, a volcano eruption or a landslide mostly causes a tsunami.

Hurricane

Hurricanes are tropical cyclone. These are low pressure winds formed over the ocean. People living close to the sea are often caught in such disasters. So, protective measures are important, e.g., shifting people to safer places, educating people about boiling water for drinking and organizing mass immunization specially for typhoid.

Drought

Drought is a prolonged dry period in the natural climate cycle that can occur anywhere in the world. It is a slow-onset disaster characterized by the lack of precipitation, resulting in a water shortage. Drought can have a serious impact on health, agriculture, economies, energy and the environment. Drought is either absence or deficiency of rainfall from its normal pattern in a region for an extended period of time.

Lightning

Lightning is a naturally occurring electrostatic discharge during which two electrically charged regions, both in

Table 19.1: India's deadliest disaster (in the last century).

Sl. No.	Name of event	Year	State and area	Fatalities
1.	Earthquake	1905	Kangra, Himachal Pradesh	20,000 deaths
2.	Cyclone	1977	Andhra Pradesh	10,000 deaths; hundreds of thousands homeless 40,000 cattle deaths. Destroyed 40% of India's food grains
3.	Latur Earthquake	1993	Latur, Marthawada, region of the Maharashtra	7,928 people died and another 30,000 were injured
4.	Odisha Super Cyclone	1999	Orissa	10,000 deaths
5.	The Kargil war between India and Pakistan	1999 May-July	Kargil district, Kashmir	
6.	Landslide	July 2000	Mumbai	—
7.	Gujarat Earthquake	2001	Bhuj, Bachau, Anjar, Ahmedabad, and Surat in Gujarat State	25,000 deaths 6.3 million people affected
8.	Tsunami	2004	Coastline of Tamil Nadu, Kerala, Andhra Pradesh and Puducherry, as well as the Andaman and Nicobar Islands of India	10,749 deaths 5,640 persons missing 2.79 million people affected 11,827 hectares of crops damaged 300,000 fisher folk lost their livelihoods
9.	Maharashtra floods	July 2005	Maharashtra State	1094 deaths 167 injured 54 missing
10.	Kashmir Earthquake	2005	Kashmir State	86000 deaths (includes Kashmir and surrounding Himalayan region)
11.	Kosi Floods	2008	North Bihar	527 deaths 19323 livestock perished 222754 houses damaged 3329423 persons affected
12.	Cyclone Nisha	2008	Tamil Nadu	204 deaths $800 million worth damages
13.	Mumbai Taj Hotel disaster	2009 January	Mumbai	—
14.	Outbreak of Swine Flu pandemic	2009	Various part of India and world	—
15.	Jaipur Oil depot fire broke out	29 October 2009	IOCL, Jaipur, India	—
16.	Cyclone Phailin	12 October 2013	Odisha, Andhra Pradesh, Jharkhand	45 deaths 3000 crore loss
17.	Cyclone Fani	3 May, 2019	Odisha (Puri and Khurdha District)	MiRs 24,176 crore
18.	Outbreak of COVID-19 pandemic	Started from December 19 in China and spread whole world subsequently	All over the world	Continuing death across the world

the atmosphere or with one on the ground, temporarily neutralize themselves, causing the instantaneous release of an average of one gigajoule of energy. This discharge may produce a wide range of electromagnetic radiation, from heat created by the rapid movement of electrons, to brilliant flashes of visible light in the form of black-body radiation. Lightning causes thunder, a sound from the shock wave which develops as gases in the vicinity of the discharge experience a sudden increase in pressure.

Blizzards

Blizzards are severe binding storms of fine snow blown by strong freezing winds. Many places in snowy regions are hit by such storms. These often cause transportation breakdown, communication breaks and isolation of the affected people from others, loss of lives and property. Thus, there will be difficulties in supplying food and other amenities to the area, and also in shifting of casualties of hospitals, etc.

Volcano

A volcano is a rupture in the crust of a planetary-mass object, such as Earth, that allows hot lava, volcanic ash, and gases to escape from a magma chamber below the surface. Volcanic eruptions cause hazards. The crystalline silica of the ash which causes possibility of silicosis. The ash can contaminate water supplies.

The wind and human activity can stir up fallen ash for moths or years presenting a long-term health and economic hazards.

Heat Waves

In summer, the heat waves cause sun stroke, shock, etc. A heat wave is a period of excessively hot weather, which may be accompanied by high humidity, especially in oceanic climate countries. Heat waves are more dangerous when combined with high humidity. The combination of temperature and humidity is measured by the heat index.

Cold Wave

A cold wave (known in some regions as a cold snap or cold spell) is a weather phenomenon that is distinguished by a cooling of the air. In the Northern Hemisphere, cold waves occur when very cold, dense air near the surface moves out of its source region in northern Canada or northern Asia. The core of a cold wave at the surface is a strong high-pressure center that forms during winter in high latitudes.

Cloudburst

A cloudburst is an extreme amount of precipitation in a short period of time, sometimes accompanied by hail and thunder, which is capable of creating flood conditions. Cloudbursts can quickly dump large amounts of water, e.g., 25 mm of precipitation corresponds to 25,000 metric tons per square kilometre.

Landslides

Landslides are a type of "mass wasting," which denotes any down-slope movement of soil and rock under the direct influence of gravity. The term "landslide" encompasses five modes of slope movement—falls, topples, slides, spreads, and flows.

Man-made Disasters

Man-made disasters are serious disruption triggered by a human-induced hazard causing human, material, economic or environmental losses, which exceed the ability of those affected to cope. The examples of man-made disasters are chemical and industrial disasters, nuclear disasters, forest fires, urban fires, mine flooding, oil spills, major building collapse, festival-related disasters, electrical disasters and fires, air, road and rail accidents, war, etc.

Industrial Disaster

An industrial disaster was defined in this review as an event which causes widespread destruction or distress and usually occurs suddenly or over a short period of time and is limited to fires or explosions in industrial settings or to chemical or radioactive releases from industrial point sources.

Nuclear Disaster

A nuclear and radiation accident is defined by the International Atomic Energy Agency as "an event that has led to significant consequences to people, the environment or the facility. Examples include lethal effects to individuals, large radioactivity release to the environment, or reactor core melt."

Oil Spill

An oil spill is the release of a liquid petroleum hydrocarbon into the environment, especially the marine ecosystem, due to human activity, and is a form of pollution. The term is usually given to marine oil spills, where oil is released into the ocean or coastal waters, but spills may also occur on land

War

- **Thermonuclear war:** It is the nuclear explosion which is a weapon used to destruct the energy by radioactive elements. In this process, both attacker and attacked suffer. The degree of destruction may be complete, severe, moderate or mild destruction. For example—the History of Hiroshima and Nagasaki.
- **Biological war:** In biological war, a purposeful contamination of food, drinking water and clothing is carried out by the enemies. This causes the suffering of both soldiers and the public with all kinds of communicable diseases, malaria, food poisoning and other water-borne diseases, plague, typhoid, etc.
- **Chemical war:** Chemical war agents, such as sulfur, mustard and chlorine gas, etc., have been used in ancient times. These agents may be in gas, liquid or solid form. These causes harms in man, animals, equipments, vegetation, etc.

Fire

Fire in hotels, shops, offices, forests and houses cause severe hazards. It may be due to careless handling of fire objects, such as throwing burning cigarettes, bidis, hot ashes, burning gas cylinders and electric sparking.

Transport Accidents

Accidents of bus, or train involve larger number of people, whereas in air crash, than the survival or injured.

Civil Conflicts

Planting of explosives by militants and terrorists for destruction of planes, ships, buses, population causes disasters. Example—bomb blast on World Trade Center in USA (2001).

Catastrophes

Toxic substances released from factories, transportation or any explosive materials causes explosion. Example—Bhopal gas explosion (1984).

Epidemiology of Disaster

Epidemiological factors of disaster included agent factors, host factors, environmental factors and psychological factors.

Agents Factors

Agent factors are again classified as primary agents and secondary agents—primary agents are the direct causes of disaster, such as falling of building, earthquakes, floods, cyclones, hurricanes, bomb blasts, epidemic outbreaks of diseases and draughts, etc. Secondary Agents are the secondary causes which affects a period later to human beings. These include bacteria and viruses that produces contamination or infection after the primary agent has caused injury or destruction.

Host Factors

In the epidemiological framework as applied to disaster, the host is human being. Host factors are those characteristics of human that influence the severity of the disasters effect. Host factors include age, immunization status, pre-existing health status, degree of mobility, emotional stability and economically stability of individuals, etc.

Environmental Factors

Physical Factors

It include the time when the disaster occur, weather conditions, the availability of food and water and the functioning of utilities, such as electricity and telephone.

Chemical Factors

Influencing disaster outcome include leakage of stored chemical into the air, soil, ground, water or food supplies.

Biological Factors

These are those occur or increase as a result of contaminated water, improper waste disposal, insect or rodent proliferation improper food storage or lack of refrigerator due to interrupted electrical services.

Social Factors

These are those contribute to the individual social support systems. Loss of family members, changes in roles and questioning of religious beliefs are social factors to be examined after a disaster.

Psychological Factors

Psychological factors are closely related to agents, host and environmental conditions. The nature and severity of the disaster affect the psychological disaster experienced by the victims. The common signs and symptoms to disaster by adults and children are:

- For adults common symptoms are extreme sense of urgency, panic and fear, disbelief, disorientation and numbing, fantasies that disaster never occurred, reluctance to abandon properly, difficulty in making decisions, night mares, anger and blaming, delayed reactions, insomnia, headache, apathy and depression, sense of powerlessness, guilt, moody and irritable, jealousy and resentment and domestic violence, etc.
- For children, the symptoms are:
  - Regressive behaviors (bedwetting, thumb sneaking)
  - Crying and clinging to parents
  - School-related problems
  - Inability to concentrate
  - Refuse to go back school

Health Effects of Disasters

The health effects of disasters may be extensive and broad in their distribution across populations. In addition to causing illness and injury, disasters disrupt access to primary care and preventive services. Depending on the nature and location of the disaster, its effects on the short- and long-term health of a population may be difficult to measure.

Disasters affect the health status of a community in the following ways:

- Disasters may cause premature deaths, illnesses, and injuries in the affected community, generally exceeding the capacity of the local healthcare system.
- Disasters may destroy the local healthcare infrastructure, which will therefore be unable to respond to the emergency. Disruption of routine healthcare services and prevention initiatives may lead to long-term consequences in health outcomes in terms of increased morbidity and mortality.
- Disasters may create environmental imbalances, increasing the risk of communicable diseases and environmental hazards.
- Disasters may affect the psychological, emotional, and social well-being of the population in the affected community. Depending on the specific nature of the disaster, responses may range from fear, anxiety, and depression to widespread panic and terror.
- Disasters may cause shortages of food and cause severe nutritional deficiencies.
- Disasters may cause large population movements (refugees) creating a burden on other healthcare systems and communities. Displaced populations and their host communities are at increased risk for communicable diseases and the health consequences of crowded living conditions.

Basic Disaster Supplies Kit

The following items are recommended for inclusion in your basic disaster supplies kit:

- Three-day supply of nonperishable food.
- Three-day supply of water—one gallon of water per person, per day.
- Portable, battery-powered radio or television and extra batteries.
- Flashlight and extra batteries.
- First aid kit and manual.
- Sanitation and hygiene items (soap).
- Matches and waterproof container.
- Whistle.
- Extra clothing.
- Kitchen accessories and cooking utensils, including a can opener.
- Photocopies of credit and identification cards.
- Cash and coins.
- Special needs items, such as prescription medications, eye glasses, contact lens solutions, and hearing aid batteries.

- Items for infants, such as formula, diapers, bottles, and pacifiers.
- Other items to meet your unique family needs.

Common Problems to All Disaster

Disasters throughout history have had significant impact on the numbers, health status and lifestyle of populations.

- Deaths
- Severe injuries, requiring extensive treatments
- Increased risk of communicable diseases
- Damage to the health facilities
- Damage to the water systems
- Food shortage
- Population movements

Health Problems Common to all Disasters

- Social reaction
- Communicable diseases
- Population displacements
- Climatic exposure
- Food and nutrition
- Water supply and sanitation
- Mental health
- Damage to health infrastructure

Communicable Diseases Disaster Management

- The risk of epidemic outbreaks of communicable diseases is proportional to population density and displacement. These conditions increase the pressure on water and food supplies and the risk of contamination (as in refugee camps), the disruption of pre-existing sanitation services, such as piped water and sewage, and the failure to maintain or restore normal public health programs in the immediate post-disaster period.
- In the longer term, an increase in vector-borne diseases occurs in some areas because of disruption of vector control efforts, particularly following heavy rains and floods. Residual insecticides may be washed away from buildings and the number of mosquito breeding sites may increase. Moreover, displacement of wild or domesticated animals near human settlements brings additional risk of zoonotic infections.
- In complex disasters where malnutrition, overcrowding, and lack of the most basic sanitation are common, catastrophic outbreaks of gastroenteritis (caused by cholera or other diseases) have occurred, as in Rwanda/Zaire in 1994.

Population Displacements

- When large, spontaneous or organized population movements occur, an urgent need to provide humanitarian assistance is created. People may move to urban areas where public services cannot cope, and the result may be an increase in morbidity and mortality. If much of the housing has been destroyed, large population movements may occur within urban areas as people seek shelter with relatives and friends. Example—surveys of settlements and towns around Managua, Nicaragua, following the December 1972 earthquake indicated that 80–90% of the 200,000 displaced persons were living with relatives and friends; 5% to 10% were living in parks, city squares, and vacant lots; and the remainder were living in schools and other public buildings. Following the earthquake that struck Mexico City in September 1985, 72% of the 33,000 homeless found shelters in areas close to their destroyed dwellings.
- In internal conflicts, such as occurred in Central America (1980s) or Colombia (1990s), refugees and internally displaced populations are likely to persist.

Climatic Exposure

The health hazards of exposure to the elements are not great, even after disasters in temperate climates. As long as the population is dry, reasonably well clothed, and able to find windbreaks, death from exposure does not appear to be a major risk among them. The need to provide emergency shelter therefore varies greatly with local conditions.

Food and Nutrition

Food shortages in the immediate aftermath may arise in two ways. Food stock destruction within the disaster area may reduce the absolute amount of food available, or disruption of distribution systems may curtail access to food, even if there is no absolute shortage. Generalized food shortages severe enough to cause nutritional problems among vulnerable population like children, pregnant or lactating women, and elderly people also.

Flooding and sea surges often damage household food stocks and crops, disrupt distribution, and cause major local shortages. Food distribution, at least in the short-term, is often a major and urgent need, but large-scale importation/donation of food is not usually necessary.

In extended droughts, such as those occurring in Africa, or in complex disasters, the homeless and refugees may be completely dependent on outside sources for food supplies for varying periods of time. Depending on the nutritional condition of affected populations, especially of more vulnerable groups, such as pregnant or lactating women, children, and the elderly, it may be necessary to institute emergency feeding programs.

Water Supply and Sanitation

Drinking water supply and sewerage systems are particularly vulnerable to natural hazards, and the disruptions that occur in them pose a serious health risk. The systems are extensive, often in disrepair, and are exposed to a variety of hazards.

Deficiencies in established amounts and quality of potable water and difficulties in the disposal of excreta and other wastes result in the deterioration of sanitation, contributing to conditions favorable to the spread of enteric and other diseases.

Mental Health

Anxiety, neuroses, and depression are not major, acute public health problems immediately following disasters, and family and neighbors in rural or traditional societies can deal with them temporarily. A group at high risk, however, seems to be the humanitarian volunteers or workers themselves. Wherever possible, efforts should be made to preserve family and community social structures. The indiscriminate use of sedatives and tranquilizers during the emergency relief phase is strongly discouraged. In industrialized or metropolitan areas in developing countries, mental health problems are reported to be significant during long-term rehabilitation and reconstruction and need to be dealt with during that phase.

Damage to the Health Infrastructure

Natural disasters can cause serious damage to health facilities and water supply and sewage systems, having a direct impact on the health of the population dependent on these services. In the case of structurally unsafe hospitals and health centers, natural disasters jeopardize the lives of occupants of the buildings, and limit the capacity to provide health services to disaster victims. The earthquake that struck Mexico City in 1985 resulted in the collapse of 13 hospitals. In just three of those buildings, 866 people died, 100 of whom were health personnel.

Nearly 6,000 hospital beds were lost in the metropolitan facilities. As a result of Hurricane Mitch in 1998, the water supply systems of 23 hospitals in Honduras were damaged or destroyed, and 123 health centers were affected. Peru reported that nearly 10% of the country's health facilities suffered damage as a result of El Niño events in 1997–1998.

DISASTER NURSING

Definition

Disaster nursing can be defined as "the adaptation of professional nursing knowledge, skills and attitude in recognizing and meeting the nursing, health and emotional needs of disaster victims."

Goals of the Disaster Nursing

The overall goal of disaster nursing is to achieve the best possible level of health for the people and the community involved in the disaster.

Based on the goal our target is:

- To meet the immediate basic survival needs of populations affected by disasters (water, food, shelter, and security).
- To identify the potential for a secondary disaster.
- To appraise both risks and resources in the environment.
- To correct inequalities in access to healthcare or appropriate resources.
- To empower survivors to participate in and advocate for their own health and well-being.
- To respect cultural, lingual, and religious diversity in individuals and families and to apply this principle in all health promotion activities.
- To promote the highest achievable quality of life for survivors.

Principles of Disaster Nursing

The basic principles of nursing during special (events) circumstances and disaster conditions include:

- Rapid assessment of the situation and of nursing care needs.
- Triage and initiation of life-saving measures first.
- The selected use of essential nursing interventions and the elimination of nonessential nursing activities.
- Adaptation of necessary nursing skills to disaster and other emergency situations. The nurse must use imagination and resourcefulness in dealing with a lack of supplies, equipment, and personnel.
- Evaluation of the environment and the mitigation or removal of any health hazards.
- Prevention of further injury or illness.
- Leadership in coordinating patient triage, care, and transport during times of crisis.
- The teaching, supervision, and utilization of auxiliary medical personnel and volunteers.
- Provision of understanding, compassion, and emotional support to all victims and their families.

Phases of a Disaster

There are three phases of disaster:

1. **Preimpact phase:**
   - It is the initial phase of disaster, prior to the actual occurrence. A warning is given at the sign of the first possible danger to a community with the aid of weather networks and satellite many meteorological disasters can be predicted.
   - The earliest possible warning is crucial in preventing toss of life and minimizing damage. This is the period when the emergency preparedness plan is put into effect emergency centers are opened by the local civil, detention authority. Communication is a very important factor during this phase; disaster personnel will call on amateur radio operators, radio and television stations.
   - The role of the nurse during this warning phase is to assist in preparing shelters and emergency aid stations and establishing contact with other emergency service group.
2. **Impact phase:**
   - The impact phase occurs when the disaster actually happens. It is a time of enduring hardship or injury end of trying to survive.
   - The impact phase may last for several minutes (e.g., after an earthquake, plane crash or explosion) or for days or weeks (e.g., in a flood, cyclone or epidemic).
   - The impact phase continues until the threat of further destruction has passed and emergency plan is in effect.

This is the time when the emergency operation center is established and put in operation. It serves as the center for communication and other government agencies of health tears care healthcare providers to staff shelters. Every shelter has a nurse as a member of disaster action team. The nurse is responsible for psychological support to victims in the shelter.

3. **Postimpact phase:** Recovery begins during the emergency phase and ends with the return of normal community order and functioning. For persons in the impact area, this phase may last a lifetime (e.g., victims of the atomic bomb of Hiroshima). The victims of disaster may go through four stages of emotional response:
   1. *Denial:* During the stage, the victims may deny the magnitude of the problem or have not fully registered. The victims may appear usually unconcerned.
   2. *Strong emotional response:* In the second stage, the person is aware of the problem but regards it as overwhelming and unbearable. Common reaction during this stage is trembling, tightening of muscles, speaking with the difficulty, weeping heightened, sensitivity, restlessness sadness, anger and passivity. The victim may want to retell or relieve the disaster experience over and over.
   3. *Acceptance:* During the third stage, the victim begins to accept the problems caused by the disaster and makes a concentrated effect to solve them. It is important for victims to take specific action to help themselves and their families.
   4. *Recovery:* The fourth stage represent a recovery from the crisis reaction. Victims feel that they are back to normal. A sense of well-being is restored. Victims develop the realistic memory of the experience.

Dimensions of a Disaster

Disasters have a number of dimensions in which they may differ—predictability, frequency, controllability, time and scope or intensity. These dimensions influence the nature and possibility of preparation planning, as well as response to the actual event.

Predictability

Some events are more easily predicated then others. Advances in meteorology, for example, have made it more feasible to accurately predict the probability of certain types of natural, weather-related disasters (e.g., tornadoes, floods, and hurricanes), while others, such as earthquakes are not as easily predicted. Man-made disasters, such as explosions are also less predictable. Whenever an event is predictable, authorities and emergency personnel have more time to prepare for situation than when an event is not foreseeable (i.e., spontaneous).

Frequency

Although natural disasters are relatively rare, they appear more often in certain geographical locations. Residents of the coastal are at greater risk for experiencing cyclone than for earthquakes, and people who live near large river systems are at greater risk for flooding than people who live elsewhere. The greater frequency of natural disasters may or may not prepare citizens for their occurrence. Some citizens become immune to repeated warnings and are less likely to seek shelter to protect themselves and their property when warned. Other citizens take each warning seriously and regularly take appropriate safety.

Controllability

Some situations allow for pre warning and control measures that can reduce the impact of the disaster; others do not. Emergency planners were able to control some of the effects of the flooding by sandbagging levees and river or sea banks to reduce the effects of water damage, and by deliberately blasting dikes and dams to divert flood waters to less populated areas. The immediate impact on people was reduced by the ability of emergency personnel to organize evacuations.

Time

There are several characteristics of time as it relates to the impact of a disaster; the speed of onset of the disaster, the time available for warning the population, and the actual length of time of the impact phase. It is more difficult to prepare for very sudden events. A flash flood for instance, may catch many unaware, while the gradual flooding allowed more time for preparation. When there is a lengthy period of warning, more protective measures can be introduced.

For example, several days' warning allows authorities in low coastal areas to evacuate vulnerable communities before a cyclone hits. Tornadoes do not offer such lengthy warning periods. The impact phase of the disaster may last for minutes, hours, or even days.

Scope and Intensity

A disaster may be concentrated in a very small area or involve a very large geographical region, usually affecting many more people. A disaster can be very intense and highly destructive, causing many injuries, deaths, and property damage, or less intense, with relatively little damage done to property or individuals. Sometimes a relatively small disaster may be extremely disruptive to a large segment of the community. For example, an explosion at a water purifying plant may cause minimal injury to property and personnel at the plant, but may reduce or eliminate the water supply for an entire community for days or even weeks.

DISASTER CYCLE AND MANAGEMENT

The Disaster Event

This refers to the real-time event of a hazard occurring and affecting the 'elements at risk'. The duration of the event will depend on the type of threat, for example, ground shaking may only occur for a few seconds during an earthquake while flooding may take place over a longer period of time.

There are four basic phases to a disaster management cycle and each phase has specific activities associated with it.

Response

The response phase is the actual implementation of the disaster plan. The best response plans use an incident command system, are relatively simple, are routinely practiced, and are modified when improvements are needed. Response activities need to be continually monitored and adjusted to the changing situation.

Wide international experience has shown that effective response depends fundamentally on two factors information and resources. Without these two vital components, the best plans, management arrangements, expert staff, etc., all become virtually useless. Bearing this fundamental premise in mind, the major *requirements* for effective response are summarised below.

Readiness of Resource Organizations

The readiness of resource organizations (both government and nongovernment) to respond to disaster situations, often at very short notice, is a very important requirement for response operations. Sometimes, failure on the part of only one designated organization may seriously upset the total response effort.

Warning

The main needs for warning are initial detection, as early as possible, of the likelihood that a disaster will occur.

- Effective means of transmitting warning information.
- Facilities to receive and assess warning information.
- Response decisions, as a result of assessing warning information.
- Dissemination of response decisions and, as appropriate, broadcast of warning information to the public. This preliminary reaction might include closing of schools, offices, and other public places, checking emergency power supplies and similar facilities and taking precautions in households to ensure supplies of food; and drinking water.

Evacuation

The evacuation of communities, groups or individuals is a frequent requirement during response operations. Evacuation is usually precautionary (in most cases undertaken on warning indicators prior to impact to protect disaster-threatened persons from the full effects of the disaster) or postimpact (to move persons from a disaster-stricken area into safer, better surroundings and conditions).

Activation of the Response System

For rapid and effective response, there usually needs to be a system for activating disaster management officials and resource organizations. It is useful to implement activation in stages. These might be alert, stand-by, and action

Coordination of Response Operations

Coordination of the action taken in response operations is very important. Good coordination ensures that resource organizations are utilized to best effect, therefore avoiding gaps or duplication in operational tasks.

Communications

As with all aspects of disaster management, good communications are essential for effective response.

Major Healthcare Activities

Activities from hospital, healthcare system, or public health agency take immediately actions during, and after a disaster or emergency occurs. After certain type of disaster, there are large number of casualties to be needed for medical treatment. Most injuries are occurred during impact, and thus the greatest need for emergency care occurs in the first few hours. The management of mass casualties can be further divided into search and rescue, first aid, triage and stabilization of victims, hospital treatment and redistribution of patients to other hospitals if necessary.

- **Rescue and first aid:** After a major disaster, the first role is rescue the victims and provide emergency services. Most immediate help comes from uninjured survivors. Mobilization of the necessary emergency services and first responders in the disaster area, such as firefighters, police and ambulance crews are important here. First responders are normally immediately overwhelmed in a mass emergency, with official response times exceeding several days. In these situations, it makes sense to mobilize organized emergency volunteers, such as nongovernmental organizations (NGOs), local Red Cross branch or St John Ambulance and community emergency response teams, etc. The emergencies during disaster are saving life, prevention of stress and protection of property but in this step first preference is to save life.
- **Field care:** Most injured persons get health facilities using whatever transport is available. In the casualty, the bed availability and surgical services should be maximized, provisions are made for food and shelters. A center is established to respond to inquires from patient's relatives and friends.
- **Triage:** Triage means rapidly classifying the injured on the basis of severity of their injuries and prompt medical intervention. The principle of *first come, first treated* is not followed in mass emergencies. Higher priority is granted to victims whose immediate on long-term prognosis can be affected by simple intensive care. Triage should be carried out at the site of disaster, in order to determine transportation priority, and admission to the hospital or treatment center, where the patient's needs and priority of medical care will be reassessed. Local health workers should be taught the principles of disaster training persons with minor or moderate injuries should be treated at their own homes.

Table 19.2: Advanced triage categories.

Class I (Emergent)	*Red*	*Immediate*
• Victims with serious injuries that are life threatening but has a high probability of survival if they received immediate care. • They require immediate surgery or other life-saving intervention, and have first priority for surgical teams or transport to advanced facilities; they "cannot wait" but are likely to survive with immediate treatment. ***"Critical; life threatening—compromised airway, shock, hemorrhage"***		
Class II (Urgent)	*Yellow*	*Delayed*
• Victims who are seriously injured and whose life is not immediately threatened; and can delay transport and treatment for two hours. • Their condition is stable for the moment but requires watching by trained persons and frequent re-triage, will need hospital care (and would receive immediate priority care under "normal" circumstances). ***"Major illness or injury;—open fracture, chest wound"***		
Class III (Non-urgent)	*Green*	*Minimal*
• "Walking wounded," the casualty requires medical attention when all higher priority patients have been evacuated, and may not require monitoring. • Patients/victims whose care and transport may be delayed two hours or more. ***"Minor injuries; walking wounded—closed fracture, sprain, strain"***		
Class IV (Expectant)	*Black*	*Expectant*
• They are so severely injured that they will die of their injuries, possibly in hours or days (large-body burns, severe trauma, lethal radiation dose), or in life-threatening medical crisis that they are unlikely to survive given the care available (cardiac arrest, septic shock, severe head or chest wounds); • They should be taken to a holding area and given painkillers as required to reduce suffering. ***"Dead or expected to die—massive head injury, extensive full-thickness burns"***		

The serious cases should be transported to hospitals of specialized treatment.

- All patients should be identified with tags stating their name, age, place of origin, triage category, diagnosis and initial treatment and also taking care of the dead is an essential part of the disaster management. So removal of the dead from the disaster place, shifting to the mortuary and reception of dead bodies by their relatives are also important in this phase. **Table 19.2** depicts the advanced triage categories.

Recovery

Once the incident is over, the organization and staff need to recover. Invariably, services have been disrupted and it takes time to return to routines. Recovery is usually easier if, during the response, some of the staff have been assigned to maintain essential services while others were assigned to the disaster response. After the disaster, the most needed thing is the healthcare facilities for the injured. Following the initial emergency phase, the food, clothing, blanket, shelter, sanitary equipment's and construction materials are required. Disaster managers must be prepared to receive large quantities of donations.

- **Epidemiological surveillance:** Disaster can increase transmission of communicable diseases by:
  - Overcrowding and poor sanitation
  - Population displacement
  - Disruption and contamination of water supply, damage to sewerage system and power systems are common in natural disasters
  - Ecological changes
  - Displacement of domestic and wild animals.

  Food water and shelter in disaster situation from new and different source. Outbreaks of gastroenteritis, respiratory infections, vector-borne disease are common after disaster. So prevention of communicable disease after some of the natural disaster are very important factor. As soon as possible public health measures taken to reduce the risk of disease transmission.
- **Vaccination:** Mass vaccination programs usually against typhoid, cholera, tetanus done to prevent some communicable diseases. Vaccination against tetanus to the injured persons.
- **Nutrition:** A natural disaster may affect the nutritional status of the population by affecting one or more components of food. Infants, children, pregnant women, nursing mothers and sick persons are more prone to nutritional problems after prolonged draught. The immediate steps for ensuring that the food relief program will be effective.
- **Rehabilitation:** Rehabilitation starts from the very first moment of a disaster. In the first weeks after disaster, the pattern of health needs will change rapidly moving from casualty treatment to more routine primary health care. Services should be recognized and restructured priorities also will shift from health care towards environmental health measures. Some of them are:
  - Water supply
  - Food supply
  - Basic sanitation and personal hygiene
  - Vector control.

Prevention/Mitigation

These are steps that are taken to lessen the impact of a disaster should one occur and can be considered as prevention and risk reduction measures. Examples of mitigation activities include installing and maintaining backup generator power to mitigate the effects of a power failure or cross training staff to perform other tasks to maintain services during a staffing crisis that is due to a weather emergency.

Emergency prevention and mitigation involves measures designed either to prevent hazards from causing emergency or to lessen the likely effects of emergencies. These measures include flood mitigation works, appropriate land use planning, improved building codes, and reduction or protection of vulnerable population and structures.

In most cases, mitigation measures aim to reduce the vulnerability of the system. Medical casualties can be drastically reduced by improving the structural quality of houses, schools and other public and private buildings. Although mitigation in these sectors has clear health implications, the direct responsibility of the health sector is limited to ensuring the safety of health facilities and public health services, including water supply and sewerage systems. When water supplies are contaminated or interrupted in addition to the social cost of such damage, the cost of rehabilitation and reconstruction severely strains the economy. Mitigation complements the disaster preparedness and disaster response activities.

Disaster Preparedness

Disaster preparedness can prevent a bad situation from becoming worse. Emergencies come in many forms and having the right checklist, supplies and kit for any possible contingency can aid in making your family safe. Planning ahead also helps everyone understand what to do should a disaster strike. In some instances, it may be several days before vital services can be prepared and surviving this period may be difficult. Disaster preparedness is highlighted every year during the month of September. When disaster strikes, having a plan of action already in place can be key to ensuring positive response and recovery outcomes. Emergency preparedness is a program of long-term development activities whose goals are to strengthen the overall capacity and capability of a country to manage efficiently all types of emergency. The objective of disaster preparedness is to ensure that appropriate systems procedures and resources are in place to provide prompt effective assistance to disaster victims, thus facilitating relief measures and rehabilitation services. Disaster preparedness is an ongoing multisectoral activity. It forms an integral part of the national system responsible for developing plans and programs for disaster management, prevention, mitigation, preparedness, response, rehabilitation and reconstruction. The system known by a variety of names depending on the country, depends on the condition of a variety of sectors to carry out the following tasks:

- Evaluate the risk of the country or particular region to disaster.
- Adopt standards and regulations.
- Organize communication, information and warning.
- Develop public education programs
- Coordinate information sessions with news media.

Effective handling of disasters requires combined efforts of the local agencies in the area., such as public and private hospitals, public health division, public welfare department, public works department, police and fire departments, red cross and civil defense services.

Adequate preparedness of the various facilities and systems which are required for response operations is also most important. Such facilities and systems usually include:

- Emergency or stand-by communications;
- A warning system, including provision of warning and information to the general public;
- A system for activating the organizational structure and its resource organizations (usually by designating stages, such as Alert, Standby, and Action);
- Emergency operation centers (which form the focal points of information management);
- A system for damage survey and assessment of needs;
- Emergency relief arrangements (for food, shelter materials, medical assistance, etc.).

Resources for Readiness

- Red cross
- Local government
- Civil defense services
- Hospital disaster planning

Disaster Management Committee: The following members would comprise the disaster management committee in hospital site:

- Medical Superintendent
- Additional Medical Superintendent
- Nursing Superintendent
- Chief Medical Officer
- Head of all department, i.e., Medicine, Surgery, etc.
- Blood bank in charge
- Officer in charge stores
- Security officers
- Dietician
- Transport officer
- Sanitary superintendent.

The disaster management committee is overall responsible for managing the disaster situation take administrative decisions, review the disasters plan and inform authorities.

- **Disaster control room:** The existing casualty would be referred as the disaster control room. It acts as reception area to receive the casualties and screen for management.
- **Local government:** They share the responsibility in maintaining law and order, determining the safety, repairing bridges, transportation maintaining health facilities and sanitation, providing safe food and drinking water.
- **Civil defense services:** Civil defense services have worked out a kind of agreement with Red Cross. The Civil defense

services provide for shelters, post-disaster services, assistance to affected community in health sanitation, maintaining law and orders, clearing debris, provision of safe drinking water, prevention and control of epidemics, etc., an emergency planning section at both Central and State Government level is established.

- **Hospital disaster planning:** Preplanning to manage disaster is very important in hospital administration. Management plan is made to fit every emergency situations, by preorganizing all aspects. Planning systematical treatment in the hospital is important to minimize confusion in receiving the injured persons. A team of well-qualified physicians and nurses at the reception at casualties makes quick decisions of the treatment. First priority area in cases of shock, fracture, burns or those requiring resuscitation.
- **Rapid response team:** The medical superintendent would identify various specialists, nurses and paramedical staff to respond within a short notice depending upon the disaster.
- **Disaster beds:** Some beds can be earmarked as disaster beds. Additional bed capacity is increased by utilization of vacant beds, day care beds, preoperative beds. Patients who can have domiciliary care or OPD management should be discharged. Utility areas to be converted into temporary wards. Additional bed capacity is done by using trolleys, folding beds and floor beds, etc.
- **Logistic support:** Separate cup boards and marked as disaster almirah should be kept in the disaster control room. All equipments, all essential medicines and surgical supplies. The disaster cup board should contain:
    - Resuscitation equipment (life-saving drugs, ambu bags, etc.)
    - IV set, syringes, vein flow, IV fluids, suturing materials.
    - Oxygen masks, nasal catheters.
    - ECG monitors, defibrillators, ventilators, etc.
    - Linen and blankets
    - Stretchers, wheel chairs
    - HIV KIT.

Figure 19.1 depicts the disaster management cycle.

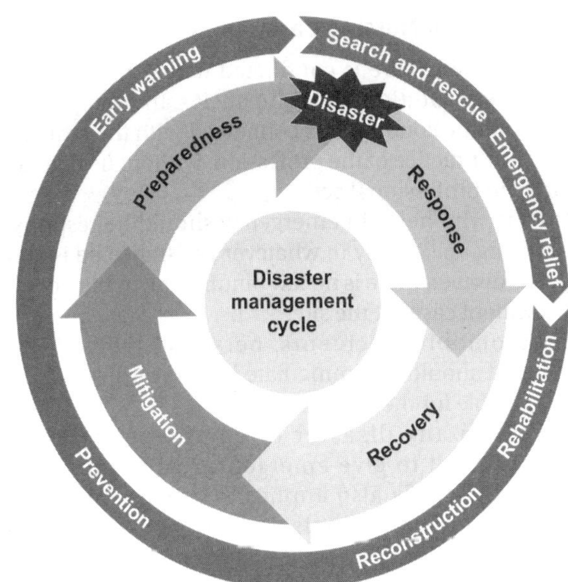

Fig. 19.1: Disaster management cycle.

Principles of Legal Aspects in Disaster Nursing

All resources professional and non-professional personnel, supplies, equipments, etc., are to be brought close to the place of disaster to facilitate immediate initial treatment.

- The treatment should continue and provide for more definite care during the period of evacuation.
- All treatment should be done in such a way that the casualty and his relation, retain their independence of care with the possible provision of medical and nursing practice.
- **Principle of triage:** This is way of setting priority. When there is a large number of victims on patients who need emergency care a system called triage is used for identifying people at greatest risk. Example—train accident, fire victims.
- Patients are classified according to the degree of emergency, such as need of immediate care and can wait for care.

In a disaster situation, this refers to sorting out casualties for immediate care in three categories:

1. **Urgent category:** Who will require life-saving measures.
2. **Serious category:** Those who are seriously injured.
3. **Minimal category:** Minor injury victims who can be attended last.

In war and thermonuclear disaster, this principle is applied in order to save largest number of casualties with simplest measures.

Basis for priority of treatment:

- Identifying minimal treatment which can be carried out by nonprofessional personnel under supervision.
- Immediate treatment to those who will have reasonable chances of survival if they receive timely life-saving measures, e.g., lacerated wound 20–40% burns, closed fractures, etc.
- Those who will need treatment as critical cases will are sorted out on the basis of multiplicity and seriousness of injury, its location, time and the qualified personnel required to treat it. Young persons are given high priority for treatment than the old people with similar injuries.

Basic of setting priority in transporting casualty to a hospital from disaster scene:

- First priority to those with airway and difficulties.
- Secondary priority to those injury cases in which application of tourniquet was essential fractures Those whose lives can be saved by delay treatment also.
- Third priority will include cases of soft wound injuries requiring debridement cases of fractured limbs, dislocations eye injuries, etc.

Legal Aspect of Nursing Care

Disaster nursing care is conducted within the framework of the state institution's health policies and the prevailing civil laws of the country. It is connected with the ethical and responsible practice of the profession, without negligence as provided in professional act.

- Anyone who helps in emergency should be responsible for acting reasonably in whatever assistance he is able to give. However, there is no law binding the public to attend to accident cases at the site.
- In automobile accidents, persons involved in the accident should get immediate help regardless who was responsible for the accident.
- Nurses in any disaster or emergency situations are expected to give emergency care practising all safeguards. This also applies to nurses employed in settings, such as schools, industries on night shifts, etc., where a doctor is not always present. The nurse works within the scope of standing order to share the physician's functions in emergency situations. If she acts with good professional judgment, complaints of negligence and related litigation are not likely to crop up. However her behavior in carrying out medical treatment, directed by physicians, in his presence and her behavior as she performs according to standing written orders in the absence of a doctor are judged favorably. Therefore, it is safe for a nurse to know the limitations imposed by such regulations in her place of work. Special attention is to be paid to procedures, such as giving intravenous parental fluids.

A nurse trained in a disaster nursing, next to a doctor, makes an important decision about the casualties. Her role gets expanded within the cope of a disaster and personnel available to help in such situations. Professional safeguards provide protection to both the nurse and the public thus these have to be adhered to while performing expanded functions. There is standing medical orders for nurses to function quickly and safely in disaster situations within the law of the country. A nurse trained in disaster nursing is in a position to give first aid treatment and take decisions to transport casualties of the hospitals.

Roles and Responsibility of a Disaster Nurse

D: Disseminate information on the prevention and control of environmental hazards

I: Interpret health laws and regulation

S: Serve yourself of self-survival

A: Accept direction and take orders from an organized authority

S: Serve the best of the most

T: Teach the meaning of warning signals

E: Exercise leadership

R: Refer to appropriate agencies

Responsibilities of Nurse in Disasters

Preparation for disasters: Disaster planning is essential for a community, business or a hospital. It involves thinking about details of preparation and management by all involved including community leaders, health and safety professionals and lay people. A disaster plan need not be lengthy.

Personal Preparation

Nurse with client responsibilities can also be a victim. So, the nurse assisting in disaster relief efforts must be as healthy as possible both physically and mentally. The following are the emergency supplies that should be prepared and stored in an easy to carry container.

- A 3-days' supply of water.
- One change of clothing and footwear per person and one blanket per person.
- A first aid kit that includes your family prescription medications.
- Emergency tools including a battery powered radio, flashlight and plenty of batteries.
- Candles and matches.
- An extra set of car keys and credit cards, cash or traveler's cheques.
- Sanitation supplies, including toilet paper soap feminine hygiene items and plastic garbage bags.
- Special items for infant's elderly or disabled family members.
- An extra pair of eyeglasses important documents should always be kept in a waterproof container.

Professional Preparedness

There should be disaster management team of nurse, psychiatric nurses, physician, surgeon, social workers and psychologists to be active and alert all the time. The team must understand the disaster plans at their workplace and community and will participate in disaster drills.

Adequately prepared nurses can function in a leadership capacity and assist others towards smother recovery phase.

Personal items that are recommended for nurses preparing to help in a disaster include:

- Copy of professional license
- Personal equipment, such as stethoscope
- Flash light and extra batteries
- Cash
- Warm clothing and a heavy jacket for weather appropriate clothing.
- Record keeping materials
- Pocket sized reference books

Shelter Management

Although voluntary health agencies take care of shelter management but the nurses because of their comfort with delivering aggregate health promotion and emotion support make ideal shelter management as a team member.

Dealing with Stress

Basic measures while working with victims dealing with stress includes, listening carefully to the victims, and telling and retelling their feelings related to disaster.

Establishing Authority, Communication and Transportation

The effective disaster plan establishes a clear of authority, develops lines of communication and delineates routes of transport. Usually, the chain is hierarchical, e.g., at the local hospital, the hospital administrator may be responsible for alerting the nurse manager to call in additional personnel. Flexibility is essential, because key authority figures may themselves be victims of disaster.

Warning and Evacuating

Disaster plans must specify the means of communicating warnings to public, as well as the precise information that should be included in warning. Information that should be communicated includes the nature of disaster, the exact geographic region affected and the action that they should take to protect themselves and their property.

Responding to Disasters

At the disaster site, police, fire-fighters, nurses and other relief workers develop a coordinative response to rescue, triage and treat disaster victims.

Immediate Treatment and Support

Disaster nurses provide treatment on site at emergency treatment stations, in shelters or at local hospitals and clinics.

Care of Bodies and Notification of Families

Identification and transport of the dead bodies should be done. Records of deaths must be made and maintained and family members should be notified.

Recovery Phase

The main objectives of disaster management in this stage is to involve all agencies and resources to restore the economic and civil life of community, e.g., construction of temporary as well as permanent houses and epidemiological services. The nurse must remain vigilant in teaching proper hygiene and making sure immunization record up-to-date as there is continuous threat of communicable diseases due to inadequate water supply and crowed living conditions.

Stages of Disaster and the Role of Nurse

Preparatory Phase

- Participate in development of community disaster plan.
- Participate in community risk assessment, such as:
  - Element of hazards, analysis of all hazard approach
  - Hazard mapping, and vulnerability analysis.
- Initiate disaster prevention measures.
- Perform disaster prevention measure.
- Identify educational and training need for all nurses.

Impact Phase

- Activation of disaster response plan
- Notification and initial responses.
- Leadership assumes control of event.
- Establish communication.
- Triage and transport the patient.
- Establish needs for the mutual hazards.
- Activate agency disaster plan.
- Integrate state and federal resources.
- Establish disease surveillance.
- Establish vector control.

Postimpact Phase

- Continue provision of nursing and medical care.
- Continue disease surveillance.
- Monitor the safety of food and water supply.
- Restore public health infrastructure.
- Evaluate the disaster nursing response action.
- Receive original disaster plan.

Organizing an Effective Disaster System

The nurse must be familiar with the personnel at the disaster scene and their roles and functions. In addition, nurse must understand the organizing of the site. A disaster scene is usually broken up into three zones.

- **Disaster zone:** It is the actual location of the incident from where patients are to be removed as soon as possible. Majority of disaster personnel are sent to this zone initially.
- **Treatment zone:** Nurses spend most of their time in this zone during a disaster, where equipment and personnel to carry out patient care are concentrated. Activities carried out in this zone include:
  - Triage of patients into treatment categories
  - Through assessment of each patient
  - Treatment of injuries
  - Preparation for transport.
- **Transport zone:** It should be situated directly next to the treatment zone, so that ambulances and other vehicles can load patients and leave for hospitals.

Role of the Nurse in Disaster at a Hospital

Disaster which occur in a care facility, such as a hospital are known as internal disasters. In addition, hospitals are often the recipients of casualties from disasters that occur in the surrounding communities, i.e., external disasters. Therefore, it is important that each hospital should be prepared for a disaster by having a simple, organized and well-defined disaster plan. A disaster committee with representation from nursing service must be formed. Frequent, planned drills are essential to the implementation of a disaster plan.

Preparation at the Emergency Department

When the emergency department is notified of the disaster, it sets in motion a series of activities. An assessment of the existing status of the patients in the department is made to take decisions concerning their care and disposition. A waiting room area for family members is located away from the emergency department so as to avoid congestion of people at the emergency. The number of patients the department can receive must be determined. Additional area can be used should be determined. Equipment should be ready. The emergency department nurses' in-charge is responsible for the following:

- Making sure as many nursing personnel as possible report for duty
- Assigning them to specific areas/rooms
- Instructing volunteers and ancillary personnel
- Providing breaks or periods of rest for triage nurse and those working in resuscitation and minor treatment areas
- Communicating the need for additional personnel to whoever concerned
- Periodic checking of supplies

Emergency department nurses are assigned to work in the following treatment areas:

- **Triage (Sorting area):** Assigning patients to appropriate treatment areas according to their severity.
- **Major treatment area (Resuscitation room):** Critical patients are placed in the resuscitation—trauma area of the department. In emergency, ICU or OT department.
- **Minimal treatment areas:** To provide first aid or basic nursing intervention is the goal of the minimal treatment area.
- **Morgue area:** Away from emergency department where the diseased can be treated with dignity.
- **Delayed area:** The staff working in this area need to reassess the patient's status and to provide comfort measures (e.g., intravenous analgesics).

Flowchart 19.1 depicts the casualty flowchart during a disaster.

Flowchart 19.1: Casualty flowchart during a disaster.

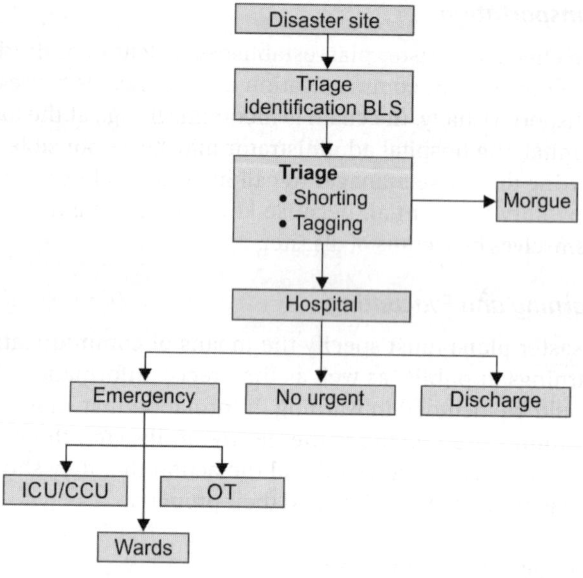

Role of a Nurse in Providing Psychosocial Care During Disaster

During disaster, people are affected in different ways and require different kinds of supports. The role of nurse is important here in community and hospital to stand with the people. The main aspects are:

- Make the client to ventilate their feelings
- Being empathic in nature
- Active listening to the patient
- Provide social support
- Provide relaxation and recreation activities
- Provide spiritual care
- Acknowledge pain, distress by leaning forward.
- Keep reminding—*i am with u.*
- Look into their eyes
- Do not ask to stop crying
- Maintain regular contact
- Do not give false promises
- Family to be encouraged to share feelings and losses.
- Mobilize contact with relatives to facilitate recovery.
- Family members to do regular activities together.
- Rituals like prayers and spiritual activities to be encouraged.
- Encouraging victims to share their feelings with one another. If it seems appropriate to do so.
- Helping victims make decisions
- Delegating tasks (e.g., reading, crafts) to teenagers and others to help combat boredom.
- Providing the basic necessities (food, clothing, rest).
- Attempting to recover or gain needed items (e.g., prescription glasses, medications).
- Providing basic compassion and dignity (privacy when appropriate and if possible).
- Referring to a mental health counselor if the situation warrants.

INDEX

Page numbers followed by *f* refer to figure, *fc* refer to flowchart, and *t* refer to table.

A

B

D

E

F

I

J

K

O

S

T

W

X

Y

Z